MATERNAL AND CHILD
HEALTH NURSING

MATERNAL AND CHILD HEALTH NURSING

A. JOY INGALLS, RN, MS
Former Instructor, Maternal and Child Health Nursing
Grossmont Vocational Nursing Program
Grossmont Health Occupations Center
Santee, California

M. CONSTANCE SALERNO, RN, MS, PNP
Professor of Child Health Nursing
San Diego State University
San Diego, California

SEVENTH EDITION

with 790 illustrations

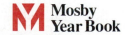
Mosby
Year Book

St. Louis Baltimore Boston Chicago London Philadelphia Sydney Toronto

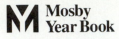

Editor: Linda L. Duncan
Developmental Editor: Joanna May
Project Supervisor: Lilliane Anstee
Design: Liz Fett

SEVENTH EDITION

Copyright © 1991 by Mosby–Year Book, Inc.

A Mosby imprint of Mosby–Year Book, Inc.

Previous editions copyrighted: 1967, 1971, 1975, 1979, 1983, 1987

Printed in the United States of America

Mosby–Year Book, Inc.
11830 Westline Industrial Drive
St. Louis, MO 63146

Library of Congress Cataloging-in-Publication Data

Ingalls, A. Joy.
    Maternal and child health nursing/A. Joy Ingalls, M. Constance
Salerno.—7th ed.
      p.   cm.
    Includes bibliographical references.
    Includes index.
    ISBN 0-8016-6231-1
    1. Obstetrical nursing. 2. Pediatric nursing. I. Salerno, M.
Constance. II. Title.
    [DNLM: 1. Obstetrical Nursing. 2. Pediatric Nursing. WY 157.3
I44m]
RG951.I5   1991
610.73'62—dc20
DNLM/DLC
for Library of Congress   90-13510
                                     CIP

GW/VH/VH 9 8 7 6 5 4 3 2

To
The bedside nurse
whatever her title

Contributors

CAROL ARCHIBALD, MPH, RN
Clinical Specialist/Research Associate-Pulmonary
University of California-San Diego Medical Center
San Diego, California

BARBARA J. COLLARD, RNC
Clinical Specialty Nurse
Women's Center/Pediatric Services
Grossmont Hospital
La Mesa, California

CAROLYN B. COLWELL, MA, RN
Lecturer, Child Health Nursing
San Diego State University
San Diego, California

JANIE FRINCKE, BS, RN
Director, Birth Center
Palomar Hospital Medical Center
Escondido, California

MARY H. INGALLS, MAEd, MT
Clinical Medical Technologist and Instructor in
Laboratory Technologies/Phlebotomy
Grossmont Health Occupations Center
Santee, California

MARGUERITE M. JACKSON, MS, RN, CIC
Director, Medical Center Epidemiology Unit and Assistant
Clinical Professor of Community and Family Medicine
University of California-San Diego Medical Center
San Diego, California

JULIE COWAN NOVAK, DNSc, RN, CPNP
Associate Clinical Professor
Director of Health Promotion Activities
Division of Family Medicine
University of California, San Diego
La Jolla, California

JUDY MILLER PETERS, MS, RN
Associate Professor of Parent-Child Nursing
Loma Linda School of Nursing
Loma Linda University
Loma Linda, California

TERI LYNN RICHARDS, MS, RN, CPNP
Pediatric Genetic Nurse Clinician
Division of Medical Genetics
School of Medicine
University of California, San Diego
La Jolla, California

Special contribution

Chapter 15
Intensive care of the newborn
JOHN E. WIMMER, Jr., MD
Associate Professor
Department of Pediatrics, Neonatology Section
School of Medicine
East Carolina University
Greenville, North Carolina

Preface

It has been said that the last decade before the "turn" of a century is especially meaningful in that it poses problems, seeks solutions and sets trends that influence the following years significantly. If this observation is true, our current agenda as citizens, nurses, and health care providers is certainly crowded with abundant content and challenge. Not that strains or stresses and deep wounds have not been in our society before, but today many people appear to have little expectation that anything can be done about them. The problems of poverty, disease, drugs and the abuse of human, environmental, and financial resources are only some of the examples of the physical, psychosocial, ethical, and fiscal dilemmas which seem to characterize the 1990s. In a way the feelings of futility and fatigue that are sometimes shared—particularly by those working in the "caring professions"—may be termed "a crisis of the spirit."

Nurses today must retain that special vision of what they can do and the difference they can make. The feeling that one can be a small but effective part of the answer to the aches and pains of the community should give us a special sense of hope and accomplishment.

This seventh edition wishes to continue to help technical and vocational nursing students as they approach a special area of national and worldwide concern—the health of mothers and their children and families. Nurses of both sexes contribute to the health care of this special grouping. It is only to avoid the awkward repetitive grammatical patterns of his or her and she or he that the feminine pronoun has been used to refer to the nurse and the masculine pronoun in most instances has been used to refer to the infant or child. The text has maintained its basic structure but has undergone extensive content revision and expansion to include topics not considered previously.

Selective examples of new topics or special areas of revision are the single room maternity care concept; a reconsideration of weight gain expectations during pregnancy; sexually transmitted diseases; the utilization of universal precautions and the concept of body substance isolation; the management of pain in children; the functions of the family and techniques of communication and discipline; recent progress in genetics and prenatal screening and diagnosis; current recommendations regarding immunization, child nutrition, and safety; and improving the child's hospital experience. Chapters 26 and 28 highlighting pediatric procedures dealing with respiration, as well as oxygenation and temperature evaluation and therapies, were almost entirely rewritten.

To assist the learner, we have included many beneficial features. Numerous new photos, drawings, and tables have been added as well as sample nursing care plans for both maternity and pediatric patients. We have also added Key Concepts as well as Discussion Questions at the end of each chapter to help students review important content. Finally, the seventh edition features a new two-color design that we believe will enhance the visual presentation. We hope that all these changes will prove to be "student helpful." A separate Study Guide, featuring many classroom and clinical activities, is also available to enhance student learning.

To assist with this revision we have had the benefit of numerous contributors, reviewers, and consultants. We wish to thank them for sharing their areas of special experience and expertise.

For this edition we have welcomed three new contributors who reviewed and helped to formulate selected portions of the text. Janie Frincke, RN, BS, and Barbara J. Collard, RNC, were particularly helpful in revising Chapters 6, 7, and 9, which deal with the childbirth experience and nursing care of the laboring mother. Carol Archibald, RN, MPH, was of great assistance as she shared her knowledge as Pulmonary Nurse Specialist to "reform" Chapter 26, Aiding Respiration and Oxygenation. The return of seven former contributors was a real asset. They deserve a special thanks. Carolyn B. Colwell, RN, MA, initiated the new section devoted to the discussion of pain control in children and again helped update Chapter 27 and other areas featuring pediatric orthopedics. Mary H. Ingalls, MT, MAEd, faithfully provided another detailed revision of Chapter 24, which considers common maternal and pediatric diagnostic tests. Marguerite M. Jackson, RN, MS, an acknowledged leader in the area of infection control, supplied important insights and information to modernize Chapter 30, now titled Infection Precautions and Childhood Communicable Diseases. Julie C. Novak, DNSc, RN, CPNP, a gifted pediatric professional, critiqued and furnished considerable content for Chapters 12 and 13 concerning the care of the normal newborn as well as the nutrition portion of Chapter 18, Preventive Pediatrics. Judy M. Peters, RN, MS, competent as always, assisted in the revision of Unit II, Chapters 4 and 5, presenting fetal development and prenatal care. Teri Lynn Richards, MS, RN, CPNP, a pediatric genetic nurse clinician, once again reviewed and updated the section on genetics in Chapter 16. John Wimmer, Jr., MD, earned our appreciation again for his careful reexamination of Chapter 15, Intensive Care of the Newborn. A notable addition to the content and style of the entire text is the thoughtful discussion questions posed for each chapter by Gloria E. Wold, RN, MSN. We thank Polly Campbell, RN, BSN, for her valuable assistance with the pediatric nursing care plans.

Reviewers and consultants also played very important parts in the production of this publication. They were most generous with their time and specialized knowledge and abilities. Listed in alphabetical order they are Laurie Blatzheim, RN, MS; William A. Brock, MD; Lorraine Carroll, RN, BSN; Jane Conner, RN, MS; Chris B. Foster, MD; Gary Friedenberg, MD; William F. Friedman, MD; Martin M. Greenberg, MD; William Griswold, MD; Barry H. Gruer, DDS, MS; Capt. Charles B. Hargrove, MC, USN; Hector E. James, MD; Evelyn Lancaster, RN, PHN; Daniel J. Marnell, MD; David G. Martin, MD; William M. McGuigan, MS, JD; Robert Novak, PhD; Nancy K. Ostrom, MD; Eli O. Meltzer, MD; Sung Min Park, MD; David F. Paa, MD; Alex F. Pue, MD; Paul Schultz, MD; Virginia Shumate, RN, BSN; Barbara Peterson Sinclair, MN, RN, OGNP; Rayburn Skoglund, MD; Capt. William Thomas, MC, USN; Cdr. Norman J. Waecker, Jr., MC, USN; Michael J. Welch, MD; and Rhea Williams, RN, PhD.

Other persons have helped to make this edition possible. The many who assisted with arrangements for pictures and the hospitals and parents that permitted use of their facilities or photographs of their children should be especially acknowledged. A special word of appreciation to Karla Barber and Linda O'Neill for their ability to see what the picture would be like before it was snapped. A "thank you" also to graphic artist Joe Ferrara who patiently responded to requests to "draw it again to show something more," and to the past and present artistry of Martha Lackey and Mary Fritchoff.

Artists of a different sort are typists who form picture paragraphs from wiggly scribbles—truly a special skill. Our gratefulness should be expressed to Marie and Melanie Steckbauer and Diane Bartlett.

We also wish to continue our recognition of Ellen Abbott Wight, former Director of the Health Occupations Center of Grossmont Adult School, for her pivotal support in the past. In addition, we desire to acknowledge the capable assistance and welcome encouragement of editors Linda Duncan, Joanna May, and Lilliane Anstee of Mosby–Year Book, Inc.

To all who have helped these pages become a book designed to help the new bedside nurses of the nineties, please accept our sincere expressions of gratitude.

A. JOY INGALLS

M. CONSTANCE SALERNO

Contents

Unit VI   Growth, Development, and Health Supervision

Unit VII   The Child, The Family, and the Hospital Setting

Unit IX   Common pediatric problems and their nursing care

Current Perspectives in Maternal-Child Care

INTRODUCTION OBJECTIVES

After studying this introductory material, the student should be able to perform the following:

1 Define the following terms: obstetrics, pediatrics, perinatology, mortality, morbidity, and neonate.
2 Discuss contributions to maternal and child health made by medical pioneers Ignaz Semmelweis, Louis Pasteur, and Joseph Lister.
3 List three main reasons for progress in maternity care leading to a reduction in infant and maternal illness and death.
4 Cite the 1987 infant mortality statistics in the United States and our present standing among developed nations reporting such statistics.

5 List three main causes of maternal death associated with childbirth and three leading causes of neonatal death.
6 Describe ways that federal governmental agencies, conferences, and legislation historically have assisted in meeting the needs of mothers, children, and youth.
7 Name two international organizations that are involved in promoting maternal-child health programs.
8 Discuss the many concerns and challenges of the nurse working in the field of maternal-child health today.

Nurses engaged in maternal and child care must be aware of current developments and goals in these fields, both locally and nationally, if they are to function meaningfully in hospitals and clinics. This brief introduction contains some definitions, important statistics, and a short historical review designed to increase the student's appreciation of the progress that has been made and the problems that remain.

That progress has been made cannot be denied. Great reductions have been realized in the number of illnesses and deaths involving both mothers and children. The overlapping disciplines of *obstetrics,* the art and science of maternal-fetal and newborn care, and *pediatrics,* the art and science of the care of infants, children, and youth, have made enormous advances in this century. Indeed, it is out of these two specialties that the new discipline of *perinatology,* the study and care of the mother, fetus, and neonate, has developed.

To help the student understand the extent of this improvement, it will be necessary to introduce some statistics; however, they need not be complicated or lengthy to tell an important story.

MATERNAL MORTALITY

Among health statistics the term "mortality" often is encountered, which means the number of persons per given population who died in a given period of time. Maternal mortality refers to the number of mothers who die per 100,000 live births for a certain period. In 1915 maternal mortality in the United States equaled 608 per 100,000; by 1983 maternal mortality had fallen to 8.0 per 100,000.

Year	Maternal mortality
1987	6.6
1986	7.2
1985	7.8

The changes in the maternal mortality rate between 1986 and 1987 were statistically significant for black women (1986, 18.8; 1987, 14.2) but not for white women (1986, 4.9; 1987, 5.1). In 1987 black women were 2.8 times more likely than white women to die of complications associated with pregnancy, childbirth, and the postpartum period. The overall *infant* mortality for 1987 also reflects the downward trend for the black and white populations (Fig. 1).

Although these figures represent a splendid reduction in the maternal death rate, it should be much lower. The national statistics for 1987 continue to demonstrate a great but narrowing difference between the maternal death rates among nonwhite mothers (12.0 per 100,000) and white mothers (5.1 per 100,000), reflecting a significant inequality in the availability or use of maternity services. Shifting centers of population, lack of education, strained and understaffed public facilities, maldistribution of services, and ineffectual health delivery systems all contribute to a higher maternal death rate than should occur in the United States.

Leading causes. The final maternal mortality statistics for 1987, cite toxemia of pregnancy, hemorrhage, and ectopic pregnancy as the three leading causes of maternal death in their order of incidence.

The statistical category labeled toxemia of pregnancy classically includes several associated signs and symptoms, such as elevated blood pressure (hypertension), albumin in the urine (albuminuria), and an abnormal amount of fluid in the tissues (edema). Symptoms of edema are swelling, rapid weight gain, headache, and, in extreme cases, convulsions. At this time there is no agreement among clinicians regarding the cause of tox-

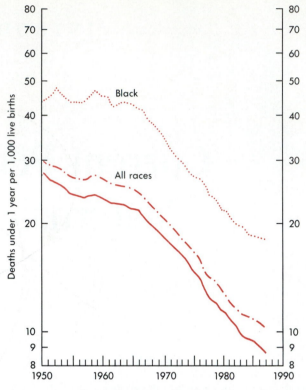

FIG 1 Infant mortality rates by race: United States, 1950-1987. *(Data from National Center for Health Statistics: Advanced report of final mortality statistics, 1987. Monthly Vital Statistics Report 38(suppl):9, 1989.)*

emic complications. Newer and preferred terminology to describe these signs and symptoms includes preeclampsia-eclampsia and pregnancy-induced hypertension (PIH).

Hemorrhage is by far the most common major maternal complication. Occasionally, hemorrhage may predispose a mother to fall victim to other difficulties, such as infection. The greatest progress in the overall reduction of maternal mortality through the years has been in the prevention of infection.

Ectopic pregnancy refers to those pregnancies that develop in places other than the normal location within the uterus. Ectopic pregnancies are often associated with significant blood loss early in gestation.

INFANT MORTALITY

Infant mortality statistics concern the number of children per 1,000 live births who die before their first birthday. In 1900 the average rate in those states reporting

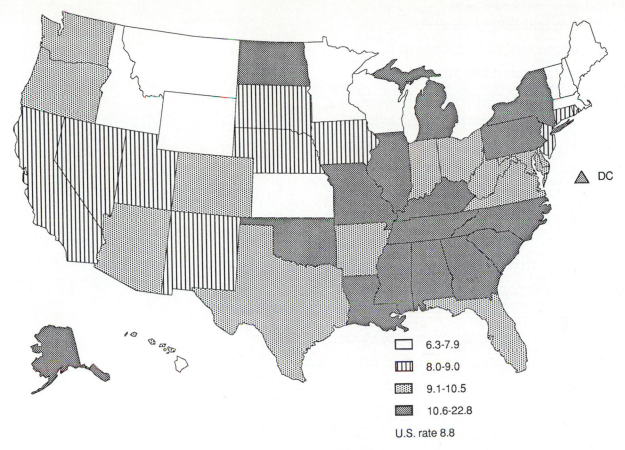

FIG 2 United States infant mortality rate per 1,000 live births, 1987. *(Data from National Center for Health Statistics: Advance report of final mortality statistics, 1987. Monthly Vital Statistics Report 38(suppl):34, 1989.)*

was 200 per 1,000; in 1987 the rate had dropped to 10.1 per 1,000 live births, the lowest rate ever recorded for the United States (see Fig. 1). However, health professionals should be aware that this figure is not consistent throughout the United States, which is positioned 20th among the nations recording such statistics (Figs. 2 and 3). Reduced to more meaningful proportions, United States infant mortality statistics mean that 1 out of every 99 babies born dies before his first birthday. The national lag in lowering infant mortality is related to the reasons cited for the rate of maternal mortality. It is no doubt caused by the many different economic, cultural, and educational backgrounds and levels found in the United States and the failure of the health care delivery system to meet the needs of these diversified groups. The country's international standing may also be influenced

slightly by the different ways in which statistics are formulated in various countries, despite attempts at standardization. However, the fact remains that, compared with the records of other nations, performance in infant mortality in the United States leaves much to be desired.

About 70% of infant deaths occur in the first 28 days of life, the *neonatal period*. Infant mortality data for 1987 reported by the US Department of Health and Human Services indicates that the leading causes of infant death were, in the order of their frequency, congenital anomalies, sudden infant death syndrome, disorders related to short gestation and unspecified low birth weight, and respiratory distress syndrome. Prematurity is the basic leading cause of neonatal death.

It will readily be seen that any method that decreases the incidence of prematurity or improves medical-nursing

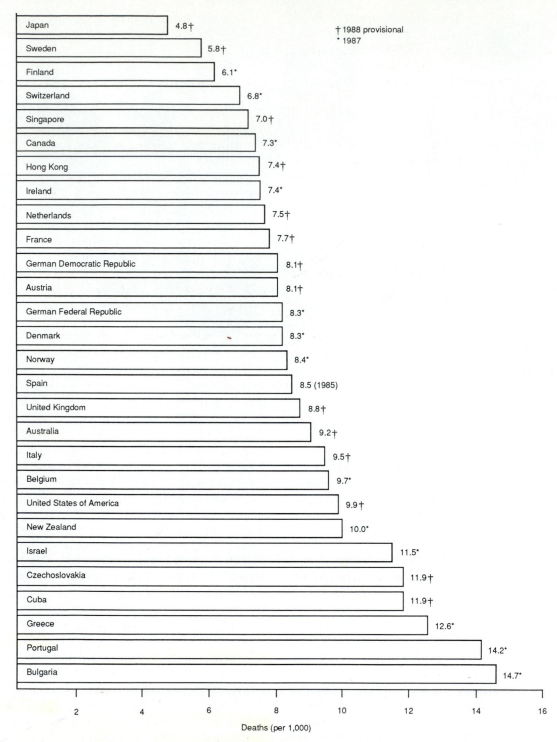

FIG 3 International infant mortality 1988. *(Data from Statistical Papers: Population and Vital Statistics Reports. New York, United Nations, 1989 Series A, 41; Demographic Yearbook, 1987, New York, 1989 United Nations.)*

management of premature infants would profoundly affect infant mortality statistics. In the past the most commonly used definition of prematurity was a birth weight of less than 5½ pounds (2,500 g), although it is recognized that not all infants of low birth weight are born before term. The current statistical definition, birth before the end of 37 weeks of gestational age, is more logical but not always verifiable (see p. 272).

Another statistical category is *perinatal mortality*. This figure includes recorded deaths of fetuses of more than 20 weeks' gestation added to those of the first 4 weeks of life (neonatal period).

CHANGE AND PROGRESS IN MATERNITY CARE

Although maternity care still could be improved a great deal, clearly conditions have changed radically for the better. It would be worthwhile for us to discuss the major reasons for this progress.

Acceptance of the germ theory

The acceptance of the germ theory led to a greater understanding of the causes of infection. Less than 100 years ago, infection was such a common companion of childbirth in some communities, notably among hospital patients, that its symptoms were termed childbed or puerperal fever (referring to the puerperium, the approximate 6-week-period after birth). Standards of cleanliness in most 19th century hospitals were nonexistent, and the suggestion that illness might be spread by the contaminated hands of physicians and medical students met with much opposition and scorn. Nevertheless, despite great difficulty and even persecution, certain individuals began to persuade the medical world that puerperal fever was really a contagion borne by many hands and common objects.

Chief among these medical pioneers was a Hungarian, Ignaz Philipp Semmelweis (1818-1865), whose sad but fascinating biography should be read by every maternity nurse. The American poet-physician, Oliver Wendell Holmes (1809-1894), is probably best remembered for his poem "Chambered Nautilus," but medical historians record his concern with maternal mortality and his widely criticized paper, entitled "The Contagiousness of Puerperal Fever." The famed French chemist, Louis Pasteur (1822-1895), confirmed that childbed fever was caused by bacteria and was contagious in character.

Improvement of techniques and teaching

Obstetric techniques and teaching have vastly improved. With the acceptance of the germ theory, new concepts of care evolved. Britain's Joseph Lister (1827-

1912), the Father of Antisepsis, began to combat infection by chemical means and new wound-dressing techniques. Students of obstetrics were given more clinical instructions at the bedside, and their "experience" was less confined to the printed page or the dissecting table. New tools, such as improved obstetric forceps, sutures, and syringes; antibiotic medications; laboratory clinical tests; transfusions; and anesthesia were developed. Hospitalization of the childbearing woman and her child became an asset.

More recently there has been the development of new laboratory methods of assessing fetal maturity and health, the wide use of ultrasonic and electronic fetal monitoring, and more aggressive techniques in treating the immature or sick newborn. Greater technologic aid is available to the mother facing high risk pregnancy and labor. These advances, along with the regionalization of maternal and infant intensive care centers, have further reduced mortality and morbidity.

Development and utilization of prenatal care

Probably most significant to the improvement of maternal and infant well-being was the development of *prenatal care* and extended obstetric services by private and governmental public health facilities. Nurses relate proudly that prenatal care began as a nursing contribution instigated by the Instructive Nursing Association of the Boston Lying-In Hospital in 1901. From one visit before childbirth, ideal prenatal care has now developed into close supervision of the expectant mother from the time her pregnancy is confirmed. Prenatal care has been extended to more and more Americans through the services of public health departments, visiting nurses, nurse practitioners, and nurse-midwives, as well as private clinics and individual physicians. However, in spite of these efforts, an alarming number of women in the United States now are not obtaining adequate prenatal care. These mothers frequently lack resources for private medical assistance and encounter or perceive numerous barriers to public maternity care. Many are young and nonwhite. A significant percentage of these women give birth to low-birth-weight babies who require extensive hospitalization for neonatal medical and nursing services. They often need long-term follow-up because of diverse disabilities. Too many of these babies become part of our infant mortality statistics and greatly increase infant morbidity statistics. Proper prenatal care would help reduce this trauma and waste.* Much analysis of health

*Cagle CS: Access to care and prevention of low birth weight, MCN 12 (4):235, 1987.

delivery systems, funding, promotional expertise, and education is still needed.

Today as never before the entire nation is experiencing the stresses of structural change and modification. These changes are reflected in numerous patterns of family organization, divisions of labor, and sexual relationships. Women who need maternity care in the United States are representatives of a mobile, pluralistic, multicultural society. They face the experience of childbearing with differing concerns, expectations, goals, and resources. Maternity nurses must increasingly be aware of the wide variety of backgrounds their patients represent, their differing needs, and the individualized care they may require.

One of the major developments of the last decade was the increasing assertiveness of consumers of health services. A growing number of expectant parents demanded to participate more actively as a family in the process of pregnancy and childbirth. For some, but not for all, this meant a birth relatively free of medical intervention. Some have sought alternatives to so-called traditional hospitalization, such as home birth or, a birth center, or in-hospital single room maternity care.

Two important statements that clearly voice these concerns are the Pregnant Patient's Bill of Rights and the Pregnant Patient's Responsibilities available from the International Childbirth Education Association. They help to identify many concerns involving modern maternity care. The declaration that childbirth is a normal rather than a pathologic event has much to commend it. Also praiseworthy are the childbearing woman's willingness to accept responsibility for the birth process and the parents' commitment to the promotion of normal childbirth. Difficulty may arise, however, when differences between normal and abnormal are not adequately appreciated in time to allow successful treatment of complications. It is extremely interesting that, as more technical and mechanical methods of detecting complications are being introduced and perfected, emphasis on humanistic values increases. The two are not necessarily incompatible; they are complementary. Indeed, maternal and child care has been described as both a science and an art.

CHANGE AND PROGRESS IN CHILD CARE

Naturally, the same factors that improved maternity care have helped to enhance the lives of children of all ages. However, pediatrics is a more recent specialty than obstetrics. Until the 1800s there was little formalized recognition of the special needs of children, the medical and surgical problems peculiar to childhood, and the different ways in which infants and children, in contrast to adults, respond to the presence of disease.

Development of pediatrics

In 1802 the first children's hospital was founded in Paris. In 1855 the first children's hospital in the United States was established in Philadelphia. But in most regions, sick, hospitalized children were often quartered with ill adults, sometimes in the same bed! Gradually, the consideration of pediatrics as a separate study was initiated. As medical schools recognized the unique qualities of the childhood period, nursing schools followed their lead and offered special classes in pediatric nursing. General hospitals established pediatric departments, and more separate treatment centers for children were inaugurated. An early leader in the recognition of the special needs of children was Abraham Jacobi, first president of the American Pediatric Society (1888) and founder of the first clinic operated exclusively for children.

Responses of a changing society to children's needs

Change in itself does not automatically guarantee progress, and certainly the vast technologic changes of the late 19th and early 20th centuries did little to improve the immediate outlook of a great number of the world's children. The new demands of the rapidly accelerating industrial revolution, often untempered by regard for the individual—child or adult—caused sudden urban congestion. Although standards of living rose for some, often the industrial laborer suffered from deprivation and exploitation. Some of those laborers working in the mills, factories, and mines were children. Two early major events, the inauguration of the White House Conferences and the establishment of the Children's Bureau, reflected a definite improvement and promotion of a better life for all children.

White House Conferences. From 1909 through 1971, close to the beginning of each decade, the very important national White House Conferences were held. These focused attention on the current prominent needs of children and youth. Delegates of private and governmental agencies at local, state, and federal levels concerned with maternal and child care, as well as selected youth representatives, convened for evaluation of these needs and the ways in which they could be met. One of the most significant documents in the history of child care was prepared at the 1930 White House Conference on Child Health and Protection. Entitled "The Rights of the Child as an Individual in the State," it has been called the "Children's Charter." The theme of the midcentury White

Pledge to children

To you, our children, who hold within you our most cherished hopes, we the members of the Midcentury White House Conference on Children and Youth, relying on your full response, make this pledge:

From your earliest infancy we give you our love, so that you may grow with trust in yourself and in others.

We will recognize your worth as a person and we will help you to strengthen your sense of belonging.

We will respect your right to be yourself and at the same time help you to understand the rights of others, so that you may experience cooperative living.

We will help you develop initiative and imagination, so that you may have the opportunity freely to create.

We will encourage your curiosity and your pride in workmanship, so that you may have the satisfaction that comes from achievement.

We will provide the conditions for wholesome play that will add to your learning, to your social experience, and to your happiness.

We will illustrate by precept and example the value of integrity and the importance of moral courage.

We will encourage you always to seek the truth.

We will provide you with all opportunities possible to develop your own faith in God.

We will open the way for you to enjoy the arts and to use them for deepening your understanding of life.

We will work to rid ourselves of prejudice and discrimination, so that together we may achieve a truly democratic society.

We will work to lift the standard of living and to improve our economic practices, so that you may have the material basis for a full life.

We will provide you with rewarding educational opportunities, so that you may develop your talents and contribute to a better world.

We will protect you against exploitation and undue hazards and help you grow in health and strength.

We will work to conserve and improve family life and, as needed, to provide foster care according to your inherent rights.

We will intensify our search for new knowledge in order to guide you more effectively as you develop your potentialities.

As you grow from child to youth to adult, establishing a family life of your own and accepting larger social responsibilities, we will work with you to improve conditions for all children and youth.

Aware that these promises to you cannot be fully met in a world at war, we ask you to join us in a firm dedication to the building of a world society based on freedom, justice, and mutual respect.

So may you grow in joy, in faith in God and in man, and in those qualities of vision and of the spirit that will sustain us all and give us new hope for the future.

House Conference was "A Fair Chance to Achieve a Healthy Personality." At this conference the "Pledge to Children" was adopted. (See box above.) The 1970-71 White House Conference focused on children and youth in the changing social scene. The White House Conferences on children scheduled for the 1980s were cancelled, but funds were made available for state-level conferences.

Children's Bureau. Principally because of the problem of child labor and a result of the support of the first White House Conference on Children and Youth, the Children's Bureau was founded in 1912. It was initially placed under the jurisdiction of the Department of Labor. When the Department of Health, Education and Welfare (DHEW) was created in 1953, the bureau became part of the responsibility of this cabinet post. In its founding legislation, as amended, the Children's Bureau was charged with the responsibility "to investigate and report on all matters pertaining to the welfare of children and child life among all classes of our people"; to carry out research, demonstration, and training functions; to help coordinate the programs for children and parents throughout the Department of Health, Education and Welfare (today known as the Department of Health and Human Services); to promote programs for youth; and to identify areas requiring the development of new projects.

The findings of studies carried out by the Children's Bureau led to the Maternal and Infant Act, also known as the Sheppard-Towner Act of 1921. This act granted federal funds, to be matched by state funds, providing the needed services to improve and promote the health of mothers and children. The Sheppard-Towner Act was opposed by many, including the American Medical Association (AMA), and was not renewed in 1929. At that time a group of physicians broke away from the AMA and founded the American Academy of Pediatrics. During this period, the country was suffering from the Great Depression, which further reduced the budgets of programs for mothers and children. In 1930 the White House Conference promoted the concept that public support was needed for a comprehensive program of medical and health care, including services for maternal and child health and for crippled children. As the federal government's responsibility for the well-being of infants and children was growing, the Children's Bureau prepared a plan that later served as the basis for the enactment of Title V legislation. Signed into law in 1935, the Social Security Act, which included the Title V programs for mothers and children, authorized federal grants to states to improve maternal and child health services. The federal responsibility for administering the programs was given to the Children's Bureau. The Children's Bureau served in this capacity until 1969 when it was revised. Health grants from the bureau then became the responsibility of the Public Health Service. What remained of the Children's Bureau was transferred to the newly created Office of Child Development where it continued to supply a wide range of technical assistance services to children and families. In 1977 the Office of Child Development was replaced by the Administration for Children, Youth and Families (ACYF). The Children's Bureau, now located in the ACYF, currently administers the National Center on Child Abuse and Neglect, established in 1974 under the Child Abuse Prevention and Treatment Act.

Social Security legislation. The Social Security Act provided for a federal-state partnership to promote maternal and child health. Title V of this legislation is the basis for extensive programs including nutrition, family planning, prenatal, and other services for mothers and children. It reinforced the principle that all people in the United States, through the federal government, share responsibility with the state and local governments for helping to provide essential community services for children. To back up this principle, the Social Security Act authorizes Congress to appropriate funds each year to be given to the states to help them extend and improve their maternal and child health, crippled children's, and child welfare services. In 1965, under Title XIX of the Social Security Act, Medicaid was authorized. With matching funds, states may receive federal aid to pay for comprehensive health care for children. Whether a child is eligible for such aid depends on his problem or diagnosis and the financial position of his family. In 1972 an extension of Title XIX provided that preventive child health services would be made available to all Medicaid recipients under age 21 years through the Early and Periodic

Screening, Diagnosis, and Treatment (EPSDT) program. The EPSDT program offers children of low-income families preventive and case-finding health services while they are in school in an attempt to correct or reduce health problems before severe handicaps develop. In 1975 a wide variety of social services was authorized under Title XX of the Social Security Act. Funds were allocated to each state to provide family planning and child care services, including foster care for needy children.

Project Head Start. Continued organized public concern for the health and welfare of children has resulted in some progress in society's efforts to protect their rights and promote their well-being.

Project Head Start is a comprehensive program launched by the Office of Economic Opportunity in the summer of 1965 and delegated to the Department of Health, Education and Welfare (now the Department of Health and Human Services) in July 1969. It is designed particularly to help preschool children from disadvantaged backgrounds develop their full potential and social competence. It provides for a daily program of learning activities, nutritious meals, medical and dental care, and psychologic, social, and economic services for these children and their families. Parental participation is a vital requirement of the program.

Child abuse and neglect. In 1978 the Child Abuse Prevention and Treatment Act Amendments and Reform Act was enacted. Federal funds provided for the National Center on Child Abuse, which had the legislative mandate to receive reports of child abuse and to disseminate information on activities and research on abuse and neglect. Federal funds were made available for demonstration projects that provided preventive, social, and medical services, as well as treatment services, for families and children at risk.

Administration for Children, Youth, and Families (ACYF). This agency administers all programs formerly in the Office of Child Development, which it replaced. The Administration for Children, Youth and Families includes three major divisions: the Head Start Bureau, the Children's Bureau, and the new Youth Development Bureau, which will have responsibility for the runaway youth program and other youth activities. ACYF coordinates and serves as an advocate for all children's programs throughout the federal government in an attempt to improve the wide range of services for children, youth, and their families. Numerous other programs concerned with the health of mothers and children are located within the Department of Health and Human Services.

Current budget reduction. Major legislative changes have reduced federal expenditures for a wide variety of health and social welfare services. In 1980 several federally funded programs were eliminated and a number of others were reduced. The Omnibus Budget Reconciliation Act passed in 1981 called for the consolidation of categoric grants-in-aid (Title V funds) with other grants into a block grant type of funding. The Title V legislation of 1935, which confirmed the commitment of the United States to provide comprehensive maternal and child health programs, continues to supply these services within the block grant funding. Federal funds in the form of block grants are allocated to the states based on several factors, including child population and financial need. Each state receiving funds must match three dollars of state money for every four dollars of federal funds. In addition the states must report to the secretary of health and human services regarding the use of these federal monies. Many of the services supported by federal and state funds are being reevaluated and reorganized.

American Academy of Pediatrics. An important analysis of health status goals for children has been conducted by the executive board of the American Academy of Pediatrics (AAP). The academy, now composed of a membership of over 17,000 pediatricians, has assumed a leadership role in establishing standards of child health care. It approved 10 health status goals for children that outline the basic requirements for good child health.

1. All children should be wanted and born to healthy mothers.
2. All children should be born well.
3. All children should be immunized against the preventable infectious diseases for which there are recommended immunization procedures.
4. All children should have good nutrition.
5. All children should be educated about health and the health care system.
6. All children should live in a safe environment.
7. All children with chronic handicaps should be able to function at their optimal level.
8. All children should live in a family setting with an adequate income to provide basic needs to ensure physical and intellectual health.
9. All children should live in an environment that is as free as possible from contaminants.
10. All adolescents and young people should live in a social setting that recognizes their special health, personal, and social needs.

Private volunteer programs. Numerous private voluntary organizations are interested in certain specific diseases or conditions and provide considerable funds for research, diagnosis, and treatment. The National Foundation is particularly interested in birth defects. The Cystic Fibrosis Research Foundation, the American Cancer Society, the Muscular Dystrophy Association, the American Heart Association, the Epilepsy Association of America, and the National Association for Retarded Children all are examples of such private voluntary groups. Other private social agencies help by providing essential community services, such as adoption, care of unwed mothers, counseling and psychiatric services, homemaking, and recreational facilities.

International organizations. On an international scale two organizations under the auspices of the United Nations immediately come to mind. The first is the United Nations International Children's Emergency Fund, called the United Nations Children's Fund since 1950, although the former initials, UNICEF, have been retained. This organization, supported entirely by voluntary contributions, was established in 1946 to relieve the distress of children caused by war. It has now greatly expanded its scope. It currently includes not only distribution of food, clothing, and medicine but also provisions for education and training of needed national workers in the health field. It is the world's largest international agency devoted to children and has received the Nobel Peace Prize for its efforts on behalf of children.

In 1956 the General Assembly of the United Nations, showing international concern for a popular topic, approved another important statement in the history of child care, "The Declaration of the Rights of the Child." Representative of UNICEF activity was its role in promoting the International Year of the Child (IYC), proclaimed by the United Nations for 1979.

The second United Nations–sponsored agency is the World Health Organization (WHO), formed in 1948. It helps coordinate efforts for disease control, provides a method of sharing new information in the fight against disease, and cooperates with UNICEF in promoting maternal and child health.

Continuing challenge

In spite of significant progress during past years, much remains to be done. Although the United States is ranked as the most affluent country in the world, many Americans continue to be burdened with poverty, hunger, illness, and despair. The concentrated urban and dispersed rural poor, changing population patterns, unevenly distributed medical care, increasing health costs, and problems affecting the allocation of resources have necessitated alterations in health care delivery.

An increased number of extended nursing roles, involving advanced preparation, has been and is now being defined. Some of these roles will include family, pediatric, and school nurse practitioners, geriatric practitioners, and nurse-midwives.

To meet the desires of consumers for more control over health care decisions and more emphasis on the promotion of health rather than the treatment of disease, new types of health insurance and prepaid medical care are being formulated. Nursing in the combined maternal-child or family care settings of the future may change in form, but its basic intent, to promote health and to cope with the threat and discomfort of disease, remains constant.

These are some of the many challenges still to be met that profoundly affect the quality of the basic unit—the family and the child it produces. Continued effort must be exerted in order to strengthen the family unit and lend stability, depth, and purpose to the daily lives of all persons so that individually and collectively they and coming generations may enjoy creatively the best that life can offer.

The present-day maternal-child nurse works in an area that demands increasing knowledge, skill, and sensitivity. Responsibilities embrace an understanding of the reproductive process, its possible complications, care of the mother and her growing child in health and illness, an ability in health teaching, an appreciation of the role of the family, and a knowledge of community resources. Each patient is an individual with particular needs. For the alert nurse there is abundant opportunity for real challenge and achievement.

═══════ INTRODUCTION ═══════

SUGGESTED SELECTED READINGS AND REFERENCES

General

Aiken LH: Nursing's future: public policies, private actions, Am J Nurs 83(10):1440, 1983.

AMA, other groups push proposals to replace some hard-to-find RNs with technical personnel, Am J Nurs 88(6):894, 1988.

Arbeiter JS: The big shift to home health nursing, RN 47(11):38, 1984.

Avant KC and Walker LO: Professionally speaking: the practicing nurse and conceptual frameworks, MCN 9(2):87, 1984.

Bishop BE: ANA's definition of nursing (editorial), MCN 8(1):1983.

Bishop BE: Did AMA do nursing a favor? MCN 13(6):393, 1988.

Bobak IM, Jensen MD, and Zalar MK: Maternity and gynecologic care: the nurse and the family, St Louis, 1989, The CV Mosby Co.

Brider P: Too poor to pay: the scandal of patient dumping, Am J Nurs 87(11):1447, 1987.

Carter ER: Quality maternity care for the medically indigent, MCN 11(2):85, 1986.

Cushing M: How courts look at nurse practice acts, Am J Nurs 86(2):131, 1986.

Damrosch SP and others: On behalf of homeless families, MCN 13(4):259, 1988.

Daria J and Moran S: Nursing in the 90s, Nursing 85 15(12):26, 1985.

DeCrosta T: Megatrends in nursing: 10 new directions that are changing your profession, Nurs Life 5(3):17, 1985.

Directory of nursing organizations, Am J Nurs 89(4):575, 1989.

Edgar AB: 200 years of childbirth, Parents 60(12):174, 1985.

Fickeissen JL: Getting certified, Am J Nurs 85(3):265, 1985.

Fleming JW: Professionally speaking: maternal-child nursing in the decade ahead, MCN 10(6):369, 1985.

Foster RLR, Hunsberger MM, and Anderson JJT: Family-centered nursing care of children, Philadelphia, 1989, WB Saunders Co.

Gale CA: Inadequacy of health care for the nation's chronically ill children, J Pediatr Health Care, 3(1)20, 1989.

Halloran E and Halloran D: Exploring the DRG/nursing equation, Am J Nurs 85(10):1093, 1985.

Huey FL: How nurses would change US health care, Am J Nurs 88(11):1482, 1988.

Joel LA: Reshaping nursing practice, Am J Nurs 87(6):763, 1987.

Lagoe R, et al: Diagnosis-related groups and regional neonatal care, Pediatrics 77(5):627, 1986.

Lesser AJ: The origin and development of maternal and child health programs in the United States, Am J Public Health 75(6):590, 1985.

LPNs widen their role; disagreement grows, Am J Nurs 90(2):16, 1990.

Mallison MB: Finally—the nation takes notice, Am J Nurs 87(8):1009, 1987.

Mallison MB: Gate crashers (editorial), Am J Nurs 90(2):7, 1990 (outcomes of care in birth centers).

Manthey M: Can primary nursing survive? Am J Nurs 88(5):645, 1988.

Mott S, Fazekas N, and James S: Nursing care of children and families, San Francisco, 1985, Addison-Wesley Publishing Co.

Omdahl DJ: Home care strictly by the rules, Am J Nurs 89(4):511, 1989.

Ostwald SK, Abanobi OC, and Kochevar LK: Nurse practitioner's perception of workplace encroachment, Pediatr Nurs 10(5):337, 1984.

Pierce C and Vandeveer D, editors: AIDS: ethics and public policy, Belmont, Calif, 1988 Wadsworth Publishing Co.

Queenan JT: Editorial: Lessons from the eastern front, Contemp OB/GYN 35(1):10, 1990.

Simon F: Childbirth through the ages, Parents 58(11):82, 1983.

Starfield B: Giant steps and baby steps toward child health, Am J Public Health 75(6):599, 1985.

Wallace HM, Ryan G, and Oglesby AC: Maternal and child health practices, San Francisco, 1988, Third Party Publishing Co.

Waters S: What happens if your hospital bills separately for nursing? RN 48(7):18, 1985.

Wegman ME: Annual summary of vital statistics, 1988, Pediatrics 84(6):943, 1989.

Wertz RW and Wertz DC: Lying-in: a history of childbirth in America, New York, 1977, Free Press.

Whaley LF and Wong DL: Essentials of pediatric nursing, ed 3, St Louis, 1989, The CV Mosby Co.

Wood D: Homeless children: their evaluation and treatment, J Pediatr Health 3(4):194, 1989.

Reproductive Anatomy and Physiology

1

Female Reproductive Anatomy

CHAPTER OBJECTIVES

After studying this chapter, the student should be able to perform the following:

1 Identify the location of all bones, landmarks, and joints described.
2 Indicate the practical significance of such measurements as the true conjugate (conjugata vera or C.V.); the distance between the ischial tuberosities (Bi. Isch. or T.I.); and obstetric stations of −2, 0, and +2.
3 Point out differences in the shape of the pelvic canal at its inlet and outlet and how they affect the mechanism of an infant's birth.
4 List four causes of distorted pelvic canals.
5 Enumerate three instances in which a study of the size and shape of the pelvic canal would be especially important.
6 Describe four ways in which pelvic size, shape, and contents may be evaluated.

7 Identify the structures of the female external genitalia (see Fig. 1-8).
8 Identify the structures shown in the midsagittal section of the female pelvis (see Fig. 1-9).
9 Describe the functions of the clitoris, urethra, vagina, uterus, oviducts, and ovaries.
10 Draw a pear-shaped uterus indicating its three main anatomic parts.
11 Name and describe the three main tissue layers that form the uterine wall.
12 Name the main or largest muscle group that helps form the female pelvic floor.
13 Define an episiotomy and explain why it may be performed. What other alternatives exist?

PELVIS: THE BONY PASSAGEWAY

To understand the events of labor and birth, the nurse must be acquainted with the first journey the fetus takes—that of a few inches through the mother's birth canal. Because this canal is shaped largely by the bones of the pelvis, we will begin with a discussion of its formation and contours.

The word *pelvis* means basin. It describes the cavity in the kidneys into which the urine drains before flowing down the ureter. It also describes the bony ring located between the trunk and thighs, joining the spine above and the femurs below. The latter is the pelvis to which we refer here.

Anatomy

The pelvis is formed by the two innominate bones and the sacrum and coccyx (Fig. 1-1, *A*). Each innominate bone is the end result of the fusion of three distinct bones: ilium, ischium, and pubis (Fig. 1-1, *B*).

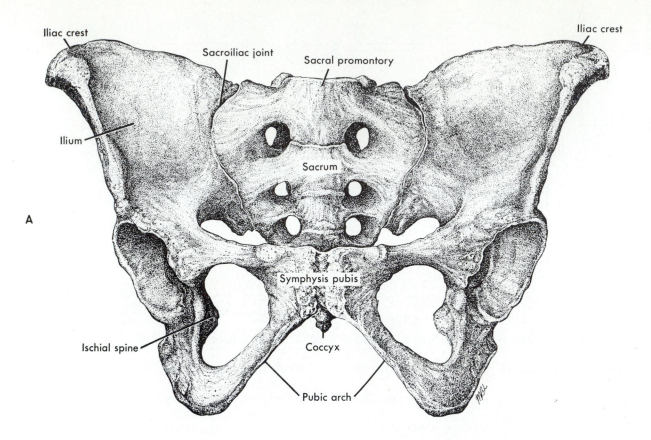

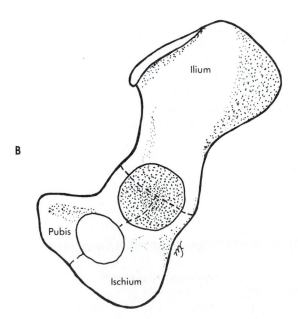

FIG 1-1 A, Female pelvis, anterior view. **B,** Schematic view of external surface of left innominate bone showing fusion of ilium, ischium and pubis.

Landmarks and joints

anterosuperior iliac spines The lower front end of the iliac crest line (Fig. 1-2).

iliac crests The hip bones. Convenient for book or baby balancing (Fig. 1-1, *A* and *B*).

iliopectineal line (linea terminalis, brim) Divides the upper or false pelvis from the lower or true pelvis (Fig. 1-2).

ischial spines (see Figs. 1-1, *A*, 1-2, and 1-3) Two important landmarks in determining the depth of the fetus in the passageway. The location of the presenting part of the fetus in the pelvic canal in relation to the ischial spines is termed its *station*. If the presenting part is at the level of the ischial spines, its station is said to be 0, or zero. If it is above the ischial spines, it is termed minus (−) so many centimeters (e.g., − 1 or − 2 cm). If the presenting part is below the ischial spines, its location is termed plus (+) so many centimeters (e.g., + 1 or + 2 cm). When a woman in labor nears full cervical dilatation and has a station of + 2 cm, the nurse must realize that, if the mechanism of labor is normal, the infant will probably be born in a relatively short time. (See also Fig. 6-6, p. 99.)

ischial tuberosities Major bony sitting support; important in measuring a transverse diameter of the pelvis (Fig. 1-3).

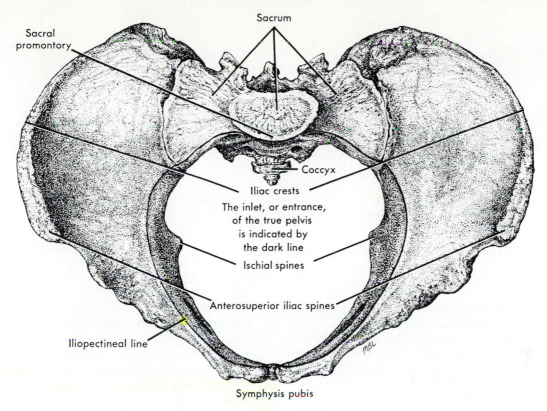

Sacrum

Sacral
promontory

Coccyx

Iliac crests

The inlet, or entrance,
of the true pelvis
is indicated by
the dark line

Ischial spines

Anterosuperior iliac spines

Iliopectineal line

Symphysis pubis

FIG 1-2   The inlet—traced by dark iliopectineal line.

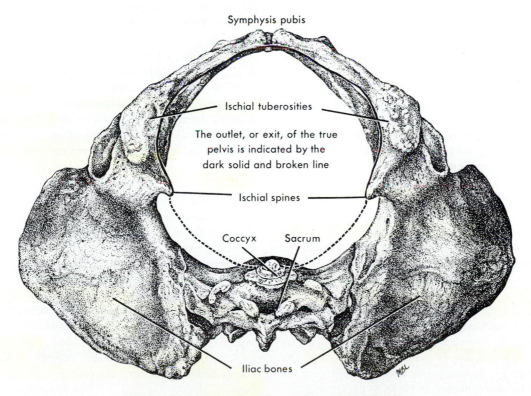

Symphysis pubis

Ischial tuberosities

The outlet, or exit, of the true
pelvis is indicated by the
dark solid and broken line

Ischial spines

Coccyx   Sacrum

Iliac bones

FIG 1-3   The outlet—traced by solid and broken dark lines.

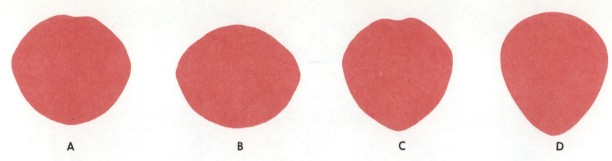

FIG 1-4 Types of pelves. **A,** Normal female pelvic inlet (gynecoid). **B,** Flattened female pelvic inlet (platypelloid). **C,** Typical male pelvic inlet (android). **D,** Ape-type pelvic inlet (anthropoid).

pubic arch Formed by the lower border of the symphysis pubis and the ischial bones (Fig. 1-1, *A*).

sacral promontory The internal junction of the last lumbar vertebra and the sacrum, important in obtaining an internal obstetric measurement, known as the true conjugate (conjugata vera or C.V.) (Figs. 1-1, *A*, and 1-2).

sacrococcygeal joint Located between the sacrum and coccyx, retains limited mobility, which may offer additional room for the passage of the fetus by bending the coccyx slightly backward possibly as much as 1 inch (2.54 cm) (Fig. 1-6).

sacroiliac joints Found at either side of the sacrum joining with the iliac bones (Fig. 1-1, *A*).

symphysis pubis Junction of the pubic bones (Fig. 1-1, *A*).

True and false pelvis. The *false pelvis,* formed chiefly by flaring wings of the iliac portions of the innominate bones, helps guide the fetus into the true obstetric canal. However, the *true pelvis* just below is the real concern of the obstetrician. In its journey the fetus must adapt to the different diameters and shapes of the true pelvis to reach the outside world successfully.

Inlet and outlet. The entrance to the true pelvis is the *inlet* (Fig. 1-2). Its shape is traced in part by the iliopectineal line. It is wider from side to side than from front to back. Therefore the head usually enters the true pelvis with its longest diameter (front to back) pointed from side to side, or in transverse position.

The exit of the true pelvis is the *outlet* and is wider from front to back than from side to side (Fig. 1-3). To pass through the outlet, the head usually must turn to accommodate its longest diameter to the longest diameter of the exit. This turning is called *internal rotation.* The canal formed by the true pelvis curves slightly near the outlet and has been likened in shape to the letter J.

Pelvic differences

Classification. No two pelves are exactly alike although they may be classified according to their measurements. The most common classification concerns the shape and dimensions of the inlet (Fig. 1-4). The typical female pelvic inlet is *gynecoid*. The typical male inlet is *android*. Unfortunately, some women have android-type pelves. A look at a male pelvis offers at least one reason why the human male could not bear children. Typically, the inlet of the male pelvis is heart-shaped and angular, and the whole pelvic structure is heavier and more confining than that of the female, with a steep and narrow pubic arch. In contrast, a typical woman's pelvis is relatively light and commodious, and the pubic arch is shallow and wide. Occasionally, a woman's pelvic inlet is abnormally flat, or *platypelloid,* with a decreased anteroposterior diameter, or it may have an *anthropoid* or apelike configuration with an enlarged anteroposterior measurement and a restricted transverse diameter. These problems may necessitate a cesarean birth (abdominal delivery). But whether a birth will terminate abdominally or vaginally depends on several factors, including the type of passageway; the size, position, and well-being of the fetus; the strength of the uterine contractions; and the condition of the laboring mother.

Causes of abnormalities. A history of certain conditions may alert the physician to expect trouble because of pelvic abnormalities. The six main causes of abnormal pelvic measurements are heredity (characteristic familial problems, dwarfism), infections (poliomyelitis, osteomyelitis, tuberculosis of the bone), poor nutrition (rickets), accidents (fractured pelves), paralysis of one or both extremities, and poor posture and exercise habits.

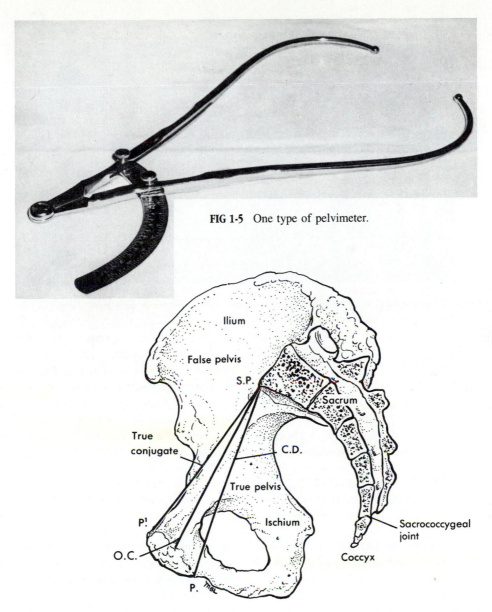

FIG 1-5 One type of pelvimeter.

FIG 1-6 Female pelvis, sagittal section. *C.D.*, diagonal conjugate; *P¹*, inner superior border of pubis; *P.*, outer inferior border of pubis; *S.P.*, sacral promontory; *O.C.*, obstetrical conjugate.

Methods of pelvic evaluation

Pelvic size, contour, and adequacy may be measured or evaluated by the methods discussed below.

External palpation. In external palpation instruments called pelvimeters (Fig. 1-5) are used to determine the most important external measurement. It reveals the distance between the ischial tuberosities (Bi. Isch. or T.I., averaging 10 to 11 cm). This measurement may help indicate the distance between the ischial spines, a critical transverse measurement.

Internal palpation. In internal palpation a lubricated gloved finger is used to determine the distance between the sacral promontory and the outer inferior border of the pubis, known as the *diagonal conjugate* (C.D., averaging 12.5 cm). From this measurement a closer estimate of the anteroposterior diameter of the inlet, referred to as the *true conjugate* (conjugata vera or C.V.) may be made. To do this, one subtracts 1.5 to 2 cm from the diagonal conjugate to compensate for the thickness and tilt of the pubic bone. The true conjugate usually

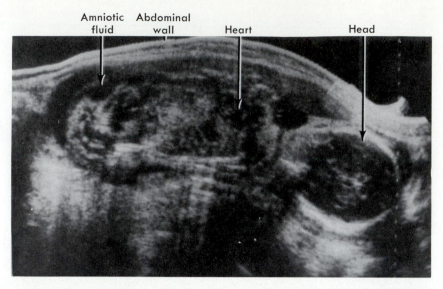

Amniotic   Abdominal
fluid   wall   Heart   Head

FIG 1-7 Longitudinal view of fetus taken using ultrasound. *(Courtesy George R. Leopold, MD, University Hospital, San Diego.)*

averages 11 cm (Fig. 1-6). The shortest distance between the posterior surface of the symphysis pubis and the sacral promontory, the *obstetric conjugate* (O.C.), like the true conjugate, is only estimated clinically.

X-ray pelvimetry. X-ray pelvimetry is now rare in most maternity settings. X-ray use has been limited because of the danger to developing fetal structures (especially in early pregnancy), the threat of subsequent childhood cancer, the possible effects of radiation to maternal pelvic contents, and the questionable usefulness of the information obtained.

However, there is on the obstetric horizon the possibility of the clinical use of computerized tomography to determine classical pelvic dimensions. CT scans also involve ionizing radiation but much less (about 20% to 30% of that required by conventional x-ray pelvimetry). These scans are simpler and safer. CT would be particularly welcome for the evaluation of breech presentations. Its cost and availability are undergoing study.*

Ultrasonography (Fig. 1-7). The use of ultrasonography to detect differences in tissue density by directing high-frequency sound waves into tissue and electrically measuring the reflected echoes from internal structures has been increasingly employed in modern obstetrics. It helps evaluate the condition of and clarify many potential problems affecting a mother and her unborn child (see Table 4-2, pp. 56-57). Although ultrasound studies cannot effectively provide traditional pelvic measurements, they do assist in the evaluation of a mother's ability to give birth through the pelvic passageway. They reveal multiple pregnancies and certain fetal positions and abnormalities of the mother or child that may complicate the pregnancy or delivery. They usually indicate the position and size of the baby's head (biparietal diameter) as well as the approximate fetal weight. With this information, along with internal and external estimates of the mother's pelvic size, a knowledge of her reproductive history, her progress during labor, and the well-being of her unborn infant, more informed decisions may be made concerning obstetric care.

During the almost 20 years in which diagnostic ultrasound has been used, no injuries to a mother or fetus have been recorded. However, this valuable tool should not be employed solely to satisfy curiosity or provide entertainment. Routine screening of all pregnancies is still controversial.* The cost-effectiveness of such screening, in the United States, has not as yet been demonstrated.

Knowledge of the structure of the obstetric passage-

*Evans MI and others, editors: Fetal diagnosis and therapy: science, ethics and the law, Philadelphia, 1989, JB Lippincott Co.

*Chervenak FA, McCullough LB, and Chervenak JL: Prenatal informed consent for sonogram: an indication for obstetric ultrasonography, Am J Obstet Gynecol 16(4):857, 1989.

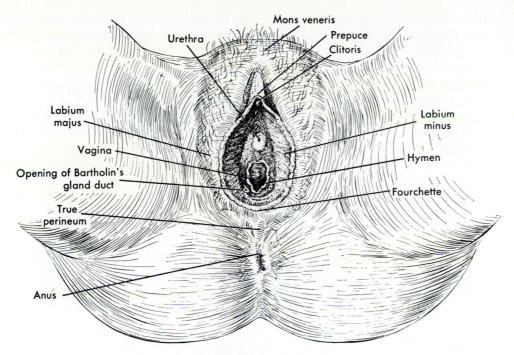

FIG 1-8 Female external genitalia.

way is essential for understanding the mechanism of labor and the problems the physician will face. So far we have reviewed the bony pelvis. We shall now discuss the soft structures involved—the muscles of the pelvic floor and the organs they support.

PELVIC CONTENTS AND SUPPORT

The fetus must pass through the pelvis, in which there are many soft tissue structures vital to normal body function. These structures are supported by layers of muscle, fibrous coverings called *fasciae,* and various ligaments and tendons. The fasciae help cushion the passage of the fetus through the hard, bony canal and direct its descent. Occasionally they impede the infant's progress, and may sustain damage at the time of birth.

External reproductive structures

When the woman is lying on her back with knees flexed, observation of the genitalia or vulva reveals the superficial relationships of many vital soft tissue organs (Fig. 1-8).

Mon veneris. The mon veneris (mount of Venus, mons pubis) is a fatty pad over the symphysis pubis which, after puberty, becomes covered with curly hair in the form of an inverted triangle extending between the legs.

Labia majora. The labia majora (larger lips; singular, labium majus) are two fleshy, hair-covered folds, extending on each side of the midline from the mons veneris almost to the anus. In a child or a woman who has not borne a child, these folds almost completely cover the structures between them. They correspond to the two halves of the scrotum in the man. Their inner surfaces are rich in oil and sweat glands.

Labia minora. The labia minora (smaller lips; singular, labium minus) are two smaller, more delicate folds of tissue, located just under the labia majora. These small folds are somewhat erectile and are also supplied with oil and sweat glands.

Clitoris. The clitoris is a small sensitive, erectile structure at the anterior junction of the labia minora. Folds of the small labia surround the clitoris; the top fold forms a fleshy hood, or *prepuce,* and the lower fold forms the *frenulum.* The clitoris corresponds to the penis as the primary anatomic center of sexual arousal.

Vestibule. The vestibule is the triangular space between the labia minora in which are the openings of the urethra, the vagina, and the Bartholin glands.

Urethral opening. * The urethra, a tissue tube about 1 to 1½ inches (2.5 to 3.5 cm) in length, leads from the urinary

*The urethral opening is not part of the female reproductive system, but it is included here because of its strategic location.

bladder to the exterior and opens in the midline between the clitoris and the vagina. This opening usually appears as a dimple or slit and after childbirth may be slightly displaced or more difficult to locate because of local swelling. On the floor of the urethra two ducts open leading to Skene's glands (also called the lesser vestibular glands), which produce a moisturizing amount of alkaline mucus.

Vaginal opening. The vagina, a large distensible tube or sheath about 3 to 4 inches (7.5 to 10 cm) long, leads down and back to the uterine cervix. The mucous membrane of its interior surface is arranged in transverse folds (rugae) that allow considerable stretching. It serves as the exit point for menstrual flow, the female organ of intercourse or coitus, and the soft tissue birth canal in labor and birth. In virgins it usually is partially covered by a membrane called the *hymen* or maidenhead. However, the hymenal membrane may be accidentally torn during childhood. The presence of the hymen is no proof

of virginity, because it may be elastic and fail to tear during intercourse. In rare cases, the hymen completely covers the vaginal opening. This condition is termed *imperforate hymen* and is relieved by a hymenectomy.

Bartholin's glands. Bartholin's glands are also known as the greater vestibular glands. These two glands produce a mucoid substance during sexual stimulation that drains into the vestibule on either side of the vagina by way of two ducts. In addition to mucoid secretion from the vaginal walls themselves, this drainage provides lubrication for intercourse.

Fourchette. The fourchette is a tissue fold below the vaginal opening, formed by the fusion of the posterior edges of the labia minora. It is often lacerated in childbirth.

Perineum. The perineum is sometimes considered to be the entire body area between a woman's legs. However, the *true* or *obstetrical perineum*, means the tissue

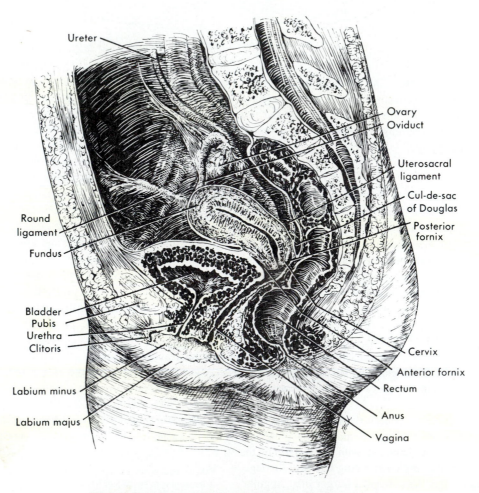

Labels: Ureter, Round ligament, Fundus, Bladder, Pubis, Urethra, Clitoris, Labium minus, Labium majus, Ovary, Oviduct, Uterosacral ligament, Cul-de-sac of Douglas, Posterior fornix, Cervix, Anterior fornix, Rectum, Anus, Vagina

FIG 1-9 Female reproductive system, midsagittal section.

block found between the posterior edge of the vagina and the anus or rectal opening. It contains the *perineal body,* a mass of connective tissue that forms the point of attachment for the muscles and fascia of the pelvic floor (see Fig. 1-11). This area is most frequently injured during childbirth. The true perineum is a critical area of pelvic support. Pelvic organs such as the vagina, uterus, bladder, and rectum may be affected by injury or inadequate repair of the perineum. Fig. 1-9 shows these internal pelvic organs and clarifies their relationships and need for support.

Internal reproductive structures

Excluding the changes that take place associated with pregnancy and childbirth, the internal reproductive organs of the adult female are usually located protectively within the pelvic cavity (Figs. 1-9 and 1-10).

Uterus. In a nonpregnant adult the uterus, or womb, is a flattened, pear-shaped hollow muscular organ about 3 inches (7.6 cm) long, 2 inches (5 cm) wide, and 1 inch (2.5 cm) thick. It protects and nourishes the developing fetus and aids in his birth. The uterine wall is composed of three layers:

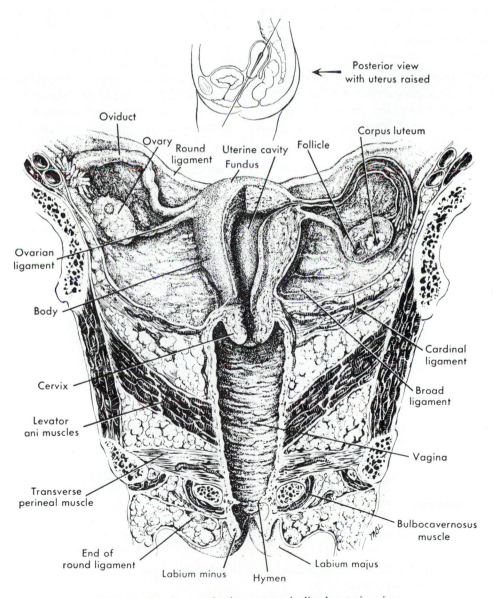

FIG 1-10 Female reproductive system, inclined posterior view.

endometrium The vascular mucus-producing inner lining that alters periodically in depth and character during the menstrual cycle.

myometrium The middle layer made up of muscular fibers that provide forceful, efficient contractions of the uterine wall during and after birth.

parametrium The outermost layer that, with the enfolding pelvic peritoneum, forms a strong connective tissue covering.

The uterus also may be divided into three main parts:

cervix (or narrow neck) Forms the main opening of the uterus.

corpus (or body) The remaining portion of the uterus.

fundus That portion of the corpus located directly opposite the cervical opening (when the uterus is raised or straightened). It is sometimes described as the rounded area found between and above the oviducts.

Normally the corpus of the uterus is tipped toward the front of a woman's body, lying above her urinary bladder. The uterine cervix dips down into the posterior portion of the vagina from above. Vaginal and cervical tissue ultimately join, forming two pouches: the anterior and the posterior fornices (singular, fornix). The posterior fornix is adjacent to a fold in the peritoneal lining of the pelvic cavity, termed the *pouch* of Douglas or the cul-de-sac. Occasionally, because of infection or bleeding in the pelvis or abdomen, pus or blood drains into this cul-de-sac and may be aspirated vaginally or rectally by a physician. (See also previous description under vaginal opening, p. 22.)

The blood supply for the uterus is derived mainly from the paired uterine and ovarian arteries. Together they form an elaborate and rich vascular network over the cervix and body of the uterus. Muscular contractions of the uterus are involuntary, guided by hormonal controls rather than motor nerves. Painful sensations that accompany contractions of the uterus and dilatation of the cervix during labor and childbirth are transmitted by sympathetic nerve fibers passing through the tenth, eleventh, and twelfth thoracic and possibly the first lumbar spinal nerves. As labor progresses and the baby descends in the birth canal, discomfort is also caused by pressure on

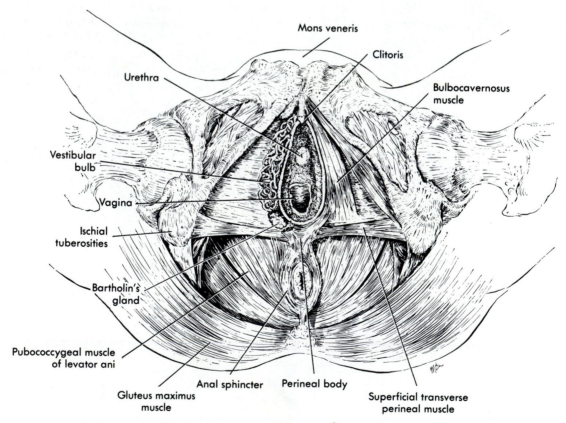

FIG 1-11 Female pelvic floor in dissection from below. Coccygeus muscle is obscured by gluteus maximus muscle.

pelvic and perineal structures outside the uterus. These sensations are transmitted by nerve fibers leading to sacral nerve pathways.

Oviducts. Uterine or fallopian tubes are paired slender, hollow tubes about 4 inches (10 cm) in length. They originate from opposite sides of the uterine cavity, just below the fundus. Their external ends terminate outside the uterine wall near each ovary with fringelike tissues called fimbriae.

Ovaries. The ovaries (female gonads) are two sex glands, sized and shaped like almonds and located on each side of the uterus beneath the open-ended oviducts. Ovaries produce the female hormones estrogen and progesterone and the female sex cells (eggs or ova; singular, ovum). At birth, an infant's ovaries contain the same number of eggs that the adult will possess—a lifetime supply. However, the eggs are immature. During childbearing years, a woman's ovaries usually release only one maturing ovum per month. When the egg is released (ovulation), it is characteristically swept up into an oviduct by the fimbriae that have hovered over the productive ovary during the maturation of the ovum. The ovum then travels through the uterine tube toward the uterus. If the ovum unites with a male sex cell (sperm) causing *fertilization* or *conception,* the event normally occurs within the oviduct. The oviducts and ovaries are often referred to as *adnexa,* or adjacent parts of the uterus.

Support of the pelvic contents

Ligaments. Not only is the uterus indirectly supported by the true perineum, it is enfolded in layers of the *broad ligaments,* which are portions of the abdominal peritoneal lining. The lower portions of the broad ligaments, sometimes called *cardinal ligaments,* are thicker. The uterus is also positioned and stabilized by other fibrous attachments such as the *round ligaments*. They lead from the uterine walls toward the front, just below the fallopian tubes, down the inguinal canals to the labia majora. The round ligaments help to hold the uterus in its forward position. The uterosacral ligaments connect the posterior cervical portion of the uterus to the sacrum. The ovaries are supported principally by the ovarian and broad ligaments (Fig. 1-10).

Muscles. The deep muscles of the pelvic floor form a type of hammock, pierced only by the urethra, vagina, and rectum. This muscle grouping, sometimes called the *upper pelvic diaphragm,* is formed by the three branches of the large *levator ani* muscle (paired pubococcygeus, iliococcygeus, and puborectalis muscles) and the coccygeus muscles.

The superficial muscles—the bulbocavernosus muscles, the transverse muscles, and the *anal sphincter*—converge in the area at the point of the true perineum, reinforcing the levator ani (Fig. 1-11). Regular, conscious exercise of the musculature of the perineal floor (particularly the pubococcygeal muscle) improves pelvic relaxation during childbirth, may help avoid or treat urinary incontinence, and may enhance sexual response. For a discussion of Kegel exercises, see p. 79.

Protection of the perineum. Various efforts are made to preserve or protect the muscles of the true perineum from tears (lacerations) at the time of birth. The head of the infant is slowly extended by external, manual pressure to force the presentation of the smallest cephalic diameter. It is delivered slowly between contractions. Many physicians, particularly in the United States, commonly perform a prophylactic perineal incision enlarging the vaginal opening called an *episiotomy*. It is an attempt to avoid an uncontrolled, jagged tear, to reduce possible prolonged pressure on the baby's head and maternal pelvic structures, and to speed delivery. Most delivery room setups routinely include the instruments and supplies needed for their execution and repair. However, routine episiotomies have become increasingly questionable. Reevaluation of birth positions, extended manual support of the perineum, and more patience during the birth process can effectively prevent many lacerations. Obvious damage to the perineal floor does not always occur as a result of childbirth. Perineal lacerations and other problems related to delivery trauma are discussed in greater detail in the chapter on labor and birth. (See pp. 138 and 141-144.)

It is well to note that in spite of the difficulties that can occur during this first human journey taken through the pelvic passageway, proper care and management prevent relatively few major problems from materializing.

Key Concepts

1. The pelvis is formed by the sacrum, coccyx, and the two innominate bones that are the end result of the fusion of the ilium, ischium, and pubis.

2. The station of the presenting part of the fetus during labor is determined by its location relative to the ischial spines.

3. The entrance to the true pelvis (inlet) is wider from side to side than from front to back; the exit (outlet) is wider from front to back than from side to side. Internal rotation enables the fetus to adapt to these differences in diameter.

4. The typical female pelvis is gynecoid. Certain pelvic abnormalities make vaginal delivery difficult or impossible. The six main causes of abnormal pelvic measurements are heredity, infections, poor nutrition, accidents, paralysis of one or both extremities, and poor posture and exercise habits.

5. Pelvic size, shape, and contents may be measured or evaluated by the following methods: external palpation, internal palpation, x-ray pelvimetry, and ultrasonography.

6. The structures of the female external genitalia are the mon veneris, labia majora, labia minora, clitoris, vestibule, urethral opening, vaginal opening, Bartholin's glands, fourchette, and perineum.

7. The female internal reproductive structures are the uterus, oviducts, and ovaries.

8. The uterine wall is composed of three layers: the endometrium, the myometrium, and the parametrium. The uterus is composed of three main parts: the cervix, the corpus, and the fundus.

9. The uterus is enfolded in layers of broad ligaments and is positioned and stabilized by other fibrous attachments such as round ligaments.

10. The pelvic floor is formed mainly by the three branches of the large levator ani muscle (paired pubococcygeus, iliococcygeus, and puborectalis muscles) and the coccygeus muscles.

11. An episiotomy may be performed to avoid an uncontrolled, jagged tear in the perineum, to reduce prolonged pressure on the baby's head and maternal pelvic structures, and to speed delivery.

Discussion Questions

1. Discuss the effects that an atypical or abnormal pelvis could have on pregnancy and delivery.

2. Identify the most common diagnostic tests related to the pelvis and reproductive organs. Is it safe to perform these tests if pregnancy is suspected?

3. How would you prepare a woman for the various diagnostic tests? What specific information should be included?

4. Many mature women are not completely familiar with the structures and functions of their body. This is also true of the reproductive system. How would you increase their knowledge and understanding? How detailed would you be in your explanation? What sort of teaching aids would you use?

5. Identify as many advantages and disadvantages of an episiotomy as you can. Discuss the implications for nursing care.

2

The Menstrual Cycle

CHAPTER OBJECTIVES

After studying this chapter, the student should be able to perform the following:

1 Define the following terms: menstruation, menses or catamenia; menarche; ovum; ovulation; follicle; corpus luteum; metrorrhagia; dysmenorrhea.
2 Describe the two different endocrine glands primarily involved with regulation of the menstrual cycle.
3 State the origins and actions of FSH, LH, estrogen, and progesterone relating to the menstrual cycle.
4 List three possible indications of ovulation and tell the practical use of these indications.
5 State when the following features occur during the menstrual cycle: proliferative phase, secretory phase, spinnbarkheit, ferning, and mittelschmerz.
6 Name four possible causes of dysmenorrhea.
7 Discuss three ways to prevent or treat the symptoms of dysmenorrhea for which no cause has been determined.

We have reviewed the anatomy of the pelvis. However, to study the physiology or function of the pelvic organs, we must discuss more than the contents of the pelvis itself.

ROLE OF THE PITUITARY GLAND

Proper functioning of the ovaries and uterus also depends on a gland located a considerable distance from the pelvic cavity but which empties its powerful products directly into the bloodstream. It exerts considerable influence on the body.

Glands that empty their manufactured products directly into the blood circulation are called *endocrine glands*. Their products are *hormones*. The gland outside the pelvis that is so important in ovarian and uterine function is the *pituitary*, located at the base of the brain. It is regulated in part by that portion of the brain called the *hypothalamus*. Some of the pituitary hormones help regulate a physiologic event universal among women called *menstruation*.

MENSTRUATION

Menstruation is the monthly elimination through a bloody vaginal discharge of a portion of the lining of the uterus that had been prepared to protect and nurture a fertilized egg in the event of pregnancy. Menstruation is also properly called menses, catamenia, and, more commonly, a period or monthly flow. Terminology that implies an undesirable condition or illness should be avoided because menstruation is not an illness but an

27

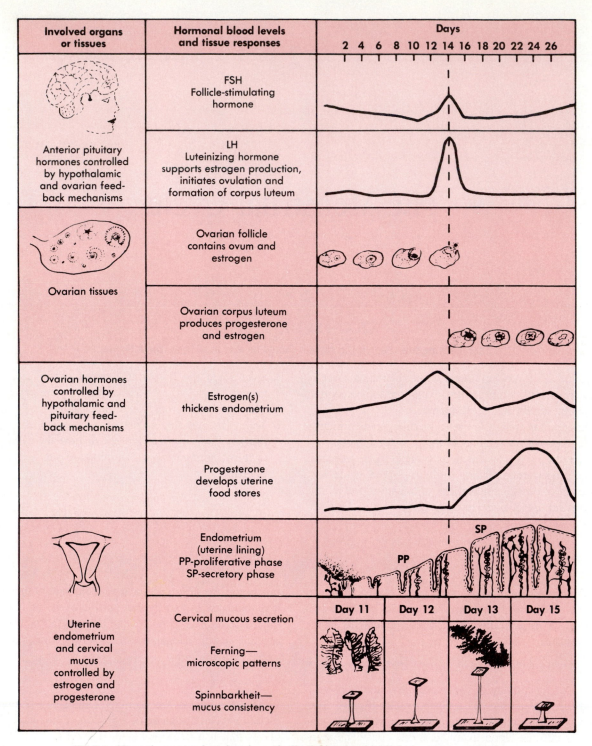

FIG 2-1 Normal menstrual cycle schematically depicted to highlight hormone production, ovulation, endometrial response, and changes in cervical mucus.

expected and necessary part of healthy mature womanhood. It may at times be inconvenient and troublesome, but it is the way all normal women function.

Menarche

The advent of menstruation in a girl is a signal of impending physical maturity. The first menses is called *menarche*. It is one of the signs of growing up. Menstruation occurs periodically throughout the childbearing years, except during pregnancy and lactation or breast feeding. The ages of onset and termination differ from person to person but seem to be affected by heredity, racial background, and nutrition.

In the United States the average age of menarche 100 years ago was 15 years of age. Today it has dropped to 12½ years of age. The earlier onset of menses is thought to be related to improved health, as demonstrated by girls in upper socioeconomic groups. Menarche is preceded by other bodily changes, such as the development of breasts, a rounding off of the many angles characteristic of the body of the preadolescent, and the appearance of axillary and pubic hair. Psychologically, a girl's interest turns toward members of the opposite sex.

The cycle

In most women menstruation occurs approximately every 28 days and lasts about 5 days. The time between the beginning of one period and the beginning of the next is called the menstrual cycle. It generally repeats itself every 4 weeks (Fig. 2-1), although variations of several days in the cycles of different women or even in the cycles of the same woman are normal. Day 1 is distinguished by the appearance of the menstrual flow.

ANATOMY AND PHYSIOLOGY

The physiology of menstruation is complex. However, a basic understanding of some relationships involved will increase an appreciation of the human body and its potential. Three organs are primarily involved: the pituitary gland, the ovaries, and the uterus. The ability to analyze the roles and interactions of these three organs and their hormonal controls has greatly improved in the last few years because of the availability of more sensitive, sophisticated research techniques and equipment. However, it should be noted that many unknowns are still encountered in the continued investigation of female reproductive physiology.

In the last decade, considerable interest has developed in a special group of fatty acids in the body now classified as hormones called *prostaglandins*. In both sexes these substances are produced by many organs of the body. However, the endometrium is especially rich in prostaglandins and they are thought to be involved in such diverse reproductive activities as ovulation, the reception and transport of ova and sperm, and the onset of menstruation. They appear to be associated with episodes of uterine hyperirritability or contraction and may be a triggering factor in the onset of labor. The far-reaching functions of prostaglandins are now undergoing extensive study.

There appears to be a wide variation in normal hormonal patterns among women. Disturbances of endocrine glands such as the thyroid and adrenals or nutritional and psychologic factors may also influence menstrual function. We will begin our explanation of menstruation with a description of the ovaries.

Ovaries

The ovaries have two basic functions. The first is the production of the hormones estrogen and progesterone. These products regulate the activities of the uterus and the pituitary gland and bring about the many body changes that help make a little girl a woman. The second basic function of the ovaries is the formation of microscopic eggs or ova that contain hereditary maternal contributions to her potential offspring (if an egg and sperm unite or *fertilization* takes place).

These eggs are stored in varying degrees of immaturity in the underlying tissues of both ovaries. Each month only one egg in the body usually develops to maturity, growing within a protective tissue envelope called a *follicle*. This follicle and other ovarian tissue are filled with estrogenic fluid, which is secreted in relatively large amounts into the blood. One of the functions of estrogen at this time is to build up or thicken the lining of the uterus. As the follicle enlarges, it pushes to the surface of the ovary to create a blisterlike bulge that may be clearly seen if the ovary is observed directly. Finally, the follicular envelope breaks open, releasing its tiny ovum from the ovary. This expulsion of the egg is termed *ovulation*. At times fleeting abdominal pain (mittelschmerz) is noted at the time of ovulation, thought to be related to peritoneal irritation caused by minor bleeding from the follicle. Ovulation characteristically occurs on the 14th day of a 28-day menstrual cycle.

After ovulation the mature egg is normally swept up into the oviduct to begin its journey to the uterus, and the empty follicle alters its function. The walls of the follicle begin to thicken and form a yellow deposit about the size of a lima bean called the *corpus luteum* (yellow body). The name *follicle* is no longer used. The corpus luteum continues to produce estrogen but, in addition, manufactures the hormone progesterone, which further prepares the uterus for pregnancy.

Pituitary gland

It is now believed that two anterior pituitary hormones, the follicle-stimulating hormone (FSH) and the luteinizing hormone (LH), help govern the ovarian and, more indirectly, the uterine cycles. Previously, a luteotrophic hormone (LTH), *prolactin,* also had been thought to be involved in maintaining the production of progesterone by the ovary. This is no longer considered to be true. However, prolactin is a hormonal stimulus in the production of maternal milk after the birth of an infant and may inhibit but not totally stop ovulation during breast feeding.

A look at the blood levels of FSH during the normal cycle discloses a moderate early elevation followed by a slight decline until the peak observed at midcycle (Fig. 2-1). This peak is followed by a gradual decrease until just before the next menses. FSH, as its name implies, is responsible for the initiation of the ovarian follicle's growth. However, it works in conjunction with LH to continue the follicle's maturation and produce the characteristic increase in estrogen production. The blood level of LH peaks at midcycle, and this surge of LH is responsible for ovulation.

Pituitary and ovarian hormonal levels inhibit and stimulate each other's hormonal secretions, using rather elaborate negative and positive feedback systems. Special neurohormones produced by the hypothalamus also are involved in these functions.

Uterus

The effect of estrogen in building up the uterine endometrium has often caused the interval between menses and ovulation to be labeled the *proliferative phase*. The second half of the cycle is frequently called the *secretory phase* because of the secretion or storage of nutrients, glycogen, and mucin in the thickening uterine wall in response to the formation of progesterone produced by the corpus luteum.

Progesterone (which means a hormone designed to promote pregnancy) helps maintain the soft nutritious wall long enough to receive any fertilized egg and to nourish it until the developing fetus is able to establish its lifeline of placenta and umbilical cord.

In addition to these changes in the uterine lining, there are alterations in the amount and type of mucus formed by the glands of the cervix. During the proliferative phase of the menstrual cycle, cervical mucus becomes typically profuse and thin. It can be pulled into long strands and suspended, for example, between two glass slides. This distensible quality is called *spinnbarkheit*. When spinnbarkheit is increased, the entry of sperm into the cervix is enhanced. Microscopic changes also are seen when the mucus is placed on a slide and dried. As the time of ovulation nears, under the influence of estrogen, special *ferning* patterns may be detected (Fig. 2-1). When progesterone is secreted in the latter part of the menstrual cycle, these ferning (or arborization) patterns disappear. If ovulation does not occur with subsequent progesterone production, ferning persists.

Knowledge of spinnbarkheit and ferning has been used in treating infertility and has been incorporated into natural family planning techniques. On the 26th day of the menstrual cycle, if pregnancy has not occurred, the corpus luteum begins to degenerate. Approximately 2 days later the thickened lining of the uterus starts to disintegrate, having lost its progesterone and estrogen support.

Menses and ovulation

The menstrual flow usually consists of a varying mixture of cellular debris, mucus, and blood. Its appearance signals the advent of another cycle. The average amount of blood lost per cycle approximates 30 ml. Losses of more than 80 ml are considered excessive and deplete the body's iron supplies. It is interesting to note that ovulation may not occur each time the menstrual cycle repeats and is not dependent on menstruation. In the absence of temperature-causing disease, ovulation can be detected by recording rectal temperatures taken before rising from sleep. Just before ovulation the temperature usually drops to the lowest level found in the menstrual cycle. This drop is followed by an abrupt rise of up to 1° F, indicating that ovulation has taken place. This information has also been used in planning pregnancies, because the most fertile period is during this temperature change (see Fig. 11-1).

ALTERATION OF OVULATION
Pregnancy

If pregnancy occurs, hormones released by the developing fertilized egg interrupt the normal menstrual cycle by maintaining the level of estrogen and progesterone and inhibiting ovulation. Secreted early in the pregnancy is human chorionic gonadotropin (hCG). Identification of this substance in the woman's urine forms the basis of some pregnancy tests.

Artificial hormonal control

Oral contraceptives (the pill) containing estrogen and progesteronelike compounds, simulate to some degree the changes in the uterine lining and the regulation of ovarian and pituitary activity during pregnancy. Ovulation is then artificially suppressed (see discussion pp. 224-225).

In some instances, ovulation is induced by the administration of hormones. For example, the fertility drug menotropins (Pergonal) may cause multiple follicles to mature and produce twins, triplets, or even larger "instant families."

PROBLEMS IN MENSTRUATION

Dysmenorrhea

The most common menstrual disturbance is dysmenorrhea, or painful menstruation. Although most women experience some discomfort (e.g., pelvic congestion, fatigue, or irritability), severe cramping and incapacitation should not be the rule. Repeated experiences of dysmenorrhea should be evaluated by a physician. Occasionally, a physical cause may be found, such as endometriosis (colonization of endometrial tissue outside the uterus), pelvic inflammatory disease, adhesions, genital tract obstruction, poor uterine positioning, presence of pelvic tumors, or possible hormonal imbalance. Dysmenorrhea may be caused or aggravated by constipation. Its probability is also increased by fatigue and emotional upset. Meticulous hygiene, proper diet, and good mental health are of prime importance to the body's total response during menstruation. Excellent teaching aids dealing with the anatomy, physiology, and hygiene of menstruation are now available through public health departments and private commercial outlets.

Treatment of dysmenorrhea depends on the cause, but moderate exercise, fresh air, a serene philosophy, prevention or relief of constipation, application of heat to the pelvis, and mild sedatives or muscle relaxants usually help discomfort. Many times dysmenorrhea is not experienced if a menstrual cycle does not include ovulation; contraceptive preparations containing estrogen or estrogen-progesterone combinations are occasionally prescribed with good results. However, if the contraceptive action of the medication or possible side effects presents problems, this method of treatment may not be appropriate. Another method of treating painful menstruation when no physical cause has been determined is the prescription of one of several medications that may inhibit the activity of body prostaglandins and therefore reduce uterine contraction. Ibuprofen (Motrin), mefenamic acid (Ponstel), and naproxen sodium (Anaprox) have been used.

Disturbances in flow

Other types of menstrual disorders should be defined. *Amenorrhea* is the abnormal absence of menses. *Menorrhagia* refers to excessive flow. *Metrorrhagia* identifies the presence of bloody vaginal discharge between periods. All these conditions should be investigated by a physician.

=== **Key Concepts** ===

1. Menstruation, also known as menses, catamenia, a period or monthly flow, is the monthly elimination through a bloody vaginal discharge of a portion of the lining of the uterus.
2. The age of menarche, the first menses, seems to be affected by heredity, racial background, and nutrition.
3. Menstruation usually occurs about every 28 days and lasts about 5 days.
4. Three organs are primarily involved in menstruation: the pituitary gland, the ovaries, and the uterus.
5. The ovaries have two basic functions: the production of the hormones, estrogen and progesterone; and the formation of microscopic eggs or ova.
6. Two anterior pituitary hormones, the follicle-stimulating hormone (FSH) and the luteinizing hormone (LH), help govern the ovarian and, more indirectly, the uterine cycles. FSH initiates the ovarian follicle's growth and works with LH to continue the follicle's maturation and produce the characteristic increase in estrogen production.
7. Estrogen causes the building up of the uterine endometrium during the proliferative phase between menses and ovulation.
8. Progesterone production results in the secretion or storage of nutrients, glycogen, and mucin in the thickening uterine wall during the second half of the cycle, known as the secretory phase.
9. Changes in cervical mucus are evidenced by spinnbarkheit and ferning patterns during the proliferative

phase. Knowledge of these changes can be used in treating infertility and implementing natural family planning.

10. Possible indications of ovulation include fleeting abdominal pain (mittelschmerz), the peak of the blood level of LH, and an abrupt rise in morning body temperature.

11. Dysmenorrhea may be caused by endometriosis, pelvic inflammatory disease, adhesions, pelvic tumors, genital tract obstructions, poor uterine positioning, hormonal imbalance, or constipation.

12. When no physical cause has been determined, dysmenorrhea can be prevented or treated with moderate exercise, fresh air, a serene philosophy, preventing or relieving constipation, applying heat to the pelvis, and using mild sedatives or muscle relaxants, oral contraceptives, or medications that inhibit the activity of body prostaglandins.

Discussion Questions

1. What role does the pituitary gland play in the reproductive cycle?

2. Earlier onset of menarche combined with changing sexual mores have contributed to an increased number of pregnancies in young teenagers. What do you think would help to change this trend?

3. A friend confides in you that her menstrual cycle has become irregular and that she has experienced increased discomfort during menstruation. What advice would you give her? On what principles would you base this advice?

4. What objective and subjective signs would give clues as to the phase of the menstrual cycle? Do you think that this information would be helpful as a means of family planning? If so, why? If not, why not?

5. Blood loss occurs during menstruation. How much loss is excessive? How would you determine the amount of blood loss? What guidance would you give the woman experiencing menorrhagia? What nursing measures could be taken to reduce the effects of this blood loss?

3

The Male Parent: His Contribution

CHAPTER OBJECTIVES

After studying this chapter, the student should be able to perform the following:

1 Identify the structures of the male genitalia in Figs. 3-1 and 3-2.
2 Indicate the functions of the testis, epididymis, vas deferens, penis, and the male hormone testosterone.
3 Name three paired male glands that add secretions to spermatozoa to form semen.
4 Define the following terms: puberty, gamete, chromosome, meiosis, and fertilization.
5 Explain the genetic mechanism of sex determination.
6 List four signs of the onset of male puberty.

The role of the mother in the creation of new life has been emphasized, but the role of the responsible father is also very important. For an emotionally, socially, and physically healthy child, both parents must make considerable contributions of time and effort. This does not mean that if these contributions are absent, the child will never achieve a happy, productive life. However, if he does, he does so *in spite of* not *because of* his early family life. The amount and type of nurturing behavior (vocal and visual stimulation, touch, and direct participation in child care activities) exhibited by fathers have grown significantly within modern Western society. But great variation is seen within families, influenced by occupational demands, cultural heritage, family structure, personality differences, and the role identification of the mother as well as the father. For the mature adult who is capable of giving as well as receiving, parenthood is not only a demanding responsibility but also one that offers a deserved sense of fulfillment and pride.

The male role in the initial creation of his offspring is relatively brief but no less miraculous because of its brevity. The male reproductive system is an intricate mechanism.

ANATOMY AND PHYSIOLOGY
Puberty

Puberty, or the maturation of the reproductive system, usually occurs late in the male (average age, 14 years) when compared with that of the female. On the average, the development of the male sex organs and secondary sex characteristics takes place 2 years later than that of the female. It involves changes such as the enlargement of the larynx and deepening of the voice, the appearance of axillary, pubic, and facial hair, the development of increased musculature, the production of semen, and the normal occurrence of nocturnal emissions or (wet dreams). Finally, the boy who could not tolerate girls suddenly finds them attractive.

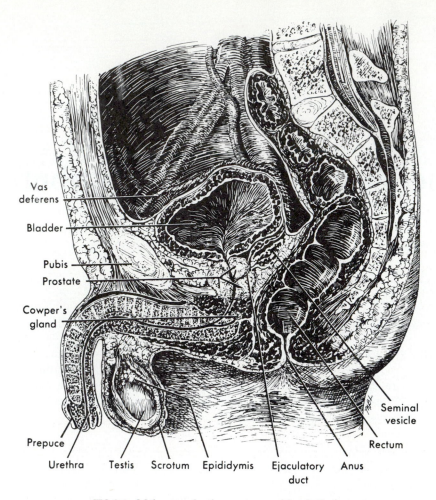

FIG 3-1   Male reproductive system, midsagittal view.

Male organs of reproduction

The male sex glands, or gonads, are two oval endo-crine organs called *testes* (singular, testis), or *testicles,* located in a fleshy pouch suspended from the abdomen called the *scrotum* (Figs. 3-1 and 3-2). The testes, which correspond to ovaries in the female, perform two main functions: the manufacture of male sex cells (gametes), or spermatozoa, and the production of several steroid hormones, primarily *testosterone*. This hormone is responsible for the appearance of male characteristics just as estrogen in the woman controls female characteristics. Testosterone is also necessary to the final stages of sperm production. The male pituitary and nearby hypothalamus help regulate events of male reproductive physiology, just as these organs in women assist in the control of female function. The male pituitary also secretes follicle-stimulating hormone (FSH) and luteinizing hormone

(LH), but these hormones in the man perform different tasks from the same hormones in a woman. FSH is responsible for promoting the maturation of spermatozoa, whereas LH, also known as interstitial cell-stimulating hormone (ICSH in the male), is involved in the production of testosterone.

The testes are found in the abdominal cavity during part of fetal development, but before birth they migrate to the scrotal sac by way of the inguinal canal. Occasionally, this migration does not occur, and a condition known as undescended testicles, or cryptorchidism, may exist. If this condition persists, sterility may occur, because the higher temperature of the abdominal cavity tends to interfere with the manufacture of sperm. If the condition continues, malignant changes are occasionally diagnosed.

Attached to the top of each testis is a coiled structure

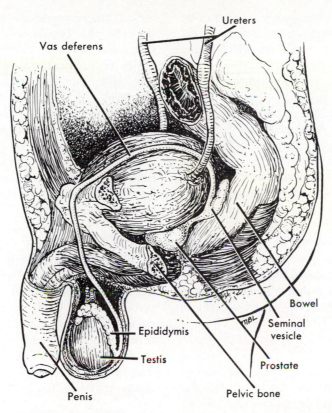

Ureters

Vas deferens

Bowel

Seminal vesicle

Epididymis

Prostate

Testis

Pelvic bone

Penis

FIG 3-2   Male reproductive system, sagittal view with partial dissection.

called an *epididymis,* which is actually an extension of the tubules of the testis in which sperm are formed. In the epididymides (plural of epididymis) the male sex cells mature. In turn, each epididymis is attached to a long tube called the *ductus deferens,* or vas deferens, which with associated nerves and blood vessels travels up the inguinal canal as the *spermatic cord*. The ductus deferens eventually loops downward in back of the urinary bladder. Attached to the ductus in this area is the *seminal vesicle*. This small pouch secretes a fluid that is added to the spermatozoa and aids the motility of the sex cell. The tube leading forward from the point of attachment of the seminal vesicle is called the *ejaculatory duct*. It joins the long urethra after passing through tissue of the *prostate gland*.

Three paired glands add secretions to the spermatozoa traveling from the testes to the exterior to form *semen,* or *seminal fluid*. These glands are the seminal vesicle, the prostate, and the bulbourethral or Cowper's gland, which opens directly into the urethra. These secretions regulate the acidity of the semen and influence the sperm's motility and life span. As a result of sexual excitement and subsequent ejaculation of 2 to 6 ml of

semen, approximately 250 to 500 million sperm are released at a time from the *penis,* the male organ of intercourse, through the urethral meatus.

When not sexually stimulated, the penis serves as the excretory organ of the male urinary system. The urethra opens at the tip of the penis in a sensitive portion called the *glans*. The glans is hooded by a fold of skin called the *prepuce,* or *foreskin,* which is slit or partially removed when a circumcision is performed.

Genetic considerations

The primary function of the reproductive systems of both sexes is the formation of a human being to ensure continuation of the species. Cells that compose living things have within their nuclei the potential of inheritance not only for the species but also for the individualized representatives of that species. Each living thing has a certain number of threadlike strands, or chromosomes, of transmittable characteristics, or genes, within the nuclei of its tissue cells. This chromosome number is constant for each species. For example, human beings have 46 chromosomes in each body tissue cell. However, because the child necessarily inherits qualities from both parents and the body tissue chromosome count must be unaltered for the species, the sex cells (gametes) of the male and female are unlike the rest of the cells found in the body. Through a special process called *meiosis,* the chromosome count in these cells is reduced by half. When male and female sex cells unite, fertilization, or conception, takes place, and the species' chromosome count is restored in the new developing embryo.

In the 1970s, another proposed method of reproduction received much publicity. This technique, called *cloning,* duplicates the genetic inheritance of an individual by substituting the nucleus of a donor's tissue cell for the nucleus of an ovum and providing an appropriate environment for growth of the developing embryo and fetus. It has been used experimentally in the reproduction of genetically duplicated frogs and mice but has not been demonstrated in the development of a human being. Certainly, perfection and use of such a technique would be accompanied by startling scientific, social, and ethical implications.

SEX DETERMINATION

Because there has been much consternation in the past concerning the sex of offspring, it should be noted that the sex of the child is determined by the type of male sex cell that penetrates the ovum or egg. Only the male sex cells, the spermatozoa, may carry the Y chromosome, and when the sperm that unites with an ovum carries the Y chromosome, a boy will result; if the sperm that fertilizes the egg carries an X chromosome, a girl will result (see Fig. 16-4, p. 323). Although research continues to explore possible ways to preselect the sex of one's offspring—such as controlling the acidity or alkalinity of the vagina or using certain techniques and timing for intercourse—the results have been highly controversial. However, as knowledge of genetic potential and control expands, preselection of one's offspring may present another ethical issue.

OUR HUMANITY

Although few people would deny that a baby is a human being, it must be agreed that the true process of reproduction of the human race does not end at conception or at birth. It only enters another phase. Just how human (in the best sense of the word) the child becomes depends on the humanity he observes and feels within his own family circle, that is, what he finds within the lives of his mother, father, and other significant persons that he values as true and lasting.

=============================== **Key Concepts** ===============================

1. Although great variation is seen within families, the amount and type of nurturing behaviors exhibited by fathers have grown significantly in modern Western society.

2. Male puberty, the maturation of the reproductive system, involves changes such as the enlargement of the larnyx and the deepening of the voice; the appearance of axillary, pubic, and facial hair; the development of increased musculature; the production of semen; and the normal occurrence of nocturnal emissions.

3. The two oval endocrine organs called testes perform two main functions: the manufacture of spermatozoa and the production of several steroid hormones, primarily testosterone.

4. Testosterone is responsible for the appearance of male characteristics and is necessary to achieve the final stages of sperm production.

5. The epididymides are extensions of the tubules of the testes, where sperm are formed. The male sex cells mature within the epididymides.

6. The vas deferens, or ductus deferens, travels from the epididymis up the inguinal canal as part of the spermatic cord.

7. The seminal vesicle, the prostate, and the bulbourethral or Cowper's gland add secretions to spermatozoa to form semen, or seminal fluid.

8. The penis is the male organ of intercourse. When not sexually stimulated, it serves as the excretory organ of the urinary system.

9. Each living thing has a certain number of threadlike strands, or chromosomes, of transmittable characteristics, or genes, within the nuclei of its tissue cells. The number of chromosomes is constant for each species.

10. Through meiosis, the number of chromosomes in the gametes (sex cells) of the male and female is reduced by half. When male and female gametes unite, fertilization takes place and the new embryo contains the correct number of chromosomes.

11. The sex of the child is determined by the type of male sex cell that fertilizes the ovum.

Discussion Questions

1. Society influences the role that the father will play in child rearing. What changes can you identify that have occurred during your lifetime and experience?
2. Discuss the physiologic and emotional changes that occur in the adolescent male. Since most nurses are females, how could they help an adolescent male understand these changes?
3. Describe the major structures of the male reproductive tract. Which structures are shared by both the reproductive and urinary systems? Is it possible for both systems to function simultaneously?
4. The sex of the child is significant to many parents. In particular many men wish for a son, and may even indicate that the woman failed in some way if the child is a girl. Is this reasonable? Why or why not?
5. Current scientific advances in the fields of genetics and biological engineering could have significant impact on conception as we know it. Identify one advance, find a current article that explains the new procedure, and discuss the ethical questions that may arise.

U N I T
I

SUGGESTED SELECTED READINGS AND REFERENCES

General

Bobak IM, Jensen MD, and Zalar MK: Maternity and gynecological care, ed 4, St Louis, 1989, The CV Mosby Co.

Fong E, Ferris EB, and Skelley EG: Body structures and functions, ed 7, Albany, NY, 1989, Delmar Publishers, Inc.

Fromer MJ: Ethical issues in sexuality and reproduction, St Louis, 1983, The CV Mosby Co.

Haughey CW: Understanding ultrasonography, Nursing '81 11(4):100, 1981.

Hole JW: Essentials of human anatomy and physiology, ed 3, Dubuque, Ia, 1989, Wm C Brown Publishers.

Jankowski CB: Radiation and pregnancy, Am J Nurs 86(3):261, 1986.

Lewis C and Mocarski V: Obstetric ultrasound: application in a clinic setting, J Obstet Gynecol Neonatal Nurs 16(1):56, 1987.

Marieb EN: Essentials of anatomy and physiology, Menlo Park, Calif, 1984, Addison-Wesley Publishing Co.

Masters W and Johnson V: Human sexual response, Boston, 1966, Little, Brown & Co.

Modica MM and Timor-Tritsch IE: Transvaginal sonography provides a sharper view into the pelvis, J Obstet Gynecol Neonatal Nurs 17(2):87, 1988.

Netter FH and Oppenheimer E, editors: The Ciba collection of medical illustrations, vol 2, The reproductive system, Summit, NJ, 1954, Ciba Pharmaceutical Products, Inc.

Samples JT and others: The dynamic characteristics of the circumvaginal muscles, J Obstet Gynecol Neonatal Nurs 17(3):194, 1988.

Thibodeau GA: Structure and function of the body, ed 8, St Louis, 1988, Times Mirror/Mosby College Publishing.

Tortora GJ and Anagnostakos NP: Principles of anatomy and physiology, ed 5, New York, 1987, Harper & Row, Publishers.

Van De Graaf KM and Fox SI: Concepts of human anatomy and physiology, ed 2, Dubuque, Ia, 1989, Wm C Brown Publishers.

Willson JR, Carrington ER, and Ledger WJ: Obstetrics and gynecology, ed 8, St Louis, 1988, The CV Mosby Co.

Menstruation

Buchmann GA: Menses topics: evaluating menstrual hygiene devices, Contemp OB/GYN 24:71, Nov 1984.

Cibulka NJ: Toxic shock syndrome and other tampon related risks, J Obstet Gynecol Neonatal Nurs 11(6):94, 1982.

Dawood MY: Adolescence: an update on dysmenorrhea, Contemp OB/GYN 23(6):73, 1984.

Delany J, Lupton MJ, and Toth E: The curse: a cultural history of menstruation, New York, 1976, Dutton Publishing Co, Inc.

Frank EP: What are nurses doing to help PMS patients? Am J Nurs 86(2):136, 1986.

Havens B and Swenson I: Menstrual perceptions and preparation among female adolescents, J Obstet Gynecol Neonatal Nurs 15(5):406, 1986.

Lublanezki N and Fischer RG: OTC-menstrual pain preparations, Pediatr Nurs 13(6):435, 1987.

Macvicar MG, Harlan JD, and Ouellette M: What do we know about the effects of sports training on the menstrual cycle? MCN 7(1):55, 1982.

Olson BR: Exercise-induced amenorrhea, Am Fam Physician 39(2):213, 1989.

Wihelm-Hass E: Premenstrual syndrome: its nature, evaluation, and management, J Obstet Gynecol Neonatal Nurs 13(4):223, 1984.

Wilson, MA: Menstrual disorders: premenstrual syndrome, dysmenorrhea, amenorrhea, J Obstet Gynecol Neonatal Nurs 13(2):112s,1984.

Fatherhood

Cath SH, Gurwitt A, and Ross JM: Fathers, Boston, 1982, Little, Brown & Co.

Fishbein EG: Expectant father's stress—due to the mother's expectations? J Obstet Gynecol Neonatal Nurs 13(5):325, 1984.

Novak J: Fathering in health and illness. In Kraft M and Denehy J, editors: Current concepts in pediatric care, St Louis, 1988, The CV Mosby Co.

Patient assessment: examination of the male genitalia; programmed medical instruction, Am J Nurs 79(4):689, 1979.

Phillips CR and Anzalone JT: Fathering: participation in labor and birth, ed 2, St Louis, 1982, The CV Mosby Co.

Reiber VD: Is the nurturing role natural to fathers? MCN 1(5):366, 1976.

Period of Gestation

4

Embryology, Fetal Development, and Signs and Symptoms of Pregnancy

CHAPTER OBJECTIVES

After studying this chapter, the student should be able to perform the following:

1 Describe the normal duration of human gestation using two measurements.
2 Define the following terms: fertilization or conception, zygote, morula, implantation, decidua, embryo, fetus, placenta, chorion, and amnion.
3 List five functions of the placenta.
4 Identify the gestational week for the following stages of fetal development or progression of pregnancy:
   a. Beginning of calcified fetal skeleton
   b. Fetal heart beat heard by ultrasound fetoscope and by conventional fetoscope
   c. Quickening felt by multiparas and primiparas
   d. First use of the term "fetus" to describe the growing child
   e. Uterine fundus at or slightly above maternal umbilicus
   f. Lightening experienced by primiparas
5 Explain the effect of the production of human chorionic gonadotropin (hCG) in pregnant women and hCG's influence on pregnancy tests.
6 Trace the normal fetal circulation pattern through the placenta, umbilical vein and arteries, ductus venosus, foramen ovale, and ductus arteriosus.
7 State eight ways that the age, size, maturity, and well-being of the fetus may be assessed in utero.
8 List six presumptive signs of pregnancy and explain other conditions that cause similar signs or symptoms.
9 Note three probable signs of pregnancy and tell why they are only probable.
10 Indicate the "see, hear, and feel" positive signs of pregnancy.

The event of *conception* (Fig. 4-1), the union of the male sex cell (sperm) and the female sex cell (ovum), sets into motion a period of growth unequaled at any other time in the life of the individual.

Just after *fertilization,* or conception, the ovum is not quite as large as the period used to complete a sentence, but within 266 days* or approximately 9 calendar months that particle of life will increase in size approximately

*The most common method of measuring complete prebirth human growth counts from the first day of the last normal menstrual period. This *menstrual* or *gestational age* (GA) expressed as 280 days, 40 weeks, or 10 lunar months is used by obstetricians. Embryologists/perinatologists often employ *embryological* or *fertilization age,* which begins 2 weeks later lasting 266 days, 38 weeks or 9.5 lunar months. Both use concepts term to include a 2-week buffer. *(Rev. 1992)*

THE MENSTRUAL CYCLE

- Menstruation
- Ovulation

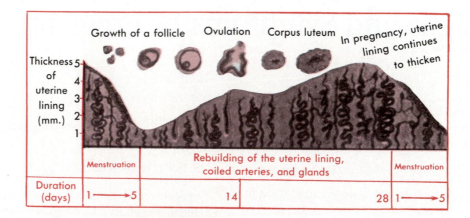

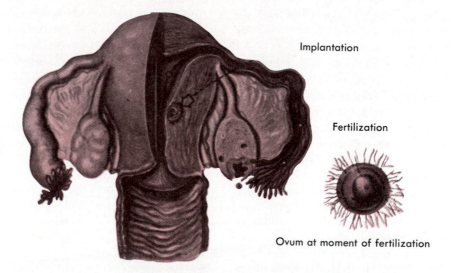

FIG 4-1   The event of pregnancy. *(Courtesy Carnation Company, Los Angeles)*

200 billion times and become the highly complex structure and personality known as a baby.

EMBRYOLOGY (Table 4-1)
Early beginnings

Conception normally takes place in the fallopian, or uterine, tube. The single cell soon divides into two, then four, then eight cells, and continues to multiply until a cell count would be impossible. The fertilized egg, or zygote, assumes the bumpy appearance of a mulberry and for that reason is called a *morula* as it journeys down the tube in search of a warm, safe place to grow. The journey from ovary to uterine cavity, where nesting or *implantation* occurs, involves about 7 days. At the end of this time the zygote, now a hollow, fluid-filled blastocyst, burrows into the soft uterine lining. Its outer surface becomes covered with finger-like tissue projections called *chorionic villi,* which aid in the process of implantation into the endometrium (known as the *decidua* during pregnancy). Implantation may cause limited bleeding, which may be reported as "spotting." The villi also manufacture the human chorionic gonadotropin (hCG) that initially signals the corpus luteum in the ovary to continue to manufacture progesterone and estrogen to prevent menstruation and additional ovulation. The aggregation of cells begins to form a definite pattern. The microscopic embryonic disc develops, and primitive beginnings of the child and his basic support system appear.

Of course, the possibility of intentional alteration in the initiation and early development of selected pregnancies exists. In 1978 an ovum obtained from a woman's ovary, fertilized by her husband's sperm in a laboratory and placed in her uterus as a blastocyst, resulted in the birth of an apparently normal, healthy infant girl. At this writing, *in vitro fertilization* has made possible the birth of many infants, including twins, to women who were denied biologic parenthood because of blocked fallopian tubes. (See also p. 230.)

Placental development and role

After implantation of a zygote, a supply and disposal system across the uterine wall is initiated through a special intermediary organ called the *placenta,* or *afterbirth.* The placenta, a miraculous structure, develops from part of the chorionic villi that extended from the outside of the egg. Attached to the uterine wall, it manufactures estrogen, progesterone, chorionic gonadotropin, and various other hormones and enzymes that apparently influence the growth and maintenance of the pregnancy and maternal preparation for birth and lactation. Using various complex molecular processes, the placenta also transports the food and oxygen necessary for fetal growth and hormones and protective substances called antibodies from the mother's blood to the fetus by way of the umbilical cord. Also, the placenta handles waste products brought to its tissues from the fetus; it allows carbon dioxide and other metabolic wastes to pass from the fetal circulation to the maternal bloodstream. The mother and fetus do not share a common bloodstream; the fetus manufactures its own blood. Normally the whole blood of the mother and that of the fetus stay within their separate, closely related channels. Blood flows from the placenta to the fetus through a large umbilical vein in the umbilical cord. The two arteries in the umbilical cord are wound around the umbilical vein and carry the waste to the placenta.

"Bag of waters"

As the embryo develops, the chorionic villi that face the interior of the uterus and are not involved in the formation of the placenta detach from the spherical covering and leave a transparent sac made up of two membranous layers called the *chorion* and the *amnion.* The inner layer, the amnion, contains a salty liquid known as *amniotic fluid,* in which the fetus may float. The amniotic fluid helps control the environmental temperature of the fetus and shield it from trauma and infection. Perhaps weightlessness is not such an extraordinary condition for mankind after all! This amniotic sac is commonly known as the "bag of waters," or the membranes. Normally, it remains intact until the time of labor and birth.

THE FETUS

From the eighth week of growth, the embryo is recognizable as a small, unfinished human and is called a *fetus,* meaning "young one." The fetus is less than 2 inches (about 3 cm) long and weighs a fraction of an ounce. Rudimentary body systems are formed and working, and the skeleton is becoming established (Fig. 4-2).

At 12 weeks. By the end of the third lunar month, the sex of the fetus is clearly discernible. Needless to say, parents are curious regarding the sex of the developing fetus. However, no *completely* safe procedure exists to determine the sex of the fetus before birth. A technique called amniocentesis makes sex identification possible before birth if this information is genetically important. Amniotic fluid is aspirated from the bag of waters and examined for cellular content and chromosome determination later in the pregnancy (Fig. 4-3).

Text continued on p. 53.

Table 4-1   Prenatal calendar

General developmental characteristics (schematically pictured)	Average weight and size	Possible maternal findings and diagnostic aids
Fetal growth measured from conception (fertilization age)		**Maternal changes measured using menstrual/gestational age (GA) (2 weeks added to fertilization age) or as indicated.**
First week		
Zygote forms: ovum fertilized in fallopian tube undergoes cell divisions (cleavage) on way to uterus 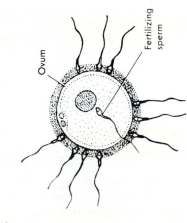	Just visible to eye	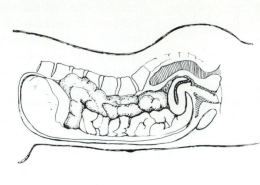
Morula forms: solid mass of about 16 microscopic cells resembling mulberry; enters uterus on third day 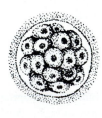		
Blastocyst: morula develops fluid-filled cavity; *trophoblast:* outer wall of blastocyst: *embryoblast:* inner cell mass from which embryo eventually forms 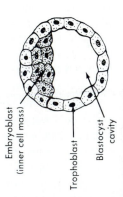		Normal female pelvis before implantation (sagittal section)

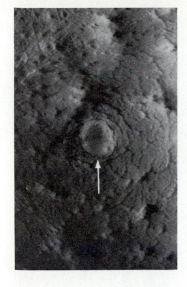

Continued.

From Hertig AT and Beck J: Contr Embryol Carneg Inst, Wash 29:127, 1941.

Implantation site of human embryo at about 12 days postconception Endometrium covers blastocyst, producing elevation or wartlike bulge on uterine surface

2 to 3 mm (1/10 inch)

Amenorrhea
Human chorionic gonadotropin (hCG) in urine beginning 10 days after conception, but tests not always sensitive
Ultrasonogram may reveal pregnancy as early as 3 to 4 weeks postconception

---

Beginning implantation of blastocyst in endometrium by invading trophoblastic tissue ±7 days

Implantation deepens and is completed; primitive uteroplacental circulation originates from enlarging trophoblast and maternal endometrial tissues
Amniotic cavity appears as opening between inner cell mass and invading trophoblast; a thin lining becomes amnion
Two-layered (bilaminar) embryo called *embryonic disc* develops, formed by ectoderm and endoderm
Yolk sac present

Thickening in midline of ectoderm gives rise to *mesoderm,* a third layer between ectoderm and endoderm forming trilaminar embryo; basic embryologic beginnings of body systems and organs

---

Embryonic stage (10 days to eighth week)

Second week

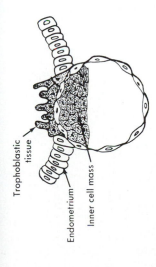

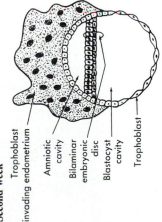

Third week

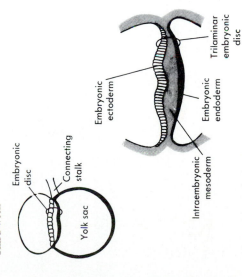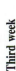

Table 4-1 Prenatal calendar—cont'd

General developmental characteristics (schematically pictured)	Average weight and size	Possible maternal findings and diagnostic aids
Three basic embryonic layers: 1. *Endoderm:* forerunner of lining of gastrointestinal tract from pharynx to rectum; epithelial parts of trachea, bronchi, lungs, liver, pancreas, and urinary bladder 2. *Ectoderm:* forerunner of mucous membrane tooth enamel, hair, nails, mammary glands, and nervous system 3. *Mesoderm:* forerunner of heart and blood vessels, spleen, blood and lymph cells, bones, and muscles Neural tube, beginning of central nervous system, forms in midline of cranial portion of ectoderm		
Cells group in mesoderm to form primitive blood vessels and blood cells; heart tube forms and contracts to circulate blood by end of third week; umbilical vessels pass through connecting stalk to placenta Flat, disclike embryo folds to form typical C-shaped cylinder Rapid development of forebrain portion of neural tube Heart prominence seen Arm and leg buds; forerunners of ears and eyes appear Primitive gut formed with incorporation of dorsal yolk sac Rudimentary lungs, kidneys	5 mm (1/16 inch)	Nausea and vomiting (?) Urinary frequency Breast tenderness, tingling, swelling Montgomery's tubercles visible Uterine enlargement Increased cervical secretion

Fourth week

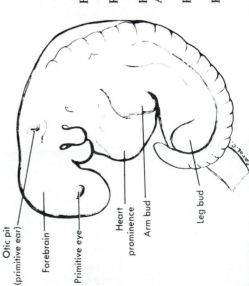

Otic pit (primitive ear)

Forebrain

Primitive eye

Heart prominence

Arm bud

Leg bud

Softening of cervix (Goodell's sign)
Softening of uterine isthmus (Hegar's sign) 6 to 8 weeks
Violet coloration of cervix and vagina (Chadwick's sign)

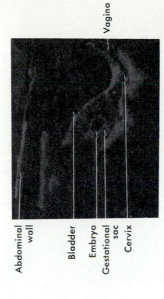

Abdominal wall
Bladder
Embryo
Gestational sac
Cervix
Vagina

Sonogram of 6 weeks' gestational sac containing embryo. (*Courtesy George R. Leopold, MD, University Hospital, San Diego, Calif.*)

3 cm (1⅛ inches)
2 g (1/15 oz)

Fifth through seventh weeks

Rapid brain development
Retina of eye forms
Heart becomes chambered
Fingers, toes, and eyes are becoming visible
Palate and upper lip forming
Gastrointestinal tract develops; part of intestine still in umbilical cord
Rapid formation of urogenital systems

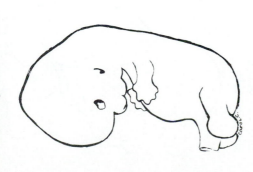

By end of seventh week all essential systems present

Fetal stage (eighth week to birth)*
Eighth through tenth weeks

Development mainly involves growth and maturation of structures begun in embryo; fetus less vulnerable to effects of drugs, most infections, and radiation
Head almost half fetal length at 8 weeks (see fetus within amniotic sac)

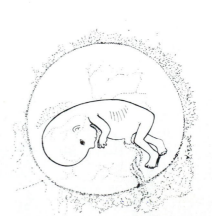

Continued.

*Some references begin the fetal stage at the end of the eighth week

Table 4-1 Prenatal calendar—cont'd

	General developmental characteristics (schematically pictured)	Average weight and size	Possible maternal findings and diagnostic aids
Eleventh through twelfth weeks	Facial features forming Eyelids present and fused Intestine retracted from umbilical cord into abdomen Palate fusion complete External sex identification possible Well-defined neck Nail beds beginning Tooth buds forming	Crown-heel length: 11.5 cm (4½ inches) 20 g (⅔ oz)	Frequent urination and nausea have usually disappeared Fetal heart tone may be detected with Doppler techniques
Thirteenth through sixteenth weeks	Rapid growth of limbs and trunk; head less prominent Active fetus Skeleton calcified on x-ray examination by sixteenth week Increasing respiratory movement detected by sonogram Approximately 150 to 280 ml amniotic fluid present Placenta distinct	19 cm (7½ inches) 100 g (3⅓ oz)	Fundus of uterus rises above pubic bone between 12 and 16 weeks Start of maternity clothing(?) Amniocentesis between fourteenth and sixteenth weeks Quickening felt at 16 weeks(?) Fundus half distance between pubis and umbilicus at 16 weeks(?)

Continued.

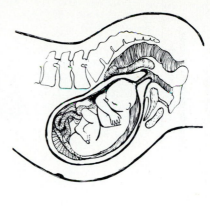

Quickening at 16 to 18 weeks
Fetal heart tone detected by standard fetoscope (18 to 20 weeks)
Secondary areola prominent
Fundus at umbilicus or slightly above at 20 weeks

Chloasma (mask of pregnancy)
Striae may develop

22 cm (8¾ inches)
300 g (10 oz)

Eyebrows, lanugo, and vernix appear
Nipples barely visible (illustration shows placental relationship)
Scalp hair visible
Fetus able to hear sounds within mother and in external world

32 cm (12½ inches)
600 g (1¼ lb)

External ear soft, flat, shapeless
Skin wrinkled, translucent, appears pink; blood in capillaries shows
Lanugo covers body

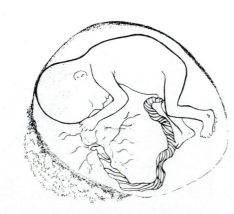

Seventeenth through twentieth weeks

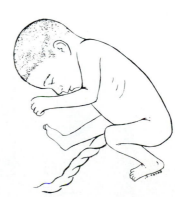

Twenty-fourth week
Only rare survivals

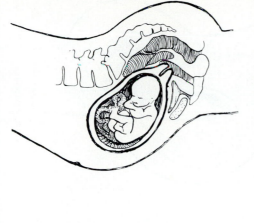

Table 4-1 Prenatal calendar—cont'd

	General developmental characteristics (schematically pictured)	Average weight and size	Possible maternal findings and diagnostic aids
Twenty-eighth week 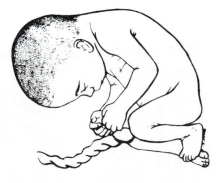	Subcutaneous fat appears, finger-nails and toenails Testes at internal inguinal ring or below Eyes open Scalp hair well developed	36 cm (14 inches) 1,100 g (2¼ lb)	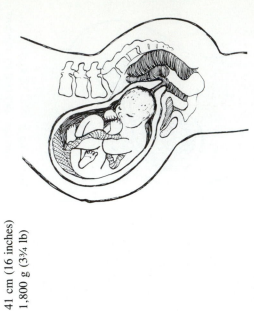
Thirty-second week 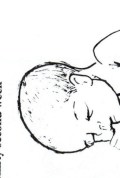	Hair fine and woolly Nails to fingertips Prominent clitoris; labia majora small and separated Skin pink and smooth 1 or 2 creases on anterior portion of soles Breast areolae visible but flat	41 cm (16 inches) 1,800 g (3¾ lb)	

Thirty-sixth week

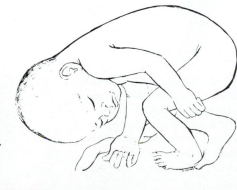

Body, limbs more rounded
Skin thicker, whiter; lanugo disappearing
Breast tissue develops under nipples
Scrotal rugae few
Testes in inguinal canal
Sole creases involve anterior two-thirds of sole

46 cm (18 inches)
2,200 g (4½ lb)

Dyspnea due to pressure on diaphragm
Lightening in primigravidas about 38 weeks
Urinary frequency returns
Increasing prominence of Braxton Hicks contractions
Colostrum may appear in breasts
In primigravida, characteristic effacement may be noted by pelvic examination

Full-term
End of thirty-eighth week
(fertilization age) (see also
p. 41, p. 272)

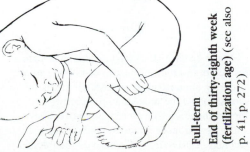

Skin whitish pink
Lanugo gone from face
Hair in single strands
Vernix decreasing
Areola 5 to 6 mm with 7 to 10 mm breast tissue
Ear well defined by outer incurving to lobe, erect from head
Testes in scrotum
Labia majora meet in midline; cover labia minora and clitoris

51 cm (20 inches)
3,200+ g
(6.6 + lb)

At term
(40 weeks, GA)

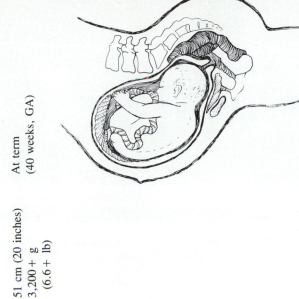

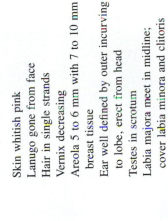

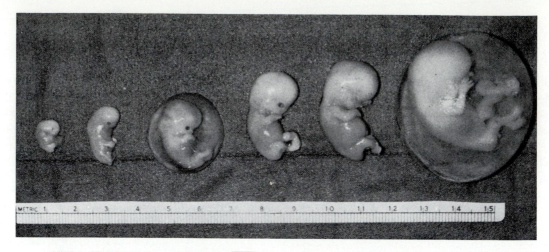

FIG 4-2 Progressive growth of the human fetus (measured in centimeters). Two amniotic sacs are pictured still intact. *(Courtesy Jeanne I. Miller, MD, Modesto, Calif.)*

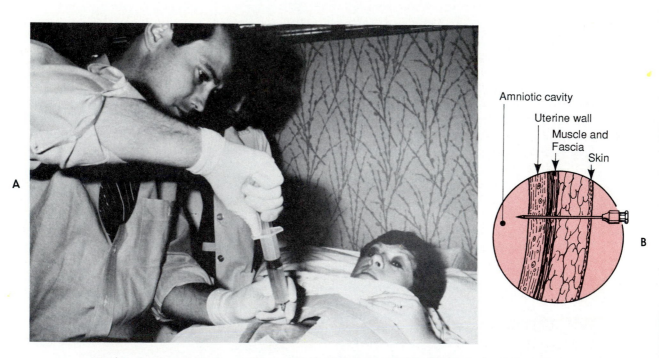

FIG 4-3 **A,** Amniocentesis—a diagnostic tool. To help lessen risk of fetal or placental trauma, ultrasound is used to locate intrauterine structures before insertion of needle. A full or partially filled bladder is now desired by some physicians during amniocentesis to push the uterus out of the pelvis and to aid in visualization. Readers should follow the procedure in their own hospitals. Amniocentesis is usually performed for genetic analysis between 14 and 16 weeks' GA. **B,** Layers of tissue through which needle must pass to reach amniotic fluid. *(Courtesy Thomas Key, MD, Dept. of Obstetrics and Gynecology, University of California—San Diego.)*

The fetus is most susceptible to malformation from the effects of maternal drug ingestion, radiation, or infection in the first trimester (the first 13 weeks of pregnancy), when basic organs and systems are being formed. It is possible for certain drugs to distort fetal development within 11 days of conception, before the woman realizes that she may be pregnant. Such an "assault" at an early gestational period usually causes fetal death. Drugs or conditions that produce fetal structural defects are termed *teratogenic*. They are currently the object of much concern and study. (See also pp. 77-78.)

At 16 weeks. At 16 weeks of intrauterine development the fetus has increased in size considerably. It is approximately 7½ inches (19 cm) long and weighs about 3⅓ ounces (100 g). The uterus is correspondingly larger, and the expectant mother may make her debut in maternity clothes. At 16 to 18 weeks GA, pregnant women usually report feelings of life, or *quickening*. Elbows, feet, and hands punch and twitch as the fetus attempts more vigorous exercise in the confining uterus.

At 20 weeks. At 20 weeks of growth, the fetus is about 8¾ inches (22 cm) long and weighs approximately 10 ounces (300 g) at this time. At 20 weeks GA, the uterus is at or slightly above the mother's umbilicus, and the fetal heartbeat is heard using a standard fetoscope.

Some state laws declare that the legal threshold of viability is 24 weeks of GA; others use 20 weeks GA as the lower limit. However, the true length of a pregnancy may be difficult to determine and can lead to moral-ethical dilemmas involving the rights and responsibilities of the parents and the community, as well as consideration for the life and well-being of the developing fetus. Infants diagnosed as less than 24 weeks of GA have made postnatal respiratory efforts. Special neonatal care units employing exceptional techniques supporting or monitoring body warmth, ventilation, cardiac function, and nutrition have been able to save fetuses of increasingly shorter gestations. Nevertheless, when all births are evaluated, such survivals must be considered a rare occurrence. (See a brief discussion of premature care on p. 272.)

The characteristics of the premature infant and his grip on life depend on his genetic endowment, the length and quality of his prenatal environment, and his immediate postnatal care. Assuming his prenatal environment and personal condition are satisfactory, each additional day the fetus is able to remain in the uterus until maturity, which is approximately 38 weeks in length, is beneficial. Each day increases his ability to withstand the demands of extrauterine life and to adjust to the tremendous circulatory, respiratory, and digestive alterations that must take place at birth. (See Table 4-1.)

Fetal circulation

A diagram of fetal circulation is shown in Fig. 4-4 to give a better understanding of the circulorespiratory changes. The umbilical vein within the umbilical cord carries blood from the placenta to the fetus and enters the body at the umbilicus. It travels upward, dividing to form a bypass of the liver called the *ductus venosus,* which eventually joins the inferior vena cava. The rich oxygenated blood from the umbilical vein mixes with the oxygen-poor blood flowing from the lower extremities and abdominal cavity toward the heart. The blood enters the heart by way of the right atrium, as in postnatal circulation. Because the pulmonary circulation is unnecessary to oxygenation, much of the blood entering the heart from the inferior vena cava crosses directly to the left atrium through the fetal shunt, or interatrial opening, called the *foramen ovale*. This blood is then guided into the usual circulation pattern, left atrium → left ventricle → aorta.

Blood from the head and upper extremities enters the right atrium via the superior vena cava, flows primarily into the right ventricle, and is eventually pushed into the pulmonary artery. However, the trip to the lungs is superfluous at this time, and another shunt, the *ductus arteriosus,* is employed. This short duct leads from the pulmonary artery to the aorta. Relatively little blood flows to the lung fields and back to the left heart by way of the pulmonary veins.

The blood that flows downward through the aorta is eventually channeled into the iliac arteries to the hypogastric arteries that join with the umbilical arteries leading to the umbilical cord and placenta.

The pulmonary circulation becomes established within a relatively short time after birth. The umbilical cord is clamped and cut, and the blood vessels it contains become occluded. Because of the changes in thoracic pressures initiated by postnatal expansion of the lungs, the foramen ovale begins to close, and the ductus arteriosus collapses and becomes a ligament within a period of days or weeks.

Methods of evaluating the fetus

Because the maturity of an infant is important to survival outside the uterus, improved techniques to determine intrauterine growth as well as general health in utero have become very helpful. Before labor, types of tests that help assess fetal age, size, maturity, and well-being

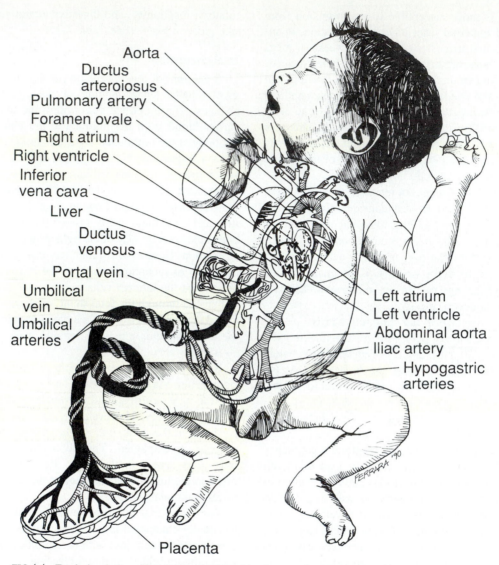

Aorta
Ductus arteroiosus
Pulmonary artery
Foramen ovale
Right atrium
Right ventricle
Inferior vena cava
Liver
Ductus venosus
Portal vein
Umbilical vein
Umbilical arteries

Left atrium
Left ventricle
Abdominal aorta
Iliac artery
Hypogastric arteries

Placenta

FIG 4-4 Fetal circulation. The darker the blood in the vessels, the greater its oxygen content. (See text for blood flow patterns.) Size of placenta has been reduced to save space. Normally, it would be more than twice the pictured size in relation to the size of infant at term. At birth the normal placenta equals about one sixth the weight of newborn. The umbilicus has been displaced to increase the visibility of the abdominal area.

have included: amniocentesis—an examination of amniotic fluid aspirated transabdominally from the amniotic sac under sterile conditions (see Fig. 4-3); ultrasonography—unlike x-ray examination, *appears* to be a safe technique for the fetus and mother at any stage of pregnancy (Fig. 4-5); maternal blood and urine analysis; chorionic villi sampling—a new test providing early diagnosis of some genetic diseases; and fetal heart monitoring. These tests are highlighted in Table 4-2. During labor the immediate status of the baby may be evaluated through simultaneous monitoring of the fetal heart rate and contraction patterns, observation of the color of the amniotic fluid, and in certain cases, by fetal blood sampling. (See pp. 56 and 57.)

Knowledge of the fetus has grown tremendously in the last decade. The intensive study of the fetus and

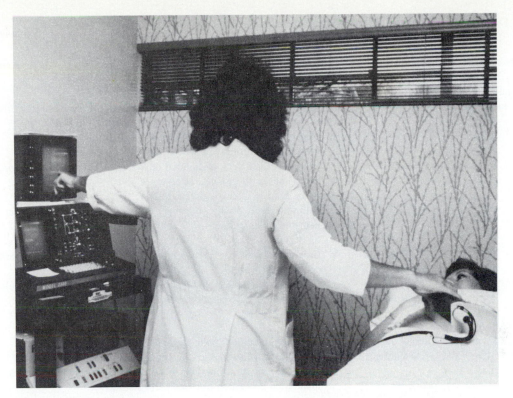

FIG 4-5 Transabdominal ultrasound examination of fetus in progress. To lift uterus from behind pelvis and provide best picture possible without causing patient unnecessary discomfort, bladder should be moderately full. Giving patient 2 to 3 cups of water (about 500 ml) before examination is usually sufficient. During the 15- to 30-minute test, mineral oil or a special gel is applied to the mother's abdomen. A smooth sensor (transducer) is then guided over the skin's surface, and a progressive series of ultrasonic images of uterine contents is obtained. Endosonography or transvaginal ultrasound imaging that utilizes a sensor introduced into the vaginal canal is becoming more available. This technique does not require a full bladder and gives better visualization for diagnosis of certain conditions, e.g., ectopic pregnancy.

newborn has developed into the growing clinical specialty of perinatology, which crosses the ill-defined borders of maternity and pediatric practice. Increasing reports of successful medical and surgical interventions used to treat the unborn have caused this small representative of the human race to gain more status as a person and a patient.

SIGNS AND SYMPTOMS OF PREGNANCY

All the activity initiated within the uterus with the onset of pregnancy cannot be kept a secret for long. Widespread changes take place in the body, creating various signs and symptoms that possess varying degrees of importance in the diagnosis of pregnancy. These signs and symptoms are usually arranged according to their accuracy into three groups: the presumptive, the probable, and the positive signs of pregnancy. However, no universal agreement exists regarding the contents of these categories. Events are noted using gestational age (GA).

Presumptive signs and symptoms

The presumptive signs and symptoms of pregnancy are those that could easily be an indication of other conditions. They usually include the following.

Amenorrhea. Although absence of menses may be an early sign of developing pregnancy, it is not always an indication. Amenorrhea may occur as a result of sudden changes in environment or occupation, emotional upset,

Table 4-2   Evaluation of the unborn infant—using gestational age (GA)

Age

Important for medical-legal considerations, e.g., dating of prospective abortion (or elective cesarean birth)

An indirect, unreliable assessment of
maturity

1. Date of first day of last normal menstrual period (Nägele's rule: count back 3 months, add 7 days to determine delivery date)
2. Fundal height (assumes normal fetal growth) (see Fig. 4-8)
3. Appearance of fetal heart tone at 10 to 12 weeks using "Doppler" fetoscope
4. Ultrasound measurements (transabdominal or transvaginal)
   a. Size of amniotic sac/uterine cavity
   b. Fetal crown to rump length
   c. Biparietal diameters, abdominal or thoracic circumferences during the second trimester for greatest accuracy
5. Amniotic fluid analysis (amniocentesis)
   a. Bilirubin levels during pregnancy uncomplicated by maternal-fetal blood incompatibilities usually reach peak at 16 to 30 weeks, then fall, disappearing by 36 weeks
   b. Creatinine levels rise as fetal urine increases; unreliable if maternal-fetal complications occur
   c. L/S ratio usually 2 at 35 weeks, but appearance of normal levels may be accelerated or retarded by maternal-fetal disorders

Maturity

Various body system development may
be monitored, but overall fetal maturity difficult to ascertain

1. Amniotic fluid analysis (amniocentesis)
   a. L/S ratio usually rises to 2 or more when lungs have matured; other biochemical tests (e.g., amount of saturated fats) increase reliability of lung maturation evaluation in complex obstetric cases
   b. Positive foam or shake test usually rules out lung immaturity
   c. Fatty cell recovery percentage—low reliability
   d. Creatinine levels may assist in assessment of renal maturity

Well-being

Indications of some specific defects as
well as clues of general fetal well-
being possible, but not all problems
identifiable

1. Ultrasound measurements
   a. Evaluation of fetal presentation; multiple pregnancy
   b. Detection of some structural abnormalities, e.g., central nervous system and genitourinary anomalies
   c. Localization of placenta; diagnosis of placenta previa
   d. Identification of excessive or diminished amniotic fluid volume: related to possible fetal abnormalities or jeopardy
   e. Motion picture (real-time techniques) may confirm fetal death
2. Amniotic fluid analysis (amniocentesis)
   a. Chromosomal studies may reveal the following:
      (1) Fetal abnormalities in chromosome number and gross structure (e.g., Down syndrome)
      (2) Sex of infant to help evaluate probability of sex-linked genetic disorders (e.g., Duchenne's muscular dystrophy, classic hemophilia)
   b. Biochemical studies may reveal the following:
      (1) Anencephaly-myelomeningocele, based on level of alpha fetoprotein
      (2) A number of metabolic and blood diseases (e.g., thalassemia)
3. Meconium-stained amniotic fluid; possible fetal oxygen lack (hypoxia)
4. Fetal movement—usually reassuring if not exaggerated
5. Fetal heart rate and contraction monitoring—external or internal
   a. Helps identify episodes of hypoxia resulting from uteroplacental insufficiency or cord compression during labor (pp. 114-121)
   b. Positive oxytocin challenge test or nipple stimulation contraction stress test may predict fetal jeopardy in true labor (p. 515)

Table 4-2 Evaluation of the unborn infant—using gestational age (GA)—cont'd

Well-being—cont'd

     c. Fetal heart rate changes in response to fetal movement without uterine contraction before labor are consistent with fetal health and form basis of *non-stress* test

  6. Fetal blood sampling (microsamples drawn from presenting part, usually scalp)

     a. Helps identify fetal hypoxia, retention of CO_2, and developing acidosis

     b. Serial samples are more meaningful

     c. pH values below 7.2 in two or more samples usually indicate need for assistance

     d. Maternal acidosis may cause misleading interpretations of fetal status

  7. X-ray examination (use of traditional films now rare because of radiation risk and availability of ultrasound)

  8. Chorionic villi sampling (CVS) at 10 to 11 weeks for genetic analysis and early detection of selected hereditary defects

  9. Maternal blood analysis helps screen alpha fetoprotein levels for possible neural tube, abdominal wall defects, or chromosomal disorders

---

malnutrition, fatigue, hormonal disorders, extensive exercise, and menopause.

Nausea and vomiting. Nausea and vomiting often occur in the morning, but are not limited to this time. Nausea and vomiting, presumably caused by changes in hormone levels in the body in the first weeks of pregnancy, are not confined to this cause, since they are a common occurrence during gastrointestinal tract irritation and emotional stress.

Frequent urination. Frequent urination, usually of small amounts, is common during the first and last weeks of pregnancy because of pelvic congestion and the particular pressure of the uterus on the bladder. Urinary frequency may also be present because of excitement, large fluid intakes, or irritation of the urinary tract. Increased urination is also associated with diabetes mellitus.

Breast changes. Tingling, swelling, and tenderness involving the breasts are also found early in pregnancy. These symptoms may also be experienced during each menstrual cycle just before menses.

Changes in shape of abdomen. Increased abdominal size and shape are usually noted the eighth to tenth week of pregnancy. However, the contour of a woman's abdomen may depend on dietary willpower rather than gestation. Increased abdominal size may also be influenced by the growth of tumors or hernias.

Changes in the skin and mucous membranes. Increased abdominal size may be accompanied by pink to purplish "stretch marks," known technically as *striae gravidarum* (Fig. 4-6). It is now thought that their presence is probably more related to increased production or sensitivity to adrenocortical hormones during pregnancy than to weight gain alone. Such skin changes are also noted in patients with Cushing's disease and, to a lesser degree, in patients with sudden weight gains not associated with pregnancy.

Another pigmentation characteristic of pregnancy is a bronze type of facial coloration called *chloasma*, or the mask of pregnancy, often seen on dark-haired women. Development of a dark line (linea nigra), extending from the sternum to the pubis in the midline is quite common. These changes in skin coloration are probably related to hormonal alterations.

Most references list the violet coloration of the vagina, cervix, and vulva, which is apparent at about 6 to 10 weeks' gestation (Chadwick's sign), as a presumptive indication of pregnancy. It is caused by increased circulation to the area and may be associated with any cause of pelvic congestion.

Quickening. Quickening, meaning the first time life or fetal movement is felt by the woman, can sometimes be imitated by peristalsis or gas and be misinterpreted. By the time quickening is felt (at approximately 16 weeks by women who have already had children and 18 weeks or more by women who are experiencing their first pregnancy), other more definite signs should be manifest.

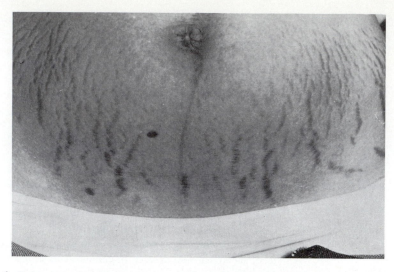

FIG 4-6 Striae (stretch marks). *(Courtesy Mercy Hospital and Medical Center, San Diego.)*

Fatigue. Fatigue, often included on the list, is a widespread complaint.

Probable signs and symptoms

The probable signs of pregnancy are more certain than presumptive signs, but not foolproof. Listed enlargement of the uterus, certain other changes in the reproductive anatomy and physiology, and positive pregnancy tests. The increasing accuracy of selected pregnancy tests has led some physicians to consider their positive results equal to positive signs.

Certain presumptive signs found in a woman who has never experienced pregnancy usually are considered *probable*. They are deepened pigmentation of the breasts, production of breast secretion (colostrum), and the presence of the linea nigra. However, these may have little diagnostic value for women who have had children recently or have been nursing their infants.

Changes in reproductive organs. Enlargement of the uterus, rather than an increase in abdominal circumference, is a definitive sign of pregnancy. Nevertheless, uterine tumors or inflammation may cause an increase in abdominal size. At 6 to 8 weeks' gestation a special softening of the region of the uterus between the body and the cervix, called the *isthmus*, occurs. It is determined by a simultaneous abdominal and vaginal examination, a bimanual maneuver illustrated in Fig. 4-7. This softening is termed *Hegar's sign*. Another softening of the uterus affecting the cervix is detected by the examiner's finger. In the nonpregnant state the cervix feels somewhat like the cartilage at the tip of a nose. During pregnancy the cervix changes in consistency to resemble the pliability of the ear lobe or lips (Goodell's sign).

Basal body temperature elevation. Basal body temperature elevation is one of the earliest diagnostic observations possible and is considered to have 97% accuracy. However, for this basal or waking temperature to have meaning, the woman must have taken her temperature consistently, using proper technique both before and after ovulation to detect the persistent relative increase in basal readings. (For interpretation of the temperature readings, see p. 222.)

Ballottement. The French term ballottement describes "tossing up a ball in the air and catching it on its return." Near midpregnancy the small fetus is enclosed in a relatively large fluid-filled sac or bag of waters. When an examiner taps the baby's head or body, it characteristically floats away and then rebounds to nudge the examiner's fingertips. Rarely this ball-like rebound may be mimicked by the movement of a uterine tumor or polyp; therefore it represents only a probable sign.

Positive biologic and immunochemical pregnancy tests. Pregnancy tests are based on the fact that the chorionic villi of an implanted ovum or of the developing placenta secrete human chorionic gonadotropic hormone (hCG), which is excreted in small amounts in urine and blood. The first pregnancy tests were biologic. A concentrated urine sample obtained from a morning specimen, voided after a period of fluid limitation, was injected into a laboratory animal. The animal was then

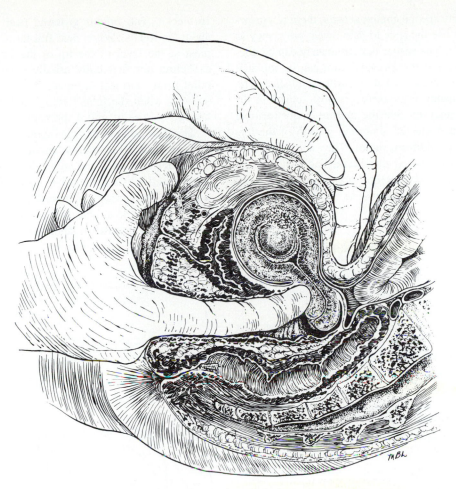

FIG 4-7 Hegar's sign.

observed for changes in its reproductive cycle. Rabbits, mice, and frogs were used. Immunochemical tests that no longer require laboratory animals are now employed.

Although the excretion of urinary hCG during pregnancy shows significant individual variations, within 48 hours of implantation hCG levels increase rapidly. Immunologic pregnancy tests have become more accurate and easier to read and have a very high level of sensitivity. Recently, *urine* tests involving the use of monoclonal antibodies have demonstrated very accurate results as early as 1 week after implantation. The use of these tests is increasing.

If pregnancy tests that have been designed for use in the home are employed, the need to follow directions carefully must be emphasized. Tests are usually done 3 days after the missed menstrual period and must be repeated if negative. A relatively low false-positive rate but a high (about 25%) false-negative result has been

reported. The use of client-performed tests continues to be controversial.*

Special *blood* tests known as radioimmunoassays (RIAs) may also be used to obtain pregnancy confirmation. The RIA for the β (beta) subunit of hCG is said to be capable of diagnosing pregnancy as early as 5 days before the first missed period.

Most pregnancy tests are only about 95% to 99% accurate, depending on when they are performed, the method used, and the presence of factors that may cause both false negatives and positives. For these reasons, "positive" results are usually considered probable and not positive signs of pregnancy. Although a firm diagnosis of pregnancy can often be made after the eighth

*Valanis BG and Perlman CS: Home pregnancy testing kits: prevalence of use, false negative rates and compliance of instructions, Am J Public Health 72(9):1034, 1982; Wasley G: Urinary pregnancy testing, Nurs Times 84(36):42, Sept 7-13, 1988.

week without any special chemical tests, there is a growing tendency to use the tests to help detect pregnancy as soon as possible. The earlier that pregnancy can be documented, the sooner that prenatal care can be initiated and an accurate estimated date of birth established. The results of pregnancy tests are especially helpful in diagnosing pregnancy outside the uterine cavity (ectopic pregnancy) or a suspected abnormal growth of the fertilized ovum (hydatidiform mole). They are strategic in planning surgery involving anesthesia; diagnostic or therapeutic radiation; prescription of medications potentially toxic to a developing pregnancy; or abortion.

Positive signs

Seeing. With ultrasound techniques, a gestation sac may be visible as early as 3 to 4 weeks after conception. Fetal form and motion become progressively more apparent with real-time sonography as the pregnancy advances.

Conventional x-ray usually reveals the skeleton of a fetus by the latter half of pregnancy. However, this method is not purposefully used today because of possible radiation injury to the fetus or the mother.

Hearing. A fetal heart tone is usually heard after 18 to 20 weeks by conventional auscultation with a standard fetoscope. Up until the 20th week the fetal heart rate is heard best at the center of the pubic hairline. Fetal heart tones are usually detected by 10 to 12 weeks after conception using ultrasonic or Doppler effect techniques.

The presence of the *funic souffle,* a rapid repetitive whistlelike sound not synchronized with the maternal pulse can be evidence of the fetal heart rate. However, this sound, caused by pulsations of blood in the baby's cord, is not always heard. Another occasional sound called the *uterine souffle,* a swishlike tone occurring at the same rate as the maternal pulse is not diagnostic of pregnancy. It originates from the mother's pulsating uterine arteries and may also be detected in the presence of large vascular pelvic tumors.

Feeling. Fetal movement is detected by a trained examiner after about 20 weeks' gestation.

Progressive fetal growth

With the growth of the embryo and fetus, as shown in Table 4-1 and Fig. 4-8, the contours and silhouette of the expectant mother change progressively. The fundus, or top of the uterus, is felt about halfway between the top of the pubic bone and the umbilicus at approximately

16 weeks. The fundus is found near the umbilicus at about 20 weeks. When near full-term, the fundus is almost at the level of the tip of the sternum. A woman expecting her first baby usually experiences a sudden relief from shortness of breath about 2 weeks before her delivery when the fetus "drops" and lightening occurs, taking pressure off the diaphragm.

The increasing size of the fundus puts greater demands on the woman's respiratory, circulatory, and urinary systems. Her intestines and stomach become crowded and compressed. Increasing size necessitates changes in wardrobe and creates a typical posture of pregnancy, which makes the simple process of tying shoes almost impossible. The onset of labor terminates the long period of waiting and is usually a welcome event.

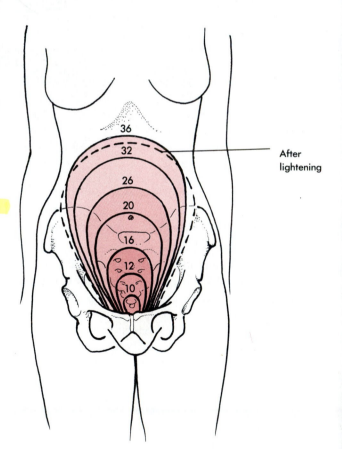

FIG 4-8 Progressive growth of fundus during pregnancy, measured in weeks. Note that fundus is lower at term than at 36 weeks' gestation.

Key Concepts

1. The fertilized egg, or zygote, is called a morula as it moves from the fallopian tube to the uterine cavity, where implantation occurs.
2. The outer surface of the zygote becomes covered with fingerlike tissue projections called chorionic villi, which aid in the process of implantation into the endometrium and manufacture human chorionic gonadotropin (hCG).
3. The placenta serves as a supply and disposal system for the developing embryo/fetus. Its functions are manufacturing hormones and enzymes; transporting food, oxygen, and antibodies from the mother to the fetus; and removing waste products from the fetal circulation to the maternal bloodstream.
4. The fetus is surrounded by a transparent sac made up of two membranous layers called the chorion and the amnion. The amnion contains amniotic fluid, which helps to control the environmental temperature of the fetus and shield it from trauma and infection.
5. From the eighth week of growth the embryo is called a fetus. Rudimentary body systems are formed and working, and the skeleton is becoming established.
6. During the first trimester the embryo/fetus is most susceptible to malformation from the effects of maternal drug ingestion, radiation, or infection.
7. At 16 weeks of growth the fetus is about 7½ inches (19 cm) long and weighs about 3⅓ ounces (100 g). At 16 to 18 weeks GA women usually report feelings of life, or quickening.
8. At 20 weeks' GA the fetal heartbeat can be heard using a standard fetoscope. Twenty to twenty-four weeks' GA is considered the legal threshold of viability.
9. The umbilical vein within the umbilical cord carries blood from the placenta to the fetus and enters the body at the umbilicus. Circulation through the fetus is very similar to postnatal circulation. Pulmonary circulation, however, is not completely established until after birth.
10. Methods of evaluating fetal status before labor include amniocentesis, ultrasonography, maternal blood and urine analysis, chorionic villi sampling, and fetal heart monitoring.
11. Signs and symptoms of pregnancy are usually divided into three groups: presumptive, probable, and positive.
12. Presumptive signs and symptoms usually include amenorrhea, nausea and vomiting, frequent urination, breast changes, changes in the shape of the abdomen, changes in the skin and mucous membranes, and quickening.
13. Probable signs and symptoms of pregnancy usually include enlargement of the uterus, basal body temperature elevation, ballottement, and positive biologic and immunochemical pregnancy tests.
14. Positive signs of pregnancy involve seeing, hearing, or feeling. Ultrasound permits visualization of the gestational sac and fetal form. Fetal heart tone can be heard using ultrasonic or Doppler technique or, after 18 to 20 weeks, with a standard fetoscope. Fetal movement can be felt by a trained examiner after about 20 weeks' gestation.

Discussion Questions

1. Discuss the importance of the placenta. How does it develop? What functions does it serve?
2. The circulation of the fetus is unique. What structures differentiate it from the mature circulation? What happens to the fetal structures after birth?
3. When the physician recognizes one abnormality, it is common to look closely for additional abnormalities. Why is this the case? If there is a problem in the gastrointestinal tract, what other structures would the physician examine carefully?
4. Your patient asks "When does my baby really look like a baby?" What would you tell her?
5. List and compare the presumptive, probable, and positive signs of pregnancy. Why do we classify the signs of pregnancy in this way? Do the signs differ in the first and in successive pregnancies?

5

Prenatal Care

CHAPTER OBJECTIVES

After studying this chapter, the student should be able to perform the following:

1 Define the following terms: viable, primigravida, primipara, multigravida, multipara, nullipara, antepartal, and prenatal.
2 List the five goals of prenatal care noted in the text.
3 Indicate five types of information that may be obtained during a woman's first pelvic examination for possible prenatal care.
4 Determine the meaning of the five-number code often used to describe a patient's obstetric history.
5 Calculate a woman's EDD (estimated date of delivery) using Nägele's rule.
6 Repeat the hemoglobin and hematocrit levels that usually signal the presence of anemia in a maternity patient.
7 Identify a protective level of rubella antibodies when evaluating the laboratory report.
8 Enumerate six signs or symptoms that should be reported by a pregnant woman to her health care provider.
9 Explain why expectant mothers are frequently weighed and routinely checked for elevated blood pressure, albuminuria, and glucosuria.
10 List five laboratory tests that are ordered fairly frequently to evaluate the status of an expectant mother.
11 Describe a diet appropriate for a woman in the last half of her pregnancy using the groupings indicated in Table 5-2.
12 Explain the origin and content of the RDAs often mentioned by nutritionists.
13 Name four foods rich in vitamin C, three foods with significant calcium content, and two foods high in iron.
14 Discuss the meaning of the phrase "empty calories" and its importance in meal planning.
15 State two considerations that may cause a health care provider to modify weight gain recommendations for a pregnant client.
16 Define the term "teratogen." List four examples of teratogens and describe problems they may cause.
17 Explain why a maternal supine resting position may not be healthy for the unborn infant.
18 Relate how Kegel exercises are performed and why they may be beneficial.
19 Share two guidelines that may be helpful in selecting appropriate exercise for a pregnant woman.
20 Indicate how a woman may need to alter her wardrobe as her pregnancy advances.
21 Identify two concerns associated with douching, especially during pregnancy.
22 Indicate a government agency that would be concerned with possible employment discrimination affecting pregnant workers.
23 Help plan clothing and furnishings for a first-born infant.
24 Compare briefly cultural differences that may affect maternal-child health practices among blacks, Hispanics, Asians, and Native American Indians.

As soon as she suspects she is pregnant, a woman should seek optimum care, even during the early months of pregnancy. Since women cannot be certain that they will become pregnant and often are not aware of a pregnancy until several weeks of gestation have elapsed, the earliest prenatal care is always the responsibility of the woman herself. Her general health habits and physical condition before a physician is ever consulted are of considerable importance. When pregnancy is established, provision for skilled prenatal supervision and assessment of her needs, preferences, and resources must be made. Care may be provided by a physician or a qualified member of a prenatal service, such as a nurse practitioner or certified nurse midwife. The licensed vocational/practical nurse (LVN/LPN) may assist in meeting patient and staff needs in this setting.

To conveniently describe an expectant mother's obstetric history and to better anticipate her needs, certain terms are used during her care. This terminology consists of a series of word roots and prefixes that help describe the number of times the woman has been pregnant and the number of times she has completed a pregnancy of a viable age. The word elements are as follows:

gravida The number of pregnancies a woman has had regardless of outcome.

para The number of *pregnancies* a woman has completed that have resulted in viable births. (The usual legal definitions of *viable* have been a pregnancy of 20 or 24 weeks or more duration, or the delivery of an infant weighing at least 500 g.) The para count does not change if an infant is living or dead; if he is born vaginally or by cesarean, or if the pregnancy produces multiple births (twins, etc.). A parturient is a woman in labor.

nul (a prefix) None. A *nulligravida* has never been pregnant. A *nullipara* has never delivered a viable child.

prim (a prefix) From primary, or first. Combined with gravida, it reads *primigravida* and means a woman who is having or has had one pregnancy. Combined with para, it reads *primipara* and technically means a woman who has completed one pregnancy of a viable age. After she is admitted into the labor-delivery suite, a woman who is carrying her first viable child but is not yet delivered is usually referred to as a primipara, or "primip," to differentiate her from a woman who has been through the birth process.

mult (a prefix) Many, or at least more than one. Combined with gravida it reads *multigravida* and means a woman who has had more than one pregnancy. Combined with para it reads *multipara*, or "multip," and technically means a woman who has completed two or more viable pregnancies. But in the labor-delivery suite the term is applied to a woman who has completed one or more, to differentiate her from a "first timer." Sometimes women who have had six or more viable births are called "grand-multips."

GOALS AND IMPORTANCE OF PRENATAL CARE

The term "antepartal or prenatal care" as used by physicians and nurses refers to the planned examination, observation, and guidance of an expectant mother. The extension of prenatal care is probably the primary factor in the improvement of maternal morbidity and mortality statistics. Society needs to appreciate its importance. The goals are as follows:

1. A pregnancy with a minimum of mental and physical discomfort and a maximum of gratification
2. A birth under the best circumstances possible
3. A normal, well baby
4. The establishment of good health habits benefiting all the family
5. A smooth, guided postpartum adjustment

For many years the overall goals of prenatal care have probably remained much the same, but interpretation of these goals and the methods for accomplishing them are undergoing continual change and accelerated expansion. During the late 1800s and early 1900s, the focus of the attending physician and nurse was on the physical needs of the parturient. Later, the psychologic aspects of her needs drew deserved attention. More recently, the physical and psychosocial needs of the entire family unit, as well as the needs of the childbearing woman, have been emphasized as health professionals concern themselves with the concept of "family-centered maternity care."*

For example, goals 1 and 2 underline the need for better health care delivery systems that would encourage socioeconomically disadvantaged urban and rural clients to receive needed care and vital health instruction. Because of financial strain, transportation difficulties, child care problems, or fear and distrust of established depersonalized and fragmented institutional management, they may not have sufficiently obtained or used these facilities. For many parents these goals also provide for more knowledge of the processes of pregnancy and childbirth and more participation in the control over these processes than were requested by recent previous generations.† For

---

*Joint position statement on the development of family-centered maternity/newborn care in hospitals, Chicago, June, 1978, Interprofessional Task Force on Health Care of Women and Children.
†McKay S: Humanizing maternity services through family-centered care, Minneapolis, 1982, International Childbirth Education Association.

some expectant parents, these goals have encouraged childbirth in settings other than the traditional hospital maternity unit. Primarily, psychologic factors have prompted their consideration of more flexible family-centered maternity care programs, alternative birth centers, or home birth. (See pp. 144-146.) Goal 3 now legally allows more choices as genetic counseling, abortion services, and, in some cases, surgical treatment of the unborn have become available. Goal 4 may encompass not only physical health but emotional well-being, knowledge and appreciation of life processes, and a sense of responsible personhood that considers individual differences as well as the common good. Today's parents do not wish to be treated all alike. They wish to have comprehensive care that will allow them certain choices, variations of expression, and informed consent. "A smooth, guided postpartum adjustment," goal 5, entails more knowledge of childcraft and parenting skills and more premeditated control of family composition.

THE FIRST VISIT

In a very real sense, prenatal care, negative or positive, has gone on in the life of a young woman before she becomes pregnant. Her basic physique was determined by her parents before her birth. Her environment has left its physical and emotional imprint. Her family circle and close friends have greatly influenced her attitude toward pregnancy and the challenges and responsibilities of motherhood. Today much controversy exists regarding the need for sex education, what should be taught by whom and at what age level. Sex education and preparation for marriage and parenthood are sometimes taught negatively, by default. Children and young people do not live in a vacuum.

What, in more detail, does formal prenatal care entail? Perhaps it would be easiest to describe the visits of the future mother to a physician's office or clinic. Usually the most lengthy visit she makes is her first.

The first prenatal visit is usually a particular time of stress. Some women are concerned because they want very much to be pregnant. Some are anxious about the nature of the examination and the tests to be made. Others may be upset because they had not planned to have a child. Family financial problems may be mounting. A number of small children may already be part of the family. Health problems at home may cause worry. Previous unfortunate obstetric experiences and half-believed gossip about pregnancy and childbirth may concern her. The marriage or relationship may be undergoing a period

of instability or even dissolution. All these possible situations tend to heighten the emotional content of the visit.

Setting and "climate"

The "climate" of the first visit as well as subsequent visits to the physician or, in some settings, nurse-midwife or nurse practitioner is all important. A nurse who has the responsibility of greeting and caring for these women has a key position in creating a cordial, respectful environment in which the woman feels personally important to the office or clinic staff and physician.

Preparation for the first prenatal visit is usually made by a telephone call. Some prenatal programs make available, through mailings or recorded tapes, extended information regarding the appointment and helpful resources. It is customary for a new patient to be asked to bring a sample of the first voided urine on the day of the appointment if her visit will be made early in the morning. When the time of the appointment arrives, it is hoped that the prospective patient will not have to wait too long. However, because of the very nature of a physician's practice, which deals with the unscheduled arrivals of babies, some waiting is almost unavoidable.

Some of this waiting time can often be put to excellent use. The nurse or receptionist can talk with the patient and make her feel welcome. Brief information cards for office use may be completed. An instructional guide "checklist" will help ensure that the learning needs of the patient and her family will be met.* Frequently changed, attractive bulletin boards may emphasize nutrition and meal planning, mental health practices, good grooming, maternity wardrobe styles, and approved courses in preparation for childbirth and child care. Up-to-date pamphlets on maternal and child care and breast-feeding literature may also be available. Not all reading material should be pregnancy-oriented, however. When waits are protracted, an offer of nutritious beverages may be appreciated. The way to the public restroom should be clearly indicated, since frequent urination is an often-encountered annoyance to the pregnant woman, and general nervousness may exaggerate this symptom. Just before the pelvic examination, the patient should have an opportunity to empty her bladder to ease the examination and to allow a more accurate measurement of the height of the fundus.

---

*Walls JL: An instruction guide for educating expectant mothers, MCN 8(4):274, 1983.

Vital signs and history

Before actually seeing the physician, the woman is usually weighed and her temperature, pulse, and respiration are checked by the nurse. In some clinics, nurses also take the blood pressures and medical and obstetric histories of new patients, but many practitioners prefer to complete the blood pressures and the histories themselves. A carefully secured history is important in determining any special care of the patient. Early detection of reproductive risk is essential to preventing maternal or fetal problems. What previous medical or surgical difficulties has she had? Any problems involving mental or emotional instability? Any family problems that may affect her toleration of the stress of pregnancy? What is her history of contraceptive use (type and timing)? What medications including vitamins is she taking? Does she smoke or use alcohol or other drugs? Is she using her automobile seatbelt properly?

A record of previous pregnancies and their outcome is important in indicating the need for special emphasis in prenatal care. One method of coding the results of previous pregnancies involves the use of five consecutive digits. The first refers to the number of pregnancies experienced, the second to the number of full-term deliveries, the third to the number of premature births, the fourth to abortions, and the fifth to children now living. Using this code, what would 6-3-2-1-5 mean? Many physicians believe that the time spent in recording the historical data is more than repaid by the greater opportunity to evaluate the childbearing woman and her child, to consider her expectations, and to establish a rapport.

Pelvic examination

The prenatal visit usually continues with the determination of the presence of pregnancy. Routines differ, but in our opinion the pelvic examination should be done first in the schedule of the physical examination to alleviate the additional anxiety of waiting and to avoid a filling bladder! The nurse, by her manner and efficiency and clear explanations can help the patient immensely.

Preparation. An adequate gown, which gives reassuring coverage but opens in such a way to facilitate a physical examination, is desirable. A drape that makes the patient feel covered, even if she is not, is a real aid. The hips should extend about 1 inch over the edge of the table with the feet supported in covered stirrups. Various drapes may be used. A nurse should always be present during the examination to reassure the patient and to protect the physician from criticism. Necessary instruments should be ready (Fig. 5-1): warmed speculum; spatula or applicator, or vaginal pipette with rubber bulb; slides and preservative for cervical cancer detection; long swabs or cotton balls; sponge sticks; both sterile and clean examination gloves; lubricant; and paper tissue wipes. A good light and a convenient stool must be provided. If the woman is able to let her knees fall outward and relax,

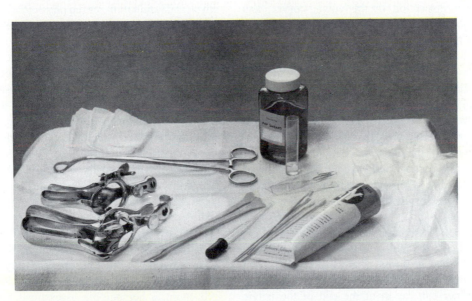

FIG 5-1 Typical pelvic tray (sterile gloves not shown). Small test tube contains physiologic saline solution for wet mount of vaginal discharge.

the examination will be less difficult. Having her breathe through her open mouth usually promotes relaxation, although there is some danger of hyperventilation in very tense patients.

Progression. The pelvic examination yields considerable information. First, the external genitalia are inspected. Next, if a Papanicolaou (Pap) smear for cancer detection is desired (and it is almost always part of the routine), a warmed bivalve speculum, lubricated with water, is inserted to reveal the cervix. Specimens of secretion may be aspirated from the posterior fornix with the pipette or secured with the applicator or spatula from the cervix and placed thinly and evenly on one or two slides. These slides must not be allowed to dry out but should immediately be placed in a fixative (usually equal parts of 95% alcohol and ether). The physician will then observe the cervix and vaginal mucosa for any abnormalities or unusual discharge; specimens of any discharge can be obtained for future study. Fungous infection caused by *Candida albicans* or infection initiated by microscopic animals, or protozoa, called *Trichomonas vaginalis,* is fairly common. Routine culture of cervical mucus for *Neisseria gonorrhoeae,* the cause of gonorrhea, has been helpful in detecting significant numbers of so-called silent infections within certain high-risk populations. The mucosa will be checked for Chadwick's sign—a violet tinge caused by increased circulatory congestion in the area.

After general inspection of the vulva, cervix, and vagina, the speculum is gently removed and a digital examination is made with the lubricated gloved hand. At this time the examiner feels the size and position of the uterus and the consistency of the cervix, and perhaps tries to elicit Hegar's sign, the softening of the uterine isthmus, through vaginoabdominal pressure. The pelvic contents are palpated to try to identify any abnormal masses or tumors. Before the examination is completed, an attempt to measure the *diagonal conjugate* to estimate the size of the pelvic canal and evaluate the position of the ischial spines and tuberosities may be made. At the end of the vaginal examination a rectal examination is usually carried out.

This time of pelvic evaluation can provide an excellent opportunity to teach the patient about her external genitalia, internal pelvic anatomy, and the normal physiologic changes that take place during pregnancy. Generally, the examiner can report at the end of the pelvic examination whether the woman is pregnant, based on a number of signs and symptoms. Many examiners include pregnancy tests as part of their initial evaluations.

Determination of delivery date

The most common method of determining the date of delivery involves a record of the menstrual cycle. The woman is asked to name the *first* day of her last *normal* menstrual period. The caregiver then counts back 3 months and adds 7 days to calculate the estimated date of delivery or confinement (EDD or EDC). (Confinement is an old term used to indicate the period of labor and birth.) For example, if a woman said her last normal menstrual period occurred between May 7 and May 12, her EDD would be February 14 of the following year. This method of calculation is called Nägele's rule. Of course, if the patient cannot remember the necessary vital statistics, then the size of the uterus may be interpreted, or the time of the intercourse that preceded conception may be known. Ultrasound evaluation may be used if it is important to estimate the age of the fetus. Occasionally *quickening* may be used as a measurable landmark, but it is not reliable. However, even Nägele's rule offers only an estimate. It is said that only 4% of all babies arrive on the predetermined date using this schedule, whereas 60% appear 1 to 7 days earlier or later. Actually, infants born within 2 weeks of the EDD calculated using Nägele's rule are still considered "full-term."

Complete examination

The first prenatal visit may continue with a complete physical examination, or the physician may only talk with the patient, giving appropriate guidance and information and making arrangements for a more detailed physical examination during the following visit.

In addition to the pelvic examination, the physician checks the woman's blood pressure; listens to her heart and lungs; examines her mouth, eyes, nose, and throat; observes and palpates her breasts for abnormalities; and inquires about her preference for feeding the infant. The breast examination should be conducted to determine whether normal breast changes are occurring and whether infection or malignancy is present. The abdomen is palpated with the knees flexed for greater relaxation of the abdominal wall, and the extremities are checked for bruises, swelling, and enlarged veins.

Usually at the conclusion of the physical examination, arrangements are made for the necessary laboratory tests. A sample of venous blood is drawn. A complete blood cell count, a hemoglobin assessment alone, or a hematocrit may be ordered to determine the amount of hemoglobin present in the blood in relation to its volume. Any pregnant woman may be or may become anemic.

Dietary deficiencies of iron are common. Although hemoglobin and hematocrit levels in nonpregnant women would be considered suspiciously low if less than 12 g/100 ml and 36%, respectively, the standards of possible anemia used during pregnancy are usually less than 11 g/100 ml and less than 33%. The differences are the result of the increased fluid content in the blood during gestation. Prenatal testing for sickle cell anemia in previously unscreened black patients is becoming more common.

A serology test for the detection of syphilis (STS) is a routine screening procedure of prenatal care. A determination of main blood group and Rh status is made to assist in maternal care in the event of hemorrhage and to detect the possibility of blood protein incompatibility, which could threaten the life of the developing fetus or neonate. If the patient is found to be Rh negative, the Rh status of the baby's father should be ascertained. Evaluation of serum antibody levels may be appropriate. (See p. 68.)

Another potential threat that can now be identified by the laboratory is rubella, or German measles. A history of the disease in childhood is not always reliable, because other conditions may have been incorrectly called rubella and the disease does not always manifest a rash. The measurement of rubella antibody level in a woman's blood has become a premarital or prenatal legal requirement in some states. The presence of antibodies in a dilution greater than 1:8 or 1:10 (depending on the manufacturer) in the hemagglutination inhibition (HI or HAI) test or a value of 1,000 or more as a result of the enzyme index assay (EIA) is said to indicate immunity. Pregnant women are *not* given the available immunization against rubella. Maximum theoretic risk of fetal damage from rubella vaccination during pregnancy is said to be 2% to 5%. However, if immunity is considered absent, the antibody titer obtained can be used as a baseline to help determine subsequent contact with the disease and the need for possible immune globulin or consideration of an abortion. New mothers at risk are immunized during the postpartum period only after reliable contraception techniques have been instituted. See discussion of rubella, p. 626.

The urine specimen brought in the same morning or secured later at the office is tested for albumin and glucose. Many physicians order a complete urinalysis initially.

In many patients, chest x-ray examination for detection of tuberculosis is being avoided through the use of Mantoux or tine skin testing. If the skin test is positive, a full-sized, conventional chest x-ray examination is recommended to rule out possible problems more easily and to avoid the higher amount of x-ray exposure involved in the use of photofluorographs or miniature films. Screening for tuberculosis, hepatitis, and malaria is becoming more important as the refugee population increases.

Some authorities suggest that all women be tested for hepatitis (HBsAg) at their first prenatal visit and again between the 28th and the 32nd weeks of gestation. If the test is positive, an immunization series would be administered to the mother as soon as possible after birth. The baby should begin treatment within the first 12 hours of life using hepatitis B immune globulin and hepatitis B vaccine.

Limiting screens of HIV only to those pregnant patients with identified risk factors is currently recommended.* However, some are advocating universal prenatal testing for HIV, since some HBsAg-positive or high-risk mothers are missed.† (See also p. 624.)

Guidance

After all these procedures have been completed, if they take place during one visit, the patient is usually tired. Lengthy instructions and explanations are not properly assimilated. Perhaps the best method of imparting needed information is through the use of some kind of prenatal instruction booklet that has been approved or written by the patient's health care provider. Some practices offer a series of teaching films that individuals or groups can view while they are waiting to see the physician. Such guidance is absolutely necessary, but all of it need not be provided on the first visit. However, some time should be spent answering questions, discussing patient expectations for the childbirth, and giving some general instructions regarding dietary requirements, risks of self-medication, smoking, and alcohol and drug consumption. Situations that should be reported promptly must be clarified.

Reportable signs and symptoms

Care givers should indicate, in a manner that is not alarming to the pregnant woman, the signs and symptoms that must be reported. These may or may not be significant, but only qualified personnel are capable of deciding their importance and must be notified of their presence.

*Barton JJ and others: Prevalence of human immunodeficiency virus in a general population, Am J Obstet Gynecol 160(6):1316, 1989.
†Rhame FS and others: The case for wider use of testing for HIV infection, N Engl J Med 320(19):1248, 1989.

They include the following:

1. Bleeding from the vagina at any time
2. Uncontrollable leaking of fluid from the vagina
3. Unusual abdominal pain or cramps
4. Persistent nausea or vomiting, especially in the second or third trimester
5. Persistent headache or any blurring of vision
6. Marked swelling of the ankles and especially of the hands and face
7. Painful or burning urination
8. Chills or fever

Then, armed with information, the woman may make an appointment for her next visit. Before her return she can jot down additional questions.

SUBSEQUENT VISITS

During the first half of the pregnancy, most expectant mothers visit their physician every 3 or 4 weeks unless special needs become apparent. After 5 months, visits are usually scheduled every 2 or 3 weeks, and in the last month, checkups may be made every 1 or 2 weeks or more often.

Examination

The subsequent visits are not as long or involved as the first. The woman is weighed by the nurse, and the blood pressure is recorded. A urine specimen is checked for albumin and glucose. The urine examination for glucose, of course, is made to detect diabetes mellitus or gestational diabetes. A glucose tolerance screen may be ordered at 24 to 28 weeks. All of the other above determinations are done to reveal the beginnings of pregnancy-induced hypertension (PIH) or preeclampsia (high blood pressure, edema, excessive weight gain and albuminuria; see p. 180). The physician or other health personnel measures the height of the uterus to see if the pregnancy is progressing at the expected rate and may repeat the pelvic examination during the first return visit.

It is essential to make careful measurements of the height of the fundus to assess the progress of the pregnancy. The use of a tape measure is recommended, though pelvimetry calipers may be used. The Doptone may be used in early pregnancy to evaluate the fetal heart rate. After about 4½ calendar months' gestation the fetal heart tone may be heard with a nonelectronic fetoscope. After 8 months' gestation the abdomen is palpated to determine the presentation of the fetus. Measurements of hemoglobin or hematocrit levels should be repeated for all pregnant women at least once late in pregnancy

(at about 32 to 36 weeks). Women who earlier had been found to have iron or folic acid deficiency anemias or other causes of hemoglobin reduction should be checked more frequently to determine their response to therapy.

If Rh incompatibility is a possibility, antibody titers should be done not only at the initial prenatal visit but also at 24, 28, 32, and 36 weeks' gestation, even if the woman received Rh immune globulin, such as RhoGAM, after previous pregnancies. Rising titers may indicate whether the baby is Rh positive and will alert the physician to developing erythroblastosis fetalis. Some cases of isoimmunization could be prevented by using *prenatal RhoGAM* administration as well. *RhoGAM* may be indicated after each amniocentesis. Adverse effects on the fetus have not been reported. A more reliable technique for evaluating fetal jeopardy related to blood factor incompatibility involves the aspiration of amniotic fluid by transabdominal needle insertion (amniocentesis) and its analysis for elevated bilirubin levels (p. 52).

Because maternal syphilitic infection may be acquired *after* a negative prenatal serology result is obtained, the prudence of securing a repeat serology test close to term should be considered. Since initial testing for maternal syphilitic infection is positive in less than 80% of patients with primary syphilis, it is essential to repeat the test near the end of pregnancy (36 weeks). Follow-up may utilize the fluorescent treponemal antibody absorption (FTA-ABS) test if the VDRL is reactive. In this instance, even though treatment has been instituted, the newborn should be tested using serum obtained from cord blood for VDRL and FTA-ABS tests, as well as IgM-specific FTA-ABS testing.

Genital herpes can be transmitted to the baby as he passes through the birth canal. When suspicious lesions are found, a test for herpes should be performed. These lesions usually first appear as tender, painful blisters (vesicles) on the vulva, cervix, vagina, anus, or buttocks. After these vesicles break, wet ulcers form, which later crust. The management of the delivery of a mother who has had genital herpes is now being reconsidered (see p. 174).

Because of the incidence of fetal and newborn problems associated with chlamydia, pregnant women should be examined and tested for this common sexually transmitted disease (p. 174).* Other laboratory evaluations of fetal and maternal health and gestational maturity are

---

*Bourcier KM and others: Chlamydia and condylomata acuminata: an update for the nurse practitioner, J Obstet Gynecol Neonatal Nurs 16(1):17, 1987.

possible but would depend on the specific problems discovered.

Guidance

During the initial and return visits a feeling of trust should be built up between the pregnant woman and the physician, other maternity team members, and office staff. The physician and nurse should be able to identify areas in which special help is required—whether the woman needs information, reassurance in her own capacity to be a good mother, possible help in organizing her household to achieve more rest and peace of mind, or simply an interested human listener.

Nutrition. The subject of nutrition has long been considered important in prenatal care. Increasing numbers of health professionals now recognize that nutrition is not only important but crucial in determining the health of the childbearing woman, her offspring, and perhaps even that of ongoing generations. It is imperative that girls and women consider themselves as possible prospective mothers by preparing themselves for the potential responsibility of such nurture long before a mate is selected. Their health, knowledge, and skills will profoundly influence the structure of any future family. A woman who furnishes her body with what it needs nutritionally to enjoy optimum personal health and who augments her diet as needed as a pregnancy progresses gives her child a better opportunity to be both well formed from his earliest days of development and wellborn as he ends his intrauterine growth period. A well-nourished mother and baby are less often the victims of obstetric and perinatal complications, such as maternal anemia, preterm delivery, infant growth retardation (small size for development dates), or significant residual neurologic damage (e.g., cerebral palsy, mental deficiency, or behavior disorders in the child).

Various aids have been devised to try to help Americans eat more nourishing food according to their body build, age, activity level, and special physiologic needs. The National Research Council periodically publishes a quantitative list of the nutrients needed. The last revision of this list, called the Recommended Dietary Allowance (RDA) was published in 1989. Table 5-1 is an abbreviated version.*

The council suggests that a normal, healthy, pregnant woman of any age be given an additional 300 calories per day during her second and third trimesters. However, calorie adjustments for special situations such as depleted body reserves or changes in activity may be needed as the individual mother is evaluated. More of almost every listed nutrient is necessary as well.

Since 1980 the requirement for ascorbic acid has been decreased from 80 mg/day to 70 mg/day for the pregnant woman. Vitamin B$_6$ recommended daily intake was changed from 2.6 mg to 2.2 mg. Zinc has been shown to affect over 70 enzymes in the human body—an important element to consider when planning the dietary intake. It is usually associated with protein foods and nuts. Selenium has been added. Sixty-five micrograms is recommended. Seafood, kidney, and liver are sources of selenium. Grains and seeds can be sources if the selenium content of the soil is adequate. The vitamin K requirement is also 65 µg per day. A green, leafy salad would meet the daily requirement of vitamin K although dairy products, liver, eggs, cereals, fruits, and vegetables are other sources.

Iron deficiency anemia is the most common anemia of pregnancy. Although the pregnant woman should increase her iron intake during pregnancy, the requirement is usually not met from dietary sources alone. The fetus needs to build an iron reserve for hemoglobin formation during the first few months of extrauterine life when the main source of nutrition is milk, which is normally iron poor. Therefore, the National Research Council advises that supplements containing 30 to 60 mg of elemental iron be taken by the pregnant woman each day. This could be continued for 2 to 3 months after delivery to help replenish the mother's iron supply. Excessive or megavitamin intake can be dangerous as well as wasteful. Routine multivitamin supplementation should not be necessary if a varied nutritious diet is consumed. However, folate (folic acid) may need to be added (400 µg/day). A specific megaloblastic anemia does occasionally occur as a result of folacin depletion in pregnancy. It is interesting to note that steroid contraceptives, which the expectant mother may have used in the recent past, may also inhibit folic acid absorption. Nondietary folic acid is often prescribed by clinicians. Prescription of prenatal fluoride has not proved to be an asset. Calcification of the permanent teeth and much of the deciduous teeth occurs after birth. The RDAs determined by the council are designed to indicate safe dietary levels of selected nutrients for a wide range of normal healthy persons. Individual differences in the dietary background or obstetric histories of pregnant women may suggest the need for variations in these allowances.

*The complete 1989 revision may be found in National Research Council (US Subcommittee on the 10th edition of the RDAs): Recommended dietary allowances, ed 10, Washington, DC, 1989, National Academy Press.

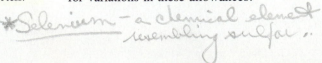

*Selenium — a chemical element resembling sulfur.

Table 5-1 Food and Nutrition Board, National Academy of Sciences—National Research Council recommended dietary allowance

Category	Age (years) or condition	Weight† (kg)	Weight† (lb)	Height† (cm)	Height† (in)	Protein (g)	Fat-soluble vitamins Vita-min A (μg RE)‡	Vita-min D (μg)§	Vita-min E (mg α-TE)‖	Vita-min K (μg)
Females	11-14	46	101	157	62	46	800	10	8	45
	15-18	55	120	163	64	44	800	10	8	55
	19-24	58	128	164	65	46	800	10	8	60
	25-50	63	138	163	64	50	800	5	8	65
	51 +	65	143	160	63	50	800	5	8	65
Pregnant						60	800	10	10	65
Lactating	1st 6 months					65	1,300	10	12	65
	2nd 6 months					62	1,200	10	11	65

*The allowances, expressed as average daily intakes over time, are intended to provide for individual variations among most normal persons as they live in the United States under usual environmental stresses. Diets should be based on a variety of common foods in order to provide other nutrients for which human requirements have been less well defined.

†Weights and heights of Reference Adults are actual medians for the US population of the designated age, as reported by NHANES II. The use of these figures does not imply that the height-to-weight ratios are ideal.

‡Retinol equivalents. 1 retinol equivalent = 1 μg retinol or 6 μg β-carotene.

§As cholecalciferol. 10 μg cholecalciferol = 400 IU of vitamin D.

‖α-Tocopherol equivalents. 1 mg d-α tocopherol = 1 α-TE.

An increasing trend (at least among some physicians) emphasizes the quality of the pregnant woman's diet with less concern about a certain total number of pounds gained. The need for quality intake is present throughout pregnancy. For a number of years the National Academy of Sciences, Committee on Maternal Nutrition has indicated that two thirds of weight gain occurs in the last half of pregnancy, paralleling fairly closely the baby's own weight gain. Quantitative increases in maternal intake have been favored for healthy, well-nourished women only after about the twentieth week.

Because a pregnant woman cannot (as yet) go to the grocery store to purchase a package labeled "60 grams of protein" and because nutritional supplements or pills are expensive, inefficient, and unsatisfying, there needs to be a way to interpret caloric and nutrient needs in terms of market basket commodities. For a long time, the concept of the four food groups and a suggested number of servings have been helpful in planning balanced family meals (Fig. 5-2). These four groups—milk, meat, fruit-vegetable, and grain—contain only those foods high in leading nutrients. (See also Table 5-2.)

In the second half of pregnancy, many women benefit from four servings from the milk group. These may include three or four cups of skimmed, lowfat (2%), or whole milk. Using nonfat dairy products reduces fat and cholesterol intake. Some fat is necessary in the diet, but it is not a scarce nutrient. Milk (and the calcium and protein it provides) is considered an important constituent of the pregnant woman's diet. However, at times its use must be modified. The woman who does not care for milk is free to use flavoring, concentrate the value of what she does drink by adding skim milk powders, use milk in cooking, or select a milk exchange of approximate equal value. For example, 1½ slices of cheddar cheese or 2 cups of cottage cheese equals approximately 1 cup of milk or yogurt.

Some adults, especially blacks and Asians, experience a digestive intolerance to the lactose found in milk and may develop abdominal cramping, intestinal gas, and diarrhea. However, they are often able to eat cheese. The harder or more aged varieties of cheese contain less lactose than processed types. Chilled dairy products, such as yogurt and ice cream, may also produce fewer symptoms.

The calcium provided in milk and its products is important. There is a tendency for calcium to be drawn from the maternal skeleton, causing *osteoporosis* and weakening its structure if dietary needs are not met. If

evised 1989 (Designed for the maintenance of good nutrition of practically all healthy people in the United States)

Water-soluble vitamins							Minerals						
Vita-min C (mg)	Thia-min (mg)	Ribo-flavin (mg)	Niacin (mg NE)¶	Vita-min B₆ (mg)	Fo-late (μg)	Vitamin B₁₂ (μg)	Cal-cium (mg)	Phos-phorus (mg)	Mag-nesium (mg)	Iron (mg)	Zinc (mg)	Iodine (μg)	Sele-nium (μg)
50	1.1	1.3	15	1.4	150	2.0	1,200	1,200	280	15	12	150	45
60	1.1	1.3	15	1.5	180	2.0	1,200	1,200	300	15	12	150	50
60	1.1	1.3	15	1.6	180	2.0	1,200	1,200	280	15	12	150	55
60	1.1	1.3	15	1.6	180	2.0	800	800	280	15	12	150	55
60	1.0	1.2	13	1.6	180	2.0	800	800	280	10	12	150	55
70	1.5	1.6	17	2.2	400	2.2	1,200	1,200	320	30	15	175	65
95	1.6	1.8	20	2.1	280	2.6	1,200	1,200	355	15	19	200	75
90	1.6	1.7	20	2.1	260	2.6	1,200	1,200	340	15	16	200	75

1 NE (niacin equivalent) is equal to 1 mg of niacin or 60 mg of dietary tryptophan.

a pregnant woman cannot tolerate milk or is having muscle cramps because of phosphorus/calcium imbalance in the blood, calcium pills may be given, but in this case a fine, relatively inexpensive source of protein is lost. Milk is also usually fortified with vitamin D, an important consideration in planning meals for women in climates with little sunshine or for those who receive inadequate exposure to sunlight.

Three servings of the meat group are usually recommended during the latter part of pregnancy. (This may include one or two eggs per day in addition to two servings of the other meat group foods listed unless an elevated blood cholesterol level is identified.) Eggs are recommended particularly for the rich iron source found in the yolk. Meat, eggs, and even fish and poultry are expensive, but they are complete proteins, containing all the amino acids necessary for growth, repair, and development. The essential amino acids (eight to ten in number, depending on age requirements) must be available to form new tissue within the mother's body, and they must be supplied in the diet. The body cannot manufacture these protein-building blocks by rearranging molecules within its own cells. Such proteins are critical to the growth of the embryo and fetus because basic body systems are formed early in pregnancy and different organs, especially the brain, undergo growth spurts in the last weeks of gestation. They are also critical for the mother to help maintain her health. But the role of deficient protein intake in causing pregnancy-induced hypertension is increasingly disputed. (See p. 73.)

If legumes such as beans or peas, corn, and nuts are used as major protein sources, they must be mixed in such a way that all essential amino acids are represented in a single meal, since none of these protein sources is complete in itself. Mixing certain incomplete proteins conscientiously or serving them with milk provides an adequate diet but is more difficult to plan. Examples of adequate protein mixes using incomplete proteins are combinations of cornmeal and kidney beans or whole wheat, soy beans, and sesame seeds. Pure vegetarian or "vegan" diets without any animal sources, dairy products, or eggs can supply adequate protein with careful planning, but other deficiencies (for example, vitamin B₁₂) may become a problem.

High-grade biologic sources of protein, such as meat, fish, poultry, milk, and eggs, contribute other nutrients as well. For example, liver, although not everybody's favorite choice, may be recommended because of its high iron content.

Fruits and vegetables are important sources of vitamins, minerals, and fiber (if they are eaten unmodified). Constipation is a real problem for many pregnant women. The increasing pressure exerted on the bowel by the enlarging uterus, diminished intestinal tone, and decreased physical exercise have all been blamed for this trouble. The use of high-fiber foods and increased fluids usually helps solve the problem. A high vitamin C (ascorbic acid) intake is advised for tissue building; the fruits and vegetables especially helpful are grapefruit, oranges, lemons, limes, tomatoes, strawberries, cantaloupes, green peppers, and cabbage. Four or more servings of fruits and vegetables are often endorsed. (In the fifth edition of *Nutrition and Diet Therapy*, Williams increased her recommendation for fruits and vegetables to

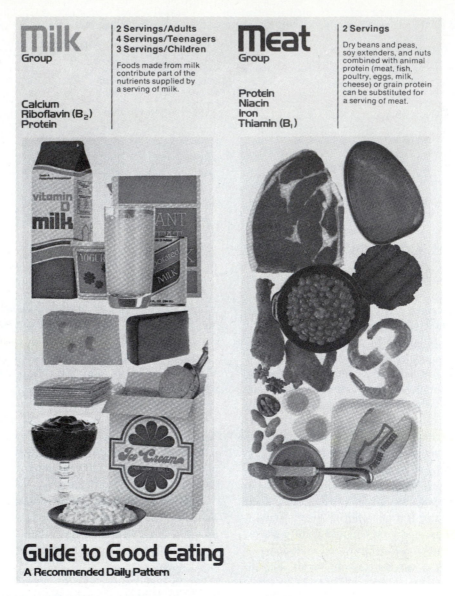

FIG 5-2 Guide to good eating indicates recommended diet for nonpregnant women and other family members. See p. 76 for modification during pregnancy. *(Courtesy National Dairy Council, Rosemont, Ill.)*

six to nine servings, depending on the sources of the servings.) Dark green and deep yellow vegetables must be included (Table 5-2).

Whole-grain or enriched breads and cereals provide sources of the B vitamins thiamine and niacin, as well as some iodine and iron. Unrefined grains, of course, also contain fiber. From four to ten servings are recommended. One slice of bread equals one serving.

Items that contribute little or no nutrient value other than calories for energy are called "empty calorie" foods. Examples of these items are candy, cake, pie, soft drinks, doughnuts, and potato chips. They add pounds but contribute nothing that would assist the pregnant woman or developing fetus except potential heat and energy. However, in some poorer malnourished populations, less costly caloric supplements may help spare available protein intake for tissue building, improving infant outcome.

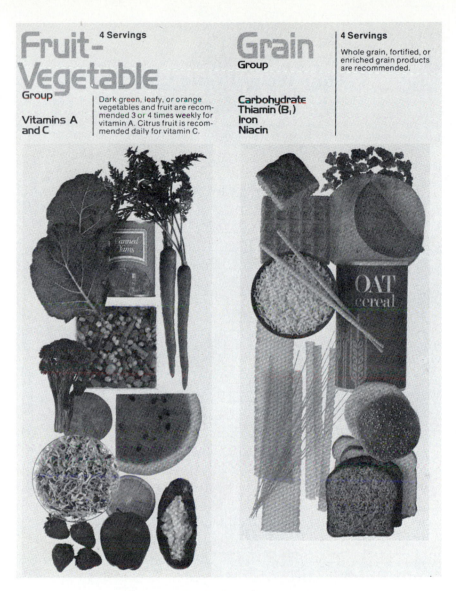

Fruit-Vegetable
Group

4 Servings

Vitamins A and C

Dark green, leafy, or orange vegetables and fruit are recommended 3 or 4 times weekly for vitamin A. Citrus fruit is recommended daily for vitamin C.

Grain
Group

4 Servings

Whole grain, fortified, or enriched grain products are recommended.

Carbohydrate
Thiamin (B₁)
Iron
Niacin

FIG 5-2, cont'd.   For legend see opposite page.

Sometimes women during pregnancy experience special cravings for unusual foods or food combinations. Generally these desires are trivial and may be humored if they do not threaten good nutrition. However, there is a type of unusual ingestion called *pica* that is characteristic of, but not confined to, lower socioeconomic ethnic groups. Women exhibiting symptoms of pica may eat relatively large amounts of substances such as laundry starch or river clay. Such ingestions interfere with good nutrition and cause anemia.

Anything that depresses good nutritional intake, whether it be nausea or vomiting, food fads, lack of finances, smoking, alcoholism, or other personal or social problems, should be evaluated and relieved or eliminated to achieve good dietary prenatal care. The pregnant woman should be cautioned not to fast during pregnancy.

The restriction of salt or sodium intake was long considered by many physicians a part of the prenatal diet. It had been advocated in an attempt to prevent and treat the symptoms of pregnancy-induced hypertension (formerly know as preeclampsia-eclampsia, or toxemia of pregnancy), a serious complication characterized by

Your Weight-Gain Chart

Weigh yourself on the same day every week during your pregnancy. Each time you weigh yourself, look on this chart and find the total number of pounds you've gained, line it up with the number of weeks you've been pregnant, and make a dot where the two lines meet on the chart. Your goal is to keep your dots inside the shaded area for your category. Don't worry if the line isn't smooth – small peaks and valleys are normal!

Name: _____   Weight-Gain Range: _____

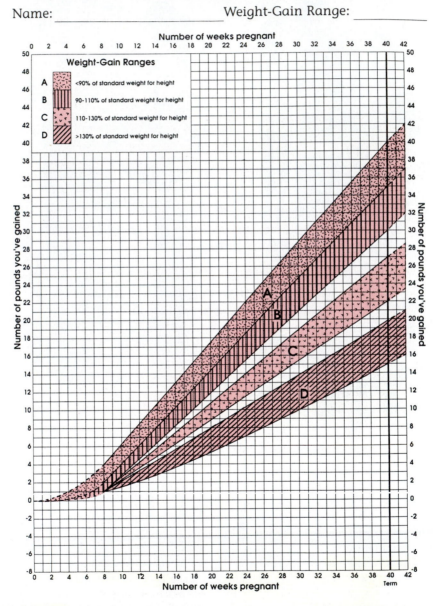

Weight-Gain Ranges

A   <90% of standard weight for height

B   90-110% of standard weight for height

C   110-130% of standard weight for height

D   >130% of standard weight for height

FIG 5-3 Prenatal gain in weight. *(Supported in part by project #MCJ 276008 from the Maternal and Child Health program [Title V, Social Security Act], Health Resources and Services Administration, Department of Health and Human Services. © Regents of the University of Minnesota, 1988.)*

Healthy Infant Outcome Project
Table for Identifying Prepregnancy Weight Status

Height (no shoes)	A Under	B Normal	C Over	D Obese
	WEIGHT STATUS CATEGORY			
	Weight in pounds (light indoor clothing)			
feet inches				
4 9	92 or less	93-113	114-134	135 or more
4 10	94 or less	95-117	118-138	139 or more
4 11	97 or less	98-120	121-142	143 or more
5 0	100 or less	101-123	124-146	147 or more
5 1	103 or less	104-127	128-150	151 or more
5 2	106 or less	107-131	132-155	156 or more
5 3	109 or less	110-134	135-159	160 or more
5 4	113 or less	114-140	141-165	166 or more
5 5	117 or less	118-144	145-170	171 or more
5 6	121 or less	122-149	150-176	177 or more
5 7	124 or less	125-153	154-181	182 or more
5 8	128 or less	129-157	158-186	187 or more
5 9	131 or less	132-162	163-191	192 or more
5 10	135 or less	136-166	167-196	197 or more
5 11	139 or less	140-171	172-202	203 or more
6 0	142 or less	143-175	176-207	208 or more
Prenatal Weight Gain Goal: (pounds)	35-40*	30-35	22-27	15-20

For twin pregnancies, the weight gain goal is 41 pounds for women entering pregnancy normal weight and 44 pounds for women entering pregnancy underweight.

Technical Notes: Weight for height ranges are calculated from the 1959 Metropolitan Height and Weight Tables for Women over the age of 25 years. A midpoint value was determined from the range of weight for height for women of "medium frame". The cut-point for underweight women is designated as a weight for height that is more than 10% below the midpoint. The normal weight range is calculated as plus or minus 10% of the midpoint for each height. The overweight range is calculated as greater than 10% through 30% above the midpoint of weight for height. The cut-point in weight for the obese category is calculated as a weight for height that is more than 30% above the midpoint of weight for height.

*The weight gain goal for women who are very underweight (20% or more below the midpoint of weight for height) may range from 40 to 45 pounds.

FIG 5-3, cont'd. For legend see opposite page.

edema of the face or hands, hypertension, and albuminuria, which could lead to convulsions and death. This complication has been a major cause of fetal, neonatal, and maternal mortality for many years. Considerable controversy continues regarding its cause, prevention, and treatment. Although the lack of enough dietary protein intake has been considered by some clinicians to be a major trigger in the mechanism of pregnancy-induced hypertension, certain studies have not supported this explanation as a primary cause. The roles of various nutritional deficiencies in the etiology of PIH appear to require further reserach before definite conclusions can be made.* Certainly, the severe weight gain and salt restrictions imposed (with good intent) on most expectant mothers 30 years ago are now considered nontherapeutic and detrimental.

*Zlatnik FJ and Burmeister LF: Dietary protein and preeclampsia, Am J Obstet Gynecol 147:345, 1983; Worthington-Roberts BS and Williams SR, editors: Nutrition in pregnancy and lactation, ed 4, St Louis, 1989, Times Mirror/Mosby, pp 85-88 and 181-184; Cunningham FG, MacDonald PC, and Gant NF: Williams obstetrics, ed 18, Norwalk, Conn, 1989, Appleton & Lange.

Table 5-2 Daily food plan for pregnancy and lactation

Food	Nonpregnant woman	Pregnancy	Lactation
Milk (skimmed or buttermilk), cheese, ice cream (food made with milk can supply part of requirement)	2 cups	3-4 cups	4-5 cups
Meat (lean meat, fish, poultry, cheese, occasional dried beans or peas)	1 serving (3-4 oz)	2 servings (6-8 oz); include liver frequently	2½ servings (8 oz)
Eggs	1	1-2	1-2
Vegetables* (dark green or deep yellow)	1 serving	1 serving	1-2 servings
Vitamin C-rich food*	1 good source or 2 fair sources	1 good source and 1 fair source or 2 good sources	1 good source and 1 fair source or 2 good sources
Good source: citrus fruit, berries, cantaloupe			
Fair source: tomatoes, cabbage, greens, potatoes in skin			
Other vegetables, fruits, juices	2 servings	4-6 servings	4-6 servings
Bread† and cereals (enriched or whole grain)	6 servings	10 servings	10 servings
Butter or fortified margarine	Moderate amount	Moderate amount	Moderate amount

From Williams SR: Nutrition and diet therapy, ed 5, St Louis, 1985, The CV Mosby Co.
*Use some raw daily.
†One slice of bread or ½ cup starch (grains or vegetables) equals 1 serving.

Studies have corroborated that protein or caloric restriction below that needed for the growth of the fetus and for preparation of the maternal system in meeting the demands of pregnancy and lactation results in a smaller infant and reduction of maternal nutritional stores. Although not all big babies are healthy babies, low-birth-weight babies make up a disproportionate percentage of infant mortality. Both maternal undernutrition and overnutrition may be hazardous to the infant. However, unless the woman's prenatal and postnatal health is threatened by the known strain exerted on body systems by obesity, weight gain in itself is not detrimental and may represent only real nutritional gain or the usual increase in body fluids associated with normal pregnancy. The problem again seems to center on the quality of food intake. One woman can gain excessive weight eating "empty calories," contributing very poor nutritional resources to herself and her child. Such a woman may be a good candidate for maternal anemia and give birth to an infant with less than optimal resources to meet his needs. Another woman may also gain more than the norm but have a diet rich in nutrients and not suffer the same complications.

A total weight gain to 10 to 12 kg (22 to 27 pounds) has long been suggested in the literature. More recently recommended is a range of 10 to 14.5 kg (22 to 32 pounds) for single pregnancies of normal weight women.

A growing number of investigators now believe that even greater weight gains may be preferable when both the health of the developing infant and that of the pregnant mother is considered. However more studies will be needed to confirm optimal levels of weight management.

The "Your Weight-Gain Chart" (Fig. 5-3) is a fairly recent effort to guide weight gain. It identifies four recommended ranges of prenatal gain for women of "medium frame" determined by their prepregnant weights (see weight for height categories on p. 75). The Chart reflects the conclusions that infant birth weights of 3,500 to 3,999 g (7 pounds, 12 ounces, to 8 pounds, 13 ounces) have consistently demonstrated the lowest perinatal mortality statistics. Using these data the maternal weight gain recommendations shown are those associated with this infant birth weight range, generated by a balanced healthy diet based on the mother's prepregnant weight.*

Weight reduction is recommended only in the interpartum period after lactation to protect the fetus from low birth weight as well as acidosis, which may be associated with maternal starvation and may have an effect on the infant's intellectual capacity. Approximate physiologic weight gain in pregnancy has been explained as below. (Greater total weight gains are said to increase the categories proportionately.)

*Brown JE and others: Report of a special panel on desired prenatal weight gains for underweight and normal weight women, Public Health Rep 105(1):25, 1990; Brown JE: Weight gain during pregnancy: what is optimal? Clin Nutr 7(50):181, 1988.

	lb		kg
Fetus	7.5		3.4
Placenta	1.0		0.5
Amniotic fluid	2.0		0.9
Uterine weight increase	2.5		1.1
Breast tissue	3.0		1.4
Blood volume	4.0		1.8
Maternal stores	4 to 8		1.8 to 3.6
Totals	24 to 28	or	10.9 to 12.7

If total weight gain is within 24 to 28 pounds, about 3 to 4 pounds is gained in the first trimester. During the remaining weeks, a weight gain of approximately 1 pound a week is considered normal. Any sudden weight gain should be suspected as a sign of developing pregnancy-induced hypertension.

Teratogens. A teratogen is an agent or factor that produces a major or minor deviation from normal structure or function in the developing embryo or fetus. Many substances and infections have proven to be teratogenic (see box). Other factors must be studied further to be proven conclusively teratogenic. However, the pregnant woman should be cautioned not to use medications unless she consults her physician. Over-the-counter medicines, such as nose drops, cold remedies, sleep medications, and diuretics, may cause problems. Certain drugs such as methotrexate and phenytoin cause fetal structural abnormalities. Others may cause hemorrhage, jaundice, neurologic symptoms, and abnormal dental pigmentation. Drugs such as cocaine, heroin, and methadone taken during pregnancy may produce addiction in the newborn. The effects that all substances prescribed to treat illness will have on the fetus have not been determined. Then, too, effects of drugs taken during pregnancy may not become obvious in the child until years later (as in the incidence of vaginal malignancy in young girls or sperm changes causing infertility in men whose mothers had received diethylstilbestrol in early pregnancy to help prevent their miscarriage). Teratogenic effects take place especially at the beginning of a pregnancy before a woman is certain she is pregnant. The stage of development determines the vulnerability of the embryo or fetus.

Smoking, alcohol, and other drugs. Smoking decreases the oxygen supply to the unborn fetus by displacing oxygen with variable quantities of carbon monoxide and decreasing intrauterine blood flow. Mothers who smoke more than 10 cigarettes a day bear smaller infants than do nonsmoking women. In some studies late fetal and newborn mortality for infants born to cigarette smokers was significantly higher than for those born to

Potential human teratogenic factors

Substances
Alcohol
Amphetamines
Cocaine
Diethylstilbestrol
Heroin
Isotretinoin (Accutane)
Lithium
Marijuana
Methadone
Methotrexate
Methyl mercury
Mysoline
Phenothiazines
Phenytoin (Dilantin)
Tetracycline
Thalidomide
Tobacco smoke
Tricyclics
Trimethadione
Valium
Warfarin (Coumadin)

Infections
Coxsackie B
Cytomegalovirus (CMV)
Rubella
Syphilis
Toxoplasmosis
Varicella?

Other
Hyperthermia
Maternal disease (as diabetes)
Maternal malnutrition
Radiation

nonsmokers. Utilization of vitamins and minerals and transport of amino acids is compromised in smoking mothers.

It is interesting to note that the smaller babies of women who smoke grow faster during the 6 months after birth than do infants of nonsmokers. This is interpreted as a response to the removal of the infant from an "inhibiting and toxic" influence in utero. However, evidence also indicates that a relationship exists between mothers who smoke excessively at home and the incidence of pneumonia and bronchitis in their babies from 6 to 9 months of age. Of course, from the perspective of general maternal health, smoking is an important factor in respiratory and circulatory disease. Pregnant women should be encouraged to decrease or stop the habit.

Intrauterine exposure to alcohol is an important teratogen. Babies born with sufficient intrauterine exposure to alcohol often demonstrate fetal alcohol syndrome (FAS). Chronic, excessive use of alcohol has been identified as a significant cause of fetal growth retardation, impaired intellect, and congenital malformation, particularly microcephaly and facial abnormalities. Both the amount and timing of alcohol consumption by the mother, as well as her own physical condition, appear to be influential. No minimum safe amounts of alcohol intake during pregnancy have been determined. Some pregnant women may need specific suggestions on how to decrease or eliminate their alcohol intake.

The use of methylxanthines (such as caffeine and theobromine found in coffee, tea, chocolate, colas, and some analgesics) by the prospective mother has been questioned. The FDA has stated that the teratogenic effects of xanthines cannot be concluded at this time. However, at normal dosage (less than 600 mg/day), teratogenic effects have not been demonstrated. The pregnant woman should be counseled to limit consumption of foods and drinks containing xanthines. A cup of coffee has 75 to 155 mg of caffeine (up to 330 mg has been reported). Caffeine does cross the placenta. Research is needed on effects of xanthines taken during pregnancy, which may affect the child after birth.* Decreased use of tobacco, alcohol, and caffeine initiated at any time during pregnancy can improve fetal outcomes.

Viruses and parasites. The fetus is particularly vulnerable to viral infections during the early weeks of development. The newborn also may be at special risk. Pregnant women should not knowingly expose themselves unnecessarily to any viral disease to which they have not proved immunity, such as rubella (German measles) or cytomegalovirus (CMV). While CMV can have teratogenic effects, it is usually more significant in the neonate as a congenital infection. Influenza is thought by some to be a teratogen in the first few weeks of pregnancy. Acquired immune deficiency syndrome (AIDS) can be transmitted to the baby through the placenta as well as during delivery if the mother has been infected. However, it is not considered a teratogen. Another potential danger to the unborn infant is a parasitic disease called toxoplasmosis, transmitted to the pregnant woman by eating or handling raw meat, drinking goat's milk, and coming in contact with cat feces. An expectant mother should not handle Tabby's litter box! In addition, she needs to be reminded to wash her hands carefully after handling raw meat, to cook meat well, to wash fruits and vegetables before eating them, and to wear gloves while gardening.

Other items that may cause teratogenic effects in the fetus include environmental pollutants, lead, and excessive use of vitamins A, D, and K.

While diagnostic x-ray films should not be taken unless necessary, no *conclusive* evidence indicates that the levels of exposure associated with *infrequent low-dose x-rays* cause fetal injury. Lead aprons and shields should be used when possible. (See also p. 20.)*

General hygiene. Good prenatal guidance involves more than information about diet, smoking, drugs, and exposure to disease. The pregnant woman will undoubtedly have questions regarding many other subjects. Sometimes she wants information regarding general hygiene—the need for rest, relaxation, and exercise. Pregnant women need to conserve their resources by getting adequate rest. They may not want actually to nap in the morning and afternoon, but at least they can sit down and put their feet up. Because the bulk of the fetus in later pregnancy may compress the inferior vena cava and crowd the diaphragm, resting in a flat supine position may interfere with venous blood return to the heart and placental circulation as well as embarrass respirations. At such a stage in her pregnancy, a left side-lying position is frequently advised. This posture provides optimal circulation to the placenta. To help prevent preterm labor, a pregnant woman should rest on either side 1 hour twice a day, drink 8 to 10 cups of fluids, and work on stress management techniques.

General exercise. Considerable research regarding the effects of exercise during pregnancy is in progress. Which sports are an asset probably depends on the health, exercise habits, and obstetric history of the individual. Some exercise is encouraged for the normal expectant mother. Curtailing the exercise of a previously active woman may be a negative factor in her physical, emotional, and mental health. Regular exercise is preferable to intermittent activity. High temperatures, strenuous activities, and dehydration should be avoided. Walking outdoors is wonderful exercise. Golfing, bowling, dancing, and swimming, when not done to the point of fatigue,

---

*Aaronson LS and Macnee CL: Tobacco, alcohol and caffeine use during pregnancy, J Obstet Gynecol Neonatal Nurs 18(4):279, 1989.

*Jankowski C: Radiation and pregnancy: putting the risks in proportion, Am J Nurs 86:261-265, 1986.

are usually endorsed. Horseback riding, skiing, long endurance exercises, and competitive tennis, especially singles, are not usually recommended for the pregnant woman until after her postpartum checkup. She should not become out of breath nor exceed 70% of her *safe maximum* attainable heart rate (SHR). SHR is usually defined as 220 minus her age.* Maternal heart rate should not exceed 140 bpm unless the woman is well conditioned before pregnancy.

Kegel exercises. Frequent exercises involving the pelvic floor (particularly the pubococcygeal muscle) may facilitate childbirth, promote healing, aid in the restoration of perineal muscle tone, and help prevent stress incontinence. The mother can best be taught these exercises during the latter part of the prenatal period and can benefit from their daily performance for the rest of her life. The pubococcygeal muscle can be identified as the one she uses to stop a stream of urine when voiding although she should not routinely practice this. (See Fig. 1-11 and p. 25.) Ask the woman to think of her perineal muscles as an elevator on the "first floor," which she should slowly raise by contraction to the "fourth floor" and lower by relaxation again. Kegel exercises should be repeated about 10 times consecutively several times a day.

Bathing. A woman is likely to perspire more heavily during pregnancy, and frequent baths and showers are needed. Bathing may become a problem in late pregnancy because of the woman's awkwardness and the risk of falls. Sponge baths may be necessary. The possibility of infecting the vaginal tract and uterus used to be a consideration, but most now consider this highly unlikely.

Hair may need special attention because of the increased activity of the oil glands of the scalp. A permanent, if desired, will "take" during pregnancy.

Preparation for nursing. If the woman is planning to nurse her baby, the physician may advise certain routines to prepare her breasts for lactation and may identify community groups such as La Leche League who can help breast-feeding mothers. If she has inverted or flat nipples, the physician may prescribe the use of a manual breast pump, teach finger compression of the breast or nipple rolling, or recommend the use of plastic breast shields, which are worn for varying intervals inside the bra, to draw out the nipple and make it easier for the newborn infant to grasp. The expression of colostrum, the early

breast secretion, may be recommended in the last 3 weeks of pregnancy to encourage milk production, to prevent engorgement, and to toughen the nipples. Because of the possibility of inducing premature labor, it is suggested that nipple preparation be done in late pregnancy, beginning about the 37th week.* Some women have caused trauma to the breast tissue by their efforts.

Often pregnant women, especially primigravidas, develop rather prominent pink marks called striae on the abdomen and breasts, probably related to hormonal increases as well as rapid weight gain. Some people think that they are not as prominent if cocoa butter is applied to the skin. Certainly it does not hurt to use it if one does not object to the odor. These lines usually retract appreciably after pregnancy and become less noticeable.

Wardrobe. Never before have expectant mothers had an opportunity for such an attractive, versatile wardrobe as they have today. Since maternity patterns are also available in fabric stores, attractive clothing need not be expensive. Maternity clothes should be lightweight, nonconstrictive, adjustable, and absorbent, and should also provide a boost to the morale.

It is especially important that the pregnant woman have good breast support to prevent fatigue and maintain a good figure. She will not be able to go through her entire pregnancy with the same size brassiere! If she plans to breast-feed her baby, nursing bras are a fine investment. A maternity corset is usually not advised. The tendency instead has been to counsel its use only for older multiparas if needed. Primigravidas and younger multiparas are usually told to practice certain exercises during pregnancy (especially the "pelvic rock, or tilt") that will improve posture and strengthen muscles. However, a light maternity girdle may be used with satisfaction. Specially designed garter belts are available. No constrictive round garters should be used because of interference in the blood's circulation from the legs.

If a woman has been accustomed to wearing high-heeled shoes, it will probably be difficult for her to descend suddenly to fairly flat heels. However, as pregnancy progresses and her center of gravity moves forward, she will find lower heels much less awkward and more flattering to her total silhouette. She will want to avoid shoe styles with ties or buckles; toward the end of her 260 plus days of waiting, tying shoes will not be easy.

*For example, a 30-year-old pregnant woman should aim for a pulse rate not higher than (220 − 30) × .7, or 133 bpm.

*Johnson FF: Assessment and education to prevent preterm labor, MCN 14(3):157, 1989; Storr GB: Prevention of nipple tenderness and breast engorgement in postpartal period, J Obstet Gynecol Neonatal Nurs 17(3):203, 1988.

Dental care. It is a good plan for the pregnant woman to have a dental checkup during the second trimester so that plenty of time is available for needed repairs as well as instruction regarding techniques in flossing and other hygiene aids. The gums may become swollen and exhibit a tendency to bleed during pregnancy. These symptoms are probably caused by the increase in estrogen and progesterone in the body and are not necessarily related to a vitamin C deficiency. Symptoms typically recede after the eighth month. The presence of gingivitis previous to pregnancy, fostered by plaque formation and malocclusion, may cause the condition to become a continuing problem without care. Some women experience an increase in salivation (ptyalism) in pregnancy.

Douching. Some women wonder whether they should douche or not. Normal vaginal secretions are usually intensified during pregnancy. Some physicians believe that douching should be done only for a specific condition with a low-pressure fountain syringe, gently introduced no more than 3 inches. Others do not recommend the practice at all.* The possible introduction of infection or incidence of air embolism is a real concern (p. 108).

Employment. Many pregnant women are employed. Whether they continue their employment and for how long depends on several factors, one of which is the type of work (heavy lifting, exposure to potential hazards of radiation or chemicals, or long hours of standing without relief). The employment of pregnant women in certain occupations is often restricted by state law, policies of the individual employer (dependent on insurance coverage, previous experience, etc), and the health of the employee (whether she is experiencing any complications).

Women have been challenging disability benefit regulations and pregnancy leave rulings that require a working expectant mother to resign her position because she has reached a certain month in her pregnancy. The Pregnancy Discrimination Act of 1978 prohibits discrimination on the basis of pregnancy in hiring, pay, conditions, or other privileges of employment. Stop and start dates are illegal. Pregnancy should be treated as any other temporary disability with regard to time off and insurance. Challenges to this act have been taken as high as the Supreme Court. Any complaints can be directed to the Equal Employment Opportunity Commission.

Travel. Sometimes pregnant women ask whether they

*Kuczynski HJ: Pros and cons of douching, J Obstet Gynecol Neonatal Nurs 9:90-93, 1980; Cunningham FG, MacDonald PC, and Gant NF: Williams obstetrics, ed 18, San Mateo, Calif, 1989, Appleton & Lange, p. 269.

should restrict travel. If a trip can be so arranged, it is best to travel during the middle trimester, because the pregnant woman is more comfortable, the danger of abortion is not as great, and the threat of premature or unprepared-for births is at a minimum as compared with later in the pregnancy. If trips must be made by car, schedules should allow for adequate rest stops and should be carefully paced. Commercial airline travel in pressurized planes is now considered as safe as other methods of transportation for this traveler. Proper use of automobile safety belts is recommended. The lap belt should be worn snug and low across the hip bones with the shoulder belt above the pregnant uterus. Last-minute protracted journeys close to term are discouraged no matter how they are made.

Sexual relations. Instructions regarding sexual intercourse during pregnancy are now much more liberal than formerly. Many physicians are now allowing most couples to have sexual intercourse until full term is reached, unless the bag of waters has ruptured or discomfort is encountered. Others, believing that orgasm may initiate painful uterine contractions or premature labor, take a more conventional approach and would limit sexual response in the last few weeks before term. If there has been a previous problem with abortion, premature birth, or bleeding during pregnancy, additional modifications in sexual life should be advised. Most couples find such privations stressful and may need counseling regarding alternative modes of mutual sexual gratification and other helpful adjustments.

Community education resources. In many communities classes are offered to help expectant parents prepare for the changes pregnancy and parenthood will bring. They may be sponsored by the local childbirth education association, American National Red Cross, YWCA, public health departments, adult education programs, postpartum support groups, hospitals, or groups of physicians. Participation in such approved groups is recommended, especially for primigravidas. Some classes concentrate on imparting an understanding of the basic anatomy and physiology of reproduction, what to expect during the "waiting months," what occurs during labor and birth, how to prepare the baby's nursery and layette, how to bathe the newborn infant, techniques of breastfeeding, and how to prepare an artificial formula. Others emphasize exercises in training the body and mind for peak performance during pregnancy, labor, and childbirth, and are usually led by a physical therapist or nurse specializing in childbirth education (Fig. 5-4). Preparation for childbirth involving techniques such as those

Women Adjusting to the Pregnant State

Selected nursing diagnoses	Expected outcomes	Interventions
Anxiety related to emotional responses to pregnancy.	Anxiety is reduced. Woman discusses her feelings and uses positive coping mechanisms to deal with her emotional responses to pregnancy.	Provide realistic reassurance that responses are normal and encourage open discussion of concerns.

Specific plans for selected problems are described below.

Selected nursing diagnoses	Expected outcomes	Interventions

A. Early phase of maternal adaptation to pregnancy evidenced by ambivalence about being pregnant.
Clinical manifestations:
  Expresses surprise at being pregnant.
  Responses to news includes mixed emotions: "Who me? Not now!"
	Woman verbalizes her concerns and exhibits positive behaviors towards pregnancy status, e.g., tells others about being pregnant, buys/wears maternity clothes.	Ask how she feels about being pregnant. Give permission to express positive or negative feeling about pregnancy, e.g., "Many women find that they do not feel quite ready when they learn that they are pregnant."
		Provide appropriate place to talk.
		Explain near universality of ambivalence in early pregnancy.

B. Alteration in self-concept: change in body image. Clinical manifestations: Feelings range from very positive to extremely negative. May worry that she is seen as fat. Feels large, heavy, and awkward as pregnancy advances.	Enlarging abdomen and other body changes are accepted as normal.	Provide information re: hormonal and uterine changes, and what outcomes can be expected, e.g., most changes revert after delivery; striae don't disappear but do fade; weight can be lost, muscle tone regained with exercise. Observe for indications that the woman is not coping well with pregnancy's impact on her body, e.g., wears constrictive clothing; repeated referral to self as "fat" or "ugly," or "look what this baby is doing to me"; overly concerned with striae or pigment changes of the skin. Arrange counseling for these women to avoid inappropriate self-care and psychologic stresses.
Altered patterns of sexual expression related to physical changes of pregnancy, changes in sexual desire, or fear of injury to fetus. Clinical manifestations: Woman may ask questions about effect of pregnancy on sexuality but, more often, will not.	Woman and partner understand the reason for these changes and concerns and will maintain a mutually satisfying sexual relationship.	Explain possible causes of discomfort or lack of responsiveness in pregnancy, e.g., fatigue, nausea, and vomiting; breast tenderness in first trimester. Fatigue and enlarging abdomen in third trimester. Determine impact on sexuality of pregnancy on woman and her partner, need of couple to share concerns. Suggest alternative sexual activities and positions. Discuss issues of safety: there is no evidence that sexual intercourse during *normal* pregnancy can cause harm to fetus. Intercourse can be safely continued until membranes rupture unless physician advises otherwise.

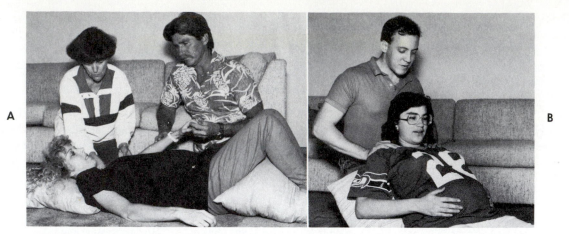

FIG 5-4 A, Childbirth education instructor teaches father to check for muscular relaxation. Such classes are available in many settings; this one is held in a home. **B,** A young couple practices relaxation, effleurage (light massage), and various breathing techniques.

advocated with Lamaze or other methods of instruction may be intensive. Attendance of the expectant parents at a series of classes with assigned practice sessions is strongly recommended. Information and exercises to promote good posture, strengthen key muscles, enhance relaxation, and lessen fear and discomfort during the birth experience are emphasized. (See also pp. 159-160.) In our opinion they are helpful to the expectant parents no matter what their preference may be regarding the use of analgesics, anesthetics, or birth procedures.

Such informal group sessions with other couples facing similar experiences, expectations, hopes, and fears guided by competent leaders are especially helpful in assisting new prospective fathers and mothers to gain needed instruction and self-esteem for their changing roles.

Pregnancy and new parenthood are developmental crises for the man as well as the woman, and new self-identities must be clarified and accepted. The crises may be changed or lessened when parenthood is repeated, but the sense of wonder, the expectations, and the strains recur. Adjustments are still to be made whether the child is the first or the fourth. The processes of role identification are more obvious perhaps in this culture for the prospective mother. Indeed, the increasingly manifest changes in her body dramatically declare a changed status in society. Psychologists who are describing the focal changes during a normal woman's pregnancy usually speak of her emotional preoccupation with self, an introversion that occurs and predominates her thinking in early pregnancy. At this time the growing fetus is part

of her and is yet to assume a real identity of its own. Consciously—or most often subconsciously—she sorts through her feelings concerning motherhood and her early experiences with her own mother. As the pregnancy continues and her body image changes, her feelings of dependency typically grow and her focus of attention generally changes to that of the father of the child as he represents protection and continuity. Later, in the third trimester, her interest is centered on preparations for the baby, who by this time has become an unknown but acknowledged individual, and on her feelings and expectations concerning labor, birth, and her ability to cope at that time with the demands of her body, her family, and society.

Pregnancy is normally characterized by feelings of ambivalence. One day the mother-to-be may be pleased and proud concerning her condition. The next day she will be fretful and even resentful regarding the disturbance in her life that the coming baby represents. Prospective mothers and fathers need to know that these contradictory feelings are normal. Men need especially to be alerted regarding the sudden mood swings and fantasies that may trouble their mates' emotional and mental equilibrium. Such knowledge will help smooth the many difficult adaptations that need to be made. Pregnancy is a developmental crisis, but it is also an opportunity for real emotional and psychologic growth. Peers and knowledgeable professional people with whom to share some of the experiences of this process are tremendous assets.

The layette. Provided finances are not too strained,

preparing the layette for the new baby can be one of the most pleasurable duties of the expectant parents. For first-timers, baby showers may also help in this regard but are not dependable. Contributors at such affairs should be told that the baby will grow, and perhaps half the group could purchase basic clothes for the 1- to 2-year-old child. If the baby is not a "firstborn," infant clothes will probably be left over from the last time. Babies usually do not wear out their clothes.

A basic layette, at least enough to start with, consists of the following items:

1. Six cotton shirts, short or long sleeves, depending on the weather (Stretch shirts cost more but can be worn by the baby longer. Long-sleeved shirts can have a fold-over cuff enclosing the hands. To purchase a 3-month size is a waste of money.)
2. Four dozen cotton gauze, bird's-eye, or flannelette diapers if diaper service is not used; 1 dozen, if it is; or disposable diapers
3. Two or three plastic diaper covers, to be used only if the baby does not have any skin irritation
4. Four or five long gowns, opening down the front with grip fasteners
5. Two or three sweaters with no more than 10% wool content to prevent allergic skin rash
6. Three or four soft, light receiving blankets
7. One square, heavy blanket for use outdoors
8. One cap
9. Booties if it is cold
10. One bunting, in a climate requiring such protection (The tendency is to overdress rather than underdress infants.)
11. Two or three waterproof squares for protecting surfaces from the baby's urine
12. Two washcloths, just for the baby
13. Six cotton sheets; two crib blankets

Basic furniture includes a bed (a bassinet, though pretty, is unnecessary), a firm mattress, and cover. No pillow should be used because of the danger of suffocation. Some type of chest of drawers for storage, a covered diaper pail, and probably a large plastic tub will be needed. A bath tray is a great convenience, but it does not have to be expensive. Any clean tray will do. Suggested items for a tray are a jar of cotton balls; a jar of safety pins; a mild soap and dish; baby lotion; and a box of paper tissues. Baby powder, especially that containing talc, is not recommended. If inhaled, it can cause serious respiratory consequences.

Even if the baby is to be nursed, there should be equipment in the home for preparing artificial feedings or for storing and feeding breast milk when the mother is away. Approved baby car seats are a necessity, and portable infant seats or baby carriers worn by the infant's caretaker can be helpful (see Fig. 18-17). Mothers can often borrow needed items.

There are many things on the market for babies, but many of those cute eye-catching gadgets and extras require money better spent elsewhere.

What to take to the hospital. The mother should have other things ready for her hospital trip before that special date comes due. Usually, the following list suffices:

Recommended articles to assist with Lamaze-type labor techniques (extra pillows, lip pomade, focal point, etc)
Two nightgowns (the short type)
Robe, slippers
Two brassieres (nursing-type if breast-feeding)
Toothbrush, dentrifice, brush, comb, cosmetics
Deodorant, shower cap
Writing materials, stamps, birth announcements, checkbook or cash for deposit at hospital, insurance identification if applicable, and a good book

Cross-cultural components influencing maternity care

When caring for a pregnant woman from another culture or ethnic group, the nurse must understand the variations in this mother's attitudes and behaviors that may result from cultural influences. Perceptions of health and illness are culturally derived. Culture definitely influences her reactions and behaviors concerning pregnancy. The care given should fit in with the prospective mother's cultural lifestyle when possible. Failure in maternity care may result from not taking into account the patient's customs and belief system. The concepts of transcultural nursing need to be applied to the planned care. For example, nutritional guidance must consider food practices and the symbolic significance of food.

In some cultures certain foods are not to be eaten (taboo) during pregnancy. Certain groups do not assign an active role to the father regarding prenatal care or labor and delivery. In some cultures grandmothers may have a primary support role during labor and later in child-rearing. The nurse teaching child health care should identify who is the principal child care provider as she works with different families and groups.

Although individuals must not be stereotyped, it is helpful to look even briefly at a few of the ethnic groups the nurse may encounter. Of course, practices and views associated with childbearing also vary with individuals, their personal values, and their economic resources. Discussing cultural influences with the mother herself will help the nurse to better plan for her special needs.

Black cultural practices. The cultural patterns of blacks in the different socioeconomic groups largely resemble the patterns of the majority of members of these groups. Extended family members typically help provide support.

Black Muslim women often follow meat-restricted diets. Their prenatal nutrition as well as that of the breast-feeding mother should be explored. They characteristically wear long modest garments and cover their hair.

Native American Indian cultural practices. The traditional Native American Indian woman often finds fulfillment through her role in pregnancy, childbirth, and rearing healthy children. Support is received from her family and community. Female family members are especially involved in these concerns.

In caring for these families it is important to be acquainted with the tribe's cultural beliefs and taboos. Many of these can be accommodated safely and with understanding. For instance, for some it is important not to palpate the baby's anterior fontanel in the presence of the family. As with other cultures, there are taboos against certain foods. American Indian women generally believe contraception should not be implemented until after the first baby.

Hispanic cultural practices. Hispanics are the largest ethnic group in the United States. They have come from many different Spanish-speaking regions of the world. Some of these families have adopted the middle-American culture, whereas others have retained the concepts and lifestyles of their Hispanic heritages. Again, extended families are common and important. The advice given by a family member may be accepted by the mother in preference to that given by a member of the health team. The "hot-cold theory" of disease and health may influence the mother's diet and compliance. Certain foods are considered hot or cold, though these concepts may have no relationship to their actual temperatures. A balance of certain foods based on this classification may be sought. Since pregnancy is viewed as normal, going to the physician may be delayed. This group is characterized by male-dominant relationships. Large families are often desired.

Asiatic cultural practices. Asian families in the United States currently represent particularly diverse cultures and socioeconomic levels. The extended family is dominant. While some taboos govern food and activity during pregnancy, pregnancy is seen as a normal, healthy process in which family members should have the major role. When caring for patients from the Asian culture, nurses should particularly protect the modesty of the patient. Male participation in the direct care of the mother is usually minimal but does not represent a noncaring attitude. Politeness and propriety characterize Southeast Asian peoples. Direct confrontation is avoided. Harmony with nature and dualist concepts of disease are part of the health beliefs and practices. The concepts of *yin* and *yang* (in some ways similar to the hot-cold theory of disease and health) and the need to balance these contrary forces in an individual's life can affect diet, hygiene, and activity, particularly in the postpartum period. Sympathetic explanations to the client and her family members are essential to nursing care.*

Arab cultural practices. Arab families feel strong family unity among extended family members and rely on them for help before going outside the family. The experience of pregnancy and birth is usually seen as an exclusively female affair. Having children, especially sons, is the important function of women. Arab women feel a special need for modesty. Often families from the Arab culture are oriented to the present; planning ahead for the care of the coming baby is not part of the culture. This should not be viewed as showing less concern for the baby, but as an aspect of the culture perhaps prompted by ancient high infant mortality rates. This emphasis on the present rather than the future should also be remembered if contraception is to be taught. Including other adult family members in health teaching is helpful. Having both husband and wife together during such discussions may increase compliance.

Perhaps socioeconomic constraints have as big a place in the outcome of the pregnancy as do cultural and ethnic variations, because nutrition plays such a vital role in the pregnancy and is affected so greatly by socioeconomic factors.

All pregnant women should have access to adequate prenatal care. However, at the beginning of the 1990s it is estimated that in the United States as many as 25% of pregnant women receive inadequate or no prenatal care.† There are financial and nonfinancial barriers to adequate

*Lee RV and others: Southeast Asian folklore about pregnancy and parturition, Obstet Gynecol 71(4):643, 1988.
†Queenan JT: Editorial: Lessons from the eastern front, Contemp OB/GYN 35(1)10: 1990; Access to prenatal care (Report of Consensus Conferences), American Nurses' Association, Kansas City, Mo, March 1987; Cagle S: Access to prenatal care and prevention of low birth weight, MCN 12(4):235, 1987.

prenatal care for all. For some women, participating in care may seem to be more costly in terms of money and effort than the benefits perceived. For others there is inadequate awareness of the community resources. Maternity nursing is addressing these issues. Our role in getting mothers to prenatal care, in assessment, nutritional and health education, stress reduction, and referral to other social support services, is highly important. We must also work with the federal and state agencies, as well as the private sector to increase the availability of adequate comprehensive prenatal health care. Ensuring that all women have access to basic life needs is essential to improving the health of pregnant women and their children. Research and evaluation of these processes and systems are a must.

PERSPECTIVE

Pregnancy is a creative, productive period in a woman's life from many points of view. It should be a happy, truly expectant interval. How a woman reacts to the challenge of pregnancy will be determined mainly by the level of her basic emotional maturity. The health team, including the nurses, clergy, and members of the community health agencies have an opportunity to help a pregnant woman and her partner mature in the understanding of themselves and their role in life at this crucial time. If these caregivers help the expectant parents, they are also helping the generation to come.

Key Concepts

1. The goals of prenatal care are as follows: a pregnancy with a minimum of mental and physical discomfort and a maximum of gratification; a birth under the best possible circumstances; a normal, well baby; the establishment of good health habits benefiting all the family; and a smooth, guided postpartum adjustment.

2. The first prenatal visit typically includes the following: taking of vital signs, health history, pelvic examination, pregnancy test, determination of delivery date, physical examination, laboratory tests, and preliminary guidance regarding pregnancy.

3. Signs and symptoms that a pregnant woman should be instructed to report to her health care provider are the following: bleeding from the vagina; uncontrollable leaking of fluid from the vagina; unusual abdominal pain or cramps; persistent nausea or vomiting; persistent headache or blurring of vision; marked swelling of the ankles, hands, and face; painful or burning urination; and chills or fever.

4. Subsequent prenatal visits are scheduled every 3 to 4 weeks initially; after 5 months, every 2 to 3 weeks; and, in the last month, every 1 or 2 weeks. These visits usually include taking of vital signs, urine examination, measurement of the height of the uterus, and assessment of fetal heart rate.

5. Good nutrition during pregnancy reduces the risk of obstetric and perinatal complications. The National Research Council's Recommended Dietary Allowance (RDA) suggests dietary adjustments for pregnancy.

6. Although routine multivitamin supplementation is normally unnecessary, supplemental iron is recommended, and folic acid may sometimes be prescribed.

7. The four food groups (milk, meat, fruit/vegetables, and grain) and the suggested number of servings provide an easy-to-follow guide for proper nutrition.

8. The suggested total weight gain during pregnancy has ranged for some time from 22 to 32 pounds (10 to 14.5 kg). Prepregnancy weight, the quality of food intake, and multiple pregnancy all may influence what is considered a healthy weight gain during pregnancy. Study of optimal gains continues.

9. A teratogen is an agent or factor that produces a major or minor deviation from normal structure or function in the developing embryo or fetus. Teratogens include smoking, alcohol, drugs, certain viruses and parasites, environmental pollutants, lead, and excessive use of vitamins A, D, and K.

10. In later pregnancy, resting in a flat, supine position may interfere with venous blood return to the heart and placental circulation, and may embarrass respirations. A side-lying position provides optimal circulation to the placenta.

11. Some exercise is encouraged during a normal pregnancy. The type and frequency depend on the woman's health, exercise habits, and obstetric history.

12. Kegel exercises may facilitate childbirth, promote healing, aid in the restoration of perineal muscle tone, and help prevent stress incontinence.

13. It is suggested that routines to prepare the breasts

for lactation should not be done until late in pregnancy because of the possibility of inducing premature labor.

14. Maternity clothes should be lightweight, nonconstrictive, adjustable, and absorbent. As the pregnancy progresses, the woman may require a larger brassiere size and may find that low-heeled shoes without ties or buckles are more comfortable and easier to put on and remove.

15. Although physicians differ in their beliefs regarding douching during pregnancy, there is a real concern about the possible introduction of infection or incidence of air embolism.

16. Whether a pregnant woman should continue her employment and for how long depends on several factors, including the type of work. Discrimination on the basis of pregnancy in hiring, pay, conditions, or other privileges of employment can be reported to the Equal Employment Opportunity Commission.

17. Participation in community education classes is recommended to help parents prepare for labor and birth and to care for their newborn.

18. Basic necessities for the newborn include the following: shirts, diapers, plastic diaper covers, long gowns, sweaters, blankets, cap, booties, waterproof squares, washcloths, bed linens, crib, chest of drawers, diaper pail, bath tray, equipment for preparing formula or storing breast milk, and a car seat.

19. The concepts of transcultural nursing need to be applied to maternity care. Cultural differences regarding childbearing influence factors such as food practices, the father's role, and the need for modesty.

Discussion Questions

1. The cost of medical care often is a reason given for delayed or inadequate prenatal care. Is this a valid reason? If you agree that prenatal care is essential, what do you think should be done to guarantee that all women receive adequate care during pregnancy?

2. Pregnancy is a normal physiologic condition, but it may require a woman to change some of her activities and in some way alter her normal lifestyle. What changes are most commonly recommended related to activity? Work? Sleep? Diet? Hygiene?

3. Identify the most frequently encountered teratogens. When are these most dangerous to the fetus? What health practices or changes in lifestyle could reduce the likelihood of the fetus being harmed?

4. Identify the most common diagnostic tests performed routinely during pregnancy. Your patient states "you keep doing these tests each time I come to the doctor." How would you explain these tests and their significance?

5. Culture plays an important part in maternal-child health practices. Select a culture other than your own that is common in your locale. Discuss the practices that are in keeping with good basic prenatal care and also those that may be harmful during pregnancy. What could you do if harmful practices are discovered?

UNIT

II

SUGGESTED SELECTED READINGS AND REFEERENCES

General

Access to prenatal care: key to preventing low birthweight. Report of consensus conference, (Pub MCH-16) Kansas City, Mo, 1987, The American Nurses' Association.

Andrews LB: Women at work: pregnant and jobhunting, Parents 57(11):36, 1982.

Arneson S and others: Automobile seat belt practices of pregnant women, J Obstet Gynecol Neonatal Nurs 15(4):339, 1986.

Bennett EC: The first trimester, J Obstet Gynecol Neonatal Nurs 13(2 suppl):93s, 1984.

Brown MA: How fathers and mothers perceive prenatal support, MCN 12(6):414, 1987.

Brown S, editor: US Institute of Medicine: Prenatal care reaching mothers, reaching infants, Washington, DC, National Academy Press, 1988.

Brucker MC and Reedy MJ: Maternity leaves and the pregnancy discrimination act, J Obstet Gynecol Neonatal Nurs 12(5):341, 1983.

Catlin AJ: Early pregnancy loss: what you can do to help, Nursing, '89 19(11):43, 1989.

Chenger P and Kovacik A: Prenatal care: dental hygiene during pregnancy: a review, MCN 12(5):342, 1987.

Dahlberg NL: A perinatal center based antepartum home-care program, J Obstet Gynecol Neonatal Nurs 17(1):30, 1988.

DeGrez SA: Bend and stretch, MCN 13(5):357, 1988.

Deutchman M: The problematic 1st-trimester pregnancy, Am Fam Physician 39(1):185, 1989.

Eastman P: The role of maternal stress in low birth weight, Contemp OB/GYN 25(5):206, 1985.

Ellis DJ: Sexual needs and concerns of expectant parents, J Obstet Gynecol Neonatal Nurs 9(5):306, 1980.

Engstrom JL: Measurement of fundal height, J Obstet Gynecol Neonatal Nurs 17(3):172, 1988.

Guidelines for perinatal care, ed 2, 1988, American Academy of Pediatrics and American College of Obstetricians.

Harmon JS and Barry M: Antenatal testing, mobile outpatient monitoring services, J Obstet Gynecol Neonatal Nurs 18(1):21, 1989.

Helton A: Battering during pregnancy, Am J Nurs 86(8):910, 1986.

Hogan LR: Pregnant again—at 41, MCN 4(3):174, 1979.

Horan M: Discomfort and pain during pregnancy, MCN 9(4):267, 1984.

Ketter DE and Shelton BJ: Pregnant and physically fit, too, MCN 9(2):120, 1984.

Lamb GS and Lipkin M: Somatic symptoms of expectant fathers, MCN 7(2):110, 1982.

Lederman R: Psychosocial adaptation in pregnancy: assessment of seven dimensions of maternal development, Englewood Cliffs, NJ, 1985, Prentice-Hall.

Longbucco DC and Freston MS: Relationship of somatic symptoms to degree of paternal-role preparation of first-time expectant fathers, J Obstet Gynecol Neonatal Nurs 18(6):482, 1989.

Mahan CS and McKay S: Let's reform our antenatal care methods, Contemp OB/GYN 23(5):147, 1984.

Merilo KF: Is it better the second time around? MCN 13(3):200, 1988.

Mueller LS: Pregnancy and sexuality, J Obstet Gynecol Neonatal Nurs 14(4):289, 1985.

Paisley JC and Mellion MB: Exercise during pregnancy, Am Fam Physician 38(5):143, 1988.

Pastorek JG II: Hepatitis B screening during pregnancy, Contemp OB/GYN 34(5):36, 1989.

Poole CJ: Fatigue during the first trimester of pregnancy, J Obstet Gynecol Neonatal Nurs 15(5):375, 1986.

Primrose RB: Taking the tension out of pelvic exams, Am J Nurs 84:72, 1984.

Rosenbaum S: Providing effective prenatal care programs for teenagers, Washington DC, 1985, Children's Defense Fund.

Tegtmeier D and Elsea S: Wellness throughout the maternity cycle, Nurs Clin North Am 19(2):219, 1984.

Winslow W: First pregnancy after 35: what is the experience, MCN 12(2):92, 1987.

Cultural differences

Bash D: Jewish religious practices related to child bearing, J Nurse Midwife 25(5):39, 1980.

Becerea RM and others: Pregnancy and motherhood among Mexican-American adolescents, Health Soc Work 9(Spring):106, 1984.

Choi EC: Unique aspects of Korean-American mothers, J Obstet Gynecol Neonatal Nurs 15(5):394, 1986.

DeGarcia RT: Filipino cultural influences, Am J Nurs 79(8):1412, 1979.

Grosso C and others: The Vietnamese-American family—and grandma makes three, MCN 6(3):177, 1981.

Higgins PG: Pueblo women of New Mexico: their background, culture and childbearing practices, Top Clin Nurs 4(1):69, 1983.

Hollingsworth AO, Brown LP, and Brooten DA: The refugees and childbearing: what to expect, RN 43(11):44, 1980.

LaDu EB: Childbirth care for Hmong families, MCN 10(6):382, 1985.

Lee PA: Health beliefs of pregnant and postpartum Hmong women, West J Nurs Res 8(1):83, 1986.

Lutwak RA: Maternity nursing and Jewish law, MCN 13(1):44, 1988.

Meleis AI: The Arab American in the health care system, Am J Nurs 81(6):1180, 1981.

Meleis AI and Sorrell L: Bridging cultures: Arab American women and their birth experiences, MCN 6(3):171, 1981.

Santopietro MS: How to get through to a refugee patient, RN 44(1):42, 1981.

Zepeda M: Selected maternal-infant care practices of Spanish-speaking women, J Obstet Gynecol Neonatal Nurs 11(6):371, 1982.

Education for childbirth

Austin SEF: Childbirth classes for couples desiring VBAC, MCN 11(4):250, 1986.

Berry LD: Realistic expectations of the labor coach, J Obstet Gynecol Neonatal Nurs 17(5):354, 1988.

Bing ED: Six practical lessons for an easier childbirth, ed 3, New York, 1983, Grosset & Dunlap.

Bonovich L: Participation: the key to learning for patients in antepartal clinics, J Obstet Gynecol Neonatal Nurs 10(2):75, 1981.

Bretschneider JU and Minetola AC: Another look at early-pregnancy classes, MCN 8(4):268, 1983.

De La Fleur TP and Payne JP: Role playing in childbirth education classes, MCN 6(5):333, 1981.

Dzurec LC: Childbirth educators: are they helpful? MCN 6(5):329, 1981.

Ewy D and Ewy R: Preparation for childbirth, ed 5, New York, 1985, The New American Library, Inc.

Faucett J and Burritt J: An exploratory study of antenatal preparation for cesarean birth, J Obstet Gynecol Neonatal Nurs 14(3):224, 1985.

ICEA position paper: The role of the childbirth educator and the scope of childbirth education, Minneapolis, Minn, 1986, International Childbirth Education Association.

Leff EW: Comparison of the effectiveness of videotape versus live group infant care classes, J Obstet Gynecol Neonatal Nurs 17(5):338, 1988.

Lesko W and Lesko M: The maternity sourcebook, New York, 1984, Warner Books.

Lieberman AB: Talking freely about pain, Genesis, ASPO/Lamaze 10(3):20, 1988.

Lindell SG: Education for childbirth: a time for change, J Obstet Gynecol Neonatal Nurs 17(2):108, 1989.

Mackay D: Teaching breathing—a new look, Int J Childbirth Ed 3(2):36, 1988.

McKay S: Assertive childbirth: the future parent's guide to a positive pregnancy, Englewood Cliffs, NJ, 1983, Prentice-Hall.

Nichols FH and Humenick SS, editors: Childbirth education: practice, research, and theory, Philadelphia, 1988, WB Saunders Co.

Patient teaching helps prevent premature births, Am J Nurs 84(3):300, 1984.

Peckham D: ICEA guide for childbirth educators, Minneapolis, Minn, 1988, International Childbirth Education Association.

Taubenheim AM and Silbernagel T: Meeting the needs of expectant fathers, MCN 13(2):110, 1988.

Todd L: Labor and birth: a guide for you, ed 2, Minneapolis, Minn, 1987, International Childbirth Education Association.

Wiles L: The effect of prenatal breastfeeding education on breastfeeding success and maternal perception of the infant, J Obstet Gynecol Neonatal Nurs 13(5):253, 1984.

Embryology and fetal assessment

Bernhardt J: Sensory capabilities of the fetus, MCN 12(1):44, 1987.

Brombate B and Oldrini A: CVS for first trimester fetal diagnosis, Contemp OB/GYN 25(5):94, 1985.

Burton BK, editor: Prenatal diagnosis, Pediatric Annals 18(11):entire issue, 1989.

Davis MS and Akridge KM: The effect of promoting intrauterine attachment in primiparas on postdelivery attachment, J Obstet Gynecol Neonatal Nurs 16(6):430, 1987.

Dickinson R and Belskie A: Birth atlas, ed 5, New York, 1968, Maternity Center Association.

Dunn P: Surgery for the unborn: a nurse's own story, Nurs Life 4(5):18, 1984.

Dunn PA, Weiner S, and Ludomirski A: Percutaneous umbilical blood sampling, J Obstet Gynecol Neonatal Nurs 17(5):308, 1988.

Ferguson HW: Biophysical profile scoring: the fetal Apgar, Am J Nurs 88(5):662, 1988.

Gaffney SE: Intrauterine fetal surgery: the ramifications for nurses, MCN 10(4):250, 1985.

Gantes M and others: The use of daily fetal movement records in a clinical setting, J Obstet Gynecol Neonatal Nurs 15(5):390, 1986.

Inturrisi M, Perry SE, and May KA: Fetal surgery for congenital hydronephrosis, J Obstet Gynecol Neonatal Nurs 14(4):271, 1985.

Knorr LJ: Relieving fetal distress with amniofusion, MCN 14(5):356, 1989.

Green D and Malin J: When reality shatters parents' dreams, Nursing 88 18(2):61, 1988.

Manning FA: Fetal biophysical profile scoring predicts trouble, Contemp OB/GYN 25(1):126, 1985.

Modica MM and Timor-Tritsch IE: Transvaginal sonography provides a sharper view into the pelvis, J Obstet Gynecol Neonatal Nurs 17(2):89, 1988.

Moore KL: Before we are born: basic embryology and birth defects, ed 2, Philadelphia, 1983, WB Saunders Co.

Nilsson L, Ingelman-Sundberg A, and Wirsen C: A child is born, New York, 1967, Penguin Books.

Rothman BK: The tentative pregnancy: prenatal diagnosis and the future of motherhood, New York, 1987, Viking Press (Penguin Books).

Sleutel MR: An overview of vibroacoustic stimulation, J Obstet Gynecol Neonatal Nurs 18(6):447, 1989.

Stringer MR: Chorionic villi sampling: a nursing perspective, J Obstet Gynecol Neonatal Nurs 17(1):19, 1988.

Tucker SM: Pocket guide to fetal monitoring, St Louis, 1988, The CV Mosby Co.

Infections

Eschenbach DA: Contending with the problem of chlamydial infection, Contemp OB/GYN 25(2):125, 1985.

Fox GN and Strangarity JW: Varicella-zoster virus infections in pregnancy, Am Fam Physician 39(2):89, 1989.

Gaffney SE and Salinger L: Group B streptococcus: the pregnant woman and her neonate, J Obstet Gynecol Neonatal Nurs 16(2):91, 1987.

Gurevich I: Counseling the patient with herpes, RN 53(2):22, 1990.

Harger JH: Improving the care of pregnant women with genital herpes, Contemp OB/GYN 26(4):85, 1985.

Marvin C and Slevin A: Chlamydia cause, prevention, and care, MCN 12(5):318, 1987.

Maslow AS and Bobitt JR: Herpes in pregnancy: exploring clinical options, Contemp OB/GYN 32(4):44, 1988.

Nettina S: Syphilis: a new look at an old killer, Am J Nurs 90(4):69, 1990.

Osborne NG and Pratson L: Sexually transmitted disease and pregnancy, J Obstet Gynecol Neonatal Nurs 13(1):9, 1984.

Pajares KF and others: Rubella vaccination, Pediatr Nurs 10(1):72, 1984.

Sacks SL: The truth about herpes, ed 3, Seattle, Wash, 1988, Gordon Soules Book Publishers, Ltd.

Sever JL: The menacing infections that spell TORCH, Contemp OB/GYN 25(2):109, 1985.

Should pregnant women routinely be tested for HIV? Am J Nurs 88(2):158, 1988.

Wendel GD: We can and must prevent congenital syphilis, Contemp OB/GYN 26(3):151, 1985.

Nutrition

Aaronson LS and others: The relationship between weight gain and nutrition in pregnancy, Nurs Res 38(4):223, 1989.

Dimperio D: Prenatal nutrition: clinical guidelines for nurses, New York, 1988, March of Dimes Birth Defects Foundation.

Dohrmann KR and Lederman SA: Weight gain in pregnancy, J Obstet Gynecol Neonatal Nurs 15(6):446, 1987.

Kliegman RM: Maternal, fetal, and neonatal consequences of obesity, Perinat/Neonat 8(4):49, 1984.

Leonard LG: Pregnancy and the underweight woman, MCN 9(5):331, 1984.

Luke B: Lactose intolerance during pregnancy, MCN 2(2):92, 1977.

Luke B: Understanding pica in pregnant women, MCN 2(2):97, 1977.

Luke B: Megavitamins and pregnancy: a dangerous combination, MCN 10(1):18, 1985.

Naeye RL: Effects of maternal nutrition on fetal and neonatal survival, Birth 10:109, Summer 1983.

Stevenson DK and Cohen RS: Overfeeding and underfeeding the fetus, Perinat/Neonat 9(6):10, 1985.

Toll-free hotline provides nutrition information for pregnant women, (1-800-MOM-4-NEWS), MCN 14(4):282, 1989.

Winick M: Nutrition and pregnancy, Pediatr Ann 19(4):235, 1990.

Worthington-Roberts BS, Yermeersch JA, and Williams SR: Nutrition in pregnancy and lactation, ed 3, St Louis, 1985, The CV Mosby Co.

Teratogens

Aaronson LS and Macnee CL: Tobacco, alcohol, and caffeine use during pregnancy, J Obstet Gynecol Neonatal Nurs 18(4):279, 1989.

Aerosol ribavirin: are nurses at risk? Nursing '89 19(9):106, 1989.

Alcohol's real effect on the fetus, Contemp OB/GYN 24(6):151, 1984.

Alexander LL: The pregnant smoker: nursing implications, J Obstet Gynecol Neonatal Nurs 16(3):167, 1987.

Barbour BG: Is fetal alcohol syndrome completely irreversible? MCN 12(6):414, 1987.

Bibbo M and Gill WB: Screening of adolescents exposed to diethylstilbestrol in utero, Pediatr Clin North Am 28(2):379, 1981.

Bingham E: Curbing cancer drugs' risks to nurses, Am J Nurs 87(6):765, 1987.

Craft K: Pregnant? Take these precautions, Nursing '89 19(1):62, 1989.

Fried PA: Pregnancy and lifestyle habits, ed 2, New York, 1983, Beaufort Press.

Maternal smoking and neonatal health care costs, Am Fam Physician 38(5):263, 1988.

No link between video terminals and birth defects, Am J Nurs 87(7):904, 1987.

Smith J: The dangers of prenatal cocaine use, MCN 13(3):174, 1988.

Stephens CJ: The fetal alcohol syndrome: cause for concern, MCN 6(4):251, 1981.

Thomson EJ and Cordero JF: The new teratogens: accutane and other vitamin-A analogs, MCN 14(4):244, 1989.

Zacharias J: A rational approach to drug use in pregnancy, J Obstet Gynecol Neonatal Nurs 12(3):183, 1983.

Parturition

6

Presentations, Positions, and Progress

CHAPTER OBJECTIVES

After studying this chapter, the student should be able to perform the following:

1 Define the following terms: presentation, position, attitude, station, effacement, dilatation, and oxytocics.
2 Use a pelvic model and fetal mannequin to depict the following fetal positions: L.O.A., R.O.P., R.O.T., L.S.A., R.M.P., and tell which position is the most common.
3 Describe three types of breech presentations.
4 Explain the origin and significance of "show."
5 List the seven movements in the mechanism of labor and delivery using an L.O.A. fetal position as an example.

6 Indicate what is meant by the four stages of labor and the approximate durations of each for primiparas and multiparas.
7 Name the two measurements of labor that may be used to graph a patient's progress when a Friedman labor curve is employed.
8 Indicate four choices that a physician makes when labor is not progressing normally.
9 Discuss the difference between a precipitate delivery and a precipitate labor and the dangers of both.
10 List four signs of the separation of the placenta from the uterine wall after delivery of the infant.

The relationship of the fetus to the obstetric passageway is of interest to both physician and nurse. It usually influences the length of labor, preparation for delivery, and type of complications possibly encountered.

Some common words are used in special ways to describe the relationship of the fetus to the obstetric passage. For example, in maternal health care one often refers to the following terms: lie, presentation, attitude, position, station, engagement, effacement, and show.

Lie and presentation

The *lie* of an infant means the relationship of the long axis of the fetus to the long axis of the uterus. If the length of the fetus is parallel with the length of the uterus,

the lie may be called "longitudinal." However, if the fetus lies crosswise in the uterus, the term *transverse lie* may be used.

Many times the term *presentation* is used synonymously with the phrase *presenting part*—the part of the baby that is coming or attempting to pass through the pelvic canal first. Headfirst placement is referred to as a cephalic presentation. Feet or buttocks presented first is termed breech. Approximately 96% of all births are headfirst, or cephalic; about 3.5% are breech. Transverse presentations account for the remaining percentage. Presentation is usually determined by abdominal palpation and rectal, vaginal or ultrasonic examinations.

A breech birth is to be avoided, if possible, because

93

it typically involves a greater risk to the infant. (See p. 149.) Today, an increasing number of obstetricians are attempting to turn selected breech presentations into cephalic. This is done by external manipulation, called *version*. Version is being used more frequently than has been the case in several years because of the simultaneous availability of electronic FHR monitoring, continuous real-time sonograms, and medications (tocolytics) that help relax the uterus. The use of these tools has substantially increased the safety and success of versions and offers another alternative to abdominal or cesarean delivery. However, a version may be contraindicated for a number of reasons, e.g., if a condition also exists that would already call for a cesarean birth (an abnormally positioned placenta), if more than one baby occupies the uterus, or if the infant is exceptionally large.

Attitude

The *attitude* refers to the degree of flexion of the body, head (Fig. 6-1), and extremities of the fetus. The normal attitude is complete flexion. A well-flexed head presents the smallest cephalic diameter and fewer mechanical problems in descent and delivery. This chin-on-chest posture makes possible the *vertex delivery* desired.

Position (Figs. 6-2 to 6-5)

The *position* is technically the relationship of a certain point of reference on the presenting part of the fetus to the pelvic quadrants *of the mother*. It gives more detailed information about fetal progress because the presenting part turns to adapt to the shape and size of the various parts of the birth canal. The maternal pelvic quadrants are identified as right and left posterior and right and left anterior (Fig. 6-2). The pelvic quadrants never change location, although the different perspectives in illustrations and diagrams can confuse the student. Sometimes the quadrants are seen from "below," that is, as they appear to the physician in front of the delivery table ready to receive the baby. Sometimes they are viewed from "above," from the vantage point of the unborn child entering the pelvis. In some other diagrams, students look directly through the abdominal wall to view the fetus within the canal. The point of reference, of course, varies according to the presenting part discussed and the amount of flexion present. In the event of a well-flexed cephalic or vertex presentation the point of reference employed is the occipital bone, or occiput. It is the most accessible bone to identify in rectal or vaginal examination. The vault of the fetal skull is made up of three paired bones and one single bone separated by tough but softer membranous seams, or sutures. It is fairly easy to follow these sutures with a gloved finger after sufficient cervical dilatation has occurred and to determine the placement of the occiput. The sutures trace a Y, and the occiput is found between the top shafts of the Y behind the triangular posterior fontanel (Fig. 6-3).

To simplify reference to the various positions, the descriptive phrase usually begins with either right or left

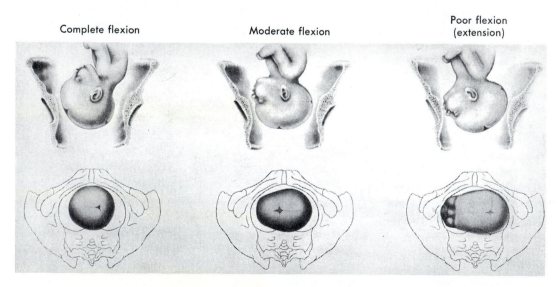

| Complete flexion | Moderate flexion | Poor flexion (extension) |

FIG 6-1 Head diameters in various degrees of flexion. (*From Phenomena of normal labor, Columbus, Oh, 1964, Ross Laboratories.*)

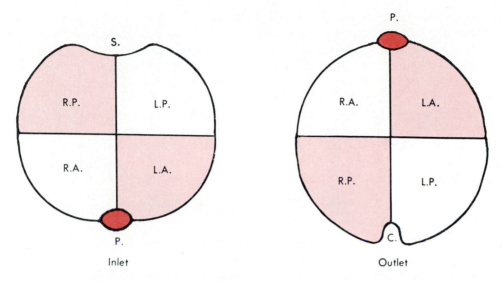

FIG 6-2 Maternal pelvic quadrants stay the same; however, the student's perspective may change. *C*, Coccyx; *P*, pubic bones; *S*, sacrum.

THE FETAL HEAD

Bones
    Frontal—2
    Parietal—2
    Temporal—2
    Occipital—1

Sutures
    Sagittal
    Frontal
    Coronal
    Lambdoid

Fontanels
    Anterior
    Posterior

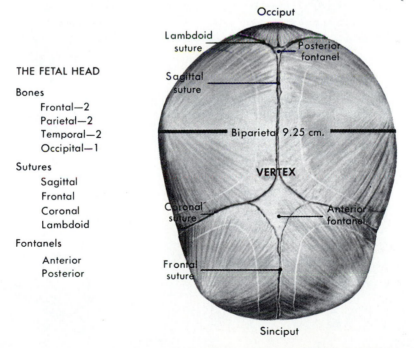

FIG 6-3 Fetal head—physician's map. *(From Phenomena of normal labor, Columbus, Oh, 1964, Ross Laboratories.)*

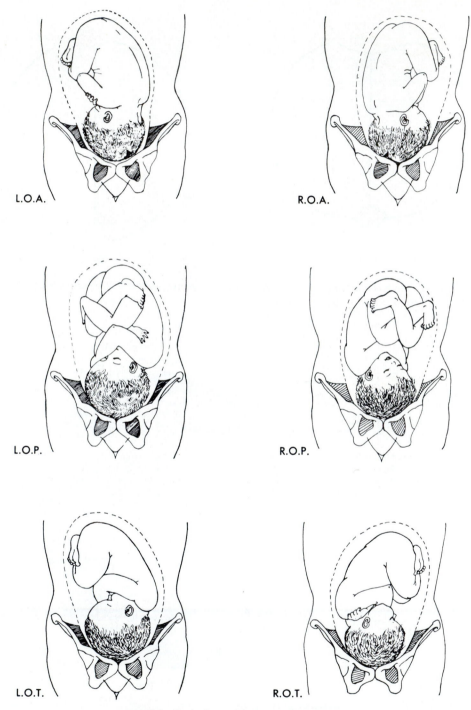

FIG 6-4 Cephalic positions—vertex type.

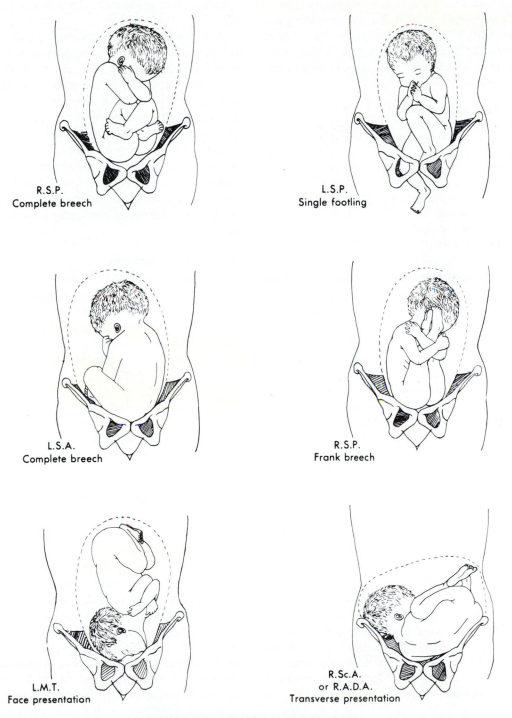

R.S.P.
Complete breech

L.S.P.
Single footling

L.S.A.
Complete breech

R.S.P.
Frank breech

L.M.T.
Face presentation

R.Sc.A.
or R.A.D.A.
Transverse presentation

FIG 6-5 Various presentations and positions.

(of the mother's pelvis), followed by the point of reference used (on the fetus) and the adjectives anterior, posterior, or transverse (referring again to the part of the mother's pelvis toward which a particular point on the fetus is directed). Thus the most common vertex position is left occiput anterior (L.O.A.). Each presenting part has the possibility of eight positions following the same pattern. Only the middle initial or code letters representing the point of reference need to be changed (Fig. 6-4). For example:

1.	Right occiput* anterior	R.O.A.
2.	Left occiput anterior	L.O.A.
3.	Right occiput posterior	R.O.P.
4.	Left occiput posterior	L.O.P.
5.	Right occiput transverse	R.O.T.
6.	Left occiput transverse	L.O.T.
7.	Occiput at sacrum	O.S.
	Occiput posterior	O.P.
8.	Occiput at the pubis	O.A.
	Occiput anterior	

Note that a transverse position is *not* the same thing as a transverse presentation, or lie. The letter "O" is usually employed only in the case of well-flexed or median vertex presentations (military). In the rare case of cephalic presentations demonstrating more deflexion, other points of reference must be sought, because the occiput is no longer available or meaningful to the examiner. In a brow presentation, the letter "F" for fronto is used, referring to the area of the anterior fontanel. Brow presentations are usually slow and difficult because of the increased diameter of the skull trying to force its way through the passageway. This presentation may require a cesarean birth. In instances of full extension of the head that results in a face presentation, the letter "M" for mentum, or chin, is used. Nowadays face presentations are rarely delivered vaginally because of a significant risk of injury to the infant's cervical spine (Fig. 6-5).

Breech presentations employ the sacrum or coccyx as a point of reference and the code letter "S" (Fig. 6-5). Characteristically, three types are described. A *complete,* or full, *breech* involves the flexion of the fetus's legs, usually tailor fashion so that the buttocks and feet appear at the vaginal opening almost simultaneously. A *frank,* or single, *breech* occurs when the thighs are flexed on the abdomen with the extended legs against the trunk and the feet against the face (foot-in-mouth posture). The

term *incomplete breech* may indicate the initial appearance of either the feet or knees. The presentation of one or both feet is labeled a *single* or *double footling,* respectively. Frank breech is commonly encountered. Breech birth is associated with a higher perinatal mortality.

A transverse lie, sometimes called a shoulder presentation, usually involves the scapula or its upper tip, the acromion; for reference "Sc" or "A" is the code. The fetus lying crosswise in the uterus may be positioned with his back toward the front or back of his mother. The fetus's scapula, posteriorly located, indicates the position of his back. Sometimes the terms *dorsoanterior* or *dorsoposterior* may be used to clarify this fetal position. A fetus whose shoulder and head occupy the right side of the mother's pelvis and whose back is toward her front is in the right acromiodorsoanterior position (R.A.D.A.). This is an impossible presentation for normal birth.

Station and engagement

Another measurement related to the location of the fetus in the passageway is *station,* which is the relationship of the presenting part to the ischial spines of the pelvis. When the presenting part is at the level of the ischial spines, it is considered engaged, and the station is said to be 0. If the presentation is above the ischial spines, it is considered high, and the station is said to be −1, −2, etc., an estimate of its location in centimeters above the ischial spines. If the presenting part is below the ischial spines, the station is coded as +1, +2, etc., making an estimate in centimeters. (A centimeter is a little less than ½ inch.) A plus station is considered low (Fig. 6-6).

Effacement and dilatation (dilation)

One should not forget that frequent and progressively stronger uterine contractions create the shortening and thinning (effacement) and dilatation (or dilation) of the cervix to an opening approximately 10 cm (about 4 inches) in diameter. It should be noted that effacement may occur "silently" as the result of unobtrusive Braxton Hicks contractions before the onset of more definitive, vigorous labor. Limited cervical dilatation (approximately 1 to 3 cm) may also take place before the onset of the formal labor period. The disappearance, or effacement, of the cervical canal as its walls move upward to become part of the lower uterine segment is expressed in percent. Primiparas (nulliparas) usually undergo 100% effacement before dilatation (Fig. 6-7). The cervix of a multipara typically undergoes effacement and dilatation

---

*Sometimes the combining form "occipito" is used instead of the noun "occiput."

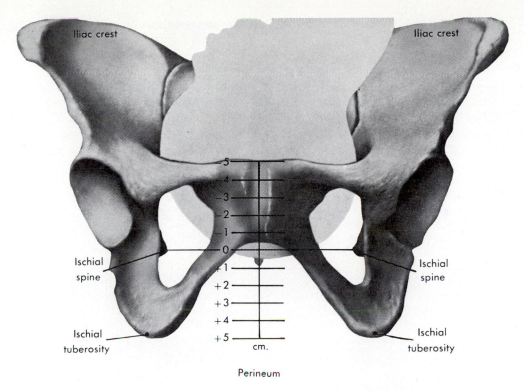

Iliac crest   Iliac crest

Ischial spine   Ischial spine

Ischial tuberosity   Ischial tuberosity

cm.

Perineum

FIG 6-6 Stations of presenting part or degree of engagement. Locations of the presenting part in relation to the level of ischial spines is designated *station* and indicates degrees of advancement of the presenting part through the pelvis. Stations are expressed in centimeters above *(minus)* and below *(plus)* the level of the ischial spines *(zero)*. The head is usually engaged when it reaches the level of the ischial spines. *(From Phenomena of normal labor, Columbus, Oh, 1964, Ross Laboratories.)*

at the same time. For a more detailed discussion of expected rates of dilatation, see pp. 102 and 104.

Show

Dilatation of the cervix is usually accompanied by what is called *show*. During pregnancy, the mucus-producing glands of the cervix have formed a deposit in the cervical canal that protects the interior of the uterus from infection. When the cervix begins to dilate, this mucus plug is discharged. As the cervix continues to dilate, small capillaries in the cervix break and stain the mucus with blood. The faster the cervix dilates and the closer it is to complete dilatation, the more abundant and red will be the "show." However, show should not assume the proportions or characteristics of frank bleeding or contain clots.

After complete dilatation both abdominal and uterine muscles contract to push the fetus through the pelvic canal. The mother has no control over the contractions of her uterus; they are under involuntary control. However, once dilatation is complete, she may push with her

abdominal muscles when her uterus contracts so that the fetus can descend in the pelvic canal.

Thus to determine the progress of the fetus, the physician is interested in the *presentation,* the body part that comes first; the *position,* the relationship of the presenting part to the pelvic quadrants; and the *station,* the depth of the presenting part in the pelvic canal. If these are known plus the relative size and shape of the pelvis and fetus, the condition of the soft-tissue uterine exit called the cervix, and the quality and frequency of the uterine contractions, the physician has a good basis to evaluate the progress of the labor and the mechanisms involved.

MECHANISM OF LABOR

Textbooks usually speak of the cardinal movements in the mechanism of labor. In the vertex delivery they usually include the following: descent, flexion, engagement, internal rotation, extension, external rotation, and expulsion (Fig. 6-8). The first *four* movements are not necessarily in order, because flexion may be present before descent and may increase thereafter. Descent and

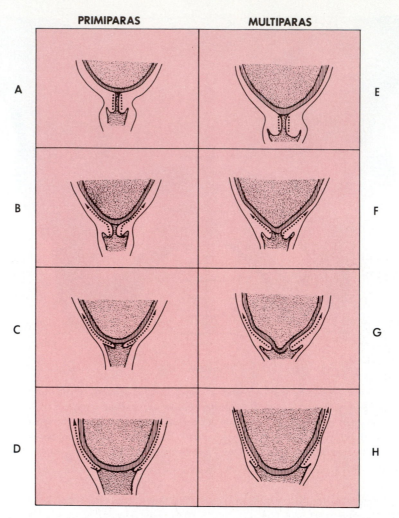

PRIMIPARAS   **MULTIPARAS**

FIG 6-7 The columns above compare the typical progress of cervical effacement and dilatation demonstrated by women in labor during their first viable pregnancies compared with that of women in labor with their second or consecutive pregnancies. **A** and **E** show long cervix. Multiparas usually have a relaxed cervical canal. **B** and **F,** Effacement or shortening of cervix begins. **C** and **G,** Cervix thins in primiparas but little dilatation occurs. Effacement and dilatation are simultaneous in multiparas. **D** and **H,** Effacement and dilatation are complete.

internal rotation also continue after engagement. These mechanisms can occur concurrently and defy a 1-2-3 order.

Descent, flexion, and engagement

In a primipara* (woman bearing her first baby), *descent* of the fetus into the true pelvis usually occurs about 2 weeks before the actual birth of the child. This descent is referred to as *lightening* and results in *engagement,* or passage of the largest diameter of the presenting part into the true pelvis. Lay people remark about this change in fetal location with the phrase "the baby has dropped." The expectant mother, with less pressure on her diaphragm, happily finds that she can breathe more easily. The increased tilt and lowered location of the fetus produce a characteristic change in the maternal figure. In a multipara, descent and engagement may not occur until dilatation of the cervix begins.

*The words "primipara" and "multipara" in this section are used from the delivery-labor room perspective. Perhaps more correct would be the terms "primigravida" or "nullipara" but these are used less frequently. Review also p. 63.

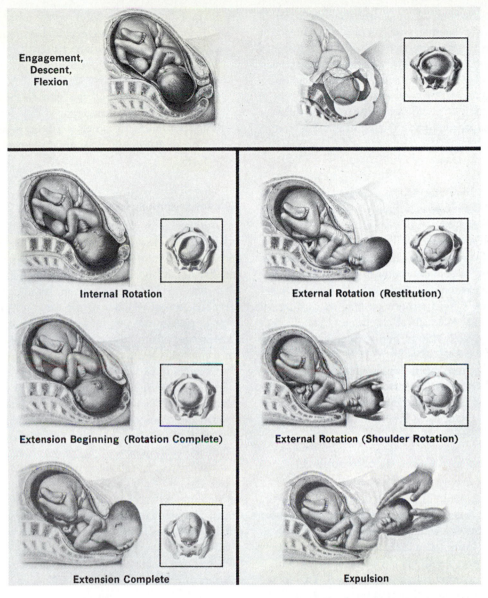

Engagement, Descent, Flexion

Internal Rotation

External Rotation (Restitution)

Extension Beginning (Rotation Complete)

External Rotation (Shoulder Rotation)

Extension Complete

Expulsion

FIG 6-8 Mechanism of normal labor, L.O.A. position showing head rotation in square inserts. *(From Nursing education aid, No. 13, Columbus Oh, 1964, Ross Laboratories.)*

Internal rotation

The amount of *internal rotation* will depend on the position of the fetus and the way the head rotates to accommodate itself to the changing diameters of the pelvis. The most common rotation is that which involves the turning of the head to occiput anterior position. If the fetus begins its descent in L.O.A. or L.O.T. position, this rotation represents only a short distance of 45 to 90 degrees. However, if the internal rotation involves moving from a posterior position, it may mean a turn of 135 degrees. For this reason posterior positions usually entail a longer labor and more lower back discomfort for the mother, who will usually appreciate firm, warm, intermittent sacral support. Occasionally, instead of rotating to an anterior position, the occiput turns to the sacrum, and the child is born in O.S. or O.P. position—a delivery that is usually slower and more dangerous to the maternal tissues. Often the occiput will complete the longer rotation from the posterior position to the pubis. Sometimes the occiput lingers unduly in the posterior position, which is called *persistent posterior,* or stops its rotation in transverse, referred to as *transverse arrest.* This can occur at almost any station or depth in the pelvic canal and may necessitate manual rotation or the use of rotation forceps by the obstetrician.

Extension

In a vertex delivery the head is delivered by *extension.* During descent the head is normally forced into a flexed attitude by the pressure of the cervix, pelvic walls, and floor. Once the occiput has rotated to anterior position and occupies the pubic arch, the head cannot make any further progress unless extension is accomplished. Because of this extension plus the natural curve of the lower pelvis, the baby's head is born pushing upward out of the vaginal canal. The rate of extension is greatly controlled by the physician. If the bag of waters (membranes) has not broken during labor, it must be broken now to prevent the baby from aspirating amniotic fluid. To avoid uncontrolled tearing of the perineum, an *episiotomy,* or surgical incision extending the soft tissue vaginal opening, may be performed just before the birth of the head. (See also p. 272.)

External rotation (restitution, shoulder rotation) and expulsion

When the perineum slides over the chin of the baby and only the neck temporarily occupies the outlet, more room is available for head movement. Usually without coaxing by the birth attendant, the back of the baby's head turns to line up with his back, revealing the baby's position before internal rotation of the head. This movement is called *restitution.* The turning movement of the head generally continues and influences the location of the back, helping to line up the unborn shoulders just beneath the pubis in anteroposterior position. This process of alignment is called *shoulder rotation.* Usually the top of the anterior shoulder is seen next just under the pubis—generally aided by the physician, who may exert gentle but firm downward traction on the head. Then the head is gently raised to clear the posterior shoulder, and the entire body follows without any difficulty. *Expulsion* of the infant is completed.

STAGES OF LABOR

Labor has been classically divided into three stages. Now a fourth stage has been identified:

Stage 1—from the onset of regular labor contractions, beginning with effacement and dilatation of the cervix to complete dilation, 10 cm

Stage 2—from complete dilation to the birth of the baby

Stage 3—from birth of the baby to the expulsion of the placenta and membranes

Stage 4—normally about a 2-hour period of transition, stabilization, and initial recovery from childbirth

Friedman labor curve

Another more elaborate way of describing labor that includes the classic first and second stages has gained prominence in the last decade. It employs what is called the Friedman labor curve. Dr. Friedman has emphasized that two measurements, when serially repeated and graphed, reveal whether or not the journey through the pelvic passageway is in preparation or process and whether satisfactory progress is being made. Those two measurements are *cervical dilatation* and *station.*

Changes in cervical dilatation. After statistical study of many thousands of birth histories, two similar S-shaped curves based on the speed of dilatation of multiparas and primiparas (nulliparas) were identified. When the rates of cervical dilatation of individual women in labor are plotted against the appropriate curve, disturbances in progress related to dilatation may be diagnosed more readily. Both curves may be divided into sections describing different phases of the labor process (Fig. 6-9). The vertical side of the graph indicates the cervical dilatation 0 to 10 centimeters and the horizontal side indicates the number of hours in labor. The length of labor is much shorter for multiparas, accounting for the variance in the curves.

Two main phases are described: a relatively slow-moving, flat first section called the *latent phase,* involving cervical softening, effacement, and early dilatation (it traces the period extending from onset of labor until more rapid dilatation manifests itself at approximately 2 to 3 cm); and a second section, the *active phase,* which is indicated by the sudden upswing and steep ascent of the tracing, ending with a brief rounding at the apex. This active phase of dilatation has in turn been divided into three phases: (1) the *acceleration phase* is the curve upward from the latent phase that first identifies cervical dilatation has increased in tempo; (2) the *phase of maximum slope* is the steepest part of the tracing; and (3) the *deceleration phase* is the rounding of the apex, which represents a slowing of the dilatation just before the pa-

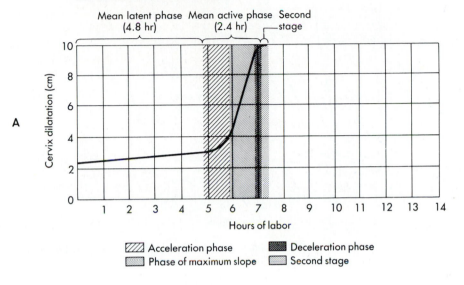

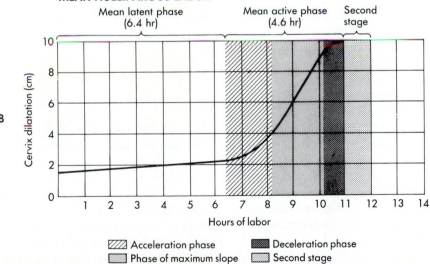

FIG 6-9 The Friedman labor curve formed by plotting the rate of cervical dilatation of the mean multiparous labor (**A**) and mean nulliparous (primiparous) labor (**B**) (*mean* indicates average). *(Based on revised mean labor statistics in Friedman EA: Labor: clinical evaluation and management, ed 2, New York, 1978, Appleton-Century-Crofts; and personal correspondence.)*

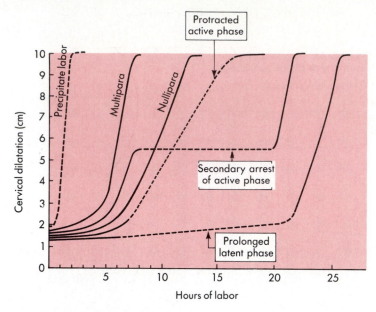

FIG 6-10 Deviations in rate of cervical dilatation (as described by Friedman). The prolonged deceleration phase is not pictured.

tient is completely dilated. Existence of the deceleration phase has been disputed, and it has often been characterized as short or absent in multiparas.

It is difficult at times to determine when the latent phase begins, since effacement and early cervical dilatation are "silent," or false labor may confuse the issue. The patient's labor graph is usually begun when a nullipara's (primipara's) contractions are experienced at regular 3- to 5-minute intervals or when a multipara attains regular contractions at 5- to 10-minute intervals.

Although the condition of the mother and the fetus is considered more important than the meticulous observation of a clock for the passage of time periods, analysis by comparison of the cervical dilatation of a maternity patient to the appropriate curve developed by Dr. Friedman may be helpful in identifying problems affecting labor. Using this standard, a labor is considered prolonged if

1. The latent phase lasts
   a. 14 hours or more for multiparas
   b. 20 hours or more for nulliparas
2. The rate of maximum slope is
   a. 1.5 cm/hr or less for multiparas
   b. 1.2 cm/hr or less for nulliparas
3. The maximum slope shows no progress in dilatation for 2 hours or more (secondary arrest—the most damaging dilatation pattern)

4. The deceleration phase lasts
   a. More than 1 hour for multiparas
   b. More than 3 hours for nulliparas

These abnormalities are shown in Fig. 6-10. When these conditions exist, the physician may decide to

1. Intensify maternal and infant assessment
2. Use sedation for the mother
3. Stimulate uterine contractions with oxytocic medication
4. Prepare for cesarean birth

Changes in station or descent. Friedman's study of the rate of descent of the fetus through the pelvic canal also produces a curve that is divided almost the same way as the dilatation curve. It is sometimes superimposed on the dilatation graph to show that the phase of maximum slope for cervical dilatation normally corresponds to the phase of acceleration for descent (Fig. 6-11).

Descent abnormalities occur alone or in conjunction with problems in dilatation. Descent is considered to be abnormally slow or arrested if:

1. During the maximum slope the rate is
   a. 2 cm/hr or less for multiparas
   b. 1 cm/hr or less for nulliparas
2. During descent labor progress is stopped for 1 hour or more

If problems in descent occur, reevaluation of fetal pre-

NULLIPAROUS DILATATION AND DESCENT CURVES

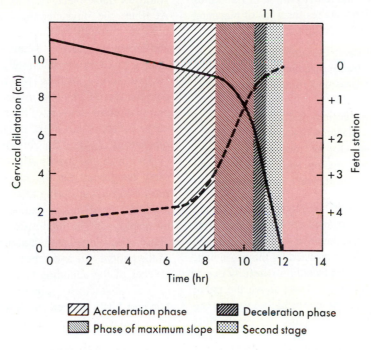

FIG 6-11   Shows approximate relationship of cervical dilatation rate to fetal descent rate in average nulliparous (primiparous) labor. *(Adapted from Friedman EA: Labor: clinical evaluation and management, ed 2, New York, 1978, Appleton-Century-Crofts.)*

Table 6-1   Usual duration of the stages of labor

	First stage	Second stage	Third stage
Primiparas (nulliparas)	10 to 12 hours	30 minutes to 2 hours	5 to 20 minutes (often aided by oxytocics or manual pressure)
Multiparas	6 to 8 hours	20 minutes to 1½ hours	5 to 20 minutes (often aided by oxytocics or manual pressure)

sentation and position and the adequacy of the maternal pelvis is made. Changes in labor posture or activity of the mother may be helpful, for example, squatting. Oxytocics may be ordered or a cesarean birth scheduled.

Note: Too rapid descent or precipitate labor (not to be confused with precipitate delivery, which means a birth without adequate preparation) can also be a prob-

lem. Too rapid descent is usually defined as a labor of less than 3 hours, which may be accompanied by maternal uterine and perineal lacerations, lowered fetal oxygenation, and infant birth injury (especially cerebral hemorrhage).

The Friedman curve is not universally employed to monitor labor progression, but it is a useful concept and tool that has added specific terminology to the analysis of childbirth.

A wise nurse or physician makes no specific predictions regarding the length of the stages of labor. However, Table 6-1 may be useful in estimating possible time intervals. Labor lengths for both primiparas and multiparas have decreased in the last generation.

Third stage: special considerations

The third stage of labor is characterized by the separation of the placenta and its expulsion.

Placental separation.   Separation of the placenta from the uterine wall is accomplished by the contraction of the uterus. The site of the placental attachment suddenly becomes reduced, but the placenta itself remains the same size, causing a separation of the two structures. The placenta slides down into the lower portion of the uterus and vagina. The physician watches for signs of placental separation, which include the following:

1. The rise of the uterus to the umbilicus or above—pushed up by the bulky placenta in the vagina
2. The increased firmness and rounded shape of the fundus
3. The lengthening of the exposed umbilical cord at the exterior as the placenta descends
4. The sudden appearance of moderate temporary vaginal bleeding originating from the site of the placental attachment at the time of separation

Placental expulsion. After the placenta is separated from the uterine wall, it is pushed out by the mother as uterine contractions resume, and she is instructed again to "bear down." Often, she is assisted by the physician, who—*after* separation of the placenta—carefully exerts abdominal pressure with one hand just above the pubic bone, momentarily pushing the uterus higher to help the placenta slip further down the birth canal. He gently pulls on the umbilical cord with the other hand (the Brandt-Andrews maneuver), causing the placenta's expulsion. At times the physician may elect to help deliver the placenta through cautious intravaginal, intrauterine, or abdominal maneuvers. Manual extraction may be a necessity in cases of abnormally retained placenta or excessive uterine bleeding. Most physicians manually palpate the uterine cavity to make sure that it is normal and empty after the delivery of the placenta. Visual inspection of the cervix is part of the usual follow-up. The expelled placenta is checked for abnormality and completeness.

The third and fourth stages of labor are probably the most dangerous for the mother because hemorrhages most often occur during this time. To lessen blood loss, *oxytocics,* medications that help contract the uterus, may be employed. The medications used will depend on the phase of delivery that their action is desired, the condition of the patient, the anesthesia used, and the personal preferences of the attending physician.

The satisfactory completion of the mechanisms of labor and birth as seen in all stages is indeed cause for congratulation for all concerned.

Key Concepts

1. The following terms are used to decribe the relationship of the fetus to the obstetric passageway: lie, presentation, attitude, position, station, and engagement.
2. The lie refers to the relationship of the long axis of the fetus to the long axis of the uterus.
3. Presentation, or presenting part, refers to the part of the baby entering the pelvic canal first. Most births are headfirst, or cephalic; about 3.5% of births are breech.
4. Attitude refers to the degree of flexion of the body, head, and extremities. The normal attitude is complete flexion.
5. The position is technically the relationship of a certain point of reference on the presenting part of the fetus to the pelvic quandrants of the mother.
6. The phrase describing fetal position comprises 3 terms: (1) right or left (of the mother's pelvis), (2) the point of reference used (on the fetus), and (3) the adjective anterior, posterior, or transverse (referring to the part of the mother's pelvis toward which a particular point on the fetus is directed). The most common vertex position is left occiput anterior (L.O.A.).
7. Three types of breech presentations may occur. With a complete or full breech the fetus's legs are flexed so that the buttocks and feet appear at the vaginal opening almost simultaneously. A frank or single breech occurs when the thighs of the fetus are flexed on the abdomen with the extended legs against the trunk and the feet against the face. Incomplete breech may indicate the appearance of either the feet or the knees.
8. Station refers to the relationship of the presenting part to the ischial spines of the pelvis.
9. Uterine contractions cause effacement (shortening and thinning) and dilatation (widening to an opening approximately 10 cm [4 in] in diameter) of the cervix.
10. As the cervix dilates, the mucus plug is discharged and becomes blood-stained as a result of the breakage of small capillaries in the cervix. This discharge is referred to as show. The faster the cervix dilates and the closer it is to complete dilatation, the more abundant and red will be the show.
11. The cardinal movements in the mechanism of labor in a vertex delivery include the following: descent, flexion, engagement, internal rotation, extension, external rotation, and expulsion.
12. When the fetus moves into the true pelvis, it is

termed descent. Descent results in engagement, or the passage of the largest diameter of the presenting part into the true pelvis.

13. The amount of internal rotation depends on the position of the fetus and the way the head rotates to accommodate to the changing diameters of the pelvis.

14. In a vertex delivery, the head is delivered by extension, with the head pushing upward out of the vaginal canal.

15. After the head has been delivered, it usually turns, helping to line up the unborn shoulders. This is called external rotation and allows for delivery of the rest of the baby, or expulsion.

16. Labor is divided into four stages. Stage 1 begins with the onset of regular labor contractions and ends with complete cervical dilatation. Stage 2 begins with complete dilatation and ends with the birth of the baby. Stage 3 begins with the birth of the baby and ends with the expulsion of the placenta and membranes. Stage 4 is the period of transition, stabilization, and initial recovery from childbirth.

17. The Friedman labor curve employs two measurements—cervical dilatation and station—to graph a woman's progress during the first two stages of labor.

18. Two main phases of cervical dilatation are described in a patient's labor graph: the latent phase and the active phase. The active phase is divided into three phases: acceleration phase, phase of maximum slope, and deceleration phase.

19. Using the Friedman labor curve, the following dilatations indicate prolonged labor: latent phase lasts longer than 14 hours in multiparas or 20 hours in nulliparas; rate of maximum slope is 1.5 cm/hour or less for multiparas or 1.2 cm/hr or less for nulliparas; or the maximum slope shows no progress in dilatation for 2 hours or more.

20. When labor is not progressing normally, the physician may decide to intensify maternal and infant assessment, use sedation for the mother, stimulate uterine contractions with oxytocic medications, or prepare for cesarean birth.

21. Fetal descent is considered to be abnormally slow or arrested if either of the following occurs: the rate during maximum slope is 2 cm/hr or less for multiparas or 1 cm/hr or less for nulliparas, or labor progress is stopped for 1 hour or more during descent.

22. Both precipitate labor, which is too rapid descent, and precipitate delivery, which is birth without adequate preparation, can be problems.

23. Usual duration of the first three stages of labor are as follows: the first stage lasts 10 to 12 hours in primiparas and 6 to 8 hours in multiparas; the second stage lasts 30 minutes to 2 hours in primiparas and 20 minutes to 1½ hours in multiparas; and the third stage lasts 5 to 20 minutes in all women.

24. Signs of placental separation include the following: the rise of the uterus to the umbilicus or above, increased firmness and rounded shape of the fundus, lengthening of the exposed umbilical cord at the exterior, and the sudden appearance of moderate temporary vaginal bleeding.

Discussion Questions

1. It is a medical fact that a breech delivery poses a significant risk to the infant. Why is this true?

2. Abnormal presentations are most common in multiple pregnancies, in cases of pelvic deformity, and in situations in which the placenta is abnormally located. Why are these all significant to fetal presentation?

3. It is desirable for the fetal head to enter the pelvis flexed in an occiput position. What would happen if the head were extended or hyperextended when entering the pelvis?

4. Is the statement "multiparas deliver more rapidly than nulliparas" true or false? What is the rationale for your answer?

5. If the progress of labor is abnormally slow, the physician may choose one or more interventions. How would you explain these to the woman in labor?

7

Labor and Birth

CHAPTER OBJECTIVES

After studying this chapter, the student should be able to perform the following:

1 List four accepted signs and symptoms of impending labor.

2 Contrast true and false labor contractions in five ways.

3 Discuss four considerations that influence when to tell a mother in labor to go to the hospital or center where she plans to give birth.

4 Explain why an expectant mother in her third trimester should avoid a prolonged supine position.

5 Indicate two reasons why a labor room enema may be ordered and two situations in which an enema should not be given.

6 Use diagrams to explain what is meant by the three classic fetal heart rate/contraction monitor patterns called early, late, and variable decelerations and their usual significance and treatment.

7 Give the probable meaning of diminished short-term variability on an FHR monitor tracing.

8 List four signs of possible fetal distress during the process of labor.

9 Define the following terms often associated with psychoprophylactic labor techniques and prenatal exercises: cleansing breaths, focal point, effleurage, sacral support, and pelvic rock.

10 Define the four stages of labor and tell how stage length may differ for women having their first babies in contrast to those who have given birth.

11 Describe the characteristics of the three classic periods of the first stage of labor as defined by cervical dilatation; discuss the recommended nursing care associated with each.

12 Note at least three factors that should be investigated or considered when the patient states that she thinks her bag of waters just broke.

13 Explain how to assist the patient and the physician with a vaginal examination and possible artificial rupture of the membranes during labor.

14 List four possible indications of the onset of the second stage of labor.

15 Consider at least two ways in which parental-infant attachment may be enhanced in the perinatal period.

16 Indicate three different forms of infant eye care that may be given after birth to prevent infection.

17 Explain the Apgar evaluation of the newborn, listing the five features observed.

18 Discuss five reasons why prospective patients may seek "alternative birth arrangements."

19 Describe major considerations involved in precipitate delivery and how one can best help the mother and newborn.

20 Enumerate five possible reasons for the induction of labor.

21 Discuss the emergency preparation of a labor patient for cesarean birth—procedures and psychologic support.

22 State three complications associated with breech birth.

23 Compare fraternal and identical twinning; indicate how preparations for a twin birth may differ from that of a single child and what complications may occur.

The following discussion of the needs of the laboring patient reflects for the most part the traditional departmentalized structure of hospital maternity care in the United States (separate labor-delivery, nursery, and postpartum areas). This pattern of care may be the one most frequently encountered by students using this text. However, it should be emphasized that many maternity services are undergoing changes and that various nursing roles are being created that overlap and extend those formerly described. Indeed, different birth settings and maternal-infant care arrangements, both within and outside hospital walls, are being sought by some parents, and the reader should be aware of the alternatives available. (See p. 144.)

Normally, the onset of labor is the anticipated climax of 9 months of constructive waiting. Under normal conditions each day has better prepared the fetus to make the transition from intrauterine to extrauterine existence smoothly, without undue strain. As the time of labor and birth approaches, the pregnant woman should be alerted to certain "get set" signs, and she should be instructed when to call the physician and/or health care provider and come to the hospital.

SIGNS OF IMPENDING LABOR

Several signs and symptoms usually precede the onset of true labor—the progressive opening of the cervix and expulsion of the baby and placenta. These hints of things to come are usually welcome. At the end of a full-term pregnancy the mother is willing to relinquish her lively and bulky boarder; however, she also has feelings of anxiety as she considers the actual period of labor and birth.

Lightening. In a woman bearing her first infant, a relative change in fetal location may be suddenly apparent about 2 weeks before birth. As the fetus "drops" into the true pelvis (a process called *lightening*) and the presenting part "becomes engaged" (the largest diameter of the presenting part passes the pelvic brim), she finds herself able to breathe more freely with less pressure on her diaphragm. Primigravidas are expected to experience lightening and engagement before true labor begins. If it does not occur, the possibility of too small a pelvic inlet or too large a presenting part (fetal-pelvic disproportion) may be considered. Women who have borne children previously may not undergo lightening until just before or during true labor.

Frequent urination. The woman may find greater pressure on her bladder and may feel the need to urinate frequently.

Energy. Many women experience a phenomenal "burst of energy" just before going into labor and want to clean the whole house. They should be advised to resist the impulse.

Uterine contractions. The uterus contracts and relaxes intermittently all during pregnancy, but its contractions are usually mild and not detected by the mother-to-be. However, in the last few weeks of waiting, these uterine contractions may become annoying and, contrary to what some texts declare, may be painful. The most discouraging aspect about these contractions of late pregnancy is that they are often only a rehearsal for the real thing. They do not serve to dilate the cervix progressively and therefore are called false labor, or Braxton Hicks contractions, after the British obstetrician who described them. Characteristics of false labor contrasted with true labor contractions include the following:

1. The duration of the contraction remains about the same, not becoming appreciably longer or more intensive as do true contractions.
2. The period between contractions remains long and irregular. True contractions are regular, with a gradually decreasing interval.
3. Pressure or pain is felt primarily in the abdomen rather than in the small of the back.
4. Walking can be tolerated during the contraction. In fact, walking may help relieve discomfort, whereas true labor contractions may be intensified by ambulation.
5. Show, or the appearance of a mucoid vaginal discharge tinged with blood, is absent in false labor but is usually present in true labor.
6. On rectal or more commonly vaginal examination, the cervix is usually found to be long and closed in false labor but is effacing or dilating in true labor.

An expectant mother should be counseled to contact her health care provider about the onset of labor if (1) contractions are regular, becoming increasingly frequent and intensive; (2) show is present; or (3) the bag of waters, or membranes, ruptures.

TRIP TO THE HOSPITAL

The time at which the woman is instructed to go to the hospital depends on her reported progress, the distance she must travel, how many babies she has had, and the history of her previous labors. Usually physicians or other designated care givers want a patient to be examined if the bag of waters is leaking or ruptures or show is increasing. If these signs are absent, admission for evaluation is often advised when the contractions of primigravidas are strong and regular at 5-minute intervals or less for about 2 hours. Women who have had one baby or more should seek professional assessment when their contractions have achieved significant strength and regularity but should not wait until a certain frequency is reached. Those who have previously experienced a full-term normal birth usually deliver more rapidly than women who have not. They are not encouraged to wait at home for a long time.

During the waiting period before coming to the hospital, if possible, a mother-to-be should be urged to take time for a shower and shampoo. She should confirm any necessary arrangements for transportation and child care needed and recheck her previously prepared suitcase contents. (See p. 83) Perhaps, she could take a nap. If labor is progressing, she should not eat any solid food and limit her intake of fluids until evaluated. In this way, she may avoid the nausea and vomiting during labor related to a slowing of the digestive process. Such precautions also may help prevent aspiration if general anesthesia is required because of an obstetric emergency.

It is hoped that the ride to the hospital will not turn into a race or be complicated with too many obstacles. Certainly it is best to be admitted without rush and confusion. Detailed planning for the journey should be made. The woman should be told by her physician or office nurse before her entry what the admission procedures involve so that she may be prepared for what will transpire.

HOSPITAL ADMISSION

Admission directly to the labor room unit with a minimum of front office procedure is desirable. Usually only one signature is needed—that of the woman herself—for permission to perform the routine procedures necessary during labor and birth. "Routine procedures" do not include a cesarean birth. The husband or chosen companion may help complete any other office admittance procedure needed while the woman is being cared for in the labor room area.

Answers to questionnaires indicate that a number of prospective fathers resent being sent to the admission desk to complete lengthy forms at a time when they feel that they can be supportive to their wives. Preadmission arrangements to obtain as much information as possible about the patient's physical, mental, and social status, as well as any expectations and desires of the parents that may affect the birth experience, are encouraged. If brief information sheets are filled out before admission by the woman and forwarded by clinic or office personnel with the current prenatal record, the individual needs and preferences of the woman and her family might be better understood and considered.

The so-called assembly-line maternity care of many hospitals has caused some women to feel more like objects than human beings. Some have so resented or feared hospitalization experiences that they seek alternatives to a hospital birth. These expectant parents may consider a home birth or may search for a birth center available in their community. However, hospitals have increasingly responded to the concerns of expectant parents by providing more options in maternity care.

All women harbor anxiety regarding their hospital experience, and some are very nervous and fearful. The nursing staff should do everything in its power to alleviate this anxiety and make the woman and her partner or family feel welcome and secure. A gracious welcome makes a lasting impression. Unfortunately, so does a rude, thoughtless, or disorganized admission experience. The expectant mother does not want to hear about the current problems of the maternity service, experiences of former patients, or the personal histories of her attending nurses. Such recitals are indiscreet, impolite, and worrisome to the woman and her family. Her chosen companion or members of the immediate family should be shown a place where they can comfortably wait during the completion of the admission procedures. If it is indicated that the laboring mother wishes to have one person remain with her during the entire admission, this desire should be honored if possible. After the admission is completed, most hospitals encourage visitation by her immediate family or companion, one or two persons at a time.

Role of the vocational or practical nurse

The prepared vocational nurse, as a part of the maternity staff, can make a real contribution to the well-being of the expectant mother and her family. Under the supervision of an experienced registered nurse, she can render valuable assistance to the department and the patient. We believe that the use of the prepared licensed vocational nurse (LVN or LPN) in nonsupervisory capacities in this department is legitimate and desirable but that it is a misuse of personnel to expect her to assume the role of a charge nurse or to delegate to her only those duties that can be accomplished by workers with less training.

The vocational nurse can provide valuable assistance

in the admittance of the patient to the labor-delivery suite. After the woman arrives at the hospital, she is usually taken by wheelchair to the labor room area. The vocational nurse helps the patient remove her clothes and put on a hospital gown. She makes special note of valuables, such as watches and eyeglasses. If the bag of waters has ruptured, the patient should remain in bed until further evaluation. If an "in bed" position is desired, she should be encouraged to rest on her side. (See p. 126.) As soon as possible the patient is properly identified, preferably by use of a careful banding technique. The vocational nurse asks the name of the attending physician and secures the patient's prenatal record if one is present at the hospital. With the supervising registered nurse, she reads the record to determine as much as possible about this patient before continuing with the admission. Important factors to check are (1) the obstetric history—the number of viable births she has had, previous difficulties, the rapidity of former labors, and Rh status; (2) the record of the current pregnancy—the expected date of birth, laboratory results, present physical or psychosocial problems, and any known allergies; (3) plans for the labor and birth—type of anesthesia, if desired, and whether she has attended childbirth education classes; (4) accommodations preferred, method selected for feeding the infant, and name of the physician who will care for the baby; and (5) marital status.

Some of the necessary admission information will, by its very nature, be absent from the prenatal record. The admitting nurse must inquire when the contractions (if any) began, if any show has been noted, and if the bag of waters is known to have broken. The staff should determine whether the patient has recently eaten. In some maternity services a voided urine specimen is routinely obtained for urinalysis at the time of admission. In others, a specimen is secured on admission only if prenatal history prompts the physician to order it. A specimen may be obtained by catheterization just before the birth. Some maternity services include weighing the patient in their admission procedure.

Although most of the time a call will have previously been received from the attending physician regarding the admission, in some situations the nurse may want to know whether the patient has contacted and been examined by the physician. She will take the patient's temperature, pulse, and respiration; determine the blood pressure, in the *absence of a contraction;* and time the duration, interval, and intensity of contractions. She will listen for and count the fetal heart rate and note the presence and character of any amniotic fluid drainage and any show. Application of external fetal and contraction monitors is often part of her care. In some settings she may perform a rectal or vaginal evaluation of the patient's progress in labor. (See p. 127.)

Role of the registered nurse

The registered nurse, who has overall responsibility for the case, greets the patient, noting any special needs. She palpates the abdomen, evaluates contractions, and examines the patient rectally or, more often, vaginally to determine the fetal station and presentation, the dilatation and effacement of the cervix, the condition of the membranes (bag of waters), and the position of the fetus. These last two are sometimes difficult or impossible to discern through the rectal-vaginal wall. If the rectum is not empty, the results of the examination may be questionable. (See also p. 98.) The position of the cervix may make the estimation of dilatation difficult. The patient's condition, progress, and reaction to labor are evaluated. The individual orders of the attending physician are consulted regarding types of analgesia and anesthesia and expected delivery setup. If no previous arrangement is known, the physician is called. The arrival of the patient at the maternity service, any unusual vital signs, pertinent information gained from the pelvic examination, and other evaluations of the patient are relayed.

Unless the presence of true labor is doubted, perineal preparation of some type is usually carried out. Whether an enema is given depends on the progress, condition, and consent of the patient and her physician's desires. If analgesia is ordered, side rails should be in place. Which staff member carries out the necessary admission procedures depends on the competencies of the personnel and the patient's condition and needs.

Procedures

Principles of the admission procedures should be discussed. It is impossible to describe in detail an admission that fits the needs of every hospital or patient. There are many ways to accomplish similar aims. However, certain principles are followed in every good maternity service no matter where it may be. We will now discuss the admission perineal "prep," the labor room enema, the timing of contractions, and the determination of fetal heart rate.

PERINEAL PREPARATION

PURPOSE: To cleanse the external genitalia in preparation for birth. This usually entails a "mini shave" of the true perineum and clipping of perineal hair. However, physicians are now more often ordering "no prep." No increase in infection has been noted because the patient has not been shaved. However, the perineum should be carefully cleansed before the birth. Cleansing does help prevent infection. Minimal shaving or clipping helps make a possible episiotomy repair and postpartum perineal observation easier.

SETUP: Provide individual equipment for each patient or equipment that is used in such a way that no cross infection can take place. Provision should be made for the following:

1. Privacy
2. Adequate lighting
3. A waterproof pad under the patient's hips to protect the bed
4. A supply of clean, warm water
5. A sudsing antiseptic solution
6. A sharp safety razor (if shaving is desired)
7. Two or three clean dry cotton balls or gauze compresses to help pull back on the skin if it is being shaved and to clean the labial folds
8. An irrigation pitcher and folded soft paper or cloth towels to help rinse off the soapy solution and dry the area
9. Several paper towels or a plastic sack to receive the waste in a convenient manner and intermittently help to clean off the razor if used
10. Clean disposable sized gloves for the nurse's use during the procedure

PROCEDURE:

1. If possible, place a light (wall or gooseneck lamp) on the side of bed opposite from where you will stand so that no shadows are cast.
2. Screen the patient. The sheet may be over the lower legs and feet; the gown is turned up to just above the perineal hairline giving adequate space to work.
3. Have the patient bend her knees and drop her legs sideways—heels toward one another. Lather the perineal hair. If shaving is ordered, create tension on the skin with a dry compress with one hand and shave with the other, placing your razor at a 30-degree angle to the skin. Cleanse away any collection of smegma (cellular debris found especially in the labial folds). Avoid getting any solution into the vagina. Wipe off prepped area with a soft towel dampened with water to remove the solution, which may be irritating. Use a different surface for each stroke (or irrigate the area) and dry with the second soft towel, using the same technique, never returning to the vulva after passing over the rectal area.
4. Before preparation of the perineal area is complete, you must turn the patient on her side to finish the perianal region. Probably the most important area to clear is between the vagina and anus, the *true perineum,* because

this is the area cut if an episiotomy is performed. Wipe off any residual solution.
5. Have your first "prep" checked so that you are certain what is expected of you. Even if it is your first "prep," you should not impress the fact on your anxious patient!
6. During the prep, if possible, try to gauge the frequency and quality of any contractions the patient may have, as well as how she is tolerating them. Report the character and amount of any vaginal discharge.

Note: No perineal pads are worn during labor to reduce the possibility of vulvar contamination resulting from the pad passing from the rectal to the vaginal area. However, the patient may have absorbent, protective bed pads under her hips.

LABOR ROOM ENEMA TECHNIQUE

PURPOSE: To empty the colon of feces in order to

1. Make descent of the fetal head easier
2. Encourage contractions
3. Facilitate rectal or vaginal examinations during labor

Note: The role of the enema in preventing infection is now considered questionable.

SETUP: More and more physicians are prescribing small, prepackaged phosphate enemas. Many are ordering no enema for those patients who have had a recent bowel movement and who can be easily examined.

CAUTIONS:

1. Enemas are not usually given to primiparas after dilatation of 6 to 8 cm or to multiparas above 4 to 5 cm dilatation to avoid expulsion of the enema during birth.
2. Enemas should not be given to a frankly bleeding patient, since this will further encourage bleeding.
3. Enemas are not usually given to patients with a high presentation (unengaged) with ruptured membranes because of the danger of prolapsed cord. Some physicians prefer that no enemas be given when membranes are ruptured even after engagement because of the increased danger of infection.

TIMING OBSTETRIC CONTRACTIONS

PURPOSE:

1. To help evaluate the efforts of the uterus to dilate the cervix and expel the baby and to aid in determining the progress of labor
2. To detect any abnormalities such as lack of uterine relaxation, which may reveal the onset of complications
3. To help detect fetal distress by simultaneous observation of contraction and fetal heart rate patterns when internal or external electronic monitors are used
4. To reassure the patient and her family by your presence and interest and, at the same time, to help her better support her labor by

a. Encouraging her and listening

b. Rubbing her back or providing sacral support as desired

c. Helping with relaxation, breathing, or pushing techniques as needed

d. Moistening her lips and offering oral hygiene

e. Changing pillowcases and replacing bed pads

f. Watching for signs of the patient's changing needs (for example, the beginning of the second stage of labor)

g. Assisting the selected labor coach to meet the patient's needs

PROCEDURE:

1. Before going to the bedside, if possible, learn the following about each patient:

   a. Number of pregnancies, viable births, living children

   b. Marital status and any special arrangements for the baby

   c. Whether she has attended childbirth education classes, specific requests regarding labor/birth

   d. Any special complications or problems anticipated

2. The fact that you are feeling her uterus, as it contracts and relaxes under the abdominal wall, to help measure her progress in labor should be explained unless she has previously had contractions timed.

3. Your hands should be clean and not too cold.

4. In the past many labor nurses have been told not to consider the word "pain" as a synonym for the contraction of the uterus because not all contractions are painful and "its use may interfere with positive maternal conditioning for childbirth." Although the term contraction may have a more neutral or constructive connotation, realistic-minded childbirth educators are now cautiously reincorporating the "p-word" into their professional vocabulary. At present, both words are being heard at the bedside spoken by both patient and nurse.

5. If the pregnancy is full-term, the fundus, where the strongest muscular contraction can be felt, will be located about four finger widths above the umbilicus. The nurse's hand should rest lightly there to best detect the uterine contractions.

6. When the uterus contracts, it gradually becomes hard. The degree of hardness is called the *intensity* of a contraction. As the uterus contracts and the uterine muscle fibers shorten, the uterus may be seen or felt to rise in the abdominal cavity. It then gradually relaxes. The time that the uterus is discernibly firm or tight is called the contraction's *duration*. Usually contractions are easier to feel on multiparas than on primiparas because of the differences in abdominal muscle tone.

7. The term *interval* in the timing of contractions is used a bit differently from what is sometimes supposed. The nurse times from the beginning of one contraction to the beginning of the following contraction when using manual assessment.

8. The time between contractions is called the *relaxation time*—a period equally as important as the interval or duration. If the relaxation time is very short or nonexistent, the baby may suffer from lack of oxygen. A continuously contracted, hard uterus may be a symptom of abruptio placentae. Between contractions the fingers should be able to depress the abdominal wall, a sensation similar to depressing a foam rubber pillow.

9. The contraction and relaxation periods and the interval have often been diagrammed as shown in Fig. 7-1. The straight line represents complete relaxation, and the curved line the actual tone of the uterine musculature.

10. Usually a relationship exists between the duration and frequency of uterine contractions and the dilatation of the cervix. It follows *somewhat* the pattern shown in Table 7-1 (1 inch = 2.5 cm).

11. Recording of observations of contractions would include duration, interval, and intensity, as well as possible patient tolerance. For example, "Contractions q 5 minutes for 35 seconds, mild in character. Using abdominal breathing effectively."

12. When electronic monitors are used, instructions for individual models must be consulted. Both external and internal contraction monitors are available. When traced electronically, the frequency of contractions is often stated as the time elapsed between contraction peaks. Monitor strips are evaluated *at least* every 30 minutes and more frequently during labor induction or active labor, or if possible signs of fetal distress occur. (See Figs. 7-5 to 7-7.)

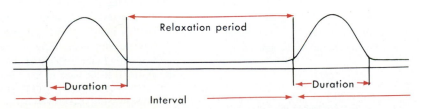

FIG 7-1   Diagram of contraction and relaxation of pregnant uterus.

Table 7-1   Common uterine contraction and dilatation relationships and possible danger signals

Cervical dilatation	Contraction	
	Duration	**Interval**
1. Fingertip to 2 cm	20–30 seconds	6–8 minutes
2. 2 cm → 4 cm	30–35 seconds	5–6 minutes
3. 4 cm → 6 cm	40–50 seconds	4–5 minutes
4. 6 cm → 8 cm	45–60 seconds	3–4 minutes
5. 8 cm → 10 cm	50–90 seconds	2–3 minutes
(Most difficult period, fatigue, nausea, vomiting, irregular, intensive contractions, "transition")		(Tends to be irregular)

Danger signals—report

Contraction duration more than 2 minutes or intensity >100 mm Hg measured by internal monitor
Relaxation period less than 30 seconds
Poor relaxation quality (intrauterine resting tone >20 mm Hg)

FETAL HEART RATE (FHR) EVALUATION

PURPOSE:

1. To help detect the presence of fetal life at the time of admission
2. To detect possible fetal distress

EQUIPMENT NEEDED: Fetal heart rate monitoring may be performed using varied equipment ranging from fairly simple hand-held fetoscopes to rather complex devices capable of continuous eletronic sensitivity and simultaneous visual and printed records. At this writing there is a revival of interest in the study and use of fetal heart monitoring employing frequent intermittent auscultation.*

The following section discusses the use of "manual" fetoscopes, as well as basic principles of simultaneous fetal heart and contraction monitoring.

Manually held monitors—used intermittently:

1. The Leffscope—a stethoscope with a large, heavily weighted bell (Fig. 7-2, *A*)
2. The DeLee-Hollis head scope (Figs. 7-2, *B* and 7-3)
3. An ordinary stethoscope equipped with rubber bands to prevent the sound distortion that results when the bell is handled directly
4. Various "lubricated" ultrasonic fetoscopes, which may amplify the FHR (Fig. 7-2, *C* and *D*), held in the examiner's hand against the abdominal wall

Note: The fetoscopes described in Fig. 1-3 and pictured in Fig. 7-2, *A* and *B*, are not used often anymore, but are included because they may be encountered and should be recognized for their past contributions.

*Freeman R: Intrapartum fetal monitoring—a disappointing story, New Engl J Med 322(9):625, 1990.

PROCEDURE:

1. Explain that you are checking the baby by listening to his heartbeat.
2. Listen to the FHR immediately following a contraction; or better yet, if your patient will allow you, listen during, as well as immediately following, the contraction to hear the heartbeat adequately. This may enable you to detect late deceleration of the heartbeat—a condition thought to be related to fetal distress resulting from uteroplacental insufficiency. (See Fig. 7-5.) However, the pressure exerted on the abdominal wall during a contraction by the manual fetoscope (especially 1, 2, or 3) may be uncomfortable and annoying to mothers and not easily tolerated by many. For this reason a monitor attached to the mother may be at times more helpful than manually held types, and listening immediately following a contraction will probably be the more frequent observation pattern used. Listen for 30 to 60 seconds, if possible. Multiply as necessary to obtain the rate for 1 minute. Every separate beat heard should be counted. It usually sounds like a little watch. At first much concentration will be needed to hear it.
3. Be sure that friction noises from the fingers or the abdominal surface do not distort the sounds. Keep your fingers off the bell. Press firmly on the abdominal wall.
4. The area where the FHR may be heard best is related to the following (Fig. 7-4):
   a. *Presentation*. In headfirst (cephalic) presentations the FHR is found in the lower abdominal quadrants, below the umbilicus. In breech presentations the FHR is usually found at the level of the umbilicus or above.
   b. *Position*. If the back of the infant is toward the mother's left (L.O.A. or L.O.P. position), the FHR will probably be heard best on the mother's left. If it points to her right, the FHR will most frequently be heard

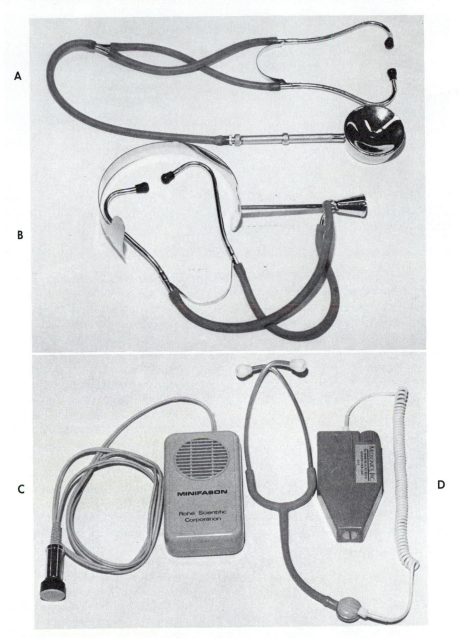

FIG 7-2 **A,** Leffscope. **B,** DeLee-Hollis head scope. **C,** Electronic ultrasound fetoscope amplifies FHR so that it may be heard by all in area. **D,** Electronic ultrasound fetoscope transmits FHR by means of ear pieces. *(Courtesy Grossmont Hospital, La Mesa, Calif.)*

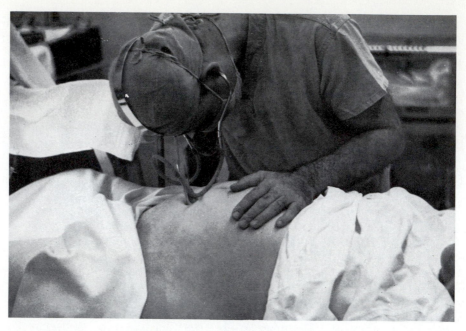

FIG 7-3 Physician listens to fetal heart rate (FHR) shortly before birth. Note location of the scope on abdominal wall. *(Courtesy Grossmont Hospital and Martin M. Greenberg, MD, La Mesa, Calif.)*

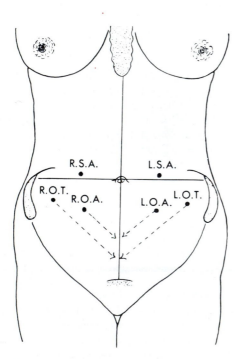

FIG 7-4 Fetal heart tone locations on abdominal wall indicating possible corresponding fetal positions and effects of internal rotation of the fetus.

best on her right. Just because an FHR can be heard in more than one place does not necessarily mean that more than one baby is involved. However, you may want to check by having another nurse listen simultaneously, using a finger-wagging technique to be sure that the pattern heard in both areas is the same.

c. *Station.* As internal rotation and descent occur, the location of the FHR changes, swinging gradually from the right or left quadrants to the midline and dropping until immediately before birth it is found just above the pubic bone.

5. It is recommended that the FHR be taken at 30-minute intervals in the first stage of labor. In the presence of risk factors, the FHR must be monitored every 15 minutes. FHR assessment must always be documented with time indications on an official record. The mother should be told at the time of admittance that a frequent check of the FHR is routine. Early in labor she or her partner may enjoy listening once, too. In the second stage of labor, the FHR of low-risk patients should be evaluated every 15 minutes. Higher-risk patients should be evaluated every 5 minutes during this period.

6. Normal FHR is usually considered to be 120 to 160 beats per minute (bpm). Rates outside this range or a rise or fall of 30 bpm from the usual level of the FHR, noted between contractions (even if still remaining within the normal range), should be reported to the supervising nurse.

Rates determined *between contractions* consistently higher than 160 or showing a 30 bpm baseline increase (fetal tachycardia) may be associated with a variety of problems (for example, maternal fever, fetal hypoxia, and prematurity). Consistent FHR of less than 120 bpm or showing 30 bpm baseline decrease (fetal bradycardia) *not associated with contraction patterns* may signal maternal hypotension. A rate that is too rapid or especially too slow may be a sign of fetal distress. A fetal heart rate under 100 bpm usually signals definite distress. However, even though the heart rate with or without the pressure of a contraction may at no time leave the normal range, significant periods of deceleration or slowing may occur undetected unless the labor is continuously monitored. Certain patterns of deceleration may indicate fetal distress (Fig. 7-5). Precise periods of FHR deceleration are difficult to determine with intermittent monitoring techniques, and therefore continuous monitoring technology has been developed.

7. Other sounds may be heard in the mother's abdomen as well. *Do not mistake them for the fetal heartbeat.*
   a. The maternal pulse may be heard. The nurse should guard against reporting the maternal pulse as the FHR by feeling the mother's radial pulse at the same time as she is listening with a fetoscope. They should be different rhythms and rates.
   b. The increased sound of the pulsation of the uterine arteries can sometimes be identified. Identification of this "sh" sound with the same rhythm as the maternal pulse does not guarantee that the fetus is alive. Sometimes the FHR can be heard at the same time in the background. Move the fetoscope about 2.5 cm (1 inch) to hear the FHR better.
   c. Rarely a sort of soft, whistling sound occurring at the same rate as the fetal heart rate can be heard. This has been called the *funic souffle,* or cord whistle. Some think it is caused by a compression of the cord. Its presence indicates fetal life.
   d. Many laboring mothers are hungry, so the nurse may hear peristalsis!

Monitors attached to mother or fetus for extended or continuous use:

1. External sensors attached to the maternal abdomen to detect the mechanical energy of the fetal heartbeat. These may produce instantaneous visual or audible signals, and when appropriately equipped, they may produce permanent written records. They may be used early in labor before significant cervical dilatation or rupture of the bag of waters. They are simple to use, and there has been no known fetal injury related to their use. However, the position of the sensors may need frequent attention as labor becomes more advanced and accuracy of the recording becomes more difficult to obtain. These FHR sensors may be combined with an externally placed dia-

phragm that is capable of recording the frequency of uterine contractions when held in place with abdominal strapping (Fig. 7-6). Examples are
   a. Small amplifying microphones (phonocardiography) used for antepartum monitoring.
   b. Ultrasonic or Doppler-type instruments that produce characteristic reflected sound waves, which are usually more clear.
2. Fetal electrocardiography to detect the electrical energy associated with fetal heartbeat.
   a. Indirect fetal electrocardiography is possible with electrodes attached to the abdominal wall. It can be used well in early labor, but considerable "electrical noise" may be generated with patient movement during advanced labor, and the recording obtained is inferior to that of direct monitoring.
   b. Direct fetal electrocardiography requires ruptured membranes, 1 to 2 cm of cervical dilatation, and a presenting part no higher than −2 station. A physician or specially trained obstetric nurse attaches the electrode vaginally to the presenting part (scalp or buttock), penetrating the epidermis by a tiny metal spiral or clip. Infection and soft tissue injury are possibilities but have not been significant problems.
3. Uterine contraction patterns interpreted by pressure exerted on a catheter inserted cervically into the uterus just beyond the parietal diameter of the fetal head may be viewed and recorded concurrently with the FHR (Fig. 7-7).

Basic definitions and concepts regarding monitor strip patterns:

1. *Baseline FHR.* The rate determined either before labor begins or during labor in a 10-minute interval exclusive of any periodic changes. Baseline rate is usually 120 to 160 beats per minute. A certain amount of beat-to-beat spacing variation is considered to be an indication of a well-developed, healthy, autonomic nervous control system. It is best evaluated by internal electrode monitors. Baseline variability of less than 5 beats per minute may be a sign of fetal jeopardy, particularly when lack of variability is found in conjunction with periods of late deceleration of the fetal heart. However, reduced variability may also be produced by the administration of certain analgesic or sedative drugs to the mother. Reduced long-term variability may also be found during 20- to 30-minute intervals of so-called fetal sleep or inactivity (Fig. 7-8).
2. *Fetal cardiac deceleration.* Three types of periodic fetal cardiac decelerations, according to their sequential relationships to uterine contractions, have been described and may be detected by continuous monitoring devices. (See Fig. 7-5 for tracings, explanations, and possible therapeutic interventions. Fig. 7-9 shows a central monitor relaying information from two patients.)

CLASSIC FETAL HEART RATE
AND CONTRACTION PATTERNS

Early decelerations (benign)
"Mirror" coincidental contractions; lowest point in
FHR corresponds to peak of contraction curve.
More common between 4 and 7 cm dilation and
second-stage labor.

Late decelerations (ominous)
Mimic somewhat shape of associated contractions,
but onset and lowest point in FHR occur after peak
of contractions. Return to FHR baseline often exceeds 20 seconds after end of contractions. Tachycardia, bradycardia and/or depressed baseline
variability poor signs.

Variable decelerations (varying significance)
Usually V- or U-shaped with abrupt fall and recovery of FHR. Severe if below 70 bpm, last for more
than 30 seconds or if recovery sloped or slow. No
consistent relationship to contraction pattern noted.
Tachycardia, bradycardia, depressed baseline variability poor signs. More common in advanced labor.

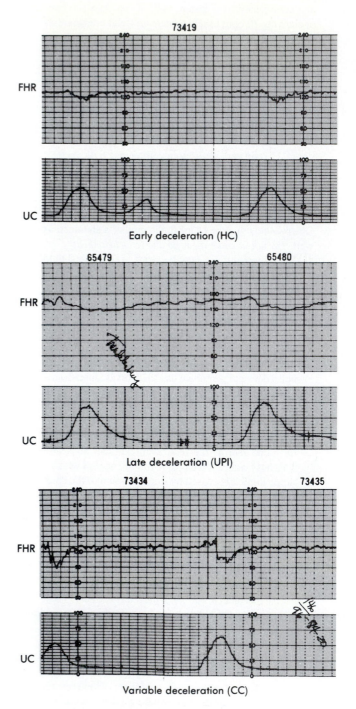

Early deceleration (HC)

Late deceleration (UPI)

Variable deceleration (CC)

FIG 7-5 Fetal heart rate and contraction patterns have been found helpful in evaluating maternal-fetal health during labor. *(Courtesy Berkeley Bio-Engineering, San Leandro, Calif.)*

Intervention

No intervention indicated

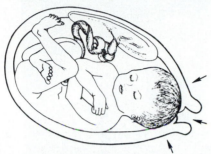

Head compression

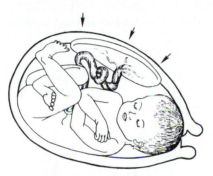

Uteroplacental insufficiency

Notify staff
Turn patient to either side
Oxygen 6 to 8 liters/min
Stop oxytocin infusion
Elevate legs
Possible fetal blood pH
Possible vaginal examination for
scalp stimulation to increase FHR

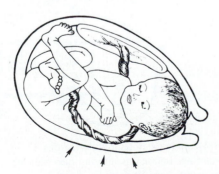

Umbilical cord compression

Notify staff
Turn patient to either side
Possible vaginal examination to
check for and protect prolapsed cord.
Possible fetal blood pH
Oxygen 6 to 8 liters/min

FIG 7-5, cont'd. For legend see opposite page.

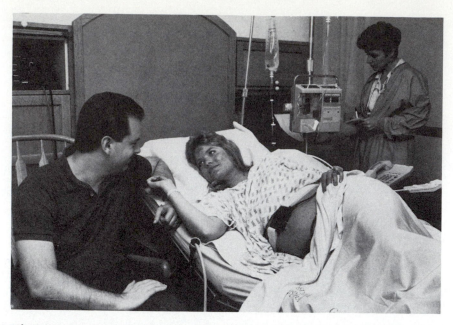

FIG 7-6 The beginning of a labor induction with oxytocin (Pitocin). Double IV set up in place. External contraction monitor positioned over fundus. External fetal heart rate monitor present but not completely visible under sheet. One room was used for all patient care. Mother and baby were discharged directly from the LDRP setting. *(Courtesy Grossmont Hospital, La Mesa, Calif.)*

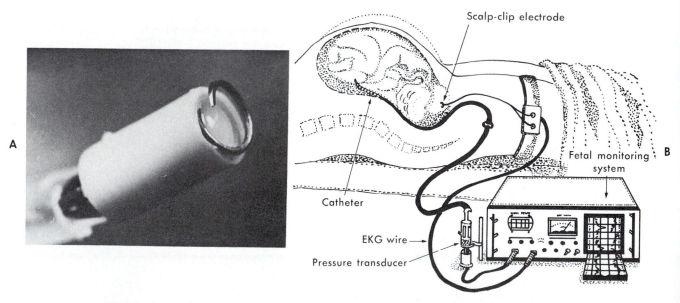

FIG 7-7 A, Spiral electrode sometimes used to attach FHR monitor to fetal presentations. **B,** Diagram of internal fetal heart and contraction monitoring. Internal monitoring may indicate fetal ECG and intensity as well as frequency of uterine contractions. It provides more information but is an intrusive procedure. *(A, Courtesy Corometrics Medical Systems, Inc, Wallingford, Conn.)*

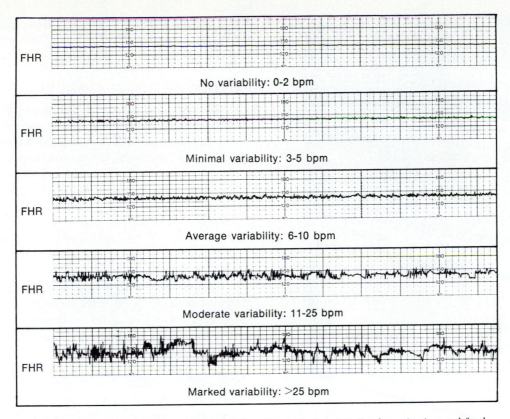

FHR
No variability: 0-2 bpm

FHR
Minimal variability: 3-5 bpm

FHR
Average variability: 6-10 bpm

FHR
Moderate variability: 11-25 bpm

FHR
Marked variability: >25 bpm

FIG 7-8 Degrees of fetal heart rate variability. *(From Tucker SM: Fetal monitoring and fetal assessment in high-risk pregnancy, ed 3, St Louis, 1983, The CV Mosby Co.)*

a. Early fetal cardiac decelerations start at the onset of a contraction and occur only at the same time as the contraction. This pattern is probably due to head compression and increase in the intracranial pressure of the infant. As far as is known, this pattern is harmless. It does not call for an intervention on the part of the obstetric team.

b. Late deceleration patterns are characterized by a slowing of the fetal heart after the peak, or acme, of the uterine contraction and by a delayed return to baseline and a regular waveform reflecting the uterine contraction. They may be found first within the normal FHR range of 120 to 160 beats per mimute. As fetal distress increases, the range and frequency of the FHR deceleration increase. This pattern is frequently associated with uterine hyperactivity caused by oxytocin administration, maternal hypotension, or various high-risk pregnancies. Obstetric interventions to decrease or eliminate fetal distress include stopping any oxytocin administration, providing oxygen by mask or cannula to the mother at 6 to 8 L/min, turning the mother to either side, and possible fetal scalp stimulation.

c. Variable deceleration patterns characterized by a pe-riodic, unpredictable slowing of the FHR that show neither a consistent sequential relationship to the uterine contractions nor a regular repetitive range or duration. The deceleration typically traces a steep-sided V or U. This type of pattern is considered to be the result of umbilical cord compression. Changes in maternal posture, to either side, oxygen administration to the mother, and possible vaginal examination are recommended interventions. A prolonged Trendelenberg position may not be appropriate in some cases, especially if the mother is receiving epidural anesthesia. Other means of decompressing a cord should be sought.

If either late or variable decelerations persist for 30 minutes after the above interventions have been carried out, the physician may consider operative termination of the labor.

3. *Fetal cardiac acceleration.* Periodic accelerations of the FHR are usually considered benign. They are often initiated by fetal movement, uterine contractions, or even maternal abdominal contractions. Indeed, accelerations of the fetal heart rate with fetal movement indicate fetal well-being and serve as the basis of the so-called non-stress test (see p. 513). However, repetitious accelera-

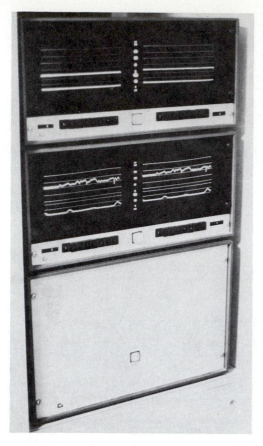

FIG 7-9   A central monitor, which might be seen at a nurse's station, displays FHR and contraction patterns of different patients in labor. *(Courtesy Corometrics Medical Systems, Inc, Wallingford, Conn.)*

tions associated with contractions may occasionally precede the development of progressive late deceleration patterns. For this reason, they should be carefully observed.

Previous comments regarding FHR range also apply with continuous monitoring techniques.*

Other signs of fetal distress. Fetal distress may also manifest itself by the passage of meconium-stained amniotic fluid when the baby is in cephalic presentation; however, this sign is not consistently reliable. Sudden exaggerated fetal movement has at times also been considered a clue of difficulty. In the presence of FHR and contraction patterns that denote possible distress, fetal scalp vein sampling may be used to confirm fetal jeopardy. The presence of an acid-base imbalance in the form of pH

---

*For more detailed discussion of evaluation of FHR patterns, students are referred to Tucker SM: Pocket guide to fetal monitoring, St Louis, 1988, The CV Mosby Co.

values below 7.20 in two or more samples usually indicates fetal acidosis requiring prompt delivery by low forceps or cesarean section.

CONTINUING CARE AND PREPARATION

After admission is completed, unless birth is imminent, a prolonged period of waiting and observation ensues in which the physical and emotional support of the woman and preparation for the birth are paramount. Usually the presence of her mother, husband, or chosen companion at the bedside is a source of support. Often the husband or companion may have trained to be the woman's labor coach and, as such, is extremely important in sustaining the morale and comfort of the parturient. If such visitation is not supportive or if it appears to antagonize or upset the patient, such observations should be reported to the charge nurse or physician. Sometimes arrangements can be made for the visitor to have a "rest"! Table 7-2 shows some of the relationships between stages of labor, patient behavior and coping techniques, and possible nursing care activities.

Several techniques make use of breathing patterns and relaxation as a method to help women cope with the discomfort of labor. Couples who have practiced these techniques in preparation for labor need only occasional reminders. Those who have no preparation benefit from the nurse's instruction and coaching.

Currently, the emphasis is on doing what feels natural versus using rigidly programmed breathing patterns. No one technique is superior to another. Use of any technique is better than using no technique. During first-stage labor, use of a psychoprophylactic technique (see p. 159) promotes relaxation of abdominal and perineal muscles. During second-stage labor, breathing patterns may be used to increase abdominal pressure and assist in expelling the fetus.

When vigorous pushing is required, the woman should not hold her breath longer than 5 to 10 seconds. When she holds her breath longer than this, the exchange of gases across the placenta is greatly reduced.

A summary of some techniques is presented in Table 7-3. Following is an explanation of the terms included:

cleansing or "welcome" breaths Deep breaths usually in through nose and out through mouth; used at beginning and end of exercises to ready body for special breathing, to help relaxation, and to restore normal breathing and gas exchange.

focal point Point or object somewhere in room used as center of visual concentration; may be coach's face, picture,

Table 7-2   The typical woman in normal labor

Stages of labor	Physical and psychologic characteristics, contraction patterns	Suggested activity, including relaxation and breathing techniques	Recommended nursing care, common physician orders
Stage I cervical effacement and dilatation to 10 cm			
Time range Primipara—10 to 12 hours Multipara—6 to 8 hours Early labor 0 to 4 cm	Cervical dilatation begins; minimal show characteristic; contractions variable, approximately 20 to 35 seconds at 5- to 8-minute intervals; possible backache; intensity of contractions increasingly strong but tolerable Alert, talkative, nervous; may welcome diversion, conversation; coach at bedside	If membranes not ruptured: may prefer to be up and about labor room or unit; when contractions cannot be ignored, slow, deep chest or abdominal breathing, and other relaxation techniques If membranes ruptured: if presenting part not engaged—confined to bed; relaxation techniques as above; if possible, turn to side, elevate head slightly; should not remain flat on back	*Admission procedures:* Welcome, orientation, individual patient assessment Review of prenatal records—TPR, BP, FHR; presentation, cervical dilatation, membranes, station, contractions, show Opportunity to void—urine specimen? enema? perineal preparation? electronic monitor application? *Follow-up nursing duties:* TPR at least every 4 hours; BP hourly? FHR, contraction pattern, show, amniotic fluid, labor tolerance every 15 to 30 minutes or less; teach breathing, relaxation IV?—check on need to void every 2 hours or less
Midlabor 4 to 8 cm	Contractions approximately 40 to 60 seconds at 3- to 5-minute intervals; intensity increasing but may still be manageable Becoming less outgoing, more introverted, concentrating on breathing patterns Increased reliance on nurse and coach	Usually confined to bed; more concentration needed; increased emphasis on breathing and relaxation techniques; accelerated shallow panting, effleurage; continued need for encouragement	*Follow-up nursing duties:* As above, evaluation of efficacy of breathing, relaxation, teach simple techniques prn; encourage and praise husband/coach and patient; need for medication? *Other possible nursing responsibilities:* Mouth care, cool cloth, back support, massage, encouragement, aid in maintaining concentration; rectal or vaginal examinations as indicated; prepare delivery room; maintain electronic monitoring, if used
Transition 8 to 10 cm	Most difficult period during labor Fatigued, perhaps nauseated; fears loss of control; contractions may be irregular, very forceful, as frequent as every 2 to 3 minutes, lasting 80 seconds or more; show increases; needs much encouragement	Switching to more intensive breathing patterns—high chest, pant-blow transition techniques	*Scheduled nursing duties:* As above plus increased emotional support, observation for onset of stage II, descent of baby, increased show, complaints of rectal pressure, desire to push, bulging perineum and caput Move multipara to delivery room at 8 cm if +1 or +2 station

Continued.

Table 7-2   The typical woman in normal labor—cont'd

Stages of labor	Physical and psychologic characteristics, contraction patterns	Suggested activity, including relaxation and breathing techniques	Recommended nursing care, common physician orders
Stage II from complete dilatation (10 cm) to birth of baby			
Time range Primipara—30 minutes to 2 hours Multipara—20 minutes to 1½ hours	Cervix completely dilated; patient desires to push; perineum bulging, anus dilated, contractions long but less frequent; show at maximum of normal Encouraged by progress made; using all resources for pushing; perhaps dozing between contractions or intensely aware and alert regarding progress of labor	Pushing patterns Rest, doze between contractions—head elevated if supine	Scheduled nursing duties Check perineum frequently during contractions for signs of progress, FHR every 5 to 10 minutes; stay with patient; move primipara to delivery room when presenting part can be seen at introitus with each contraction; sterile perineal prep; assist physician Possible anesthesia offered; subarachnoid, epidural, pudendal block, local, or general
Stage III from birth of baby to delivery of placenta			
Time range Primipara—5 to 20 minutes Multipara—5 to 20 minutes (time depends on techniques employed)	Excited, extremely anxious and curious about infant; reactions vary according to individual and type of birth preparation and anesthesia received Possible resumption of contractions Separation and delivery of placenta	Inspection and touching of newborn, possible breast-feeding; may recommence pushing to deliver placenta when separation occurs Resting, visiting with husband or companion and baby	Oxytocics as ordered; care for infant, allowing parents to observe; check for abnormality, warmth, eye prophylaxis, identification, cord, Apgar evaluation; assist physician in obtaining cord blood, preparing to suture lacerations or episiotomy as needed; observe mother for relaxed fundus, hemorrhage, problems in delivery of placenta, and interaction with infant
Stage IV from delivery of placenta to postpartum "stabilization"			
Time range 2 to 4 hours	Fundus firm, at or below umbilicus Lochial flow moderate Relieved that labor has ended Animated or exhausted; great individual differences seen	Quiet, recovery period Visit with husband or companion and baby, if possible Refreshing bath Light meal?	Transfer to postpartum recovery area; admission temperature check Provide period for more interaction with infant if desirable BP, P,R, lochial flow and fundus check every 15 minutes for at least 2 hours; ice pack to perineum? Observe for voiding problems Observe response to type of analgesia, anesthesia

Table 7-3 Summary of some suggested breathing and relaxation techniques

Labor phase	Breathing-relaxation techniques, instructions to patient	Suggestions and diagrams
Stage I		

Early
  0 to 4 cm
	Practice distraction
	When contractions cannot be ignored, use deep chest or abdominal breathing
	  1. Cleansing breath
	  2. Focal point
	  3. 6 to 9 slow breaths/min (in nose, out pursed lips)
	  4. Effleurage?
	  5. Cleansing breath
	Possible pelvic rocking, sacral support
	Relaxation checks
		If possible (membranes intact), stay up—walk, play games, plan a vacation, make out the grocery list, etc.
		
		30 to 40 second contraction
		Inhale
		Exhale ⊢——1 minute——⊣
		∧∨ Deep, cleansing breath
		∧∧∧ Deep breathing, 6 to 9/min

Midlabor
  4 to 8 cm
	Begin when needed:
	Accelerated-decelerated shallow panting
	  1. Cleansing breath
	  2. Focal point
	  3. Rhythmic slow acceleration-deceleration with contraction
	  4. Effleurage
	  5. Cleansing breath
	Sacral support
	Relaxation checks
	Increasing coach support
		Mouth care
		Cool cloth
		
		40 to 60 second contraction
		∧∧ Shallow breathing

Transition
  8 to 10 cm
	Begin when needed:
	Pant-blow breathing
	  1. Cleansing breath
	  2. Focal point
	  3. 4 to 6 shallow breaths, then short blow during length of contraction
	  4. Cleansing breath
	Intensified coach support
		Mouth care
		Cool cloth
		
		60 to 90 second contraction
		∧∧∧∧ Pant/blow breathing

Continued.

Table 7-3 Summary of some suggested breathing and relaxation techniques—cont'd

Labor phase	Breathing-relaxation techniques, instructions to patient	Suggestions and diagrams

Stage II

From complete dilatation to birth of baby

Breathing techniques that enhance bearing down efforts

Natural	Vigorous
Begin when urge to bear down is present	Begin when completely dilated
Use any position preferred	1. Cleansing breath
1. Push only when urge to push is felt	2. Elevate head and back; second deep breath
2. Push only during expiration with glottis open	3. Hold no longer than 5 to 10 seconds, trapping air in chest; bend and drop knees to side; pull on thighs, knees, or bed rails while pushing down; keep hips motionless on bed
3. Push no longer than 5 to 6 seconds	4. Take another breath
4. Do a series of short pushes with each contraction	5. Repeat 3 and 4 until contraction is over
Recommended to avoid fetal hypoxia and maternal fatigue	6. Cleansing breath
Indicated when fetus is at risk (compromised)	Rest; doze between contractions
	Recommended to shorten second stage when necessary and when regional block is used

furniture, etc; serves to maintain cerebral input; patient should preferably not close eyes during contraction.

effleurage Light, patterned abdominal massage usually done with tips of fingers

sacral support Counterpressure exerted to lift sacrum slightly off bed if patient is supine, or firm lower back pressure; may use hands, towels, rolling pins, etc.

pelvic rock Alternately increasing and flattening the lumbar sacral curve of the back

Early labor

The woman in early labor (usually defined as up to 4 cm dilatation) is characteristically alert, talkative, and nervous. She is generally most eager to cooperate with the physician and nursing staff in attendance and responds readily to a calm, cheerful nurse who seems genuinely interested in her welfare. Her contractions, though perhaps uncomfortable, are tolerable. If her membranes are not ruptured, her contractions are not very frequent or intensive, and show is not remarkable, she will probably appreciate being up and around for a while and not automatically confined to her bed just because she has been admitted to the hospital. It has been found that when she does rest in bed, there is less interference with maternal and fetal circulation, increased urinary function, and greater uterine efficiency if she reclines on her side. However, it is true that a number of nursing observations and procedures (manual fetal heart rate determination and

checking the dilatation or perineum) may be more easily carried out if the patient turns to the supine position intermittently. Later in labor, during transition and while the mother is pushing, a semisitting position may be preferred. However, other postures, upright or squatting, may be used in some settings.

If the patient is going to be supine for an appreciable length of time, the head of the bed should be elevated approximately 30 degrees to prevent circulatory and respiratory disturbances. She should conserve her physical and nervous energy for the more demanding period of labor to come. Her temperature, pulse, and respiration should be documented at least every 4 hours and more often if individual history or indications warrant it. Blood pressure should be recorded routinely every hour. Fetal heart tones should be checked at 30-minute intervals or less during the first stage of labor and with increasing frequency as labor progresses. (See p. 116.) The amount and character of any show or amniotic drainage, if present, should be noted. At times a question of whether the bag of waters has broken may exist. It is important to try to determine the time of its rupture, since the possibility of uterine infection after rupture becomes greater as the hours go by before birth. Such a situation may be detrimental to both mother and child. To find out whether any vaginal leakage is amniotic fluid, the nurse (before any antiseptic or lubricant other than water is used on the perineal area) may gently insert a sterile applicator or gloved finger into the vaginal canal to be moistened by the fluid present. It is then pressed against a strip of phenaphthazine (Nitrazine paper). If the paper turns blue indicating alkaline drainage, the moisture is probably amniotic fluid—if it is uncontaminated by blood. A yellow or acidic reaction usually indicates urine.

RUPTURE OF THE MEMBRANES (SPONTANEOUS)

If the bag of waters breaks at any time while the patient is in the labor area (if not ruptured before admission), she should be instructed not to get out of bed or sit up completely. The nurse inspects the perineum for signs of a prolapsed cord or, in the case of advanced labor, evaluates signs of the advance of the presenting part (bulging perineum, appearance of the fetal scalp) and the amount and color of the amniotic fluid.

Normal fluid is very light yellow. If there is any meconium (infant stool) in the fluid, staining it a brownish yellow to gray-black, it should be reported immediately. Meconium-stained amniotic fluid during cephalic presentations is considered a sign of fetal distress—the response of the fetus to oxygen lack. Such staining during a breech presentation is usually not considered significant, since the pressure exerted on a breech during its passage through the pelvic canal may cause the discharge of meconium, and no real fetal distress may be involved. The appearance of red-tinged amniotic drainage, old, dark blood, bright red, frank bleeding, or blood clots at any time during labor should also be reported. Fetal heart tones should be checked immediately after the rupture of the membranes to try to detect possible cord prolapse and compression. The fact that the bag of waters appears to have ruptured should be reported to the charge nurse immediately. Contractions should be frequently evaluated, depending on the progress the patient seems to be making.

Evaluation of progress

Rectal or vaginal examinations. Proof of the labor progress may be gained through rectal or vaginal examinations. Vaginal examinations have been increasingly employed because of the greater accuracy and helpfulness of the information obtained and the lack of infectious complications observed when they are performed appropriately. (In most maternity departments, the rectal examination has been abandoned.) Pelvic examinations should be kept to a minimum because of the discomfort to the patient and the possibility of introduction of infection. Student nurses are not routinely taught the techniques of rectal or vaginal examinations. To instruct all students in the techniques would be useless because unless these techniques are practiced frequently, the ability to interpret what is felt is never learned or is easily lost. In addition, the patient would have the discomfort of duplicate examinations.

Vocational nurses or practical nurses (LVN/LPN) frequently assist the physician and patient during rectal or vaginal examinations. Whether or not a LVN/LPN performs either evaluation would depend on the state and agency rulings governing practice.

The patient is usually supine with head elevated slightly for either rectal or vaginal examination. The attending nurse prepares and assists the patient and helps her to relax during the examinations. If a rectal approach is to be used, only clean gloves and lubricant are needed. If a vaginal examination is desired, preparatory procedures differ from institution to institution and physician to physician. In some instances the patient is cleansed and draped as for delivery, and the physician may scrub his hands with a brush before putting on sterile gloves. In other hospitals the preparation may not be so elaborate. However, certain principles should always be observed. The vulva should be cleansed. The examiner's hands should be carefully washed. A sterile examining glove should be used. A sterile lubricant and disinfectant per physician's order should be poured over the gloved fingers and vulva. Care should be taken in inserting the fingers not to touch anything but the actual vaginal canal so that organisms from anal or other areas are not introduced into the canal. Usually it helps if the patient drops her knees toward the outside and breathes deeply through her open mouth during the digital examination. Holding the nurse's hand seems to give some patients great comfort, too.

After the examinations, the patient's perineal area should be cleansed of any remaining lubricant or antiseptic, and dried and she should be encouraged and reassured. A vaginal examination can reveal information not detected by a rectal examination because the cervix and presenting part are felt directly by the fingers and not through the rectovaginal wall. It may help greatly in the determination of the type of presentation, the position, and the condition of the bag of waters. Pelvic evaluations should not be performed routinely if abnormal vaginal bleeding is observed, because such examinations may increase blood loss.

Rupture of the membranes (artificial). At times, in an effort to induce or hasten labor or to apply an internal monitor lead, the physician artificially ruptures the membranes during a vaginal examination. This is done, however, only under certain conditions. The cervix should be effaced, and some dilatation must be present. The head should be engaged. The physician ordinarily uses a sterile instrument with a small clawlike end, such as an Allis, Iowa, or special plastic hook. The membranes are ruptured between contractions, and the fluid flow is controlled to avoid the cord being swept out of place by a sudden gush of "water." Prolapse of the cord and its subsequent pinching between the presenting part and the bony pelvis is a serious complication for which one must watch. As always, immediately after the membranes have ruptured, the fetal heart rate should be checked to determine any distress of the fetus.

The actual rupture of the bag causes no pain because there are no nerves in the membranes, but the pressure exerted to perform the vaginal examination and to position the instrument may cause some discomfort. The patient should be encouraged especially during this period. If rupture of the membranes is anticipated at the time of a vaginal examination, the patient should be placed on several bed-protecting pads to catch the drainage. Some advocate placing the patient on a bedpan; however, the patient's discomfort is usually increased in such a position. The approximate amount (small, moderate, or large) of fluid expelled and its color should be noted and recorded. Remember, the appearance of meconium in the amniotic fluid during a head presentation is interpreted as a sign of fetal distress. After the examination the patient should be made as comfortable as possible. The excess lubricant should be wiped from the vulva, using good technique (wiping from front to back with no return of a used sponge to the vaginal region). Dry protective bed pads should be in place. If the presenting part of the baby is tight against the cervix and the physician so orders, the laboring mother may be allowed to ambulate.

Intensified labor: characteristics and care

As labor progresses, more frequent and intensive contractions are experienced. More and more, the woman's attention is focused on meeting the demands of these contractions on her physical and psychologic resources. If she has had training in relaxation and breathing techniques, these usually are of great aid. Some abdominal and high chest breathing exercises are described in Table 7-3. If a laboring patient has had no previous training in these techniques, she may still benefit from some simple instruction in abdominal breathing. This usually eases the discomfort significantly. Rapid breathing techniques

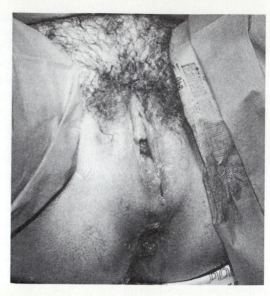

FIG 7-10 Note bulging of perineum and appearance of fetal head (caput). *(Courtesy Grossmont Hospital and Martin M. Greenberg, MD, La Mesa, Calif.)*

can also be taught; but if the woman is unfamiliar with the method, she is likely to hyperventilate, and the normal proportion of oxygen to carbon dioxide in the blood will be upset. She may feel light-headed, and her fingers may begin to tingle. Such side effects should be avoided. If they appear, it may help if she breathes into a paper bag or places the sheet momentarily over her nose. The patient should be especially encouraged, and signs of her progress and condition should be frequently shared with family members.

Probably the most difficult period of labor is that called *transition,* lasting approximately from 8 to 10 cm dilatation. The laboring patient is now fatigued and usually discouraged. She wonders if she is ever going to have her baby and worries about her performance when she does. Her contractions may be irregular, at times seeming to come "one right after another." Nausea and vomiting are common. She is usually most grateful for the presence of the nurse or labor coach, who can help tremendously by offering firm back rubs, sacral support, cool, fresh pillowcases, damp clean gauze sponges to ease the dry mouth, oral hygiene, or a cool cloth on the forehead. The husband or the chosen companion can often help with these simple methods of relieving distress. The nurse should offer the bedpan at intervals to be sure her bladder does not become distended. Distention may delay descent or traumatize the bladder, causing edema of the trigone area and inability to void in the postpartal period.

Signs of the second stage of labor. During this period the patient needs to be evaluated frequently concerning the possibility of the onset of the second stage of labor, the period of expulsion. The physician and other delivery room personnel should be kept informed of the patient's progress. The second stage will ordinarily be heralded by (1) an increase in show, (2) an involuntary urge to push or bear down with each contraction as the presenting part escapes the uterus and descends, (3) the fetal heart tone usually being heard just above the pubic bone in head presentations, and (4) late signs, including the bulging of the perineum, the dilatation of the anus, and the appearance of caput, or the fetal scalp (Fig. 7-10). It is fervently hoped that a multipara will be adequately prepared for the actual birth before these last signs manifest themselves. Usually, multiparas are transferred to the delivery room at about 8 cm dilatation to avoid a last-minute race. However, women bearing their first babies are often not transferred to the delivery room proper before these last signs appear, since the period between complete dilatation and the birth of the infant may be relatively protracted for a primipara. One reason the "birthing room" concept is popular is that it avoids transfers of patient from one room to another for different stages of labor. Such transfers can be quite difficult at times.

Most hospitals in the United States now allow fathers or the expectant mother's chosen companion in the delivery room, especially those who have attended childbirth education classes. The excitement and wonder of the occasion are appropriately shared with these significant persons. The father sits at the head of the delivery table, encouraging the mother in her efforts and watching with her the progress of the birth in an overhead mirror. For most couples, sharing the moment of birth together appears to create a "natural high" that they never forget. However, the father or companion will have previously agreed to leave in the event of problems when his presence is thought to compromise the best interests of the mother. Not all men want to see their children born, but for those who do, it seems to be a memorable, positive experience.

Pushing. Although she may wish to do so, a woman usually should not be urged by the nurse to bear down or push before complete dilatation of the cervix is determined. To do so could cause greater fatigue for the mother, greater strain on the fetus, and possible swelling

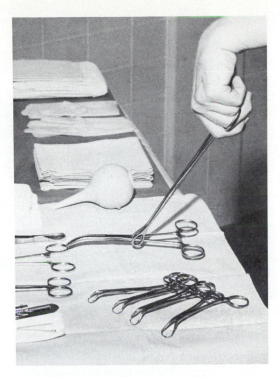

FIG 7-11 Lifting sterile instruments. For beginners this is a good grip. The instrument is balanced and the hand is far from surface of table. Sterile supply tables may also be prepared using sterile gloves instead of sterile transfer forceps. *(Courtesy Grossmont Hospital, La Mesa, Calif.)*

and injury to the cervix. After complete dilatation and preparations for the birth are made, pushing is usually recommended. Most women are relieved by pushing and cooperate well in following instructions if they are not confused by too many instructors. (See Table 7-3.)

Preparation of the delivery room
(Figs. 7-11 to 7-14)

Before the second stage of labor is reached, the delivery room should be prepared for the actual birth of the baby. The responsibility of its preparation may be that of a trained vocational nurse. Hers is an important responsibility. To execute it correctly, she must have a clear concept of the principles of sterile technique, know where supplies are kept, and know the patient's special needs and the attending physician's desires. She should have some idea when the room will be needed so that she can plan her work. The actual preparation of the delivery room will vary in different maternity services,

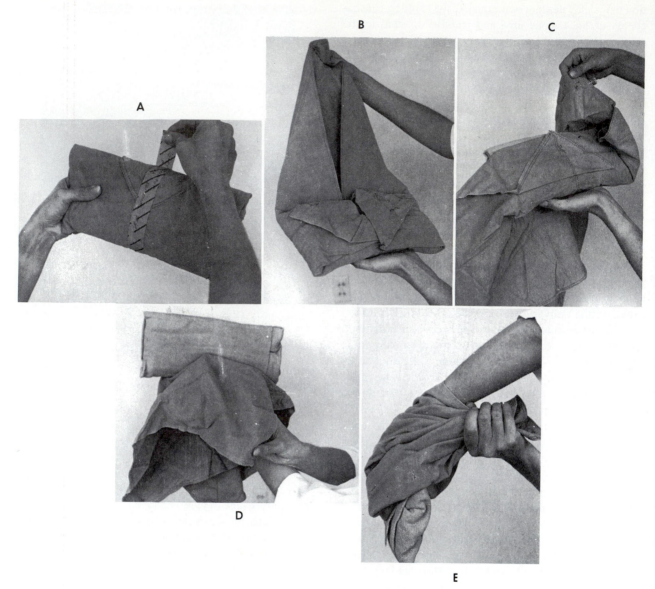

FIG 7-12 Opening sterile packages. **A,** Remove heat-sensitive tape closing package, checking tape for color change, label, and date. Start unwrapping package with point of the wrapper facing you. In this way the part of package next to you will remain covered and protected for longest period possible. **B,** Pull back the point and let it drop down after assuring yourself that outside of dangling wrapper will not contaminate any nearby sterile surface. **C,** Pull back two side folds by little turnbacks designed for your use. Uncover the end on side of supporting hand first, then the side next to active hand. If you are preparing inner package for drop onto sterile surface, stabilize pack by bringing your thumb over top of wrapper before completely exposing inner pack. **D,** Pull back the last fold covering inner wrap to expose sterile surface. The inner pack can now be picked up by gloved associate or it can be "scooted" onto sterile table while the ends of outer wrapper are held back to prevent contamination. **E,** if hand-thumb grip is used, the pack can be dropped in manner pictured. Care must be taken not to get too close to sterile table or field while adding supplies. *(Courtesy Grossmont Hospital, La Mesa, Calif.)*

but the basic needs to be met and the principles employed will be the same.

Capsule review of principles and practice of aseptic technique. The practice of asepsis is not really difficult if the appropriate equipment and supplies are available and if conscientious, knowledgeable persons are involved in their use and care. It is, however, a serious responsibility that involves evaluation of the area environment, including the nurses' dress and personal health problems that may threaten the safety of the patient. Four simple rules sum up aseptic technique:

1. Know what is sterile.
2. Know what is not sterile.
3. Keep the two apart.
4. Remedy contamination immediately.*

Using transfer forceps. The use of transfer forceps, or "pickups," in the handling of sterile supplies is as safe as the techniques employed for their care. Because wet forceps often become contaminated, their use has all but disappeared. When used, any wet forceps should be held so that the grasping ends are pointed downward. If wet forceps are used, care should be taken not to touch the ends of the instrument on any exposed inner side of the holding canister. The area above the level of solution cannot be considered sterile because of prolonged exposure to the air. In some areas a fresh, dry, sterile canister and forceps may be used for each birth setup (Fig. 7-11). Transfer forceps should not be held below the level of the waist or above the shoulder. Today, the nurse commonly wears sterile gloves to set up the delivery supply table.

General considerations. Review the methods of unwrapping and placing supplies (Fig. 7-12). When approaching a sterile field to add sterile supplies, take care to avoid accidentally brushing or touching the area. When passing a sterile field, keep a safe distance away and, if possible, face the field. Never turn your back on a sterile area. Avoid turning your back toward an associate who is gowned in a sterile manner.

If contamination of a sterile area does occur, the event must be immediately reported. It is no terrible sin to contaminate. It is dangerous and irresponsible to contaminate a sterile field, to know it, and to do nothing about it when something can be done. No one at the time may see the lapse of asepsis, but ultimately the patient may suffer from its results. The medical-nursing team should be glad to have breaks in technique or inadvertent

*Hoeller ML: Surgical technology: basis for clinical practice, ed 3, St Louis, 1974, The CV Mosby Co.

contamination called to their attention so that they may correct the situation.

DELIVERY ROOM SETUP REMINDER
(Figs. 7-13 and 7-14)

PURPOSE: The purpose of this procedure is threefold:

1. To provide an aseptic field for the anticipated birth and subsequent newborn and maternal care
2. To ensure the convenient placement and operation of all necessary articles to promote safety, speed, and confidence on the part of the staff in behalf of the physical and emotional care of the mother and child
3. To aid in the necessary legal and statistical recording of the event

SETUP:

1. Personal preparation
   a. Secure information.
      (1) Which physician (for glove size, etc.)
      (2) Which delivery room
      (3) Type of anesthesia to be used, if any anticipated
      (4) Special problems involving the patient (Rh-negative, preeclampsia, varicosities of the extremities, etc.)
      (5) Approximate time the room is needed
   b. Put on mask. Be sure all your hair is covered by a cap.
   c. Wash hands.
   d. Review in your mind the principles of sterile technique.
2. Open necessary sterile packs. Check outside tapes on packs for proof of sterilization if this type of tape is used. Check dates on packs to avoid outdated materials. Usually included are
   a. The basic delivery pack with drapes and materials used on the patient or for the delivery
   b. The instrument pack (unless instruments are taken directly from a sterilizer)
   c. The basin-set pack, used to provide a sterile basin for the placenta and a sterile basin for lubricating obstetric forceps, rinsing gloved hands, or cleansing the patient
   d. The perineal preparation tray may provide
      (1) A cleansing solution
      (2) Sterile gauze sponges
      (3) Sterile gloves or sponge sticks
      (4) An antiseptic for the skin after the cleansing of the area (This is not always used.)
   e. The anesthesia supplies (if appropriate)
   f. Any indicated obstetric forceps are usually placed conveniently (still wrapped) in the room until called for, except Piper forceps used in breech deliveries for the aftercoming head. Piper forceps are usually unwrapped previously and placed on the supply table.

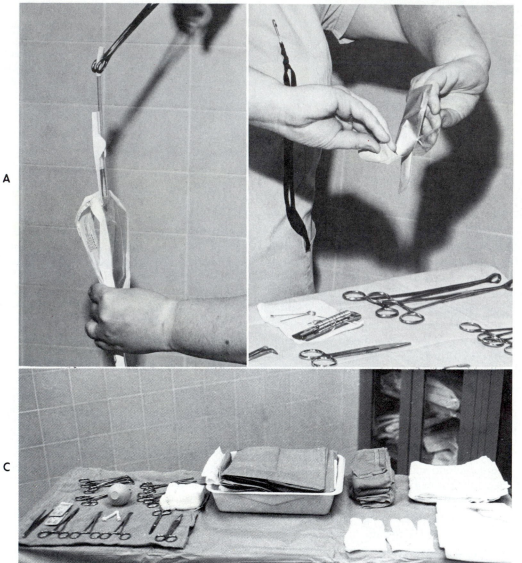

FIG 7-13 **A,** Extracting sterile catheter from commercially prepared peel-back package. **B,** Dropping sterile suture from commercially prepared peel-back package. **C,** One way to set up basic delivery room table. *(Courtesy Grossmont Hospital, La Mesa, Calif.)*

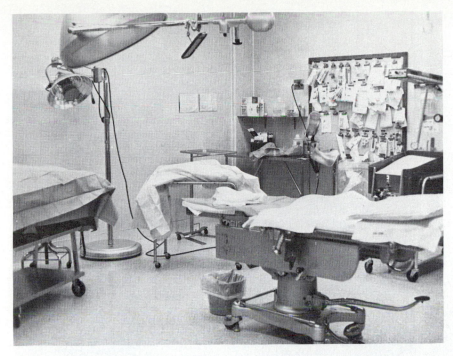

FIG 7-14 View of so-called traditional delivery room. The patient labors elsewhere and is transferred to the delivery room when birth is expected fairly soon. After giving birth she is transferred again to receive care in a recovery or postpartal area. Not seen are anesthetic machine and maternal and fetal monitors.

3. Check infant care equipment and supplies (warmer, suction, oxygen and bulb syringe, blankets, nurse's gown, and examination gloves).
4. At the time of the birth the necessary records are brought into the room for completion, and the identification procedures for mother and child are carried out.

Transfer and immediate predelivery care

The transfer of the patient to the delivery room should be as smooth as possible. If the patient has a strong desire to push and it is not appropriate activity at the time, she should be advised to pant through her open mouth. Care should be taken in the transfer of the patient. She can usually help considerably in the move to the delivery table if the staff is able to wait until a contraction is not present. It is imperative that observation and recording of maternal pulse and blood pressure as well as FHR patterns continue in a consistent manner (at least every 15 minutes) after the patient has been transferred to the delivery room, whether a vaginal or cesarean birth is expected.

While the patient is being prepared in the delivery room, the physician may be dressing and scrubbing for the administration of the spinal anesthesia, if used, or for the delivery itself. Many obstetric units currently have anesthesiologists on staff to assist with deliveries. The circulating nurse uncovers the sterile table and basin set and turns on the necessary lights. If no spinal anesthesia is used, the physician generally advises the staff when the patient should be placed in dorsal lithotomy position with her legs in supports, if this position is used.

Positioning. Ideally, two nurses assist in lithotomy positioning, although it can be accomplished by one. To prevent strain on the patient's back, both legs should be raised or lowered at the same time. Coaching her to bend her knees as her legs are raised helps. If crutch or stirrup-type leg supports are used, the supports must be fitted to the patient, not the patient fitted to the supports! Most delivery tables have some method of dividing in half, temporarily eliminating the foot portion of the table to allow the buttocks to hang over the end of the upper part of the table and the physician to stand directly in front of the perineum. As soon as the patient's legs are adequately secured in the supports, the table is so adjusted.

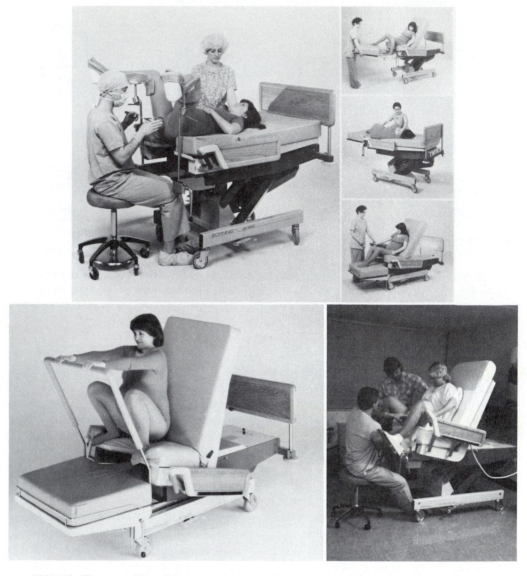

FIG 7-15 The versatility of the maternity bed called "Genesis" and specialized maternity furniture (beds, tables, and chairs) are popular now. Some maternity services remove the head board permanently to allow easy access to the patient's head by an anesthesiologist. *(Courtesy Borning Corporation, Spokane, Wash.)*

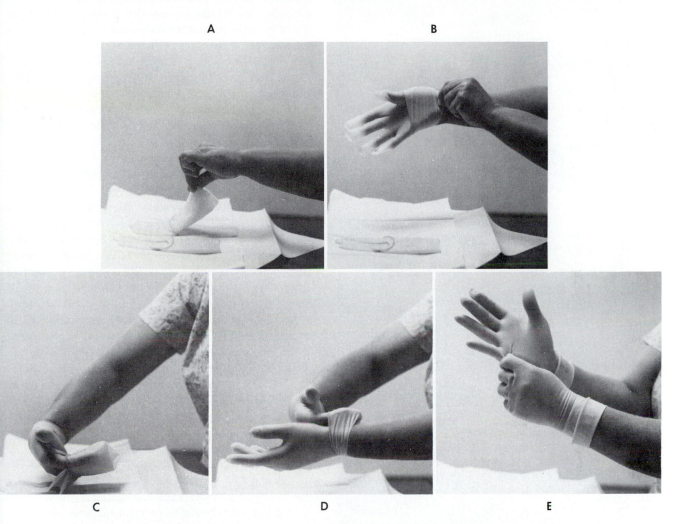

A   B

C   D   E

FIG 7-16 Gloving procedure. **A,** Sterile gloves usually lie side by side with thumbs on top at outside edges, the left glove on left and the right glove on right. Pick up glove by pinching cuff folded down over palm of glove. If right-handed, slide right-hand glove on first. Your bare fingers may touch any area of the glove that represents inside of glove. **B,** Slide your hand in with rotating motion while pulling on turned-down cuff. **C,** Pick up second glove with gloved hand by sliding your sterile fingers *under* turned-down cuff. **D,** Place your other hand into glove, sliding and rotating your hand as you pull out and up against inside of cuff with your gloved fingers. Keep your thumb back out of the way. Remember, your arm and top of cuff are contaminated and must not be touched with your fingers. When only gloves are worn, it is permissible to retain narrow cuffs at tops of gloves, but they are not sterile and should not be treated as such. **E,** After you are gloved, you may adjust fingers. Learning to glove takes time, patience, and usually more than one pair of gloves. (*Courtesy Grossmont Hospital, La Mesa, Calif.*)

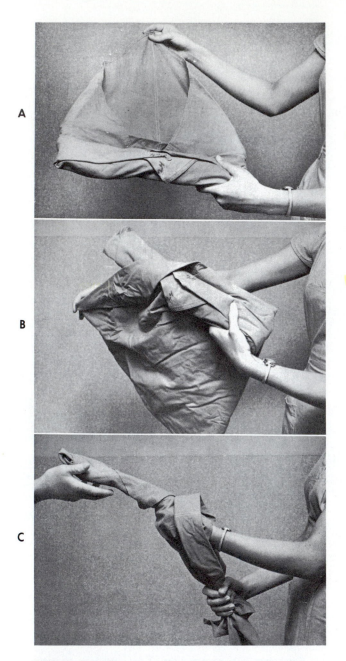

FIG 7-17 Steps in unwrapping sterile forceps to hand to physician. **A,** Grasp one end of package, remove outer tape, and unwind outer wrapper. **B,** Pull back inner turnback at top of package and continue to uncover inner wrap (like peeling a banana!). **C,** Grasp carefully all dangling ends of outer wrap and pull them out of the way toward your wrist. Do not touch inner wrap. *(Courtesy Grossmont Hospital, La Mesa, Calif.)*

This is called "dropping" or "breaking" the table.

Giving birth in lithotomy position is not an anatomic necessity, but it is the position that is associated with the use of spinal or general anesthesia and is the most familiar to many physicians in the United States. In England, a modified side position is often used. In some cultures the mother gives birth in a squatting position. In parts of Europe a modified Fowler's position is typically used, with flexion and abduction of the lower extremities. These last two postures allow gravity to aid the mother in her efforts to push the baby to the outside world. Special adjustable combination labor-delivery beds or chairs are now available that assist the mother to maintain a more physiologic birth position (Fig. 7-15).

Sterile perineal preparation. As soon as the table is "dropped," the circulating nurse cleanses the abdomen, thighs, and complete perineal area with a soap or antiseptic solution. This procedure is the so-called sterile prep. Again, it is carried out in different ways in different institutions. It may involve sterile gloving or the use of sterile forceps or sponge sticks (Fig. 7-16). The principles are the same: to help prevent infection and to increase the visibility of the area involved. In performing the prep to prevent contamination of the birth canal, care should be taken to ensure that no sponge is used in the anal-rectal area and then returned to the vulvar region. Usually the first sponge is used to cleanse side to side from the pubic bone to the umbilicus. It is then discarded. The second and third sponges are used in cleansing the thighs with an up-and-down motion from the labia majora to the midthigh. Each is discarded directly after use. The fourth and fifth sponges are used to clean the labia on the right and left of the vagina, avoiding the rectum, and then discarded. The last cleansing sponge passes directly over the vagina and anus.

The patient may be rinsed and dried in a similar manner and perhaps sprayed or painted with an antiseptic. The purpose of the prep should be kept in mind. The object is not to go through so many prescribed motions but to clean the skin. On the other hand, it must be performed rather swiftly, or the baby may be there before one is finished. The gowned physician is usually ready to drape for delivery as soon as the nurse is finished. Care must be taken to see that the physician's hands and gown are not contaminated as the nurse completes the prep.

Draping. During the draping procedure, the circulating nurse provides a stool for the physician, pushes the sterile supply table and double basin rack into position,

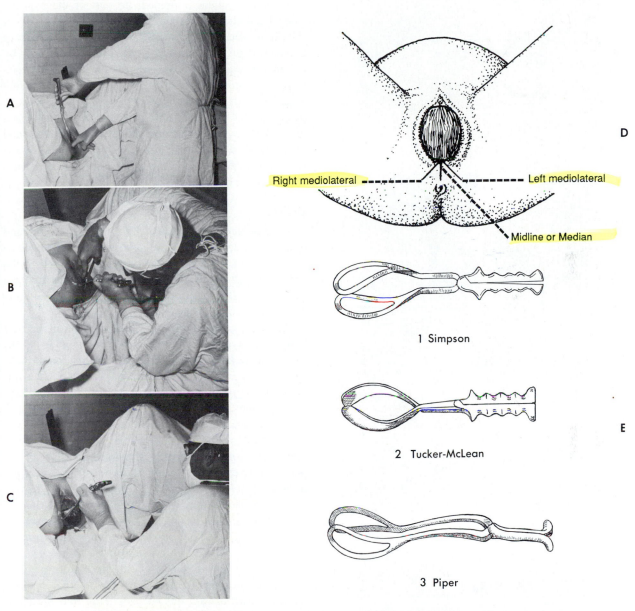

Right mediolateral

Left mediolateral

Midline or Median

D

1 Simpson

2 Tucker-McLean

3 Piper

E

FIG 7-18 **A,** Insertion of one forceps blade. **B,** Midline episiotomy (one blade of the forceps has been inserted). **C,** Use of outlet forceps. **D,** Various types of episiotomies. **E,** Three kinds of obstetrical forceps: *1,* Simpson; *2,* Tucker-McLean; *3,* Piper (sometimes employed to deliver after-coming head of breech presentation). *(A to C, Courtesy Wayne B. Henderson, MD, San Diego.)*

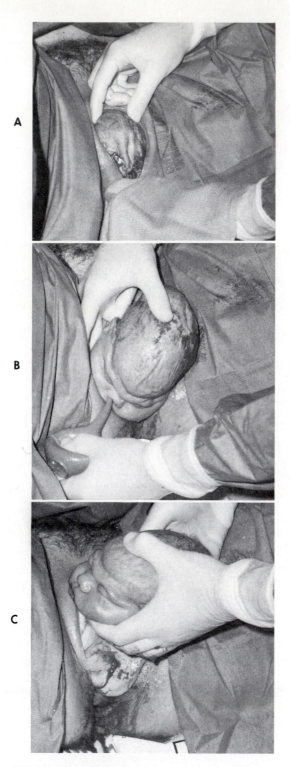

FIG 7-19 Delivery sequence L.O.A. **A,** Crowning. **B,** Delivery of head and clearing of airway, mouth, then nose. **C,** Delivery of posterior shoulder. *(Courtesy Grossmont Hospital and Mark A. Treger, MD, La Mesa, Calif.)*

adjusts the light and mirror (if being used), unwraps the forceps if they are desired, secures any needed additional supplies, and begins her record of the delivery.

After the patient is draped, no part of the exposed side of the sterile linen (or paper) covering the patient should be touched by anyone not properly gloved or gowned. If pressure must be exerted on the abdomen by a "nonsterile attendant" for any reason, she must reach under the sterile drape, avoiding the exposed perineum to accomplish her task. After the baby is born, if he is placed on his mother's abdomen, the nurse may reach under the covering drape and, using the drape as a hand guard, hold on to an infant arm or leg to help give support while his airway is aspirated or the cord is tied. Babies can be very slippery.

Delivery

Forceps and episiotomies. After the sterile prep and draping are complete, if the mother's bladder needs to be emptied or a special urine specimen is necessary, the physician will perform a catheterization before the birth of the baby. But the procedure is no longer as common before delivery as it once was.

At times, especially if the mother is bearing her first baby, the physician may use *outlet forceps* (Fig. 7-18) to lift out the baby's head. Judicious application of these forceps may shorten the second stage of labor considerably if the mother is finding it difficult to push effectively or the baby's or mother's condition makes more rapid delivery advisable. However, the use of outlet forceps just to save time is questionable. Forceps are usually applied in conjunction with a planned incision of the perineum to enlarge the vaginal opening called an *episiotomy.*

An episiotomy may be performed without the use of forceps. It is done to prevent lacerations or damage to the perineum, to avoid possible prolonged pressure on the infant's head, and to hasten delivery. There are two main types of episiotomies: (1) the midline or median, which features an incision from the vaginal opening straight down toward but not extending into the anus, and (2) the mediolateral, which begins at the midline above the anus but angles to the left or right. (Fig. 7-18, *D*). The midline type is said to be easier to repair and more comfortable for the mother but occasionally it may extend during the birth, tearing the anal sphincter. The mediolateral type of episiotomy is designed to prevent this complication but is considered more difficult to repair and usually is more painful during the postpartum period. The *routine* use of outlet forceps and/or episi-

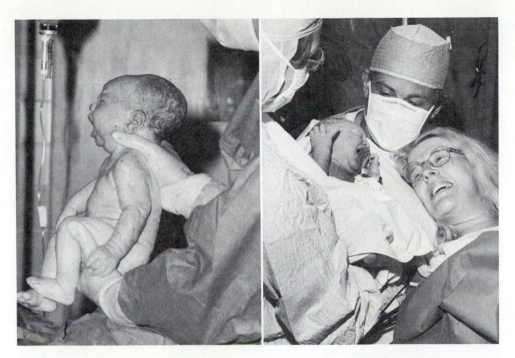

FIG 7-20   A long-awaited personal introduction! It's good to have Father there for this special moment. *(Courtesy Grossmont Hospital, Mark A. Treger, MD, and Martin M. Greenberg, MD, La Mesa, Calif.)*

otomy is controversial and has stirred considerable debate.* The birth of many babies does not involve the use of either forceps or episiotomy.

Rather rarely, other types of forceps may be used to achieve progress at delivery associated with head rotation or midforceps application. High forceps (historically applied before engagement has taken place) are never recommended in modern obstetrics.

Delivery mechanisms (Figs. 7-19 and 7-20). If forceps are not used for the complete delivery of the head, it may be delivered manually between contractions by slow gentle extension. If the mother is able, she may be asked to bear down between contractions to facilitate the actual passage of the head from the vaginal canal. After the head is delivered, the physician checks to see whether the umbilical cord is wound around the baby's neck. If it is, it must be slipped over the baby's head or clamped and cut to avoid strangulation or excessive pulling. Even before the entire body of the baby is delivered, the mouth may be aspirated to clear the airway. To deliver the shoul-

ders, the physician usually turns the baby's head to the side so that the occiput lines up with his back. The physician may then gently but firmly pull down to deliver the top (anterior) shoulder and then gently pull up to deliver the bottom (posterior) shoulder. Scarcely before one realizes it, all of the baby has been born. Further aspiration of the airway may be necessary. Usually the infant cries very soon after birth. His umbilical cord is clamped in two places and cut between the clamps. He is then handed to the nurse for further care in a way that protects the physician's gloves from contamination and makes a safe transfer. Increasingly, the baby is being given to the mother or father to hold soon after birth. Mother-infant skin-to-skin contact is believed to promote attachment and assists in maintaining the baby's body temperature.

The baby

Immediate care. The nurse caring for the newborn infant should wear a clean overgown. Freshly washed hands should be covered by disposable gloves until all fluid is removed from the baby's skin. Review the implementation of universal precautions (see p. 615). To

*Simpson D: Examining the episiotomy argument, Midwife Health Visit Commun Nurse 24(1):6, 1988.

Table 7-4 Modified Apgar scoring chart to evaluate newborn status 1 and 5 minutes after birth

New name	Traditional sign	0	1	2
A Appearance	Color	Blue, pale	Body pink Extremities blue	Completely pink
P Pulse	Heart rate	Absent	Slow (below 100)	Over 100
G Grimace	Reflex response (e.g., to catheter in nostril)	No response	Grimace	Cry, cough, or sneeze
A Activity	Muscle tone	Flaccid	Some flexion of extremities	Actual motion
R Respiratory effort	Respiratory effort	Absent	Slow, irregular	Good, crying

Total score: 1 min _____

5 min _____

Severely depressed	0 to 3
Moderately depressed	4 to 6
Vigorous	7 to 10

This Apgar scoring chart incorporates a concept first introduced at the University of Kentucky Medical Center, Lexington, Kentucky, by Robert Beargie, MD. Modified from Campbell SJ: New use for the APGAR name, Point of View/Ethicon 17:6, 1980.

avoid the metabolic problems brought on by cold stress, the first step in the management of the newborn infant is to prevent the loss of body heat. This can be an especially critical factor in a newborn who needs resuscitation. Heat loss is prevented by placing the infant under a radiant heat source and quickly drying him. These two steps, which should be done for all infants following delivery, require only a few seconds to accomplish and can prevent the infant from becoming cold-stressed as a result of evaporative, convective, and radiant heat losses. Even healthy term infants are limited in their ability to produce heat when exposed to a cold environment, especially during the first 12 hours of life.

An overhead radiant heater allows access to and full visualization of the infant. Do not cover the infant because this prevents the radiant heat waves from reaching the skin. Place the infant under the warmer and using a warm towel or blanket gently and quickly dry the head and body to remove the amniotic fluid and prevent evaporative heat loss. The stimulation that this activity provides may initiate or help maintain respiration. Remove the wet towel or blanket from the bed.

Many adjustments must be made in the newborn's body to fit him for his new environment. He should be placed on his side and carefully and frequently observed. The nurse must provide warmth (usually in the form of an incubator, heated blanket, or a radiant infant warmer), observe his color and breathing pattern, and attach the identification approved by the hospital. During the same period of time, she usually performs the prophylaxis prescribed to prevent gonorrheal infection of the eyes (although some neonatologists state that it may be safely delayed up to an hour after birth when that time is desired to enhance the maternal-infant attachment process and early breast-feeding).

The American Academy of Pediatrics has termed acceptable the instillation of 1% silver nitrate ($AgNO_3$) solution, erythromycin 0.5% in single use tubes, or sterile ophthalmic ointment containing tetracycline 1% into the newborn's eyes for the prevention of ocular gonorrheal infection.* Many hospitals have been using erythromycin, which has been thought to be more effective against chlamydial infection and does not cause the eye

*American Academy of Pediatrics: Report of the Committee on Infectious Disease, ed 20, 1986, Elk Grove Village, IL, AAP.

irritation associated with the application of less costly silver nitrate. However, reports of a recent large research study indicate that erythromycin may not be significantly more effective than silver nitrate in preventing chlamydial infection.* Saline or water irrigations following the installation of AgNO₃ unfortunately do not reduce the incidence of chemical conjunctivitis and may curtail the efficacy of the solution.

Apgar evaluation. If the Apgar method of evaluating the newborn infant is used, the infant should also be scored for heart rate, respiratory effort, muscle tone, reflex irritability, and color, 1 and 5 minutes after birth. This scoring may be done by the physician, anesthesiologist, or nurse; but the nurse is thought by some to be the more "impartial and available" observer, especially for the 5 minutes' evaluation. The Apgar score is used in follow-up studies of the child and is reviewed in many research inquiries. Infants receiving a score of 7 to 10 are considered vigorous. Scores of 4 to 6 denote mild to moderate depression, whereas 0 to 3 indicates severe depression. The highest score that can be given is 10. Dr. Apgar believed that few newborn infants conscientiously scored deserve a first rating totaling 10. She believed that few babies are completely pink 1 minute after birth (Table 7-4).

The birth experience and immediate treatment of the newborn have been critiqued provocatively by the French obstetrician Frederick Leboyer in his book and film, *Birth Without Violence*. His dramatic writings certainly highlight a facet of maternity care that heretofore has received less attention. His call for more consideration of the sensory needs of the newborn seems to be legitimate, although his methods have stirred much comment. For normal births he stresses the following: a quiet, dimmed atmosphere, support for the infant's spine, maternal-child skin-to-skin contact, an intact umbilical cord until pulsation has ceased, newborn body massage, and a gentle body temperature water bath followed by warm wrapping and breast-feeding. Objections most often voiced regarding his techniques involve the dimmed environment, which may inhibit an adequate ability to observe, and the additional time and space that is needed to carry out his recommendations in busy maternity services. Some couples are seeking out physicians sympathetic to Leboyer's principles. Most labor-delivery units will use this technique if parents request it. Cord infection is not increased.

*Hammerschlag MR and others: Efficacy of neonatal ocular prophylaxis for prevention of chlamydial and gonorrheal conjunctivitis, N Engl J Med 320(12):769, 1989.

Third stage of labor

Use of oxytocics. In most cases some form of oxytocic is ordered after the birth of the baby or after the delivery of the placenta. After the delivery of the placenta, oxytocin is frequently employed to promote uterine contraction.

Delivery of the placenta (Fig. 7-21). After it has separated from the uterine wall, the placenta may be delivered through the bearing-down efforts of the mother if she is awake, or it may be expressed by the physician. This must be done very carefully and only when the placenta has separated and the fundus is firm; otherwise the grave complications of hemorrhage or inversion, a turning inside-out of the uterus, may occur. Signs of placental separation are (1) the rising of the uterus to or above the umbilicus, (2) the rounding out and firming up of the fundus, (3) the lengthening of the umbilical cord outside the vulva, and (4) a small gush of blood to the exterior. The placenta should be inspected to see if it was delivered in its entirety. Most physicians also perform an internal palpation of the uterus to assure themselves of its condition.

The placenta is a unique and valuable organ even after delivery. In some hospitals, placentas that have not become contaminated with stool or were not born of women whose pregnancies were complicated by infectious disease, fever, or premature rupture of the membranes are saved and later processed by a pharmaceutical concern to extract the immune globulin they contain. The cords of these placentas have also been evaluated and processed to provide vascular grafts to patients with circulation problems. The retrieval of surfactant from amniotic fluid obtained during cesarean operations is benefiting infants with respiratory distress syndrome.

Immediate postpartum care

Lacerations. After the delivery of the placenta, any necessary perineal repair can be made (Fig. 7-22). Generally, if an anesthetic was used for a delivery, the same one can be employed. Sometimes a local anesthetic is administered. If this is used, the physician will need a syringe (usually Pitkin), some infiltration needles, and the local anesthetic of choice, as well as the usual materials involved in a perineal repair. A seat and good light should be provided.

In spite of precautions, lacerations or episiotomy extensions occasionally occur. Some maternal tissues tear more easily than others. Very large babies or unusual positions are a special threat to the perineum. Lacerations of the perineum are described as first, second, third, and

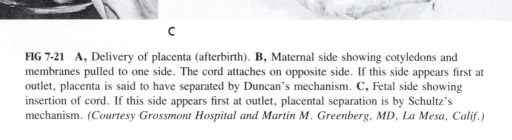

FIG 7-21 A, Delivery of placenta (afterbirth). **B,** Maternal side showing cotyledons and membranes pulled to one side. The cord attaches on opposite side. If this side appears first at outlet, placenta is said to have separated by Duncan's mechanism. **C,** Fetal side showing insertion of cord. If this side appears first at outlet, placental separation is by Schultz's mechanism. *(Courtesy Grossmont Hospital and Martin M. Greenberg, MD, La Mesa, Calif.)*

fourth degree. First-degree lacerations, involving a tear in the mucous membrane and skin only, are fairly common and usually of no permanent consequence. Second-degree lacerations include a tear into the muscles of the perineal block but exclude the rectal sphincter. Adequately repaired, they usually heal well with little problem. However, third-degree lacerations, which by definition involve the circular anal sphincter muscle, are more difficult to repair and may result in permanent dam-age to the perineum and sphincter (review the anatomy of the pelvic floor). Fourth-degree lacerations also involve the rectovaginal wall. To avoid third- and fourth-degree lacerations or episiotomy extensions that are uncontrolled and more difficult to repair, some physicians are purposely cutting the rectal sphincter (performing an episioproctotomy also known as a proctoepisiotomy) when the perineum is endangered. Lacerations may involve areas other than the true perineum. Tears of the

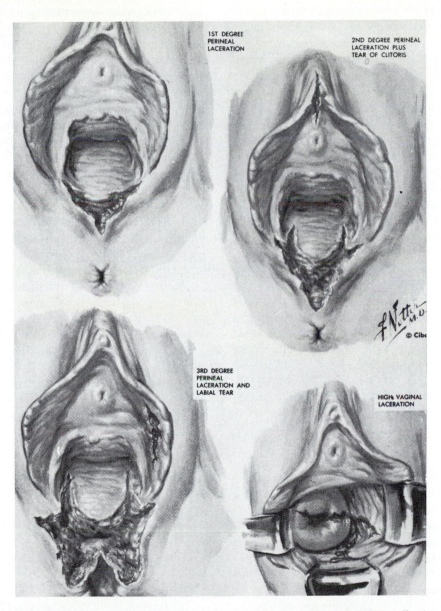

1ST DEGREE PERINEAL LACERATION

2ND DEGREE PERINEAL LACERATION PLUS TEAR OF CLITORIS

3RD DEGREE PERINEAL LACERATION AND LABIAL TEAR

HIGH VAGINAL LACERATION

FIG 7-22 Obstetric lacerations—vagina, perineum, and vulva. *(From the CIBA collection of medical illustrations, by Frank H. Netter, MD, Copyright CIBA.)*

labia, interior vaginal wall, and cervix are not uncommon. All these areas should be inspected for such tears after a birth.

If repair is nonexistent, inadequate, or improper, the patient is soon a possible candidate for hemorrhage, hematoma, and infection. As weeks and years pass, certain pelvic displacements and malfunctions may show themselves. The woman may be troubled with urinary or fecal incontinence, or she may suffer from a sagging of the pelvic musculature. When the tissue wall between the bladder and the vagina becomes abnormally relaxed, usually because of previous injury, the bladder drops out of place and pushes the anterior vaginal wall backward. The resulting abnormal condition is called a *cystocele*. A similar hernialike abnormality involving the rectovaginal wall and a falling forward of the rectum is known as a *rectocele*. Small rectoceles or cystoceles are usually asymptomatic and are not surgically repaired. Large abnormalities of this type, however, may cause complaints such as a "dragging sensation" in the pelvis and conditions such as stress incontinence, urinary retention, and cystitis in the case of cystocele or constipation and hemorrhoids in the case of rectocele. A vaginal repair of these difficulties, or colporrhaphy, may be performed. If both a bladder and a rectal prolapse are surgically treated, the procedure is often called an A and P (anterior-posterior) repair. *Prolapse,* or a falling out of place of the uterus, often accompanies these other displacements. Occasionally abnormal canals or tracts between two body cavities or a body cavity and the exterior develop as a result of obstetric injury. These tracts, most often found between the vagina and the urethra or between the vagina and the rectum, are termed *fistulas* and are difficult to eliminate. An adequate early repair of any obstetric injuries to the birth canal or its supports is important to continuing good health.

After birth the baby is shown or given to the mother. The infant may remain with her and her husband or companion for a more extended period designed to promote attachment, or he may be taken to the nursery with his birth records after only a short interval. If the mother is not alert, definite arrangements should be made for her to see the infant later as soon as she is able.

With the termination of any repair and the cleansing of the perineum, the head and foot of the delivery table are again realigned and the patient's legs removed from the stirrups or supports. Before the perineal pads are attached, if an episiotomy or laceration has occurred an ice pack may be ordered and applied to the patient's perineum to help prevent swelling and discomfort. The perineal pads are attached, and a warm, clean hospital gown replaces the one worn by the patient during the birth. She is covered by a warm blanket.

In some maternity services any initial preparation of the breasts of nursing mothers is done at this time also. Some mothers nurse their babies while still on the delivery table or in the delivery room if the baby is in good condition and free of excessive mucus and the new mother is alert and so wishes. The nursing of a baby directly following delivery of the placenta has a physiologic basis, since stimulation of the breasts causes the uterus to contract and helps prevent blood loss when other means of control are not available (something to remember in a disaster situation). The early establishment of an intimate mother-child relationship involving touch and nourishment is also considered one way to promote positive maternal emotions or maternal attachment. For some mothers who are not troubled by the relative lack of privacy and are not too tired, this opportunity may be cherished.

Observation. Throughout this early postpartum period, often called the fourth stage of labor, the patient is being observed for excessive bleeding and signs of shock. The blood pressure and pulse are frequently determined and the respirations observed. The uterus is palpated frequently to discover any relaxation of the fundus. If an intravenous infusion is in place (often used in conjunction with spinal anesthesia), it is carefully watched for rate of administration and possible infiltration. Many of these infusions contain an oxytocic and should not be given rapidly. Great care should be exercised to ensure that the needle is not dislodged during the transfer of the patient from the delivery table. Several hands may be needed for this project if the patient has an intravenous infusion and is temporarily unable to use her legs properly because of the lingering effects of spinal anesthesia. However, the staff may be fortunate in having a mechanical aid for the patient transfer. The new mother may remain in the delivery room suite for a specified time for close observation near equipment that may be needed, or she may be transferred to a special postpartum recovery room. At the time of her various changes in location, special attention should be given to the transfer of her personal belongings. Family members should see her as soon after the birth as is appropriate.

Alternative childbirth arrangements

The labor-delivery procedures just described could be called a "modified traditional" hospital maternity experience, although different hospitals incorporate their own

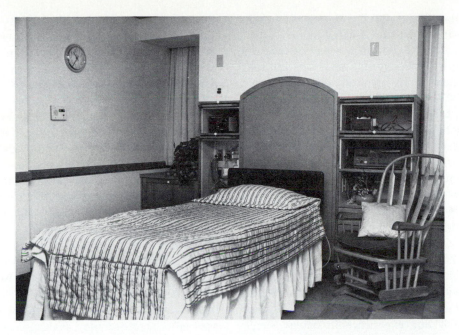

FIG 7-23 Single room maternity care is increasingly available for those who wish the safety of hospital facilities and the convenience and privacy of labor, delivery, recovery, and postpartum care in one area. This LDRP room has most of the equipment needed for a normal delivery. *(Courtesy Grossmont Hospital, La Mesa, Calif.)*

variations. Within the last few years a growing number of couples have wished to investigate alternatives to birth in traditional hospital settings. Several reasons are given for their search for other childbirth arrangements. They include a desire for a more relaxed, "personal" atmosphere and more flexibility in the types of care offered with the possible presence of other family members and friends (including, in some instances, sibling observation of the event); a perceived in-hospital attitude that childbirth is an abnormal or pathologic process; a wish for a birth with less medical intervention (for example, obligatory fetal monitoring, administration of drugs, artificial rupture of the bag of waters, routine transfer from the labor area to a "delivery room," episiotomy, and forceps application); an expressed need to have the newborn near at hand; disappointment in the organization or lack of rooming-in accommodations; concern over possible infant contact with "hospital germs"; lack of rest; and the high cost of hospitalization.

It is important that hospital administrators, physicians, and nurses examine and evaluate these reasons. Consumer discontent may be valid and unnecessary in many instances. The rationale of some hospital routines may be questioned. The alternatives that some families have

chosen may not sufficiently recognize that, although childbirth is a physiologic process, it can be complicated by unexpected considerations that call for decisions based on professional expertise and experience.

Alternatives to so-called traditional hospital birth vary in availability and safety. Some parents have decided to give birth at home. The birth attendant may be a physician, certified nurse-midwife, lay-midwife, friend, or father. The legality and proficiency of the attendant differ, depending on locale and circumstances. Although a minority of physicians will attend home births for selected "low-risk" women, many will not. They contend that, although other developed countries such as Great Britain and the Netherlands offer home birth to certain women, the health care system in the United States is not organized to render such care routinely with safety. They cite the small but important percentage (5% to 10%) of mothers and infants who, although not considered high risk, develop problems during the labor-birth period. They are concerned about professional backup in the event that they cannot attend the birth and about the threat of malpractice judgments. They are also influenced by the accessibility of hospital facilities and perinatal centers.

Another method of meeting the objections to traditional childbirth is the use of a birthing room or an alternative birth center (ABC), which is part of or near a hospital or clinic where emergency equipment and staff are available if needed. It is typically designed to care for uncomplicated births in a homelike setting. The room serves for labor, birth, and early postpartum care. Such centers have liberal visitation policies and usually discharge the mother and baby several hours after birth. Early follow-up nursing visits are made to the home. Most of these centers have been in operation a relatively short time. They may use nurse-midwives as well as physicians to monitor the labor and assist at the birth.

Still another alternative in maternity services is Single Room Maternity Care, currently being called the "wave of the 90s" (Fig. 7-23).* The long-used traditional hospital labor and delivery unit is based on the surgical transfer model with mother being moved from room to room, often during the most critical biologic or psychologic moments of the birth experience. In contrast, Single Room Maternity Care provides for the labor, birth, recovery, and initial postpartum care in one location. Mother, baby, and her support person stay in one or, at the most, two rooms during the entire hospital stay. This concept combines the science and safety of modern medicine, the knowledge of the caregivers, and the needs of the family into one package. Now hundreds of hospitals across the United States have initiated one of the two types of care described in the following text.

LDR (Labor, Delivery, Recovery). The mother is admitted to a birthing suite and remains there for her labor, delivery, and recovery. The rooms often are decorated much like hotel rooms but all necessary medical equipment is readily available. Although alternative birthing rooms were never completely successful, they did prove that good outcomes are still possible in less than sterile environments. Now hospitals are able to meet consumer demand for more "humanized services" in a medically safe environment with the initiation of Single Room Maternity Care.

Following recovery, the mother and her infant are moved to a Mother-Baby Unit, where the goal is to enable one nurse to care for the mother and baby together. There are many advantages to this type of nursing care. It encourages both parents to get to know their baby and begin functioning as a family unit under the guidance of skilled maternity personnel. Nursing is less fragmented. Assessments, treatments, and teaching are more easily coordinated when one nurse knows the status of both patients. It decreases chances for error, minimizing the number of people receiving a report on each patient. The risk of infection can also be decreased when mother and baby remain together.

LDRP (Labor, Delivery, Recovery, Postpartum). LDRP is essentially the same as the LDR except that the mother is not required to move to another unit following recovery, but continues to be cared for in the same room.

Unlike other alternative birth options no "screening out" is needed for this system. Because the mother and her baby are in a hospital setting with all available equipment and personnel, all women who are having vaginal deliveries can be taken care of in the Single Room Care System.

It will be extremely interesting to observe how maternity care services in the United States will be structured in another 10 years. Certainly they are undergoing a period of intense scrutiny, evaluation, and change. Families are so diverse in their expectations, desires, and needs; perhaps a "cafeteria of options" (without sacrificing valuable maternal and neonatal safeguards) can be developed to provide true family-centered maternity care.

Special situations

We now consider some special situations that occasionally arise in the labor-delivery sequence.

Precipitate delivery. First to be considered is "precipitate delivery." This means a birth that occurs with such speed and in such a situation that proper preparation and medical supervision of the event are lacking. A multipara with a relaxed perineal floor may have an extremely short period of expulsion. Two or three powerful contractions may cause the baby to appear. In this instance the nurse may be the only one at the bedside or delivery table to assist the patient. In no instance should she leave the patient alone. If it is obvious that the baby would be born before the delivery room is reached (for example, the patient has had three children [para 3] and the head is almost delivered), the nurse should do the best she can with what she has at hand. The call light should be turned on.

Birth of the head. There is seldom time for washing and putting on gloves in a precipitate delivery, although this would be ideal. The baby's head should not be forcibly held back, since this may cause fetal distress and aspiration, but it is important to maintain flexion of the fetal head to avoid trauma to maternal periurethral and perineal tissue. This restraint can usually be achieved by

*Machol L: Single-room maternity care gains converts, Contemp OB/GYN 34(5)62, 1989.

allowing the baby to emerge slowly against a guiding hand placed on the top of the advancing head. The fingers of the nurse should not enter the vagina. If the bag of waters is not broken, it must be pinched or torn to release the fluid and protect the baby from aspiration. The actual delivery of the head should be accomplished between contractions, with the mother panting or lightly bearing down. As soon as the head is born, the nurse should wipe off his face and, if possible, suction the baby's mouth and nose. She should also check to determine whether the cord is around the neck. If it is, she should slip it over the head or shoulders to prevent choking. Rarely it may be too tight to slip over with the fingers. If this happens, it is hoped that sterile clamps and scissors are available in the labor room or that a staff member has answered the light and brought the emergency pack containing the clamps and scissors necessary to cut the cord. The mother should be firmly instructed to pant through her open mouth and not push during this interval.

External rotation and expulsion. After the head is delivered, the face wiped, suction employed, and the location of the cord determined, frequently the rest of the child's body emerges without further assistance. However, if there seems to be no further progress and the back of the head has not already turned toward the mother's thigh, it can be turned in the direction of least resistance to line up with the child's back. There is no need to hurry. Next, the head should gently but firmly be directed downward to deliver the top shoulder. After the top shoulder is expelled, the baby is lifted up toward the pubic bone to release the bottom shoulder. The rest of the child is delivered without any particular problem. Before the birth of the baby, it is sometimes helpful if the mother's hips can be elevated (or the foot portion of the table lowered a few inches) by another person to give more room for perineal support and the gentle up-and-down maneuvers described and to help keep the baby's face free of vaginal and anal drainage.

Immediate care of the baby. As soon as possible, the infant's airway should be cleared. If a suction bulb is available, it is usually quite effective. (See Fig. 13-1.) The baby should not lie in a puddle of amniotic fluid where aspiration can take place. His body should be supported on the nurse's hand and arm at the level of the mother's uterus and tilted to "drain" without any tension being placed on the umbilical cord. After the airway is clear, he may be gently stimulated to cry, if necessary, and placed on his side—head slightly lower than his body—on his mother's abdomen. (Most of these babies

cry immediately.) He should be wrapped in a towel or blanket for warmth. There is no haste to cut the cord or, for that matter, to deliver the placenta. The cord can wait until proper sterile equipment is available. The nurse should wait for delivery of the placenta unless professional aid is very long in arriving or excessive bleeding occurs. However, if no professional help is forthcoming, if the signs of separation of the placenta have occurred, if the uterus is firm, and if the mother experiences a return of contractions, she may be asked to bear down to deliver the placenta. It should be supported as it is expelled so that the membranes are not torn. It should be saved for later evaluation by a physician. Usually the physician, who in the meantime has been contacted by the staff, completes the delivery of the placenta and repairs any lacerations.

A calm, reassuring manner on the part of the nurse (even if she does not really feel calm) is helpful to the mother and all concerned. Usually no great permanent harm results from a precipitate delivery, but every effort should be made to prevent its occurrence. All patients should be evaluated frequently for progress during labor. Signs of the approach of the second stage of labor should not be ignored. In such births the advantages of antisepsis and asepsis are largely lost, and there is greater danger of injury to the maternal tissues, of aspiration and injury to the baby, and embarrassment for the patient, not to mention the nurse.

Induction of labor. At times in the labor suite there may be admitted a pregnant woman who has come on appointment to have her labor artificially initiated or induced.

Reasons for induction. Indications for an induction of labor may include: (1) a problem with erythroblastosis fetalis (isoimmunization), (2) prolonged rupture of the membranes after 37 weeks' gestation without spontaneous onset of contractions, (3) increasing symptoms of preeclampsia, (4) postmaturity (baby *definitely* late in arriving), (5) maternal diabetes mellitus, or (6) fetal death without labor onset. Induction planned for the convenience of the patient or the physician is seldom considered a valid reason. Induction to produce abortion is discussed in Chapter 11.

Methods and care. Candidates for induction of labor must be selected carefully, since it is not a procedure totally without risk to the mother and baby. Today, labor is most often induced by intravenous administration of the synthetic pituitary hormone oxytocin (Pitocin or Syntocinon). Unless the cervix is ready, labor will not occur. The cervix must at least be partially effaced and soft and pliable. One method used fairly often today to prepare or "ripen" a cervix to make it more likely to respond to oxytocin is the application of prostaglandin E_2 gel within the cervical canal. At times, the application of prostaglandin E_2 gel alone may initiate labor.

If the membranes are artificially ruptured and labor does not begin within 24 hours, the increased possibility of introducing infection must be faced. Posterior pituitary hormone is powerful and can cause violent uterine contractions that can lead to premature detachment of the placenta, uterine rupture, and fetal hypoxia. For this reason oxytocin (usually 10 units per 1,000 ml of Ringer's Solution) should be given only in small amounts per infusion pump. Another liter of fluid without oxytocin should be included in the IV setup (piggyback) allowing the nurse to discontinue the uterine stimulation if necessary while still maintaining access to the vein. The labor of the induction patient should be electronically monitored. A strip showing the FHR pattern before introduction of the oxytocin should be obtained. During induction, it is usually recommended that the FHR, the maternal blood pressure and pulse, and the frequency and duration of any contractions, as well as the quality of the uterine relaxation period, be assessed and documented every 15 minutes. Uterine contractions lasting more than 60 seconds or occurring more than every 2½ to 3 minutes, exaggerated uterine tone and poor relaxation, and signs of FHR abnormalities usually indicate that the infusion of oxytocin should be slowed or stopped. Rules regarding use of oxytocin for induction need to be determined and followed. The physician should be readily available in the event of problems.

Cesarean birth. With the decreasing risk involved in the performance of cesarean birth (removal of the child through incisions in the abdominal and uterine walls), the operation is used more frequently in modern obstetrics. In fact, in 1980, many hospitals in the United States were reporting that approximately 20% of their births were by cesarean. The rise in cesarean births has been attributed to (1) a more aggressive approach to poor progress in labor, (2) an increased tendency to use cesarean for breech birth delivery, (3) a rise in repeat cesarean patients, and (4) the medical malpractice climate. Electronic fetal monitoring may be a factor, especially when first introduced to an obstetric service.

Reasons for cesarean birth. The most common reason for cesarean birth in the United States has been a previous cesarean birth. However, some physicians now are less reluctant to consider a trial labor and vaginal birth if the reasons for the former cesarean birth do not persist, if

the mother so wishes, and if the previous uterine incision was not vertical in direction. Others think that the possibility of uterine rupture is too great.

Needless to say, a mother entering the hospital for a repeat cesarean is usually not enduring the stress of an unexpected surgery hastily arranged because of the appearance of an obstetric complication. However, sometimes women who are admitted to the labor area suddenly demonstrate symptoms that suggest the emergency use of the procedure: conditions such as abruptio placentae, placenta previa, fetal-pelvic disproportion, abnormal presentations, prolapsed cord, uterine inertia (failure of the uterus to contract sufficiently to continue progress in labor), or signs of fetal distress. Conditions that indicate acute fetal distress or maternal jeopardy demand the prompt and rapid preparation of the patient once the condition has been discovered and the course of action determined. A patient scheduled for an emergency cesarean delivery is subjected to many procedures in a few minutes. Everything should be done as calmly and quickly as possible. The patient's morale should be supported because, if she is alert, she will probably be frightened.

Preparation. The following procedures are routinely carried out:

1. Signing of the operative permit by the patient or responsible party
2. An abdominal-perineal prep, which starts at the nipple line and includes the entire abdomen from side to side as well as the perineal area visible when the legs are parallel
3. Insertion of an indwelling catheter—sometimes done in surgery after anesthesia
4. Blood type and crossmatch and hemoglobin determination
5. Removal of any hairpins or hard objects from the hair; application of a surgical cap; removal of cosmetics, any extra jewelry, glasses, contact lenses, etc, to be given to the family; taping of wedding and engagement rings to the fingers without impeding circulation
6. Removal and safekeeping of any dentures
7. Preoperative medications as ordered
8. Removal of nail polish so that nailbeds may be checked for cyanosis is infrequently requested now because of the increasing availability of the oximeter, the vogue of artificial nails, and the recognition that nail cyanosis is a relatively late sign of poor oxygenation

The patient is given nothing by mouth from the time cesarean birth is contemplated, if this restriction has not been instituted previously. If not already in progress, an intravenous infusion is started.

Patients may be transferred to an operating room suite for surgery, or a delivery room may be prepared for the procedure. During all the busy preparations, any family members present should not be forgotten, and provision should be made for them to wait in as much mental and physical comfort as possible. Some hospitals permit the fathers to stay with the mothers during the section if general anesthesia is not used. In many areas, classes are now available to parents anticipating or interested in cesarean birth.

Breech presentation. A breech presentation is another situation that may be part of labor-delivery experience.

Incidence. Approximately 3% of all births are breech. There is currently renewed interest in trying to change a breech presentation to that of cephalic. (See p. 94.)

Complications. Although a breech presentation would probably not be considered an abnormality, it involves more risk to the infant than a cephalic birth, and the mother is likely to have a longer and more tiring labor. As a rule there is greater possibility of prolapse of the umbilical cord during breech labor, and during the delivery of the baby it may be compressed against the pelvic outlet. The baby may try to take a breath before his head has been born and aspirate tenacious vaginal secretions. Occasionally trouble is encountered in the extraction of the arms. Sometimes an unexpectedly large head may cause concern, and cerebral damage may occur. Although few maternity services today routinely provide a sterile scrub nurse in the delivery room, many physicians appreciate and request the help of such a nurse at the time of breech birth. Such an attendant usually helps support the baby's body or may, when instructed, apply fundal pressure when it comes time for the delivery of the head. A special type of forceps called Piper's forceps, applied to the aftercoming head, may be used at the time of a breech birth. It should always be on the sterile supply table when a breech birth is anticipated. The head is often delivered so that the baby almost seems to do a guided half somersault over the mother's abdomen. A rather deep episiotomy is customary in breech births. The baby may have edematous or bruised genitalia. Today the physician may elect to perform a cesarean birth because of the increased fetal mortality and morbidity (10% to 15%) of a vaginally delivered breech. However, many of these breech births involve premature infants—another factor to consider when evaluating the statistics.

Twins or multiple births. Twins are another interesting occurrence in an obstetric department. They occur about once in every 90 pregnancies. There are two types of twins—fraternal and identical (Fig. 7-24). Fraternal twins are the result of two simultaneous pregnancies developing from the fertilization of two separate ova by two distinct spermatozoa. They do not resemble one another any more than siblings resemble one another. They

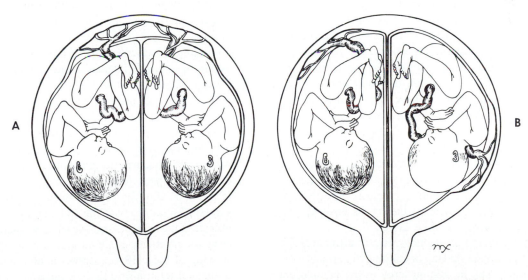

FIG 7-24 **A,** Identical twins. **B,** Fraternal twins. Note differences in construction of amniotic sacs.

may be of the same sex or of opposite sexes. The placental circulation of each fetus is separate, although the adjoining placentas may be fused. Each fetus develops within its own amniotic and chorionic sac.

Identical twins result from the division of one fertilized ovum into two identical halves that develop into two similar individuals of the same sex. The placental circulation is shared by the attachment of two umbilical cords. Each infant is encased in a separate amniotic sac but shares the chorionic sac with his twin. Fraternal twins are more common than identical. Approximately 54% of twins are premature, and the risk of intracranial hemorrhage, developmental respiratory distress syndrome, and other neonatal difficulties is high. Mortality for a second-born twin is about three times higher than it is for the first-born sibling, probably because of a greater incidence of malpresentations. Thus the nursery should be alerted when a twin birth is anticipated. Occasionally such an event is not anticipated, and the family, physician, and nurse are surprised to receive a "bonus baby."

Preparations and complications. When twinning is expected, two sets of identification should be ready with double newborn record sheets. Two sterile baby receiving blankets, two cord clamps, and two aspirator bulbs should be available. In almost one half of all twin births, both infants are cephalic presentations, but any combination of presentations and positions may exist. Occasionally, the babies' relative positions cause problems in their birth. Mothers of twins are more likely to suffer from preeclampsia and placenta previa and, because of the greater distention of the uterus, are more often victims of postpartum hemorrhage.

The nurse's experience in the labor-delivery room area can be a highly satisfying, rewarding type of nursing. If skilled in human relations and the observations and procedural techniques necessary to care for her patients, she can play an indispensable, gratifying role in a crucial period in a family's life. The alert student in this area can learn much and gain an appreciation of and reverence for life that she will never forget.

Key Concepts

1. Signs and symptoms of impending labor include the following: lightening, frequent urination, burst of energy, and uterine contractions.

2. Characteristics of false labor compared with true labor include the following: the duration of contractions remains the same in false labor, but becomes longer in true labor; the period between contractions remains long and irregular in false labor, but is regular in true labor; pressure or pain is felt primarily in the abdomen during false labor, but in the small of the back with true labor; walking can be tolerated during false labor, but intensifies contractions in true labor; show is absent in false labor, but is usually present in true labor; and the cervix is usually found to be long and closed in false labor, but is effacing or dilating in true labor.

3. Considerations that influence when the woman in labor should be instructed to go to the hospital are the following: her reported progress, the distance she must travel, how many babies she has had, and the history of her previous labors.

4. Perineal preparation includes careful cleansing and may also include shaving or clipping of perineal hair.

5. An enema may be administered in the labor room to make descent of the fetal head easier, to encourage contractions, and to facilitate rectal or vaginal examinations during labor. Enemas are not usually given to primiparas after dilatation of 6 to 8 cm or to multiparas above 4 to 5 cm; nor should they be given to a frankly bleeding patient or to a patient with a high presentation with ruptured membranes.

6. Obstetric contractions are timed to help determine the progress of labor, to detect abnormalities, to help detect fetal distress, and to reassure the patient and family.

7. Recording of observations of contractions includes duration, interval, intensity, and patient tolerance.

8. Normal fetal heart rate (FHR) is considered to be 120 to 160 beats per minute.

9. Three types of fetal cardiac decelerations may be detected by continuous monitoring devices. Early decelerations start at the onset of a contraction and occur only concurrently with the contraction. Late deceleration patterns are characterized by a slowing of the FHR after the peak of the contraction and by a delayed return to baseline and a regular waveform reflecting the contraction. Variable deceleration patterns are characterized by a periodic, unpredictable slowing of the FHR that shows neither a consistent sequential relationship to the contractions nor a regular repetitive range or duration.

10. Possible signs of fetal distress during labor include

the following: the passage of meconium-stained amniotic fluid when the baby is in the cephalic position; sudden exaggerated fetal movement; baseline FHR variability of less than 4 bpm; late or variable deceleration patterns. Repetitious FHR accelerations should be carefully observed.

11. Several techniques make use of breathing patterns and relaxation as a method to help women cope with the discomfort of labor.

12. The first stage of labor is characterized by three classic periods: early labor (0 to 4 cm dilatation), midlabor (4 to 8 cm), and transition (8 to 10 cm).

13. When the membranes rupture the nurse should do the following: inspect the perineum for signs of a prolapsed cord, evaluate signs of the advance of the presenting part, assess the amount and color of the amniotic fluid, check the fetal heart rate, and report that the membranes have ruptured to the charge nurse.

14. During a vaginal examination the attending nurse prepares and assists the patient and helps her to relax. If the physician elects to rupture the membranes artificially, the woman should be placed on several bed-protecting pads. After the membranes have been ruptured the FHR should be checked and the woman made as comfortable as possible.

15. Indications of the onset of the second stage of labor include the following: an increase in show, an involuntary urge to push with each contraction, the fetal heart tone is heard just above the pubic bone in cephalic presentations, and late signs that include bulging of the perineum, dilatation of the anus, and appearance of the fetal scalp.

16. To properly prepare the delivery room for birth, the nurse must understand the principles of aseptic technique, know where supplies are located, and be aware of the patient's special needs and the physician's specific requirements.

17. In preparation for delivery, the nurse assists with transferring the woman to the delivery room, positioning her, and cleansing the perineal area. The doctor usually drapes.

18. Forceps, which are sometimes used to lift out the baby's head, are usually applied in conjunction with an episiotomy, although an episiotomy may be performed when forceps are not used.

19. Immediately after birth, the nurse must provide warmth for the infant, observe his color and breathing pattern, and attach identification per hospital policy.

20. Three types of prophylactic measures to prevent gonorrheal infections of the eye can be administered: 1% silver nitrate solution, erythromycin 0.5%, or sterile ophthalmic ointment containing tetracycline 1%.

21. Using the Apgar score, the newborn's heart rate, respiratory effort, muscle tone, reflex irritability, and color are recorded 1 and 5 minutes after birth. Infants receiving a score of 7 to 10 are considered vigorous; scores of 4 to 6 denote mild to moderate depression; and a score of 3 or less indicates severe depression.

22. Lacerations of the perineum are described as first, second, third, and fourth degree. First-degree lacerations involve a tear in only the mucous membrane and skin and are usually of no permanent consequence. Second-degree lacerations include a tear into the muscles of the perineal block and usually heal well if adequately repaired. Third-degree lacerations involve the circular anal sphincter muscle and may result in permanent damage. Fourth-degree lacerations also involve the rectovaginal wall.

23. Parent-infant attachment may be promoted by maternal-infant skin-to-skin contact immediately after birth; delay of up to 1 hour before administration of eye prophylaxis may help the mother and/or father to relate to a more responsive newborn and facilitates breast-feeding shortly after birth.

24. Couples may seek alternatives to birth in traditional hospital settings for various reasons, including the following: a desire for a more relaxed atmosphere, a perceived in-hospital attitude that childbirth is an abnormal process, a wish for a birth with less medical intervention, a need to have the newborn near at hand, concern over infant exposure to "hospital germs," lack of rest, and the high cost of hospitalization.

25. Alternatives to traditional hospital birth include the following: home birth, birthing rooms or alternative birth centers (ABCs), and single room maternity care.

26. If precipitate delivery is imminent, the nurse should remain calm and reassuring and do the following: turn on the call light, guide the emerging head, break the bag of waters (if not already ruptured), make sure the cord is not around the infant's neck, clear the infant's airway, help deliver the body, and wrap him in a towel or blanket.

27. Indications for induction of labor include the following: a problem with erythroblastosis, prolonged rupture of the membranes after 37 weeks' gestation

without spontaneous onset of contractions, increasing symptoms of preeclampsia, postmaturity, maternal diabetes mellitus, and fetal death without onset of labor.

28. Preparation for emergency cesarean birth should include the following: signing of the operative permit; abdominal-perineal prep; insertion of an indwelling catheter; blood type and crossmatch and hemoglobin determination; removal of hairpins, cosmetics, jewelry, glasses, dentures, and the like; application of surgical cap; and preoperative medications.

29. Complications that may be associated with breech birth include the following: longer labor, prolapse of the umbilical cord, aspiration of vaginal secretions, difficulty in extracting the arms or head, and cerebral damage.

30. In preparation for the delivery of twins, two of each of the following should be readied: identification sets, record sheets, sterile receiving blankets, cord clamps, and aspiration bulbs.

31. Mothers of twins are more likely to suffer from preeclampsia, placenta previa, and postpartum hemorrhage.

Discussion Questions

1. You are working in a prenatal clinic. What signs of impending labor would you discuss with your patients? How could you explain the difference between true and false labor?

2. Modern obstetric care has changed dramatically in the past few years. Locate individuals who gave birth within the past few months, 5 years ago, 10 years ago, 20 years ago and as far back in time as you care to go. Discuss the differences in preparation for childbirth, physical care in labor (such as enemas, perineal preps, and so on), delivery/birthing rooms, presence of significant others, length of hospital stay and any other areas that you feel are significant.

3. Coaching is important throughout labor. How can the nurse assist the spouse or significant other in this role?

How can the nurse provide the necessary care during labor without detracting from the couple's personal experience of birth?

4. You are monitoring a patient in labor and everything appears to be progressing normally. Suddenly the fetal heart rate begins to decrease. What action would you take first? Next? Explain your reasons. It has been determined that a cesarean birth is necessary. How would you physically and psychologically prepare the mother?

5. It has been found that parental-infant attachment is best established immediately after delivery. How may medical interventions such as Apgar scoring, eye prophylaxis, and other care impact this bonding?

8

Pain Relief during Labor and Birth

CHAPTER OBJECTIVES

After studying this chapter, the student should be able to perform the following:

1 Define the following terms: analgesic, sedative, hypnotic, anesthetic, and amnesic.
2 Indicate at least three different factors that influence the timing and dosage of analgesia given during labor.
3 Name an analgesic commonly given during labor and indicate why it is often given with tranquilizers.
4 Differentiate between subarachnoid (spinal or saddle) and epidural regional anesthesias in timing of administration, effect on the patient, possible complications, and nursing care.
5 Describe the use of local anesthesia and pudendal blocks for the alleviation of pain and explain their safety and effectiveness.
6 Explain the philosophy on which psychoprophylactic preparation for childbirth is based.

METHODS OF PAIN RELIEF

The subject of modern childbirth would be incomplete without at least a brief discussion of the most common methods being used to make the experience of labor and birth easier and more comfortable for the mother. The physiologic origin of labor pain has not been adequately explained. It results partly from intermittent muscular contractions of the fundus and stretching of muscle fibers of the cervix, lower uterine segment, and vagina. (Review the involved sensory nerve pathways on p. 24.) The amount of painful stimuli produced is also influenced by the individual patient's pelvic anatomy, the size and flexion of her baby's head, the strength, duration, and frequency of her uterine contractions, and the presence or absence of certain obstetric deviations or complications.

Within the last few years it has been found that a person's pain threshold also may be significantly altered by the level of available *endorphins*, morphinelike hormonal substances in the body. These special proteins appear to interfere with the transmission of pain-producing impulses to the brain or the brain's sensitivity to those impulses. The endorphin level falls in the presence of anxiety, tension, fatigue, or extended negative stimuli. This phenomenon may offer a physiologic basis for the observation that a woman's perception of pain and her resulting behavior are greatly influenced by her interpretation of what is occurring, the training she has received, her cultural background, and the emotional support she gains from those about her.

Therefore methods of pain relief during labor and birth involve more than the administration of drugs; they also include ways available to help the patient understand the process of childbirth and to cooperate consciously with what her body is trying to accomplish. Usually a clean, calm, quiet, attractive environment, attention to techniques of relaxation, application of counterpressure to the mother's back, possible position changes, close supervision and encouragement from a concerned nursing staff and physician, and the companionship of those she loves greatly decrease the need for administration of analgesic and anesthetic medications. Methods of relief depend on the patient's special needs and wishes, the availability of desired agents or equipment, and the expertise and willingness to utilize them. Incorporated in their selection also should be the important considerations of risk versus benefit and financial constraints.

Key vocabulary

Five words are defined before a discussion of pain-relieving drugs or procedures is attempted.

amnesic A technique or medication that causes memory loss of varying degrees

analgesic A technique or medication that reduces or eliminates pain

anesthetic A technique or medication that partially or completely eliminates sensation or feeling. It may be a nerve-blocking type (local or regional anesthesia) or a sleep-producing type (general anesthesia)

hypnotic A technique or medication that causes sleep

sedative or tranquilizer A technique or medication that relieves anxiety and quiets the patient

Obstetric analgesia (first and second stages of labor)

The prescription and administration of analgesic drugs during the first stage of labor must be carefully considered and performed. Actually, the physician is caring for two patients. It must be realized that all analgesics may have a hypnotic effect not only on the mother but also on her fetus. Dosage and time of administration must be calculated so that the baby will not be too sleepy at the time of birth to breathe on his own. Before birth, sleepiness of the fetus is not crucial because he does not have to breathe; he gets all his oxygen from his mother. But after birth, this oxygen supply is no longer available. Failure to breathe, or respiratory depression, results in a condition known as asphyxia neonatorum. If a premature birth is expected, the mother is encouraged to continue her labor with a minimum amount of analgesia because the premature infant does not detoxify drugs well and may exhibit respiratory depression at birth. Some antagonistic medications (for example, naloxone hydrochlo-

ride [Narcan]) are now available to counteract the depressant action of drugs containing narcotics on the newborn infant's respiratory system. Naloxone is very effective, although its dose may need to be repeated. It has no known detrimental action in newborns except when used to treat addicted newborns. Then it may precipitate acute withdrawal symptoms.

Another consideration in the administration of drugs during the first stage of labor is the possible effect of the medication on the progress of the labor. Given too soon during the latent phase, many analgesics may unnecessarily slow down or even stop contractions. Most physicians do not wish to give any drug before active labor has been established or approximately 4 cm of cervical dilatation has been achieved. Many patients will not need medication before or even after this dilatation has been reached.

Analgesics, hypnotics, and amnesics: effects and side effects. An analgesic commonly used in labor is the narcotic meperidine (Demerol). This drug is frequently given in combination with a tranquilizer such as hydroxyzine (Atarax or Vistaril) or promethazine (Phenergan). These combinations are more effective because they increase the analgesic effect and counteract the nausea often associated with the narcotic.

Intermittent inhalation analgesia used in the latter portion of the first and during most of the second stage of labor has had considerable popularity in certain areas of the world. The patient breathes anesthetic gases through a mask or a mouthpiece. When these gases are properly administered in low concentrations, the patient does not become unconscious but benefits from a real reduction in discomfort. Nitrous oxide may be self-administered by the patient using a specially designed dispenser, or it may be administered by an anesthesiologist or nurse-anesthetist using an anesthesia machine. It is important that such analgesia not become anesthetic in depth, since regurgitation and aspiration can become a real and deadly complication. Instructions for the use of various types of gases and equipment must be carefully followed. Inhalation analgesia usually does not provide sufficient relief for the entire second stage of labor. Often its analgesic effects are augmented by a pudendal block or infiltration of the perineum with a local anesthetic.

Obstetric anesthesia (first, second, and third stages of labor)

Anesthesia is the province of a trained physician, anesthesiologist, or nurse-anesthetist. Nurses should not attempt to function in this area without skilled advanced training. Administration of anesthesia is not a nursing function.

General anesthesia. In obstetrics a general anesthetic may be inhaled or administered intravenously. General anesthesia in obstetrics is used less often than formerly for normal births. This is because regional anesthetics are safer and parental participation in the birth process is being emphasized.

Special considerations. When a general anesthetic is planned, it is important to know when the labor started and how recently the patient has eaten, because a real danger of aspiration, obstruction of the airway (asphyxiation), and pneumonia exists. The patient should be given nothing by mouth unless it is ordered, because during labor digestion stops and recent meals may remain in the stomach. Even if a woman in labor has not eaten recently, her highly acidic gastric secretions may still pose the threat of acid aspiration pneumonitis (Mendelson's syndrome). To counteract this possibility, some physicians order oral administration of 15 to 30 ml of an antacid such as sodium citrate every 3 hours during labor, and most order one dose just before a scheduled cesarean birth. Chilling the liquid antacid may increase its acceptance. In case of vomiting, the patient's head should be turned to the side or, if possible, she should be placed on her side. Chewing gum or dentures are removed from the mouth before administration of anesthetic.

Some anesthetic gases used in the past were either flammable (ether, chloroform) or explosive (cyclopropane). Now, other effective gases are available that do not present safety hazards, and older anesthetic gas products have been essentially phased out or banned. This has eliminated the need to be concerned with the buildup of static electricity in personnel and other safeguards against explosion, and has facilitated the use of the cautery during abdominal deliveries.

Other considerations are also important when using general anesthetics. During the period when a patient is being anesthetized (the period of induction), the delivery room should be as quiet as possible to make the induction smooth without patient distraction. Undue confusion and noise should also be avoided at the time of emergence.

Because all anesthetics cross the placenta and, if given in sufficient concentration, produce symptoms in the child, they should not be started too far in advance of the expected birth. When the condition of the fetus requires emergency cesarean birth or when rapid uterine relaxation is needed for various obstetric maneuvers, general anesthesia may be favored. It does not cause the maternal hypotension that sometimes accompanies re-

gional conductive anesthetics and may be administered rapidly with good results. Usually general anesthesia is induced by an intravenous injection of a sleep dose of thiopental (Pentothal) and a paralyzing dose of succinylcholine (Anectine). This is followed by rapid placement of a cuffed endotracheal tube into the trachea. The nurse may be asked to help at this time by pushing on the cricoid cartilage of the larnyx (just below the "Adam's apple"). This helps close off the esophagus. Both cricoid pressure and endotracheal intubation help prevent aspiration. The anesthesia is then maintained with nitrous oxide, oxygen, a muscle relaxant, and perhaps halothane. Once the baby is delivered, a narcotic and a tranquilizer are usually given intravenously to complete the anesthetic. Oxygen must always be mixed with gas anes-

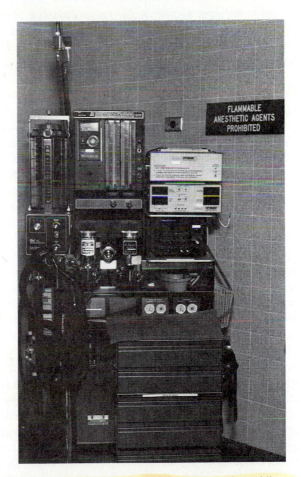

FIG 8-1 General anesthesia machine capable of providing a number of gas anesthetics. Most hospitals no longer use flammable gases. *(Courtesy Alex Pue, MD, and Donald N. Sharp Memorial Community Hospital, San Diego, Calif.)*

thetics to supply the body needs of the mother and her unborn child (Fig. 8-1).

Thiopental (Pentothal) produces a rapid induction by intravenous injection. If thiopental is given for only brief periods, the brain of the fetus is bypassed and little neonatal depression is seen.

Nitrous oxide (laughing gas) is often given for analgesic effect in the period of expulsion during contractions. Administered in low concentrations, it relieves the mother's pain but still allows her to bear down with her contractions. When nitrous oxide is used as an anesthetic, care is needed to prevent maternal respiratory and neonatal depression. Nitrous oxide may support combustion but is nonexplosive.

Halothane (Fluothane) and *isoflurane* (Forane) are anesthetic gases that are useful in producing rapid uterine relaxation when needed. (In low concentrations they can be used to decrease awareness during the early stages of operative deliveries if a light general anesthetic is desired.) Both anesthetic gases can cause uterine hemorrhage and hypotension if concentrations become too high.

Ketamine hydrochloride (Ketaject), given by intravenous injection, produces rapid anesthesia and is used primarily for emergencies in obstetric anesthesia. It is useful when blood pressure tends to be low. It should not be used with hypertensive patients, and may be associated with dreamlike episodes and hallucinations. Reduced stimulation during emergence is recommended.

Regional (conductive) anesthesia. Regional or conductive anesthetics have become popular in recent years.

Subarachnoid block. The use of a subarachnoid block, commonly called a spinal or saddle, has been particularly successful for vaginal deliveries. The patient is supported in a sitting position on the edge of the delivery table or lies on her side with her curved back facing the physician. Next, a thin sterile spinal needle (with or without a larger introducing needle) is inserted between the vertebrae at about the level of the iliac crests. Its tip is placed in the subarachnoid space below the spinal cord, identified by the appearance of cerebrospinal fluid dripping from the needle's hub. Between contractions an anesthetic that is heavier than the cerebrospinal fluid such as lidocaine (Xylocaine) is injected into the subarachnoid space. The patient is then positioned on her back with her uterus displaced to her left side. Her head and shoulders are elevated and her legs placed in stirrups (Fig. 8-2).

Classically, a saddle block is supposed to affect only those areas of the body that would be touched by a saddle if a person were riding a horse. In practice the anesthesia is usually more extensive. Low spinal anesthesia com-

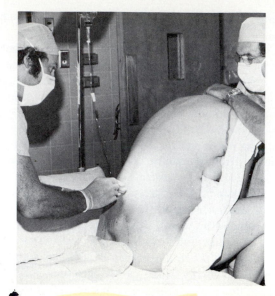

FIG 8-2 Administration of subarachnoid (spinal or saddle) anesthetic. *(Courtesy Grossmont Hospital, and Martin M. Greenberg, MD, La Mesa, Calif.)*

monly numbs the abdominal and pelvic areas below the umbilicus, affecting the abdomen, perineum, legs, and feet. It takes effect immediately and gains maximum potency in 3 to 5 minutes. How long it lasts (1 to 3 hours) depends on the medication used. For cesarean birth a subarachnoid block that is designed to go higher (up to the nipples) is frequently used. Because of vertebral abnormalities, or past back surgery not all women can have spinal anesthetics. A very few women are allergic to the type of medications usually injected. Sometimes lack of time or qualified medical personnel precludes the use of this type of anesthetic.

Much has been said about the aftereffects of subarachnoid anesthesia. The so-called spinal headache is a complication often feared by patients. Actually the incidence of spinal headache has been estimated as less than 5%, and it is decreasing. The use of an intravenous infusion to promote better hydration of the patient and the use of only small-bore needles to cut down on the possibility of cerebrospinal fluid leakage has reduced the incidence of postdelivery spinal headaches. It is debatable whether keeping the patient flat during the postdelivery period is helpful. Subarachnoid block anesthesia does entail certain other inconveniences, however. The mother must sit quietly while the procedure is carried out. This is difficult to do during the second stage of labor, even with the support of an understanding nurse. Subarachnoid block

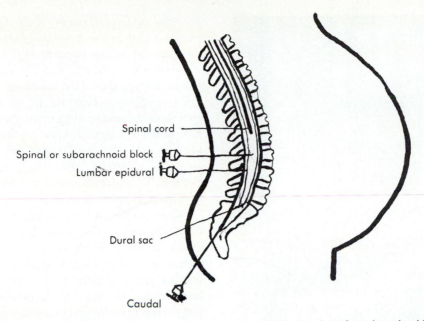

Spinal cord

Spinal or subarachnoid block

Lumbar epidural

Dural sac

Caudal

FIG 8-3   Types of regional anesthetics. External sites for needle insertions for subarachnoid and lumbar epidural may be the same, depending on the patient and the extent of anesthesia desired. The difference in the two approaches is depth of needle placement. Epidural injection does not enter dural sac; a subarachnoid injection does.

anesthesia does not stop contractions, but the patient does not feel them. The patient may find it difficult to push properly, and usually outlet forceps are used. Occasionally a patient's blood pressure may drop, possibly affecting the baby's oxygen supply, or the patient may have trouble breathing because of a high level of anesthesia. In the immediate postpartum period the patient may find it more difficult to void spontaneously. (See also Postpartum Care.)

Many practitioners believe that the positive aspects of subarachnoid anesthesia outweigh the negative aspects. The baby is not in danger of being put to sleep and of having a difficult time breathing at birth because of the anesthetic. The mother is awake. She may see her baby being born. She can hear his first cry—a real thrill. The regional anesthetics are safer than gas anesthetics for obstetric patients. Nausea and vomiting during and after use of regional anesthetics are minimal. The patient is awake and less likely to choke or aspirate, even if she vomits.

Recently very thin catheters capable of passing through a spinal needle have become available. They allow continuous administration of a spinal anesthetic. In certain situations, this procedure may offer the benefits of more versatility, less side effects, and more safety

than the "single shot" spinal or the continuous epidural anesthetic discussed below.

Epidural anesthesia techniques. Other types of regional anesthetics are available (Fig. 8-3). In considerable vogue some time ago was continuous *caudal anesthesia,* or one-shot caudal. This technique introduced local anesthetic agents into the sacral canal, where significant nerves travel outside the meninges or spinal cord coverings. It is rarely used today.

Another kind of regional anesthesia, less difficult to administer than caudal is called a *lumbar epidural block.* The drug is injected into the epidural space, usually between the second and third or the third and fourth lumbar vertebrae, while the mother lies on her side or is supported in a sitting position. Following careful identification of the desired location, a nylon or plastic catheter is threaded through the needle at the insertion site and the needle is removed (Fig. 8-4). The catheter is conscientiously secured in position with tape. After a small test dose, cautious instillation of the anesthetic is begun. Currently bupivacaine (Marcaine), 2-chloroprocaine (Nesacaine), and lidocaine (Xylocaine) are the most frequently used local anesthetics.

The patient should be informed about what she may experience during the initiation of the epidural. She may

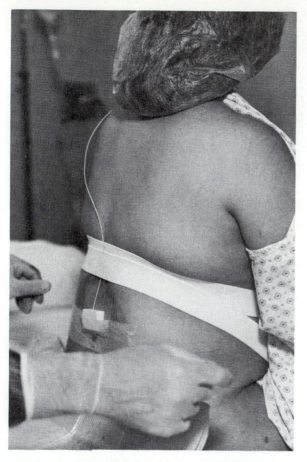

FIG 8-4 The epidural catheter has just been inserted and is taped securely in place. The white belts help support the external fetal heart and contraction monitors. *(Courtesy Alex Pue, MD, and Donald N. Sharp Memorial Community Hospital, San Diego, Calif.)*

detect a burning or stinging sensation at the site of the injection of the local anesthesia before the insertion of the needle and cannula, local pressure during insertion, and a "crazy bone" feeling in her leg, hip, or back if the flexible catheter touches a nerve as it advances into the epidural space. During the 5-minute period after the test dose is injected, she should be observed for the appearance of hypotension and questioned regarding lower extremity sensory changes and loss of ability to move her legs. These symptoms may indicate unwanted penetration through the dura mater into the subarachnoid space. This is to be avoided, since the larger amounts of anesthetic routinely used during epidural techniques could cause dangerously high anesthesia, compromising res-

pirations and oxygen supply. A dural puncture could also predispose the mother to spinal headache. (See preceding discussion of subarachnoid block.)

Another complication that can occur is the rare unintentional injection of the anesthetic into a blood vessel. The patient may indicate ringing in the ears, light-headedness, circumoral tingling or numbness, and the sudden recognition of a metallic taste. Convulsions may follow, at which time the patient is placed in a side position, the airway is preserved, and oxygen is given. Diazepam (Valium) or thiopental sodium (Pentothal) may be administered to stop the seizure.

When epidural dosage is administered during labor, the patient may remain on her side with her head slightly raised, or she may be placed in a modified supine position with a firm wedge-shaped pillow under her right hip so that her uterus is tilted to the left. These postures are assumed to help control the level of anesthesia obtained and to prevent the weight of the uterus from compressing the maternal aorta and vena cava. When the compression of these vessels interferes with the circulation of the blood in the mother and eventually deprives the fetus of oxygen, the resulting signs and symptoms have been called the *aortocaval* or *supine hypotensive syndrome*. One must always be alert for developing maternal hypotension. An epidural block may also cause hypotension by blocking certain sympathetic nerve fibers in the epidural space.

The anesthetic may be infused through the catheter in small continuous amounts using an infusion pump or given intermittently when the analgesic action lessens. Usually pain relief begins within 3 to 5 minutes after injection, and full effect is obtained in 8 to 15 minutes. According to one study* about 85% of the women receiving epidurals are free of pain, 12% experience partial relief, and a remaining 3% do not benefit at all. Many women will still confirm sensations of abdominal or perineal pressure and note weakness or numbness in their legs. Because of the loss of normal pelvic sensation together with routine intravenous hydration, many are prone to urinary distention. They should be asked to empty their bladders before the epidural is begun and should be watched carefully for difficulty in voiding. The patient may need to be catheterized. For a cesarean birth, the effects of an epidural block may be extended by injecting more local anesthetic until the level of numbness is felt up to the nipple line.

Contraindications to using an epidural anesthesia in-

*Crawford JS: Continuous lumbar epidural analgesia for labor and delivery, Br Med J 1:72, 1979.

clude current anticoagulant therapy, a history or presence of hemorrhage or shock, septicemia or local infection in the area of the proposed injection, and various spinal problems.

Epidural techniques can be used to good advantage in the latter part of the first stage of labor and continued into the second and third stages. The patient is typically alert and comfortable. Those women wishing medication during their labors are usually enthusiastic regarding the method. However, epidural anesthesia requires the supervision of an anesthesiologist, special apparatus, and continuous maternal-fetal monitoring and support by the nurse. It is very important to detect signs of maternal hypotension and to evaluate the duration and quality of uterine contractions, progress in labor, and fetal heart rate response. The mother's urge and ability to push may be impaired, and forceps deliveries are more common than in patients who have received no anesthesia before delivery. Use of epidurals is growing in most areas of the United States.

It is now becoming a fairly common practice in some hospitals to inject narcotics along with local anesthetics into the subarachnoid (spinal) or epidural spaces to manage pain during both vaginal and cesarean births and to provide postoperative pain control. One technique uses long-lasting morphine (Duramorph) and/or other shorter-acting narcotics such as fentanyl (Sublimaze). It can provide very effective analgesia. However, side effects such as itching, nausea, and vomiting occur frequently when narcotics are used in this way. Urinary retention also may occasionally result. The major concern is a rare but potentially fatal complication—delayed respiratory depression.* Because of the possibility of this problem when narcotics are injected into the subarachnoid or epidural spaces, the respiratory patterns of the patient must be carefully monitored over an extended period. Protocols for special observation and care should be in place.

Local anesthesia and nerve blocks

Pudendal block. Local anesthesia by direct infiltration of the perineal tissues or infiltration of those nerves that serve to relay sensation initiated in the perineal area to the brain is probably the safest anesthesia for both mother and baby available today. A popular technique called pudendal block stops sensory impulses from the pudendal nerve by infiltration of a local anesthetic into specific areas with a long needle. With its use, an episiotomy

---

*Ross BK and Hughes SC: Epidural and spinal narcotic analgesia, Clin Obstet Gynecol 30(30):561, 1987.

may be performed. It may be used satisfactorily in conjunction with nitrous oxide. However, some women do not experience the relief they desire.

Paracervical block. Another type of analgesic technique is called a paracervical block. It features injections of local anesthetic into the lateral fornices of the vagina at the junction of the vaginal wall and the partially dilated cervix. Although it may relieve discomfort from contractions, the technique in most instances is not sufficient to meet the total needs of most patients during delivery. Even more important, the paracervical block has been associated with episodes of fetal bradycardia and a few fetal deaths. For all these reasons, this type of block is infrequently undertaken today.

EDUCATION FOR CHILDBIRTH

In the mid-20th century few mothers in the United States remembered much of the experience of labor or delivery. Most, in the hospital setting, were given types and doses of drugs designed to relieve pain, which also produced at least partial amnesia of the event. These medications too often were associated with the birth of infants whose respirations were depressed at birth.

Modern trends in obstetrics favor a more alert patient during labor who is able to participate with dignity in her experience of childbirth. To this end greater efforts have been made to educate the woman for her role, both psychologically and physically. Many different courses have been instituted to teach helpful techniques in posture, breathing, and relaxation, as well as to impart basic information about labor and birth to the expectant mother. Husbands or chosen companions are encouraged to attend the sessions to understand and aid their partners.

The late English obstetrician Dr. Grantly Dick-Read probably popularized the term "natural childbirth" in his book *Childbirth Without Fear*. In his writings and lectures he stressed that much of the fear pregnant women feel is caused by a lack of knowledge of what is really happening and an ensuing feeling of helplessness. He declared that fear builds tension and that tension eventually produces pain. Because of this, much of his effort was spent in educating the future mother and prescribing exercises to condition her body for labor and birth.

In 1952 the French obstetrician Fernand Lamaze became intrigued with the labor and delivery techniques based on Pavlov's theories of conditioned response that he had observed during a visit to the Soviet Union. When he returned to Paris, he introduced psychoprophylactic concepts into his practice to prepare his patients for their maternity experiences and to assist them in a conscious, rewarding participation in the birth of their children. Much of what Dr. Lamaze emphasized was also stressed by Dr. Read. However, the relaxation taught by Dr. Lamaze is based on the principle that a high level of concentrated cerebral activity can inhibit the reception of other stimuli. That is, the mind (psycho) could be induced to prevent (prophylaxis) the reception of unpleasant and painful sensations. The patient is educated (conditioned) to respond neuromuscularly to specific verbal cues. Intense preoccupation with certain muscular tension and release patterns, respiratory movements, and massage may help attain these goals. A specially prepared labor coach, sometimes called a monitrice, may be assigned to assist and support the patient in her efforts to utilize her training.

Frequently, the husband or chosen companion of the expectant mother fills the role of labor coach. The coach and the labor-delivery room staff should work as a team for the realization of a constructive, dignified, aware, satisfying parturition. The attending nurses should be calm, cheerful, and knowledgeable concerning the aims of the techniques employed. The methods used may differ, but it is helpful if the nurses acquaint themselves with the different types of programs that may be available in their communities and the ways in which expectant mothers have been taught.

Today, at the beginning of the 1990s many childbirth educators are emphasizing the need for increased flexibility and individualization in the labor techniques offered to their clients. In this broader teaching perspective more consideration is given to the wide range of normal physiologic responses found in women, their varying cultural backgrounds, and different personalities. These considerations affect their perception and tolerance of pain and the selection of coping skills and has led to the support of more types of maternal behavior during labor. This broad teaching perspective relieves a certain rigidity (reflected especially in past teaching of certain respiratory patterns to coincide with contractions), which was helpful to some, but not to all.

Women trained for labor need nursing support and encouragement from a nurse who will enhance their efforts; help evaluate and aid relaxation; render sacral support or pressure as directed; share information regarding progress in labor; and be sincerely complimentary of the idealism and efforts manifested by the patients and their partners. In addition, the nurse should render the other nursing care services and observation that all laboring women require. Occasionally symptoms of hyperventilation may be associated with some of the rapid-breathing techniques used. The patient may complain of tingling hands and feet, which cause annoyance or loss of concentration. Slowing respirations or breathing into a paper bag helps relieve these problems. Symptoms related to hyperventilation are not frequent because rapid-breathing patterns have been modified to include slower acceleration and deceleration periods and shallower respirations.

The absence of all forms of drug-induced analgesia or anesthesia is not a prerequisite of either the Read or Lamaze method, although this interpretation has been made. However, some women do not use any analgesic or anesthetic drugs. With the greater availability of epidural anesthesia in many areas of the United States, more women are currently using the various nonmedical techniques learned in classes during early labor and completing their labor and birth experience with epidural anesthesia.

Those who have evaluated psychoprophylactic techniques (used them or cared for patients who were prepared as recommended) generally believe that they are of real value. The breathing and relaxation exercises, patterned light massage (effleurage), visual focal point or imagery, and mental and physical conditioning that such team efforts involve represent helpful tools that many mothers can profitably employ as they face the task of childbirth. If a laboring woman decides to use other alternatives (such as analgesia, tranquilizers, or anesthetics), she should not feel herself to be a failure or guilty of betraying a concept. She is not a competitor in a contest. She is a participant in an experience.

The main problem in using psychoprophylactic techniques seems to be in securing enough time and personnel to prepare the woman adequately. She may find it difficult to attend instruction classes. Many people do not agree that these methods of caring for the childbearing woman are truly natural childbirth. They look on them as intensive education and preparation for childbirth. Some women respond very well to the conditioning offered. Others have personal histories or personality structures that make constructive participation in psychoprophylactic labor and birth, such as Read, Lamaze, and others have recommended, difficult or impossible. These methods are advised only for those undergoing a normal labor and birth. For patients seeking a sympathetic practitioner and undertaking the preparation involved, such management of labor and birth can bring many enduring rewards, not the least of which is a characteristically noisy, vigorous new member of the family.

More information regarding childbirth education can be obtained from the American Society of Psychoprophylaxis in Obstetrics, Inc. (ASPO/Lamaze), 1840 Wilson Blvd., Suite 204 Arlington, VA 22201 (202-362-9188); or the International Childbirth Education Association, P.O. Box 20048, Minneapolis, Minnesota, 55420-0048 (612-854-8660).

Hypnosis and acupuncture. No discussion of obstetric analgesia and anesthesia can be undertaken without mentioning hypnosis and acupuncture. Hypnosis, an intense altered state of receptive concentration, is greatly enhanced by high motivation. The psychoprophylactic method of preparation for childbirth incorporates certain aspects of this technique. The ability to attain a trancelike state can be measured by use of the Hypnotic Induction Profile.* A trance may be induced by another person or self-induced. Training for this type of pain relief has been

*Spiegel H: Obstetrics, pain and hypnosis. In Cosmi E, editor: Obstetric anesthesia and perinatalogy, New York, 1981, Appleton-Century-Crofts.

typically time consuming and expensive. The use of group sessions has made hypnosis more accessible. However, it still has not become a popular form of pain control for maternity patients.

The use of acupuncture for vaginal deliveries has received mixed reviews. In a preliminary study, Cosmi and Vellay found that acupuncture associated with electric stimulation (electroacupuncture) in the dorsolumbar and lumbosacral areas may eliminate painful sensation during labor. It also has been proposed that acupuncture releases endorphins (morphinelike compounds) from the pituitary gland and midbrain. Surely these forms of pain relief and control are worthy of more study and research.

No perfect means of pain relief applicable to all women and situations has been found. But physicians have at their disposal many agents of worth that, when used judiciously and backed up by good nursing care, will assist the patient tremendously.

Key Concepts

1. Dosage and time of administration of analgesics during labor are affected by the following factors: the need to ensure that the baby will be alert enough to breathe at birth, the maturity of the infant, and the possible effects on the progress of labor.

2. The narcotic meperidine (Demerol) is frequently given in combination with a tranquilizer because the combination increases the analgesic effect and counteracts the nausea often associated with the narcotic.

3. Drugs used for general anesthesia include thiopental (Pentothal), nitrous oxide (laughing gas), halothane (Fluothane), isoflurane (Forane), and ketamine hydrochloride (Ketaject).

4. A subarachnoid (saddle) block is administered during the second stage of labor and commonly numbs the abdominal and pelvic areas below the umbilicus, affecting the abdomen, perineum, legs, and feet. Possible complications include spinal headache, difficulty in pushing, a drop in blood pressure, respiratory difficulty, and problems with spontaneous voiding postpartum.

5. Epidural anesthesia can be administered during the latter part of the first stage of labor and continued into the second and third stages. Normal pelvic sensation

is lost, but many women still confirm sensations of abdominal or perineal pressure and note weakness or numbness in their legs. Possible complications include urinary distention, hypotension, and decreased urge and ability to push.

6. A pudendal block stops sensory impulses from the pudendal nerve by infiltration of a local anesthetic into specific areas with a long needle. Some women do not experience the desired relief.

7. Paracervical block involves injections of local anesthetic. This technique is rarely sufficient to meet the total needs of most patients during delivery and has been associated with a few fetal deaths. It is infrequently used today.

8. Psychoprophylactic preparation for childbirth is based on the principle that a high level of concentrated cerebral activity can inhibit reception of unpleasant and painful sensations. Knowledge of the birth process reduces stress and anxiety. Conditioning exercises during pregnancy and breathing and relaxation techniques during labor can reduce physical discomfort.

9. Hypnosis and acupuncture are infrequently used methods of pain relief during labor.

===== **Discussion Questions** =====

1. Locate articles and books used in preparation for childbirth classes or attend a childbirth education class. How do the methods such as Lamaze, Read, and others you identified differ? How are they similar? What do you feel is the greatest benefit of preparation for childbirth?

2. Types and amounts of analgesic medication used during labor have changed in recent years. Why is there a trend toward minimizing the amount of analgesic given to a woman during labor?

3. There is a wide variety of anesthesia used during labor and delivery. Identify the most common types of anesthesia and discuss the advantages and disadvantages of each.

4. What maternal and fetal factors should the nurse monitor and observe most carefully when analgesics are administered during labor? Why are these significant?

5. What is meant by the statement, "The timing of the administration of analgesics can have an impact on the progress of labor?"

9

Complications Associated with Pregnancy and Childbirth

CHAPTER OBJECTIVES

After studying this chapter, the student should be able to perform the following:

1 Indicate ways of preventing, lessening, or treating the following so-called "minor" discomforts of pregnancy: nausea and vomiting, heartburn, constipation, lower extremity varicose veins, hemorrhoids, and muscle cramps.

2 Compare two vaginal inflammations, trichomoniasis and candidiasis, considering causative agents, signs and symptoms, treatment, and prevention.

3 Discuss two problems associated with douching and why some physicians do not advocate this procedure even by the nonpregnant woman.

4 Outline the needs of the pregnant woman with diabetes regarding insulin dosage, urine testing for ketones, and blood glucose monitoring.

5 Indicate four analyses or procedures used to help evaluate the status of a diabetic mother's unborn child.

6 Explain efforts to protect mother and unborn child from syphilis, indicating methods of transmission, disease identification, and treatment.

7 Identify three dangers of gonorrheal infection and why this infection affects reproductive capacity.

8 Discuss dangers posed by the herpes simplex virus to the unborn infant.

9 Define the various types of abortion: spontaneous,

induced, threatened, inevitable, complete, incomplete, habitual, and "missed."

10 Describe the major threat to the mother's life during the rupture of a tubal-type ectopic pregnancy and note the signs and symptoms of such a situation.

11 Contrast in three ways the two obstetric abnormalities associated with the attachment of the placenta to the uterine wall, placenta previa and abruptio placentae.

12 List at least five nursing considerations that must be remembered when caring for a maternity patient experiencing abnormal bleeding.

13 Cite the three major signs of preeclampsia (now known as pregnancy-induced hypertension [PIH]) and state four indications of worsening patient status. (See Table 9-1.)

14 Indicate four categories of expectant mothers who statistically are more likely to develop PIH.

15 Explain why a maternal side-lying position is advantageous to the fetus.

16 Note the action and uses of magnesium sulfate in the treatment of preeclampsia–eclampsia, as well as its side effects and the antidote recommended.

17 Point out four types of labor patients who have a higher incidence of the obstetric emergency "prolapse

Continued.

of the cord" and explain what should be done as soon as the problem is identified.

18 Indicate four reasons why a premature birth should be avoided and two methods that may be employed to halt labor.

19 Discuss reasons for the high rate of teenage pregnancy in our society and the problems this condition may pose for the community.

20 Tell how the labor of a teenager may differ from that of an older mother.

MINOR PROBLEMS OF PREGNANCY

A French obstetrician named Mauriceau once declared that pregnancy was a disease of 9 months' duration. Today health professionals and prospective parents do not like the term "disease" applied to normal pregnancy, but it is conceded that a number of minor discomforts may be associated with this period of waiting. Some were mentioned in Chapters 4 and 5. Let us take a more detailed look at those discomforts and others not previously discussed.

NURSING CARE PLAN

Women with "Minor Problems" Associated with Pregnancy

Selected nursing diagnoses	Expected outcomes	Interventions
Knowledge deficit related to self care strategies for coping with minor discomforts of pregnancy.	Women verbalizes understanding of discomforts and utilizes self-care measures to lessen their impact.	Explain cause of condition and provide anticipatory guidance for self care throughout pregnancy.
	Specific plans for selected problems are described below.	

A. Alteration in urinary elimination pattern related to physical changes of early and late pregnancy.
Clinical manifestations:
   Patient complains of fullness, frequent urination.
	Sleep pattern is undisturbed by nocturia.
	Maintains adequate fluid intake.
	Recognizes and reports symptoms of urinary tract infection.
		Collect additional information concerning urinary complaint to distinguish normal condition from possible urinary tract infection.
		Teach patient signs of urinary tract infection such as burning on urination, fever, flank pain, cloudy urine, urgency. Explain importance of reporting promptly to physician if they occur.
		Advise patient to:
		   Void when urge occurs—minimize urinary stasis (potential for infection).

Selected nursing diagnoses	Expected outcomes	Interventions
		Eliminate fluid intake after 6 PM (be sure to maintain adequate intake during day).
		Empty bladder immediately before going to bed.
		Reduce intake of beverages high in caffeine, e.g., tea, coffee, cola, which acts as a urinary irritant.

B. Alteration in comfort related to varicose veins of the lower extremities, vulva or anus. Previous history or family history of varicosities.
 	
Clinical manifestations:
    Visible, distended, superficial veins.
    Discomfort varies from mild to severe; throbbing pain.
	Varicose veins are prevented or their severity lessened.
	Discomfort from varicosities is reduced.
		Explain cause of varicose veins during pregnancy: high hormone levels result in relaxed vein walls; enlarging uterus, long periods of standing or sitting, straining with bowel movements and constrictive clothing.
		If varicosities common in family, patient should follow preventive measures before signs or symptoms appear.
		Teach patient self-care measures to prevent or treat discomfort:
		  1. Wear support stockings—apply in AM before rising.
		  2. Rest with hips and legs elevated.
		  3. Avoid constricting garments.
		  4. Change standing or sitting positions frequently.
		  5. Prevent constipation by intake of increased fluid and dietary fiber.
		  6. Support vulvar varicosities with peripad held snugly in place by belt or maternity panty girdle.

C. Alteration in comfort and potential alteration in nutrition related to nausea and/or vomiting during early pregnancy.
 	
Clinical manifestations:
    Transient nausea and/or vomiting: commonly called "morning sickness" but may occur at any time.
	Nausea and vomiting resolves after first trimester.
	Adequate nutritional status is maintained.
	Woman is able to continue with usual daily activities.
		Collect additional information regarding severity and timing of nausea and vomiting. If they are continuous or severe, notify physician.
		Explain cause of nausea and vomiting during pregnancy: hormonal changes cause slowed gastric emptying, slowed peristalsis.
		Advise dietary modifications:
		  1. Eat high carbohydrate food before arising (soda cracker, dry popcorn).
		  2. Avoid greasy or spicy food.
		  3. Eat six small meals rather than three large meals.
		  4. Avoid foods or odors identified as causing problems.
		  5. Avoid drinking liquid with meals.

Digestive difficulties

Nausea and vomiting. Probably the first discomfort noted by many pregnant women is nausea and vomiting—particularly in the morning, although it may occur at any time. Remember that it is a presumptive signal of pregnancy. This temporary condition is experienced by approximately 50% of pregnant women in the first trimester. It is said to be linked with the great hormonal changes in the body at the onset of pregnancy or a decreased blood glucose or glycogen reserve. Emotional factors may also enter into the cause-and-effect relationship. The most successful preventative seems to be eating more frequent, small meals instead of three large meals as is customary. Liquids are tolerated better if taken between, instead of with, meals. Eating something dry and high in carbohydrate value, like a few crackers or a piece of toast, 15 minutes before getting up also seems to help. If the nausea persists and becomes severe, threatening the nutrition of the mother, it is considered a serious complication called *hyperemesis gravidarum*. It may ne-

cessitate hospitalization, administration of intravenous feedings, and, in some instances, psychiatric counseling.

Heartburn. Heartburn, or *pyrosis,* an uncomfortable burning sensation felt behind the sternum, often accompanied by gas and acid regurgitation into the esophagus, has nothing to do with the heart. It only feels that way. Heartburn becomes more common as pregnancy advances and is related to decreased peristalsis and the pressure of the growing fetus, which cause stomach acid reflux and secondary esophagitis. For this reason, lying flat directly after eating is not recommended. Since the ingestion of fat inhibits the secretion of stomach acid, a small amount of milk or cream taken about 20 minutes *before* eating might merit some consideration. Heartburn can also be prevented or lessened if gas-forming foods, such as cabbage, cauliflower, brussels sprouts, onions, cucumbers, radishes, turnips, and dried beans, are avoided. More frequent, smaller, leisurely meals are also recommended. With the physician's approval, an antacid such as Maalox (a mixture of magnesium and aluminum

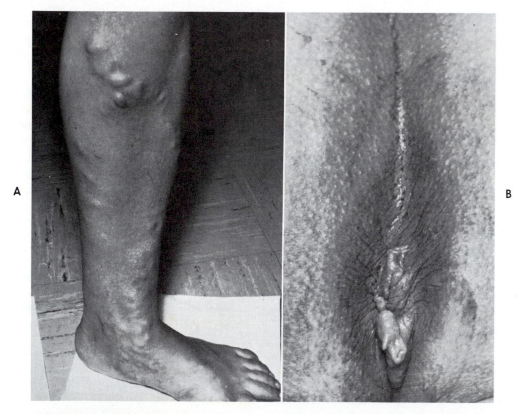

FIG 9-1 **A,** Varicose veins of lower extremity. **B,** Varicosities of rectal area (hemorrhoids). *(Courtesy Mercy Hospital and Medical Center, San Diego, Calif.)*

hydroxides) may be used, especially before bedtime. Sodium bicarbonate or other products high in sodium often considered for such distress, should be avoided.

Constipation. Constipation may also be a problem, especially if the woman has had such difficulty before pregnancy. Four things may help: a diet that includes plenty of roughage, abundant fluids, regular exercise, and a consistent time of day set aside for evacuation when she does not have to hurry. Mild laxatives may also be used, but an expectant mother should check with her physician regarding the type and frequency of such medication. Taking a laxative is one way labor might be initiated.

Circulatory difficulties (Fig. 9-1)

Varicosities. Many pregnant women suffer from *varicosities,* also called varices, or varicose veins. They most often occur in the lower extremities and rectal area but occasionally also involve the vulva and groin. These are surface veins, the walls of which are thin and greatly enlarged. Their prominence during pregnancy is especially common because of increased blood volume, edema, and obstruction in venous return from the lower extremities that accompany gestation. Increased hormone levels may also cause relaxation of the smooth muscles in the walls of veins. They may appear as a swollen, purple, knotted network just under the skin. Affected lower extremities tire easily. The swollen veins may be more than a cosmetic problem, since occasionally they may be injured, may rupture, and may bleed or become the point of origin for a blood clot (thrombus). Most patients find relief by wearing support hose or applying bandages that stimulate return circulation to the heart. If elastic bandages are used, they should be applied from the foot up, with an even tension so that they themselves will not become obstructions to circulation. Ideally, support hose or bandages are used after the patient has had her legs elevated several minutes to drain the swollen veins. Swelling and fatigue will be less if the pregnant woman avoids standing for protracted periods and especially if she lies down at intervals and elevates her feet above the level of her head. Round garters or knee- or calf-length elastic-topped hose should never be worn. Pooling of blood in the lower part of the body plus dilatation of the surface blood vessels may be one cause of the faintness experienced by many pregnant women.

Hemorrhoids. Rectal varicosities are termed hemorrhoids. They may be external or internal and are produced or aggravated by the pressure of the developing fetus or constipation. They can be painful and occasionally may become thrombosed or may bleed. Most of the time surgical treatment is not contemplated during pregnancy because the condition usually disappears or vastly improves after childbirth. Attention should be paid to the prevention of constipation. Witch hazel compresses, analgesic ointments, such as dibucaine (Nupercainal), special suppositories, and sitz baths may help.

Muscle cramps

Muscle cramps are often experienced during pregnancy; they usually involve the calf muscle and can be agonizing. They result from a calcium and phosphorus imbalance in the body, causing a form of *tetany.* Immediate treatment consists of straightening the leg by pushing down on the knee and pulling the ball of the foot up toward the knee. Preventive therapy for muscle cramps includes increased calcium intake in the form of calcium lactate or gluconate, with increased vitamin D intake. Some physicians using this regimen may limit the woman's intake of milk because of its high phosphorus content. Others continue to recommend a quart of milk a day but prescribe small quantities of aluminum hydroxide gel (Amphojel) in the diet to prevent the assimilation of excess phosphorus. The patient should be advised to avoid fatigue, cold legs, and pointing her toes when stretching. She should lead with her heels when walking.

Leukorrhea

During pregnancy the hormonally stimulated cervix produces more mucus than is normal during ovulation or before or after menstruation. This physiologic discharge, termed leukorrhea, is unpreventable and may be bothersome. Women should be advised not to douche. Treatment includes cleanliness of the perineum, avoidance of occlusive underwear, wearing of pads, reassurance, and the recommendation to report the following; foul odor, change in color or character of the discharge, and vulvovaginal itching.

When leukorrhea has the characteristics just mentioned, the discharge may be caused by a vaginal or vulvar infection. Descriptions of common vaginal infections follows.

Trichomoniasis. *Trichomonas vaginalis,* a microscopic protozoon, is a common cause of leukorrhea (Fig. 9-2, *B*). This organism may inhabit the vaginal canal without causing noticeable symptoms. However, during pregnancy the increase in alkalinity of the vagina may cause *T. vaginalis* to multiply rapidly and create annoying signs and symptoms. Typically these symptoms are an

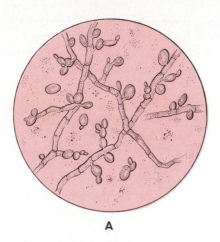 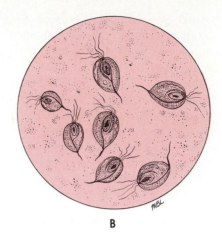

FIG 9-2 Microscopic views. **A,** *Candida (Monilia) albicans,* a fungus. **B,** *Trichomonas vaginalis,* a protozoan or microscopic animal.

irritating, profuse, thin, foamy yellow malodorous vaginal discharge and vulvovaginal itching or burning. The motile organism may be identified under the microscope in hanging drop slide preparations. Sometimes a simple glass slide with cover slip allows visualization of the motile parasite. *Trichomonas* is difficult to combat locally because of the structure of the vaginal folds. Metronidazole (Flagyl), administered orally or vaginally, has proved effective and is now the drug of choice. Formerly, its use during the first trimester of pregnancy was not recommended. However, research involving 1020 women who were given metronidazole during the first 3 months of pregnancy has demonstrated no increased frequency of birth defects.* The sexual partner should be treated concurrently.

Candidiasis vulvovaginitis. Candidiasis is an infection caused by a yeast or fungus called *Candida albicans,* or *Monilia albicans.* It is easily diagnosed by direct microscopic examination of the discharge or by culture techniques (Fig. 9-2, *A*). A *Candida* vaginal infection produces a cheesy, whitish discharge and beefy red vulvar irritation. Like *Trichomonas, C. albicans* can inhabit the body without producing any apparent signs or symptoms, or it may spread tremendously and be quite notable. Candidiasis is seen frequently in pregnant women, diabetics (treated and untreated), women using broad-spec-

trum antibiotics (for example, penicillin, tetracycline, and erythromycin), and women living under stressful conditions. Stress is thought to affect the acid-base balance of the vaginal mucosa. Treatment includes the careful prescription of fungicidal agents applied locally in the form of vaginal suppositories and creams such as miconazole nitrate 2%, clotrimazole, or nystatin (Mycostatin). Nystatin also may be given by mouth to prevent monilial overgrowth when broad-spectrum antibiotics are prescribed or to treat an oral infection. *C. albicans* in the oral cavity produces thrush, discussed on p. 242. Intermittent cool tap water compresses applied to the vulva may prove soothing to the patient.

Other causes. Gonorrhea, unfortunately a very common infection that may produce vaginal or urethral discharge, will be discussed under "major problems," p. 174. Most often gonorrhea is asymptomatic in women. Mixed infections of the vaginal tract may be encountered that are especially difficult to treat.

Many physicians do not advise douching during pregnancy. Even in the nonpregnant state, evidence indicates that douching usually should not be done; bacteria may be forced in a retrograde fashion through the cervix, uterus, and tubes, causing endometritis and salpingitis. Besides causing an increase in pelvic infections, douching washes away the normal vaginal flora, leading to an overgrowth of hostile bacteria. As an alternative to douching, sitting in a warm tub of water and allowing the water to gently rinse the vaginal vault is recommended.

---

*Rosa FW, Baum C, and Shaw M: Pregnancy outcomes after first trimester vaginitis drug therapy, Obstet Gynecol 69(5):751, 1987.

Some conditions or characteristics that constitute increased risk for a mother and her unborn child

1. Low socioeconomic, educational status (influencing especially nutrition, prenatal care supervision, and compliance)
2. Little or no prenatal care
3. Maternal age less than 18 or more than 35 years old
4. More than four pregnancies (especially if more than 35 years old)
5. Conception within 2 months of last delivery
6. Living at high altitude
7. The presence of coincidental maternal disease or significant health problems involving
   a. Cardiovascular disease
   b. Renal disease
   c. Diabetes mellitus
   d. Tuberculosis or other pulmonary disease
   e. Herpes simplex, syphilis, viral infections
   f. Hereditary anomaly or possible carrier state (for example, sickle-cell anemia, myelomeningocele, cystic fibrosis, osteogenesis imperfecta)
   g. Use of drugs: alcohol, nicotine, and street drugs
   h. Ingestion of fetotoxic medication, exposure to radiation or toxic chemicals
   i. Obesity (more than 20% greater than standard weight for height)

8. Previous obstetric complications that may recur, such as
   a. Preeclampsia-eclampsia (pregnancy-induced hypertension)
   b. Severe anemia, clotting problems, intrapartum or postpartum hemorrhage
   c. Cephalopelvic disproportion
9. Previous poor fetal outcome (repetitive fetal loss, stillbirth)
10. Deviations in the current pregnancy such as
    a. Twinning or other multiple pregnancies
    b. Premature or small-for-date fetus
    c. Postmature fetus (more than 42 weeks)
    d. Breech presentation
    e. Polyhydramnios or oligohydramnios
    f. Preterm or prolonged rupture of membranes
    g. Any of the complications noted in Section 8 above
    h. Obstetric complications (placenta previa, abruptio placentae, abnormal presentation, Rh or blood group sensitization)

MAJOR PROBLEMS OF PREGNANCY AND CHILDBIRTH

High-risk pregnancies

Certain characteristics or conditions of the prospective mother or her child cause jeopardy. Some of these can be detected at the onset or shortly after the beginning of gestation. Such pregnancies are often termed high risk. However, the amount of risk involved includes more than the presence of a specific condition. It also involves the general health of the individual and other related psychologic and social factors. Because it is difficult to accurately rate all the situations noted, the box above highlights factors constituting *increased* risk. Some of these patients are being referred to regional obstetric intensive care centers, or perinatal centers, where specialists and sophisticated equipment are available. These centers are commonly associated with neonatal intensive care units, capable of caring for the endangered newborn in the best manner possible. The maternal, fetal, and infant mortalities for many of these conditions have decreased with the use of these facilities.

Diabetes mellitus. Nearly one in 300 pregnancies is complicated by diabetes mellitus, an endocrine disorder characterized by high levels of blood glucose owing to insufficient insulin production by the pancreas. Prior to the implementation of insulin therapy, few diabetic women conceived, and many of those who conceived, did not survive pregnancy. Insulin improved fertility and decreased maternal mortality, but perinatal mortality remained high (about 40%). In recent years technologic advances have dramatically altered the management of diabetic pregnancies. Today, mothers receiving optimal care who demonstrate diabetes before their pregnancy experience a perinatal mortality of about 5%. Those who only show signs of diabetes during pregnancy have no greater perinatal morality than those without this condition. Only with intensive care are such outcomes possible.*

Not all women are aware that they are diabetic.

*Gabbe SG: Diabetes mellitus: ways of individualizing care, Contemp OB/ GYN 36(1):68, 1990.

NURSING CARE PLAN

Psychosocial Nursing Care of the High-Risk Patient during Labor and Delivery

Selected nursing diagnoses	Expected outcomes	Interventions
Fear and anxiety related to specific high-risk condition and uncertainty of outcome for mother and baby. Clinical manifestations: Expresses concern for condition of baby and self. Increased verbalization and questions or withdrawn and uncommunicative. Crying, restless, irritable, trembling. Difficulty in concentrating when directions given. Unable to relax and control breathing without continual reminders.	Patient will use effective coping mechanisms: Able to cooperate during procedures. Verbalizes understanding of risks to baby and self and rationale for plan of care.	Stay with woman. Indicate concern with eye contact, touch, as well as verbal communication according to patient's cultural background. Speak slowly and clearly. Provide simple, accurate explanations of procedures to woman and family. Allow her to express feelings in her own way: talking, crying, moaning. Help her to focus on relaxation breathing. Praise her for positive efforts. Offer information on condition and progress: emphasize hopeful findings (e.g., FHR within normal limits) but avoid false reassurance. Recognize needs of support person/family: demonstrate support techniques, provide respite if needed. Need for food, sleep, shower? Explore possible family desires for added spiritual support, involvement of clergy, prayer.

Screening for hyperglycemia begins with the first antenatal visit and continues throughout pregnancy. This screen includes risk assessment, urinalysis to detect glycosuria (each prenatal visit includes a urinalysis for glucose), and additional laboratory analysis when indicated. Some physicians are recommending that all prenatal patients have a 1-hour glucose screen between 24 to 28 weeks of gestation. The following risk factors warn that diabetes may develop during the stress of pregnancy: prior delivery of a larger than 9-pound infant or an infant with anomalies, previous stillbirth, history of polyhydramnios, recurrent monilial vaginitis, family history of diabetes mellitus, and obesity.

Tests used to diagnose diabetes mellitus are the glucose tolerance test, fasting blood sugar determination, and 1-hour postprandial evaluation of blood sugar. A presumptive diagnosis is based on the presence of glycosuria, but definitive diagnosis depends on the results of other laboratory tests.

The hormonal changes of normal pregnancy cause resistance to insulin utilization, which increases blood sugar. High blood levels of glucose cause increased insulin output, which increases the rate of fat breakdown and protein synthesis. In this manner, additional amounts of glucose and amino acids are made available for fetal consumption, and an alternative source of fuel—free fatty acids—is provided for maternal energy requirements.

Effect of pregnancy on the diabetic state. Pregnancy does not worsen the diabetic state, unless the diabetes is poorly controlled, but it significantly affects insulin control of the disorder. Also, women with marginally productive pancreatic cells may exhibit diabetes during pregnancy (gestational diabetes) but have normal blood sugar levels after delivery.

The diabetic woman's need for increased amounts of injected (exogenous) insulin varies during pregnancy. Until about 18 weeks of gestation, insulin needs are reduced. After that time the developing placenta produces increasing amounts of hormones that cause resistance to insulin utilization so that from 20 weeks until term insulin needs both fluctuate and increase. Immediately after the expulsion of the placenta, insulin needs drop abruptly and remain low for a period of time. Less insulin is required by the nursing mother.

Effect of diabetes upon pregnancy. Chronic hyperglycemia has vascular effects. These vascular changes also affect the placenta, and the result is placental insufficiency of varying degrees. Hyperglycemia early in pregnancy may cause abortion or adversely affect embryonic development. Fetal anomalies are five to six times more common. Hyperglycemia later in pregnancy is associated with intrauterine death (especially after 36 weeks), large but physiologically immature infants (above 9 pounds), and various types of neonatal illnesses. Poorly controlled diabetes (hyperglycemia) increases the woman's risk of infection, especially pyelonephritis and monilial vaginitis. The probability is higher that she will experience pregnancy-induced hypertension or polyhydramnios, with their attendant risks of placental detachment, amniotic fluid embolism, and disseminated intravascular coagulation (DIC).

Drug therapy. Insulin is secreted by the islets of Langerhans in the pancreas. Failure of these cells to produce insulin results in hyperglycemia because insulin is required to carry glucose across the peripheral cell membranes.

Two types of medication are used to correct hyperglycemia. One is the administration of exogenous insulin. The other is an oral hypoglycemic medication that lowers blood sugar by stimulating the pancreatic cells to produce more insulin. However, any previously prescribed oral hypoglycemics are discontinued during pregnancy because this class of medication may be teratogenic and produce neonatal hypoglycemia.

Management of the insulin-dependent diabetic woman. Just as insulin is the key to lowering maternal mortality, appropriate blood sugar levels (euglycemia) are the key to bettering perinatal outcome. Maintaining euglycemia *before conception* is important if the embryo is to be protected in the early weeks before pregnancy is suspected or diagnosed.

Both obstetrician and endocrinologist usually monitor the diabetic woman's pregnancy. Home control and management include these five aspects: urine testing for ketones; blood glucose monitoring; insulin administration by infusion pump or subcutaneously; diet control; and exercise modified to gain control. (For a discussion of diet and exercise requirements for the individual diabetic see pp. 757-759.)

Urine testing. Ketosis is monitored by testing the urine for the presence of ketones. Urine sugar is not a reliable indicator during pregnancy; therefore blood sugar should be monitored directly. To ensure accuracy, urine used for testing should not have been standing in the bladder for a period of time. For this reason the urine used for testing is the second voided specimen. This means the individual voids and, one half hour later, voids again; the specimen tested is taken from the second voiding.

Blood glucose determination. At home blood glucose determination can be done by either of two methods: color-stable strips or the use of Glucostix and a reflectance meter. The latter method is associated with fewer hospitalizations for blood sugar stabilization.

Insulin management. Insulin administration may be by subcutaneous injection or by use of an insulin pump. Insulin may be infused continuously by using one of two insulin pump systems available for home use. When insulin is administered subcutaneously, split doses are usually necessary.

Perinatal evaluation and care of the infant. Fetal surveillance intensifies after 26 weeks' gestation and is essential for judging the most favorable time for delivery. Ultrasound examinations estimate fetal size, fetal growth rates, and the volume of amniotic fluid. Amniocentesis is used to obtain amniotic fluid specimens for measures of pulmonary maturation (L/S ratio). Stress and nonstress tests evaluate placental sufficiency.

Among the factors that influence perinatal survival are the severity of the diabetes, control of the diabetes during pregnancy, placental function, the occurrence of obstetric complications or congenital abnormalities, and prematurity. See p. 307 for discussion of the care of infants of diabetic mothers.

When labor occurs, insulin is infused continuously with an infusion pump; hourly blood sugar assessment is used to compute insulin dosage; and the fetus is monitored electronically. After delivery, blood sugar levels continue to be the basis for determining insulin dosage. Breastfeeding mothers require more calories and less insulin. When acetone is present in the urine, breast-feeding must be suspended, the infant formula-fed, the breasts pumped, and the physician contacted for supervision.

Lowering perinatal mortality and morbidity is a team effort and is brought about by internist, obstetrician, pediatrician, nurse (including at times a nurse specialist in diabetes), and diabetic mother working together.

Cardiac problems. The incidence of heart disease in obstetric patients varies from 0.5% to 2.0%. Individuals with heart disease are classified according to the amount of activity that causes disability or distress. During pregnancy the cardiac output is increased by more than one third, the heart rate accelerates by 10 beats per minute (bpm), and the blood volume is expanded by one third. After birth, readjustment in vascular volume occurs. The periods of maximum cardiovascular stress and the times that some measure of decompensation most likely will occur are after 14 weeks, especially during labor and in the hours immediately following birth.

Signs and symptoms of decompensation are heart rate greater than 100 bpm and respirations greater than 28 per minute, which is associated with dyspnea, coughing, rales at the base of the lungs, and pallor or cyanosis. Decompensation must be treated to avoid overt heart failure.

When cardiac disability is minimal, maternal and perinatal mortality are only slightly increased. With marked degrees of cardiac disease, the maternal mortality is 1% to 3%, and the perinatal mortality is about 50%.

Urinary problems. The pregnant patient with urinary tract disease is a challenge to medical management, especially when kidney function is impaired. Pregnancy puts a strain on the urinary system. The developing uterus may pinch or kink the ureters (particularly on the right because the growing uterus rotates to the right during pregnancy). Stoppage of normal urinary flow predisposes the system to infection (pyelonephritis). Infections are often caused by colon bacilli, but other organisms may also be responsible. If the kidneys are already damaged by a previous pathologic condition, the added strain imposed by the excretion of fetal waste may be significant. Infection of the kidney and urinary tract may manifest itself in several ways: chills and fever; lower back pain; pain on voiding; and a urinalysis of a clean-catch specimen characterized by the presence of numerous white blood cells, bacteria (100+ colonies per ml), and perhaps red blood cells and albumin. Recurrent infection may necessitate urologic tests to rule out urinary tract obstruction or other non-pregnancy-related causes. Untreated infection may prompt premature labor and delivery.

Infection of the kidney usually responds well to measures such as bed rest, forced fluids, urinary sedatives or analgesics, and antibiotic therapy based on sensitivity studies. When hospitalized, these patients are routinely on intake and output measurement and undergo frequent blood pressure and daily weight determinations. Daily urinalysis is often ordered. Renal disease may be inflammatory or degenerative. It is closely connected with the condition of the blood supply to the kidneys, and any continuous process that interferes with this supply will present symptoms in time. Conversely, any significant damage to the kidney will reflect itself in a change in the circulatory system, particularly an elevation of the blood pressure, as more and more pressure is exerted in an attempt to maintain adequate filtration. The onset of significant hypertension is related to a worsening prognosis for both fetus and mother. Patients whose renal disease is not caused by a current infection (for example, glomerulonephritis) receive much the same nursing care as those with a diagnosed bacterial invasion, and antibiotics are often given prophylactically. Chronic or advanced renal disease should be frequently evaluated by renal function tests. It may pose a real threat to both the mother and her unborn child.

Syphilis. A complete prenatal examination should always include a serologic test for detection of syphilis (STS) (see p. 68). In the 1950s it was believed that the problem of syphilis had been largely solved because of these prenatal precautions and the successful introduction of antibiotics in its treatment. Many "L clinics," so named for lues, another word for syphilis, were closed. Education of the public and the related necessary casework regarding venereal diseases or conditions that are primarily sexually transmitted (at that time principally syphilis and gonorrhea), which were responding so well to penicillin therapy, were not continued with the same diligence. Health workers were concerned to find later that national morbidity for syphilis had risen sharply. The reported cases of gonorrhea had also increased alarmingly. These increases were caused in part by the ill-founded sense of security regarding these diseases and by the cutbacks in federal, state, and local budgets helping in its control. These increased incidences were also symptoms of the growing restlessness, lack of purpose, family breakdown, and increase in sexual activity that have become major problems of 20th century society. Syphilis is most common in urban areas in the sexually active population aged 15 to 29.

Transmission. The infectious agent, a corkscrewlike organism, or spirochete, called *Treponema pallidum,* invades the mucous membranes or skin, or both. Though primarily a sexually transmitted disease (STD), syphilis may be acquired through accidental inoculation by contaminated needles or exposure to infectious skin lesions by professional personnel or other contacts. Transplacental syphilis infection of the unborn infant may occur at any time during pregnancy. Because young fetuses are unable to manifest a readily detectable response to early invasion of syphilis, they formerly were inaccurately considered to be safe by virtue of a special placental barrier until approximately 18 weeks' gestation. The techniques of electromicroscopy and immunofluorescence have proved this concept to be in error. The infective organism cannot live for more than a few hours in an environment deprived of moisture and is destroyed by drying. It is also killed by many chemicals, including soap.

Stages. The disease has been divided into three different stages of development, or progression. The first stage—the period of initial body response—usually manifests itself from 10 to 90 days after exposure. The average time is 3 weeks. Classically, the characteristic lesion of the first stage of the disease is a relatively hard, raised, painless area crowned by a craterlike depression found at the site of entry known as a *chancre*. This lesion is not always seen, however. Sometimes it actually seems to be absent; at other times it is present, but hidden from view in the folds of the vaginal or urethral canals. Rarely the chancre may develop on the lips or breast. It is highly infectious. The spirochete may be identified in its secretions in dark-field microscopic studies. However, at this time the findings of the serology test are usually negative. The chancre disappears after 3 to 5 weeks. The uninformed victim may think the problem has also disappeared, but such is not the way of syphilis. The organisms have been multiplying and spreading throughout the body. Usually not long after the chancre vanishes, the person discovers other difficulties, and their advent signals the beginning of the second stage of the infection.

The second stage of syphilis is characterized by a bronze- or rose-colored flat or raised scaly rash that may be quite faint, appearing on different body areas but most significantly on the palms of the hands and soles of the feet. This eruption is often accompanied by enlargement of the lymph nodes. Flattened, moist, wartlike lesions called *mucous patches,* or *condylomata lata,* may also appear on the skin and mucous membranes. These are highly infectious, containing the spirochete. The person does not feel well and may have a headache, sore throat, and aching joints and muscles. There may be a spotty loss of hair. These signs and symptoms may fade away

after several weeks, never to return in the same way, or they may reappear at irregular intervals for a period of up to 4 years. During the second stage of syphilis the serology test is routinely positive.

The third stage of the disease may occur anywhere from 2 to 20 years after the initial contact with the spirochete. Although the disease is present, it may produce no visible symptoms. It is then considered to be latent. About 30% of those patients in the tertiary stage develop widespread serious disorders that interfere greatly with life. Soft tumors called *gummas* develop in the tissues and may ulcerate or form abscesses. Vital centers, such as the brain, spinal cord, large blood vessels, and heart, are often damaged. There may be gastrointestinal symptoms. Infected persons may become mentally ill. They may be unable to walk normally because of central nervous system disease causing a typical body-jarring gait. They are usually not infectious at this stage. Routinely the serology test is positive.

Adequate treatment of syphilis with penicillin in the first or second stages brings an optimistic prognosis. Results of treatment in the third stage are questionable.

Congenital syphilis. Although initial prenatal maternal serology examination can be successful in identifying most potential cases, the incidence of congenital syphilis has continued to reflect the rising incidence of maternal and secondary syphilis. The problem has increased because of a growing number of women who for various reasons are not receiving prenatal care or who are not receiving adequate serologic testing, treatment, or response to treatment. Some physicians repeat blood tests later in pregnancy to combat new, developing infection and fetal damage, since previous maternal infection and treatment do not produce immunity or protection of the fetus.

The syphilitic baby may not be born alive. The untreated syphilitic mother characteristically has a high spontaneous abortion rate. If born alive, the affected child may suffer from various problems. Probably the most common characteristic of the syphilitic infant is the presence of a thick, almost continuous, sometimes blood-tinged nasal discharge associated with a sniffling sound on respiration. For this reason the manifestation is called *snuffles*. The skin, especially over the palms of the hands and soles of the feet, may be blistered and peeling. There may be sore fissures around the lips and anus. The joints are sometimes very tender. The liver and spleen are usually enlarged. The causative organism has been found in lesions of the skin and mucous membranes. All syphilitic infants should be isolated until at least 24 hours after adequate treatment is begun. (Drainage/secretion and universal precautions should be in place. See discussion, p. 155.) More permanent but later-appearing signs indicating the prior presence of congenital syphilis are notched teeth (Hutchinson's teeth) and a so-called saddle nose. Penicillin is again the drug of choice in the treatment of congenital syphilis. (See also p. 307.)

Gonorrhea (GC). In many communities gonorrhea has now reached epidemic proportions, particularly among the teenage and young adult population (see Fig. 30-5). Many city and county health departments accept minors for free, confidential STD diagnosis and treatment, without parental consent, relying on their right under law to care for persons of all ages suffering from communicable diseases. However, not all states have laws that permit private and hospital physicians to treat minors for venereal disease without parental consent.

Gonorrhea is caused by a coffee bean-shaped diplococcus, *Neisseria gonorrhoeae.* In females it may produce an irritating, purulent, infectious vaginal discharge, and, since it often infects the Skene glands, may initiate burning on urination. The disease may spread into the reproductive tract and cause inflammatory changes. It may produce abnormal narrowing of the fallopian tubes and may be responsible finally for ectopic pregnancy (a pregnancy that develops outside the normal uterine placement) or sterility. In males it generally produces a urethral irritation or discharge. However, asymptomatic carriers of either sex are possible. Gonorrhea may also become a more generalized infection, spreading through the bloodstream and lymphatic system. It is not innocuous, occasionally causing serious complications, spreading abscesses, arthritis, and other inflammations in both sexes.

Previous disease confers no immunity in the event of additional exposures. The incubation period extends from 1 to 14 days. Recommended medications have been aqueous penicillin or ampicillin in conjunction with probenecid to prolong antibiotic activity. A resistant strain of the gonococcus does not appear to respond characteristically to this routine treatment. Spectinomycin (Trobicin) has been successfully used, but the safety of the drug has not been established during pregnancy.

Chlamydia infection. Today, the bacterial microorganism, *Chlamydia trachomatis* (CT) is considered to be the cause of the most common sexually transmitted disease in the United States in which over 4 million new cases are estimated to occur each year. It easily surpasses gonorrhea in the number of persons affected, although it shares some of its characteristics and outcomes.

Like gonorrhea, CT is often present without creating noticeable signs or symptoms, but is also able to produce much pain and anguish. In men, it may be associated with urethritis, epididymitis, and possibly sterility. In women, it may initiate pelvic inflammatory disease (PID), leading to ectopic pregnancies and infertility. Women under 20 years of age who have recently become sexually active and who have multiple sex partners are especially at risk for acquiring CT disease. Almost 50% of these women diagnosed as infected with CT also have gonorrhea. Penicillin or spectinomycin is usually effective in treating gonorrhea but not chlamydia. It has been recommended that patients with either disease receive treatment for both. Extended erythromycin therapy has been advocated for chlamydia infections during pregnancy. (See also p. 307 for neonatal impact.)

Herpes genitalis. Herpes simplex virus type 2 (HSV-2), a sexually transmitted disease, characteristically infects the lower genital tract. The lesions are similar to those of the related common fever blister caused by herpes simplex type 1 (HSV-1). Type 1 may also cause genital lesions but not as commonly as HSV-2, although rates worldwide appear to differ considerably. Regardless of the agent's type, the lesions often involving the vulva, perineum, and cervix are painful blisters that rupture to reveal shallow ulcerations that later crust. Healing of primary lesions is usually complete in 2 to 4 weeks.

The first episode of infection typically is accompanied by fever, dysuria, lymphadenopathy, and flulike symptoms. Recurrent lesions are not as painful and last about 10 days; often these infections are asymptomatic. Infected persons shed the virus irregularly and indefinitely. The virus is identified by tissue culture of scrapings from the base of a lesion or by detection of typical giant cells in a Papanicolaou smear.

During early pregnancy a first attack of herpes genitalis may be responsible for an increased incidence of spontaneous abortion. Later in pregnancy such a primary infection increases the risk of premature birth. The infant born vaginally of a mother suffering from primary genital herpes has about a 50% chance of neonatal infection. However, the risk of neonatal infection in the case of *recurrent* maternal disease is much lower—4% to 5%. When neonatal infection occurs, the probability that an infant will die is over 50%. An infant who survives may exhibit significant neurologic damage. These are frightening statistics.

In the past many obstetric management protocols have been proposed including extensive prenatal monitoring by cultures and clinical observation of patients with a history of genital herpes. Such monitoring has proved to be expensive and does not produce information that can reliably predict when a newborn will be infected or if cesarean delivery would avoid neonatal infection. In 1988, the American College of Obstetricians and Gynecologists and the American Academy of Pediatrics recommended that "expeditious" or rapid cesarean delivery be undertaken for patients "who have *active* lesions near or at term and who are in labor, or who have ruptured membranes." The fact that the patient may have had confirmed active genital lesions previously during the pregnancy was not thought to be sufficient cause to perform follow-up cultures or schedule cesarean delivery.*

After delivery, depending on the patient's labor/delivery history and on hospital policies, the infected mother and infant may be cared for in a private room. The mother is taught the principles and procedures of drainage and secretion precautions to protect her baby and others from the infection. She may breastfeed.

Acyclovir (Zovirax) is usually considered the most effective drug in hastening the healing of primary lesions. Its use during pregnancy has not been adequately studied and is not recommended. Sitz baths and/or heat lamps may be comforting.

Herpes virus type 2 is associated with later cervical dysplasia and may be linked with the development of cervical cancer. Follow-up observation is essential.

Acquired immune deficiency syndrome (AIDS). For a brief outline of the cause, description, importance, mode of transmission, and nursing care of patients with this diagnosis see pp. 615 and 624.

Tuberculosis. Tuberculosis (TB) is still an important health problem throughout the world. In the United States, 23,495 new cases were reported in 1989. It is frequently associated with poverty, overcrowding, and poor nutrition. Of particular concern has been the relatively high rates of disease affecting black and Hispanic Americans, recent immigrants to the United States, and persons infected with both TB and human immunodeficiency virus (HIV).

Tuberculosis is spread through air-borne TB germs from the coughs or sneezes of a person with infectious tuberculosis. A susceptible person who shares the same air for a prolonged period of time may eventually breathe in TB germs and become infected. Only 5% of *newly* infected people progress to active disease within 1 to 2 years after infection. The other 95% control the infection,

*American Academy of Pediatrics/American College of Obstetricians and Gynecologists: Guidelines for perinatal care, ed 2, 1988, p 145.

are *not* infectious, but for the rest of their life remain at risk of progressing to active disease. From this group, another 5% progresses to active disease if they do not complete a full course of preventive therapy.

Persons with a positive tuberculin skin test (Mantoux) should receive a chest x-ray and be evaluated for preventive therapy with isoniazid (INH). INH is taken for 6 to 12 months to prevent progression of infection to active disease. Preventive therapy for pregnant women is usually postponed until after delivery.

General symptoms of TB are fever, weight loss, fatigue, and night sweats. Symptoms of pulmonary disease include these same general symptoms with the addition of cough, sputum production, hemoptysis, and chest pain. Treatment for active disease must include a minimum of two to three antituberculosis drugs. A pregnant woman with active disease needs effective drug treatment to protect herself and her fetus. Length of treatment varies depending on the regimen to which the patient is assigned, drug susceptibility results, and patient response to treatment. Regimens vary from a 4-drug/6-month protocol to a 2-drug protocol lasting 18 months or more. Current recommendations from the Centers for Disease Control/American Thoracic Society are available at the local Health Department Tuberculosis Control Program.

Diseases associated with pregnancy

The following complications are so grouped because they are of major importance and are associated only with pregnancy, labor, and birth. They are not always preventable or predictable.

Hemorrhagic complications. The threat of hemorrhage is a very real consideration during all periods of pregnancy, birth, and even after delivery. In the months of gestation, vaginal bleeding is always considered to be a potential menace to both the fetus and the mother. As mentioned previously, hemorrhage is the most common complication of pregnancy.

Abortion. Spotting or bleeding during the early months is often related to abortion, defined as loss of the fetus before viability.

Types. Abortions may be *spontaneous,* without any premeditation (called miscarriages by the public), or they may be *induced.* Most communities identify two types of induced abortion: legal abortions, which are done after medical consultation following definite prescribed protocols, and criminal abortions, which have no legal sanction. The problems of sepsis, hemorrhage, and unequal availability to all women are some of the factors that have brought about changes in the laws governing le-

NURSING CARE PLAN

Admission of Pregnant Patient with Acute Third Trimester Bleeding—An Obstetric Emergency

Selected nursing diagnoses	Expected outcomes	Interventions
A. Potential fluid volume deficit related to hemorrhage.	Harmful effect on mother and infant will be minimized.	*No routine enema, vaginal or rectal exam on admission*—such manipulation can worsen bleeding.

B. Potential altered fetal tissue perfusion—oxygen deficit.
Clinical manifestations: diagnosis?
If abruptio placentae:
Vaginal bleeding (dark red) may or may not be present.
Possible portwine colored amniotic fluid.
Abdominal pain—mild to severe.
Uterus firmly contracted and tender to palpation.
Vital sign changes—increased pulse and decreased blood pressure
(Changes may be greater than amount of visible bleeding would indicate.)
Fetal heart rate and pattern changes.
Increased fetal activity.
If placenta previa:
Vaginal bleeding (bright red), varies in amount.
No abdominal pain or tenderness, uterus soft between contractions if in labor.
Vital sign changes—increased pulse and decreased blood pressure depending on amount of bleeding.
Fetal heart rate and pattern changes.
	Delivery of infant with Apgar of 7 or above.
	Maternal vital signs, hematocrit within normal limits.
		Notify physician promptly of admission and initial assessments.
		Review obstetric history—course of present pregnancy.
		Keep patient NPO and on bedrest.
		Frequent observation of:
		  Level of consciousness; behavior
		  Vital signs
		  Skin color and temperature
		  Urinary output (possible Foley catheter)
		  Fetal heart rate and (if present) contraction patterns electronically monitored
		  Vaginal bleeding—note color-presence of clots; count or weigh blood-stained pads.
		  Other abnormal bleeding—petechiae, purpura, epistaxis, bleeding gums (possible signs of DIC).
		  Localized abdominal pain.
		Uterine contractions?
		Evaluation for need of analgesia.
		Patient response to administration of IV fluids and acceptance and preparation for blood products as ordered.
		Expect follow-up blood and coagulation studies.
		Assist physician with ultrasound and other medical, diagnostic and therapeutic interventions.
		Alert pediatrician and nursery staff of impending delivery, possible C-section. Review preparation, secure permits as needed.

C. Anxiety related to potential life-threatening situation (see Nursing Care Plan on p. 170).		Provide emotional support to woman and family.

galized abortion. The problem of induced abortion continues to be a controversial issue in our society.

Other terminology is also used in describing an abortion. Physicians and nurses often use the adjectives "threatened" and "inevitable." A *threatened abortion* may possibly be halted. It may declare itself by uterine cramping or intermittent backache and spotting, but the loss of blood is relatively small, and the cervical opening remains closed. An *inevitable abortion* is characterized by severe or persistent contractions, moderate to abundant blood loss, and dilatation of the cervix. Loss of the fetus cannot be prevented. An *incomplete abortion* refers to the retention of some of the products of conception, most commonly a portion of the placenta. The uterus usually must be emptied by a mechanical dilatation of the cervix and gentle scraping of its walls by a curet. Such a procedure is called a dilatation and curettage, or "D and C." If abortion must take place at all, a *complete abortion* is desirable. In a complete abortion, all the products of the pregnancy are eliminated from the uterus. Patients with the diagnosis of inevitable abortion are admitted to the gynecologic service. However, if the viability of the fetus is debatable, the patient may be referred to the obstetric service.

Women who have lost more than three pregnancies at about the same stage of development are said to be victims of *habitual abortion*. Sometimes a very young fetus will die in the uterus and remain there 2 months or longer before it is expelled, through either spontaneous processes or medical or surgical intervention. Such a situation is declared a *missed abortion*. In such cases the placenta usually has remained attached to the uterus for an extended period of time, and the amniotic fluid has been gradually absorbed, producing a type of fetal mummification or even petrification.

Nursing care. The nursing care of a woman who is threatening spontaneous abortion would routinely include bed rest; avoidance of stress; observation for uterine cramping and loss of amniotic fluid; temperature, pulse, and blood pressure records; careful determination of the presence and amount of vaginal bleeding (the physician may wish all pads and soiled linen to be saved to evaluate extent of blood loss or frequent hematocrit and hemoglobin checks); and watchfulness to secure any passed tissue for diagnosis. Periodic checks for fetal heart tone should be performed if normally it should be heard. Vigilance for an elevation of temperature should be maintained. Iron medication or blood transfusions may be indicated. Sedatives and antibiotics may be employed. Inevitable abortion may be speeded by use of certain drugs (oxytocics) to stimulate the uterus to contract or by surgical intervention, especially in the presence of hemorrhage. A patient who aborts must continue to be closely observed for complications for several hours or days, depending on her general condition and the circumstances of her loss.

About 50% of all threatened abortions terminate as abortions. A large percentage of such fetal loss is associated with some defect in the developing child. Spontaneous abortion seems to be one way that nature tries to rectify a basic error. Attention to certain health measures may at times prevent fetal death from abortion. General improvement of maternal health, previous immunization against infectious diseases, and proper prenatal care are all valuable. If loss after the first trimester is caused by premature dilatation of the cervix (incompetent cervix), the cervix may be closed by various suturing techniques and released only when the fetus is ready for birth (for example, Shirodkar and Würm and Lash procedures). It would appear that spontaneous abortion during the first trimester is not caused by climbing stairs, jogging, exercise, activity, or intercourse. About 10% to 15% of all pregnancies end in spontaneous abortions with no known causes.

The nursing care of a patient undergoing a voluntary legal abortion in the hospital setting will be determined by her condition, the length of her pregnancy, and the method used by the physician to terminate her pregnancy. Termination is most often secured by dilatation and curettage, aspiration techniques, or prostaglandin administration; see Chapter 11.

Because of changes in the interpretation and content of abortion laws, nurses working in gynecologic, delivery, and operating room areas may be requested more frequently to assist in the process of legal abortion. If a nurse's scruples dictate that she not participate, she may decline to offer her services, if by so doing she is not jeopardizing the immediate health or life of a mother. (For example, she could secure another nurse to assist for whom abortion did not pose the same ethical problem.)

Ectopic pregnancy. The term ectopic pregnancy refers to any pregnancy that does not occupy the uterine cavity. In the majority of pregnancies the migrating egg is fertilized by the sperm in the fallopian tube and usually nests or implants in the lining of the uterine wall. Sometimes the tubes are abnormally narrowed, stenosed from inflammation, tumor, or congenital origin; then the tube may allow the sperm to ascend but be too narrow to allow the passage of the fertilized egg into the uterus.

The egg develops in the tube and soon causes rupture. Rarely, the embryo may continue growing as an abdominal pregnancy, which in unusual cases produces a full-term child who may survive if delivered through an abdominal incision. Pregnancies have also been found trying to develop in the ovary. The danger of hemorrhage in ectopic pregnancy is extremely serious. The amount of vaginal bleeding observed does not always reveal the true condition of the patient, since much blood loss can be hidden within the abdominal cavity. An ectopic pregnancy is most often tubal. A higher incidence of ectopic pregnancies is associated with failure of intrauterine contraceptive devices.

Symptoms. If tubal rupture or abortion occurs, the patient, who may or may not consider herself to be in early pregnancy, characteristically suffers severe knifelike pain in either lower abdominal quadrant. This may or may not be followed by spotting or bleeding. Shoulder pain from blood irritating the diaphragm or the urge to defecate are classic symptoms. A mass in the cul-de-sac may be palpated or bloody fluid may be aspirated by the physician. Ultrasound studies may aid diagnosis.

The signs of shock that develop are out of proportion to the amount of blood loss apparent. The patient may exhibit the classic signs of circulatory shock: pallor; cold, clammy skin; rapid, weak pulse, which will slow if shock deepens; falling blood pressure (a systolic reading of 90 mm Hg or under is usually considered "shock," depending on previous readings obtained); apprehension; loss of consciousness; and dilated pupils. Rapid surgical treatment and blood-loss replacement are generally indicated. Estimates vary, but ectopic pregnancy is more common than is usually supposed, occurring approximately once in 200 pregnancies. It terminates almost invariably with fetal loss, and the maternal mortality in the United States approaches 1 in 800 cases.

Placenta previa (Fig. 9-3, *A*). Two main types of obstetric hemorrhage are associated with the location of the placenta and its attachment. In the condition known as placenta previa, the placenta implants low on the interior

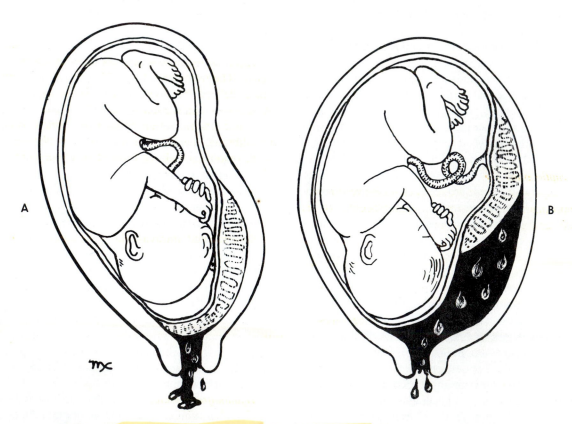

FIG 9-3 **A,** A type of total placenta previa. **B,** Abruptio placentae, or separation of normally inserted placenta.

of the uterine wall. (A *total placenta previa* will cover the cervical opening; a *partial* or *incomplete placenta previa* impinges on but does not cover the cervix; and a *marginal placenta previa* is low-lying, close to the dilating cervix.) In the latter part of pregnancy, the uterine contractions, which are always taking place to some degree though not always felt by the mother, may loosen the attachment of this abnormally positioned placenta and cause bright red, painless bleeding. The presence of placenta previa in other cases may not be detected until the onset of true labor and the dilatation of the cervical canal. Because of the relative safety of cesarean birth today, it is usually the treatment of choice. However, if the placenta is not implanted too low, if bleeding is minimal, and if the fetus is well but premature, some obstetricians may adopt a "wait-and-see" attitude and eventually deliver the patient vaginally. The use of electronic fetal monitors may be of real aid in detecting fetal problems in this instance.

Infection and emboli are other possible complications of placenta previa that should be considered. Hospitals may practice the "double set up technique" when treating a patient with placenta previa. Because vaginal or rectal examinations may worsen any bleeding present but may be considered necessary for the physician to obtain a proper evaluation, these procedures are delayed until preparations are completed for either a cesarean or a vaginal delivery in the same location as needed. Detection of a low placental insertion by the use of ultrasonic techniques is helpful. Placenta previa is more common in women who are multiparous. It occurs once in approximately 200 births.

Abruptio placentae (Fig. 9-3, *B*). The other type of hemorrhage related to placental attachment results from abruptio placentae, also called ablatio placentae or premature separation of the placenta. In this condition the placenta is implanted in the correct place, but for some reason—high blood pressure, sometimes as part of the preeclampsia-eclampsia syndrome or glomerulonephritis, possible dietary deficiency, local injury, rapid changes in intrauterine pressure, fetal pressure on the maternal vena cava, or other factors—it becomes detached. Although its name implies that the detachment occurs suddenly, this is not always the case. Separation of the placenta from the uterine wall may occur over a period of time. Detachment may occur first at the center of the placenta, resulting in hidden hemorrhage at first, or it may begin at the rim or outer portion, causing vaginal bleeding of varying amounts. Old blood, which has been trapped behind the separating placenta, appears dark when it finally escapes from the vaginal canal. Fresh bleeding usually is bright red (amniotic fluid may become portwine colored). Bleeding from a premature separation of a normally implanted placenta may be severe enough to cause rapid maternal circulatory shock, death, or brain damage to the infant because of lack of oxygen, and even danger of maternal mortality.

Symptoms. The first sign of abruptio placentae during labor may be an alteration in the contraction pattern. The contractions become very strong and almost constant. Little relaxation period, if any, may be detected. The uterus becomes tender and boardlike if enlarged with retained hemorrhage. There may or may not be external bleeding from the vagina. The symptoms of shock may be greater than the amount of visible bleeding would indicate. The fetal heart rate is either greatly accelerated or slowing. Late decelerations on the fetal monitor indicate diminishing placental function. The use of electronic monitoring techniques is encouraged, especially in suspect cases. The fetus, in its struggle to obtain more oxygen, may be very restless and active. If the amniotic sac, or bag of waters, is ruptured, meconium may be seen in the amniotic fluid—another sign of fetal distress. As shock from blood loss develops, the blood pressure falls, and the pulse increases and weakens. Abruptio placentae in its more severe forms is an obstetric emergency. The treatment often, although not inevitably, includes delivery by cesarean birth and blood replacement. A serious complication of abruptio placentae that has been encountered often enough to warrant mention is hypofibrinogenemia, an abnormally low fibrinogen level in the blood that makes normal blood clotting impossible. Treatment may include fibrogen replacement or use of cryoprecipitate (containing both fibrinogen and clotting factor VIII). A rare but serious associated complication, possible in other obstetric and medical settings as well, is disseminated intravascular coagulation (DIC). This problem begins with the triggering of coagulation mechanisms, probably by incidents such as the introduction of unusual clot-forming substances from the detaching placenta or its associated blood clot into the maternal circulation. Paradoxically, difficulties related to an opposing overprotective anticoagulation response by the body may lead to hemorrhage. Expert medical management and intensive nursing care are needed in these precarious circumstances. (See also p. 186.)

Hydatidiform mole. Another complication that may produce hemorrhage, although it is characterized by a much more unusual series of signs and symptoms, is called hydatidiform mole (usually shortened to hydatid mole). It is fairly rare in the United States but relatively common in parts of Asia. In this condition, for some unknown reason, the developing embryo and placenta deteriorate and usually lose their identity. Instead, a mass of abnormal, rapidly growing, trophoblastic tissue develops. It is theorized that formation of the mole is preceded by the death of the embryo and the disappearance of fetal circulation, while maternal circulation continues to sustain residual trophoblastic tissue. However, a mole can exist with a normal pregnancy. At times this tissue may resemble a cluster of small grapes, or it may be of tapioca consistency. Its presence may be suspected when the growth of a pregnancy seems abnormally rapid (a 3-month pregnancy may equal the size of a 5-month gestation), when no fetal heart tone or movement is detected, and when nausea and vomiting are excessive or persistent. Vaginal bleeding may be intermittent. Quantitative chorionic gonadotropin levels in the urine are greatly elevated. Ultrasonic diagnosis is possible. No fetal skeleton is demonstrated. If part of the abnormal tissue is expelled from the uterus, pathologic examination is indicated. This growth rarely may erode the uterus and cause rupture. It occasionally becomes malignant, spreading to the lungs and other body parts. After the mole's removal, pregnancy tests are continued to see whether any trophoblastic tissue is still active in the body and producing hormones. In the event of the diagnosis of hydatid mole, physicians may consider the advisability of removal of the uterus (hysterectomy) because of the possibility of the development of a malignant tumor, choriocarcinoma. Spreading choriocarcinoma, fortunately, is often curable by the use of anticancer chemicals such as methotrexate and actinomycin D.

Other causes. The causes of obstetric hemorrhage previously discussed—abortion, ectopic pregnancy, placenta previa, abruptio placentae, and hydatidiform mole—are those that most often occur during pregnancy or early labor. However, they are not the only causes of significant blood loss associated with childbirth. Obstetric laceration—vaginal, perineal, or cervical—and postpartal uterine atony (abnormal postpartal relaxation of the uterus) leading to excessive bleeding from the site of former placental attachment can be important intrapartal and postpartal complications.

Care of the bleeding patient. Before leaving the topic of blood loss during pregnancy and labor, let us review the care of patients who are bleeding. Presented below are some important dos and don'ts that all nurses should know. Although licensed vocational or practical nurses (LVNs or LPNs) should not have the total responsibility

for such patients, they should understand the following basic considerations:

1. Never give a bleeding patient an enema as part of the "routine admit." Never examine a bleeding patient rectally or vaginally. The physician performs any needed pelvic examination. Unnecessary manipulation of the area may increase the bleeding (especially in patients with placenta previa). Institute a regimen of bed rest and give the patient no food or fluids until ordered otherwise.
2. Observe the patient carefully and frequently:
   a. Take frequent pulse and blood pressure determinations. Compare, if possible, the results obtained with the patient's blood pressure reading on her prenatal record. Check for falling blood pressure and rising pulse.
   b. Check for type and amount of vaginal bleeding or amniotic drainage. If it is possible, save the evidences of bleeding for evaluation by the physician.
   c. Apply the fetal heart monitor routinely in any situation in which fetal stress or distress is a potential problem.
   d. Monitor also the character of any contraction and relaxation period by frequent observation. Check for any special uterine tenderness or rigidity and for poor or absent uterine relaxation.
3. Keep the charge nurse and physician informed of changes in the patient.
4. Expect possible orders for intravenous fluids, blood analyses, and cross match for blood transfusion. Record intake and output. Know if any religious scruples would preclude transfusion (for example, if the patient is a Jehovah's Witness).
5. Maintain a calm, supportive manner.

Pregnancy-induced hypertension (PIH) (preeclampsia-eclampsia syndrome, toxemia of pregnancy)

Definition and importance. Traditionally, toxemia of pregnancy, preeclampsia-eclampsia, or, using its newer name, pregnancy-induced hypertension (PIH), has been described as a serious, statistically important disorder characterized by the development after the 20th week of gestation of *hypertension,* with *albuminuria* or *edema* or both. These symptoms should be progressive in severity to actually make the diagnosis of PIH. If coma or seizure—not caused by coincidental neurologic disease—occurs, it is then called *eclampsia* (Fig. 9-4).

NURSING CARE PLAN

Admission of a Primipara with Pregnancy-Induced Hypertension (PIH)

Selected nursing diagnoses	Expected outcomes	Interventions
Potential for injury: A. Maternal, related to organ dysfunction as a result of generalized vasospasm.	Decreased maternal blood pressure, proteinuria, and edema.	Maintain patient on bedrest in left or right lateral position to increase blood flow to fetus and kidneys.

B. Fetal, related to impaired maternal placental perfusion.
Clinical manifestations:
  Rising blood pressure.
  Increasing proteinuria.
  Hyperactive reflexes.
  Complaints of headache, visual disturbances, epigastric pain.
  Decreased urinary output.
  FHR changes indicating distress.
	Absence of convulsions or coma.
	Safe delivery of viable infant.
		Monitor progress:
		  Blood pressure frequency depends on severity of condition/orders
		  Record hourly urine output, via catheter; report if <30 ml/hr.
		  Test for urine protein every hour or as ordered.
		  Weigh daily and assess edema, especially in sacral area.
		  Record intake and monitor IV fluids and infusion site.
		  Assess response to magnesium sulfate therapy.
		Monitor fetal well-being:
		  Continuous FHR monitoring.
		  Assist with assessment of fetal welfare and maturity (NST, ultrasound, amniocentesis).
		Maintain seizure precautions, quiet, darkened room, emergency tray with airway, oxygen, and suction immediately available, padded side rails.
		Observe for spontaneous onset of labor—need emergency delivery pack.

Preeclampsia affects approximately 5% of the entire maternity population in the United States, although in some areas, particularly the Southeast, and in some other parts of the world, the incidence is considerably higher. About 5% of those demonstrating preeclampsia develop eclampsia. Approximately 8% of those mothers who become eclamptic succumb to the disease or its compli-cations. Preeclampsia-eclampsia, or the older term "toxemia of pregnancy," has long been listed among the first three causes of maternal mortality. Chief causes of maternal death associated with preeclampsia-eclampsia are aspiration (pneumonia), cerebral hemorrhage, cardiac failure with pulmonary edema, or obstetric hemorrhage associated with premature separation of the placenta. A

CLASSIC SIGNS OF PREECLAMPSIA-ECLAMPSIA

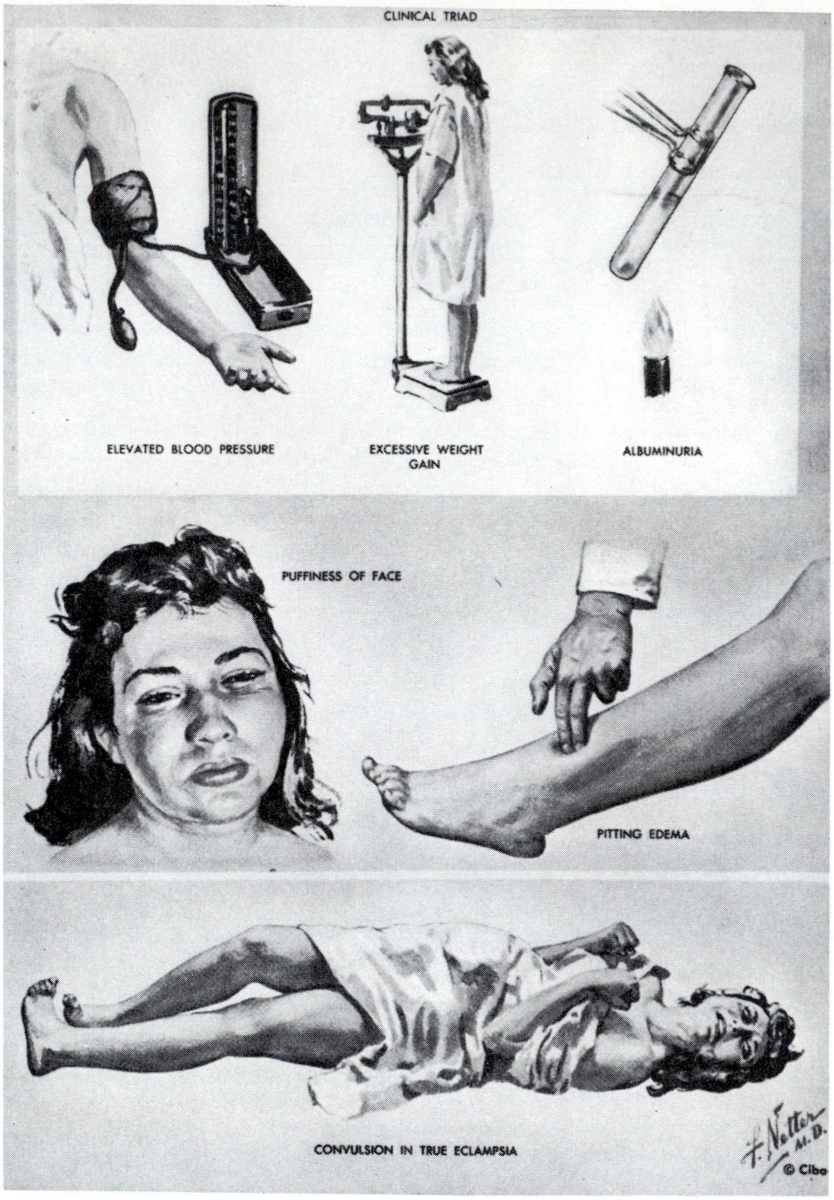

CLINICAL TRIAD

ELEVATED BLOOD PRESSURE   EXCESSIVE WEIGHT GAIN   ALBUMINURIA

PUFFINESS OF FACE   PITTING EDEMA

CONVULSION IN TRUE ECLAMPSIA

FIG 9-4   Symptomatology of preeclampsia and eclampsia. *(From The CIBA collection of medical illustrations, by Frank H. Netter, MD, Copyright CIBA.)*

surviving infant may suffer from intrauterine growth retardation. A perinatal mortality of about 20% has been reported for North America.

Different types of pathologic conditions, especially cardiovascular and renal disorders, may mimic certain aspects of preeclampsia. Considerable effort has been made in recent years to tighten its definition to advance the treatment of the patient and to aid in promoting accurate statistical reporting and analysis. Indeed, when any of the three classic signs of preeclampsia (hypertension, albuminuria, or edema) occur singly during a pregnancy, use of the term *preeclampsia* is not usually rec-

Table 9-1   Comparison of signs and symptoms of mild and severe preeclampsia-eclampsia (PIH)*

Characteristics	Mild preeclampsia	Severe preeclampsia
Blood pressure	Greater than 140/90 but less than 160/110 mm Hg 30 mm Hg systolic rise; or 15 mm Hg diastolic rise over baseline readings of early pregnancy (Above readings obtained after rest in a sitting position 2 times at least 6 hours apart.)	Blood pressure greater than 160/110 mm Hg
Proteinuria (albuminuria)	300 mg/L/24 hours or 2 separate random daytime specimens 6 hours apart (true clean catch) of 1+, 2+	5 g or more per 24 hours, 3+ in true clean-catch or catheterized specimen
Edema	Weight gain of more than 3 lb (1.4 kg) per week or 6 lb (2.72 kg) per month—any sudden weight gain is suspicious	Weight gain advances at accelerated rate
	Generalized visible edema 1+, 2+	Edema more pronounced, especially of hands, face 3+ (as condition worsens, edema of lungs, brain, and other organs)
Urine output	Not below 500 ml/24 hours	Oliguria less than 500 ml/24 hours
Neurologic signs and symptoms	Absent or only occasional headaches, blurred vision, or spots before eyes	More persistent headaches, blurred vision, and spots before eyes—retinal arteriole spasms on ophthalmic examination
	Normal peripheral reflexes	Hyperactive knee jerk and other tendon reflexes
		Irritability, tinnitus
Other organ involvement		Liver involvement causing epigastric or right upper quadrant abdominal pain, nausea, vomiting (often said to precede convulsion/coma or onset of eclampsia)
		Pulmonary edema manifested by respiratory distress, rales, cyanosis

*These criteria are not uniformly accepted by experts in the field.

ommended. Instead, current usage advises that the modifier *gestational* precede these signs, denoting a transient condition worthy of interest and consideration but not the label "preeclampsia." Hypertension that predates the 20th week (except in multiple coexistent or molar pregnancies) is usually not considered to be indicative of true preeclampsia either—although later the trio of signs may be superimposed on a preexisting chronic hypertension causing a particularly dangerous variety of the disorder. Concurrent edema and albuminuria with hypertension are not necessary to a diagnosis of preeclampsia. For example, a patient may be quite ill and manifest significant edema but not spill any protein in her urine.

Signs and symptoms. The signs and symptoms of pregnancy-induced hypertension may, of course, extend beyond the classic three manifestations. Table 9-1 includes more possible findings that help determine the relative seriousness (mild or severe) of the disorder and therefore influence the types of treatment advised. However, some authorities favor abandoning the terms "mild" and "severe," since all preeclampsia is potentially life-threatening. It should be pointed out also that a number of clinicians do not consider the usual criteria of hypertension (a blood pressure at or above 140 systolic or 90 diastolic) to be appropriate during pregnancy because blood pressure levels normally are reduced—especially during the second trimester. In midpregnancy, blood pressure readings greater than 120/80 are considered elevated by some investigators. Blood pressures in mild preeclampsia as described in Table 9-1 are better indications of hypertensive states in pregnancy. The definition of a 30 mm Hg systolic elevation or a 15 mm Hg diastolic rise, obtained two different times at least 6 hours apart after a period of rest, is often used.

When reviewing only some of the possible signs and symptoms of preeclampsia, one is struck by the total body involvement that this potentially lethal progressive disorder may demonstrate. The kidneys, heart, lungs, liver, and brain may become prominent direct and indirect targets of the disease process, which is characterized by erratic narrowing of the microscopic arteries. This pervasive vasospasm of the arterioles probably accounts for many of the abnormalities found. However, its onset may be very subtle, with no remarkable initial signals that a patient may notice. Pregnant patients should be asked to report any swelling of the hands (tight rings) or puffiness of the face, headache, or visual problems such as blurred vision or "spots before eyes." However, these clues of difficulty usually appear late. Regular and frequent prenatal supervision is needed for verification or interpretation of hypertension, albuminuria, and weight gain. Sudden weight gain, often signaling edema, is also associated with a rising hematocrit as more fluid from the blood transfers to the tissue spaces. As fluid leaves the bloodstream, less blood is processed by the kidneys, and a fall in urine production occurs. Albuminuria, often the last sign of the three classic clinical findings to be noted, is thought to appear as blood vessel spasm and hypertension affect the kidneys. Some investigators have described unique microscopic renal changes that usually disappear after delivery. Abnormal neurologic signs and symptoms are probably related to lowered blood oxygen levels to the brain, minimal to massive cerebral hemorrhages, and edema. Abdominal pain is said to be associated with swelling and vascular involvement of the liver. This pain and nausea and vomiting are often noted before the onset of seizure or coma, as is pulmonary edema. The appearance of fever indicates a general worsening of the patient's status.

Possible etiology. Many theories have been formulated regarding the causes and the mechanisms of preeclampsia-eclampsia. A limited list includes explanations involving uterine overdistention; lack of normal blood supply to uterine and placental tissues; uterine ischemia; the presence of superabundant chorionic villi or the first exposure to such tissue; malnutrition; hormonal changes; autoimmune mechanisms; and genetic considerations. Most references state that the cause is unknown.

Identification of women at risk. Though much debate still exists regarding the causes of preeclampsia-eclampsia, it is generally agreed that certain groups of mothers are more likely to develop the condition. These include young teenage and older nulliparas (primiparas); those with multiple pregnancy; those with a history of renal, vascular, or hypertensive disease; diabetics; and those who develop hydatidiform mole. Victims demonstrate an apparent familial tendency toward the disorder.

Some researchers think certain tests help predict the onset of preeclampsia later in pregnancy. One test is the so-called rollover or supine pressure test (SPT), performed between the 28th and 32nd week of gestation. Upper extremity blood pressure is measured while the expectant mother lies flat on her side. The patient is then rolled over to a supine position. Her blood pressure measurement is repeated immediately and again in 5 minutes. A diastolic *rise* of 20 mm Hg or more *after* the woman has turned to the supine position has been said to be a significant prognostic sign. However, inconsistent responses to this maneuver have caused it to lose some support. Tests that have been based on an abnormal rise in blood pressure after an infusion of the substance angiotensin II also continue to be controversial.

Treatment and nursing care. Treatment of preeclampsia depends on the severity of the symptoms encountered, the philosophy of the physician, and the understanding and compliance of the patient. She and her family deserve careful teaching regarding her problem, its observation, and its treatment. Regular, adequate prenatal care is the best insurance for control of the complication.

In *mild* forms of preeclampsia, if a patient is conscientious in carrying out her physician's instructions, all treatment may be possible on an out-patient basis, but many physicians prefer to hospitalize these patients until symptoms are controlled. Treatment is directed toward relieving the edema and hypertension and restoring normal kidney function. Bed rest in a side-lying position to increase placental blood flow is usually helpful in decreasing high blood pressure. Bed rest is often very difficult for a mother to maintain at home, especially if she has small children. Attention must be paid to her sources of help and support, or this important ingredient in her care will be lost. Improvement of the diet, emphasizing high-quality protein, vitamin, and mineral intake, and avoidance of empty calories, is to be encouraged. Salt restriction below normal dietary levels (4 to 6 g/24 hours) is usually not recommended. Diuretics, except in select cases, are considered to be of little value and may cause harm to the patient and the fetus.

When preeclampsia patients are hospitalized, a bed rest regimen in a quiet room is usually advised. Bed rest patients should be observed particularly for sacral edema. Blood pressure and fetal heart rate are taken at least every 4 hours. A daily weight determination and urinalysis are common. Twenty-four-hour urinary protein levels may be ordered, and creatinine clearance tests to measure renal function are favored. Intake and output should be observed. The patients are questioned regarding the appearance of any symptoms, such as headache, blurred vision, abdominal pain, or nausea. Intermittent tests of fetal maturity and well-being (see p. 57) may provide information needed to direct the care of the unborn infant and his mother. Although for many physicians the treat-

Use of magnesium sulfate (epsom salts, MgSO₄) in treatment of preeclampsia-eclampsia (PIH)

Action and uses	Reduces transmission of nerve impulses from brain to muscles. Used primarily to prevent or treat convulsions. Some vasodilation and smooth muscle relaxation observed but not used chiefly for these effects.
Intent	To administer enough to prevent convulsions but avoid dangerous *nervous system* and *respiratory depression* caused by excessive magnesium serum levels in the body—either respiratory or cardiac arrest could occur.
Administration	May be ordered by IM (now rare) or IV, intermittent or continuous drip. Introductory (bolus) and maintenance dosages prescribed based on clinical observations and serum levels. *Extreme care* must be used to be sure the concentration and volume of solutions to be given are understood. IM dosages should be given with long (3-inch) needles using Z track technique. With physician approval, lidocaine may be injected with MgSO₄ to relieve pain.
Antidote	10% solution calcium gluconate 10 to 20 ml, given intravenously, injected slowly (over 3 minutes to prevent ventricular fibrillation).
Monitoring side effects and patient response	Blood pressure, pulse, respiration every 15 to 30 minutes while on continuous IV infusion; before and after on varying schedules for intermittent IV or IM therapy; an initial decrease in blood pressure may be noted because of vasodilation. Patient may complain of generalized warmth, exhibit diaphoresis. Level of consciousness: anxiety may become disorientation, drowsiness, slurring of speech, coma. Frequency and intensity of uterine contractions may diminish. Repeat doses should not be given and physician should be notified if any of the below exist: 1. Patellar knee-jerk absent 2. Respirations below 14/minute 3. Urine output for previous 4 hours less than 100 ml 4. Signs of fetal distress 5. Elevated magnesium serum levels—above 10 mg/dl (therapeutic levels 4 to 10 mg/dl)

ment for this disease currently remains almost as controversial as its proposed causes, all agree that the birth of a viable child as soon as possible is the best therapy. The rationale of treatment is to improve the condition of the mother to allow a vaginal or abdominal delivery at term. However, if her condition continues to deteriorate, induction of labor or a cesarean birth may be carried out.

Severe preeclampsia. Preeclampsia has been defined as "severe" if one or more of the following signs and symptoms are present: blood pressure of 160/110 mm Hg or more, albuminuria 3 + or more, urinary output of less than 500 ml/24 hours, persistent cerebral or visual disturbances, pulmonary edema, or cyanosis.

For a patient with severe preeclampsia, the room should be quiet and dimmed, and an emergency tray should be close at hand, containing the following equipment: airway, percussion hammer (to test reflexes), and perhaps a padded tongue blade. (A tongue blade or "bite block" is still standard equipment in most hospitals, but

unless it can be inserted without force, its use is to be avoided. The tongue heals—teeth do not.) The tray also includes medications: emergency anticonvulsants, sedatives, antihypertensives, diuretics, and heparin-containing drugs, with appropriate equipment for their administration. Probably the most commonly used medication in the tray is magnesium sulfate. Rules regarding its use and that of its antidote, calcium gluconate, are highlighted in the above box. An oxygen mask or cannula, a suction apparatus, and possibly emergency delivery equipment should be nearby.

Fortunately the occurrence of seizure is rare today. Increase in blood pressure, severe headache, abdominal pain, apprehension, twitchings, and hyperirritability of the muscles often precede seizures. As soon as the seizure manifests itself, the patient's entire body or head should be turned to the side. Suctioning is rarely necessary, but aspiration is a danger. (See discussion of tongue blade use, p. 661.) During the periods of rigidity and muscle contraction (tonic and clonic phases), the patient should be restrained only enough to keep her from hurting herself or rolling off the bed. The sides of the bed should be padded with pillows. Be aware that labor may progress rapidly and that babies have been suddenly born during a convulsive episode.

To measure urinary output and character more accurately, an indwelling catheter is inserted and attached to a urinometer. The blood pressure cuff is left in place. Frequent blood pressure, pulse, and respiration checks are made. Typically the patient is heavily sedated. An intravenous infusion is instituted for therapy as needed. Electronic fetal monitoring should be ongoing. A severely preeclamptic or eclamptic patient should never be left alone. Certain patients may convulse in response to loud noises, jarring of the bed, or bright lights. Conversation should be minimal. Routine bed baths, unnecessary procedures, or patient stimulation should be avoided.

As soon as the patient's convulsions are controlled, the condition of the fetus (if the seizures occur before birth) is ascertained, and plans for the birth are considered. The patient may deliver spontaneously. If the progress of labor is sufficient and the conditions of the patients (mother and fetus) are satisfactory, vaginal birth may be the procedure of choice. After birth the possibility of convulsion diminishes with the passage of time, and convulsion 72 hours after birth is rare. Intensive nursing must continue during the early postpartal period, but improvement is usually rapid.

Rupture of the uterus. Rupture of the gravid uterus may occur during late pregnancy but is most often reported during labor and birth. The nurse should know under what circumstances this emergency is most likely to occur, the signs and symptoms most often seen, and the usual treatment pursued.

Uterine rupture is most frequently associated with previous uterine surgery (for example, cesarean births with classic uterine incisions, myomectomies), injudicious use of obstetric forceps or oxytocin, a tempestuous or prolonged labor (for example, fetal-pelvic disproportion), or grand-multiparity.

Typically the patient experiences a period of strong, almost unremitting contractions that, in spite of their force, produce little progress in the descent of the fetus in the birth canal. The uterus becomes extremely tender, and a weakening of its lower segment may cause a distention above the pubic bone, which may simulate the appearance of a full bladder. At the moment of rupture the patient may exclaim that she experienced a sharp pain

and "felt something giving way." If rupture is complete—that is, the wall of the uterus is torn through—contractions suddenly cease. However, partial ruptures are more common. These may not be detected until postpartal intrauterine palpation.

Classically the patient, after experiencing momentary relief from pain, develops signs of profound circulatory shock resulting from intra-abdominal hemorrhage. Some of this blood loss may be visible vaginally. Signs and symptoms of rupture depend on the extent and depth of the tear, the location of the fetus, and the stage of labor in which the complication occurs. Occasionally, the onset of symptoms will be delayed. Almost all the unborn babies and one third of their affected mothers die when a classic rupture occurs.

Treatment of severe cases usually consists of immediate laparotomy, possible hysterectomy, antibiotics, and massive blood transfusions.

Amniotic fluid embolism. A complication that few women survive involves the spontaneous, accidental infusion of amniotic fluid into the endocervical or uterine veins after the bag of water has ruptured. This may occur anytime during the labor-delivery or immediate postpartum period but has been most often reported near the end of the first stage of labor. Amniotic fluid containing particles of meconium, vernix, and lanugo may enter the large blood sinuses in the placenta through defects in the placental attachment. These emboli gain access to the mother's general circulation and lodge in the lungs. Although the entire disastrous mechanism is not clear, it would seem that this foreign matter also produces profound shock and disseminated intravascular coagulation (DIC), leading to lowered fibrinogen levels in the blood and subsequent hemorrhage. This complication is more frequently associated with tumultuous uterine contractions and has been described in a disproportionate number of cases in which oxytocin has been administered to initiate or stimulate labor.

Symptoms manifest themselves suddenly. The patient may complain of chest pain or dyspnea and become extremely restless and cyanotic, occasionally expectorating frothy, blood-tinged mucus. Profound circulatory shock from hemorrhage may occur rapidly. Fetal death may result, and maternal death is almost always the outcome. Fortunately this complication is rare—occurring only once in several thousand births.

Emergency care includes intravenous administration of fibrinogen, blood, and other substances that will help restore normal clotting mechanisms, which paradoxically in DIC may include heparin, epsilon-aminocaproic acid

(EACA) and oxygen therapy. If the baby is not yet born, he is delivered as soon as possible.

Prolapse of the cord. When the umbilical cord precedes the presenting part of the fetus during labor so that the blood circulating within the vessels of the cord may be clamped off against the pelvis by the continued advance of the fetus down the birth canal, an obstetric emergency exists. This condition, termed prolapse of the cord, occurs in approximately 0.4% of labors. The nurse should be aware that this complication is more common during labors involving multiple pregnancies, an unengaged fetal presenting part, footling breech or shoulder presentations, or small fetuses. It is more common when pelvic distortion or asymmetry is present. To prevent prolapse of the cord, patients in labor whose fetal presentations are not engaged should not ambulate or sit up steeply after cervical dilatation is advanced. Enemas should not be given routinely to these patients. A sudden gush of amniotic fluid may push the cord down into the vagina or to the exterior. This is one of the reasons why the fetal heart tone is always taken after the bag of waters ruptures spontaneously or is ruptured artificially by the physician. Sometimes the cord is clearly visible outside the vaginal canal. In other instances it has prolapsed but is not visible; it may only be felt. As long as pulsations are detected, blood is flowing in the cord. Periodic checks of the fetal heart tone are necessary and continuous monitoring of the fetal heart rate is probably preferable, since any compression of the cord would usually cause detectable, abnormal alterations in its rhythm or rate. A constantly monitored patient with cord compression may characteristically reveal variable deceleration patterns. Other signs associated with fetal distress could be the passage of meconium during a cephalic presentation and sudden agitated fetal activity.

Treatment is directed toward removing any real or potential pressure on the prolapsed cord by applying vaginal or abdominal pressure to push the baby away from the cord. A head-down position for the mother may also be considered. Close observation of the fetal heart tone is maintained. The nurse should never attempt to replace the cord into the birth canal. Oxygen may be administered to the mother; it will not cause harm and may be helpful to her and the infant. Usually the only feasible treatment is cesarean birth, carried out as quickly as possible.

Premature labor and birth. A baby born before the end of the 37th week of gestation is considered premature. Prematurity involves about 10% of all babies. The incidence of a baby born "before its time" represents a special threat to the life or future health of the infant, special physical, psychologic, and economic stress on the family, and a challenge to community resources. Premature babies are more likely to suffer trauma during birth, to be victims of respiratory distress syndrome and other problems, and to require longer supportive hospital care.

For these reasons, in most cases, attempts are made to prevent or halt a premature labor, unless continuing the pregnancy would jeopardize the mother or fetus or the labor is considered to be inevitable. If evidence exists of intrauterine infection, hemorrhage, rupture of the bag of waters, or cervical dilatation beyond 3 or 4 cm, these efforts would not be appropriate. Bed rest may inhibit progression. Certain drugs that may be used to quiet uterine contractions are terbutaline sulfate (Brethine), ritodrine (Yutopar), or magnesium sulfate ($MgSO_4$). All the drugs mentioned for suppression of labor have important side effects. Patients receiving them should be carefully observed, especially for hypotension and tachycardia. A maternal cardiac monitor may be appropriate.

If labor cannot be terminated, little analgesic medication is given because the premature infant's body cannot detoxify drugs well, and his respirations at birth must not be depressed. The administration of a glucocorticoid, betamethasone (Celestone), to the mother will hasten maturity of fetal lungs by promoting earlier formation of lung surfactant. This may enable the infant to avoid respiratory distress syndrome. However, some concern has been expressed over possible subsequent neurologic changes in the baby's brain that may affect his intellectual potential. A type of spinal anesthesia may be given at delivery. A deep episiotomy may be performed to minimize head compression at expulsion. The nursery must be notified of an impending premature birth. Ideally a pediatrician particularly skilled in the immediate care of immature newborns (neonatologist) is present at the birth. Transport to a special intensive care nursery may be indicated.

Special attention to the psychologic needs of the mother is essential. Her labor is all the more demanding and difficult because her body is not prepared for the event, the outlook is precarious, and analgesic aids are minimal.

Teenage parenthood

Other problems meriting consideration by nurses may be related to special circumstances surrounding the events of pregnancy, birth, and the responsibilities of parenthood. They may not be physiologic or anatomic problems

NURSING CARE PLAN

Admission of a Multipara in Early Preterm Labor

Selected nursing diagnoses	Expected outcomes	Interventions

A. Knowledge deficit related to potential for premature labor and delivery.
 Clinical manifestations:
   Gestation of more than 20 but less than 37 complete weeks.
   Contractions every 10 minutes or less, lasting more than 30 seconds for more than 1 hour.
   Cervical dilatation less than 4 cm (greater dilatation indicates imminent delivery).
   Rupture of membranes?
   Absence of maternal medical condition, i.e., (PIH).
   Absence of maternal fever or foul vaginal drainage (signs of intrauterine infection)?
   Patient frightened and asking questions about her condition.
	Labor is arrested.
	 Pregnancy is maintained as long as possible with maternal and fetal benefit.
	 Patient demonstrates understanding of situation and management plan.
		Help patient maintain bedrest. Patient should try to remain on side on flat bed, with only small pillow to enhance blood flow to the fetus and decrease pressure on the cervix.
		 Adjust external monitor for FHR and uterine contractions.
		 Explain treatment plan (patient should be given written instructions for hospital and home.)
		 Administer fluid PO or IV as ordered. I & O maintained. Adequate hydration needed but avoid overhydration.
		 Assist with diagnostic examinations, cultures to r/o cervical or urinary tract infection which may cause uterine irritability.
		 Test clear vaginal drainage, if alkaline may be amniotic fluid, membranes ruptured—more possibility of infection and early delivery.
		 Monitor maternal temperature-intrauterine infection precludes tocolysis.
		 Monitor following unit protocol response to tocolytic medication used. Notify MD if signs and symptoms below are noted.
		   Magnesium sulfate:
		     Respirations less than 14
		     Urinary output less than 30 ml/hr
		     Reflexes absent
		     Hypotension develops
		   Ritodrine (Cardiac monitor may be applied).
		     Maternal tachycardia, over 100; irregular pulse.
		     Severe anxiety, tremors, palpitations.
		     Respiratory distress, chest pain.
		     Nausea, diarrhea, epigastric distress.

Selected nursing diagnoses	Expected outcomes	Interventions
		Turbutaline sulfate: Nervousness, hypertension, palpitations, muscle cramps, weakness, continuous nausea/vomiting. If unable to stop labor, assist with preparation for delivery. If labor stops, prepare patient for discharge (see B and C).
B. Potential noncompliance with treatment regimen related to lack of knowledge and lack of support at home.	Patient verbalizes understanding of risk recurrence and treatment plan.	Nurse should explain risks of recurrence and treatment plan—expect anger, guilt, anticipatory grief. Avoid false reassurance.
C. Potential alteration in family processes related to decreased maternal activity and concern for fetal well-being. **Home plan** Patient to be discharged at risk for recurrence of preterm labor. Medical orders include restriction of activity, medication, monitoring for uterine conditions.	Patient follows recommendations to identify and treat premature labor. Family and significant others will share feelings and provide mutual support to minimize stress.	Teach patient self-care: 1. Recognition and prompt reporting of warning signs of labor.* 　Palpate uterus for contractions 　Menstrual like cramps 　Low dull back ache (constant or intermittent) 　Increased pelvic pressure 　Increase or change in vaginal discharge 　Abdominal cramping with or without diarrhea 　Patient should report any of the above if present for more than 1 hour. Early intervention may prevent the birth of "premie" needing care in ICU. 2. Maintain adequate hydration and elimination. Dehydration and/or full bladder may stimulate uterine contractions. Patient should drink 2-3 quarts of water or juice each day and void every 2 hours. 3. Limit activity as ordered, possible bedrest with only BRP or rest periods 2-3 times/day. 4. Avoid sexual stimulation (stimulation of breasts or genitalia may cause uterine contractions). Discuss needs with partner. 5. Take oral tocolytic medication as ordered, monitor self for side effects. 6. Identify support system—she may need help (child care, or household assistance). 7. Consider appointment with social worker to learn of community resources or deal with other family problems.

*Some services are evaluating the home use of external contraction monitors.

per se, but they represent situations that may be associated with certain obstetric complications and may profoundly affect the entire experience of the patient and her future adjustment to life's challenges. One such situation that continues to create concern in American society is teenage parenthood. Teenagers make up approximately 18% of sexually active women capable of becoming pregnant. However, they account for about 46% of all out-of-wedlock births. In 1985, 1,031,000 teenagers became pregnant; of these 31,000 were younger than 15. Forty percent of the teenage pregnancies were terminated by induced abortion. Women under 20 accounted for 26% of all abortions and 15% of all births in the United States.* Most single teenage mothers are keeping their babies with or without family assistance. Those who receive support from their own families and remain at home fare better educationally and financially than those who live alone.

Numerous teenage marriages take place after pregnancy or birth has occurred. The divorce rate for these unions is very high. This is not meant to imply that no successful marriages begin in the teenage years. It does, however, reveal that the chances for a satisfactory, continuing family relationship are slim. Unfortunately, teenage marriages in modern American society often are an attempt to solve or escape problems too serious and complex to be corrected by a wedding ring.

Many factors are related to the incidence of early marriage or out-of-wedlock births. These factors most often involve family conflicts, social and economic deprivation, individual psychologic problems, and lack of education and appreciation regarding the role and responsibilities of sexuality in the family and society. Communities are now becoming more aware of the needs of the young parent, married or not. A number of programs have been instituted that make it possible for the pregnant girl's formal education to continue. These programs also may supervise prenatal care; prepare girls for their experiences during pregnancy, labor, and birth; provide education in mothering skills; and assist them with

*Wallis C: Children having children, Time 126(23):78, Dec. 9, 1985; Henshaw SK and Van Vort J: Teenage abortion, birth and pregnancy statistics: an update: Fam Planning Perspect 21(2):85, 1989.

needed personal and vocational planning. Attempts are made to avoid repeat pregnancies by unmarried teenagers. Often, though not without exception, such situations involve failure to complete education, dependency on government welfare, and family instability. A few agencies work with the unwed father, as well as the mother. Much is still to be done to prevent or treat the personal and community stress caused by teenage pregnancy.

Physicians and nurses are learning more about the needs of the pregnant teenager, both in and out of the hospital setting. Needless to say, most teenage maternity patients need a great deal of supportive care, careful instruction, and explanation to enable them to gain constructively from their experiences. A punitive attitude toward these patients from the nursing staff does not aid the individual or solve the larger problems involved.

The nurse should realize that the incidence of preeclampsia-eclampsia is higher in teenagers, especially girls in their early teens from lower socioeconomic backgrounds. This increased incidence may be related to the poor nutrition exhibited by many of these young girls. These patients also have an especially large number of low birth weight babies. The delivery room nurse will be interested to know that teenage multiparas are more susceptible to precipitate labor than any other group of obstetric patients. For the unmarried pregnant teenager or teenager who has experienced a forced marriage, the trauma of the situation is mainly psychosocial. Her misdirected search for identity, freedom, love, or recognition places her in a role for which she is ill-prepared, faced with decisions that will unavoidably influence the rest of her life.

• • •

This chapter, with its dismal recital of the minor and major complications of pregnancy and labor, may seem frightening to the student anticipating marriage and founding a family. However, it is the purpose of a text to point out the unusual as well as the commonplace. It is the business of a nurse to know about the possibility of these problems, although some of them may never be encountered—either personally or professionally.

Key Concepts

1. The most successful method of preventing nausea and vomiting is eating more frequent, small meals. Eating something dry and high in carbohydrate value 15 minutes before getting up is also helpful.

2. Heartburn can be prevented or decreased if gas-forming foods are avoided. More frequent, small, leisurely meals are recommended and antacids can be sometimes used.

3. Four things may relieve constipation: (1) a diet that includes plenty of roughage, (2) abundant fluids, (3) regular exercise, and (4) a consistent time of day set aside for evacuation.

4. Varicose veins in the lower extremities are usually relieved with the use of support hose or the application of bandages. Swelling and fatigue will be lessened if the woman avoids standing for protracted periods and if she periodically lies down and elevates her feet.

5. Hemorrhoidal discomfort may be relieved by witch hazel compresses, analgesic ointments, special suppositories, and sitz baths.

6. Preventive therapy for muscle cramps includes increased calcium intake, avoiding fatigue and cold legs, and avoiding pointing the toes when stretching.

7. During pregnancy the increase in alkalinity of the vagina may cause *Trichomonas vaginalis* to multiply rapidly and result in an irritating, profuse, thin, foamy, yellow malodorous vaginal discharge that is accompanied by vulvovaginal itching or burning. Treatment should first be attempted with topical agents. Orally administered metronidazole (Flagyl) has proven effective but should be used with caution.

8. Candidiasis is caused by *Candida albicans* and produces a cheesy, whitish discharge and beefy red vulvar irritation. Treatment includes fungicidal agents applied locally or nystatin taken orally.

9. Douching may cause an increase in pelvic infections and may lead to an overgrowth of hostile bacteria.

10. The diabetic woman's need for injected insulin varies during pregnancy. Until about 18 weeks of gestation, insulin needs are reduced; from 20 weeks until term, insulin needs both fluctuate and increase.

11. Ketosis in the pregnant diabetic is monitored by testing the urine for the presence of ketones. Blood glucose determination can be done at home with color-stable strips or with a Glucostix and a reflectance meter.

12. Ultrasound examinations, amniocentesis, stress, and nonstress tests are helpful in evaluating fetal status in the diabetic pregnant woman.

13. Syphilis may be acquired through sexual contact or by accidental inoculation by contaminated needles. Transplacental syphilis infection of the fetus may occur at any time during pregnancy. Presence of the disease can be determined by a serologic test. Adequate treatment with penicillin in the first or second stage of the disease is usually effective. Results of treatment in the third stage are questionable.

14. Gonorrheal infection may produce abnormal narrowing of the fallopian tubes in females and may be responsible for ectopic pregnancy or sterility.

15. A first attack of herpes genitalis during early pregnancy may result in spontaneous abortion. Later in pregnancy such a primary infection increases the risk of premature birth. The infant born vaginally of a mother with primary genital herpes has about a 50% chance of neonatal infection. More than 50% of infected newborns die.

16. Abortions may be spontaneous, without any premeditation, or induced. A threatened abortion may possibly be halted; loss of the fetus cannot be prevented with an inevitable abortion. An incomplete abortion refers to the retention of some of the products of conception, while a complete abortion involves elimination of all products of pregnancy. Women who have experienced more than three abortions at about the same stage of development are said to be victims of habitual abortion. A missed abortion occurs when a very young fetus dies in utero and remains there 2 months or longer before being expelled.

17. The danger of hemorrhage in ectopic pregnancy is extremely serious. If tubal rupture occurs, the woman characteristically experiences severe knife-like pain in the lower abdomen which may or may not be followed by spotting or bleeding. Shoulder pain and the urge to defecate are classic symptoms.

18. In placenta previa the placenta implants low on the interior of the uterine wall. Bright red, painless bleeding may occur late in pregnancy, or the condition may not be discovered until the onset of true labor. Cesarean delivery may be the treatment of choice.

19. With abruptio placenta the placenta is properly placed but becomes detached. The first sign of this occurrence during labor may be strong, almost con-

tinuous contractions with or without external vaginal bleeding. Treatment often includes cesarean delivery and blood replacement.

20. When caring for a maternity patient experiencing abnormal bleeding, the nurse must remember the following: never administer a routine enema; never examine the patient rectally or vaginally; observe the patient carefully and frequently; keep the charge nurse and physician informed of changes; expect possible orders for IV fluids, blood analysis, and cross match for blood transfusion; record intake and output; and maintain a calm, supportive manner.

21. The three classic signs of preeclampsia are hypertension, albuminuria, and edema.

22. The following women are more likely to develop preeclampsia-eclampsia: young teenage and older nulliparas, those with multiple pregnancy, those with a history of renal, vascular, or hypertensive disease, diabetics, and those who develop hydatidiform mole.

23. Mild forms of preeclampsia may be treated on an out-patient basis. Bed rest in a side-lying position to increase placental blood flow usually helps to decrease blood pressure.

24. Magnesium sulfate reduces transmission of nerve impulses from brain to muscles and is used primarily to prevent or treat convulsions. The antidote for magnesium sulfate is calcium gluconate.

25. Prolapse of the cord is more common during labors involving multiple pregnancies, an unengaged fetal presenting part, footling breech or shoulder presentations, and small fetuses.

26. If prolapse of the cord occurs, immediate treatment is directed toward removing any real or potential pressure on the prolapsed cord by applying vaginal or abdominal pressure to push the baby away from the cord.

27. Premature babies are more likely to suffer trauma during birth, to be victims of respiratory distress syndrome, and to require longer supportive hospital care. The birth of such an infant places psychologic and economic stress on the family and presents a challenge to community resources.

28. Bed rest may inhibit progression of premature labor. Certain drugs are also used in an attempt to quiet uterine contractions.

29. Factors related to teenage pregnancy include family conflicts, social and economic deprivation, individual psychologic problems, and lack of appreciation regarding the role and responsibilities of sexuality in the family and society. These pregnancies often involve failure to complete education, dependency on government welfare, and family instability.

Discussion Questions

1. Many discomforts are common during pregnancy. Discuss those most common in each trimester of pregnancy. Identify nursing measures that will help reduce each problem. Develop a method for explaining these discomforts to a primigravida.

2. Preexisting maternal health conditions such as diabetes mellitus and a variety of infectious diseases present a risk to both mother and fetus. What diagnostic tests are used to identify these conditions? What medical treatments are typically instituted? What are the nursing responsibilities in these situations?

3. Loss of a pregnancy places physical and psychologic stress on a woman. Identify the various types of abortions. What symptoms would a woman manifest in each type? What nursing care measures should be

instituted? How would you deal with the psychologic needs of these individuals?

4. The placenta supplies oxygen and nutrients to the fetus. If there is an abnormal placement of the placenta or premature separation of the placenta from the uterine wall problems may occur. How would you recognize these conditions? What nursing measures should be instituted in suspected abruptio placenta? In suspected placenta previa?

5. Which women are likely to develop pregnancy-induced hypertension? Other than elevation of the blood pressure, what signs and symptoms should the nurse recognize as significant? What medical and nursing measures are instituted in cases of PIH?

UNIT
III

SUGGESTED SELECTED READINGS AND REFERENCES

General

Alley NM: Morning sickness: the client's perspective, J Obstet Gynecol Neonatal Nurs 13(3):185, 1984.

Berkowitz RS and Goldstein DP: Complications of molar pregnancy, Contemp OB/GYN 24(2):57, 1984.

Campbell B: Overdue delivery: its impact on mothers-to-be, MCN 11(3):170, 1986.

Chagnon L and Easterwood B: Managing the risks of obstetrical nursing, MCN 11(5):303, 1986.

Collea JV: Reducing mortality from breech presentations, Contemp OB/GYN 25(1):171, 1985.

Conley NJ and Ohshanshy E: Current controversies in pregnancy and epilepsy: a unique challenge to nursing, J Obstet Gynecol Neonatal Nurs 16(5):321, 1987.

Foster CA: The pregnant trauma patient, Nursing '84 14(11):58, 1984.

Galvan BJ, Van Mullem C, and Broekhuizen FF: Using amnioinfusion for the relief of repetitive variable decelerations during labor, J Obstet Gynecol Neonatal Nurs 18(3):222, 1989.

Halperin ME and Enkin M: Induction of labor in post term pregnancy, ICEA Rev 12(1):1, 1988.

Haq CL: Vaginal birth after cesarean delivery, Am Fam Physician 37(6):167, 1988.

Horan M: Discomfort and pain during pregnancy, MCN 9(4):267, 1984.

Howe CL: Dealing with third-trimester bleedings, RN 48(2):29, 1985.

International Childbirth Education Association: ICEA position statement: cesarean section and VBAC, Minneapolis, Minn, 1989.

Jones LC and Bennett M: Human immunodeficiency virus (HIV) during pregnancy, Int J Childbirth Educ Assoc 5(1):21, 1990.

Kobert LJ: Dilemmas in practice: are universal precautions changing the "nurture" of obstetrical nursing? Am J Nurs 89(12):1609, 1989.

Kucyznski HJ: Support for the woman with an ectopic pregnancy, J Obstet Gynecol Neonatal Nurs 15(4):306, 1986.

Lagrew DC: Strategies for managing emboli in pregnancy, Contemp OB/GYN 35(1):113, 1990.

Leach L and Sproule V: Meeting the challenge of cesarean births, J Obstet Gynecol Neonatal Nurs 13(3):191, 1984.

Loos C and Julius L: The client's view of hospitalization during pregnancy, J Obstet Gynecol Neonatal Nurs 18(1):52, 1989.

Loveman A, Colburn V, and Dobin A: AIDS in pregnancy, J Obstet Gynecol Neonatal Nurs 15(2):91, 1986.

Maloney R: Childbirth education classes: expectant parent's expectations, J Obstet Gynecol Neonatal Nurs 15(3):245, 1985.

Marshall C: The art of induction/augmentation of labor, J Obstet Gynecol Neonatal Nurs 14(1):22, 1985.

Maslow AS and Bobitt JR: Herpes in pregnancy: exploring clinical options, Contemp OB/GYN 32(4):44, 1988.

Miller CF and Sutter CS: Vaginal birth after cesarean, J Obstet Gynecol Neonatal Nurs 14(5):383, 1985.

Morning sickness may be a good sign, Am J Nurs 86(6):647, 1986.

NAACOG: Nursing responsibilities in implementing intrapartum fetal heart rate monitoring: NAACOG statement, Washington DC, 1988.

Pridham KF and Schultz ME: Parental goals and the birthing experience, J Obstet Gynecol Neonatal Nurs 12(1):50, 1983.

Rosenfeld JA: Renal disease and pregnancy, Am Fam Physician 39(4):209, 1989.

Snyder DJ: Peer group support for high-risk mothers, MCN 13(2):114, 1988.

Sodhi VK and Sausher WF: Dermatoses of pregnancy, Am Fam Physician 37(1):131, 1988.

Stephany T: Supporting the mother of a patient in labor, J Obstet Gynecol Neonatal Nurs 12(5):345, 1983.

Tucker SM: Pocket guide to fetal monitoring, St Louis, 1988, The CV Mosby Co.

Whitaker CM: Death before birth, Am J Nurs 86(2):157, 1986.

Wiley K and Grohar J: Human immunodeficiency virus and precautions for obstetric, gynecologic and neonatal nurses, J Obstet Gynecol Neonatal Nurs 17(3):165, 1988.

Young JT and Poppe CA: Breast pump stimulation to promote labor, MCN 12(2):124, 1987.

Anesthesia and analgesia

Bruker MC: Nonpharmaceutical methods for relieving pain and discomfort during pregnancy, MCN 9(6):390, 1984.

Henrikson ML and Wild LR: A nursing process approach to epidural analgesia, J Obstet Gynecol Neonatal Nurs 17(5):316, 1988.

International Childbirth Education Association, Inc: ICEA positon paper: epidural anesthesia for labor, Minneapolis, Minn, 1987, The Association.

Lieberman AB: Easing labor pain, New York, 1987, Doubleday.

McLaughlin M and Taubenheim AM: Epidural anesthesia for obstetric patients, J Obstet Gynecol Neonatal Nurs 10(1):9, 1981.

Powell AH and Bova MB: How do you give continuous epidural fentanyl? Am J Nurs 89(9):1197, 1989.

Richart RM and others: Paracervical block-anesthetic hazard to the fetus, Contemp OB/GYN 17(4):97, 1981.

Rimar JM: MCN Pharmacopoeia: epidural anesthesia with bupivacaine, MCN 10(6):407, 1985.

Roberts JE: Factors influencing distress from pain during labor, MCN 8(1):62, 1983.

Slavazza KL and others: Anesthesia, analgesia for vaginal childbirth: differences in maternal perceptions, J Obstet Gynecol Neonatal Nurs 14(4):321, 1985.

Sosa R and others: The effect of a supportive companion on perinatal problems, length of labor, and mother-infant interaction, N Engl J Med 303(11):597, 1980.

Vadurro JF and Butts PA: Reducing anxiety and pain of childbirth through hypnosis, Am J Nurs 82(4):620, 1982.

Birthing alternatives

Boyd ST and Mahon P: The family-centered cesarean delivery, MCN 5(3):176, 1980.

Chute GW: Expectation and experience in alternative and conventional birth, J Obstet Gynecol Neonatal Nurs 14(1):61, 1985.

Coursin ML: Reflections: the good "new" days in OB, Am J Nurs 84(4):580, 1984.

Dodge JR: When childbirth is a family affair, RN 48(12):20, 1985.

Gerlach C and Schmid M: Second skill educational development of personnel for a single-room maternity care system, J Obstet Gynecol Neonatal Nurs 17(6):388, 1988.

Gimbel J and Nocon JJ: The physiological basis for the Leboyer approach to childbirth, J Obstet Gynecol Neonatal Nurs 6(1):11, 1977.

International Childbirth Education Association, Inc: ICEA position paper on planning comprehensive maternal and newborn services for the childbearing year, Minneapolis, Minn, 1985.

Johnsen NM and Gaspard ME: Theoretical foundations of a prepared sibling class, J Obstet Gynecol Neonatal Nurs 14(3):237, 1985.

Leboyer F: Birth without violence, New York, 1976, Alfred A Knopf, Inc.

Machol L: Single-room maternity care gains converts, Contemp OB/GYN 34(5):62, 1989.

May KA and DiTolla K: In-hospital alternative birth centers: where do we go from here? MCN 9(1):48, 1984.

McKay S: The assertive approach to childbirth—using communication and information strategies to increase birthing options, Minneapolis, Minn, 1986, International Childbirth Education Association, Inc.

Peddicord K, Curran P, and Monshower C: An independent labor-supporting nursing service, J Obstet Gynecol Neonatal Nurs 13(5):312, 1984.

Reed G and Schmid M: Nursing implementation of single-room maternity care, J Obstet Gynecol Neonatal Nurs 15(5):386, 1986.

Waryas FS and Luebbers MB: A cluster system for maternity care, MCN 11(2):98, 1986.

Labor and birth

Bernardini JY, Maloni JA, and Stegman CE: Neuromuscular control of childbirth prepared women during the first stage of labor, J Obstet Gynecol Neonatal Nurs 11(6):105, 1982.

Bloom KC: Assisting the unprepared women during labor, J Obstet Gynecol Neonatal Nurs 13(5):303, 1984.

Cogan R and Hinz R, editors: Support during labor: good common sense, ICEA Rev 8(1):entire issue, 1984.

Cohen WR: Steering patients through second-stage labor, Contemp OB/GYN 24(1):122, 1984.

Epperly TD and Breitinger ER: Vacuum extraction, Am Fam Physician 38(3):205, 1988.

Friedman EA: Failure to progress in labor, Contemp OB/GYN 34(6):42, 1989.

Friedman EA: Labor: clinical evaluation and management, New York, 1978, Appleton-Century-Crofts.

Glazer G and Hulme MA: Prostaglandin gel for cervical ripening, MCN 12(1):28, 1987.

Kintz DL: Nursing support in labor, J Obstet Gynecol Neonatal Nurs 16(2):126, 1987.

McKay SR and Mahan CS: Laboring patients need more freedom to move, Contemp OB/GYN 24(1):90, 1984.

McKay SR and Roberts J: Maternal position during labor and birth: what have we learned? Int J Childbirth Educ 4(3):19, 1989.

McKay SR and Roberts J: Second stage labor: what is normal? J Obstet Gynecol Neonatal Nurs 14(2):101, 1985.

Neher JO: Prostaglandin E$_2$ induction of labor, Am J Nurs 38(2):223, 1988.

Roberts JE and Kriz DM: Delivery position and perineal outcome, J Nurse Midwife 29(3):186, 1984.

Shannahan MK and Cottrell BH: The effects of birth chair delivery on maternal perceptions, J Obstet Gynecol Neonatal Nurs 18(4):323, 1989.

Whitley N and Mack E: Are enemas justified for women in labor? Am J Nurs 80(7):1339, 1980.

Yeates DA and Roberts JE: A comparison of two bearing down techniques during second stage labor, J Nurse Midwife 29(1):3, 1984.

Young D: Crisis in obstetrics—the management of labor, Int J Childbirth Educ 2(3):13, 1987.

Complications: diabetes

American Academy of Pediatrics/American College of Obstetricians and Gynecologists: Guidelines for perinatal care, ed 2, 1988.

Bobak IM, Jensen MD, and Zalar MK: Maternity and gynecologic care: the nurse and the family, St. Louis, 1989, The CV Mosby Co.

Engel NS: Insulin therapy in pregnancy, MCN 14(1):19, 1989.

Erik M and Washington J: An overview of gestational diabetes, Int J Childbirth Educ 1(2):7, 1986.

Gabbe SG: Diabetes mellitus: ways of individualizing care, Contemp OB/GYN 36(1):68, 1990.

Good-Anderson B: Home blood glucose monitoring in the pregnant diabetic, J Obstet Gynecol Neonatal Nurs 11(2):89, 1982.

Reece EA and Hobbins JC: Ultrasound's role in diabetic pregnancies, Contemp OB/GYN 23(2):87, 1984.

Strock E: Gestational diabetes: what the childbirth educator should know, Int J Childbirth Educ 4(3):32, 1989.

Zigrossi ST and Riga-Ziegler M: The stress of medical management on pregnant diabetics, MCN 11(5):320, 1986.

Complications: pregnancy-induced hypertension (preeclampsia-eclampsia)

American Academy of Pediatrics/American College of Obstetricians and Gynecologists: Guidelines for perinatal care, ed 2, 1988.

Brengman SL and Burns MK: Hypertensive crisis in L&D, Am J Nurs 88(3):325, 1988.

Hoffmaster JE: Detecting and treating pregnancy-induced hypertension: a review, MCN 8(6):398, 1983.

Poole JH: Getting perspective on HELLP syndrome, MCN 13(6):432, 1988.

Wheeler L and Jones MB: Pregnancy-induced hypertension, J Obstet Gynecol Neonatal Nurs 10(3):212, 1981.

Zuspan FP and Zuspan KJ: When your patient has pregnancy-induced hypertension, Contemp Obstet Gynecol 22(4):36, 1983.

Complications: preterm labor

Aumann GME and Blake GD: Ritodrine hydrochloride in the control of premature labor: implications for use, J Obstet Gynecol Neonatal Nurs 11(2):75, 1982.

Engel NS: Erythromycin for idiopathic preterm labor, MCN 14(4):277, 1989.

Few BJ: Indomethacin for treatment of premature labor, MCN 13(2):93, 1988.

Gill PJ and Katz M: Early detection of preterm labor: ambulatory home monitoring of uterine activity, J Obstet Gynecol Neonatal Nurs 15(6):439, 1987.

Gill PJ, Smith M and McGregor C: Terbutaline by pump to prevent recurrent preterm labor, MCN 14(3):163, 1989.

Johnson FF: Assessment and education to prevent preterm labor, MCN 14(3):157, 1989.

Koehl L and Wheeler D: Monitoring uterine activity at home, Am J Nurs 89(2):200, 1989.

Payne P and Nance N: Preterm labor, Int Childbirth Educ Assoc Rev 12(2):entire issue, 1988.

Complications: teenage pregnancy

Burke PJ: A community health model for pregnant teens, MCN 8(5):340, 1983.

Ewy D and Ewy R: Teen pregnancy: the challenges we faced, the choices we made, Boulder, CO, 1984, Pruett Publishing Co.

Fullar SA and others: A small group can go a long way, MCN 13(6):414, 1988.

Hall T: Identification and prevention of adolescent pregnancy, Int J Childbirth Educ 2(3):10, 1987.

Howard JS and Sater J: Adolescent mothers: self-perceived health education needs, J Obstet Gynecol Neonatal Nurs 14(5):399, 1985.

Osofsky HJ: Mitigating the adverse effects of early parenthood, Contemp OB/GYN 25(1):57, 1985.

Penn F and Armstrong C: Tanya was 11 years old and pregnant, Nursing '89 19(5):52, 1989.

Rhodes AM: Options and issues for pregnant adolescents, MCN 13(6):427, 1988.

Rose J: Teaching pregnant teens in standard childbirth education classes, Int J Childbirth Educ 2(3):34, 1987.

Sewall KS: Peer-group reality therapy for the pregnant adolescent, MCN 8(1):67, 1983.

Sherline DM: When the mother is a child herself, Contemp OB/GYN 24(6):83, 1984.

Slager-Earnest SE, Hoffman SJ and Beckman CJA: Effects of specialized prenatal adolescent program on maternal and infant outcomes, J Obstet Gynecol Neonatal Nurs 16(6):422, 1987.

Wallis C: Children having children, Time 126(23):78, 1985.

Postpartal and Population Problems

The Postpartal Period

The postpartal period, or puerperium, is usually considered the interval extending from the birth of the baby until 6 weeks after. This interval is characterized by the development of lactation and the return of the reproductive organs to their approximate prepregnant positions. Of course, some mothers, not wishing to or unable to nurse their babies, do not experience the full development of lactation. The return of the reproductive organs to the nonpregnant state is called the process of *involution*. The postpartal days are numbered starting with the first day after birth. Today, the average patient's postpartum in-hospital stay has been greatly abbreviated, posing new challenges and opportunities for nurses.

ADMISSION
Preparation and transfer

The basic care of the postpartum patient is an extension of the care given in the delivery or birthing room after childbirth. If the concept of continued care in one setting is followed, the patient may labor, give birth, and receive her postpartum nursing care in the same room. However, many maternity services include a special postpartum recovery room where a new mother is closely observed and cared for during the first 2 to 4 hours after birth or until her condition is considered stabilized. The patient who is transferred to a postpartum area is put in a unit previously prepared for her. The bed is turned down, and bed protectors are placed to catch extra vaginal drainage. Near at hand are a sphygmomanometer, stethoscope, and individual unit equipment, such as towel and washcloth set, wash and emesis basins, soap, bedpan, back care lotion, breast and perineal pads, perineal irrigation equipment, and newspapers or paper bags for discarding pads. If the patient has an intravenous infusion, support for the bottle also is needed.

The transfer of the patient from the stretcher to the bed may require two or three persons, depending on her condition and the equipment available. When planning to move her, it is important to know the type of delivery (vaginal or abdominal) experienced, the kind of anesthesia employed, if any, and the status of her recovery. Women who have delivered in an LDR (Labor, Delivery, Recovery) setting may be transferred by wheelchair. Before the delivery room nurse leaves the area, she checks the patient's fundus and vaginal flow to determine whether the uterus is firm and raises side rails, if appropriate. When transferring records, she makes sure that any pertinent information concerning the patient, her delivery, and the status of her infant is related to the postpartum charge nurse. The patient's personal effects are carefully transferred so that nothing is lost in the move. The description of care that follows relates particularly to the patient who delivered vaginally.

Immediate postpartum or recovery period

The postpartum nurse checks and records the mother's *pulse, respirations,* and *blood pressure* at least every 15 minutes during the first hour and thereafter until her condition is stable. During this same period, the mother's *temperature* should be recorded once. The nurse must also check and appropriately document

1. Consistency and location of the fundus every 15 min
2. Type and amount of vaginal discharge (lochia) and the appearance of the perineum every 15 min
3. Signs and symptoms of distention of the urinary bladder every 15 min (intake and output should be recorded carefully during this period)
4. Rate of flow and condition of any infusion present, and amount and type of medication
5. General condition of the patient: color, feel of her skin (warm or cold, dry or clammy), level of consciousness (drowsy, apprehensive, unresponsive), and presence of nausea or vomiting
6. Emotional status: depression, any special complaints (pain) or requests (need to see husband and infant, interactions with infant, family, and friends)
7. Recovery from anesthesia, if any (return of motion, sensation, or consciousness)
8. Nutritional and fluid status

Observation for signs of hemorrhage

Blood pressure, pulse, and general condition. Occasionally the blood pressure is elevated at the time of transfer. This condition may be the result of the excitement of the birth and seeing the baby. It may be related to the type of oxytocic the patient received or is still receiving by intravenous infusion. It may be a sign of preeclampsia or may be caused by the presence of pain or urinary retention. It is important to know the patient's baseline vital signs and what they have been since the birth. Blood pressures over 130 mm Hg systolic or 90 mm Hg diastolic should be reported to the charge nurse.

The mother's blood pressure may be low. Any pressure of 100 mm Hg systolic or below should definitely be reported. Other pressures that are higher but not hypertensive compared with the patient's baseline and that continue to fall should be reported for evaluation. Many patients with a systolic reading of 90 mm Hg or below are going into circulatory collapse or shock. Such a falling blood pressure is accompanied by an initially rising pulse. However, if the patient continues into shock, the pulse will gradually slow, weaken, and have a thready quality. Abnormally dilated pupils, pale, cyanotic, or clammy skin, apprehension, and unconsciousness are also signs of shock.

Some postpartum patients have a relatively slow pulse, but it is of good quality and is not associated with other signs of shock. This pulse rate (usually in the 60s) is not significant.

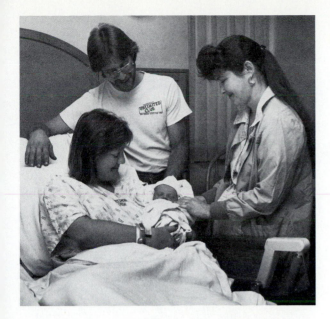

FIG 10-1 This young couple welcomes a sleepy new member of the family. One nurse in each shift is responsible for postpartal care as well as for the baby's well-being. Meeting the infants needs at the bedside provides many teaching-learning opportunities for both the nurse and the family. Such organization of client care has been called *mother-baby care*, *dyad maternity nursing*, or *couplet care*. (*Courtesy Grossmont Hospital, La Mesa, Calif.*)

Lochia. The attending nurse is also interested in the amount and character of vaginal drainage, or lochia. As she examines the patient's drainage, she must check under the patient's hips because much of the drainage may not be on the perineal pad but may seek lower dependent areas. Immediately after birth the lochia should be moderate in quantity and dark or bright red—a quality called *rubra*. (About 2 days later the lochia changes to pinkish brown, called *serosa*). The fresh drainage normally has a fleshy but not foul odor. The presence of clots should be reported. The patient usually wears two perineal pads (peripads) that must be changed once or, at most, twice during her first 2 hours postpartum. These should always be removed and applied from front to back to avoid contamination of the perineum.

Accurate visual assessment of the amount of lochial flow is often difficult. Estimating the amount by measurement of the stain on the peripad may be complicated by the different types of pads used and how often they are changed. However, saturation of one peripad within 1 hour is usually considered heavy drainage. When es-

timating blood loss and its significance, the nurse must also consider the size and condition of the patient.

Fundus. The first consideration related to blood loss is the condition of the uterus. Is the fundus firm and contracted? Is it at or below the umbilicus? If a fundus is large, soft, or boggy (seems to contain excess blood), it should be gently massaged with a circular motion until firm while one hand is held against the top of the pubic bone to prevent the uterus from being inverted or prolapsed. If clots are suspected, once the fundus is firm it may be gently grasped and positioned in the middle of the abdomen. Pressure is then exerted in the direction of the pelvic canal to push out the clots that were emptied from the uterus into the lower uterine segment and vagina during the massage. The uterus can be overstimulated by excessive manipulation, leading to its relaxation and possible hemorrhage. Students should not attempt to express clots alone until instructed individually. In the event of excessive vaginal bleeding, massage is the first measure employed to control vaginal hemorrhage.

It is surprising how quickly the uterus responds to simple massage in most cases. The nurse can easily feel the uterine muscles tighten. This tightening of the uterine muscle to make a firm fundus is essential. It pinches off the large vessels that brought blood to and from the placental sinuses before the placenta separated and was delivered. A nursing baby will also stimulate the uterine muscles to contract.

Postpartum hemorrhage. When the uterus does not contract or remain contracted, the presence of placental fragments in the uterus is suspected. If bleeding continues to be excessive and the uterus remains firm, a cause other than uterine relaxation must be sought to explain the blood loss. Excessive bleeding may develop because of a previously undetected cervical or vaginal laceration or a defective suture or repair. An abnormally bleeding patient may be returned to the delivery room for inspection of the uterus and vaginal canal. In some cases a dilatation and curettage of the uterus or the insertion of vaginal or, more rarely, uterine packing is undertaken. If no lacerations or abnormal tissue retention is evident, treatment is usually confined to the administration of additional oxytocics, such as oxytocin, synthetic injection (Pitocin, Syntocinon), ergot, or its modification, methylergonovine (Methergine). Such treatment combats the lethargy of the uterine muscles known as *uterine inertia*. Blood transfusions may be required. Patients who have had many children, multiple or frequent pregnancies, large babies, long or induced labors, uterine dystocia, or preeclampsia should be especially observed for uterine inertia.

The location and consistency of the fundus are important. A high, soft fundus suggests uterine bleeding; a high, firm fundus more often indicates urinary retention. A distended bladder, located just below the uterus, causes the fundus to rise (usually to one side and most often to the right). This is an important cause of postpartal hemorrhage. After the completion of the third stage of a normal full-term labor, the fundus should be found below or possibly just at the umbilicus. Any higher position is suspect.

The position of the fundus is usually coded by counting finger widths above or below the umbilicus in the following manner. If the fundus (which usually feels somewhat like a large cantaloupe through the abdominal wall) is two finger widths above the level of the umbilicus, it is recorded as +2. If it is located one finger width below the level of the umbilicus, it is recorded as −1. A recording of 0 may indicate that the fundus is found at the level of the umbilicus, but usually nurses write "@ umbilicus." A typical record of the condition of the fundus would be "Fundus: firm −2 midline." On the first postpartal day the fundus is usually felt at the umbilicus or below at −1 or even −2 position. The location of the fundus may be influenced by the size of the patient's baby, the condition of her uterine muscle, the content of the urinary bladder, and abnormal conditions such as retained placental fragments and the development of uterine infection. Normally the uterus undergoes involution at the rate of about one finger width a day. At the end of 10 days it is usually down behind the pubic bone again and not palpable (Fig. 10-2).

Multiparas often complain of "aftercramps," caused by the contraction of the uterus in the process of involution. They are more often bothered by cramping than are primiparas, who usually possess better muscle tone. Nursing mothers may experience more aftercramps because of the stimulation of the uterus during the process of nursing. Mild analgesics usually relieve the discomfort.

Observation for signs of urinary distention. The most common cause of a high fundus is a full bladder. Even if a woman is catheterized just before birth, she may have a full bladder fairly soon after admittance to the postpartum area, especially if she is receiving or has had intravenous infusions. Catheterization just before birth, which was once routine, is now relatively infrequent.

Other signs of urinary distention are a puffy area just above the pubic bone, complaints by the patient that she feels she should void but cannot, or the voiding of small amounts—less than 200 ml. This is called *dribbling* and

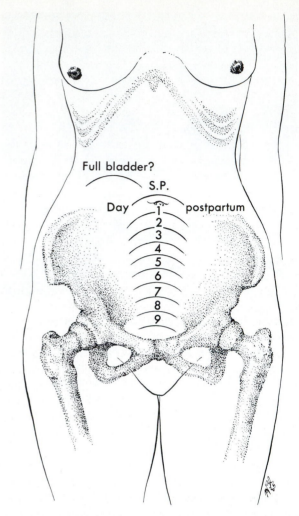

FIG 10-2 Involution of uterus, showing various positions of fundus. *S.P.,* Level just after separation of placenta from uterine wall before its delivery.

usually indicates a full bladder that can contract only partially to release limited amounts of urine. A distended bladder jeopardizes normal bladder tone and may lead to the development of residual urine, an amount that routinely remains in the bladder and is not voided. Residual urine is an excellent medium for bacterial multiplication. A distended bladder may also interfere with the normal contraction of the uterus and predispose the patient to hemorrhage. The condition can be painful and add to the aftercramping experienced by some patients.

Encouraging voiding. Voidings of postpartum patients are usually measured until two voidings of over 300 ml are recorded and a fundus check after the voidings indicates that the patient is emptying her bladder well. Thereafter patients are encouraged to void every 3 to 4 hours and to report any associated pain, burning, or difficulty. To check the efficiency of a bladder, the physician sometimes orders a catheterization for residual urine. It is important that all the equipment necessary be at the patient's bedside before she voids so that the catheterization proceeds without delay.

If a patient is suspected of having a full bladder, every effort should be made to help her void without resorting to catheterization, which may cause inflammation even in the best of circumstances, especially if repeated. Several techniques to encourage voiding may be useful.

If the patient cannot get up to go to the bathroom because of her general condition or because she has had spinal anesthesia and does not as yet have an ambulation order, the problem of initiating natural voiding is particularly difficult. Many patients find it difficult to use the bedpan. The time that physicians allow their patients to ambulate postpartum differs widely. Patients who have received subarachnoid spinal (saddle block) anesthesia may be confined to bed, flat or with only one pillow, for 8 to 12 hours after the birth. The restriction of ambulation and posture is chiefly to prevent the leakage of spinal fluid through the puncture site in the dura, causing a decrease of fluid and pressure related to the onset of "spinal headache." New mothers who have had epidural anesthesia usually may ambulate with assistance when the anesthetic has "worn off." They often feel dizzy the first time they sit up in bed. Those rare patients who have had a general anesthetic usually may get out of bed at the end of 8 hours. Those who have had local or no anesthetic usually are allowed to rise with aid as soon as they wish. Sometimes if a physician knows that a choice must be made between catheterization and probable success in voiding, he orders earlier ambulation. Patients who have had saddle block or epidural anesthesia also experience more problems voiding because they have lost normal feeling in the bladder area.

If a metal bedpan must be used, it should be warmed. Patients who have had a subarachnoid block are raised just enough so that their hips are not higher than their heads while positioned on the pan. Privacy should be maintained, and, if possible, water should be left running into a washbowl to provide psychologic stimulation. If an order is available, giving an analgesic such as oxycodone (Percodan) or acetaminophen (Tylenol) and codeine about 20 minutes before the bedpan is offered often solves the problem. Having the patient blow bubbles through a straw into a glass of water or pretend to blow up a balloon while she is on the bedpan sometimes relaxes the sphincter muscle. Some nurses report that placing a few drops of spirits of peppermint or an open ampule of spirits of ammonia in the bedpan relaxes the urinary sphincter and safely stimulates a void. Pouring a measured amount of warm water over the perineum, using a sitz bath, or taking a shower, if approved, may help the patient void. If not, it helps clean the area before catheterization. Encouraging the patient to drink amounts of fluid exceeding normal requirements before she voids usually adds to rather than relieves the problem and is not recommended.

The height of the fundus should always be determined after voiding or catheterization to evaluate, by change in the position of the fundus, the efficiency of the emptying process and other possible problems with fundal relaxation.

Catheterization technique. If none of the preceding methods brings about the desired result, catheterization must be carried out. The nurse should know whether a specimen should be saved for laboratory analysis. The technique of catheterization and the materials used differ from hospital to hospital. The following instructions are general to make allowances for the different setups used, but they include principles that should be understood, as well as review information for the student.

Individual differences of opinion still exist regarding how much urine should be removed from the bladder during the catheterization of a postpartum patient. The most common practice is to empty the bladder completely but slowly, even after more than 700 to 1,000 ml of urine is obtained. Although there could be a mild sympathetic response of slightly lowered blood pressure when more than 1,000 ml is removed, this could result from decreased maternal anxiety caused by the pressure of a full bladder. Lowered blood pressure has not been found to be significant in this type of patient.* If urine remains in the bladder, the problems that may be encountered usually outweigh any mild sympathetic response.

CATHETERIZATION: POSTPARTUM AREA

Use hospital procedures, bearing the following principles in mind:

1. Check the physician's order regarding catheterization.
2. Explain in simple terms what is going to be done for the patient and that she will feel better as a result of the procedure.
3. Provide privacy and lighting.

*Sands JP: Bladder pressure and its effect on mean arterial blood pressure, Invest Urol 10:14-18, 1972.

4. Get sufficient exposure to identify the urethral meatus, but be gentle. Some patients have stitches in the vagina and true perineum.

5. Some of the newly delivered "saddle" patients have little feeling in the area; others are very sensitive.

6. Once a nurse's hand has touched the patient, the hand is contaminated.

7. Sometimes holding the labia back with a cotton ball under one supporting finger helps maintain the position.

8. Technically, if the labia close after the crucial area has been washed with antiseptic, the area must be rewashed, since it has been contaminated by the enfolding tissue; thus it is important to maintain the labia in the drawnback position.

9. The female urethra is about 1½ inches long. No more than 4 inches of the catheter should ever be inserted, to avoid bladder puncture. If obstruction is encountered, the catheter should never be forced. There may be an abnormality of the canal (presence of a tumor, stricture, etc), or the meatus may not be properly identified.

10. A slight downward incline of the catheter may aid insertion as the urethral canal slopes downward when the patient is in dorsal recumbent position.

11. Always measure the amount of urine obtained and record it. Note also the color of the urine. Note whether a catheter was left in place and if a specimen was obtained and sent to the laboratory.

12. Assure the patient that the inability to void is usually temporary.

Emotional status. The patient's emotional status can be an early indication of psychologic or physical problems. Also, this is an important time for the patient to begin the development of *maternicity,* which supplies her with the emotional energy needed for feeling that her infant occupies an important part of her life. This is a time for developing bonds of affection. The postpartal woman must have her own needs met so that she may meet those of her baby. She must control her own body before she can best undertake the mothering tasks ahead.

The labor experience is often one of the most demanding periods for a woman. To use it instructively in her life, she will need to talk about it and relive it. (See also p. 216.)

Assessment for pain. Although most patients are able to describe discomfort, it is important to make a systematic assessment of the presence, cause, type, and location of pain. Changes in the patient's blood pressure and pulse may also indicate the existence of pain. Perhaps nursing measures, such as emptying the bladder, comfort and cleansing procedures, or positioning, will ease the discomfort. Applications of cold or heat, as ordered, may

be indicated. And, of course, analgesics will be used when needed, as ordered. The success of every measure in relieving the pain must be evaluated and documented.

CONTINUING CARE

Good aseptic technique during all procedures in the postpartum area is needed because, within the uterine cavity, easily accessible to microorganisms from the exterior, is an open "wound," the former place of placental attachment. This diminishing but still easily infected area is well supplied with veins and arteries. It provides an ideal entry into the general body circulation and the possibility of septicemia. Infection is still a threat if nurses are not enlightened and conscientious in their techniques.

Perineal care

During the last 50 years postpartum perineal cleansing has been given in countless ways in maternity services across the nation. Techniques have ranged from the use of separate sterile irrigation setups by a masked nurse each time the procedure was needed to teaching the mother which way to wipe with a clean washcloth. The acceptance of a technique should be based on its safety, adequacy, simplicity, expense, and aesthetic satisfaction for all concerned. The principles involved in perineal care should be the same whether it is done by the nurse or the patient herself.

Perineal cleansing. Perineal cleansing is performed to prevent infection, eliminate odor, observe the area and lochial flow, and ease the patient. Any equipment used by one patient should be absolutely clean and should not be used by another. Reusable equipment should be sterilized between patients. Hands should be washed before and after care. Nurses should use gloves. Care should be taught in cleansing the perineum and in removing and applying perineal pads so that soil cannot be introduced to the vulva. This means, for both nurse and patient, wiping from front to back once only with each cleansing surface. The nurse rountinely removes and applies perineal pads from front to back and does not touch the surface that is next to the perineum.

At least once each shift the perineum of the patient who gave birth vaginally should be observed for signs of infection (redness, swelling, or unusual discharge) and for signs of trauma. A hematoma in the area may develop slowly. Sufficient light should be provided to see the area clearly. The perineal pad should be changed each time the toilet is used. Some maternity services issue plastic squeeze bottles for antiseptic solution or warm tap water plus cellulose wipes to each mother for self-care. Water

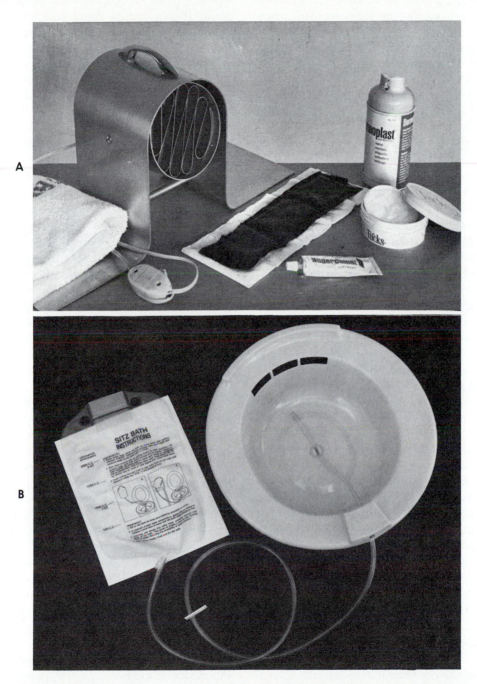

FIG 10-3 A, Aids in relieving perineal discomfort through local application: perineal lamp (hood is draped with towel when used), perineal ice pack (unwrapped for better view), Nupercainal anesthetic ointment, Dermoplast antiseptic-anesthetic spray, and Tucks (lightweight witch hazel-impregnated compresses). **B,** Sitz bath easily portable for use in hospital or home. *(Courtesy Grossmont Hospital, La Mesa, Calif.)*

temperature should be tested on the thigh or wrist to promote comfort and prevent burns. Other services issue pitchers and furnish appropriate solutions. Still others provide individually wrapped, moist towelettes impregnated with rapid-drying antiseptic. The use of a clean washcloth when showering is appropriate, with the mother using only the front-to-back motion.

In most instances the mother is taught perineal cleansing for use after each trip to the bathroom. This should be continued at least twice a day until the lochial flow has stopped. If a bed rest regimen is necessary, the patient may be placed on a bedpan and warm water poured over her perineum, taking care to avoid entering the birth canal with the water. Then she may be patted dry front to back with clean tissue.

Episiotomy and first- and second-degree lacerations. For patients who have episiotomies or laceration repairs, perineal care usually involves more than just cleansing. Many hospitals provide an antiseptic, analgesic benzocaine perineal spray such as Dermoplast or Americaine. The physician may also order sitz baths to increase circulation and ease discomfort in the perineum. Maternity services may also offer a perineal lamp ("Peri light") several times a day for 20-minute intervals to improve circulation, promote healing, and ease discomfort. Lamps and sitz baths are usually not offered until 12 hours after birth. If given too early, they may stimulate additional bleeding. This consideration may mean that many mothers will be discharged before any such treatments are received. When perineal lamps are used, care must be taken that they are no less than 18 inches (41 cm) from the perineum. A 25- to 40-watt lamp is used. The thighs of blondes, redheads, and other fair-skinned women should always be draped before the lamp is used. This is a good time to observe the perineum.

Patients with standard episiotomies and first- and second-degree lacerations usually respond well to the combination of cleansing, heat lamp or sitz bath, and analgesic spray. However, at first many such women still would prefer to stand rather than sit. Advising the mother to tense her buttocks and tuck in her pelvis before sitting down often lessens the pull and discomfort of the perineum.

Other local analgesics may also be ordered, such as dibucaine (Nupercainal) ointment and witchhazel compresses such as Tucks (Fig. 10-3).

Third- and fourth-degree lacerations. Mothers with third-degree perineal laceration (extending into the rectal sphincter) may need more help. Great caution must be exercised in giving patients who have such problems any type of enema, suppository, or cathartic if they are ordered. If the anterior rectal wall has also been torn (fourth-degree laceration), even more care is needed. Oral and topical analgesics may be ordered.

Application of cold to the perineum. Occasionally, swelling of the perineal tissues is likely in a certain patient. An order for the application of cold compresses or ice packs may be written. An ice pack should be wrapped with clean, waterproof material and a fairly thin, absorbent outer layer and intermittently applied directly to the perineum. It may be held in place by its own attachments or by an encircling sanitary pad. Various commercial clean and sterile perineal ice packs are now available. They need to be fairly comfortable, durable, and able to provide cold for reasonable periods. If no such pads are available to the nurse, she may fill a rubber glove with cracked ice and water, close it tightly, and wrap it in a light, disinfected plastic covering and a clean towel. Ice packs must be changed often. The perineal area should be observed frequently for developing hematoma or increased swelling. Application of ice is usually limited to the first 24 hours, when it is most effective in preventing edema (see p. 144).

Ambulation

As previously stated, the ambulation of the postpartum patient is determined by the orders of the attending physician and depends on the type of anesthetic given during delivery and the general condition of the patient. (See p. 203.) Early judicious ambulation of postpartum patients lessens the incidence of respiratory, circulatory, and urinary problems, prevents constipation, and promotes the rapid return of strength. When the patient is first allowed out of bed, *the nurse should not leave her alone.* These patients often become dizzy and faint. If the patient does become faint, she should be eased onto a chair, her bed, or even gently to the floor. She should never be left alone. If she is on a chair, the nurse can support her while she lowers her head to her knees. No matter how many days postpartum, the nurse should always evaluate her ambulating patient.

The first time the postpartum patient gets up she may experience a sudden, temporary gush of vaginal discharge. If it is dark red, it is probably not significant. It reflects the patient's change in posture after being recumbent for several hours when the uterine drainage was not as efficient. However, the patient should be evaluated for shock.

Bathing and breast care

Although a postpartum bed bath for patients who have delivered vaginally is not routinely done in all hospitals, cleanliness, comfort, and observation for infection must be prime considerations for the newly delivered mother. The postpartum patient is likely to perspire heavily. It is one way in which the body rids itself of excess fluids. A bed bath or shower should be offered in a timely manner.

If a bed bath is to be done, special attention should be given to the two areas that are easily infected—the breasts and the perineum, which leads to the internal reproductive tract. If the patient delivered by cesarean, the incision line would constitute a third area susceptible to infection.

Postpartum bathing procedures. Whether the mother is to shower or to have a bed bath, she should be instructed in care of her breasts. Usually only clear water is used in washing the breasts. Soap may have a drying effect and cause cracked nipples.

1. Wash in a circular manner from the nipple outward.
2. Dry the area carefully; if the mother is nursing, exposure of her nipples to air for short periods, (15 minutes) will help maintain healthy tissue.
3. Apply brassiere. All patients should have some type of adequate breast support and breast pads if needed.
4. Be sure the brassiere is large enough. The breasts should not be pushed down against the chest wall. They should be elevated and lifted toward the opposite shoulder.

While giving a bed bath, do not massage or rub the mother's feet or legs vigorously because of the danger of emboli. Perineal care is done as a separate procedure following the bath. At this time the principles of perineal self-care may be taught.

Anatomy of the breasts. A brief description of the anatomy of the breast permits a greater understanding of the basics of breast care, the technique of nursing an infant, and the principles involved in pumping the breasts.

The breasts, or mammary glands, are divided into segments, or lobes, which in turn are divided into lobules (smaller lobes). These contain the actual milk-producing glands known as *acini,* or alveoli (Fig. 10-4). The breasts are richly supplied with blood vessels, lymphatics, and nerves.

Each segment of the breast radiates from the central colored portion, known as the *areola,* which in turn rings the sensitive erectile tissue known as the *nipple*. Milk ducts from the acini travel toward the areola and open out onto the surface of the nipples. Usually each nipple has 15 to 20 such openings.

As each major milk duct approaches the areola, it widens temporarily, forming a small reservoir, or sinus. When the baby begins sucking, oxytocin from the posterior pituitary is released. Its action stimulates the contraction of muscles around the milk ducts, allowing the milk to flow into the sinus to be readily available to the baby. This physiologic response is called the *letdown reflex*. It may be accompanied by a tingling or shivering sensation. It occurs in both breasts, even though the baby is only nursing at one. The oxytocin also stimulates the uterine muscles to contract, thus lessening the possibility of hemorrhage and increasing the rapidity of involution. When a mother pumps her breasts manually, she obtains the best flow if she first presses the breast tissue back with her thumb and fingers and then squeezes the breast. Properly holding the breast with one hand during nursing not only allows the baby to breathe more comfortably but also encourages secretion of milk. For more on breast-feeding see pp. 256-260.

Breast engorgement. Breast engorgement may occur about the third day postpatrum and is often regarded by mothers as the result of the milk "coming in." However, the tenderness and swelling do not result entirely from the presence of more milk. Engorgement results, for the most part, from the increased venous and lymphatic congestion in the breast tissue.

Engorgement may be avoided or lessened by breast massage techniques and manual expression of colostrum during the prenatal period. It also will be greatly reduced or eliminated by frequent early (on-demand) feedings of the newborn. With engorgement the breasts may feel hard and nodular. Lay people have called this "caked breasts." This uncomfortable and painful condition is sometimes eased for nursing mothers by the manual expression of a small amount of milk. Good breast support worn continuously, warm, moist compresses, a warm shower, or the use of an oxytocin nasal spray prescribed to enhance the letdown reflex and the flow of milk may be helpful. Analgesic drugs may also be prescribed to relieve the pain. Many medications can pass through the milk to the nursing infant with varying effects. A nursing mother should always check with her physician before taking medication.

Nonnursing mothers may be made more comfortable

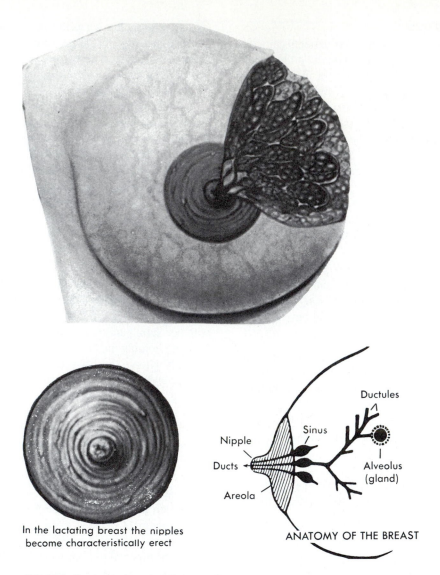

In the lactating breast the nipples
become characteristically erect

Nipple

Ducts

Areola

Sinus

Ductules

Alveolus
(gland)

ANATOMY OF THE BREAST

FIG 10-4   Lactating breast. *(Courtesy Carnation Company, Los Angeles, Calif.)*

by snug breast binders, supportive bras, the application of ice "caps" to the breasts, and analgesics. The prescription of oral estrogenic compounds, such as stilbestrol and chlorotrianisene (TACE), to suppress lactation is now infrequent and not recommended. The incidence of painful engorgement experienced by nonnursing mothers who did not receive such medications is low, and other means of treating the discomfort are preferable. Research indicates that a causal relationship may exist between the later development of endometrial cancer and the use of such substances. An increased occurrence of thromboemboli following the use of estrogens, especially after cesarean birth, has been reported; therefore informed patient consent is required by the Federal Drug Administration before estrogens are given.

A nonhormonal drug, bromocriptine mesylate (Parlodel), which suppresses lactation by preventing the secretion of prolactin, is sometimes prescribed. However, it has been associated with sudden episodes of hypotension, nausea and vomiting, and other side effects.

Many physicians believe that the best therapies available to relieve the discomfort of the nonnursing mother are the mechanical aids previously described plus the "tincture of time."

Pumping the breasts. When the order is given for a mother's breasts to be pumped, it is usually done to

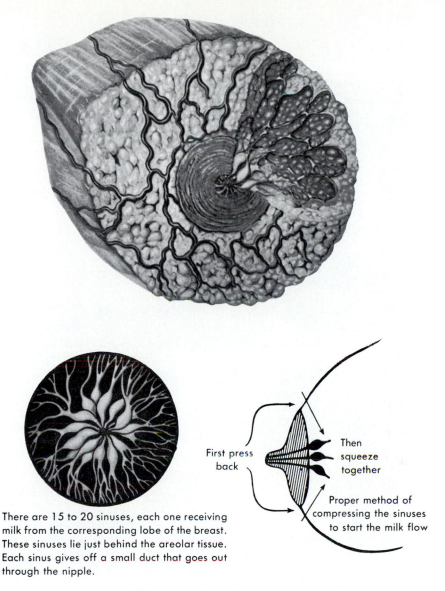

There are 15 to 20 sinuses, each one receiving milk from the corresponding lobe of the breast. These sinuses lie just behind the areolar tissue. Each sinus gives off a small duct that goes out through the nipple.

First press back

Then squeeze together

Proper method of compressing the sinuses to start the milk flow

FIG 10-4, cont'd Lactating breast.

maintain or encourage her milk supply. This procedure is not advised routinely to relieve engorgement in nonnursing mothers, because emptying the breasts stimulates more milk production.

A mother may pump her breasts manually as described or use a hand or electric pump as shown in Fig. 10-5. Whatever method is used, she should be supported comfortably in a sitting or side position with her hands and breasts freshly washed. Any equipment that touches her breasts should be sterilized before use. If the milk is saved for the baby, it should be collected in a sterile container, using aseptic technique. The mother should be instructed on how to empty her breasts using the method that is ordered or preferred. If the electric breast pump is used, the nurse must make sure that the suction is not too great. It should be increased *gradually*. A record of the amount of milk obtained should be kept in the patient's chart. Mothers sometimes are distressed by the color of their milk. They should be assured that although human breast milk looks more bluish than cow's

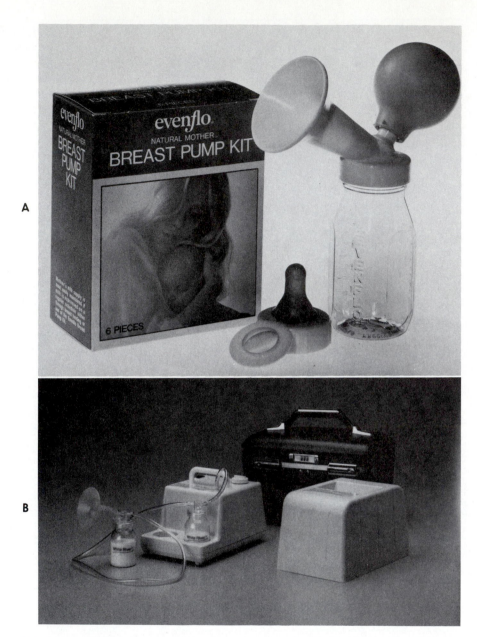

FIG 10-5 A, Manual breast pump-bottle combination. **B,** The White River Breast Pump and Breast Pump Kit features a flexible cup and a pumping action which simulates a nursing neonate. It weighs under 10 lbs. *(A, Courtesy Evenflo Products Company, Ravenna, Ohio. B, Courtesy Elena Grant, Natural Technologies, Laguna Hills, Calif.)*

milk, it is perfectly suited for the baby. Colostrum, the first secretion from the breast, is more creamy or orange in appearance.

Breast infections. Infections of the breast are not as common today as formerly, but occasionally they still occur. Most infections are introduced at the nipple area,

which may be fissured or cracked because of poor nursing techniques or exceptionally fragile breast tissue. Because of early discharge practices, such a complication is usually not found while the patient is in the postpartum area. It becomes the subject of an office call and, rarely, an admission to another part of the hospital for excision and drainage of an abscess. Fortunately, most cases of mastitis do not progress as far as abscess formation. The nurse should always observe the patient's breast or inquire about their condition. Signs of inflammation or cracked and bleeding nipples should always be reported. Breast infections are most often caused by the organism *Staphylococcus aureus*. The application of cold or heat to the breast may be ordered. The treatment prescribed depends on the stage of the infection and any organism cultured. Systemic antibiotics are commonly given. Nursing the infant is usually continued, although opinions differ regarding the advisabilty of continuing breastfeeding until the infection subsides. An antibiotic is chosen that is not harmful to the infant.

Elimination

Constipation, caused by diminished intestinal and abdominal muscle tone, may be a problem to the postpartum patient. Physicians often order a mild laxative the evening of the first or second postpartum day. If this medication does not produce results, a suppository or a gentle enema is often scheduled. Since many of these patients have hemorrhoids or adjacent episiotomy or laceration repairs, one must be careful when inserting the suppository or well-lubricated enema tip. Early ambulation, increased fluids, and a diet containing roughage and cereal food fiber may prevent constipation. If stools are difficult to pass, a stool softener may be prescribed. During the second day the patient may experience diuresis with a urinary output as high as 3,000 ml.

Supportive care and educational opportunities

Aims of postpartal hospitalization. The postpartal hospital stay should ideally provide safety, rest, constructive encouragement, and instruction for the recent parturient, as well as opportunities to initiate parent-infant attachment. However, in some areas the actual hospitalization period is so brief that it is difficult to realize the ideal. Discharge on or before the second postpartum day is almost routine in many parts of the United States, and short stays of 24 hours or less are frequent. The pendulum has swung a long way from 40 years ago, when 5 to 10 days passed before the new mother stirred from her bed.

The need for a swing in the pendulum of postpartum management is not debated. Certainly early ambulation and self-care techniques have reduced the incidence of many complications associated with prolonged bed rest, such as thrombophlebitis, pneumonia, and subinvolution of the uterus. However, the shortened postpartal stay necessitates a prenatal reevaluation of the needs of the new mother and her provisions for help in the home setting. The average primipara has had less opportunity than her counterpart of past generations to learn the art of child care in her own family circle while growing up. Often her first responsible contact with a newborn infant arrives the day she takes her own baby home from the hospital unless she has had the benefit of rooming-in with her baby. Many times she has adequate and loving help at home. Too many times she does not.

Educational resources. There do not seem to be enough hours in the hospital day to teach a new mother what she needs to know about herself and her baby and to give her sufficient time to regain her strength and composure. Of course, for multiparas, perhaps education needs are not as great, but in these days of early discharge most primiparas cannot gain the desired assurance even if hospital classes and practice sessions could be held all day long and they could attend them all.

At present one answer seems to lie in the introduction of parentcraft courses into the regular school curriculum. Also, greater use of the prenatal and postnatal courses offered by such community agencies as adult school programs, childbirth education associations, YWCA, Red Cross, and public health departments and greater involvement by the visiting nurse should be encouraged. More single room care facilities in hospitals, an increased awareness by all postpartum staff members of their teaching roles, and the possibility of family telephone contacts and home visitations with postpartum and nursery representatives following discharge are needed.

Parent education needs or teaching topics

1. Recognition of postpartum complications and what is normal
2. Perineal and breast care
3. Fluid needs, nutrition, and weight loss
4. Rest and exercise
5. Birth control concerns (if wished)
6. Anticipating and dealing with "postpartum blues"
7. Physician's appointments
8. Prevention of infection
9. Infant care and feeding (Chapter 13)
10. Prevention of accidents
11. Coping mechanisms—support groups

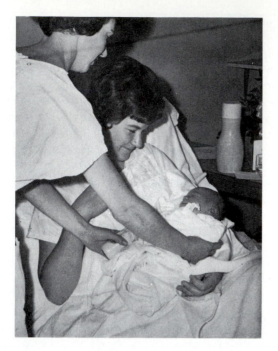

FIG 10-6 Nurses can do a great deal to reassure new mothers. *(Courtesy Grossmont Hospital, La Mesa, Calif.)*

The vocational nurse may not find herself involved in any formalized classroom teaching, but the quality of nursing care given, the importance she places on personal hygiene (her own and her patient's), and the skill she develops in observing, listening to, and responding to her patient's needs will make her an important teacher nonetheless. With the use of primary nursing and care of the mother and infant together, opportunities for teaching a mother to care for her own infant are increased.

Of course, in places where postpartum stays are longer and facilities and staff are available, actual classes in baby care, bathing, formula preparation, and nursing techniques may be offered to mothers. Some maternity departments have started closed-circuit television classes. If the prerequisites are present, the maternity department should not neglect its opportunity (Fig. 10-6).

At her arrival on the postpartum unit, the mother's needs should begin to be assessed. It is important to focus on the individual mother's needs, since the time available is often short. The box on p. 211 offers areas of teaching needs. After teaching, it is important to gain feedback from the mother to evaluate what she has learned. Listening to the mother describe lessons in her own words or observing her as she performs the skill are two ways to evaluate her learning.

Family-centered postpartum care makes it possible for both parents to get to know their baby and to begin functioning as a family unit under the guidance of skilled maternity nursing personnel. This is also an especially adaptable method for providing learning opportunities for the mother and whatever extended family is present. Because the baby is cared for at the mother's bedside, she has an opportunity to observe and ask questions of the nurse. Both the father and the mother (when she feels strong enough) may choose to participate in the care of their child. Visiting regulations vary in different hospital settings; however, siblings and other family members are often encouraged to visit and hold the new family member. Careful attention must be paid that good handwashing is done by anyone touching the baby. Cover gowns may or may not be used, as dictated by hospital policy. Multiple studies have shown no increased infection rate when gowns are not used.*

Family-centered care, unlike the rooming-in concept, is a flexible concept of individualized care, which permits the parents to share the childbearing experience and to have access to their baby during the postpartum period to the extent they desire. This does not preclude the baby from being taken to a nursery when the parents so wish.

Continued care and support. The new mother usually has many questions, some of which the nurse will be able to answer immediately. Others she must refer to the physician.

One of the first things the mother wishes to investigate after she has seen her baby and recovered some of her strength is her own weight loss. She is usually dissatisfied with her initial loss the first time she steps on the scale. She needs to be reassured that under normal conditions she will approximate her prepregnant weight in about 1 month. However, to regain a good figure, she must regulate her caloric intake to her metabolic needs. The weight gained during pregnancy in normal conditions is caused by the size of the infant, the weight of the placenta (about 1 pound), the amniotic fluid (about 2 pounds), the increased size of the uterus (about 2 pounds), breast enlargement (about 3 pounds), and increased circulating and tissue fluids and reserves.

Sometimes students are taken aback when they see postpartum patients ambulating for the first time. They confide to one another that Mrs. Smith does not look as though she has delivered yet. Multiparas, because of the

*Renaud M: Effects of discontinuing cover gowns on a postpartal ward upon cord colonization of the newborn, J Obstet Gynecol Neonatal Nurs 12(6):399, 1983.

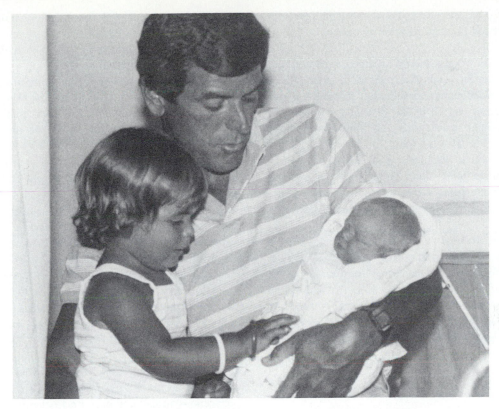

FIG 10-7   Siblings now are often encouraged to visit their new brother or sister in the hospital.

repeated stretching of the abdominal muscles, particularly need time and effort to regain a nonpregnant shape. Occasionally a hernia develops because of the separation of the rectus abdominis muscles, which are supposed to support the abdominal contents. This condition adds to the "pregnant look." A number of years ago the use of straight or many-tailed scultetus abdominal binders for support were common. Now they are seldom ordered unless the abdomen is particularly pendulous. If the scultetus binder is ordered in the postpartum period, it should be applied upside down with the wrapping starting at the top to avoid forcing the uterus up and out of place.

Nowadays it is thought better to rely on the abdominal muscles for support and to build up their strength instead of advocating indiscriminate use of abdominal binders. Various postpartum exercises are recommended to restore muscle tone as well as improve circulation, promote involution, and regain general strength. These exercises are graded according to difficulty, ranging from deep breathing and gentle range of motion to pelvic tilts, leg lifts, and modified sit-ups. The progression of exercises should be directed by the attending physician because

some may be too strenuous or even dangerous if done too early. (The knee-chest position done in early puerperium has been associated with a few cases of air embolism.)

Mothers often ask what they may do when they return home. They should be advised to increase their activities gradually and to avoid fatigue, lifting heavy objects and older children, and climbing stairs. They should be encouraged to have midmorning and midafternoon rest periods and arrange to have extra help at home. Newly delivered mothers have a tendency to try to do too much and then to regret it. Even while mothers are in the hospital the provision for rest is sometimes limited. Nurses should make every effort to provide their patients with a restful environment and periods of relaxation. Showers and shampoos at home are allowed as soon as desired. Many physicians allow tub bathing equally as early. Douching should be deferred until after the routine partpartum examination by the physician in 3 to 6 weeks, *if it is resumed at all*. (See p. 168.) The physician's advice should be sought regarding resumption of sexual intercourse. Couples are usually asked to wait until lochial discharge has stopped and discomfort has been minimized. Methods of contraception may need to be discussed.

In the interim women should be encouraged to contact their health care providers if any problems arise. Accessible and knowledgeable nursing staff members, a good physician-patient chat, and the distribution before discharge of printed instructions and hints for a smooth adjustment to life with the baby solve some of the predictable difficulties. Problems that should be reported when the patient notes them include pain or localized tenderness in the legs, increased vaginal flow, painful breasts or cracked nipples, painful urination, backache, and fever.

In nonnursing mothers, menses usually return in 5 to 8 weeks. The nursing mother may not experience menstruation until several weeks after the weaning of her infant. This does not mean, however, that she cannot become pregnant during this period. Success in nursing the infant may be enhanced by support groups such as La Leche League and the federally sponsored food supplementation program for Women, Infants, and Children (WIC).

Discharge

The discharge of the mother and child from the maternity service is an exciting time for the family. A calm and, literally, collected patient the morning of discharge is the exception despite all efforts to smooth the departure. Before the patient leaves, any instructions that are to be carried out after discharge concerning the mother or baby must be clarified. Great care should be taken that all her belongings leave with her.

The baby is identified again and dressed for the short trip outdoors to the car. The mother is usually discharged in a wheelchair. For maximum safety, the baby should ride home in an approved infant seat, not in his mother's arms.

SPECIAL CONSIDERATIONS

Postpartum hemorrhage, the most common serious problem in the postpartum period, has been previously discussed on p. 201. Preeclampsia-eclampsia has been discussed on pp. 180-186.

Cesarean birth patient

If a cesarean birth is anticipated, the mother may be admitted initially to the postpartum unit and prepared for surgery by its staff. For a review of what this preparation entails and other related information, see p. 148.

Nursing care postsurgery. The physical care of the post-cesarean-birth patient is similar to that of any patient who has had abdominal surgery. However, in addition, this patient has become a mother. She requires special attention to her postpartal needs.

Immediate observation. Blood pressure, pulse, and respiration rate should be taken at least every 15 minutes for a minimum of 2 hours and until stable. A falling blood pressure and a rising pulse are among the first signs of difficulty. Other signs of shock include pallor, cold, clammy skin, apprehension, disorientation or unresponsive behavior, and dilated pupils. But do not wait to observe all the classic signs of shock before seeking help. The dressing should be observed for drainage and any staining reported. The lochia must be observed and evaluated. As a rule cesarean birth patients have less lochial flow. After the placenta is extracted during surgery, the uterus is inspected and gently sponged, emptying the cavity of some of the drainage that would otherwise be expelled vaginally. The fundus may be gently palpated after surgery to determine its position, but it should not be massaged routinely.

The patient usually receives intravenous fluids during the first 24 to 48 hours. The first ordered fluids may contain an oxytocic to cause the uterus to contract. The intravenous infusion should be frequently observed for rate of flow and signs of infiltration. An indwelling Foley catheter is usually maintained for 12 to 24 hours or until the IV fluids are discontinued. The catheter should be checked for rate of flow and the type of urine being expelled. The tubing must be stabilized, without dependent loops. Routine temperature checks are resumed.

Pain control and psychologic postpartal support. Timely analgesia makes the recent cesarean birth patient much more comfortable. The nurse must be attentive to the patient's needs. A variety of medications and methods of administration may be used. Intermittent intramuscular injections have been traditional. However, today, patient-controlled analgesia (PCA) by intravenous route or epidural narcotic administration just before the removal of the indwelling epidural catheter following surgery may be alternatives. (See also p. 159.)

Although the initial physical care of the new cesarean birth mother is perhaps the primary priority, the emotional and maternal needs of the patient must not be forgotten. According to her strength and desires, she should be given opportunity to see, handle, and nurse her infant. Communication with the nursery should be frequent. If the infant can be brought to the bedside for care, perhaps this should be recommended. Often this patient feels very isolated and fearful regarding her offspring.

Dietary considerations. Although orders may vary considerably, at first the new cesarean birth patient is usually given nothing by mouth, and then she is gradually given a progressive surgical diet based on her toleration of oral feedings. This means progressing from sips of water to a clear liquid, to a soft diet, and then to a regular diet, over a period of approximately 2 to 3 days. Because of their reputations as gas-formers, milk, ice water, and citrus juices are often omitted from the diet along with other notorious foodstuffs such as green peppers, cauliflower, and brussels sprouts. Some observers believe that drinking through straws may also increase flatus. A new surgical patient or one with an IV infusion or an indwelling catheter should have intake and output determinations taken and recorded.

Ambulation. Although orders to ambulate the patient may not be written until the day after cesarean birth, planned movement in bed should be carried out. The patient is periodically encouraged to breathe deeply and cough as soon as she is put to bed from surgery. She is turned at least every 2 hours. How long she remains flat depends on the anesthetic used, her general condition, and her physician's orders. When she is first allowed out of bed, she should briefly dangle her feet and then stand and march in place only; during the second attempt, she should walk with the nurse's support. Walking the patient to a chair two steps away for a 15-minute period of sitting is not considered the best interpretation of "ambulate the patient." The sitting position does not aid the circulation in the lower extremities. It is important to follow orders for progressive ambulation. Just because a patient is hesitant does not mean that ambulation should not be carried out. The nurse does not need to reiterate all the complications the physician seeks to avoid by early ambulation. Usually if the nurse simply states that it will help the patient feel stronger faster and prevent or relieve flatus, this provides the needed motivation.

Some physicians are allowing some cesarean section patients to shower relatively soon after delivery, with a plastic protector over their abdominal dressings.

Abdominal distention. Abdominal distention caused by trapped flatus can be distressing to any patient who has undergone abdominal surgery. Frequently, it is the chief complaint of the cesarean birth patient. Although medications such as morphine or meperidine hydrochloride (Demerol) may be used for postoperative pain, it is still better to prevent or eliminate the distention. As part of her care, the nurse evaluates the condition of the abdomen. Is the area just above the dressing hard, bloated, and tender, or is it soft and relatively flat? Ambulating the patient may relieve distention—so may intermittent, small enemas, the Harris flush technique, or insertion of a rectal tube. Also helpful are suppositories, laxatives, or the use of neostigmine. Occasionally, strange to say, the use of carbonated drinks allow the patient to "bring up air" more easily and gain relief. In severe cases a nasal gastric tube connected to suction may be inserted.

Sutures. The cesarean patient receives perineal irrigations for cleanliness and comfort, but no sprays or heat lamps are used, since no suturing or trauma occurred in the perineum. Abdominal sutures, clips, or adhesive "butterflies" are usually removed about the fifth or sixth postoperative day.

Complications. Cesarean births result in a relatively low maternal mortality. Neonatal mortality, however, is higher. The results depend on the condition of the mother and the fetus, the equipment available, and the skill of the operator and nursing staff. Related maternal problems reported include sepsis, hemorrhage, thrombus formation, embolism, and complications of anesthesia. Occasionally afibrinogenemia, causing bleeding problems, complicates the recovery. (See also the discussion of puerperal infection p. 216.)

The sorrowing mother

Not all mothers admitted to the postpartum area leave with healthy babies. Some leave without a child because the infant did not survive birth or died in the early hours of life. Some leave alone because their infant is premature or has some abnormality. It is especially sad when a new mother who has waited for her child with anticipation finds that for all her waiting and care she has either no child or a child with gross deformities. Parents need each other at this time. For the nurse to give parents the support they need in this crisis, she must acknowledge her own feelings. Only then can she really begin to understand the parents' reactions. Nurses are in a position to give a great deal of help and support to parents during infant sickness or death. Most parents have an overwhelming need to talk about the experience and should be allowed to do so with whomever they choose. Some of the things a nurse can do to facilitate the parents' acceptance of the deformity or death are showing concern, allowing the parents to cry, relaxing visiting hour regulations, supporting the parents in their need to see and touch the infant, providing adequate and appropriate information, and allowing expressions of anger (recognizing these to be part of the grief process). Listening is probably the most important part of emotional support; platitudes are not helpful. Groups of bereaved parents are being organized in some settings to allow parents to share feelings and benefit from group counsel. Supportive nurses who are available, who listen, who recognize the stages of mourning, and who respond to the patient's cues, by touch or voice, will be much appreciated.

Some mothers leave the maternity area without babies because they are not keeping their infants. If a mother is planning to give up her baby for adoption, the nursing staff should be alerted regarding her wishes for infant care and comfort. An emotionally healthy mother with support of friends and family may work through the crisis better when given an opportunity to perform caretaking activities for her baby.

Nurses on the postpartum unit should be in contact with the nursery when a baby is not "doing well." Team members need sharing of information by everyone working with the family. Early parental contact with the infant usually should be encouraged. Referral to helping agencies may be needed.

Maternal postpartal challenges and tasks

It has been said that all postpartum patients, regardless of their different individual backgrounds and specific strengths and problems, must respond successfully to certain challenges related to changes in body image, roles, and responsibilities before they can develop a satisfactory sense of progress, wellness, and fulfillment. Ramona Mercer, in her excellent article "The Nurse and Maternal Tasks of Early Postpartum,"* speaks of the mother's need to review and integrate her childbirth experience into her total self-concept and to put aside the fantasies that she may have entertained regarding her unseen baby by identifying, claiming, and learning to care for her real infant. Mercer indicates that as the mother adapts to the reality of her changing body and her new role as both mother and mate, she is performing a type of necessary "grief work." The nurse can be an important force helping the mother cope with these changing perceptions and developing "duties" in a realistic and successful manner.

Postpartum blues

As the body hormonal levels change and the responsibilities of an enlarging family and infant care suddenly make themselves felt, many new mothers experience some degree of transitory depression, commonly called "postpartum blues." The nurse may enter a patient's room for a routine check and find the previously exuberant

*Mercer RT: The nurse and maternal tasks of early postpartum, Am J Matern Child Nurs 6:341, 1981.

mother wiping away tears. While providing tissues and gently asking what she may do to help, the nurse is often told that the patient does not really know why she is crying. "The tears just come." The knowledge that many mothers sometimes are a bit depressed during the week after childbirth is usually reassuring to the patient.

Postpartum depression and psychosis

Labor and birth often comprise a physically and emotionally exhausting period even for the normal, healthy woman. For a small but seemingly growing minority of women, the weeks following delivery represent a special period of unresolved stress that can result in progressive symptoms of mental disorder. For some the intensity of their distress may eventually bear the label of "postpartum psychosis." These mothers become withdrawn and uninterested or belligerent and suspicious. They are often victims of unreasonable fears. In severe cases they may become dangerous to themselves and others.

Because of increasingly early discharge practices, the nurse in the hospital setting rarely sees the anxiety and developing delusions described. The causes of these disturbances are probably long-standing and multiple, including physiologic and psychosocial factors. The crises of parenthood may serve as only the triggering mechanism for the maladaptive patterns of behavior observed. Often these patients have had histories of previous emotional instability or illness. The fourth postpartum week is a common time for the onset of signs and symptoms. Much more needs to be learned about this condition and its origins.

Puerperal infection

The term "puerperal infection" may be used to describe any infection of the reproductive tract during the puerperium. In the past, a patient has been considered to have a puerperal infection if she has a temperature of 100.4° F (38° C) or more on 2 successive days during the first 10 days postpartum, excluding the first 24 hours—unless another source of the temperature is determined. Now with early discharge and frequent use of antibiotics, some authorities define a puerperal infection differently using various criteria (such as temperature elevations of more than 101° F after the second day, signs and symptoms of infection, or a positive culture).

The appearance of a puerperal infection is always a serious development. It may involve the perineum proper, the uterine lining (endometritis), or the pelvic area outside the uterus (parametritis). It may extend by means of blood vessels and lymphatics to areas relatively far removed, as in the case of septic thrombophlebitis of the leg. It is most often localized, but it can become a generalized peritonitis or septicemia.

Although the classic causative organisms implicated are the streptococci and *Staphylococcus aureus,* puerperal infections may be caused by multiple organisms. Many times the bacteria that invade the uterine wound at the former site of the placenta and produce infection are those also commonly found in the intestines or colonized on the cervix, vagina, and perineum of the patient without causing any local tissue invasion or damage.

The incidence of puerperal infection is thought to be influenced by numerous factors, including the length of time the bag of waters has been ruptured before delivery, the number of cervical examinations performed, the types and number of incisions and lacerations, and the general health of the mother. Delivery by cesarean section has been associated with higher rates of infection than vaginal birth. The use of prophylactic antibiotics before and/or after surgery has decreased infection rates markedly.

If puerperal sepsis is diagnosed in the cesarean birth patient, all efforts should be made to determine the original source of the infection. This would involve a knowledge of the patient, the personal health of attending personnel and visitors, and nursing and medical techniques used. Careful handwashing and aseptic techniques continue to be an important priority.

Accompanying signs and symptoms. Along with the appearance of fever, pelvic infection is often accompanied by abdominal tenderness or pain, foul-smelling lochial drainage, an abnormally large uterus, and the presence of chills. The patient may complain of general malaise and lack of appetite and display a rise in pulse rate. Such signs and symptoms should be reported immediately. Detection of a puerperal infection should initiate isolation procedure and perhaps even the removal of the patient from the maternity service proper. Such a diagnosis may also affect the nursing procedures in the care of the infant.

Treatment of a case of puerperal infection depends on the extent of involvement. Antibiotics to which the causative organisms are sensitive are ordered. In cases of pelvic infection the patient most often is placed in Fowler's position to encourage drainage of the affected area.

Extension of infection. Observation for signs of the extension of the infection or generalized peritonitis should be constant. Such indications are increased abdominal tenderness and distention, and nausea and vomiting, as well as those previously listed.

Thrombophlebitis. Not all cases of thrombophlebitis involve the presence of infection, but many do. Clots may form anywhere in the body where a slowdown in circulation, a repair of damaged tissue, or a plugging of bleeding vessels occurs. During the postpartum period, clots or thrombi may form in the pelvis or the lower extremities. They may localize and interfere with local circulation, set up areas of inflammation, or actually become foci of infection. Rarely, they may break away from the original site of formation and travel about in the circulation. Then they are called *emboli.* These clots are particularly dangerous because they may enter some small but vital vessel and cause grave damage or sudden death. This most often occurs in the case of an embolus or emboli to the lung field or brain.

Fairly common sites of deep vein thrombophlebitis are the calf or the thigh. The patient may experience calf pain when her foot is firmly dorsiflexed while her leg is supported in an extended position (positive Homans' sign). Sometimes circulation is so impeded that the leg swells considerably, is extremely painful, and may demonstrate red streaks or locally inflamed areas. The skin may be so tense that is appears lighter in color. Signs and symptoms may vary considerably.

Treatment of thrombophlebitis usually involves bed rest with elevation of the affected leg, analgesics, and the possible application of heat with a heat cradle. Antibiotics may be indicated. Some physicians may prescribe anticoagulants to cut down on the formation of further thrombi. The nurse must recognize that use of anticoagulants for a postpartum patient significantly increases the possibility of postpartum hemorrhage. Observations of any abnormal bleeding must be quickly reported. Blood pressure should be taken periodically. Prothrombin determinations by the laboratory are expected.

After the acute phase when ambulation is approved, an order for support stockings is common. Applied correctly, they help speed the venous circulation back to the heart and discourage the formation of clots. No massage of the legs is permitted for fear of dislodging previously formed clots. Ambulation is ordered only after assessment of the day-by-day progress of the patient, revealed by the presence or absence of fever and her general condition. Thrombophlebitis may occur in all degrees of severity. As a preventive measure, some physicians automatically order that elastic stockings be applied to the legs of their patients who have had difficulties with varicosities.

• • •

The postpartum hospital stay is brief in many parts of the United States. However, the nurse can do much, even in this short interval, to help the patient face her increased responsibilities with added knowledge, skill, energy, and assurance.

Key Concepts

1. The postpartum period, or puerperium, is usually considered the interval extending from birth until 6 weeks after birth. During this period the reproductive organs return to the nonpregnant state. This process is called involution.

2. During the recovery period the nurse should monitor the patient for the following: vital signs, consistency and location of the fundus, type and amount of vaginal discharge, appearance of the perineum, signs and symptoms of distention of the urinary bladder, rate of flow and condition of any infusion present, general condition, emotional status, recovery from any anesthesia, and nutritional and fluid status.

3. Vaginal drainage after delivery is called lochia. Immediately after birth lochia should be moderate in quantity and dark or bright red. The presence of clots should be reported.

4. After the completion of the third stage of a normal, full-term labor, the fundus should be found below or possibly just at the umbilicus. The location of the fundus may be influenced by the size of the infant, the condition of the uterine muscle, the content of the urinary bladder, and abnormal conditions such as retained placental fragments and the development of uterine infection.

5. The position of the fundus is usually recorded by counting finger widths above or below the umbilicus. The consistency of the fundus is usually described as soft, firm, or boggy.

6. If the fundus is large, soft, or boggy, it should be gently massaged with a circular motion until firm while one hand is held against the top of the pubic bone to prevent uterine inversion or prolapse.

7. The acceptance of a particular technique for perineal cleansing should be based on its safety, adequacy, simplicity, expense, and aesthetic satisfaction for all concerned. Techniques have ranged from the use of separate sterile irrigation setups by a masked nurse to teaching the woman how to properly cleanse herself with a clean washcloth.

8. Patients with standard episiotomies and first- and second-degree lacerations usually respond well to a combination of cleansing, heat lamp or sitz bath, and analgesic spray. Mothers with third-degree (those extending into the rectal sphincter) or fourth-degree (those extending into the anterior rectal wall) lacerations require special care. Great caution must be exercised in giving these patients any type of enema, suppository, or cathartic. Oral and topical analgesics may be ordered.

9. Early judicious ambulation of postpartum patients decreases the incidence of respiratory, circulatory, and urinary problems; prevents constipation; and promotes the rapid return of strength.

10. After delivery, a bed bath or shower should be offered in a timely manner. Special attention should be given to the areas that are easily infected: the breasts, the perineum, and, if the patient was delivered by cesarean, the incision line.

11. Breast engorgement results, for the most part, from increased venous and lymphatic congestion in the breast tissue. Nursing mothers experiencing breast engorgement may find that the following measures provide relief: manual expression of a small amount of milk, good breast support worn continuously, warm, moist compresses, a warm shower, and the use of an oxytocin nasal spray to enhance the letdown reflex. Nonnursing mothers may be made more comfortable by snug breast binders, supportive brassieres, the application of ice "caps" to the breasts, and analgesics.

12. Constipation may be a problem for the postpartum patient. Early ambulation, increased fluids, and a diet containing roughage and cereal food fiber may prevent constipation. If constipation occurs, a mild laxative, suppository, or enema may be prescribed.

13. Postpartum parent education needs include the following topics: recognition of normal postpartum course and complications; perineal and breast care; fluid needs, nutrition, and weight loss; rest and exercise; birth control; postpartum "blues"; physician's appointments; prevention of infection; infant care and feeding; prevention of accidents; and coping mechanisms.

14. The physical care of the postcesarean birth patient is similar to that of any patient who has had abdominal surgery. She usually receives intravenous fluids during the first 24 to 48 hours and has an indwelling

Foley catheter for 12 to 24 hours. She is gradually given a progressive surgical diet based on her tolerance of oral feedings. Abdominal distention is frequently the chief complaint of these patients. Sutures, clips, or adhesive "butterflies" are usually removed about the fifth or sixth postoperative day.

15. Puerperal infection may be demonstrated by temperature elevations of more than 101° F after the second day, signs and symptoms of infection, or a positive culture. Signs and symptoms may include abdominal tenderness or pain, foul-smelling lochia, an abnormally large uterus, chills, general malaise, lack of appetite, and elevated pulse rate.

16. Possible signs and symptoms of thrombophlebitis include calf pain, swelling, red streaks, locally inflamed areas, and tense skin that appears lighter in color. Treatment usually involves bed rest with elevation of the affected leg, analgesics, and application of heat. Antibiotics and anticoagulants may also be prescribed.

Discussion Questions

1. When performing early postpartum checks, you discover that the uterus is "boggy," 2 cm above the umbilicus, and displaced to the side. What nursing measure would you institute first? Next? After that? Give rationales for your choices.

2. Special care of the breasts is recommended for all postpartum women. How does the care differ for nonnursing and nursing mothers? What should be done if engorgement occurs in the nonnursing mother? In a nursing mother?

3. With early discharge becoming increasingly common, postpartum observation by a nurse may last only 1 or 2 days. Identify the signs and symptoms that might indicate maternal complications. Discuss how and when you could best communicate these danger signs to a new mother.

4. Changes in body image, fatigue, and emotional swings are common in the postpartum patient. How could you help a new mother cope with these?

5. A primigravida has prepared for childbirth by attending a series of natural childbirth classes. Due to cephalopelvic disproportion she delivers by cesarean. What feelings may she be having regarding the birth experience? What would be the best methods to help her deal with her feelings?

11

Population, Ecology, and Reproduction

CHAPTER OBJECTIVES

After studying this chapter, the student should be able to perform the following:

1 Discuss three problems associated with continuing world population growth.
2 State three main types of contraception, and discuss the ways they prevent the formation or early development of a fertilized ovum.
3 List five methods of preventing *fertilization* and the advantages and disadvantages of each.
4 Indicate what are considered the three most reliable methods of contraception.
5 Identify three side effects of the "pill."
6 Explain what is meant by "natural family planning."
7 Discuss three aspects of the 1973 U.S. Supreme Court decision regarding abortion: permissions necessary, conditions under which the procedure may be performed, and the age of the fetus.
8 Identify the probable impact of the decision rendered by the U.S. Supreme Court in *Webster v. Reproductive Health Services* in 1989.
9 List four surgical interventions performed to limit childbearing through sterilization and why they should be considered carefully.
10 Define infertility and discuss what may be done if failure to conceive is due to blocked fallopian tubes.
11 Discuss philosophic considerations that may influence a person's attitude toward birth control.

Any modern maternal and child health text would be neglecting a crucial area of concern and controversy if it did not include at least a brief consideration of population growth, natural resources, and environmental protection. These subjects are vitally linked with maternal and pediatric interests such as genetic counseling, birth planning, abortion, sterilization, fertility, and adoption. Because discussion of birth planning has often been part of postpartal counseling, these topics are included in this unit. However, the student can readily understand that these represent a much broader area of concern, involving more than this particular interval in a woman's life.

For many centuries some of these subjects were deemed irrelevant, irreverent, or simply outside the possibility of human control. The idea that the entire earth could become impoverished or poisoned by mankind was foreign to most human thought. A simple optimism existed encouraging the belief that, as one resource became scarce, another would be prepared to take its place. Problems of ecology such as the balance of nature were considered to be largely theoretic or curiosities of only local importance.

Today, human beings are increasingly aware of the changing ecologic balance and their role in it. Complex ecologic issues are concerns at both local and international levels. In many areas legislation has been affected. The impact of this focus on impending ecologic crisis is beginning to have a wide range of effects on individual and collective life-styles in the Western world.

To be deemed responsible ancestors by future generations, this generation must realize that although the earth's resources are finite, or limited, the demands for its bounty are steadily increasing.

The world's population currently stands at approximately 5.2 billion, with a projection of 6 billion at the end of the century. Although population projections are extremely difficult to construct, the following observation is indeed sobering. It took the earth's human inhabitants until approximately 1850 to form a living group of 1 billion persons; only 80 years passed before a second billion was present. Forty-five years later, the population had doubled to 4 billion.

The predictable impact of a population growth of this magnitude on food supply, natural resources, and political stability is ominous. A nation whose population is rapidly increasing and whose vital resources are curtailed frequently becomes a militant nation. As populations double and triple, goods, services, and natural resources are stretched to the point where they can no longer meet basic human needs, and increased mental and physical illness is anticipated. Is mankind expecting famine, war, and disease to automatically solve the population problem? There must be other more acceptable alternatives!

The options would all seem to involve a conscious, orderly limitation of the number of persons who inherit the earth. Such a limitation may be achieved in various ways, and much debate focuses on the efficiency and ethics of the techniques employed. The basic methods, all of which have been used at some time, are (1) abstinence, (2) contraception, (3) planned abortion, (4) sterilization, (5) infanticide, and (6) adult murder.

Of these methods infanticide and adult murder are unacceptable to all modern societies. Abstinence, though highly efficient when practiced, would be difficult to implement. Its use within the context of marriage, except under special circumstances for agreed periods, may be questioned. Alarm that the world is rapidly becoming overpopulated and recognition of the right of individuals to control their fertility have resulted in a considerable modification of attitudes, both public and private, concerning the desirability and methods of birth planning. Three methods seem to have gained some acceptance by segments of today's society. They are contraception, abortion, and sterilization. Many governmental agencies—local, state, national, and international—have been obligated to provide birth control services for those who desire them and cannot otherwise obtain them. This is a far cry from former years, when many public institutions, by inaction if not by proclamation, effectively impeded birth control practices.

Not all human beings accept the same explanation of the origin and meaning of life, nor do they agree concerning the order of life's priorities. Philosophic differences in viewpoint cause various groups or individuals to endorse, tolerate, or condemn certain techniques of population control or family planning. These philosophic considerations include convictions regarding (1) the ultimate purpose and potential of the individual and mankind as a whole, (2) how the developmental state of the unborn child affects his status as a person or soul, (3) the rights of the unborn versus those who have already begun extrauterine existence, (4) the purposes of the marriage relationship and sexual intercourse, (5) the responsibility and ability of the individual to make and implement decisions involving personal conduct, and (6) the role of Deity in the affairs of human beings.

In the area of birth control the function of the health professional is to counsel, reassure, and inform, allowing an individual to decide his or her own course of action. Each potential set of parents should consciously make the decisions whether or not to have children and which method of birth control they will employ. This decision should be appropriate for them and in accordance with their own personal, societal, and religious values and beliefs.

CONTRACEPTION

Contraception techniques or methods used to prevent conception temporarily are usually considered to fall into three main categories: (1) those that prevent fertilization, (2) those that prevent ovulation, and (3) those that prevent implantation. Strictly speaking, the last is not a method of contraception, since the egg may be fertilized but unable to embed itself into the uterine lining to maintain life. A brief description of these methods follows.

Methods used to prevent conception

Natural methods

Coitus interruptus. Coitus interruptus is probably the oldest type of birth control practiced. The method employed is that of premature withdrawal of the penis before ejaculation during intercourse. Although this method is used by many couples, its reliability is low because sperm are emitted in varying quantities in the normal lubricating

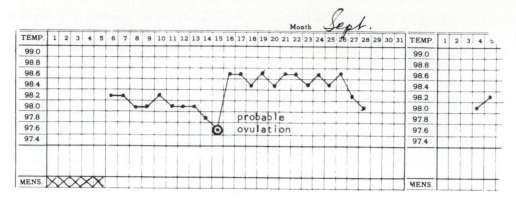

FIG 11-1 Basal body temperature (BBT) graph. Ovulation may be signaled by a drop in basal body temperature 12 to 24 hours before the postovulation rise of about 0.4° to 0.8° F. However, not all women demonstrate this initial dip in temperature readings. The BBT elevation usually continues until about 2 days before menstrual flow reappears. If pregnancy occurs, temperature remains within a relatively high range. Basal body temperatures must be taken consistently, either rectally or vaginally before *any* activity directly on awakening each morning.

fluid secreted before and during intercourse.

Rhythmic abstinence. The human ovum is susceptible to fertilization for approximately 18 to 24 hours after ovulation. Sperm deposited in the vagina are ordinarily capable of fertilizing the ovum for no more than 72 hours. These are the principles underlying the various "rhythm methods" for preventing pregnancy.

Calendar rhythm. Use of mathematical calculations to predict the probable time of ovulation is the basis of this method. If the menstrual cycle was consistently 28 days in length, ovulation would predictably occur at midpoint. Ovulation most often takes place about 14 days before the onset of the next menstrual period. Unfortunately, there is little consistency in the number of days between the onset of the last menstrual period and ovulation. Thus, since menstrual cycles differ so much from woman to woman and, indeed, at various times in the experience of any one woman, use of a calendar alone to estimate the time of ovulation to avoid the period of greatest fertility if unreliable and reduces protection considerably.

Temperature rhythm. The temperature rhythm method relies on slight changes in basal body temperature (BBT) that begin just before ovulation (Fig. 11-1). An extended, careful calendar history of menses and daily basal body temperature patterns do not predict ovulation but try to identify the "safe" luteal phase of the menstrual cycle when intercourse would be least likely to produce a pregnancy. Some women commonly ovulate as early as day 7 following onset of menses. A woman should consider that she may be fertile from the beginning of her cycle

(or no later than day 4, if her cycles are longer than 25 days) until the slight increase in basal temperature (usually from .4° to .8° F) is maintained for at least 3 consecutive days.*

Potential problems with this technique stem from the fact that basal body temperature may vary with sleeplessness, illness, digestive disturbances, immunizations, alcohol ingestion, fever, emotional upset, and medications to induce sleep. Participants must be carefully instructed to secure the results desired.

Cervical mucus rhythm. The cervical mucus rhythm method (also called "Billings" or "ferning" method) depends on identifying fertile periods by awareness of "dryness" and "wetness" in the vagina as the consequence of changes in amount and kind of cervical mucus formed at different times in the menstrual cycle.

Symptothermal method. The symptothermal method is the newest of the rhythm methods and has been actively promoted by an organization called Couple to Couple League (CCL). Its effectiveness depends on periodic abstinence during fertile periods identified by a combination of factors. Records are kept of menstrual cycle, basal temperature, changes in vaginal mucus, disturbances in normal routine, and many other items (spotting, pains, moods, cervical softening, and other secondary signs). Testing urine for luteinizing hormone (LH) may also be combined with monitoring of BBT.

*Hatcher RA and others: Contraceptive technology 1988-1989, ed 14, New York, 1988, Irvington Publishers, Inc, p 358.

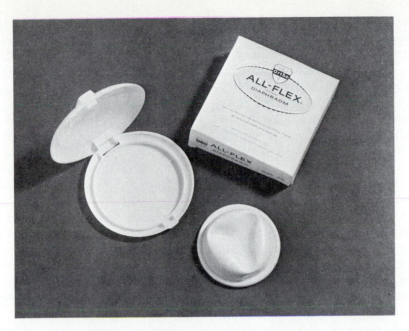

FIG 11-2 Rubber spring diaphragm with case.

Natural family planning (NFP) is characterized by avoidance of intercourse during fertile periods, and the "fertility awareness method" (FAM) employs a barrier method of birth control during fertile intervals. A helpful resource for those persons wishing to use any natural method of contraception is *The Fertility Awareness Workbook.**

Local barrier methods

Condom. The most widely used birth control device in the world, the condom was probably first employed to prevent the spread of sexually transmitted diseases. Today, it is being recommended widely for the same purpose. Largely because of the fear of acquired immune deficiency syndrome (AIDS), the public acceptance of condoms has increased markedly. However, transmission of herpes, chlamydia, gonorrhea, and syphillis is also reduced by condom use. The most protective condoms appear to be those made of latex containing effective spermicide. Shaped like a finger cot, the condom is worn over the penis during intercourse to prevent semen from entering the vaginal canal. It must be applied carefully to the penis after erection. To prevent the condom from ripping during ejaculation, a half-inch space or "pocket" should be maintained at its end. Petroleum jelly should

never be applied to a condom because it weakens rubber. However, it can be used in conjunction with chemical contraceptives, which may also serve as lubricants. Condoms should be stored away from heat and should never be reused.

Cervical caps and diaphragms. Use of cervical caps and diaphragms as known today was first reported in the 1800s. Popular in Europe, cervical caps typically have been made of rubber, metal, or plastic and fit closely over the cervix. In 1988, the FDA approved the importation and use of the Prentif cavity-rim soft rubber cervical cap in the United States. It is available in three sizes. Instructions state that prescriptions should be limited to women with normal Papanicolaou tests and that users should return to their health care providers for repeat Pap tests after 3 months of intermittent use. Four percent of cap users experience abnormal changes in results of their Pap tests. If such changes occur the use of the cap is to be discontinued.

Diaphragms are latex domes with spring rims (Fig. 11-2). They are positioned over the cervix between the pubic bone and the posterior vaginal wall. Both devices must be used in conjunction with spermicidal cream or jelly. They hold these chemicals in place over the mouth of the uterus.

Caps and diaphragms must be fitted by a physician or technician. The woman's ability to insert them properly must be checked, and detailed education regarding their

*Kass-Annesse B and Danzer H: The fertility awareness workbook, Atlanta, 1986, Printed Matter, Inc (PO Box 15246, Atlanta, Ga 30333).

use is necessary. Because of anatomic differences, not all women can be fitted satisfactorily. Some women find it distasteful to insert the device. These barriers are probably most effective when inserted no longer than 1 hour before intercourse, since the spermicidal application becomes less powerful with the passing of time. It is usually recommended that they remain in place at least 8 hours after intercourse but no more than 24 hours at one time.

Vaginal sponge. Another type of barrier contraceptive, the vaginal sponge was approved for use in 1983 and since then has achieved considerable popularity. Made of soft polyurethane (like that used in the body for biomedical purposes), the mushroom-shaped device contains 1 g of the spermicide nonoxynol-9. It prevents pregnancy in three ways: by slow but constant release of spermicide, by blocking the cervical opening, and by absorption of semen and subsequent destruction of sperm. It is sold over the counter in a single size, 2 inches (5.1 cm) in diameter and ¾ inch (1.9 cm) thick. The device is relatively easy to insert over the cervix, and an attached loop aids in its removal. The manufacturer's instructions should be consulted. After intercourse the sponge must be left in place at least 6 hours and removed within 24 hours following insertion.

The recommended 24-hour limit for cervical caps, diaphragms, and vaginal sponges is designed to reduce the complications of tissue injury, infection, and toxic shock syndrome (TSS). These methods of contraception should not be used during menses or when abnormal vaginal discharge is noted.

Women should be informed regarding symptoms of TSS, a rare but serious sickness, in order to seek appropriate, timely medical care. TSS is caused by a toxin produced by the microorganism *Staphylococcus aureus*. Danger signs include a temperature of 101° F or more, diarrhea, vomiting, muscle aches, and a sunburnlike rash typically occurring at the time of or immediately following menstruation.

Other intravaginal contraceptives. Other substances available in the form of creams, jellies, suppositories, foams, aerosols, and foam tablets provide both a physical barrier to sperm penetration and chemical spermicidal action. Many spermicides give the best protection when applied no more than 30 minutes before intercourse. However, some products remain active longer and may be inserted up to 6 hours before intercourse. With the exception of suppository or pellet formulations, no waiting period after application is needed before the spermicide becomes effective. All substances need to remain in the vagina for 8 hours after intercourse. Be sure to read product labels carefully.

A newer type of intravaginal contraceptive introduced to the United States recently has been marketed in Europe for 10 years as C-film. A small 2-inch square of paper-thin spermicidal (VCF) film is inserted over the cervix no less than 5 minutes before intercourse to allow it to dissolve releasing nonoxynol-9.

Intravaginal spermicidal/barrier agents sometimes cause local irritation or fail to melt or foam as designed. Some couples object to the foaming activity. Higher pregnancy rates are thought to be attributable chiefly to inconsistent use rather than to failure of this category of contraceptive.

Douches. Vaginal irrigations are not recommended as a means of contraception. Sperm may enter the cervix 10 to 90 seconds after ejaculation. Douching may help to force sperm into the uterus.

Methods used to prevent ovulation: oral contraceptives (OCs)

In recent years various combinations of estrogens and progesteronelike compounds have been introduced in tablet form which, when taken orally as directed, are designed to prevent the escape of the ovum from the ovary. They simulate pregnancy in this regard. Another associated action of these substances that helps to prevent pregnancy in the rare instances when ovulation is not inhibited involves (1) the decrease in and the thickening of cervical mucus, making the uterus less hospitable to spermatozoa and (2) the altered maturation of the uterine endometrium, rendering it inappropriate for successful implantation. "The pill" was first accepted for general use by prescription in the United States in 1960. It is now one of the most popular methods of contraception in this country.

If the standard technique of administration is followed, a woman is given a special dispenser to help her keep a record of her medication. There are basically two types of pills and programs that may be prescribed. One type of tablet (the combination), including both estrogens and progesterones, is taken daily for 3 weeks and omitted for 1 week. (More frequently today packets are prepared with 28 pills [21 active and 7 inert] so that a pill is taken every day). When no medication or the inert tablets are taken, withdrawal uterine bleeding usually occurs. Correctly followed, this method of contraception is more than 99% effective.

The second type is the all-progestin "mini pill" (norethindrone), which is taken every day. Perhaps technically it should not be placed in this category, since it does not necessarily inhibit ovulation but seems to prevent sperm transport by causing cervical mucus to thicken. One of three patterns of menstrual response may occur: (1) no change in menstruation may be experienced—and ovulation will still take place; (2) irregular menstrual-type bleeding may occur associated with lack of or reduced ovulation; or (3) the woman may become completely amenorrheic. If menstrual flow seems excessive or prolonged or if pregnancy is suspected, a physician should be consulted. The method is claimed to be 96% effective.

The so-called morning-after pill, designed to be taken after unprotected intercourse, often contains diethylstilbestrol in large doses. Its effectiveness has been established, but because of diethylstilbestrol's suspected role in causing cancer, the advisability of its use is seriously questioned at this time. Combined birth control pills have also been used for postcoital contraception. Ethinyl estradiol 50 μg and norgestrel 0.5 mg are taken within 72 hours of intercourse, and the same dosage is repeated exactly 12 hours later.

Frequently reported problems associated with oral contraception include nausea, occasional vomiting, breast tenderness, acne, headache, increased weight gain, and irregular vaginal bleeding. Certain vascular phenomena that are induced or enhanced by oral contraceptives, though rare, can be serious. In various studies the risk of increased incidences of blood clot formation and embolism were estimated to be 3 to 11 times greater in women who used oral contraceptives than in similar women who did not. However, these studies involved medication in higher dosages than prescribed currently.

The risk of problems occurring in women using OCs is dramatically increased among women who smoke—especially those over 35 years of age. Also, a small number (less than 5%) of women using oral contraceptives have developed hypertension. For most this side effect is mild and reversible; the blood pressure returns to normal in 1 to 3 months after discontinuation of the pill. Supporting the need for continued research has been the finding that OCs appear to be associated with a rise in serum cholesterol in some patients. The possible relationship of the use of OC to the detection of breast cancer continues to be investigated. Several studies have reported that OC users have a decreased risk of ovarian and possibly endometrial malignancy.*

Oral contraceptives have a number of disadvantages: the patient must have the ability and motivation to take them faithfully; they are expensive; and they may interfere with lactation, causing insufficient milk supply and absorption of the drug by the baby. However, some physicians are prescribing low-dose contraceptives to lactating mothers. Probably the best hormonal contraceptive during lactation is progestin alone, which appears to have no effect on the milk supply. Advantages of "the pill" include its high reliability, the fact that its use does not interrupt the sex act, and the woman's ability to easily stop therapy when she chooses to conceive.

Because of their convenience and high level of effectiveness, oral contraceptives will probably continue to be a popular form of reversible contraception. Careful screening to determine which women are at risk, the use of the lowest acceptable dosage pill for each woman, and careful follow-up help to prevent any developing problems. It must be emphasized, however, that the use of OCs does not prevent sexually transmitted diseases. Many couples are reevaluating their sexual practices in the light of this consideration.

Methods that may prevent implantation: intrauterine devices

Authorities do not agree about how intrauterine devices (IUDs) control pregnancy. The mechanism involved interferes in some way with the fertilization process, the readiness of a fertilized ovum to implant, or the ability of the uterine wall to receive the egg. IUDs inserted in the early 1900s often caused tissue damage and infection because of their placement or design. Their use was largely abandoned by physicians. However, in the 1960s and 1970s, with the advent of polyethylene and improved designs, including the tiny 7-shaped, copper-containing "Cu 7" IUD, they were a particularly popular method for controlling birth in populations who lacked the finances, skill, or opportunity to use other techniques. (Fig. 11-3). IUDs must be positioned by a proficient physician or technician.

The use of IUDs is associated with uterine cramping, bleeding, and in rare instances infection and perforation. According to studies sponsored by the National Institute of Child Health and Human Development, women who have never delivered an infant of viable age (nulliparas) are at greatest risk for developing infertility related to pelvic inflammation associated with IUD use. The research indicates that the IUD should not be the contraceptive method of first choice for women who have not borne a child. In addition, use of an IUD is not advisable for women who have had pelvic infections or who are

*Hatcher RA and others: Contraceptive technology 1988-1989, ed 14, New York, 1988, Irvington Publishers, Inc, pp 225-227. Cunningham FG, MacDonald PC, and Gant NF: Williams obstetrics, ed 18, San Mateo, Calif, 1989, Appleton & Lange, pp 924-929.

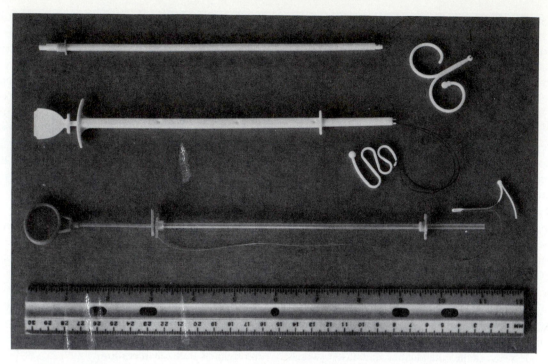

FIG 11-3 Types of intrauterine devices (IUDs) with their inserters which have been used in the past: *(top)* Saf-T-Coil, *(center)* Lippes Loop, and *(bottom)* Cu 7. Use of intrauterine devices is now undergoing considerable reevaluation primarily because of litigation in progress.

not involved in a mutually monogamous (faithful) relationship.

IUDs may be spontaneously expelled. However, they require little care after insertion and, unless expelled, they may remain in place for months or years without untoward symptoms. Ectopic pregnancies occur more frequently among wearers of IUDs than among pregnant women in general, not because the device causes these abnormally placed pregnancies but because it prevents uterine pregnancy much more efficiently than it does extrauterine gestation. If intrauterine pregnancy does occur, it is recommended that the IUD be removed as soon as possible to prevent the risk of septic abortion.

In the 1980s there were numerous lawsuits against selected manufacturers related to the use of IUDs. Because of this, most manufacturers have discontinued these products and many physicians, fearful of involvement in litigation, have abandoned their use. At this writing, only two IUDs are being marketed in the United States. Long, detailed, signed consent forms are typically required.

Reliability of contraceptive methods

An evaluation of the efficiency or reliability of the various methods of contraception is difficult to present in statistical terms because in some instances data collection and analysis have posed particular problems. Contraceptive techniques can be ranked for effectiveness as follows with the recognition that more research is needed:

Most reliable

"The pill"
Condom used with spermicidal agent

Highly reliable

Intrauterine devices
Condom
Diaphragm used with spermicidal agent
Cervical cap used with spermicide
Vaginal sponge

Moderately reliable

Aerosol vaginal foam
Rhythm, using basal body temperature, cervical mucus indicators, or combination techniques

Intravaginal agents alone
  Gels or creams
  Suppositories
  Tablets (foaming and nonfoaming)
  VCF film

Less reliable

Coitus interruptus
Calendar rhythm

Several exciting prospects are being explored for future contraceptives. They include synthetic substances, corresponding to a luteinizing hormone-releasing hormone (LHRH), which are being considered for both male and female contraceptive control and time-release contraceptive implants or microcapsules.

Clearly no perfect method exists that is applicable to all persons and circumstances, and research continues. Equally clear is that a method must be used consistently to be effective. It is important to note that the maternal death rate associated with pregnancy and childbirth is greater than that associated with the use of any of the types of contraceptives previously discussed and with legal first-trimester abortion.

ABORTION

If a pregnancy occurs that for medical, psychologic, economic, or social reasons is unwanted by those who would have the responsibility of bearing and caring for the child, the possibility of terminating the intrauterine life before it is supposedly capable of extrauterine survival is sometimes considered. From the mid-1800s when abortion was outlawed until 1967, the only way that a woman could procure a legal abortion in most states was through a statement of medical agreement that continuation of the pregnancy would be a threat to her life. (A few states also considered the *health of the mother* in the wording of relevant legislation.) Laws condemning abortion were written more than 100 years ago when the operation was dangerous even under the best auspices, and, in unskilled hands, was often catastrophic. Community concepts concerning population growth, roles of women and children, and meanings and rules surrounding sex, pregnancy, and childbirth also influenced this legislation. In the time between 1967 and 1973, several states modified their statutes to include other reasons for abortion: the mother's physical and mental health, probable serious deformity of the baby, and cases of incest or rape. A few made abortion, with certain reservations, a private decision between a woman and her physician.

In January 1973 the U.S. Supreme Court ruled that the decision to have an abortion in the first trimester of pregnancy rests only with the woman in consultation with her physician. In the second trimester before viability of the fetus the state recognizes a vested interest in the health of the woman and can regulate the conditions under which an abortion is performed but cannot prohibit the procedure. After "viability" which is variously considered to be after 20 or 24 weeks gestation, the state may prohibit abortion based on its interest in the life and health of the fetus. Most states do prohibit such abortions except to save the life or health of the pregnant woman.

The judicial decision has not been unchallenged, and practical compliance with the law appears uneven, although 25 attorneys general simply declared their former state legislation "null and void." Organizations such as the Right to Life Committee and the National Youth Pro-Life Coalition, which favor abortion only when the mother's life is in danger, are supporting efforts to overturn the Supreme Court decision by a constitutional "Human Life" amendment. They also support other antiabortion legislation such as states' rights laws that would allow each state's legislature to determine its own abortion regulations. Meanwhile, the National Abortion Rights Action League (NARAL) and the National Organization for Women are groups working to maintain the impact of the 1973 court action.

In 1989 the U.S. Supreme Court decided in the case of *Webster v. Reproductive Health Services* that a state's decision to forbid public money and facilities for abortion places no governmental obstacles in the way of a woman who chooses to terminate her pregnancy. The action was considered to be similar to a situation in which a state may decide not to subsidize other medical costs. However, the ruling will affect those women and their unborn who do not have financial access to private care or the ability to seek public abortion services elsewhere. The issue of the legal availability of the option of abortion in our society is indeed complicated and controversial. The 1973 *Roe v. Wade* case has not been overturned, but through individual state legislation, its action may be limited.

Medical and nursing personnel must be familiar with the laws regulating abortion in the area in which they practice. Legal sanctions and funding regulations regarding this problem are undergoing rapid change.

The question of professional participation in abortion when not done for obvious health needs of the mother is, for many, emotionally charged, morally disturbing, and legally complex. As the legal abortion rate has risen, maternal and infant mortality rates have dipped, but reported embryonic and fetal deaths have, of course, climbed.

The following methods of abortion are employed in hospital clinic or office settings if the pregnancy is of less than 3 months' duration:

1. *Aspiration*. The uterine contents are dislodged by the use of a specially designed suction catheter or vacuum apparatus. The procedure is rapid (approximately 5 minutes), and blood loss is minimal. It is now the most common method used and has the fewest complications.
2. *Dilatation and curettage*. The cervical canal is progressively dilated, and the products of conception are gently scraped from their uterine attachments.

Note: The progesterone-antagonist RU-486, the so-called abortion pill developed in France in 1980, is not available in the United States.

Methods used if the pregnancy is of greater than 3 months' duration are as follows:

1. *Dilatation and evacuation*. This procedure, performed under local anesthetic between the 13 and 20 weeks of pregnancy, involves a gradual dilatation of the cervix and removal of the fetus by alternating suction and curettage. This is currently the most common method used in the second trimester.
2. *Prostaglandin (PG) administration*. Prostaglandin E_2 or F_2a can effectively cause the uterus to contract and the cervix to soften and dilate, resulting in the eventual expulsion of the fetus and other products of conception. PGE_2 in the form of vaginal suppositories or gels applied to the cervical canal has become increasingly available. PGF_2a may be injected into the amniotic sac. These methods of administration reduce but do not eliminate the nausea, diarrhea, and fever experienced when oral or IV routes of prostaglandin administration had been employed. Lomotil or Compazine may be prescribed to help control these problems. A rare but very distressing possibility associated with prostaglandin abortions is the delivery of a live abortus.
3. *Other intra-amniotic instillations*. Because of the potential for severe life-threatening maternal complications, saline intra-amniotic instillations are rarely performed today. However, solutions of hypertonic urea may be instilled with more safety into the amniotic sac (with or without PGF_2a) after partial withdrawal of amniotic fluid. The urea definitely kills the fetus and the prostaglandin helps ensure expulsion.

4. *Laminaria "tents" used followed by PG or oxytocin administration or surgical evacuation*. Laminaria are compressed seaweed cervical inserts that gradually swell in place causing cervical dilatation with less trauma than other mechanical means.
5. *Hysterotomy*. A type of cesarean birth, a hysterotomy is performed when a nonviable fetus is judged present. It usually involves a hospitalization and recovery period similar to that of a cesarean birth patient.

Obviously, termination of a pregnancy after 3 months is a more difficult and hazardous procedure. The incidence of second-trimester abortions has dropped dramatically with increased public awareness of abortion availability. Of women seeking abortions, 90% do so in the first trimester. In 1985 over 1.6 million women in the United States obtained abortions.

The psychologic impact of abortion, though perhaps not immediately apparent, is an important consideration. Clearly, contraception is a better solution than abortion. Other nursing concerns regarding a patient having an abortion are discussed briefly on p. 177.

STERILIZATION

In some instances an individual or couple, for health, genetic, social, or personal considerations, may wish to permanently discontinue the capacity to have children. Any process that produces this result is termed *sterilization*. Many couples in the United States now complete their desired families at an early age. Rather than long-term use of contraception, more couples are now requesting sterilization after they have had their desired number of children. Procedures for permanently discontinuing the capacity to have children may be performed on either the man or the woman. Such procedures do not interfere with the ability to participate in sexual relations nor do they diminish any masculine or feminine characteristics previously present.

Over the years many advances have been made in the techniques and social acceptance of female sterilization. Following is a brief description of the three broad types of procedures:

1. *Sterilization using a laparotomy approach* or "mini-laparotomy," involves abdominal incisions to visualize and ligate or otherwise occlude the fallopian tubes.
2. *Sterilization using a laparoscope* ("Band-Aid") surgery has been widely publicized and accepted as an inexpensive, safe, and effective method of sterilization. Under general or local anesthesia the

physician observes the operative site through a laparoscope introduced into the abdominal cavity through a small incision at the base of the umbilicus. The fallopian tubes may be occluded by electrocoagulation or the placement of several types of clips or rings. This procedure may be performed in a hospital or surgi-center on an inpatient or outpatient basis.

3. *Vaginal tubal sterilization* may be performed by entering the peritoneal cavity through the posterior vaginal fornix (colpotomy) with or without a scope similar to the laparoscope. The basic sterilization procedure is as described for the laparoscopy technique. This technique is associated with an increased risk of infection.

Sterilization of the man by *vas ligation,* or vasectomy, is accomplished without entry into the abdominal cavity. It may be an office procedure. Twin surgical incisions are often made in the area where the scrotum joins the body, just over the vas. The ducts are tied and separated. Portions may be excised. After the operation the man does not become sterile immediately, and follow-up sperm counts should be made to determine when contraceptive techniques are unnecessary.

Although sterilization procedures are intended to be permanent, occasionally a man or woman may regret his or her decision. In some cases the tubes may be rejoined and reproductive ability regained, but sterilization should be viewed initially as a lasting intervention. Occasional spontaneous failures of sterilization techniques have been reported, but attempts to provide temporary sterility using various devices have been disappointing.

GENETIC COUNSELING

Advances in understanding genetic disorders have been rapid in the last few years, and with them the need and desire for genetic counseling have grown. Genetic screening offers the possibility of reducing suffering resulting from genetic defects. Large screening programs have been initiated to detect people who may be carriers of harmful genes, such as those of Tay-Sachs disease and sickle cell anemia. There is no coercive action associated with the information given. What persons do with the knowledge they gain is a personal choice. Through the use of the services of a genetic counselor, the genealogy of the client or couple may be investigated. Such a study is particularly helpful when a hereditary problem has been identified in a person's family but the potential incidence of the defect is unknown. The investigation may include pedigree analysis and tissue studies to determine chromosomal patterns and biologic constituents. Genetic screening may also be of value in cases of possible alteration or damage of an individual's genetic components.

Whether the subjects of screening tests are found to be carriers of genetic problems or not, psychologic problems may confront them, and the nurse must be aware of this. Regional genetic counseling is available in most areas to aid the client who has difficulty in understanding the concept of probability, psychologic defense reactions, and differences in individual values. A wide range of psychologic, ethical, and financial considerations are involved in genetic counseling (See also p. 325.)

SUBFERTILITY OR INFERTILITY

In a world where population increase is a major problem, it seems inconsistent to be concerned about the inability of a man and woman to conceive. Yet the capacity to have children of one's own lineage is particularly desired by and meaningful to most persons, even if they are not ruling monarchs! Some authorities have stated that a marriage may be regarded as infertile when pregnancy has not occurred after a year of periodic intercourse without the use of contraception.

Couples who come to a fertility clinic have two outstanding needs. The first is for education about reproduction and about procedures used to evaluate fertility. The second is for counseling to help them maximize their potential for conceiving. Knowledge about reproduction provides the client with a basis for understanding the circumstances necessary for conception and reasons for evaluating fertility.

The first step in evaluating the infertile couple is a complete history and physical examination of both the man and the woman to rule out related endocrine problems, emotional conditions, or disease entities that may be interfering with conception.

The next step is usually an evaluation of the reproductive capacity of the man. Recent semen samples are examined microscopically to detect abnormalities in number, form, and motility of his sperm. If few or no sperm are found, hormone analysis, testicular biopsy, and x-ray studies may determine whether the spermatozoa are manufactured but lack transport because of a blockage in his reproductive system. If this is the case, surgery to relieve the obstacle is sometimes possible. If sperm are not being produced or are limited in quantity, hormonal therapy may be helpful.

Evaluation of the female's capacity to conceive is more complex because of the difference in anatomy. A complete physical examination is usually followed by a determination of the ability of the woman to ovulate. Several methods may be used; these include detection of a characteristic pattern of basal body temperature readings (see Fig. 11-1), urine testing to determine a preovulatory rise in luteinizing hormone (LH) levels, microscopic examination of a biopsy of the endometrium, or lining of the uterus, and investigation of the viscosity of the cervical mucus. If ovulation is established, examination of the patency of the fallopian tubes through dye and gas studies may be performed. The uterine cavity, the vaginal canal, and the type and action of cervical and vaginal secretions may also be investigated.

If ovulation does not occur, hormonal therapy as well as general measures to improve health may be helpful. One example of a hormonal product that stimulates ovarian function is a follicle-stimulating hormone called menotropins (Pergonal). Another medication that has been used to promote pregnancy is clomiphene citrate (Clomid). Perganol in particular has been known to promote the maturation of more than one ovum during the menstrual cycle, causing the development of multiple births (for example, quadruplets and quintuplets). Since these infants are usually of low birth weight and very fragile, multiple births are a mixed blessing to even the most eager parents.

Surgical intervention to open blocked passageways that must be traversed by the ascending sperm or the descending egg may also be performed with varying success, depending on the area treated. Sometimes the diagnostic procedures used to detect fallopian tube obstruction also serve as therapy, causing the removal of minor blocks in the oviducts. Medical treatment of pelvic inflammatory disease may enable conception to occur.

The 1978 birth of the first "test tube" baby added yet another alternative for selected clients previously unable to conceive because of oviduct defect. A "test tube baby" is a fetus that is conceived by a process known medically as *in vitro fertilization* (IVF). An egg is removed from the mother-to-be approximately 2 weeks after her last menstrual period has occurred. This is done through a process that is known as laparoscopy, or more recently, transvaginal aspiration under sonography. The egg is then placed in specialized culture fluid and kept in an incubator. At an appropriate later time a specific quantity of sperm from the father-to-be is introduced into the fluid containing the egg in the incubator.

Under these circumstances, fertilization occurs. The zygote is then removed from the fertilization fluid using a microscope and placed in a fresh culture fluid for a day or two to allow time for growth and division. The microscopic multicellular embryo is then transferred into the woman's uterus.

In 1984 an important modification was developed involving transfer of egg(s) and sperm into the distal end of a patent fallopian tube directly after aspiration. This procedure is called gamete intrafallopian transfer (GIFT). In major centers where there is extensive experience with the IVF procedure, the pregnancy rate is about 20%. The GIFT technique may increase a couple's possibility of parenthood beyond this percentage. This expensive technology is rapidly advancing and changing.

How intensively solutions for infertility will be sought depends on the ages of the couple, their continued interest, cooperation, the technology available, and financial resources. At times, persistent failure to conceive because of certain male defects can be circumvented through artificial insemination techniques using the husband's sperm. More rarely, semen from an anonymous, healthy, normal man may be employed. Instances of so-called surrogate motherhood have also been reported. This is a legally precarious and controversial arrangement whereby the sperm of the husband of a barren wife is inseminated into another woman who carries the resulting fetus to term.

The conventional methods of formal adoption or foster parenthood, though sometimes not available to couples and often involving long waiting periods, may be a satisfying solution. There are certainly many children already on earth who need loving care.

●　●　●

Never before in the history of this world have the questions of population, ecology, and reproduction appeared more critical than in this last half of the 20th century. All persons should be informed concerning the problems to be faced and their possible solutions. All those engaged in the provision of maternal and child health, whether within or without the hospital setting, need to be especially involved in striving to increase the possibility that a newborn boy or girl will not only be well and well-formed, but also welcome.

Key Concepts

1. Problems associated with continuing world population growth include food supply, natural resources, and political stability.
2. Methods to control fertility are contraception, abortion, and sterilization.
3. Contraceptive methods that prevent fertilization are coitus interruptus, rhythmic abstinence, local barrier methods, and oral contraceptives. Intrauterine devices (IUDs) also help prevent pregnancy.
4. The most reliable methods of contraception are oral contraceptives ("the pill") and condoms used with spermicidal agents.
5. Frequently reported problems associated with oral contraceptives include nausea, occasional vomiting, breast tenderness, acne, headache, increased weight gain, and irregular vaginal bleeding.
6. Natural family planning (NFP) is characterized by avoidance of intercourse during fertile periods. The fertility awareness method (FAM) employs a barrier method of contraception during fertile intervals.
7. The 1973 U.S. Supreme Court decision regarding abortion specifies that the decision to have an abortion in the first trimester of pregnancy rests only with the woman in consultation with her physician. In the second trimester the state can regulate conditions under which an abortion is performed, but cannot prohibit the procedure before viability. The state may prohibit abortion in the third trimester except to save the life or health of the mother.
8. In 1989 the U.S. Supreme Court decided in the case of *Webster v. Reproductive Health Services* that a state's decision to forbid public money and facilities for abortion places no governmental obstacles in the way of a woman who chooses to have an abortion.
9. Four types of surgical interventions result in sterilization: (1) sterilization of the woman using a laparotomy approach, (2) female sterilization using a laparoscope, (3) vaginal tubal sterilization, and (4) sterilization of the man by vasectomy.
10. Some authorities consider a couple to be infertile when pregnancy has not occurred after a year of periodic intercourse without the use of contraception. If infertility is the result of the absence of ovulation, hormonal therapy may be helpful. Surgical intervention to open blocked fallopian tubes may be performed with varying success.

Discussion Questions

1. Discuss the "natural" (requiring no medications or barriers) methods of birth control. What are the major advantages and disadvantages of these methods?
2. Discuss the advantages and disadvantages of the other methods of contraception. As a nurse what do you think your role should be in family planning?
3. Elective abortion is a national issue. Some individuals are pro-life and others are pro-choice. Do research on material in magazines and newspapers that present both sides of this issue. Discuss the issues raised.
4. Elective sterilization is possible for both males and females. If a couple chooses this option, which spouse do you think should be sterilized? Why? What are the risks involved in sterilization?
5. Infertility is a serious issue to those affected. What help (related to technology) is available to infertile couples? Is this available in your area? If so, explore the costs involved. Is adoption always an alternative for infertile couples?

UNIT
IV

SUGGESTED SELECTED READINGS AND REFERENCES

The postpartal period

Bastin JP: Action stat! Postpartum hemorrhage, Nursing 89 19(2):33, 1989.

Berchtold N: Depression after delivery—help from the childbirth educator, Int J Childbirth Educ 4(3):14, 1989.

Bucknell S and Sikorski K: Putting patient-controlled analgesic to the test, MCN 14(1):37, 1989.

Collins C and Tiedje LB: A program for women returning to work after childbirth, J Obstet Gynecol Neonatal Nurs 17(4):246, 1988.

Curry MA: Variables related to adaptation to motherhood in "normal" primiparous women, J Obstet Gynecol Neonatal Nurs 11(6):115, 1982.

Gruen DS: Babies and jobs, Seattle, Pennypress, 1986.

Hale JF and Wade DS: One way to cure postpartum charting blues, Am J Nurs 87(8):1044, 1987.

Hampson SJ: Nursing interventions for the first three postpartum months, J Obstet Gynecol Neonatal Nurs 18(2):116, 1989.

Hawkins JW and Gorvine B: Postpartum nursing: health care of women, New York, 1985, Springer Publishing Co, Inc.

Hill PD: Effects of heat and cold on the perineum after episiotomy/laceration, J Obstet Gynecol Neonatal Nurs 18(2):124, 1989.

Hiser PL: Concerns of multiparas during the second postpartum week, J Obstet Gynecol Neonatal Nurs 16(3):195, 1987.

Inglis T: Postpartum sexuality, J Obstet Gynecol Neonatal Nurs 9(5):298, 1980.

Inturrisi M, Camenga CF, and Rosen M: Epidural morphine for relief of postpartum, post-surgical pain, J Obstet Gynecol Neonatal Nurs 17(4):238, 1988.

Jacobson H: A standard for assessing lochia volume, MCN 10(3):174, 1985.

Jankowski H and Wells SM: Self-administered medications for obstetric patients, MCN 12(3):199, 1987.

Jansson P: Early postpartum discharge, Am J Nurs 85(5):547, 1985.

Lockhart B: When couples adopt, they too need parenting classes, MCN 7(2):116, 1982.

Martell LK and Mitchel SK: Rubin's "puerperal change" reconsidered, J Obstet Gynecol Neonatal Nurs 13(3):145, 1984.

Mercer RT: The nurse and maternal tasks of early postpartum, MCN 6(5):341, 1981.

NAACOG Committee on Practice: NAACOG OGN nursing practice resource: mother-baby care, Washington, DC, 1989, NAACOG.

Petrick JM: Postpartum depression: identification of high-risk mothers, J Obstet Gynecol Neonatal Nurs 13(1):37, 1984.

Ramlee D and Roberts J: A comparison of cold and warm sitz baths for relief of postpartum perineal pain, J Obstet Gynecol Neonatal Nurs 15(6):471, 1986.

Reed BD: Postpartum hemorrhage, Am Fam Physician 37(3):111, 1988.

Wadd L: Vietnamese postpartum practices; implications for nursing in the hospital setting, J Obstet Gynecol Neonatal Nurs 12(4):252, 1983.

Wilkerson NN and Barrows TL: Synchronizing care with mother-baby rhythms, MCN 13(4):264, 1988.

Population, ecology, and reproduction

Beeman PB: Peers, parents, and partners; determining the needs of the support person in an abortion clinic, J Obstet Gynecol Neonatal Nurs 14(1):54, 1985.

Brown MA: Adolescents and abortion: a theoretical framework for decision making, J Obstet Gynecol Neonatal Nurs 12(4):241, 1983.

Chez RA and Keith L: Clinical dialogue: fitting a diaphragm, Contemp OB/GYN 22(2):181, 1983.

Cohen L: Whose right to life? MCN 13(2):83, 1988.

Contraceptive counsel from teenage peers, Am J Nurs 84(5):590, 1984.

Ehrlich PR: The population bomb, New York, 1968, Ballantine Books, Inc.

Frye BS: Nurses and abortion, J Obstet Gynecol Neonatal Nurs 18(3):193, 1989.

Greenberg MJ: Vasectomy technique, Am Fam Physician 39(1):131, 1989.

Hatcher RA and others: Contraceptive technology 1988-89, ed 14, New York, 1988, Irvington Publishers, Inc.

Heaton CJ and Smith MA: The diaphragm, Am Fam Physician 39(5):231, 1989.

Janowski MJ: The road not taken, Am J Nurs 87(3):334, 1987.

Kennedy BJ: Dilemmas in practice: I'm sorry, baby, Am J Nurs 88(8):1067, 1988.

Kurtzman C and Block DE: Family planning: beyond contraception, MCN 11(5):340, 1986.

Lane C and Kemp J: Family planning needs for adolescents, J Obstet Gynecol Neonatal Nurs 13(suppl):61s, 1984.

Lindsay JW: Pregnant too soon: adoption is an option, Buena Park, Calif, 1987, Morning Glory Press.

Lindsay JW: Parents, pregnant teens and the adoption option: help for families, Buena Park, Calif, 1988, Morning Glory Press.

Loucks A: A comparison of satisfaction with types of diaphragms among women in a college population, J Obstet Gynecol Neonatal Nurs 18(3):194, 1989.

Maine D and Wray J: Population: effects of family planning on maternal and child health, Contemp OB/GYN 23(3):122, 1984.

Monier M and Laird M: Contraceptives: a look at the future, Am J Nurs 89(4):496, 1989.

Moore ML: Recurrent teen pregnancy: making it less desirable, MCN 14(2):104, 1989.

Neidhardt A: Why me? Second trimester abortion, Am J Nurs 86(10):1133, 1986.

New bedfellows: "Good" lipids and the pill, Am J Nurs 88(5):634, 1988.

Pace-Owens S: Gamete intrafallopian transfer (GIFT), J Obstet Gynecol Neonatal Nurs 18(2):93, 1989.

Panzarine S and Gould CL: Knowledge about contraceptive use and conception among a group of urban black adolescent mothers, J Obstet Gynecol Neonatal Nurs 17(4):279, 1988.

Rhodes AM: The rights of minors, MCN 13(4):28, 1988.

Schneider TB:Voluntary termination of pregnancy, J Obstet Gynecol Neonatal Nurs 13(2 suppl):77s, 1984.

Wall EM: Development of a decision aid for women choosing a method of birth control, J Fam Pract 21(5):351, 1985.

Wall-Hass CL: Women's perceptions of first trimester spontaneous abortion, J Obstet Gynecol Neonatal Nurs 14(1):50, 1985.

Welzritchie C: Adoption: an option often overlooked, Am J Nurs 89(9):1156, 1989.

The Newborn Infant

12

The Normal Newborn Infant

CHAPTER OBJECTIVES

After studying this chapter, the student should be able to perform the following:

1 State average birth weight and length of newborns by sex.
2 Define or describe the following features involving the baby's head: molding, overriding sutures, fontanels, caput succedaneum, cephalhematoma, and cradle cap (seborrheic dermatitis)
3 Indicate the normal range of the head circumference of a newborn, the fraction of a baby's total length that his head represents, and the normal time range of closure for the anterior fontanel.
4 Describe common newborn skin manifestations such as vernix caseosa, lanugo, erythema toxicum, Mongolian or Asiatic spots, petechiae, milia, and acrocyanosis.
5 Contrast physiologic and pathologic jaundice in the newborn according to the usual time of onset and the maximum level of serum bilirubin by the fifth day of life.
6 Note the normal axillary temperature range for the neonate expressed in centigrade and Fahrenheit, the typical apical pulse range, the typical respiratory range (regardless of activity), and the average blood pressure at birth.
7 Explain what is meant by respiratory retractions and their significance.
8 List three reasons why it is important to burp an infant.
9 Describe the normal stool cycle of a formula-fed newborn and how the stools of breast-fed babies usually differ.
10 Recall two neonatal conditions that are responses to the passage of maternal hormones across the placenta to the infant.
11 Discuss the ability of the newborn to respond to touch, sight, taste, and smell.
12 List and describe five inborn or primitive reflexes.

The newborn infant is a marvelous creation, the result of approximately 40 weeks of intensive growth and development never to be equaled at any subsequent period of his life. A passive participant in the drama of birth, the infant, for the present and near future, is almost totally dependent on the physical care, emotional support, and mental stimulus given his inborn potential by his immediate environment. The human newborn does little for himself. In his egocentric way he waits impatiently for his needs to be met by others as if no other needs exist, and indeed, as far as he knows, they do not.

Although all newborn infants have occupied similar environments during their 9 months of prenatal life, even this basic experience is not identical. True, all lived in the warm, watery environment of the amniotic sac, but not all infants receive identical portions of nourishment or oxygen. Their genetic backgrounds differ, greatly influencing basic body strengths and weaknesses. The stresses and strains of each pregnancy and birth are rarely duplicated. Babies are individuals. Each is different, and a wide range of shapes, sizes, and behavior patterns must still be labeled "normal." So although one often speaks of the typical newborn infant, it must be realized that such a child exists only within the pages of textbooks.

QUALIFICATIONS OF NURSERY PERSONNEL

The nurse caring for the newborn infant has a tremendous responsibility. Because of the newborn's inability to verbalize his needs, the nurse must be a keen observer. Technique, skills, and a gentle approach must be based on sound scientific principles and high ethical standards. The nurse's health must be evaluated frequently to verify the absence of infection.

THE TYPICAL NEWBORN INFANT

Having explained that a baby is really an individual, we will now describe the general appearance, anatomy, and physiology of the "representative" newborn infant. For unknown reasons approximately 106 male infants are born for every 100 female infants. However, the male newborn infant appears to be more fragile than the female, with a higher mortality. The average male newborn infant at birth weighs about 7½ pounds (3.40 kg), whereas the average female weighs about ½ pound less, or 3.18 kg. The average male length is 20 inches (50.8 cm), ½ inch longer than his female counterpart. Of course, these figures are just averages, and much depends on the heredity of the child. Blacks and Asians usually have smaller babies, whereas Caucasians and Hispanics tend to have larger children.

When uninitiated persons first see a newborn infant, certain reactions are fairly standard: "He seems to be all head." "Where is her chin?" "Nurse, my baby has flat feet!" "Boy! She sure is red." "Will his sku!l always be that shape?"

The head

The head of a newborn infant represents one fourth of its total length (Fig. 12-1), but in adulthood the head equals only one eighth of the individual's total height. The newborn infant's occipital-frontal head circumference (OFC) normally ranges from 13 to 14 inches (33 to 35.5 cm). The head's rate of growth averages 1 cm

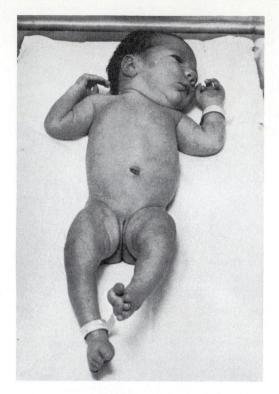

FIG 12-1 Representative newborn infant, 3 days old. Note size of head relative to total length. *(Courtesy Grossmont Hospital, La Mesa, Calif.)*

each month during the first year. It usually exceeds that of his chest by 2 cm. No wonder the relative size causes comment!

The shape of the baby's head can also cause a mother or father needless concern. Cesarean-born babies and even breech babies usually have rounded, "normal-appearing" heads. But infants who are born vaginally in cephalic presentations, particularly those who are first-born, usually undergo considerable head sculpture, or *molding*. This molding is caused by the compression of the head in the birth canal during labor. The infant skull, because of the soft membranous seams separating the skull bones, can become shaped in its journey through the canal. In response to the pressure of the cervix and bony pelvis, the head usually elongates, and the skull bones may even overlap in places. This phenomenon is called *overriding sutures*. The molding lasts for about a week.

The *fontanels,* or soft spots, where sutures cross or meet, are particularly noteworthy. Two are easily felt and identified: the anterior diamond-shaped fontanel, through

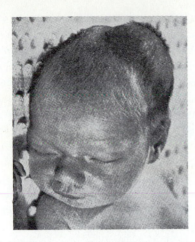

FIG 12-2 Cephalhematoma over parietal bone. *(From Davis ME and Rubin R: DeLee's obstetrics for nurses, ed 17, Philadelphia, 1962, WB Saunders Co.)*

which a pulse is sometimes visible (fontanel means "little fountain"), and the smaller posterior fontanel just above the occiput. The larger fontanel closes at 9 to 18 months of age. Occasionally it is the site of "cradle cap," or "milk crust," also called seborrhea. This occurs when the parent or nurse is fearful of cleaning this soft area, and secretions from the oil glands and cellular debris build up. Actually the cartilage covering the fontanels is tough. The parent should be assured that no harm will come from shampooing the area well. The posterior fontanel is so small, averaging 1 cm, that it is closed by 6 weeks of age.

Two other temporary conditions involving the head may manifest themselves and cause parental anxiety. These are usually caused by the continued pressure of the undelivered head against the partially dilated cervix. The first and less important is called *caput succedaneum,* or caput. Caput is an abnormal collection of fluid under the scalp on top of the skull that may or may not cross suture lines, depending on its size. The accumulation is usually absorbed over a period of days and requires no treatment. The second condition is *cephalhematoma* (Fig. 12-2), caused by a collection of bloody fluid under the first covering layer (the periosteum) of a flat cranial bone. It is normally restricted to one bone. If it crosses a suture line, a skull fracture may be suspected. It usually develops when labor is particularly prolonged and the passageway is tight in relation to the needs of the passenger, causing bruising against the pelvis. As a result of the trauma, small blood vessels under the periosteum break. A cephalhematoma may not be apparent at the time of birth because of the presence of a more inclusive caput. Like caput, cephalhematoma, although temporarily disfiguring, is not harmful and requires no treatment. However, it is important to note the infant's blood values, since excess bleeding into the cephalhematoma may cause some lowering of hemoglobin and hematocrit levels.

General body proportions

Parents are often amazed to see the small size of the infant's face compared with the total head size. The facial bones are underdeveloped, and the chin is almost nonexistent. The baby's neck is usually short and creased and difficult to clean unless the head is tipped backward and unsupported while the child is held at the shoulders. The torso of the normal newborn infant displays a relatively small thorax and a soft, rather protuberant abdomen. The genitalia are small but may be swollen. The extremities are short in relation to body length. The feet are always flat because of the presence of a fatty pad that normally disappears by the time a child has been walking for 6 to 12 months.

Ears and eyes

The ears may be folded and creased and may seem out of shape initially because of positioning while in the uterus. They soon return to their normal shape. The infant should respond to sound at birth.

The eyes may not track properly and may cross (strabismus) or twitch (nystagmus). These symptoms are usually not considered significant unless they persist beyond the first month of life. The irises of caucasian neonates are slate blue, and true eye color is seldom determined until 3 to 6 months of age. It is difficult to tell what a baby is able to see. The pupils react to light, and the infant can focus on objects (for example, on another person's eyes) at about 12 inches (30 cm) away. Recent research shows that they can see faces, shapes, and colors. Blinking is an inborn protective reflex. The lacrimal glands evidently function only minimally at birth, and the newborn infant's cries are characteristically tearless. Occasionally, an eye discharge is apparent, caused by eye irritation initiated by the prophylactic against *ophthalmia neonatorum* (a condition that results from a gonorrheal infection in the mother). The prophylactic, which is required in most states, may be silver nitrate, 1%, an ophthalmic ointment containing tetracycline, 1%, or more commonly erythromycin, 0.5%. Because of sensitivity problems, penicillin is seldom used for this purpose. The reason for the eye irritation or conjunctivitis should be explained to the parents. It is important to note the time of onset of neonatal conjunctivitis to help determine its cause. Any exudate from the eyes that persists should be cultured to exclude bacterial conjunctivitis. (See also p. 140.)

Skin

The skin of the newborn infant is subject to numerous conditions and manifestations that almost always elicit questions.

Vernix caseosa. The skin of the fetus is protected from its watery environment by a soft, yellowish cream named vernix caseosa, or "cheesy varnish." This is an accumulation of old cutaneous cells mixed with an early secretion from the oil glands. Sometimes the baby is thickly covered with vernix at birth. Sometimes it is found in abundance only in the body creases.

The skin of the newborn infant is thin. The more immature the baby is, the less developed will be the layer of subcutaneous fat. For this reason babies who are a few hours old, when oxygenation is optimal, tend to be red. The smaller the baby, the more tomato-colored he tends to be—especially when upset and crying. Nurses should be aware that black babies are light-colored at birth and darken gradually.

Lanugo. A relatively long, soft growth of fine hair called lanugo is often observed on the shoulders, back, forehead, and cheeks of the newborn infant. In fact, some infants may seem to have sideburns. The more premature the infant, the more conspicuous this extra growth of hair tends to be. This hair falls away and disappears early in postnatal life.

Erythema toxicum. Another skin manifestation that can be puzzling but is considered harmless is a condition known to the nursery staff as "newborn rash," or erythema toxicum. The adjective "toxic" perhaps should not be used because no poison has ever been proved to be the cause. In fact, the cause is unknown. The lesions consist of red blotches that may become hivelike elevations and may later develop tiny blisters in the center containing clear fluid. Smears and cultures reveal eosinophils but no bacteria. These lesions may appear on the day of birth and persist for hours or days. They are most often seen on the trunk but may appear elsewhere. They are not contagious and are most frequently seen on vigorous, healthy babies. No treatment is needed.

Mongolian spots. About 90% of babies of African, Indian, Asian, or Mediterranean ancestry and 10% of Caucasian babies exhibit blue-black colorations on their lower backs, buttocks, anterior trunks, and, rarely, fingers or feet. These spots are not bruise marks or signals of ill treatment, nor are they associated with mental retardation. These so-called mongolian or Asian spots fade in early childhood but may persist indefinitely.

Jaundice. The skin of the infant on about the third day may begin to take on a yellow cast. This icterus, or jaundice, is not usually considered to be of pathologic origin but is thought to be associated with the destruction of red blood cells that are no longer needed in as great a number as when external respiration by means of the lungs was impossible in utero. However, if jaundice is present before 24 hours of age, it is considered pathologic, and the possibility of Rh factor, blood group incompatibility (ABO), or hepatitis should be recognized and determined. Indeed, no matter what the age of the baby, the fact that the baby is jaundiced should be reported and evaluated because the number 24 is not magical, and occasionally difficulties may occur later. The jaundice caused by the expected erythrocyte destruction, seen to some extent in almost all newborn infants, has been termed *physiologic jaundice*, and is characterized by a rise in the serum bilirubin to a maximum level of 12 mg/100 ml by the fifth day of life.

Petechiae. Another possible signal of skin trouble that usually turns out to be a false alarm is the presence of petechiae, small blue-red dots on the body caused by the breakage of minute capillaries. If present, these dots are usually seen on the face as a result of pressure exerted on the head during a difficult or rapid birth. Nevertheless, if petechiae are accompanied by jaundice or begin to increase measurably after birth, one may consider a diagnosis of hematologic disease. True petechiae do not blanch on pressure.

Milia. Small pinpoint white or yellow dots are common on the nose, forehead, cheeks and chin of the newborn infant. They are clogged sweat and oil glands that have not yet begun to function normally and are called milia. They disappear with time, and under no circumstances should they be expressed.

Birthmarks. Small reddened areas are sometimes present on the eyelids, midforehead, and nape of the neck. They are probably the result of a local dilatation of skin capillaries and thinness of the skin. Because of the frequent involvement of the nape of the neck, they are sometimes called "stork bites." Other terms are *salmon patch* and *telangiectasia*. In contrast to port-wine stain or nevus flammeus, stork bites are lighter in color, blanch on pressure, and fade during early childhood. Some are noticeable only when the person blushes, is extremely warm, or becomes excited.

Other birthmarks are sometimes seen. The so-called strawberry mark may not be present at birth but may develop days or weeks later. It is characterized by a dark or bright red, raised, rough surface. Since it is formed by a collection of capillaries at the skin's surface, it may be classed as a blood vessel tumor, or *hemangioma*. The first signs of a strawberry mark may be a grouping of red dots that eventually coalesce, forming the clear-cut raised lesion. Most often this mark disappears spontaneously in early childhood without treatment. However, if severe hemorrhage, recurrent infection, or rapid growth causes pressure on a vital structure (such as a nerve or the trachea), therapy designed to reduce or remove the strawberry mark may be indicated. Although rarely used, the application of dry ice at brief intervals, injection of a substance to destroy the involved blood vessels, or actual surgical excision, depending on the location of the strawberry mark, are methods of removal. A "wait-and-see" attitude is advocated, because most lesions regress spontaneously, and all methods of removal cause scarring.

Additional birthmarks that may sometimes cause concern are various flat or raised, frequently pigmented irregularities of the skin that are generally termed moles, or *nevi* (singular, nevus). These lesions are usually benign. However, change in color, rapid growth, or increased irregularity of the border of the nevus warrants a dermatology referral. There is one type of blue-black mole that is considered precancerous, and any such lesion must be evaluated by the physician to ascertain its true character.

Vital signs in the newborn infant

Temperature. Before birth the temperature of the fetus is about 1° F higher than that of the mother. With exposure to the outside world the newborn infant's body temperature immediately drops. If care is not taken to dry the infant and keep him warm his temperature can drop to a subnormal range. The internal organs of the neonate are poorly insulated, and the skin is relatively thin. The newborn infant's heat-regulating center and circulatory system have not yet matured, and his body temperature rapidly reflects that of his environment.

The newborn does not raise or maintain body temperature by shivering but is aided in his efforts to increase body temperature by a special tissue found only in neonates called *brown fat*. It is located principally between the scapulae, in the neck region, behind the sternum, and near the adrenals. This tissue produces a chemical, noradrenaline, which helps burn fats in the presence of oxygen to increase heat. When the neonate is placed in a warm incubator or wrapped in warm blankets, his temperature usually stabilizes in the "normal range" within 8 to 12 hours. Axillary temperatures should range from 36.5 to 37.0° C (97.7 to 98.6° F). Maintaining body warmth as much as possible in the immediate postnatal period may be critical to the well-being of an infant; therefore special efforts have been initiated to provide warmth to newborns in many delivery rooms. (See also p. 579.) A newborn infant's feet and hands are bluish (acrocyanotic) for about 6 to 12 hours after birth, and circulation is particularly poor in the extremities. For this reason one should not attempt to judge an infant's temperature by feeling the feet or hands. Evaluating the warmth of the trunk is more accurate. Newborn infants are sometimes overheated by overzealous nurses or parents who put too much clothing or bedding on or around them. The newborn infant is not yet able to perspire effectively as the sweat glands are not functioning adequately. The baby may break out in a pinpoint reddish rash that is called *prickly heat,* or *miliaria*.

Pulse. It is very difficult to take a radial pulse on an infant. For this reason all pulse readings are routinely taken with a stethoscope over the heart (precordial) region through the chest or possibly the back. The reading is called an *apical pulse* (AP). Newborn infants' pulse rates usually range between 120 and 160 beats per minute (the same as the fetal heart rate).

Respirations. A newborn infant's respirations are irregular and usually abdominal or diaphragmatic in character, typically ranging from 30 to 80 breaths per minute, depending on the baby's activity. If respirations at rest are persistently 45 or more per minute, the rate is usually considered abnormal, and further respiratory evaluation is required. At no time are costal or sternal retractions considered normal in the newborn infant. Retraction, or a sucking in of the chest wall in the rib or sternal area on inspiration, is an indication of respiratory distress. (See Fig. 26-3.)

Blood pressure. In many hospitals the blood pressure of the newborn is recorded routinely following birth. Measured with a cuff 1-inch wide, the average blood pressure at birth is 80/46 mm Hg. If blood pressure is abnormal, the physician is notified and serial determinations are made. If available, a Doppler blood pressure device should be used because it is the most accurate method. Otherwise, a systolic reading may be obtained by noting the pressure when palpating the return of the brachial pulse if the blood pressure is inaudible using standard techniques. Students should know that as a person grows older, pulse and respiratory rates decrease, whereas blood pressure readings rise.

Survey of the newborn infant's body systems

Gastrointestinal system

Mouth. The newborn infant's mouth is of great interest to parent and physician and should be carefully examined for gross abnormalities such as cleft lip and palate. However, certain small structural differences in the normal newborn infant may need to be explained to the first-time parent to alleviate anxiety. Near the center of the hard palate little white glistening spots may occasionally be observed. These are called *Epstein's pearls*. They mark the fusion of the halves of the palate and will disappear in time.

Sometimes the mother has heard of an oral infection called *thrush* and thinks that Epstein's pearls are an indication of this infection. Thrush, or oral moniliasis, caused by a fungus called *Candida (Monilia) albicans,* is a coating on the tongue and cheeks that looks something like milk curds (Fig. 12-3). It does not disappear when water is given to the infant as do true milk curds. The white patches adhere to the mucous membrane, but when they are forcibly lifted by an applicator, a raw, red, sore surface is revealed.

The gums of the newborn infant may at times appear somewhat jagged, and the rear gums may be whitish. Although the primary teeth are semiformed, they are not

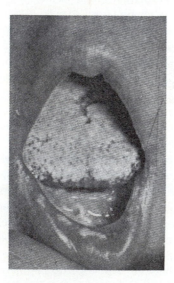

FIG 12-3   Thrush. *(From Potter EL: Pathology of the fetus and the newborn, ed 3, Chicago, 1975, Year Book Medical Publishers, Inc.)*

erupted. If a tooth is present at birth, it usually is an "extra," which has little root. These so-called rice teeth are sometimes pulled to prevent aspiration when they loosen.

The cheeks of the newborn infant have a chubby appearance because of the development of fatty sucking pads that persist until use of the cup is well established.

Parents may be worried about the possibility of tongue-tie, or a restrictively short frenulum at the base of the tongue. Actually problems in food manipulation or speech because of this condition are rare.

Stomach and intestines. The fetus has no need for a digestive system of its own. All its food is provided predigested by the placental circulation. A good share of the waste products created are eliminated through the same circulation. After birth, however, digestion is a different story.

The capacity of the newborn infant's stomach at birth probably varies from 1 to 2 ounces (30 to 60 ml) and increases rapidly. The feeding usually begins to leave the stomach before the total is taken. It is common for infants to swallow air as they feed, especially when bottle-fed. Swallowed air in the stomach may cause difficulty in continuing the feeding, or it may cause vomiting later. Air passing into the intestines may cause colic (abdominal cramping). Bottle-fed babies need to be burped frequently. Newborn infants are usually burped after every ounce of formula. The older infant is burped once halfway through the feeding and again at the end of the feeding. Nursing babies are usually burped once or twice during a feeding. Immediately after the feeding, a small amount of milk (less than an ounce) may come up with a bubble. This is termed a "wet burp," spitting up, or a small regurgitation. Within limits this is a natural occurrence. It usually subsides by 8 to 9 months of age as the gastrointestinal tract matures.

The first stool of the newborn infant is meconium, a greenish black, tarry, odorless, but very tenacious material. It consists of old lining cells of the gastrointestinal tract, swallowed amniotic fluid debris, and early tract secretions. The first stool should appear in a maximum of 24 hours. If it does not, malformation of the gastrointestinal tract is strongly suspected. Meconium continues to be the normal stool for about 2 days, then the products of ingested milk begin to change the color of the stool. It becomes first brown and then yellow-green and more loose in consistency. These are the *transitional stools.* Later the stool will become yellow as more milk-product digestion takes place. The stools of formula-fed babies are characteristically lemon yellow and curdy. The stools of breast-fed babies have a more yellow-orange color, are usually softer, and during the first few weeks are more frequent. The wide range of normal stool patterns should be explained to the mother.

Circulatory system. In fetal life the circulatory system serves also as a modified respiratory system, since oxygen is not obtained through the breathing of air into the lungs but through the successive pulsations of the vein in the umbilical cord leading from the placenta attached to the uterine wall. Carbon dioxide is also eliminated through this attachment by way of the two umbilical arteries.

At birth, of course, this type of respiratory function is not continued, since the cord is cut or the placenta soon becomes detached. The fetal circulation, which is designed to channel blood flow to functioning organs and largely avoid the lung fields, is rerouted after birth. (See discussion of fetal circulation, p. 53.) The two fetal shunts that direct blood flow away from the pulmonary circulation normally close, apparently because of changes in internal pressures and vascular reflexes resulting from loss of the maternal oxygen source and subsequent lung expansion. The opening between the two atria of the heart, the *foramen ovale,* shuts, closing off the blood flow to the left atrium from the right heart and forcing more blood into the right ventricle. The *ductus arteriosus,* the fetal vessel between the pulmonary artery and the aorta, collapses, obliging the pulmonary artery to send its total contents to the lungs.

The circulation of blood in the baby at birth is not at the same stage of development throughout the body. The hands and feet are typically blue, a condition termed *acrocyanosis.* At times the entire body of a baby at birth may be blue because the fetal blood has a relatively low oxygen content, and a momentary disturbance of the placental circulation may occur before expansion of the lungs is possible. However, as soon as the airway is cleared and a healthy cry is elicited, the skin "pinks up" dramatically. Although significant, color is the least important of the characteristics or vital signs to be considered when using the Apgar scoring method in evaluating a newborn infant's need for resuscitation. (See Table 7-4.) If a newborn infant is chilled or inactive for a period of time, a mottled pattern may be seen on the skin—particularly on the extremities. This purplish mottling, called *cutis marmorata,* is transitory in nature and soon disappears.

For a discussion of newborn infants' blood pressure readings and pulse rates, see p. 241.

Vitamin K is routinely given to newborn infants in many nurseries to prevent hemorrhage because of the natural low prothrombin level in this period of life. It is especially recommended for those suffering from hemorrhagic disease of the newborn, infants born of complicated deliveries, or premature infants. However, it has been found that too high a dosage (usually over 5 mg) may be accompanied by an increase in jaundice and in some cases kernicterus (the yellow staining of the basal ganglia of the brain, causing possible cerebral damage).

Three blood vessels are found in the umbilical cord—one vein and two arteries. These are fairly easily seen in the cut umbilical stump. Considerable interest has developed in counting these vessels at the time of the nursery admission because, if only two vessels are found, there is significantly increased incidence of internal congenital defects (malformed kidneys, heart, etc).

The vessels of the umbilical cord are fairly soon occluded by clot formation and shrinkage. However, if the cord is manipulated often, the clot may become dislodged, and bleeding through the cord stump may occur if the ligature or cord clamp is loose. Large cords that contain a great amount of gelatinous connective tissue, called *Wharton's jelly,* must be especially watched for bleeding, since the cord will shrink in diameter and the clamp or ligature may become ineffective. The cord has no sensory nerves; the baby does not feel it when the cord is clamped or cut. The umbilical cord drops off, and the place of attachment heals in about 7 to 10 days.

Respiratory system. Although the fetus normally begins breathing movements in utero, the lungs serve no respiratory function because the oxygen supply is secured through the placental circulatory system from the mother. The birth process stimulates a series of events that transform the fluid-filled lungs into organs capable of gas exchange. Some of the lung fluid is squeezed out during the passage through the birth canal, and the rest is rapidly absorbed as the lungs fill with air. Initially the newborn may need some assistance in clearing the upper airway, because thick mucous secretions may lead to obstruction. Newborn respiratory rates and patterns are discussed on p. 241.

Babies normally are nose breathers during early infancy and do not breathe through open mouths. Lint or dried mucus in the nose may make the infant sneeze or breathe loudly. Cyanosis other than of the hands and feet, costal or substernal retractions, flaring nostrils, and expiratory grunts heard with or without a stethoscope all are possible signs of respiratory distress.

In the United States the most common cause of respiratory difficulty in the first few minutes or hours of birth has been the too liberal use of sedatives, tranquilizers, analgesics, and anesthetics, which not only affect the mother but also pass over the placenta to the baby, making the newborn sleepy and disinclined to take a first breath. Because of this, a real effort has been made in the last few years to reduce the use of these agents.

It is not known exactly why a baby takes that first breath, but the following factors are believed to be significant:

1. The buildup of carbon dioxide in the fetal bloodstream caused by the beginning separation of the placenta from the uterine wall and the pressure of the uterine contractions
2. The decrease of oxygen in the fetal bloodstream
3. The rapid change in the baby's environment at the moment of birth
4. The direct handling of the baby for the first time in his life

Urinary system. The newborn infant's renal system does not have the ability to concentrate urine to the degree of the older child or adult. Water is not reabsorbed as freely by the nephrons, and a newborn infant may become dehydrated rather easily. A newborn infant with profuse diarrhea or vomiting is in imminent danger of dehydration.

Uric acid is found in relatively large amounts in the urine of the newborn infant. Occasionally this substance may "crystallize out" as it cools in the diaper, leaving a pink stain like "brick dust."

All infant voidings in the newborn period should be recorded. Although newborn infants may not void a large amount or often at first, it is important to note that they are able to void normally.

Endocrine system and genital area. The endocrine system of the newborn infant is supplemented by maternal hormones that have crossed the placental barrier. These maternal contributions—presumably the estrogenic hormone, luteal hormone, and lactogenic hormone—when withdrawn from the baby through the act of birth, bring about certain phenomena that may cause parents concern and should be explained. The maternal hormones crossing to the fetus may affect the breasts of both male and female infants, causing swelling, which is particularly noticeable about the third day of life. The breast secretion sometimes seen has been given the interesting name of *witch's milk*. The breasts may continue to be edematous for 2 to 3 weeks, but gradually the congestion subsides without treatment. The breasts

should not be squeezed; this only increases the possibility of infection and injures the tender tissue.

Maternal hormones acting on the miniature uterus of the female newborn infant may set the stage for *infantile menstruation*. The hormones help thicken the infant's tiny endometrial lining. Withdrawn at the time of birth, these hormones no longer maintain this thickened uterine lining, and a tiny menstrual flow may be observed. Usually only a few blood spots are seen on the diapers. The entire process may terminate in 1 or 2 days. This bleeding should not be profuse, and any considerable blood loss may be an indication of hemorrhagic disease. White mucoid vaginal discharge in the newborn infant is also thought to be stimulated by maternal endocrine secretions. The genitalia of both the boy and the girl may be swollen. Hymenal tags that regress spontaneously may be seen on girls. Breech infants may have particularly swollen genitalia because of the prolonged pressure on the area. In male infants the scrotum most often contains the testes, although sometimes the descent of one or both is delayed. The foreskin of the uncircumcised infant is normally tight. Few are retractable at birth, and only about 50% are retractable at 1 year. They should not be forced. If adherence of the prepuce (phimosis) persists, circumcision may be advised to facilitate gentle cleansing.

At birth the thymus gland, located under the sternum and above the heart, is larger than a baby's fist. The thymus, long a mysterious lymphoid tissue difficult to classify, is now considered to be an endocrine gland. It seems that a hormone, thymosin, has been identified, which in cases of the lack of a thymus can be administered to help prevent or control infection. It is now thought to initiate the body's complex immune reactions by producing special defensive cells that are distributed to the spleen, bone marrow, and lymph nodes. After puberty, however, the thymus atrophies, and the change in the gland's size is thought to either stimulate or reflect the development of sexual maturity. Pressure on the respiratory tract from a large thymus has, in the past, been cited as a rare cause of infant suffocation. This has not been adequately substantiated. Although many theories have been advanced, including sleep apnea and excessive parental smoking, the primary cause of so-called crib death, or sudden infant death syndrome (SIDS), is still unknown.

Neuromuscular system. The nervous system of the normal newborn infant is immature. Essential activities for maintenance of life and protection are largely reflex in character—inborn reactions making life possible until

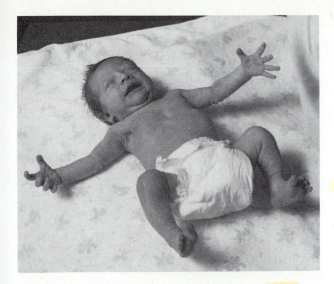

FIG 12-4 This baby is demonstrating the classical Moro reflex initiated when his head was brought forward and then allowed to fall back suddenly (30 degrees) against a padded table. His head is in the midline; both arms are abducted at the shoulder, elbows are extended, and hands are opening.

the nervous system and associated muscles can "grow up" to the demands of more complex living. Inborn, or primitive, reflexes that normal newborn infants possess include the rooting, sucking, and swallowing reflexes employed in eating and the protective reflexes, such as coughing, sneezing, gagging, blinking, and perhaps crying. Other muscular reactions in newborn infants are also reflex.

The most commonly tested muscular reflex is a total body response known as the Moro reflex, normally present during the first 3 to 4 months of life. This response is probably elicited when the baby senses a loss of support. When the infant's head is brought forward and then allowed to fall back suddenly (about 30 degrees), abduction of the upper extremities at the shoulder, extension of the elbows, and opening of the hands follow (Fig. 12-4). The startle reflex initiated by a loud noise or sudden movement or jarring may be considered part of the Moro reflex consisting of flexion of the extremities and palmar grasping. These are two distinct movements, since one can occur without the other. When testing for the Moro reflex, make sure the baby's head is in midline position. Either the absence of the Moro reflex or an asymmetric response in the newborn infant may indicate brain damage.

Another often seen reflex position is called the asymmetric tonic neck reflex (ATNR). The child assumes a modified fencer's position while on his back. The arm and leg on one side of the body are extended while the opposing arm and leg are flexed. The fists are shut and the toes curled. The head is turned toward the extended arm, which incidentally is usually the dominant side. This reflex position may be commonly seen until the infant is about 6 months of age and must disappear before the infant can crawl. Grasping, a primitive reflex, should be elicited by placing a finger in the ulnar side of the infant's palm. (See Figs. 17-1, *A*, and 17-2, *A*.)

The immaturity of the nervous system is demonstrated by the unstable temperature regulation of the newborn infant and his limited ability to pursue purposeful activity. A newborn may turn his head, blink, or grimace in response to sound but be unable to sort out the sound

Table 12-1 Newborn behavior states

State	Description	Characteristics
1	Deep sleep	Eyes closed, no eye movement under lids
		Respirations regular
		Occasional jerky movements at regular intervals
2	Light sleep	Eyes closed, rapid movement under lids
		Respirations irregular, occasional sucking movements
		Random but smoother movements
3	Drowsy	Eyes open or closed, eyelids fluttering
		Activity level variable, movements are smooth
4	Alert	Eyes open, bright look, attention focused on source of stimulation
		Minimal activity
5	Active	Eyes wide open, considerable activity
		Thrusting movements of arms and legs
6	Crying	Intense, difficult to break through
		High activity

Adapted from Brazelton TB: Neonatal behavioral assessment scale. In Clinics in developmental medicine, no. 50, London, 1973, MacKeith Press.

and make it meaningful. The sense of taste and smell are well developed. Newborns show a preference for some tastes and smells over others. Within a few days they show a preference for the smell of their own mother's breast milk over that of another nursing mother. Cutaneous sensation is highly developed. Pressure, temperature, and pain are increasingly felt by the infant. The newborn reacts to cuddling, caresses, and skillful, gentle handling with greater relaxation and acceptance of care. At first he sleeps about 20 hours a day, waking to be fed, bathed, changed, repositioned, and briefly entertained.

A baby's level of consciousness ranges between deep sleep and crying. The so-called quiet-alert state (4 on Table 12-1) affords an especially rewarding opportunity for infant-parent interaction. It is usually first observed sometime during the first hour following birth. The order of peripheral nervous system development and muscular coordination proceeds from the head region to the arms and then the legs. Later, the finer activities of the hands and feet are perfected.

Usually a newborn infant stays in the position in which he is placed, since he doesn't have the ability to turn himself. However, a baby should never be left alone on a table or bed. Accidents can happen!

Intellectual development is difficult to assess in the newborn, but it is reassuring when the primitive reflexes are present and symmetric. There is cause for concern when a baby fails to suck well, lacks good muscle tone, or is lethargic and unresponsive to care.

• • •

All in all, the newborn infant is quite an invention, and the succeeding months of his life will include some of the most perplexing, exasperating, and wonderful hours ever experienced by any family lucky enough to welcome him into their home.

Key Concepts

1. The average male at birth weighs about 7½ pounds and is 20 inches in length. The average female newborn weighs about 7 pounds and is 19½ inches long.

2. Infants born vaginally in cephalic presentations usually undergo considerable head sculpture, or molding, which is caused by the compression of the head in the birth canal during labor. The phenomenon of overriding sutures occurs when the head, in response to the pressure of the cervix and bony pelvis, elongates and the skull bones overlap.

3. Two of the fontanels, where sutures cross or meet, are easily felt and identified: the anterior diamond-shaped fontanels and the smaller posterior fontanel just above the occiput. The larger fontanel closes at 9 to 18 months of age; the posterior fontanel is closed by 6 weeks of age.

4. Common newborn skin conditions and manifestations include the following: vernix caseosa, an accumulation of old cutaneous cells mixed with an early secretion from the oil glands; lanugo, a relatively long soft growth of fine hair; erythema toxicum, red blotches that may become hivelike elevations; mongolian spots, blue-black colorations on the lower back, buttocks, and anterior trunk; petechiae, small blue-red dots on the body; and milia, small pinpoint white or yellow dots on the nose, forehead, cheeks, and chin.

5. Jaundice that is present before the newborn is 24 hours old is considered pathologic. Physiologic jaundice is characterized by a rise in the serum bilirubin to a maximum level of 12 mg/100 ml by the fifth day of life.

6. The normal range of the newborn's vital signs are as follows: axillary temperature, 36.5° to 37.0° C (97.7° to 98.6° F); apical pulse, 120 to 160 beats per minute; respirations, 30 to 80 breaths per minute; and blood pressure 80/46 mm Hg.

7. Respiratory retraction, which is a sucking in of the chest wall in the rib or sternal area on inspiration, is an indication of respiratory distress.

8. Infants need to be burped because they frequently swallow air as they feed. Swallowed air in the stomach may cause difficulty in continuing the feeding, or it may cause vomiting later. Air passing into the intestines may cause abdominal cramping.

9. The stools of formula-fed infants are characteristically lemon-yellow and curdy. The stools of breast-fed babies have a more yellow-orange color, are usually softer, and during the first few weeks are more frequent.

10. Maternal hormones crossing to the fetus may cause swelling of the infant's breasts, breast secretions, female infantile menstruation, and swollen genitals.

11. Inborn reflexes that newborn infants possess include the rooting, sucking, and swallowing reflexes employed in eating, and the protective reflexes, such as coughing, sneezing, gagging, blinking, and possibly crying.

1. If possible, survey at least six normal newborns. Identify as many normal variations as possible. Did any of the newborns *not* have any normal variations? Did some have more than others? Did the mothers verbalize any concern about these normal variations? Identify the variation and the correct teaching that would apply.

2. Jaundice is considered pathologic if it occurs within 24 hours of birth, usually not if seen after 24 hours. What factors can contribute to the likelihood of jaundice? What laboratory tests measure the level of RBC destruction? Can the severity of the problem be determined by observation?

3. Discuss the normal progression of stools observed in the newborn. How does the stool of breast-fed babies differ from the stool of bottle-fed babies?

4. A new mother is concerned that the baby might regurgitate and choke if put down too soon after a bottle feeding. What feeding and burping techniques are recommended to prevent these problems? How would you position an infant after a feeding? Why?

5. New parents are discussing whether their baby can see, hear, and smell. What would you tell them? They express interest in ways they can enhance positive stimulation for the baby, such as mobiles, or other crib toys. What suggestions would you make? Why?

13

Care of the Normal Newborn Infant

CHAPTER OBJECTIVES

After studying this chapter, the student should be able to perform the following:

1 List the nine universal needs of the newborn.
2 Enumerate four ways in which an infant's airway may be cleared during or after birth.
3 Identify three instances in which supplemental oxygen should be administered to the newborn.
4 Indicate four reasons why it is important to keep the newborn infant warm.
5 Note two situations in which newborns must be observed closely for the development of bleeding.
6 List at least six ways to protect the newborn from infection.
7 Discuss 10 conditions the nurse is looking for during the newborn inspection bath.
8 Explain three safety factors when lifting or carrying an infant.
9 List five advantages of breast-feeding.
10 State dietary modifications a nursing mother may need to make for herself or her baby.
11 Compare the contents of cow's milk and human milk, regarding calories, protein, carbohydrates, fat, and minerals.
12 Develop a mini-lesson plan incorporating basic techniques of breast-feeding, which could be taught to mothers preparing to nurse their infants.
13 Develop a mini-lesson plan that would incorporate the basic techniques of infant formula preparation and feeding for mothers planning to bottle-feed their infants.
14 Indicate four main methods of evaluating the nutritional status of an infant.
15 List five signs of dehydration in the infant that could relate to inadequate fluid intake.
16 Describe five aspects of postcircumcision newborn nursing care.
17 Identify eight areas of potential parent education that the nurse may explore with a new father and mother during her contacts and bedside care.

UNIVERSAL NEEDS

Since the 1960s the trend in the United States in the care of the newborn is toward specialization. The branch of medicine specializing in the care of the newborn is called *neonatology,* and specialists are found primarily in centers that serve a large high risk maternity or infant population. Today, one encounters recovery or transition nurseries devoted to the care of infants less than 24 hours old or newborn surgical patients; neonatal intensive care units (NICU) designed for small, premature, or sick infants (Chapter 15); and intermediate or progressive care units for those infants whose nursing needs are not as intensive. Such care opportunities now make possible the survival of many babies who formerly would have died or suffered severe damage. Along with the trend toward specialization, there continues to be a growing emphasis on family-centered maternity care. It is now recognized that normal healthy newborns need not be separated from their mothers. In some hospitals a mother and her baby are seen as a unit and are cared for by one nurse. This is referred to as mother-baby nursing or couplet care. Many hospitals provide opportunity for the baby to "room-in" with the mother and for the father to visit and participate in infant care. Some centers permit other healthy siblings and grandparents to see and hold the baby as well. Even when the infant is sick and must be in a NICU the parents are encouraged to spend time with their baby. But no matter what the circumstances or locale of birth or the type of care facilities available, all newborn infants have certain needs that must be met for them to thrive and take their place in society. Some of these needs take priority, some can be met simultaneously, and still others are important but need not be rushed. Following are listed nine universal needs of the newborn infant:

1. A clear airway
2. Established respiration
3. Warmth
4. Protection from hemorrhage
5. Protection from infection
6. Identification and observation
7. Nourishment and fluids
8. Love—parent-infant attachment
9. Rest

A clear airway

The first two needs must be met immediately or the baby will not survive, and no amount of oxygen, mouth-to-mouth resuscitation, or intermittent positive pressure will stimulate a newborn infant to breathe if its airway is not open. Conversely, if the airway is not clear but filled with amniotic fluid, meconium particles, or blood, and the infant does try to take a breath and inhale, the respiratory tract may become plugged, irritated, or contaminated. The airway may be cleared by using these methods:

1. Wiping off the child's nose and mouth at the time of the birth of the head
2. Gently suctioning first the mouth and then the nose with a small, soft, short bulb aspirator or a soft catheter attached to a trap and low wall suction before birth is complete (Fig. 13-1)

3. Holding the child's head down to drain immediately after birth while gently compressing the throat toward the mouth to milk out secretions
4. Visualizing the larynx with a laryngoscope and suctioning the trachea by trained personnel for unresponsive infants

Established respiration

With the introduction of closed-chest cardiac massage techniques and appliances to stimulate the heartbeat electrically, perhaps "established respiration" should read "established respiration and heartbeat." However, for this discussion it will be assumed that heart action is present and adequate. (For cardiopulmonary resuscitation of the newborn infant see Table 26-3.) If respiration does not occur spontaneously after the airway is clear, the child should be stimulated to cry. Many infants respond to gentle rubbing of the back or gentle suctioning of the nose with a soft catheter. More vigorous stimulation consists of slapping the heels or rubbing the sternum. If breathing is not initiated soon after stimulation, methods of breathing for the infant must be employed. Sometimes this means the use of intermittent positive pressure by means of orotracheal tube or mask and bag. Sometimes the operator will blow directly through a patent endotracheal tube. No matter what method is used, it should be emphasized that an airway must be maintained through proper head positioning and/or the use of a small oropharyngeal airway to keep the infant's tongue from falling back and obstructing the pharynx.

When a child is being resuscitated, is breathing poorly on his own, has generalized cyanosis, or has a heart rate under 100 beats per minute, supplementary oxygen should be administered.

Warmth

Newborns may suffer from depressed body temperature or hypothermia not because they produce heat poorly but because they are so vulnerable to heat loss. They lose heat easily because the body surface area is so great in relation to weight, and they have relatively little subcutaneous fat to provide insulation. Heat is provided for the infant in most delivery room settings through the use of unenclosed infant warmers, which provide easy accessibility for care by utilizing overhead radiant heat panels. The baby should be dried immediately after birth with a warm towel or blanket to decrease heat loss. (See p. 139.) An interesting study by Phillips, comparing heat loss in heated cribs with heat loss in the mother's arms, confirmed that the mother is a reliable

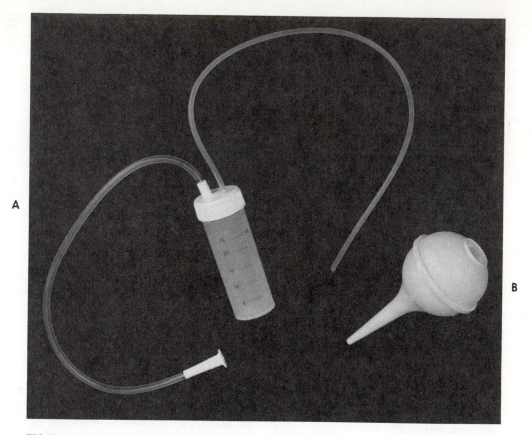

FIG 13-1 A, DeLee-type mucus trap. One tubing leading to little bottle or trap is suction catheter; other tube may be attached to low wall suction. (Since more precautions against AIDS have been instituted, oral suction has been discontinued.) **B,** Aspirator or suction bulb, is frequently used to clean a baby's mouth and nose even before rest of body is delivered. Bulb *must* be compressed before tip of aspirator is placed where suction is desired, or opposite effect will be produced!

source of heat for the normal, dry, wrapped infant placed on the mother's chest.* This has implications for early maternal-infant attachment processes.

The importance of maintaining an infant's body heat immediately after birth and in the extended neonatal period has been emphasized because the temperature of the infant affects the number of calories the baby must burn to keep warm, as well as his oxygen consumption, the incidence of apnea, and the acid-base balance of his blood. When the infant is sick, the provision of appropriate heat is critical. (See also p. 581.)

The way in which the baby is dressed depends on the temperature of the nursery or rooming-in area. Current

*Phillips CRN: Neonatal heat loss in heated cribs vs mother's arms, J Obstet Gynecol Neonatal Nurs 3:11, 1974.

recommendations are that nursery air temperature be maintained at 24° C (75° F) with a relative humidity in the range of 35% to 60% for personnel comfort. Some babies are perfectly warm in only a cotton shirt and diaper, covered by a light cotton blanket. Except for an initial rectal temperature reading when a check is made for imperforate anus, 3-minute axillary temperature determinations are now advocated. An electronic thermometer may be employed. Axillary temperatures for the normal newborn should range from 36.5° to 37.0° C (97.7° to 98.6° F).

Protection from hemorrhage

Today most babies born in hospitals have their cords clamped with some type of compressive band. These commercial clamps have proved to be satisfactory, and although the cord must still be frequently observed for bleeding, incidents of difficulty are extremely rare. When a ligature of any kind is being used, it is usually tied twice approximately 1 inch from the abdominal wall in a depression in the cord made by a previously placed hemostat, if one is available. The tie is secured by a square knot for stability and checked frequently during the first few hours to detect any loosening or bleeding.

Protection from hemorrhage in the newborn infant also becomes important when caring for the male infant after circumcision, to be discussed later in this chapter.

In an effort to decrease the possibility of abnormal cerebral pressure and subsequent intracranial bleeding, newborns are not placed in a prolonged head-down position.

Vitamin K to decrease coagulation time is routinely administered in most hospitals (p. 243).

Protection from infection

Protecting the newborn infant from infection is a constant challenge to delivery room and nursery nurses. It involves the entire environment of babies and the techniques used in handling and nourishing them. It even can be said to reach back to the prenatal period when efforts are made to prevent any contamination of the fetus by organisms that are able to pass over the placental barrier (viruses, spirochetes). The baby, while in the hands of the delivering physician or nurse midwife is considered and maintained sterile. The cord is clamped and cut aseptically. Then the baby is usually handed to a circulating nurse who, having carefully washed her hands and put on clean gloves and overgown, receives him for further care.

In most states of the United States, protection of the infant from infection involves the use of some prophylactic against ophthalmia neonatorum caused by the gonorrheal organism. The prophylactic agent may be drops of silver nitrate 1%, or an ophthalmic ointment containing tetracycline 1% or most commonly erythromycin 0.5%. Although the agent should be instilled shortly after birth, a delay of up to 1 hour is acceptable. This delay may facilitate the initial maternal-infant attachment by allowing the newborn unimpaired eye contact with the mother. Care must be taken in administering the drops or ointment; no pressure should be put on the eyeball itself. Occasionally, if the eye area has not been previously touched, shading the baby's eyes from the light will cause them to open spontaneously, making instillation comparatively easy. If this helpful reaction does not occur, the nurse pulls down on the lower lid to instill

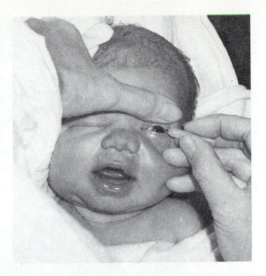

FIG 13-2 Nurse stabilizes head with one hand and pulls down on conjunctival sac with one finger of other hand while dropping in silver nitrate. *(Courtesy Grossmont Hospital, La Mesa, Calif.)*

the agent into the conjunctival sac (Fig. 13-2). All the while the nurse guards the child from cold and continues to observe skin color and respiration patterns. Parents should be told that the eyedrops may cause some swelling and drainage within the next 24 hours. (See also p. 140.)

A central nursery for normal newborn infants and a separate postpartum area for mothers have been the principal pattern of hospital infant care for over 50 years, and this chapter recognizes that many hospitals are still organized in this way. However, a growing number of hospitals are offering mother-baby care units or have initiated single-room maternity care. In these settings one nurse cares for the needs of both mother and baby. (One of the benefits of these newer types of hospital maternity care is the reduction of the risks of infection.) No matter how patient care is organized, all hospital personnel must be aware of the potential hazard of sepsis.

After birth the infant has his own individual bassinet and should also have his own bath equipment, supply of linen, and layette (Fig. 13-3). Infants should be bathed in their own beds and not on a common bathing table. The scale used for determining weight should be protected and balanced and handled in such a way that no cross-infection could take place. Any instruments or appliances that must be used for more than one infant because of lack of supply must be carefully disinfected or sterilized after use. This would apply to stethoscopes,

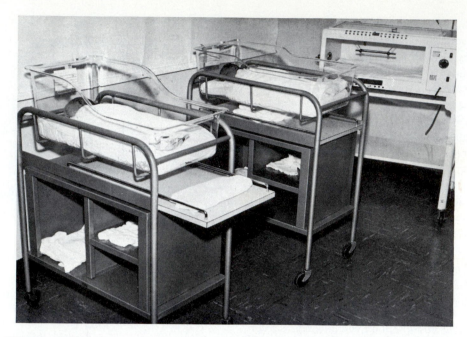

FIG 13-3 Individual nursery unit reduces possibility of cross-infection. *(Courtesy Grossmont Hospital, La Mesa, Calif.)*

circumcision boards and instruments, resuscitators, and other equipment.

Staff members should wear simple, hospital-supplied and laundered clothing on duty, keep their fingernails short, restrict jewelry, and evaluate their own health. No personnel should assume responsibility of caring for newborns while suffering from a contagious respiratory condition, skin infection, or diarrhea.

Personnel entering the nursery usually wash their hands and arms above the elbow with an antibacterial product such as povidone-iodine (Betadine) before starting patient care. Handwashing is mandatory after the care of each baby or individual unit and in the care of the same baby after changing a soiled diaper and proceeding with further needs. The hands should always be washed before treating the cord, since it can become the site of serious infection. It should be observed for signs of inflammation and drainage. A nurse who leaves the maternity area should wear a cover gown to protect her clean nursery gown. If her gown should become soiled in the nursery with urine, emesis, or stool at any time, it should be changed. Unless wrapped in a protective blanket or on a protective cover, the infant should be held away from the nurse's gown during care and feedings to protect the nurse's dress from becoming a source of cross-contamination to other infants. Precautions not

necessary at home are essential when many infants from many backgrounds and families are being cared for in a small area, such as the hospital nursery.

Parents and ancillary staff (e.g., x-ray personnel) should also be taught the importance and technique of good handwashing when visiting the nursery or caring for infants in the mother's hospital room or in the home.

Professional organizations such as the American Academy of Pediatrics, hospital accreditation boards, and local public health and safety officials take an active part in making recommendations and requirements governing the construction, maintenance, and operation of the nursery as well as other parts of the hospital. They are concerned about the floor space available, distance between bassinets, type of ventilation, control of temperature and humidity, provision for adequate lighting, safety of electrical appliances, elimination of possible fire hazards, appropriate dressing and handwashing facilities, and safe formula preparation as well as optimum techniques.

Identification and observation

Identification of the infant may be accomplished in various ways, but it should always be done beyond doubt before the baby leaves the delivery room. In multiple births the infants should be identified immediately after birth to avoid confusion. Identification that can be easily counter-checked—the use of double or triple bands—is recommended.

Admission bath. Most infants have their admission bath in the nursery after being checked in, identified, weighed, and measured. Many infants are not bathed completely until several hours after birth when the body temperature is higher. Newborn infants are covered with varying amounts of vernix and blood. They may also be soiled with meconium. During the admission bath the nurse reaffirms identification, inspects the infant more carefully than was possible in the delivery room, takes his temperature, dresses him appropriately, and places him in a warm incubator or bed depending on his body temperature and observational needs. An admission bath usually employs a mild soap solution or an antibacterial product. The following description outlines procedures for the admission bath, although details may differ from hospital to hospital. The nurse's hands are carefully washed before starting. Depending on the circumstances of the birth and the condition of the baby the nurse may wear gloves. (See p. 615.)

ADMISSION BATH

MATERIALS:

1. Basin of warm water
2. Mild soap or antibacterial product
3. Paper mesh squares
4. Sterile cotton balls
5. Triple dye, Bacitracin, or alcohol, 70% for cord care
6. Applicators for cord care
7. Two towels or soft diapers for covering and drying
8. Individual thermometer
9. Small plastic comb
10. Laundry hamper
11. Appropriate clothing, diaper, shirt, and receiving blanket

PROCEDURE:

1. The temperature is taken.
   a. Axillary temperature is taken by placing a thermometer deep in the axilla while holding the arm gently but firmly against the chest.
   b. Usual time is 3 minutes or until the mercury stops rising.
   c. If the infant is cold, the bath is delayed until the temperature reaches the normal range.
2. The newborn infant is usually partially wrapped with a towel or blanket to prevent chilling.
3. The eyes may be wiped with cotton balls moistened with water. Irrigation or wiping starts at the nose and proceeds outward to prevent unwanted drainage from the inner canthus of the eye from entering the lacrimal duct leading to the nose. (One cotton ball is used for each wipe.)
4. The face is cleaned with a paper mesh square or cotton balls dipped in clear water. No soap is used, since it may be drying to the skin.
   a. If necessary, the opening of the nose is cleared with water-moistened, firmly twisted wisps of cotton as babies are nose breathers.
   b. The external ears may be gently wiped with water-moistened cotton balls, but the canal is never probed.
5. The head is gently but efficiently sudsed and rinsed over the washbasin.
   a. A football hold on the baby is best.
   b. A small comb, gently used, helps to lift out particles of vernix that are difficult to dislodge.
6. The bath is continued by washing, rinsing, and drying the neck, chest, arms, hands, abdomen, and back.
   a. The recently clamped cord and its base are usually avoided until later when an antiseptic is applied. Nurseries today put no gauze dressing on the cord and have found that it dries much faster and has no greater incidence of infection for having been left exposed.
   b. Vernix caseosa may be thick and difficult to remove, particularly from the creases. To avoid skin irritation only what wipes off easily should be removed. Special attention should be paid to the neck creases.
   c. After turning the baby on his side to wash, rinse, and dry, a partially folded towel may be placed under the washed portion of the infant to be completely unfolded when the "bottom half" is clean.
   d. A small undershirt may be put on at this time, rolled up away from the cord to conserve warmth until the bath is completed.
7. The bath is continued, washing the legs, feet, and then the buttocks and perianal region.
8. The nurse's hands are again washed, and any ordered antiseptic is applied with an applicator to the cord end and the inner rim of the skin cuff surrounding the base of the cord. The vessels in the cord may be counted at this time.
9. The genitalia are inspected and cleansed with cotton balls previously moistened with clear water.
   a. For a baby girl the cotton balls may be wiped gently from front to back between the labia, never using a ball more than once.
   b. For an uncircumcised baby boy pediatric urologists do not recommend attempting to retract the foreskin of the newborn until about 5 months of age—since most are adherent. The glans that is visible should be gently cleansed with a moistened cotton ball.

10. The diaper is put on, and the infant tucked into bed. The crib identification card is checked against the infant's personal identification.
    a. Newborn infants are frequently propped on their right sides with a rolled blanket. For the older infant a right-side position is better because of the aid that gravity gives to the flow of food from the stomach and because any air or bubble remaining will rest near the entrance of the stomach and be more easily expelled.
    b. No newborn infant should be left unattended on his back because of the danger of aspiration.
    c. In some hospitals the newborn infant is not dressed until shown to the parents and waiting relatives.
11. Notations regarding voidings, stool, or any pertinent observations should be appropriately recorded.

Throughout the bath procedure the nurse is inspecting and evaluating the infant. As she cleans the eyes, she watches for discharge, conjunctival hemorrhage, or areas of opacity. As she feels the head, she checks the contour, the relative size of the fontanels, and the presence of areas of swelling. Pushing down on the chin, she peers into the mouth. Continuing the bath procedure, the nurse evaluates respirations, counts and separates fingers, and judges skin turgor and muscle tone. As she washes each part, she inspects the infant. She wants to be able to report significant findings so that the pediatrician or family practitioner may be called if necessary. Every new baby should be completely examined by a physician or nurse practitioner within 24 hours of birth, and the condition of some may necessitate a much earlier examination.

Inspection bath. On the following days the bath of the newborn infant serves two main purposes—inspection and stimulation. An example of this procedure follows. Details of possible eye care and genital cleansing are similar to those observed during the admission, both described previously.

DAILY INSPECTION BATH

MATERIALS:

1. Each infant should have its own individual unit including
   a. Thermometer
   b. Diapers, shirts
   c. Linen supply
   d. Blankets
2. Paper mesh squares or two washcloths
3. Mild soap or tap water alone
4. Alcohol 70%, triple dye, or other cord antiseptic
5. Applicators for cord care

6. Scales and scale paper if baby has not been weighed earlier
7. Scratch paper and pencil
8. Laundry hamper
9. Disinfectant for equipment cleanup

PROCEDURE:

1. Wash hands; check crib for needed materials.
2. Identify the baby.
3. Undress the baby as necessary to take temperature and drop clothing into hamper.
4. Take the temperature (axillary or rectal) following appropriate technique.
5. Weigh if necessary, placing the baby on a clean paper on the scale.
6. Replace the baby in the crib on the scale paper.
7. Apply alcohol or other ordered antiseptic to the cord at the base by the skin margin and at the tip.
8. Wash the face with a paper mesh square and clear water. Wash the rest of the baby with mild soap and water solution or plain tap water in the following order: external ears, head, neck, arms, front of body (avoiding the cord), back, legs and feet, lower back, and anus. Pat dry. (Genitalia are cleansed as necessary with newly washed hands and a separate paper mesh square or cotton ball.)
9. Dress the baby and change the bed as necessary.
10. Place the baby on his abdomen, head to one side. Tuck one or more blankets over the infant.
11. Record weight, temperature, general condition, stool, and urine on work paper as appropriate. Loose, watery stools should be reported.
12. Hands should be washed before and after each baby's care and after caring for the anal-genital area before proceeding with additional tasks with the same child. Hands should also be washed before removing a cord clamp when the cord is dry. Students should not remove cord clamps without appropriate supervision.
13. Avoid chilling the baby during the procedure.
14. All equipment that becomes contaminated while weighing should be washed with disinfectant before it is reused. Scales, cart, and all equipment are washed with disinfectant at the end of daily care.
15. As the infant is bathed, inspect for the following:
    a. Color—jaundice, cyanosis, pallor
    b. Rash
    c. Petechiae
    d. Bruise marks
    e. Edematous area on the head
    f. Condition of the mouth—excess salivation
    g. Condition of the eyes (cleaned only if a discharge is present)
    h. Condition of genitalia
    i. Condition of the cord (signs of inflammation, discharge, bleeding)

j. Signs of possible paralysis or spasticity
k. General level of alertness and activity
l. Indications of respiratory distress
m. Possible congenital malformations

Lifting and holding. The positioning, handling, and transporting of young babies can sometimes be alarming to new or beginning student nurses. Both need to be reassured of their ability to learn to care for their charges and to learn comfortable and safe methods of handling a baby. A baby does not break, and knowledge of certain principles will help to give the infant greater support and confidence.

The newborn infant usually tries to maintain a fetal position. With a little coaxing, the child usually readily assumes his unborn posture. This is sometimes useful to the pediatrician or family practitioner who is trying to evaluate the placement of a foot or the line of a mandible.

The newborn infant has one continuous anteroposterior spinal curve and no real control of head movements, although in the prone position the baby may raise its head slightly and briefly. Whenever the baby is lifted or transported, the head, being so large and heavy in relation to the rest of the body, must be supported for comfort and to prevent muscle strain. For safety all lifts must have at least two contact points so that if one fails, another is still available. Babies, even small ones, can be wriggly and sometimes slippery. Following is one of the most common methods of lifting an infant on his back from a bed:

1. Facing the soles of the feet, lift the legs and buttocks slightly with one hand by grasping the feet, ankles separated by a finger.
2. Slide the opposite hand, palm up, under the full length of the baby until finally the entire back and head are supported.

A second method follows (Fig. 13-4):

1. Facing the baby's side, slide one hand from the side under the head and neck to grasp the outside arm. The head is supported by the forearm, or the head and neck may be supported by the grasping hand.
2. With the other hand reach under the legs to grasp the farther thigh, or grasp the feet holding one finger between the ankles. This is a good lift for weighing the baby or putting him into a tub.

A baby should not be lifted by the arms. When head stability is attained at about 3 months of age, the child may be lifted by grasping the trunk with both hands below

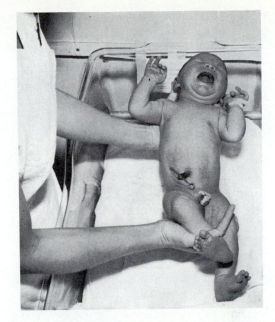

FIG 13-4 One method of lifting baby, starting from side position. Head and upper back are supported by one hand, legs by other. Note that baby is gently grasped. *(Courtesy Grossmont Hospital, La Mesa, Calif.)*

the arms. A newborn infant should not be left alone flat on his back. The baby may be propped with a rolled blanket along his back to maintain a side position or may be placed on its abdomen with the head turned to one side. Some newborn infants, when placed in this position for protracted periods, seem to object and rub their knees up and down on the linen, causing reddened shins. Baby beds should have firm mattresses regardless of the style. No pillow should be used. A child should not always be placed in the same position, since this can distort the shape of his head or chest or cause localized baldness.

Babies have been carried in many ways: some methods are more comfortable for the one who carries and others give the baby a greater sense of safety and support. Three ways are common in the United States and are recommended:

1. The traditional cradle hold (Fig. 13-5): the child's head is cradled in the bend of the elbow; the forearm reaches around the outside of the body to grasp the outer leg with the fingers. The nurse's opposite hand and forearm helps support the back and buttocks. This additional support may be momentarily withdrawn if the hand is needed for a task.

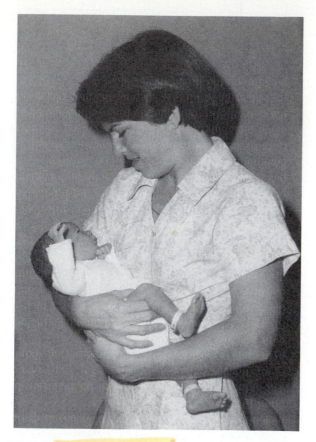

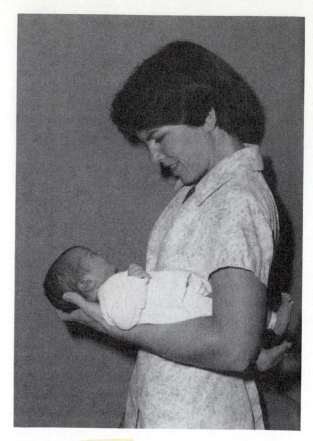

FIG 13-5 Traditional cradle hold. This baby was a wiggler! (Figs. 13-5 through 13-7 show a baby who would normally be wrapped in a blanket and a nurse who would normally wear a cover gown. However, both protective devices were removed to more clearly illustrate the holds.) *(Courtesy Grossmont Hospital, La Mesa, Calif.)*

FIG 13-6 Football hold. *(Courtesy Grossmont Hospital, La Mesa, Calif.)*

2. The football hold (Fig. 13-6): About half the length of the baby's body is supported by the nurse's forearm with the head and neck resting in her palm. The rest of the body, legs, and buttocks are firmly wedged between the nurse's elbow and hip. This is a fine secure hold, and it was definitely designed to provide the parent or nurse with a free hand. However, one should not carry the baby in this position, since the head is somewhat unprotected.
3. The shoulder hold (Fig. 13-7): The baby is held up against the chest and shoulder. The palm of one hand supports the baby's buttocks. The other hand keeps the head and back from sagging. Two hands are needed to support the baby's back correctly. This is the hold used often for burping the baby.

Most newborn infants love to be cuddled, and the way they are handled, touched, and fed is how nurses and caregivers can show love and respect for them as individuals and as important members of humanity.

Nourishment

Nourishment, though not the most pressing of a newborn infant's needs, eventually becomes paramount. In modern society there are two ways of meeting this need—breast-feeding and formula feeding.

Breast-feeding. Breast-feeding, of course, has an ancient biologic basis and is still the most universally recommended way of providing an infant with nourishment. A mother should carefully consider the advantages of breast-feeding when deciding how she will feed her infant. A father who is supportive of breast-feeding will influence the mother's success. Therefore, he should also be given information regarding the advantages of breast-feeding.

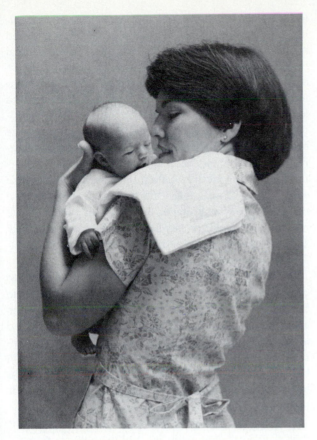

FIG 13-7 Shoulder hold. *(Courtesy Grossmont Hospital, La Mesa, Calif.)*

Advantages. Putting the baby to breast contributes to the mother's well-being in that the stimulation of the infant's nursing causes the recently emptied uterus to contract and helps in the return of this organ to its proper size and position, a process called involution. A further benefit is the relaxing effect that prolactin, the milk-producing hormone, has on the mother. Many investigators believe that the baby receives certain immune factors through the breast milk that help protect the baby against diseases to which the mother may have been previously exposed. It is agreed that as a general rule breast-fed babies have fewer respiratory tract infections and alimentary tract disturbances. Certainly, when environmental hygiene is poor, breast-feeding is preferred over the great possibility of contaminated artificially prepared feedings because breast milk is normally sterile.

The observation that cow's milk was first designed for calves, whereas mother's milk is specifically designed for babies, is indisputable. The curd of human milk is softer than that of cow's milk and is easier for a baby to digest. Breast-fed babies have fewer allergy problems. At first, breast-fed babies have more frequent stools than formula-fed infants. The stools are yellow-orange and aromatic but not offensive. Later on they may have fewer stools than their formula-fed counterparts. No prolonged preparation time is necessary, and in the long run, successful nursing is less expensive. Obesity is seen less often in children who have been breast-fed. If the mother nurses her baby, the return of menstruation may be delayed until several weeks after weaning, but nursing is no guarantee that pregnancy will not occur. However, the nursing mother may experience such a sense of closeness to her baby, fulfillment, and motherliness that this becomes the primary reason she continues to nurse.

Contraindications. Even though some mothers may want to nurse, occasionally the condition of the mother or baby makes it inadvisable. Maternal illness that is particularly protracted, severe, or contagious in nature may preclude breast-feeding. A mother who is in a high risk group for acquired immune deficiency syndrome (AIDS) (for example, has used intravenous drugs) should receive a HIV blood test before nursing. Mothers who have newly diagnosed active tuberculosis should be separated from their newborn infants until they have received appropriate medications and are judged noncontagious (usually 2 or more weeks). The mother then will be individually evaluated regarding her own health, and the condition of her infant. A woman with cardiac disease or established renal disease may be discouraged from nursing because of the demands on her own body resources that nursing may make. Mentally disturbed mothers may not be allowed the close contact needed for feeding their infants either artificially or by breast unless closely supervised.

Other considerations. The nursing mother must have a good diet to maintain her resources and provide sufficient nourishment for her infant. She produces about 25 ounces of milk when lactation is fully established. In the second half of the first year, production typically drops about 20%. She needs more calories—approximately 500 to 1,000 more calories per day—than when she is not pregnant nor breast-feeding. Some of these calories can come from the stores of maternal fat built up during pregnancy. Therefore, an additional 500 calories per day is adequate unless the mother is underweight.

She also needs increased fluid intake to maintain her milk production. Her diet should include at least 1½ quarts (4 to 5 glasses) of skimmed or low fat milk in liquid form or cooking mixtures a day to protect her personal calcium supply and to avoid possible *osteoporosis,* or weakening of the bony skeleton. Calcium in the form of medication can be supplied if necessary, but a balanced diet containing calcium-rich foods would give her other healthful nutrients, benefit the whole family, and eliminate the need for pills.

The new Recommended Dietary Allowances (RDAs), revised in 1989, indicate two different levels of nutritional requirements reflecting the higher needs of the first 6 months of lactation compared with the normal moderate decrease in milk production typical of the second 6 months. It is suggested that the nursing mother maintain a daily protein intake of about 65 g in the first period and about 62 g in the second. The recommended intake during pregnancy is 60 g.

During the first 6 months the RDAs of vitamins A, most B complex, C, and E in addition to the minerals zinc, iodine, and magnesium are expanded above those advised during pregnancy. In the second 6 months, requirements for these same nutrients remain above or at the level recommended during pregnancy. Only the recommendations for folate, iron, and vitamin B_6 are lower during lactation than during pregnancy. (See the RDAs for lactation on p. 70.)

Some foods eaten by the mother have been said to cause the nursing baby abdominal distress, such as cramping or diarrhea, and in the past women have been given lists of foods to avoid while nursing. There is no scientific basis for limiting "gassy" foods to prevent gas in a breast-fed baby. Many babies do not seem aware of any deviation in the mother's diet. However, while some babies do not seem to tolerate certain foods, no one food affects every baby. Examples of foods that have caused problems are "strong" vegetables, such as cabbage, brussels sprouts, asparagus, and onions, and certain fruits such as prunes. By omitting the suspected food from her diet for a day or two and observing the baby's response, a mother can usually determine whether the baby is reacting to that food. Fussiness also has been reported in babies whose mothers drink large amounts of coffee or cola drinks.

Most, if not all, drugs taken by the mother may pass through the milk to the baby. The drug thiouracil used in treating hyperthyroidism actually becomes more concentrated in the maternal milk and may affect the infant severely. Certain laxatives are as effective on the baby as on the mother and should be avoided or used only judiciously. Common medications to be avoided include cascara, Epsom salts, and Ex-Lax, but not inert mineral oil. It is wise to counsel mothers to remind their physicians that they are nursing when receiving new prescriptions. Concern has been expressed regarding the amount of DDT and other environmental contaminants found in some human milk samples. However, discontinuation of breast-feeding is not recommended by authorities unless the level of DDT is judged to be high.

Some cultures teach that an intake of low-percentage beer or, for those more affluent, the addition of champagne to the diet increases milk production. The benefits from these are probably caused by increased fluid intake and a feeling of relaxation. It is true that a tense, worried mother may have difficulty in maintaining an adequate milk supply. However, alcohol does pass into breast milk and its consumption should be discouraged while breast-feeding.

More and more mothers who must or who prefer to work outside the home are successfully continuing to breast-feed. This requires extra effort because to maintain a milk supply the breasts must be stimulated and emptied at fairly frequent intervals. A nursing mother may manually empty her breasts when unable to feed her infant because of separation, but this procedure may not always be convenient. Electric or manual breast pumps may be preferable.

The nursing mother needs good breast support. The typical nursing bra, with the liftdown cup, is efficient and easily used. Many mothers use freshly laundered or paper handkerchiefs or soft-cellulose pads strategically placed to absorb leakage.

A mother with severely cracked nipples, mastitis, or breast abscess is no longer required to terminate nursing. Many authorities recommend continuation of breast-feeding while antibiotics and other remedies are used. With proper initial management and frequent nursing such conditions are avoidable.

The condition of the baby may influence the decision of whether to nurse. Small premature infants usually do not have the strength to suckle at breast, but they may benefit from the expressed maternal milk. For this reason, mothers of premature infants may wish to maintain their milk supply for the immediate use of the baby in the hospital (to be given by means of gavage) and for later use when the baby goes home. Other babies, unable to suckle, may benefit from maternal milk; a child with a cleft lip or palate may be able to breast-feed, depending on the extent of the defect. If household freezing techniques are used, maternal milk may be stored for 1 to 2 weeks. Longer storage necessitates quick-freezing and deep-freezer storage.

To be completely successful, most nursing mothers must really want to nurse, have supportive family members, be convinced of its advantages, and receive prenatal instruction regarding the care and normal function of their breasts, as well as encouragement and assistance in the postpartum period. If a woman has flattened or inverted nipples, they may be treated during this preparation period by prescribed nipple stretching exercises, use of special breast cups, or suction. (See also p. 79.) In some localities groups of mothers particularly interested in promoting breast-feeding have formed organizations to help the new mother or mother-to-be. La Leche League International, founded in Illinois in 1956, is an organization that is dedicated and active in this field. The League's address is 9616 Minneapolis Avenue, Franklin Park, Illinois 60131.

Techniques. Some babies nurse well from the start; others take a little while to get the idea of what they are supposed to do. However, with breast-feeding the nurse and mother have some powerful allies—inborn reflexes and hunger. By using his own natural behaviors and reflexes the baby can be assisted to begin nursing at the

breast. In preparation for breast-feeding the mother first washes her hands. Then she and her baby should be comfortably positioned. The mother needs to be in good body alignment and well-supported in the position of her choice. If sitting up in bed or in a chair, she usually finds it more comfortable to place the baby on a pillow in her lap. This brings the infant closer to the breast with less strain. She may lie on her side with her lower arm cradling the baby if the baby has no history of ear infections.

To empty the breast effectively and to preserve the nipple in good condition the baby must nurse with the areola in his mouth and not just the nipple. This is important because, if the baby is allowed to chew on the end of the nipple, painful, cracked, or fissured nipples may result. The following will help the baby to get a good grasp. While in a comfortable sitting position the mother holds the infant using the cradle hold (see Fig. 13-4). The infant should then be turned onto his side so that his entire body faces his mother and his lower arm can be tucked underneath him or around his mother's waist. In this position he does not have to turn his head or strain to reach the breast, and he is close enough to

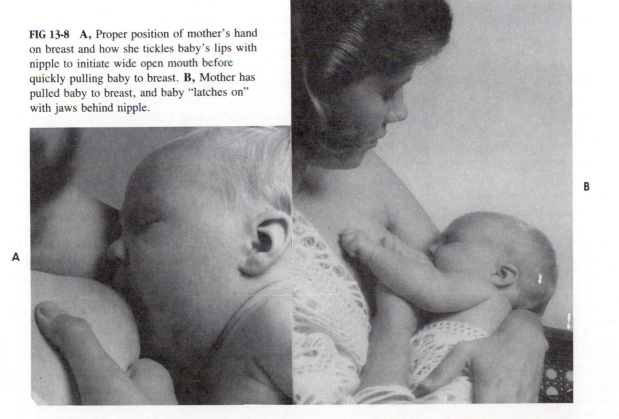

FIG 13-8 A, Proper position of mother's hand on breast and how she tickles baby's lips with nipple to initiate wide open mouth before quickly pulling baby to breast. **B,** Mother has pulled baby to breast, and baby "latches on" with jaws behind nipple.

A

B

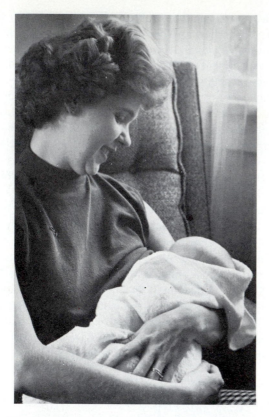

FIG 13-9 It is possible to nurse infant unobtrusively.

fit his open mouth well back onto the areola. Now the mother can support her breast, using her free hand, by placing her fingers under the breast and her thumb above in preparation for the infant's mouth. By lightly tickling the baby's lips with her nipple, the mother can stimulate the baby to open his mouth. After a few moments of tickling the baby will open his mouth wide. While the mouth is open wide, the mother quickly pulls the baby toward her as closely as she can. The tip of the baby's nose should touch her breast. If he needs more room to breathe, her thumb is conveniently there to press the breast gently away from his nose (Fig. 13-8).

The same steps apply to a mother who is nursing lying down, except that the infant is placed on the bed so that he is lying on his side facing his mother. It is possible to nurse infants using various modifications as necessary (Fig. 13-9).

Sometimes if the baby has difficulty getting started or is new at the breast, gently expressing a drop of milk on the tip of the nipple will serve as an appetizer and help give the baby the basic idea. If the breasts are engorged, expressing some milk before beginning to nurse will re-

lieve tension of the breast and make it easier for the baby to grasp the areola. Nipples should be allowed to air dry after feeding. Soaps and antiseptics should not be used. Washing the breasts and nipples once a day with clear water is sufficient. Repeated washing of the nipple even with clear water removes the protective oils and predisposes it to cracking. Therefore the use of creams or ointments that need to be washed off before nursing should be avoided.

When removing the baby from the breast, the nurse should remember that babies are capable of considerable tenacity. To convince an infant that it is best to let go, the nurse can gently pull down on the chin or insert a finger into the corner of the infant's mouth between the jaws to release them and break the suction.

The first few days the baby obtains an "introductory milk," called colostrum, which has a laxative effect and contains protective antibodies. Maternal milk becomes "complete"—that is, possesses its characteristic content—several weeks later.

It must be emphasized that the greatest aid to milk production is frequent stimulation and emptying of the breasts. If the breasts are not emptied, milk production may dwindle. Probably the ideal maternity accommodations for a nursing mother, particularly if the child involved is her first, is the rooming-in plan or a modification of rooming-in. In this setting the baby may be put to the breast as desired and is not limited to the 4-hour feeding schedules followed by many hospitals without family-centered postpartum care programs. Babies seem to do the best when allowed to feed on demand without limitations as to frequency or length of feeding. Nursing infants are often fed every 2 to 3 hours when breast-feeding is initiated. The length of the feeding varies considerably from baby to baby and is usually somewhere between 10 to 30 minutes. Limiting the time the baby nurses at the breast is no longer considered effective in preventing sore nipples. It is generally recommended that a mother nurse from both breasts at each feeding. Perhaps the most important consideration is that the breast be emptied. If it is not emptied by the baby, the mother should empty it manually or with the aid of a pump to maintain milk production. For a brief presentation of breast anatomy and more details of breast care, see the section on postpartal care (pp. 207-211).

Breast-fed babies, like formula-fed babies, must be burped to remove swallowed air. Sitting the infant up or holding him over a protected shoulder while gently rubbing his back, in addition to patience, produces results for both breast and bottle babies.

Artificial feeding. Today, with present knowledge of nutrition and increased understanding of food processing and preservation, the bottle-fed baby need not be threatened with malnutrition or disease in developed countries. Although mothers should be told the advantages of breast-feeding, they should not be considered or made to feel like maternal failures if they cannot or choose not to nurse. To assume such a position is unrealistic and unkind. To force a mother to nurse against her will may cause an unhappy cycle of rebellion, failure, and regret and may make those few mothers who cannot or should not nurse feel lacking in maternal virtue. Some have schedules that are difficult to combine with nursing; some are concerned that their youngsters are not getting enough to eat; and some have felt like failures in past nursing experiences. For others the process of nursing is physically unattractive and may lack approval from their mates. Many healthy children have been formula fed in this society. A loving mother cuddling her baby while tilting a milk-filled bottle need not consider herself a "poor mother."

The primary health care provider should guide the selection of formula. The American Academy of Pediatrics recommends that nonbreast-fed infants receive iron-fortified formula during the first year of life. Numerous commercially prepared proprietary formulas that contain the necessary iron and vitamins are available (see Table 13-1). These may come in liquid or powder form. Directions must be carefully followed since some are ready to use and others must be diluted or mixed. Their use saves preparation time and bother. The cost involved differs with the type, form, and vendor. The less modification needed before use, the more expensive the product. A number of companies are manufacturing disposable prefilled nursing units. Most hospitals use commercial baby formula.

Preparation of formula. If the more costly ready-to-feed bottle formula is not purchased, the most frequently recommended method of formula preparation today is the so-called tap water method, using prepared formula in the form of liquid concentrate, or powder.

TAP WATER METHOD—FORMULA PREPARATION

This method of formula preparation has become popular because of its simplicity. Used conscientiously, it is safe. Abused by lack of cleanliness or improper technique, it may be associated with infant illness.

MATERIALS:

Capped formula bottle
Nipple
Bottle brush
Soap or detergent
Sauce pan
Can opener
Spoon
Formula as prescribed: ready to use, liquid concentrate, powder

PROCEDURE:

1. Use a clean formula bottle that has been *meticulously washed* in warm, sudsy water, rinsed in *hot* water, and air dried.
2. Use a nipple that has been carefully washed and rinsed. Make sure that the nipple holes are open. (Some references also recommend boiling the clean nipple 3 to 5 minutes).
3. Measure the ingredients needed for one feeding into the bottle. Be sure that you understand what dilution (if any) is to be made because formula is sold in many different forms and concentrations. Read the directions! Babies have become ill and even died because caretakers have not realized this. Add warm water from the tap to the bottle in the amount the formula directions indicate. (Boil tap water that is unapproved.) Mix with clean spoon.
4. Feed *immediately;* do not save formula from one feeding to the next or for more than an hour.

Special handling of infant formula is necessary because milk is such an ideal medium for the nourishment and growth of other living things in addition to human babies. Microorganisms that are not at all compatible with the baby's digestive system may multiply rapidly in milk if it is improperly bottled or is left open to air and warmed for an extended period. Typhoid organisms were fairly common contaminants of milk and milk products before pasteurization became widespread. Because of the baby's susceptibility, certain methods of disinfection or "sterilization" of the formula (aseptic or terminal) were considered necessary until the last decade. Now it is believed that in most instances a conscientious clean technique is sufficient unless formula must be prepared in advance and stored. However, hospitals usually use sterile precautions until an infant has reached 3 months of age. Plastic bottles employed for older infants who hold their own, if reused, should be sterilized between patients.

Techniques of feeding. Feeding an infant his formula can be an enjoyable experience. The hands should be clean; the milk usually should be tepid (no sensation of hot or cold) falling on the inside of the parent's or nurse's wrist.

Experiments using cold formula for feeding the new-

Table 13-1 Composition of milk and selected infant formulas*

	Common usage	Calories per oz	Nutrient source		
			Protein	Carbohydrate	Fat
Human milk					
	First 12 months or longer	20	Casein, lactalbumin	Lactose	Human milk fat
Whole cow's milk					
	After first 12 months	20	Casein, lactalbumin	Lactose	Cow's milk fat
Cow's milk base formulas					
Similac with iron	Normal infant, breast milk unavailable	20	Nonfat cow's milk	Lactose	Soy oil, coconut oil
Enfamil with iron	Normal infant, breast milk unavailable	20	Nonfat cow's milk, whey	Lactose	Soy oil, coconut oil
SMA with iron	Normal infant, breast milk unavailable	20	Nonfat cow's milk, demineralized whey	Lactose	Oleo, coconut oil, soy oil
Soy base formulas					
Isomil	Infants with allergy to cow's milk	20	Soy protein isolate	Corn syrup solids, sucrose	Soy oil, coconut oil
Prosobee	Infants with allergy to cow's milk	20	Soy protein isolate	Corn syrup solids	Soy oil, coconut oil
Nursoy	Infants with allergy to cow's milk	20	Soy protein isolate	Sucrose	Soy oil, safflower oil, coconut oil
Transitional formula					
Advance	Interim between breast milk/formula and whole milk	16	Nonfat cow's milk, soy	Lactose, corn syrup solids	Soy oil, corn oil
Special formulas					
Enfamil premature	Premature infants	24	Nonfat cow's milk, demineralized whey	Lactose, corn syrup solids	Corn oil, MCT† oil, coconut oil
Similac PM 60/40	Infants with renal and cardiac disease	20	Nonfat cow's milk, demineralized whey	Lactose	Safflower oil, soy oil
Pregestimil	Infants with fat or carbohydrate malabsorption	20	Casein hydrolysate	Corn syrup solids, modified to tapioca starch	MCT† oil, corn oil
Nutramigen	Infants with soy and milk protein allergies	20	Casein hydrolysate	Sucrose, modified to tapioca starch	Corn oil
Portagen	Infants with fat malabsorption	20	Casein	Modified tapioca starch	MCT† oil, corn oil, lecithin

*Commercially prepared formulas are vitamin fortified. Consult individual labels for detailed vitamin content.
†Medium-chain triglycerides.

Nutrients				Minerals				
Protein (g/100 ml)	Carbohydrate (g/100 ml)	Fat (g/100 ml)	Whey:casein ratio	Sodium (mEq/L)	Potassium (mEq/L)	Calcium (mg/100 ml)	Phosphorus (mg/100 ml)	Iron (mg/100 ml)
1.1	6.8	4.5	60:42	6.5	14.1	34	14	0.1
3.5	4.9	3.7	18:82	22.0	40.2	123	96	0.05
1.5	7.3	3.6	18:82	10.0	20.5	51	39	1.2
1.5	7.0	3.7	60:40	9.1	17.6	47	32	1.27
1.5	7.2	3.6	60:40	6.5	14.3	44	33	1.26
2.0	6.8	3.6	—	13.9	19.7	70	50	1.2
2.0	6.9	3.6	—	12.7	20.0	63	50	1.3
2.0	6.9	3.6	—	8.7	18.9	63	44	1.25
2.0	2.7	5.5	—	10	23	51	39	1.2
2.4	8.9	4.1	60:40	13.6	22.7	95	48	0.12
1.6	7.5	3.5	60:40	7	15	40	20	0.26
1.9	9.1	3.2	—	13.8	19	63	42	1.27
2.2	8.8	2.6	—	15.7	17.5	63	48	1.27
2.4	7.8	3.2	—	13.8	12.6	63	48	1.27

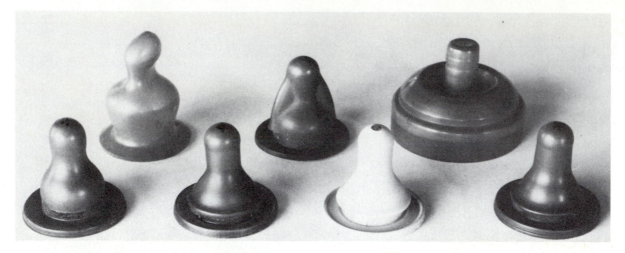

FIG 13-10 Various types of nipples. *Back row, left to right:* Nuk, winged, Platex. *Front row:* regular three-hole, cross-cut, cereal (large-hole), and soft rubber for premature infants.

born have demonstrated no undesirable effects, even on premature babies. However, it is psychologically difficult to give a young infant a *cold* meal. Many nurseries have discarded formula warmers because of problems with elevated bacterial count on the equipment. Feedings are offered at room temperature. The rate of nipple flow should be almost one drop per second when the bottle is inverted. Nipple holes may be enlarged by a hot needle mounted on a cork. Vigorously sucking babies should be given a resistant nipple. Babies who tire easily and premature babies do better with a soft, pliable nipple (Fig. 13-10).

Be sure the nipple is on top of the tongue, and do not push it too far back—it may stimulate the gag reflex. Babies seem to drink best when held closely on a definite incline. Studies indicate that such positioning minimizes the possibility of retrograde infection through the eustachian tubes to the middle ear and helps prevent aspiration. (Fig. 13-11.) The neck of the bottle should always be tipped so that it is full of milk. Air in the baby's stomach may cause pain, decrease appetite, or promote regurgitation. Bubbles may be expelled by rubbing the baby's back in an upright position. This may be done after each ounce with newborn babies or halfway through and at the end of the feeding for older babies. It may be best to burp some babies, particularly finger suckers and those who have been crying, before feedings as well. (Fig. 13-12.) Newborns should be carefully observed before and during feedings for indications of any abnormality in the digestive or respiratory tracts. Prefeeding coughing, cy-

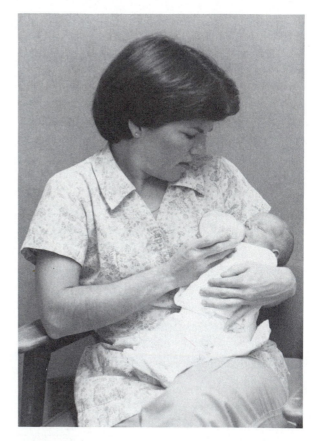

FIG 13-11 Nipple should always be full of formula and infant preferably upright. *(Courtesy Grossmont Hospital, La Mesa, Calif.)*

anosis, and excessive mucus may be associated with anatomic abnormalities. Regurgitation of a feeding through the nose and mouth should be reported at once. Many babies are offered water before they are put to the breast or fed formula to evaluate their ability to drink without difficulty.

After feeding, the infant may need to have his diaper changed. He should be placed on his right side or abdomen to sleep. The amount taken should be recorded in nursery records. The newborn infant may take only 1 ounce the first day and 2 or 3 ounces per feeding on the second and third days. Newborns usually are fed every 3 or 4 hours. See Table 13-2 for average formula amounts and number of feedings.

Evaluation of nutritional status. There are numerous ways of judging whether a newborn infant, either formula-fed or breast-fed, is receiving enough to eat.

1. Observing his behavior—does he seem content,

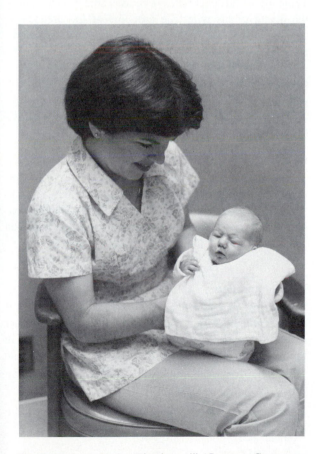

FIG 13-12 Let's hear a "thank you!" *(Courtesy Grossmont Hospital, La Mesa, Calif.)*

or is he a short sleeper and irritable? (Note that babies cry for reasons other than hunger pangs; for example, if they are wet, too tightly bundled or too warm, have gas pains, or want to be held.)

2. Watching for signs of dehydration from poor fluid intake:
   a. Fewer than 6 to 8 wet diapers per day
   b. Dark, concentrated urine; dry, hard stools
   c. Dry mucous membranes
   d. Dry skin with little "bounce" (poor turgor)
   e. Low-grade fever (Note that the most common cause of low-grade fever is dehydration, although the nurse shouldn't overlook the possibility of infection.)
   f. Elevated specific gravity (above 1.020)
   g. In severe cases, sunken fontanels
3. Measuring intake:
   a. This is routine with bottle-fed babies.
   b. If measuring is ordered, breast-fed babies are weighed dressed and wrapped directly before the feeding and directly after the feeding, before any diapers are changed with the same clothes and blankets (1 g = 1 ml).
   c. Intake should be evaluated in terms of a 24-hour period and not individual feedings.
4. Measuring weight gain:
   a. This method is of little use currently because of the short hospital stays of most newborn infants in the United States (sometimes less than a day).
   b. All babies lose weight directly after birth, which should cause no concern unless the weight loss approaches 10% of the birth weight. Bottle-fed babies regain their birth weight more rapidly than most breast-fed babies.
   c. After weight gain is reestablished, a gain of about 1 ounce a day is average, equaling about 6 ounces a week. At the end of 5 months most babies have doubled their birth weight.

Love—parent-infant attachment

The birth of a child is a special occasion, and although the child needs to be protected against infection and overhandling, the way that the child is introduced to the parents and siblings is of great importance. If possible, both the father and the mother should have an opportunity to see and handle the infant without hurry directly after birth. (See Fig. 10-7.)

The importance of this early postpartum period to the formation of positive mother-child and mother-father-

Table 13-2 Suggested schedule on an approximate 4-hour basis for average-weight bottle-fed infant

Age	Milliliters per feeding	Ounces per feeding	Number of feedings	Time of feedings
First week	60-90	2-3	6	6,10,2,6,10,2
2 to 4 weeks	90-150	3-5	6	6,10,2,6,10,2
2 to 3 months	120-180	4-6	5	6,10,2,6,10
4 and 5 months	150-210	5-7	5	6,10,2,6,10
6 and 7 months	210-240	7-8	4	6,10,2,6
8 to 12 months	240	8*	3	7,12,6

Modified from Williams SR: Nutrition and diet therapy, ed 4, St Louis, 1981, The CV Mosby Co, p. 409.
*In midafternoon 120 ml (4 ounces) milk may be given.

child relationships is being explored attentively. The newborn has been reported to be often more alert during the first hour after birth than in the immediate subsequent hours. Many researchers agree that birth and the immediately postpartum period when the baby is first seen, touched, and cared for are sensitive periods in the development of attachment. If the mother is also alert and willing and the circumstances of the labor and birth are conducive, an early parent-child interaction followed by frequent visits appear to help young parents develop gratifying maternal-paternal identities.

Long-term studies of maternal attachment to normal and high-risk infants in the early postpartum period, its manifestations, and long-term influence on the child are now under way.* The nurse is in an excellent position to assess and facilitate attachment. Numerous investigators have described the typical initial exploratory behavior of human mothers and fathers. Gentle fingertip touching of the hands and feet progresses to massagelike motions of the palm on the baby's trunk. Eye-to-eye contact is remarkable, and a characteristic "en face" position is often demonstrated (the mother's face poised directly in front of and in line with that of her infant). This eye-to-eye observation helps establish the newborn's identity as a person and provides rewarding feedback to the mother. However, many parents establish strong attachments to their infants without having experienced early "hands on" contact. If for some reason such early interaction is not provided, it should be remembered that human beings are very adaptable. Future relationships can still be rewarding and meaningful. The results of the studies now in progress will be interesting.

Nurses must recognize that many expectant fathers

*Klaus MH and Kennell JH: Parent-infant bonding, ed 2, St Louis, 1981, The CV Mosby Co; Lamb M: Second thoughts on first touch, Psychol Today 16:9, 1982.

want to be involved not only in the preparation for parenthood but in the actual birth and care of the infant. Mothers must be helped in understanding that just as they have many adjustments to make, so do new fathers. A father often has a need to handle and touch his newborn. Typically he has experienced various concerns including the health of his wife, the outcome of the pregnancy, changes in sexual practices, and increased financial responsibility.

If the newborn's siblings, grandparents, and other family members visit, they should be able to see the baby and visit with the new mother according to her wishes. Newborn infants may receive all other things, but if they do not receive true love, they will not thrive.

Rest

Although it is important for newborns to receive stimulation, they also need times of relatively little input to "organize" their world and to grow. Overstimulated babies are likely to be more nervous, with shorter attention spans.

SPECIAL NEEDS
Parent education

The new parent will have a lower level of anxiety if she is equipped with a comprehensive knowledge of her child. Although she is in the hospital for a brief time in the postpartum period, it is the nurse's responsibility to initiate or build on teaching in the following areas:

Importance of stimulation
Developmental milestones
Possible sibling rivalry
Infant care
    Bathing
    Skin care
    Cord care
    Circumcision care

Nutrition
  Breast-feeding
  Formula preparation
  Introduction to solids
Sleep patterns
Elimination patterns
Safety
  Car seats
  Never leaving child unattended
  Cool vs hot mist vaporizer
  Pacifiers
  Cribs
Available community resources

Additional teaching can be begun or continued in high school family education classes, prenatal and postnatal parent education programs, clinic and office waiting rooms, and well-child visits.

Baptism

Sometimes other occasions of special meaning and deep significance occur in the nursery. Catholic parents and occasionally Protestant families may request baptism of their child while the baby is in the nursery. Efforts should be made to comply with the religious practices of parents of any faith. When the child is in no immediate danger, a member of the clergy involved should always be called. Most hospitals have appropriate utensils available. If doubt exists concerning what should be in readiness, the clergy may always be consulted. Some bring their own articles. Most require only a pitcher of pure water. If the child is a member of a Catholic family and appears to be in immediate danger of death, a nurse may baptize the baby. It is preferable that a nurse of the Catholic faith should do this task, but any adult may do so. In performing the baptism, she should pour water on the head or face of the child while saying, "I baptize you in the name of the Father, and of the Son, and of the Holy Spirit." A record of the baptism should be made in the nurse's notes and the parents notified. This simple but deeply meaningful act can be of great comfort to the family.

Circumcision

Circumcision involves the slitting or surgical removal of all or part of the foreskin, or prepuce, of the penis. Advocates of the procedure believe that it makes hygiene easier, decreases irritation of the area from an accumulation of cellular debris (smegma) under the foreskin, and may help to avoid urinary tract infection and cancer. Other practitioners declare that circumcision is unnecessary and a possible source of infection, hemorrhage,

and meatal stenosis. The outcome of this surgery appears to depend a great deal on the skill and technique of the operator. The American Academy of Pediatrics has stated that there are no valid medical indications for circumcision in the newborn period. Routine circumcision of all male infants appears to be decreasing.

The circumcision of a Jewish infant has religious import. Among Orthodox Jews it is undertaken by an ordained circumciser called a "mohel." This ceremony, called the brit or bris, is usually performed after the child leaves the hospital on the eighth day of life. The child is then officially named.

Physicians usually have individual preferences regarding the technique used, but the following setup list and procedure may be helpful.

CIRCUMCISION PROCEDURE

MATERIALS:

1. Sterile setup including
   a. One circumcision drape
   b. Two 4 × 4 squares (flats or gauze compresses)
   c. Two cotton balls
   d. Three small hemostats (mosquito clamps)
   e. One Yellen (Gomco) clamp, 1.3 to 1.1 cm in diameter
   f. One scalpel handle and added blade
   g. Possibly, needle holder, needle, and suture materials (chromic 3-0)
   h. One grooved director and probe
   i. One thumb forceps
2. Sterile gloves, appropriately sized
3. Ordered antiseptic for skin preparation such as povidone-iodine (Betadine)
4. Dressing materials
   a. Petrolatum-impregnated gauze
   b. Tincture of benzoin application
5. A circumcision board, diapers, pins, or special restraining halter that ties over the board
6. Lidocaine HCL 1% (Xylocaine), 1 ml, without epinephrine if anesthesia is used
7. Syringe, 1 ml, with 27 gauge, 0.5 inch (1.2 cm) needle if anesthesia is used

PROCEDURE:

1. Preliminary
   a. Obtain a signed informed consent from parent before procedure.
   b. Properly identify the baby. Check for possible reasons for not proceeding with the operation (presence of inflammation, tendency to bleed). Clean diaper area.
   c. Restrain the baby gently but firmly on a padded or plastic circumcision board.
   d. Ensure good light. A stool or chair may be appreciated by the operator.

e. Use of a pacifier may comfort the baby during the procedure.

2. Technique
   a. The technique of circumcision differs considerably from physician to physician. Local anesthetic is being used more frequently as the entire question of pain perception in infants and small children is being reexamined.*
   b. The Yellen (Gomco) clamp may be used to cut off circulation, and the foreskin excised. Sutures may or may not be used.
   c. The foreskin may be freed from the glans with probe, cut away, and bleeders controlled and sutured.
   d. A nonconstrictive dressing is applied. Petrolatum-impregnated gauze is often used.

3. Aftercare
   a. Notice of the recent circumcision should be attached to the crib.
   b. Frequent checks should be made to determine possible swelling and bleeding.
   c. Voidings, especially the first after the procedure, should be carefully charted. There is a danger of urinary retention.
   d. The area should be kept clean, soiled or displaced dressings should be replaced with clean materials.
   e. The infant is positioned on his side.

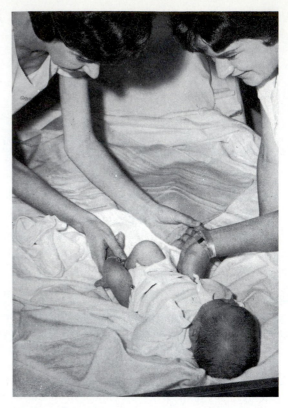

FIG 13-13   Identification of baby before hospital discharge using double-banding technique. *(Courtesy Grossmont Hospital, La Mesa, Calif.)*

Sometimes circumcisions are performed not long before the baby's discharge home. In this event the parents should be carefully instructed regarding observation and care of the area.

DISCHARGE PROCEDURE

Discharge is an exciting, somewhat trying time for most parents. Before the actual time of departure, the physician's order for discharge is checked and home orders are reviewed. The mother's belongings are packed, and clothes are put out for the infant. Mothers should have ready at least 2 diapers, pins (or 2 disposable diapers), a baby shirt, kimono, and receiving blanket or comparable wardrobe. Identification should be estab-

lished, and the baby viewed and dressed in his own clothes (Fig. 13-13). The discharge record should be signed and witnessed. If the mother has chosen to bottle-feed, a supply of formula may be available to take home. (Some people believe that sending formula home with breast-feeding mothers; sets them up for failure.) Before saying goodbye to the family, the nurse should make sure discharge instructions are understood and preferably written out, with any questions answered. Ideally, the baby's first car ride home from the hospital should be in an approved automobile safety restraint. Many hospitals and insurance plans are making this item available to new parents.

Before leaving the infant, the nurse should take one last peek at his face to assure herself of his condition and wish him well.

*Engel NS: Lidocaine dorsal penile nerve block for circumcision, MCN 14(5):311, 1989; Stang HJ and others: Local anesthesia for neonatal circumcision: effects on distress and cortisol response, JAMA 259(10):1507, 1988.

Key Concepts

1. The nine universal needs of the newborn infant are a clear airway, established respiration, warmth, protection from hemorrhage, protection from infection, identification and observation, nourishment and fluids, love (parent-infant attachment), and rest.

2. The infant's airway may be cleared using the following methods: wiping the nose and mouth when the head has been delivered, suctioning the mouth and nose, holding the head down while gently compressing the throat toward the mouth, and visualizing the larnyx with a laryngoscope and suctioning the trachea.

3. Supplemental oxygen should be administered when an infant is being resuscitated, is breathing poorly on his own, has generalized cyanosis, or has a heart rate under 100 beats per minute.

4. It is important to keep the newborn warm because the infant's temperature affects the number of calories he must expend to keep warm, his oxygen consumption, the incidence of apnea, and the acid-base balance of his blood.

5. The nurse should frequently check the infant's clamped umbilical cord for bleeding. Protection from hemorrhage is also important when caring for the male infant after circumcision.

6. Protecting the newborn from infection involves eye prophylaxis; provision of an individual bassinet, bath equipment, supply of linen, and layette; disinfecting or sterilizing instruments or appliances used for more than one infant; ensuring that nursery staff are not infected with any communicable disease; using separate gowns in the nursery; and good handwashing technique.

7. During the inspection bath the nurse assesses for the following: color; rash; petechiae; bruise marks; swellings on the head; condition of the mouth, eyes, genitalia, and cord; signs of possible paralysis or spasticity, general level of alertness and activity; indications of respiratory distress; and possible congenital malformations.

8. When lifting or transporting the infant, the head must be supported for comfort and for prevention of muscle strain. All lifts must have at least two contact points so that if one fails, another is still available. A baby should never be lifted by the arms.

9. Advantages of breast-feeding include the following: nursing causes the mother's recently emptied uterus to contract and promotes involution; prolactin has a relaxing effect on the mother; the baby may receive certain immune factors through breast milk; breast milk is easier to digest; breast-fed babies have fewer allergy problems; and obesity is seen less often in children who have been breast-fed.

10. The breast-feeding mother needs an additional 500 calories per day, should increase her fluid intake, consume at least 1½ quarts of skimmed or low fat milk per day, and increase the amount of protein in her diet. She may also require increased amounts of some vitamins.

11. The greatest aid to milk production in the breast-feeding mother is frequent stimulation and emptying of the breasts. It is generally recommended that a mother nurse from both breasts at each feeding.

12. Numerous commercially prepared formulas that contain the necessary iron and vitamins are available in liquid or powder form. Special handling of infant formula is necessary because milk is an ideal medium for microorganisms.

13. The infant's nutritional status can be evaluated by observing his behavior, watching for signs of dehydration, measuring intake, and measuring weight gain.

14. Signs of dehydration from poor fluid intake include the following: fewer than six to eight wet diapers per day; dark, concentrated urine; dry, hard stools; dry mucous membranes; dry skin with little "bounce"; low-grade fever; and elevated urine-specific gravity.

15. Areas of potential parent education include the importance of stimulation, developmental milestones, possible sibling rivalry, infant care, nutrition, sleep patterns, elimination patterns, safety, and available community resources.

16. Care of an infant following circumcision should include attaching a notice of the recent procedure to the crib, checking frequently for swelling and bleeding, charting voidings, keeping the area clean, and positioning the infant on his side.

Discussion Questions

1. Hypothermia is a serious problem for the newborn. How is body temperature best measured? How often should the temperature be taken? Discuss the various ways in which heat is lost. What measures can the nurse take to minimize heat loss?

2. Why is a newborn at increased risk for infection? What procedures are used in your hospital to reduce the risk of neonatal infections?

3. Soon after delivery the new mother wants to nurse her baby. She is unsure of technique and awkward handling the baby. You are her nurse. What would you do?

4. Compare and contrast breast- and bottle-feeding. What are the advantages of each method? The disadvantages? If you were asked which is "better" for the baby, what would your response be?

5. Circumcision is performed both as a religious ritual and as a hygiene practice. What risks are increased with this procedure? What nursing interventions should be instituted before and after a circumcision? Discuss the issue of pain in the newborn. (Anesthesia is not consistently administered for a newborn circumcision.)

14

Infants with Special Needs: Prematurity and Abnormality

CHAPTER OBJECTIVES

After studying this chapter, the student should be able to perform the following:

1 Define these terms as they apply to the newborn: preterm or premature; term, postterm, or post-mature; small for gestational age (SGA); appropriate for gestational age (AGA); large for gestational age (LGA); and low birth weight infants.

2 List five factors that should be considered when determining the status of a small newborn.

3 Cite the incidence of prematurity in the United States and its impact on infant mortality statistics.

4 Contrast the appearance and other characteristics of the premature infant and the full-term infant in at least four different ways.

5 List six signs of possible increasing intracranial pressure in the infant.

6 Note three types of shunts being used to treat hydrocephalus, and discuss the postoperative care of the infant who has undergone a shunting procedure, including observation, positioning, nutrition, and two complications that may be encountered.

7 Indicate three known causes of mental retardation and its incidence in the general population.

8 Describe a child with standard trisomy-21 including five characteristic signs.

9 Compare the problems associated with the spinal abnormalities meningocele and myelomeningocele.

10 State the rule of tens often used to determine the optimal time for the repair of a cleft lip.

11 Discuss the postoperative nursing care of children with cleft lip and cleft palate repairs and how it differs for each.

12 Define the following congenital abnormalities: tracheoesophageal fistula (TEF), imperforate anus, omphalocele, hypospadias, syndactyly, polydactyly, and talipes equinovarus.

13 Discuss the mechanism, prevention, and treatment of erythroblastosis fetalis associated with Rh incompatibility.

14 Describe three maneuvers that should be avoided while caring for newborns because they may cause a complete hip dislocation in unidentified infants at risk.

15 Describe the most effective device for treating congenital dislocation of the hip (CDH) during infancy.

This chapter is included to help students appreciate some of the more common abnormalities or conditions encountered during their practical experience and to help them assist more intelligently in the care of infants who have these conditions. Some of the conditions discussed are found and treated in the nursery and pose few or no problems later. Other anomalies by their very nature call for prolonged therapy and correction long after the neonatal period, infancy, or, indeed, childhood has passed.

THE PRETERM (PREMATURE) INFANT

(Figs. 14-1 and 14-2)

Among those babies with special needs, the first to be discussed are the preterm or premature infants. In the past the most common definition of prematurity was based on weight. For a long time, babies having a birth weight under 5½ pounds (2,500 g) were considered premature. However, in reality some of these babies had completed a term gestation and were underweight because of genetic or intrauterine factors. In fact, the term *premature,* referring to the infant born before the end of the 37th week of gestation, is now often being replaced by the more accurately descriptive adjective *preterm*. In this chapter the two words, preterm and premature, are used synonymously. Infants who are small at birth for other reasons are called small for gestational age (SGA). Babies may be of *low birth weight* because of an abbreviated gestation, unfavorable prebirth conditions, or both. The following is a more complete, newer classification of newborns based on gestational age (calculated from the first day of the last normal menstrual period) and birth weight (gestational age is 2 weeks longer than fertilization age):

preterm or premature Any infant born before the end of 37 weeks' gestation regardless of weight.

term Any infant born between the beginning of the 38th week and the end of the 42nd week of gestation regardless of weight.

postterm or postmature Any infant born after the end of 42 weeks' gestation regardless of weight.

small for gestational age (SGA) Any infant weighing less than 90% of the babies of the same gestational age.

appropriate for gestational age (AGA) Any infant weighing less than the heaviest 10% and more than the lightest 10% of the babies of the same gestational age.

large for gestational age (LGA) Any infant weighing more than 90% of babies of the same gestational age.

low birth weight infants Any preterm and small for gestational age infant weighing less than 2,500 g, or 5½ pounds.

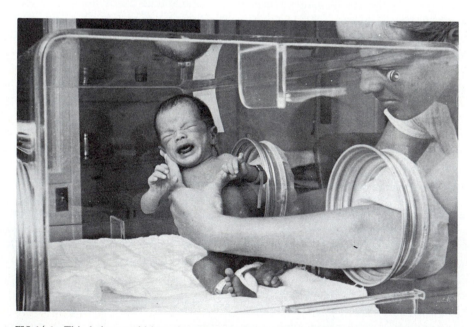

FIG 14-1   This baby would have been technically premature if only birth weight were considered. However, Asian ancestry influenced size; he was probably a "finished product," although he weighed less than 5½ pounds (2,500 g). *(Courtesy Grossmont Hospital, La Mesa, Calif.)*

Actually, in determining the status of the small infant, birth weight, heredity, possible length of gestation, clinical appearance, and behavior all must be considered. Although some babies cannot be classified as premature by the scale or calendar, they are judged underdeveloped and treated as "premies."

The mortality percentages related to birth weight and gestational age have improved significantly in modern perinatal centers as a result of advanced knowledge, sophisticated equipment, and increasingly skilled personnel. However, survivals of 26-week gestations or infants weighing less than 750 g are very rare. Prematurity accounts for approximately two thirds of infant mortality. The incidence of prematurity in the United States varies with the population studied. In general, it approaches 7%. In the black population it is between 10% to 11%.

Role of the nurse

The student nurse who wishes to work with premature babies should seek more supervised advanced training than is possible in her basic course. The nursery care of these infants must be extremely gentle, deft, and precise, and the ability to evaluate their behavior and reactions properly takes an extended period of time to acquire. However, although as a student she may not have the opportunity to be involved in the direct nursing of many premature infants, she should understand the nature of the problems encountered in such nursing. Some of these babies are cared for in an intensive care setting, others in the pediatric area. The leading cause of neonatal mortality, remember, is prematurity.

Causes

The causes of low birth weight infants are not always known. However, it is recognized that low birth weight infants are more frequently born to mothers of lower socioeconomic status. This may be related to the nature of prenatal care, the obstetric complications encountered, nutrition, and general health practices. Young teenage mothers also have a higher rate of low birth weight babies. Multiple births are almost always associated with prematurity. Heavy smoking seems to be an etiologic factor of prematurity.

Appearance and activity

The typical premature infant has a "wrinkled old man" appearance resulting from a lack of subcutaneous fat. The baby has a good supply of long, soft body hair called *lanugo,* the head and abdomen are relatively large, and the thorax is small. There is little molding of the skull (Fig. 14-3). Respirations are usually irregular, and the premature infant may be surprisingly active (Table 14-1).

Nutrition

Sucking and swallowing reflexes may be weak or absent in very small infants, necessitating feedings by gavage (insertion of a stomach tube), by intravenous feedings, or both. Intravenous feedings are now commonly given, especially to infants weighing less than 1,200 g or classified as "sick" prematures. These feedings may be given by umbilical catheter or peripheral veins. Stronger "premies" may do well when fed with a soft rubber nipple.

Premature feeding schedules and techniques are controversial at the present time. However, after a period of evaluation of an infant's tolerance for glucose water, oral feedings generally progress to formulas richer in calories than those normally fed to full-term infants. These calorie-rich formulas are necessary because of the premature infant's lack of nutritional reserves and great need for rapid growth. Often breast milk is used. Later the diet is supplemented by iron administration. Often the premature infant is also given vitamin E, which is believed to help protect lung structures, prevent eye problems such as retrolental fibroplasia, and preserve red blood cell integrity.

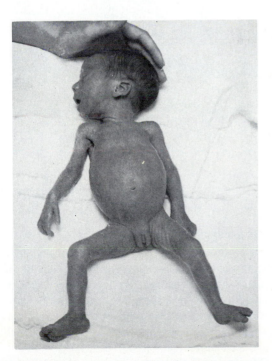

FIG 14-2 Typical premature infant. *(Courtesy Grossmont Hospital, La Mesa, Calif.)*

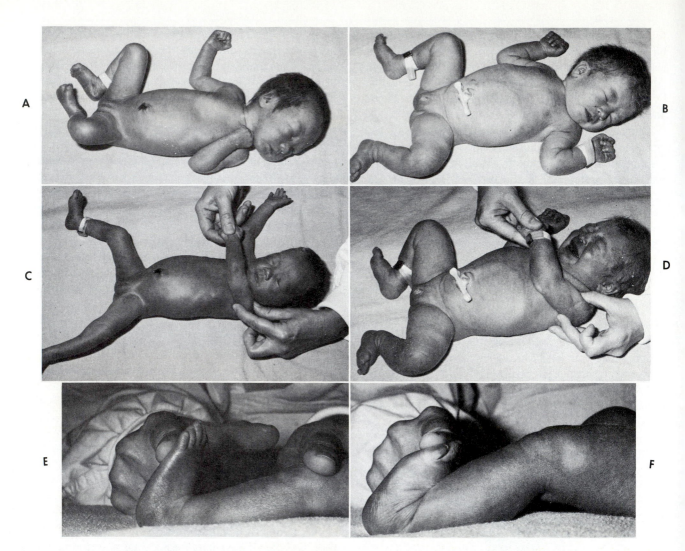

FIG 14-3 Illustrations on left show premature infant; those on right show mature infant. **A** and **B,** Typical body contours and postures. **C** and **D,** Scarf sign: immaturity seen when elbow passes midline. **E** and **F,** Prematurity is seen when heel cord is short and sole crease is scanty. *(Courtesy Naval Hospital, San Diego, Calif.)*

Most premature infants are put on a 2- or 3-hour feeding schedule. Nourishment is offered in very small amounts of 1 to 5 ml at a time, since the danger of overfeeding the premature baby is real. Overfeeding may increase abdominal distention, cause respiratory embarrassment, and trigger vomiting, which may induce aspiration. The infant must be burped frequently. After a feeding the baby's head and chest are elevated by tilting the incubator mattress tray, and the infant is positioned on his side to discourage emesis and aspiration.

Special needs

The maintenance of body temperature is a real challenge in the care of premature infants. Because of the immaturity of the temperature-regulating center in the brain, little stability is seen. The baby must be specially assisted in his efforts to keep warm. This aid may be provided by the open-type infant warmer or an enclosed plastic incubator.

Oxygen levels above that of room air (21%) may be required to meet the infant's metabolic needs. The most

Table 14-1 Postnatal estimation of fetal age based on signs of maturity assuming normal growth (gestational age)

	28 weeks	32 weeks	36 weeks	40 weeks
Skin	Thin, red, gelatinous	Smooth, dark pink; many vessels visible	Pink, tender; few vessels visible	Pale pink; no vessels
Breasts	Flat, areolae barely visible	Well-defined areolae	Areolae raised: 1 to 2 mm breast tissue	7 to 10 mm breast tissue
Sole creases	None	One anterior transverse crease	Creases on anterior two thirds of sole	Creases on heels
Ears	Pinna soft, flat; stays folded	Slight incurving at top; returns slowly from folding	Incurving upper two thirds; springs back from folding	Incurving to lobe; firm, stands out from head
Genitalia				
Male	Testes undescended; scrotum smooth	Testes high in canal; few scrotal rugae	Testes high in scrotum; more rugae	Testes low in pendulous scrotum; rugae complete
Female	Labia majora widely separated; clitoris, labia minora prominent	Labia majora and labia minora more equal in size	Labia majora becoming closer, nearly cover labia minora	Labia majora completely cover labia minora
Neurologic posture	Hypotonic, arms and legs extended	Partial leg flexion	Froglike; flexion all limbs	Hypertonic
Recoil	None	Partial leg recoil	Partial arm and leg recoil	Prompt recoil

accurate way to evaluate a baby's oxygen status is through the use of intermittent arterial blood gas determinations. Although some babies may approach oxygen toxicity levels when the environmental oxygen reaches 40%, others with diminished respiratory function will need higher levels of environmental oxygen to achieve correct blood concentrations. Environmental oxygen concentrations together with blood gas analyses are important. They are monitored to evaluate the infant's general condition in response to therapy and to prevent the blindness or visual loss called *retrolental fibroplasia* (RLF). This condition can be produced by extended high oxygen concentrations in the blood, causing the immature blood vessels in the retinas of the eyes to hemorrhage. The retinas partially or completely detach from the inner surfaces of the posterior chambers of the eyes and become fibrous masses behind the lenses, unable to receive visual stimuli.

Premature infants are especially susceptible to injury and must be handled with extreme gentleness and discretion. (They need their rest to grow!) They are particularly susceptible to injury at the time of birth and may suffer from intracranial hemorrhage and brain damage. A large percentage of cerebral palsied children, who exhibit some form of spasticity or lack of muscle control were premature. Mental retardation and lack of muscular coordination may stem from brain injury or prolonged lack of oxygen caused by delayed or interrupted breathing

at the time of or subsequent to birth. They may also be caused by bilirubin deposits in the brain tissue resulting from the inability of the immature liver to handle red blood cell breakdown satisfactorily. Jaundice is a significant finding.

Premies, because of their abrupt debut, are deprived of the antibody protection given by mothers to full-term infants. They are also less prepared to manufacture their own antibodies. They become easy victims of infection and must be scrupulously guarded.

Significant immaturity of the respiratory system is an often encountered finding. Some of these infants require a ventilator to assist them with breathing for a prolonged period of time. Failure of lung tissue to expand, or atelectasis, is frequently reported. *Hyaline membrane disease,* or *respiratory distress syndrome* (RDS), is found in a high percentage of premature babies, particularly those delivered by cesarean section, and in children of diabetic mothers. (These babies, though large, appear to be physiologically immature and should be treated similarly to premature infants.) RDS is the most common cause of death in premature infants. It is discussed on pp. 303-305.

•   •   •

Care of the premature infant is a heavy responsibility; life is enclosed in a fragile package. Yet some of the celebrated figures of history, who have made vast contributions to mankind, entered the world in just such an unfinished state—such men as Sir Isaac Newton and Sir Winston Churchill. Do not underestimate the "premie"!

ABNORMALITIES OF THE NEWBORN INFANT

One wishes that each baby would be perfect in every detail—physically, intellectually, and emotionally ready to meet the challenge of life without an initial obstacle or defect. Sadly, such is not the case. Approximately 1 in 14 of all children is born with some kind of abnormality, causing disfigurement or resulting in physical or mental handicaps or a shortened life, although not all these problems may be noted at birth.

The birth of a handicapped or ill child is always a distressing time for the family. Feelings of failure, anxiety, guilt, frustration, anger, and exhaustion are common. Parents at first may be unable to believe that their child is abnormal, and when the realization comes, grief may be intense. Problems in organizing the family to meet the unexpected demands created by the necessary trips to the hospital, physician, and therapist and the extra financial burden can seem almost without end to the often perplexed and unprepared parents.

Although the vocational nurse is not in a position to give professional guidance to mobilize the total resources of the family and community to meet the needs involved, she should recognize the pressures under which the family is operating. She should know how much has been told the parents regarding their child and be extremely discreet in her conversations. She should be supportive in allowing the parents to express themselves and in relaying any problems that seem to be causing worry to the charge nurse or physician. It is *important* that the parents not feel alone in their attempt to adjust to the reality of their child's imperfection. In an attempt to prevent such feelings the nurse can be a vital liaison between the family and medical staff, clergy, and community resource personnel. Guided participation in the care of their child usually helps reduce feelings of isolation.

Birth injuries

Intracranial hemorrhage. The most common type of birth injury is *intracranial hemorrhage*. As noted previously, it is most often seen in premature infants but can be diagnosed in full-term babies as well, particularly those who had a traumatic passage to the external world. Symptoms or signs of hemorrhage within the skull may manifest themselves suddenly or gradually and may vary according to the location and extent of the hemorrhage.

These include irritability, listlessness or cyanosis, marked irregular respiration, varying degrees of paralysis, lack of appetite or poor sucking reflex, tremors, convulsions, projectile vomiting, unequally dilated pupils, tense or bulging fontanels, and a high, shrill cry. These kinds of symptoms could arise from other causes, such as intracranial abscess, cerebral edema, tumor, or developing hydrocephalus—in fact, from anything that would increase the pressure within the skull. Diagnosis is usually made through the history and observation of the infant or by computed tomography (CT) or computed ultrasonography (see Table 24-5). Sometimes the bleeding is mild and stops spontaneously, and the child recovers with little or no effects. Sometimes pressure is so intense that it must be relieved by aspiration of the subdural space or by surgery. Sometimes brain damage is permanent, or death results from the condition.

The infant is usually placed in an incubator with his head slightly elevated in an attempt to relieve pressure. Rarely, a spinal tap may be done for the same reason or as a diagnostic aid. Vitamin K to relieve bleeding tendencies may be prescribed. Sedatives such as phenobarbital may be ordered for tremor. It is important for the nurse observing the infant to be able to describe accurately the type of tremor, convulsion, or abnormal behavior pattern seen; her description of the part of the body affected—one or both sides—how long it lasted, and what event, if anything, occurred just beforehand may help the physician localize the area of bleeding. The child is kept as quiet as possible.

Fractures. Fractures may occur at birth. The most frequently broken bone is the clavicle, or collarbone. It usually heals without treatment. Fractures of long bones are uncommon; they may be splinted. All broken bones normally heal rapidly during infancy.

Facial paralysis. Temporary or even permanent paralysis occasionally results from nerve injury during childbirth. Facial paralysis may be caused by forceps pressure. The affected side of the face does not move, and the eye may remain open. This condition usually disappears gradually.

Erb's palsy. Injury to the brachial plexus, the network of nerves that branches to supply the nervous control of the upper extremities, may cause the arm on the affected side to hang limply from the shoulder and rotate internally. With this condition, called Erb's palsy, the Moro reflex is asymmetric. The infant cannot raise his arm. This injury, is usually not permanent. Treatment consists of immobilizing the arm in an abducted, externally rotated position with flexion at the elbow.

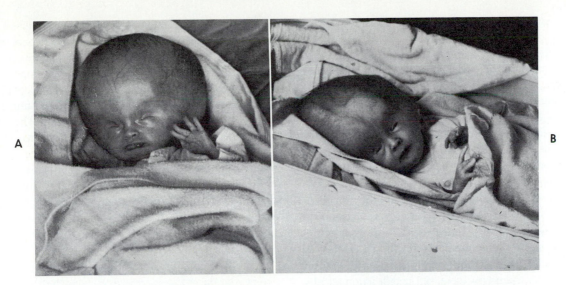

FIG 14-4 A, This baby with advanced hydrocephalus was 4½ weeks old. He was delivered 7 weeks early by cesarean section. **B,** Same child at 3 months of age. Cranium had collapsed. He died at 5½ months of age. (Shunting procedures available today would have prevented such enlargement.)

Developmental disabilities

Several studies have indicated that about 15% of all infants manifest developmental dysfunctions or demonstrate a potential for difficulties of this type. This number of children demands attention. Developmental disabilities are associated with conditions such as prematurity, hydrocephalus, meningomyelocele, cerebral palsy, phenylketonuria, mental retardation of undefined origin, and slow achievement of skill and growth milestones.

Emphasis is on early identification to minimize problems and to foster growth and development. Public Law 94-142 has been established for children with developmental disabilities in school, giving them the right to a multidisciplinary assessment and a plan to meet their educational, developmental, and health care needs. Some programs are federally- or state-supported, such as Head Start or the Regional Centers for the Developmentally Disabled. State institutionalization of patients has been reduced by home or community integration. The nurse assumes a primary role in the health assessment and follow-up ensuring that any health care problem interfering with function receives appropriate care.

Hydrocephalus. Hydrocephalus is a defect that results from the accumulation of abnormally large amounts of cerebrospinal fluid within the cranium, causing abnormal enlargement of the immature skull (Fig. 14-4).

Types. There are a variety of causes of hydrocephalus. The condition may result from an impairment of the circulation of cerebrospinal fluid (CSF) within the ventricular system. This may be a congenital structural defect or may be due to a space-occupying lesion within the ventricular system. This type of obstruction produces what is commonly known as *noncommunicative hydrocephalus* (obstructive hydrocephalus), indicating that the impairment of flow is within the ventricular system. Occasionally, the impairment is within the subarachnoid space; therefore CSF communicates from the ventricles to the subarachnoid space but cannot reach its primary sites of reabsorption in the arachnoid villi. This form of hydrocephalus is called *communicating hydrocephalus*. It may follow intracranial hemorrhage, such as occurs in prematurity or head trauma, or infections, such as meningitis.

Early recognition and treatment. The infant responds to mounting cerebrospinal fluid pressure by an abnormal symmetric increase in head size. Other manifestations noted shortly after birth include bulging of the fontanels, separation of sutures, distended scalp veins, irritability, and vomiting. A downward displacement of the eyes and skin tension, giving the pupils a "setting-sun" appearance, is a late symptom.

Early reduction in ventricular size is essential if the child is to have the best chance of becoming a useful individual. The treatment of hydrocephalus is influenced by the degree of intracranial pressure, the level of obstruction, and any associated major congenital defects found.

Hydrocephalus is usually treated by insertion of a tube or shunt that drains the ventricular fluid into a body space outside the skull. The well-being of the child depends on the continuous functioning of the shunt. The most commonly employed shunt systems are the ventriculoperitoneal and lumboperitoneal shunts. When a ventriculoperitoneal or lumboperitoneal shunt can no longer function correctly, a ventriculoatrial shunt is employed.

Ventriculoperitoneal (VP) shunt. The ventricular catheter is inserted into the lateral ventricle through a small burr hole. The distal catheter is passed beneath the skin down the neck and may tunnel across the front of the chest to enter the abdominal cavity. Several inches of coiled catheter are left in the peritoneal cavity in an effort to provide the necessary increased length automatically as growth proceeds. The ventriculoperitoneal shunt is the most commonly employed shunt in infants because additional tubing can be placed in the abdominal cavity to allow for growth (Fig. 14-5).

Lumboperitoneal shunt. The proximal catheter is placed in the lumbar subarachnoid space. The distal catheter passes from the lumbar subarachnoid space to the peritoneum and empties into the peritoneal cavity, as does the ventriculoperitoneal shunt. The lumboperitoneal shunt is employed in those forms of hydrocephalus in which there is a communication between the lumbar subarachnoid space and the ventricular system. The advantages of the lumboperitoneal shunt are that it avoids surgery in the cranium and has a lower incidence of infection. It requires less revision for development, since most of the growth of the child is vertical and not transverse. If the spinal subarachnoid space is spacious enough to accept shunt tubing, the lumboperitoneal shunt is performed.

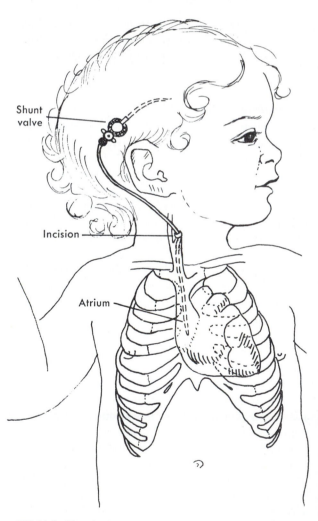

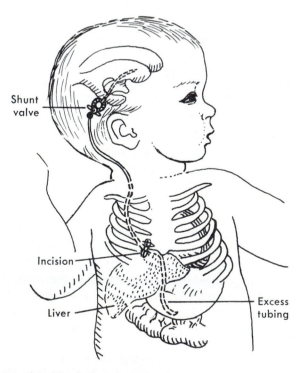

FIG 14-5 Ventriculoperitoneal shunt drains cerebral spinal fluid from ventricles of brain into peritoneal cavity where it is absorbed.

FIG 14-6 Ventriculoatrial shunt drains cerebrospinal fluid from ventricles of brain to right atrium.

Ventriculoatrial (VA) shunt. The insertion of tubes and valves that allow one-way flow of fluid has led to the successful shunting of cerebrospinal fluid into the right atrium as well as the peritoneal cavity. A burr hole is made in the skull, and a small tube is directed into the lateral ventricle of the brain. Through a small neck incision the cardiac tube is inserted into the right atrium by way of the internal jugular vein (Fig. 14-6). Both VP and VA shunts are connected to the reservoir situated beneath the skin and behind the ear. The entire device is covered with skin. Under normal operating conditions cerebrospinal fluid flow is unobstructed. The flushing devices differ on the various tubes used. In the Pudenz-Mishler double-lumen device, both the ventricular and distal tubes are flushed when the reservoir is compressed. Pumping the functioning shunt permits highly effective flushing in both directions. Obstruction of the ventricular tube, the most common cause of shunt malfunctions, may be cleared by occluding the easily felt distal catheter with finger pressure and compressing the reservoir. Thus the flushing device serves a dual purpose: it flushes and checks the operation of the entire system. In postoperative care a check by manually depressing the skin (pumping) over the reservoir of the flushing device and watching for refill may determine if the shunt is functioning properly.

Postoperative care. When the infant is wide awake, dextrose in water is offered by mouth. If it is tolerated, breast milk or formula may be given. It is important that the nurse observe the baby before the shunting procedure to compare and evaluate his postoperative condition. To avoid respiratory complications, the child must have his position changed at least every 2 hours. His head should be placed carefully to avoid pressure on the cranial wound, which might predispose the skin to breakdown. The fontanel should be less tense and slightly depressed. If the fontanels are sunken, the child is kept flat. If the fontanels are full or bulging, his head is elevated. Pulse and respiration determinations and pupil equality checks are done frequently. The nurse must be constantly alert for any signs of increased intracranial pressure, such as slowed pulse and respirations, lethargy, irritability, vomiting, and tense fontanels. Head circumference should be measured daily at the widest diameter. Any abnormalities detected by those observations, signs of faulty functioning of the flushing device, or an elevated temperature indicating a postoperative infection should be recorded carefully and immediately called to the attention of the attending physician.

Complications. Infections continue to be the major problem in shunts. Despite all methods of parenteral antibiotic therapy, including injections into the spinal canal, bacteremia can be cleared only by the replacement of a new shunt mechanism in a different site. Debilitated infants seem to be susceptible to infection. Other problems include obstruction of the shunt system caused by tubing plugged by debris at the ventricular end, thrombus formation at the cardiac end, and adhesion formation at the peritoneal end. Improved methods of controlling this problem continue to be sought.

Continued care. When surgical intervention cannot be considered, nursing care of the child with advanced hydrocephalus takes considerable gentleness and patience. The head may be extremely large with widely separated cranial bones, broad sutures, and bulging fontanels. Despite the plasticity of the infant skull, injury to the brain usually causes some degree of mental retardation. There may be wide swings in body temperature, tremors or convulsions, lack of appetite, or vomiting. The tension of fontanels and other signs of increasing intracranial pressure should be checked daily.

Attention must be given to preventing pressure sores on the scalp by frequent turning and soft pillow supports. When not being supervised directly, the child should be positioned on his side or abdomen with his head turned to the side to prevent aspiration. Support for the head must always be given during feedings, and the nurse may find it more comfortable for the baby and less tiring for herself to place a pillow on her arm for head support and to rest her elbow on a chair arm. After feeding and burping, the infant should be left as quiet as possible to prevent vomiting. Malnutrition and infection are common complications for these unfortunate babies.

Cranial stenosis

Other congenital deformities of the skull may be found, but happily they are rare. The sutures of the skull may prematurely close (cranial stenosis), causing abnormal pressure on the brain and possible mental retardation, as well as an asymmetric distorted appearance of the head, if unrelieved. Very rarely a child may be born without a developed brain and lack the typical cranial covering of the brain. This condition is called *anencephaly* and is fatal.

Mental retardation

Mental retardation is an extremely common problem. It affects approximately 2% of the general population. Good prenatal and delivery care helps prevent some of the possible causes (birth injury, anoxia). Some types of

Table 14-2 Intelligence classifications*

Classification	Intelligence quotient (IQ)	Performance level
Profound retardation	0-24	Unable to attend to personal needs; always requires supervision; 0- to 2-year-old intellectual ability
Severe retardation	25-50	May be trained to meet personal needs but not self-sustaining; 3- to 7-year-old intellectual ability (trainable mentally retarded)
Moderately severe retardation	50-79	Self-sustaining in simple jobs with supervision; 8- to 11-year-old intellectual ability (educable mentally retarded)
Dull normal	79-89	
Average	90-110	What most of us are
Above average	110-130	What most of us would like to be
Gifted	130-150	May have problems in adjustment, emphasizing that both social compe-
Genius	150 and above	tence and intellectual ability contribute to individual success in society

*One of many classifications of intelligence used.

mental retardation can be prevented or improved by dietary supervision, hormonal therapy, or genetic counseling.

Intelligence classifications. Because of the many problems found in trying to determine a person's intellectual capacity by testing devices, the concept of IQ, or intelligence quotient, has lost much of its former significance. The mental age score attained by an individual in testing may be influenced by motivation and environment, as well as the test presentation itself. Nevertheless, IQ scores are still often obtained. They represent a special testing score (mental age) divided by the individual's chronologic age multiplied by 100. Table 14-2 shows certain ranges of IQ, indicating various degrees of intelligence.

Down syndrome. A common (1 in 650 live births) type of mental retardation, which is associated with certain physical characteristics and has undergone considerable investigation, is that of Down syndrome, or mongolism. The most common type of Down syndrome "standard trisomy 21," is associated with an abnormal chromosome count in all the baby's body cells. (See p. 324.) Retardation is mild to profound.

Infants with Down syndrome are usually identified in the nursery, but some are diagnosed later. Characteristically, these infants are short; they have relatively small skulls, flattened from front to back; their birth weights are usually low; and their behavior is lethargic. The most reliable signs of Down syndrome are exaggerated epicanthic folds, which make the eyes slant up and out; short hands and fingers with the little finger bent in (clinodactyly); a deep, horizontal crease across the palm (simian crease); and a large space between the great and

small toes. Physicians examine the eyes in an effort to detect small white dots on the iris, which, when present, are helpful in confirming diagnosis. Decreased muscle tone and excessive joint mobility are also significant findings (Figs. 14-7 and 14-8).

After the newborn period, other signs manifest themselves, such as delayed eruption of teeth, fissured tongue, and retarded intellectual and physical development. These infants often have congenital heart malformations, umbilical hernias, and duodenal atresia. If they survive long enough, they usually possess affectionate, placid personalities. Frequently, depending on home circumstances and the individual needs of the child, he can remain with the family, and care outside the home community is not necessary. No one knows the true cause of this condition, but standard trisomy 21 is found most often in cases in which the mother is near the end of her reproductive life. The translocation type of Down syndrome may be hereditary.

Phenylketonuria. Another less common type of mental retardation is produced by an inherited error in metabolism of a certain essential amino acid, or protein, called *phenylalanine*. Phenylketonuria, called PKU, is an autosomal recessive condition. Phenylalanine hydroxylase, which catalyzes the conversion of the essential amino acid phenylalanine to tyrosine, is absent in the liver of affected infants. Unless appropriate measures are taken, phenylalanine builds up in the bloodstream and after a few months, the toxic effects begin to produce noticeable damage to the brain. A high level of phenylalanine can be detected in the blood serum of the newborn infant, but a few weeks are usually needed before urinary phenylketones present. The detection of PKU is achieved

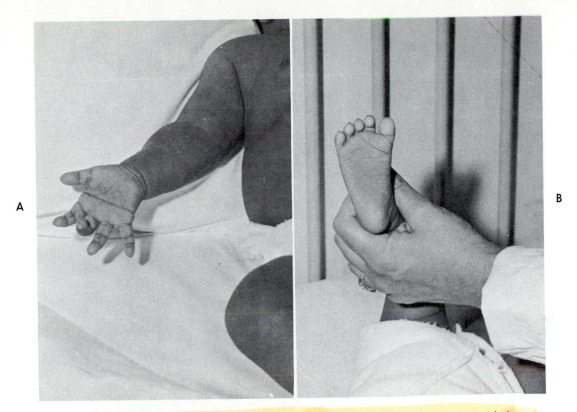

FIG 14-7 A, Hand of infant with Down syndrome. Note deep, straight palmar crease (simian line). **B,** Same infant's foot. Note exaggerated space between big and little toes. *(Courtesy Naval Hospital, San Diego, Calif.)*

by mandatory screening of newborn blood. Measurement of blood phenylalanine (Guthrie test) obtained by heel puncture should be done after 72 hours of life but before 7 days.

Treatment of PKU consists in eliminating as much of the offending protein as possible from the diet for an indeterminate period of time. Since phenylalanine is found in many protein foods, the diet is extremely curtailed. Lofenalac formula plus supplemental protein is instituted to maintain low plasma levels of phenylalanine. Mental retardation can be prevented without impairment of physical growth when dietary restriction of phenylalanine is initiated before the infant is 30 days of age.

Galactosemia. This rare inherited disorder of galactose metabolism also leads to mental retardation, as well as failure to thrive, liver disease, and cataracts in untreated children. A galactose-free diet must be initiated immediately and continued throughout life. (See p. 750.)

Congenital hypothyroidism. Inadequate production of thyroid hormone, which may be due to any number of causes including cretinism, agenesis of the thyroid gland, or other genetic disorders of the thyroid is a serious problem in the newborn. Delayed treatment results in irreversible mental retardation and developmental and physical disabilities. Clinical signs of hypothyroidism develop gradually in the infant and may not appear until the infant is several months of age or older.

The typically affected baby has a large tongue that, because of its size, may protrude from the mouth, causing problems in feeding. The child's cry is hoarse; the hair is coarse; the skin is dry (no perspiration is observed); constipation is a continuous problem; and growth is retarded if the condition is untreated. The degree of mental retardation depends on the time of diagnosis and the initiation of treatment. If hypothyroidism is diagnosed early and hormone replacement therapy is undertaken, the infant usually progresses fairly normally. Routine newborn screening occurs in all 50 states. It includes T_4 and/or TSH blood analyses to diagnose and treat hypothyroidism, thereby reducing the incidence of mental retardation and thyroid problems.

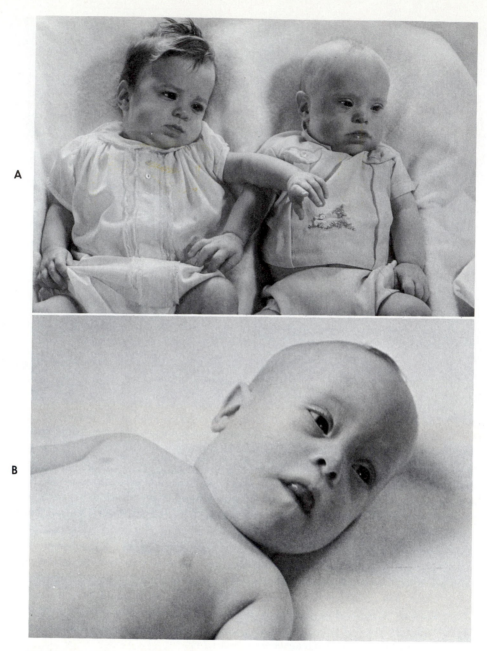

FIG 14-8 A, These children are brother and sister (fraternal twins). Boy manifests Down syndrome; his sister is unaffected. **B,** Close-up of male twin. Note large tongue and typical eyes.

About 15% of retardation results from brain injury associated with birth or from infection in utero. Another 5% is caused by chromosomal abnormality such as Down syndrome or specific single gene defects like PKU. The remainder, or about 80%, results from unfavorable polygenetic combinations from the general gene pool. This group accounts for most of the milder forms of retardation whereas the more severe forms are usually caused by brain injury, chromosomal abnormalities, or single gene factors producing metabolic disorders.

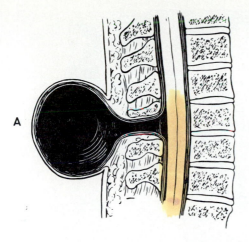 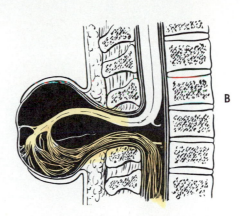

FIG 14-9 A, Section of spinal cord and vertebral column showing meningocele. Note that no nervous tissue protrudes through defect into sac. **B,** Section of spinal cord and vertebral column showing a myelomeningocele. Nervous tissue is found in herniated meningeal sac. *(From Benz GS: Pediatric nursing, ed 5, St Louis, 1964, The CV Mosby Co.)*

Spina bifida

Spina bifida, a condition briefly noted in the discussion of hydrocephalus, may exist in several degrees of severity. The term "spina bifida" simply means divided spine, or that a portion of the posterior wall of the spine is missing. Spina bifida is a genetic condition with a multifactorial pattern of inheritance (pp. 322-323). It is identifiable in utero through analyses of maternal serum as well as of amniotic fluid. Most states now require that the maternal alphafetoprotein (AFP) serum detection test be offered to women pregnant between 16 and 18 weeks.

Types. The defect may be so small that is offers no difficulty and is discovered only when an x-ray examination of the spine is done for other reasons. This type of defect is called *spina bifida occulta,* or hidden divided spine. The spina bifida occulta detected by x-ray examination is without symptoms in 25% of the cases. However, there is a syndrome of spina bifida occulta in which not only this radiologic abnormality is noted but varying degrees of orthopedic deformities or urinary tract dysfunction. This is caused by pressure on the nerve roots on the lower part of the spine or pressure on the lower spinal cord itself. Such a condition is diagnosed with spinal ultrasonography in infancy.

Another type is termed *spina bifida cystica* because it exhibits a cystlike structure. There are two kinds of spina bifida cystica. A *meningocele* involves a protrusion of only the covering meninges of the spinal cord and cerebrospinal fluid. The child usually develops normal urinary and intestinal control and has no paralysis, but the sac, until removed, is a cosmetic problem, and its possible injury always poses the problem of infection of the nervous system. The second and more serious kind of spina bifida cystica is called *myelomeningocele* or *meningomyelocele* (Figs. 14-9 to 14-11). In this condition the meninges protrude through the spinal opening, and nerve tissues are also found in the herniated sac. Since spina bifida cystica occurs early in the pregnancy with a poor migration of the nerves involved in the defect, there are varying degrees of weakness of the legs, sensory disturbance, and impairment of rectal and urinary sphincter function. If the lesion is high in the spine, the degree of paralysis is severe. If it is low, for instance, in the sacral spine only, the child has minimal weakness of the lower extremities but significant urinary and bowel control problems. Hydrocephalus is frequently seen in patients with myelomeningocele, depending on the position of the myelomeningocele in the spinal canal. Thus infants with myelomeningocele at a thoracic level will have an incidence of 90% to 95% of hydrocephalus. Those with a sacral myelomeningocele have only a 45% chance of hydrocephalus.

Nursing care. The nursing care of the child with either meningocele or myelomeningocele is challenging. Before surgery the sac, or mass, as it is sometimes called, must be protected from injury and infection. The child must be adequately nourished and should be assured of loving care. To protect the sac, the child is usually positioned on his abdomen or carefully propped on his side. Because of the usual position of the sac, no diapers are

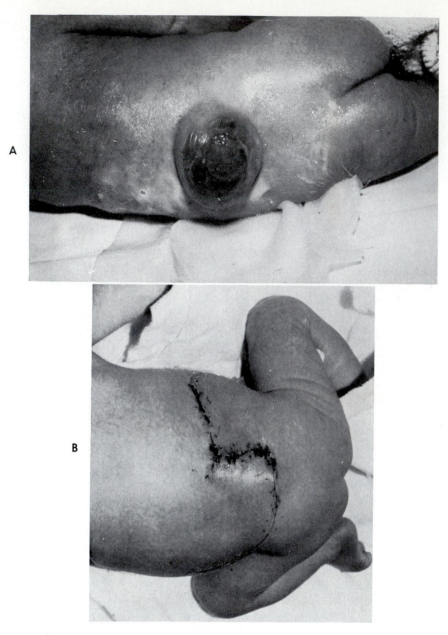

FIG 14-10 A, Myelomeningocele before surgery. (An antibacterial dressing was used.) **B,** Repair of same patient. *(Courtesy M.C. Gleason, MD, San Diego, Calif.)*

pinned in place. To avoid putting strain or pressure on the sac, the nurse must be extremely careful in lifting the infant. Slipping her hands and forearms, palms up, under the leg and chest area to grasp the farther thigh, arm, and shoulder seems to be a safe, effective way of lifting and moving the smaller infants. Caution must be taken when putting these children in a sitting position, even if no direct pressure is exerted on the sac. Sometimes the sac is so low on the spine that the sitting position puts too much tension on the area.

A positioning device called a Bradford frame may be used for infants with meningocele, consisting of a metal framework that rests on the bed and elevates the baby on a divided, padded canvas support. The perineal area

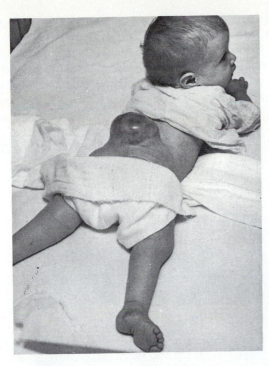

FIG 14-11 This youngster's myelomeningocele was repaired shortly after photograph was taken. (*Courtesy Children's Hospital and Health Center, San Diego, Calif.*)

and sac are placed directly over splits in the canvas, and a bedpan is positioned directly underneath. Plastic strips hanging from the opening of the frame help direct urine and feces into the pan. This device helps protect the area from soil and pressure.

For feeding, the infant may be propped on his side with his head elevated, held by one nurse with his head over her shoulder and fed by another nurse holding the bottle. However, if the child's condition permits, he may be held in a sitting position with no pressure on the sac.

Meticulous skin care must be given and pressure areas prevented. Occasionally, to avoid infection, the sac may be covered by sterile gauze moistened by saline. A foam rubber ring with a hole large enough to admit the sac may be placed over the sterile compresses and wrapped in place with an elastic bandage. Treatment depends on the size, location, and condition of the sac, but surgical closure is usually planned early to avoid the problem of infection. The sac should be observed for variance in size and tenseness as well as ulceration. Any leaking of fluid should be reported immediately. The head of a child with myelomeningocele usually is regularly measured to

detect developing hydrocephalus. The sensation and movement of the lower extremities are evaluated as care is given.

After surgery (usually a flap-type procedure), the prone position is maintained, at least until the sutures are removed. There may be no dressing over the incision, and a dry incision and body warmth may be maintained by a carefully positioned gooseneck lamp or the use of an incubator. Although surgery rarely improves function, it certainly improves the child's appearance and facilitates care. In these patients the effects of gravity, the lack of supportive muscles and, occasionally, uneven growth make a straight spine difficult to achieve. Without the use of external support and in some cases surgery, a patient may literally sit with his rib cage resting on his thighs. The lower extremities may also be affected; hips often are subluxed or dislocated, and the feet may be clubbed.

Urinary tract complications are frequently seen because the majority of these children have neurogenic bladders. When the child with spina bifida is about 3 years of age, parents are taught clean intermittent catheterization techniques. The risks and consequences of inadequate bladder drainage far exceed those of infection. Intermittent catheterization several times a day has become a standard management tool for children with neurogenic bladders. This technique has resulted in satisfactory continence in older patients who are, for the first time in their lives, free from odor, shame, and discomfort. The care of a patient with spina bifida, complicated by a herniation of nerve tissue elements, continues for life. The child needs constant psychologic and emotional support, as well as physical assistance, to become a healthy personality capable of giving to as well as receiving from his environment. To meet the various specialized needs of these patients, many communities have multidisciplinary clinics.

Cleft lip and cleft palate

Cleft lip and cleft palate are common congenital malformations, appearing approximately once in every 1,000 births. They constitute a failure in the embryonic development of the child, and a hereditary factor is often found to be significant. Cleft lip is found more often in males, whereas females more often have cleft palates. Cleft lip, sometimes called harelip, may vary from a simple notching of the border of the lip to a deep split extending through the lip to or into the nose. It may exist on only one side of center or be found on both sides. It usually does not create a problem in feeding. The major problem involves the infant's appearance. For this reason a cleft lip is usually repaired as soon as the child's condition is sufficiently stable or when the infant is 10 weeks of age, weighs 10 pounds, and has a hemoglobin of 10 g (the rule of tens). A second repair may be necessary when the child is 4 or 5 years of age to correct scar irregularities and nasal asymmetry.

A cleft palate may constitute a lack of fusion of only part of the hard or soft palate or may extend along the entire roof of the mouth. Cleft palate is repaired at about 12 to 18 months of age or according to the child's individual needs.

Before taking their baby home to await surgery for cleft palate, the parents must receive detailed instructions regarding the infant's care and have several opportunities to feed the infant with supervision. The baby with a cleft palate sometimes has difficulty sucking normally, as he cannot create the necessary vacuum in his mouth. The child may be fed slowly with a rubber-tipped medicine dropper or syringe, no faster than the baby's capacity to

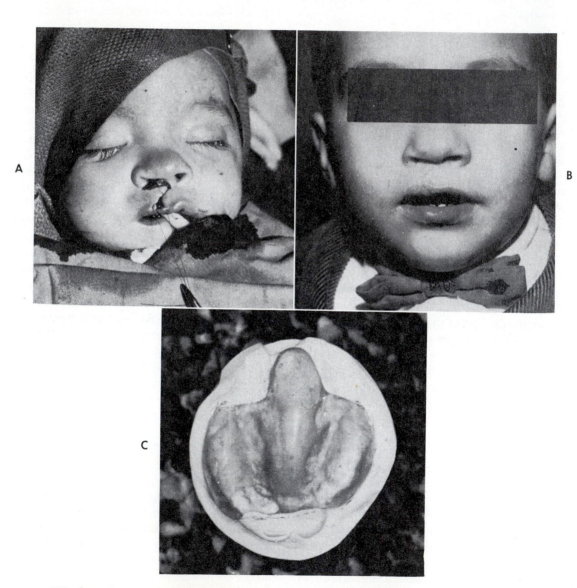

FIG 14-12   A, Closure of unilateral complete cleft lip. B, Same child, 13 months later. C, Palate prosthesis resting in plaster-of-Paris mold. Prosthesis is used until child is old enough for optimal palate repair. (*Courtesy M.C. Gleason, MD, San Diego, Calif.*)

swallow. Rarely, a specially molded cleft-palate nipple with an extra built-in hump that fits the cleft in the palate and makes sucking possible is employed. Occasionally soft, long lamb's nipples are tried, or the child may be fed from the end of a small spoon. Sometimes the defect is so placed or is so small that a regularly shaped soft nipple may be used. The baby is fed in an upright position to help prevent aspiration and regurgitation through the nose. The method of feeding that is most successful and closest to that used by a normal baby is the method of choice. Since these babies swallow more air than usual, they should be burped frequently. This will lessen the possibility of emesis or unattended "wet burps" and subsequent aspiration. Some children with cleft palate are fitted early with a prosthesis to guard against nasal regurgitation, aid in the formation of speech patterns, and maintain anatomic relationships important to the final repair.

The success of plastic surgery depends on the extent of the defect, the developmental stage of the individual, the repair techniques available, the skill of the surgeon, the standard of nursing care, and the cooperation of the parents. A cleft palate is difficult to repair, and the child may have to undergo several procedures at different ages (Fig. 14-12).

Postoperative care of the child with cleft lip. After surgery for a cleft lip the infant's arms should be restrained to prevent damage to the suture line. Elbow restraints may be used to prevent the infant from rubbing the repaired lip with his hands. (See Fig. 23-4, *A*.) The nurse can adequately restrain the arms of very young infants by pulling their long shirt sleeves past their hands and pinning the sleeves to their diaper. Periodically these restraints should be removed one at a time to provide needed exercise and inspection of the arms. Placing the baby upright in an infant seat also helps protect his suture line from trauma.

The suture line should be kept clean, and no crust should be allowed to form because crusting can enlarge the scar. Various solutions are used for cleaning, depending on the physician's preference. Tightly wrapped, sterile cotton applicators saturated with hydrogen peroxide, warm sterile water, or physiologic saline solution may be used to remove the blood or crust. Such maneuvers must be done gently but persistently. Soaking the area for a brief period with a saturated applicator or sponge before any motion over the area is attempted helps considerably. Afterward the lip should be gently dried. Sometimes an antibiotic ointment may be left on the suture line.

Every effort should be made to keep the child happy because a happy child cries less and puts less strain on the repair. The parents should be encouraged to cuddle the infant and, as soon as feasible, participate in feedings under supervision. Water is offered first, and formula feedings soon follow. The child may be fed by a small medicine cup or a rubber-tipped medicine dropper and graduated to a soft nipple when sucking is allowed. Whichever method of feeding is used, the infant should be held in a sitting position, fed slowly, and carefully burped.

Postoperative care of the child with cleft palate (Fig. 14-13). A cleft palate is a much more serious defect than a cleft lip, considering the impairment of function it produces. Not only is feeding difficult, involving possible problems of aspiration and dental placement, but speech is often nasalized, and infections of the respiratory tract and middle ear are common. The child who has undergone palate surgery is usually fed from a cup or side of a spoon. Nothing is introduced into the mouth that may endanger the suture line, and unless the child is old enough to understand and cooperate, arm restraints must be used. The diet progresses from clear liquid to full liquid to soft food over a period of approximately 2 weeks. The mouth should be rinsed with water at the end of a meal.

The problems of the child with cleft lip, cleft palate, or both are occasionally so complex that the combined therapy of a plastic surgeon, pediatrician, orthodontist, speech therapist, child psychiatrist, and medical social worker may be needed. For this reason, clinics for those with cleft lip and palate are found in most large cities.

Other digestive tract abnormalities

Other abnormalities of the digestive tract are found with enough frequency to merit mention, especially since they are so serious in nature.

Esophageal atresia and tracheoesophageal fistula (Fig. 14-14). Esophageal atresia refers to the congenital absence or closure of the esophagus at some point. The upper portion usually ends in a blind pouch. Tracheoesophageal fistula represents an open connection between the trachea and the esophagus. A frequent association exists between esophageal atresia and tracheoesophageal fistula as a result of the nature of embryonic development.

Several varieties of these malformations are known, but the three major types are (1) tracheoesophageal fistula with esophageal atresia (80% to 95% of cases) in which the upper esophagus ends in a blind pouch and the lower esophageal segment connects with the trachea; (2) esoph-

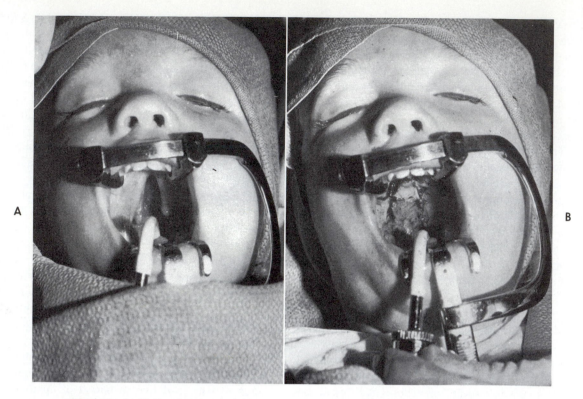

FIG 14-13 **A,** Cleft palate just before surgery. **B,** Closure of cleft palate. *(Courtesy M.C. Gleason, MD, San Diego, Calif.)*

ageal atresia alone; and (3) tracheoesophageal fistula alone. These anomalies are relatively common. About 25% of the infants with digestive tract abnormalities are premature. Another 25% usually have associated defects (congenital heart defects and gastrointestinal malformations, such as imperforate anus). Maternal polyhydramnios is frequently noted in these infants as a result of the inability of the fetus to dispose of swallowed amniotic fluid. The malformations are slightly more common in male infants.

Symptoms. The infant with esophageal malformation usually cries at birth, breathes well, and becomes a normal, healthy color. Soon, however, saliva accumulates in the pharynx and mouth, and the infant froths or drools. The mucus is thick and seems excessive, but it is actually a normal amount of mucus that simply cannot pass through to the stomach and therefore pools in the esophageal pouch. Respirations become noisy, gurgling, and rapid. The cry is hoarse. Respiratory difficulty increases, and cyanosis occurs. If the infant is fed, he will repeatedly cough, gag, and regurgitate. Feeding is usually followed by aspiration of breast milk or formula into the lungs, which leads to pneumonia and often to atelectasis. All the pulmonary symptoms are caused by the drainage of secretions into the lungs from the stomach or mouth by way of an esophageal fistula or overflow from an esophageal pouch.

Diagnosis. Diagnosis can be easily made in the delivery room or nursery by the inability to pass a catheter into the stomach. X-ray films positively confirm the diagnosis of an esophageal malformation.

Treatment. For the infant with tracheoesophageal fistula, a gastrostomy is performed as an emergency measure. This is to prevent over-distention of the stomach with air, leading to regurgitation of gastric contents into the tracheobronchial tree. Antibiotics are administered to treat the pneumonia. Once the infant's condition is stable, usually within 7 to 10 days, surgical repair is done. The chest is opened, and the tracheoesophageal fistula is tied off (ligated). Connection of the esophageal segments is also performed, if possible; otherwise, this is accomplished at 1 to 2 years of age.

Nursing care. Preoperative care is directed toward prevention of aspiration and stabilization of the infant.

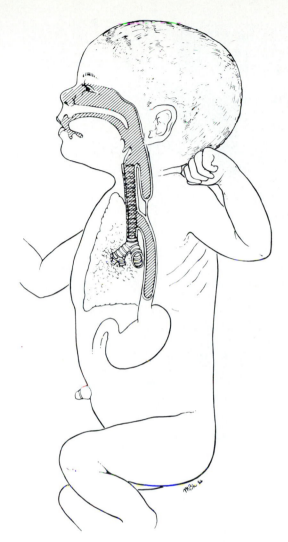

FIG 14-14 Most common type of esophageal atresia involves upper esophageal segment ending in a blind pouch and lower tracheoesophageal fistula. There is great danger of aspiration.

open. An esophageal sump tube is not used postoperatively—suctioning is performed very gently only as needed.

Prognosis depends largely on the initial condition of the infant at the time of diagnosis, degree of prematurity, presence of other malformations, and whether or not feedings had been given. After the surgical repair is complete and recovery has taken place, these infants generally develop normally. They do, however, have a higher incidence of pulmonary infections during their first year and usually a harsh cough for some time. Continued medical supervision is essential.

Imperforate anus. Occasionally the infant's rectum ends as a closed or blind pouch or connects to an adjacent canal (urethra, vagina) by means of a fistula (Fig. 14-15). The possibility of this defect is one reason that observation of the stools of the newborn is so important. Often a temporary colostomy, an abdominal exit for the contents of the colon, must be made. Later the creation of a normally placed functional rectal opening will be attempted surgically.

Abdominal hernias. An absence of the normal abdominal wall in the region of the umbilicus that allows a portion of the intestinal contents to be clearly observed, virtually unprotected, and subject to herniation and strangulation is called an *omphalocele* (Fig. 14-16). The defect may be small or exaggerated. Its repair is usually considered a surgical emergency. Another type of hernia, involving the abdominal contents and causing respiratory distress as well as digestive problems, is the *diaphragmatic hernia*. In this condition an abnormally large opening is present in the diaphragm that allows part of the contents of the abdominal cavity to displace upward into the chest. Sometimes the entire stomach, as well as portions of the intestine, is found in the thorax, crowding the heart and lungs. This situation, too, is a surgical emergency.

Hypospadias

A fairly common malformation of the urinary system that is found in male infants is hypospadias (Fig. 14-17). The urethra, instead of traveling the entire length of the penis, opens out of the underside of the penis, either at its base or at varying distances from the tip. Sometimes the presence of hypospadias, coupled with other irregularities of the external genital organs, leads to confusion in determining the sex of the infant, and cell studies and exploratory operative procedures may be necessary. The repair of hypospadias by the extension of the urethral canal is preferably accomplished between 2

The baby is kept in a head-up position and given oxygen with humidification to help relieve respiratory stress; constant or intermittent gentle suction is applied to the esophageal pouch by means of a specialized (sump) tube. The baby is handled minimally and receives nothing orally. Fluids are administered intravenously by way of a peripheral vein or by umbilical catheter. Postoperative care is much the same but includes proper care of the surgical incision, chest tube, gastrostomy, and frequent turning. Initially the gastrostomy is allowed to drain freely into a collection bag. When feedings are begun through the gastrostomy in 2 to 3 days, the tube is elevated and left

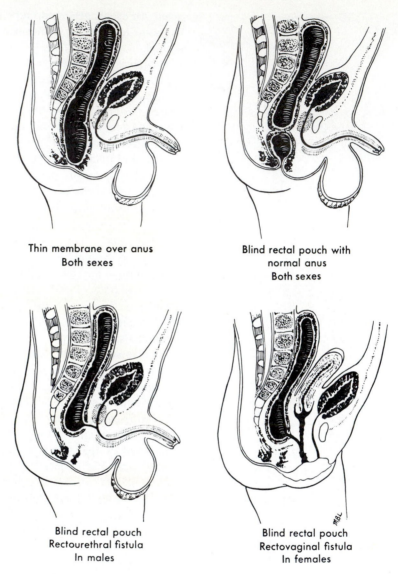

Thin membrane over anus
Both sexes

Blind rectal pouch with
normal anus
Both sexes

Blind rectal pouch
Rectourethral fistula
In males

Blind rectal pouch
Rectovaginal fistula
In females

FIG 14-15 Types of imperforate anus in the newborn infant.

and 3 years of age. Minor positional deviations of the urethral meatus may not require treatment.

Congenital heart deformities

Congenital cardiac conditions frequently stem from the persistence of some part of the fetal circulation pattern, so it would be of benefit to review the basic circulation that is present before birth (Fig. 4-4). The foramen ovale may fail to close, resulting in an *atrial septal defect*. The ductus arteriosus may persist. However, real structural deviations may also exist in many different combinations. (See pp. 718-720 for more detail.) Open-heart surgery, with the use of the heart-lung machine, now gives more hope for survival and the possibility of a more normal life for victims of congenital heart defects.

Hemolytic disease of the newborn infant

A number of conditions can cause blood destruction in the fetus or newborn infant. Probably the most well-known cause is Rh factor incompatibility, which may initiate the condition *erythroblastosis fetalis*. The Rh fac-

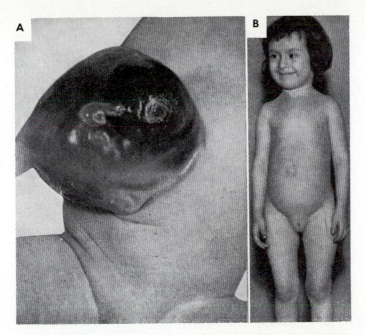

FIG 14-16 Omphalocele before repair **(A)** and after corrective surgery **(B)**. *(From Potter EL: Pathology of the fetus and newborn, Chicago, 1952, Year Book Medical Publishers, Inc.)*

tor was first identified in the blood of Rhesus monkeys. Actually the Rh factor has been found to be a group of related protein antigens that under certain conditions may be capable of causing the formation of potentially dangerous antibodies. The two antigens that seem to cause difficulty clinically are D and its genetic variant D^u. Approximately 85% of the white population and higher percentages of the nonwhite population have these substances in their blood (Fig. 14-18).

Rh incompatibility. If a woman who lacks the Rh protein in her blood marries a man who also lacks it, no problem will exist for their offspring because of the Rh factor. However, if her husband is Rh positive and their child inherits Rh-positive blood from his father, trouble may occur.

Probable mechanism. Some of the baby's blood cells carrying the Rh protein may pass through a microscopic tear in the placental barrier and reach the mother's bloodstream. The mother's body automatically manufactures antibodies (protective substances) designed to destroy the foreign protein in her body. These antibodies may then find themselves in the fetal circulation. There, they do just what they were designed to do: they destroy the Rh protein, or factor, and, in so doing, also destroy the red blood cell to which it is attached. The fetus suffers from the effects of anemia. Making a valiant effort to supply

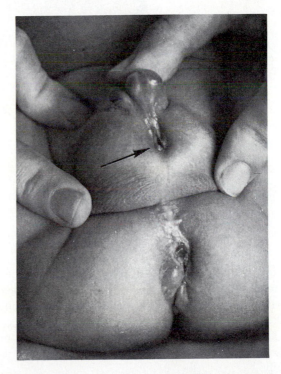

FIG 14-17 This infant suffers from multiple congenital anomalies. Arrow indicates opening of urethra at base of penis (hypospadias). An imperforate anus was previously repaired.

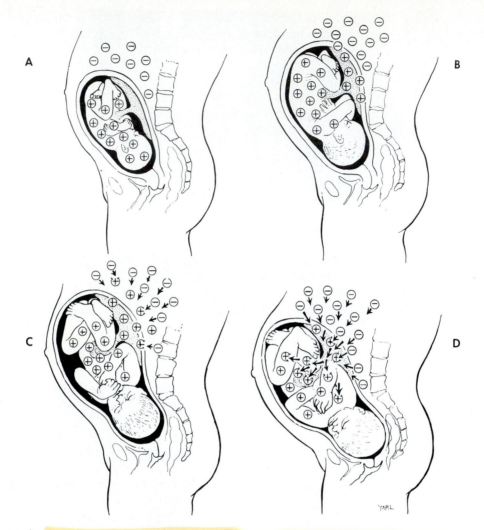

FIG 14-18 Mechanism of erythroblastosis fetalis, which is caused by Rh incompatibility. **A,** Rh-positive child is carried by Rh-negative mother. **B,** Rh protein crosses placental barrier and invades mother's bloodstream. **C,** Mother's system manufactures antibodies to destroy foreign Rh protein. **D,** Antibodies cross back over placenta and destroy baby's blood cells, which are intimately associated with Rh protein.

more red blood cells, he forces out into his bloodstream immature, inadequate forms of red blood cells called erythroblasts. This is the reason that the resulting disease is termed *erythroblastosis fetalis*. In severe cases congestive heart failure associated with enlargement of the spleen and liver occurs. The infant is in great jeopardy.

Shortly after birth, toxicity caused by the large amount of red blood cell breakdown products (chiefly bilirubin) circulating in the baby's body may lead to brain damage known as *kernicterus*. This condition causes neurologic impairment, such as spasticity, deafness, mental retardation, or death. One of the first clinical manifestations of Rh factor sensitivity in the infant is the appearance of jaundice within 24 to 36 hours. The baby with a more severe case may be lethargic, suck poorly, and manifest spasticity.

However, not all mothers with Rh-negative blood have such ill babies. Sometimes the baby is also Rh negative and no such problem arises. Sometimes the number of antibodies the mother has produced in response to the baby's cells in her bloodstream is so small that no damage to the baby is detected. Usually trouble is not encountered until the second or third infant. After several pregnancies the titer of antibodies in the blood usually increases greatly. This titer may be measured during pregnancy; also, the progress of the disease may be estimated by analyzing amniotic fluid aspirated from the sac surrounding the baby. These tests allow the physician to evaluate the health of the fetus and plan for the baby's birth and care.

Treatment. When the presence of erythroblastosis fetalis is determined in a newborn infant, exchange transfusion is carried out. The umbilical vein is used to achieve access to the baby's bloodstream by means of a polyethylene catheter. A carefully measured amount of blood is slowly withdrawn and discarded by a syringe equipped with a complex of stopcocks. Then crossmatched, Rh-negative donor blood without an Rh antibody titer, warmed to room temperature, is pushed slowly by syringe back into the baby's body as a replacement. This process is repeated many times until complete replacement is estimated to have occurred. During the procedure, close observation of the baby's vital signs and the blood volume exchange is essential. The baby must be kept warm, and oxygen may be administered. This treatment must occasionally be repeated, but the results are usually highly successful, and a child born in good condition and receiving prompt transfusion when needed has an excellent prognosis.

Intrauterine transfusion of those unborn infants, who show signs of not being able to survive until viable, is now available at a few research centers. It is not without risk but may be considered when no other hope for the fetus exists.

The exposure of infants with elevated blood bilirubin levels to blue or fluorescent light to reduce the amount of circulating bilirubin is now frequently used. The naked infant, positioned under the lamps with protective eye shields in place, is turned periodically to increase body surface exposure, and is given increased fluids.

Prevention. For the Rh-negative mother who has never been sensitized (that is, formed detectable levels of Rh antibodies) because of a previous contact with the Rh protein, protection is now available that, when properly used, is essentially 100% effective in preventing the detrimental effects of Rh incompatibility. Passive immunization or ready-made antibody protection, given within 72 hours after the birth of an Rh-positive infant or abortus destroys the invading Rh protein and inhibits the natural formation of antibodies of the mother. This special passive immunization, Rh immune globulin, first

marketed as Rho-Gam, unfortunately does not aid Rh-negative women who have already actively developed their own immunization against the Rh factor.

Rh immune globulin must be administered to the woman at risk *after each exposure* to Rh-positive blood. In certain instances fetal-to-maternal hemorrhages take place that are too large for the normal dose of 300 μg of Rh-immune globulin to provide adequate protection. The number of fetal cells in the maternal circulation can be estimated by the use of the Kleihauer-Betke test or the more recent commercially available Fetaldex technique and the dosage increased as necessary. Some physicians, in an effort to protect a small but important group of Rh-negative women who have unknown antepartal bleeds that may cause early sensitization, administer the immune globulin to all Rh-negative women at 28 weeks' gestation as well as after amniocentesis and birth.

A mechanism similar to the Rh problem, but usually of a less serious nature, can operate when the mother has type O blood and the baby has type A, B, or AB. Such a situation is called "ABO incompatibility."

Orthopedic abnormalities

Orthopedic abnormalities are common in the newborn nursery. As a general rule, the earlier they are treated the better the prognosis.

Congenital dislocation of the hip (CDH). There are two main types of congenital dislocations of the hip: (1) *teratologic,* which develops during life in utero and is commonly associated with other orthopedic problems, and (2) *typical,* which occurs just before, during, or shortly after birth, probably caused by the softening effects of the maternal hormone relaxin on the baby's ligaments and the stress of labor and birth. The hip joints of every newborn should be examined within 24 hours of birth for congenital dislocation. They can usually be successfully treated by simple manipulation. There are 1.5 cases of CDH per 1,000 live births. It affects girls eight times more frequently than boys. Dislocation, or luxation, is present when the femoral head is completely displaced from the socket, or acetabulum. Subluxation, or partial displacement, is more common, occurring in approximately 1 in 60 births. A subluxated hip may become completely dislocated during a baby's care unless certain types of maneuvers are avoided. These infants should never be lifted by their feet for diapering. Their legs should never be pulled, nor should their hips be completely extended when wrapped in a blanket. Since one does not always know which child may have incipient hip problems, these cautions should apply to the care of

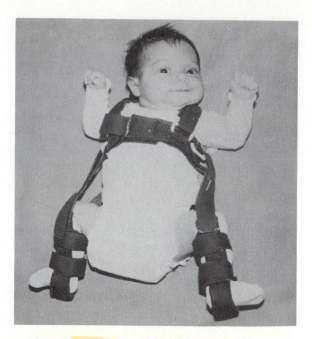

FIG 14-19 Pavlik harness is indicated in treatment of congenital subluxation or dislocation of hip in newborn or infant up to 8 months. Chest halter is positioned at nipple line and fastened with Velcro closure. Leg and foot are placed in stirrup and fastened by Velcro closure. Front stirrup straps are connected to halter. Straps are adjusted so that hip is flexed above a right angle. (Courtesy Scott J. Mubarak, MD, San Diego, Calif.)

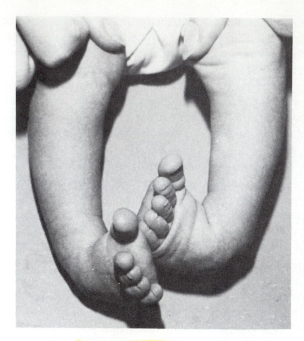

FIG 14-20 Talipes equinovarus. (Courtesy William C. McDade, MD, San Diego, Calif.)

all babies. Barring complications, the subluxated hip of 88% of the affected newborns becomes normal by 2 months of age.

Physical findings that the nurse can detect include asymmetry of the thigh folds, limited abduction of the affected hip, and shortening of the femur when the knees and hips are flexed at right angles and when abduction is attempted with the child lying supine on a firm table. The diagnosis is usually confirmed by x-ray examination. Since the socket becomes progressively more distorted if reduction is delayed, the goal of treatment is the immediate return of the femoral head to the acetabulum. A normal hip joint can be obtained when treatment is begun in the first few weeks of life. Reduction of the hip is not difficult and involves maintenance of the hip in a stable position of flexion and abduction. Semirigid abduction devices are more practical and preferred for treatment of infants with CDH. The best and most popular device for treating CDH is the Pavlik harness (Fig. 14-19). This allows flexion and abduction but prevents extension or adduction. The child's orthopedic condition is frequently evaluated on an outpatient basis. Early treatment may

reduce therapy to about 3 months' duration. If the child's x-ray film indicates normal location of the hip at 2 years of age, the condition may be considered cured. Treatment after 6 months of age varies. It may involve traction for a few weeks followed by casting or operative reduction. However, when CDH is diagnosed at 2 years of age, the outcome is seldom optimal. In children over 8 years, even the most extensive operative procedures cannot produce a functionally satisfactory hip. About one third of the degenerative hip joint disease found in adults is caused by the residual effects of CDH. In adults such conditions may be helped by a total hip arthroplasty.

Clubfoot (talipes). Clubfoot is the most common congenital anomaly of the lower extremity. In the most common form of this condition (talipes equinovarus), the anterior half of the foot is adducted and inverted. The medial border of the foot is concave, the lateral border is convex, and the heel is drawn up (Fig. 14-20). The cause of clubfoot is unknown, but it has been postulated that it results from arrested or abnormal development of a particular part of the germ plasm during embryonic life. One or both feet may be involved. It is twice as common in males as in females.

The feet of the newborn infant must be carefully evaluated. Not all apparent deformities are true clubfoot. Some distortions are simply caused by intrauterine positions and not real structural differences. These feet can be corrected to neutral position in all elements of the deformity by manipulation during examination. A true clubfoot cannot. Both, however, need careful follow-up.

The treatment of clubfoot should be started as soon as the baby's condition is stable. Treatment may be divided into three stages: (1) correction, (2) maintenance of correction, and (3) long-term follow-up. Correction usually consists of stretching and strapping or casting. Casting is changed as often as every 3 to 7 days over a period of about 10 weeks. Follow-up must continue for several years after completion of active treatment to guard against recurrence of the deformity and a less than satisfactory outcome. Surgery is often necessary to fully correct the clubfoot deformity.

Syndactyly and polydactylism. Syndactyly, or webbing of the fingers or toes, is a very interesting anomaly, usually responding well to surgical separation. Syndactyly may accompany another digital abnormality called *polydactylism,* or the presence of extra fingers or toes. At times, these extra digits have no bony connection with the hand or foot and, when a ligature is tied around the fleshy stalk and cuts off circulation, the digit soon drops off. When a bony connection exists, surgery is necessary.

Effect of contagious diseases

The effect of contagious diseases on the fetus and newborn infant is discussed in Chapters 9 and 15. Those considered are syphilis, gonorrhea, chlamydia, tuberculosis, rubella (German measles), toxoplasmosis, cytomegalovirus and herpes simplex virus infections.

• • •

Many abnormalities are possible in the newborn infant, but considering the intricacies of life, the miracle is that more of them do not occur.

Key Concepts

1. In determining the status of the small infant, birth weight, heredity, possible length of gestation, clinical appearance, and behavior all must be considered.

2. The incidence of prematurity in the United States varies with the population studied; in general it approaches 7%. Prematurity accounts for about two thirds of infant mortality.

3. The typical premature infant lacks subcutaneous fat; has a good supply of lanugo; has a relatively large head and abdomen, and a small thorax; has little molding of the skull; irregular respirations; and may be surprisingly active.

4. Sucking and swallowing reflexes may be weak or absent in very small infants, necessitating supplemental nutrition. The danger of overfeeding is very real.

5. Special needs of the premature infant may include the following: maintenance of body temperature, provision of appropriate level of oxygen, protection from injury and infection, and assistance with respiration.

6. The most common type of birth injury is intracranial hemorrhage. Symptoms include irritability, listlessness or cyanosis, marked irregular respiration, varying degrees of paralysis, lack of appetite or poor sucking reflex, tremors, convulsions, projectile vomiting, unequally dilated pupils, tense or bulging fontanels, and a high, shrill cry.

7. Hydrocephalus results from the accumulation of abnormally large amounts of cerebrospinal fluid within the cranium. Three types of shunts used for treatment are ventriculoperitoneal, lumboperitoneal, and ventriculoatrial. Infection is the most common complication following shunting.

8. Mental retardation affects about 2% of the general population. Causes include birth injury, infection in utero, chromosomal abnormalities, and unfavorable polygenetic combinations.

9. Infants with Down syndrome are characteristically short; have relatively small skulls, flattened from front to back; usually have low birth weights; and exhibit lethargic behavior. Reliable signs include exaggerated epicanthic folds, short hands and fingers with the little finger bent in, a deep, horizontal crease across the palm, and a large space between the great and small toes.

10. Spina bifida is a genetic condition in which a portion of the posterior wall of the spine is missing. A meningocele presents a cosmetic problem and possible injury of the sac poses the problem of infection of the nervous system. A myelomeningocele results in varying degrees of weakness of the legs, sensory disturbance, and impairment of rectal and urinary sphincter function.

11. Cleft lip and palate occur about once in every 1,000 births. A cleft lip is usually repaired when the infant is 10 weeks old, weighs 10 pounds, and has a he-

moglobin of 10 g. Cleft palate is usually repaired at about 12 to 18 months of age.

12. Nursing care after cleft lip surgery includes restraining the infant's arms, cleaning the suture line, careful feeding, and keeping the infant as happy as possible. Following cleft palate surgery, the child is usually fed from a cup or side of a spoon; nothing is introduced into the mouth that may endanger the suture line; and arm restraints are usually used. The mouth is rinsed with water after each meal.

13. Tracheoesophageal fistula represents an open connection between the trachea and esophagus. A gastrostomy is performed as an emergency measure. Surgical repair is done after the infant's condition has stabilized.

14. An infant with imperforate anus may require a temporary colostomy before the surgical creation of a normally placed functional rectal opening.

15. The omphalocele and diaphragmatic hernia are both considered surgical emergencies.

16. Hypospadias is a fairly common malformation of the male urinary system. Surgical repair is usually accomplished by a series of operative procedures before the child reaches school age.

17. Rh factor incompatibility may initiate the condition erythroblastosis fetalis. This occurs only when the fetus of an Rh-negative woman inherits Rh-positive blood from the father. Treatment involves an exchange transfusion. Administration of Rh immune globulin prevents the detrimental effects of Rh incompatibility in the newborn. It must be administered to the woman at risk after each exposure to Rh-positive blood.

18. There are two main types of congenital dislocations of the hip (CDH): teratologic and typical. They can usually be successfully treated by simple manipulation. Reduction of the hip involves maintaining a stable position of flexion and abduction.

19. To avoid completely dislocating an unidentified subluxated hip, infants should never be lifted by their feet for diapering, their legs should never be pulled, nor should their hips be completely extended when wrapped in a blanket.

20. Treatment of clubfoot may be divided into three stages: (1) correction, (2) maintenance of correction, and (3) long-term follow-up.

Discussion Questions

1. In light of what you have studied regarding fetal growth and development, why is length of gestation a more significant measure of maturity than size or weight?

2. With technologic advances it is now possible to save many infants with abnormalities who would formerly not have survived. Many of these infants will have developmental disabilities and require special care for the rest of their lives. What significance does this have for nurses?

3. Many of the more sophisticated tests such as amniocentesis and ultrasound enable the physician to detect abnormalities before birth. As a nurse, how would you respond and provide care to a woman who knows before delivery that the child will not be normal?

4. In what ways would you modify nursing care if the infant or child is physically handicapped? Mentally handicapped?

5. Hemolytic disease in the newborn is most often related to blood incompatibilities. Which combinations are most likely to cause hemolytic problems? What diagnostic tests are used to monitor the fetal/neonatal condition? What, if anything, can be done to prevent these problems?

15

Intensive Care of the Newborn

CHAPTER OBJECTIVES

After studying this chapter, the student should be able to perform the following:

1 State the main objective of neonatal intensive care units (NICUs).
2 Indicate three main types of diagnoses encountered among the newborns admitted to an NICU.
3 List five responsibilities of the comprehensive regional perinatal center.
4 Discuss four ways that health care personnel can reduce the anxiety of parents whose infants are transferred to a regional NICU.
5 Identify at least six maternal risk factors that should alert the maternity staff to possible neonatal difficulty.
6 Discuss the potential for increased heat loss by the premature neonate.
7 Describe how output is monitored (measured and analyzed) for the typical NICU patient.
8 Enumerate five kinds of analyses that must be a constant concern of the nurse caring for a newborn who is receiving oxygen-enriched ventilatory support.
9 Explain the increased need for fluid of the premature or low-birth-weight infant and four ways the hydration of these babies can be monitored.
10 State two reasons why overfeeding a premature infant may be particularly dangerous and two methods that can be used to evaluate the infant's ability to digest what is offered.
11 Describe four methods that can be employed to provide nourishment to newborns depending on their condition and needs.
12 Discuss methods of maintaining a patent airway and avoiding further respiratory problems for the infant receiving ventilatory assistance.
13 Discuss three problems associated with the use of umbilical catheters and possible signs of such difficulties.
14 Indicate the major developmental problem of infants with RDS and its prenatal assessment of risk.
15 Identify normal values for pH, Po_2, and Pco_2 levels in arterial blood after the first few hours following birth.
16 Indicate three nursing considerations when caring for an infant receiving phototherapy.
17 Discuss the infections identified by the acronym TORCHES and their impact on the fetus.
18 Describe three aspects of the treatment and nursing care of the newborn infant undergoing withdrawal symptoms because of maternal drug addiction before his birth.
19 Emphasize the need to teach that maternal alcohol consumption during pregnancy may negatively affect the unborn infant.
20 Describe the potential problems faced by infants of diabetic mothers, and stress the need for close observation for their detection.

NEONATAL INTENSIVE CARE UNIT

Neonatology, the study and treatment of the newborn, has rapidly become a highly specialized area of pediatrics. Continuing advances in detection, prevention, and treatment of disorders of the newborn have led to the development of specialized neonatal units with highly trained personnel. Basic nursing courses do not attempt to prepare the vocational nurse to work in these units. However, with further training and education, selected licensed vocational-practical nurses may be part of these specialized units. Students may have a period of observation and closely guided participation during their obstetric or pediatric experiences. This chapter is designed to help these students better understand the types of patients, conditions, and procedures they may encounter, and to help nurses better comprehend the histories of small patients who are transferred from special care areas to other sections of the hospital.

Objectives and characteristics

The main objective of the neonatal intensive care unit, (NICU) is to provide the earliest and maximum degree of medical and nursing care for the infant at risk so that each infant attains the best possible outcome. As neonatal mortality is reduced, continuing efforts must also be made to decrease the incidence of long-term problems

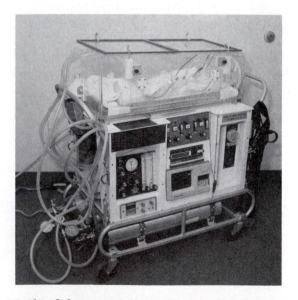

FIG 15-1 Infant transport incubator equipped with built-in ventilator, cardiorespiratory and blood pressure monitor, intravenous infusion pump, and transcutaneous P_{O_2}/P_{CO_2} monitor. *(Courtesy John Wimmer, MD, East Carolina University.)*

such as chronic lung disease, intestinal disorders, and neurodevelopmental handicaps. Awareness of the causes and prevention of residual damage is therefore necessary for the NICU nurse.

Prematurity and its various complications are the most frequently encountered problems in the NICU. Other patients have birth defects, infection, jaundice, hypoglycemia, perinatal asphyxia, or one of many less common disorders. Furthermore, since most hospital recovery rooms are poorly equipped and staffed to care for small infants, the NICU must provide postoperative care for neonates recovering from general anesthesia and various surgical procedures.

NICU patients require many types of specialized care to meet their needs. Mechanical ventilation, intravenous fluid therapy, continuous monitoring of vital signs, body temperature regulation, and even mundane tasks such as feedings require specially trained physicians and nursing personnel and sophisticated biomedical equipment. The NICU nurse must become comfortable with handling tiny, fragile infants and proficient with the many mechanical aids used in their care.

The regional perinatal center

Because intensive care facilities are very expensive and are seldom necessary in smaller general hospitals, the concept of the regional perinatal center has evolved. In addition to the NICU, such a center provides an obstetric-perinatal service for both outpatient and inpatient care of high-risk mothers and their unborn babies. The center usually serves a defined geographic region, accepting referrals of patients with complicated conditions from other hospitals. It often operates a newborn transport system to bring critically ill neonates born elsewhere to the NICU.

Other responsibilities of the comprehensive perinatal center include the supervision of continuing education for health professionals of the region, long-term follow-up of infants treated in the NICU, and ongoing research in perinatal-neonatal medicine. Many perinatal centers are associated with schools of medicine, nursing, and other health professions.

Neonatal transport

When neonatal problems are anticipated, the mother should be transferred to the perinatal center for delivery if possible. Such an "in utero transport" is not only safer for the infant but also prevents the undesirable separation of mother and baby. However, since many infants with serious problems are born at hospitals without neonatal intensive care facilities, the regional center must be able to provide safe, immediate transfer to the NICU when necessary. The neonatal transport team usually consists of a pediatrician or a neonatal nurse clinician or practitioner, a respiratory therapist, and one or more NICU staff nurses. Reliable ambulance and, in some areas, helicopter or airplane service is necessary. Special equipment is needed, including a transport incubator (Fig. 15-1) capable of maintaining the infant's body temperature, a portable monitor, intravenous infusion device, and ventilation equipment to provide care in transit.

The infant must be evaluated quickly. Laboratory tests, x-ray examinations, or procedures may be necessary. Intubation, umbilical catheterization, chest tube placement, administration of antibiotics, glucose, or fluids, and warming or other maneuvers may be required. Infants should always be adequately stabilized before departing for the NICU.

Before the transport team leaves the referring hospital, they should talk with the infant's parents, telling them about the child's condition and what will be done in the NICU. Visiting hours should be discussed and telephone numbers given, as well as directions to the NICU. If at all possible, both parents should be allowed to see and handle the infant, and a photograph of the baby should be given to them. They should be encouraged to visit their infant as soon and as frequently as possible.

Supportive care of the parents

Separation of an infant from its parents in the immediate postpartum period, although necessary to provide adequate treatment for critically ill babies, can be extremely disruptive to the establishment of normal parent-infant interaction. For this reason the NICU personnel must be extremely supportive of the parents and make every effort to help them adapt to this stressful situation. Visiting should be restricted only when absolutely necessary, e.g., for example, while procedures are performed, while the medical staff is making rounds, or during emergencies. Parents should be encouraged to touch and hold their infant as much as possible, and they should help with bathing, feeding, giving vitamins, and other daily routines as soon as the infant's condition permits.

Ominous terms such as "brain damage," "cerebral palsy," and "blindness" should not be used. Parents whose children have suffered setbacks should be informed and counseled appropriately, but the practice of telling them to "expect the worst" can severely interfere with the parent-infant attachment process. Most patients cared for in the NICU survive with minimum, if any, permanent handicaps, so parents should usually be en-

couraged. Open lines of communication between parents and staff should keep them aware of their child's progress and alleviate unfounded apprehensions. Although the parents' presence in the NICU and frequent questions can sometimes be a nuisance, their feelings must be respected. In this way the psychologic trauma of having their baby in the unit may be minimized.

Staffing in the NICU

Because of the critical nature of the NICU patient's condition, constant vigilance is necessary to anticipate crises—preventing them, if possible—and to be prepared when they occur. Early detection of deterioration improves the chances for successful intervention. The nurses work closely with the physicians, some of whom must be immediately available at all times.

Since potentially life-threatening conditions may be heralded by subtle changes in the patient's behavior or appearance, the nurse must develop astute powers of observation. A clear understanding of each infant's disease process is imperative, and preparation must be made for any emergency situation that might result from the disease itself or from the treatment (for example, a pneumothorax that develops in an infant receiving mechanical ventilation). The nurse must also be familiar with the biomedical equipment, such as monitors and ventilators, and be able to interpret alarms and spot malfunctions quickly.

The ideal nurse-patient ratio is 1:1 for infants who are critically ill or in an immediate postoperative phase (Fig. 15-2). The average ratio is 1:2 for most sick infants and up to 1:4 during the convalescent phase. Some hospital settings provide a separate progressive care unit where the staffing ratio can be increased.

Nursery personnel use a separate covergown technique for each infant. Handwashing is of major importance; personnel wash meticulously before and after handling any infant or piece of equipment. Caps and masks are not used. Cover gowns are worn by physicians, parents, and other personnel. In some hospitals persons may freely enter the NICU without gowning or washing as long as no infant or equipment is touched.

CRITICALLY ILL NEONATE
Anticipation of the need for care

Prompt recognition and treatment of the sick infant are of utmost importance in obtaining the best possible outcome. The majority of patients are the products of a relatively small number of high-risk pregnancies. Therefore knowledge of predisposing factors often allows anticipation and early treatment when appropriate, includ-

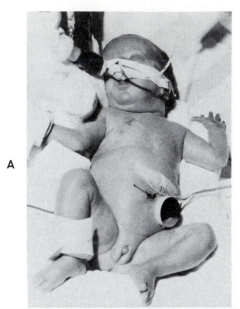

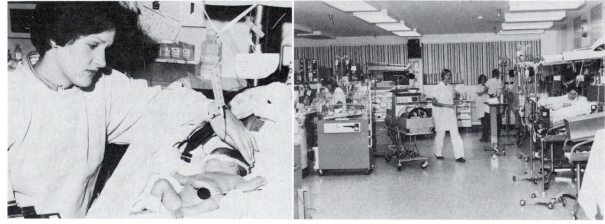

FIG 15-2 Neonatal intensive care unit or special care nursery from three perspectives. **A,** This tiny infant was 1 month old when photograph was taken. Born weighing 2¼ pounds (1,022 g), she was first ventilated mechanically because of respiratory distress syndrome. Heat sensor and umbilical catheter are present. She had patent ductus arteriosus repair when 6 days old. **B,** Mother came in almost every afternoon. She progressively participated in care of her daughter as child improved. **C,** One corner of busy NICU showing mother at side of her baby who was receiving maximum care. *(Photography by Bob Burgen; courtesy Children's Hospital and Health Center, San Diego, Calif.)*

ing transfer of the mother to the perinatal center for delivery. An increased incidence of neonatal disease is seen in infants whose mothers have any of the following risk factors: (1) lack of prenatal care, poor nutrition, or other socioeconomic problems; (2) previous history of obstetric complications, such as abortion, stillbirth or neonatal death, premature delivery, prolonged infertility, pregnancy-induced hypertension (PIH), placenta previa, placental abruption, or blood group incompatibilities; and (3) medical illnesses, such as diabetes mellitus, cardiac or renal disease, infection, or alcoholism or drug addiction. Complications of labor and birth may also adversely affect the infant. These include premature labor, premature rupture of membranes, abnormal presentation or fetal size, multiple births, meconium staining of amniotic fluid, and inappropriate maternal analgesia or anesthesia.

These infants deserve special attention, usually including the presence of the pediatrician at the birth and frequently requiring a period of observation in the NICU.

Maintenance of body temperature

Attention to temperature regulation is an important part of the nursing care of sick neonates. Many neonates, especially low birth weight premature infants, have difficulty maintaining body temperature. They have thin skin that is not insulated by the subcutaneous fat characteristic of full-term infants. Small babies also have an increased proportion of body surface area to body mass, and immature central nervous system temperature regulation centers. For these reasons they have increased heat losses caused by conduction, convection, radiation, and evaporation. Keeping the infant's environmental temperature in the neutral thermal range allows normal body temperature to be maintained with the least expenditure of energy. This decreases the baby's requirements of oxygen, calories, and fluid. It is an extremely important measure, particularly in the small premature infant with little reserve capacity. (See also pp. 580-581.)

Skin temperature is continuously monitored by a sensor attached to the baby's chest or abdomen (Fig. 15-2, A). Axillary and/or rectal temperature should be checked with a thermometer and recorded periodically. Fluctuations in temperature or discrepancies between skin and core temperature may indicate infection or other problems and should be reported promptly.

Open radiant warmer beds provide easy access to infants requiring frequent intervention and close observation. Treatments, procedures, and nursing care can be performed without disturbing the thermal environment. The bed can be tilted up or down. Special enclosed infant care units (incubators) are used for infants who need to be isolated or do not require such frequent direct contact.

Monitoring the NICU patient

Heart rate and respirations are monitored continuously by an electronic cardiorespiratory monitor with audible alarms for apnea, tachypnea, bradycardia, and tachycardia. Blood pressure is measured by the Doppler method, by a standard infant blood pressure cuff, or by means of a pressure transducer connected to an indwelling arterial catheter (usually umbilical). Pulse oximeters may be used to monitor oxygen saturation, and transcutaneous oxygen and carbon dioxide monitors may be helpful with patients with respiratory problems. With each voiding the infant's urine is measured and tested for blood, glucose, protein, pH, and specific gravity. Urine output can be measured using disposable diapers, which are weighed (in grams) before use and again after the infant has voided on them. Alternatively, plastic urine collection bags can be used, but they may cause skin trauma and collection is sometimes difficult, especially from females. Stools should be described and checked for occult blood. Accurate intake and output charts must be maintained and must include blood withdrawn for diagnostic tests. Daily weights should also be recorded. Small infants with fluid balance problems are sometimes weighed every 12 hours.

Infants with respiratory problems require particularly careful observation. The oxygen content of the inspired air-oxygen mixture ideally should be monitored continuously or at least checked hourly. For patients receiving ventilatory support (either continuous positive airway pressure or mechanical ventilation), the ventilator settings, endotracheal tube position, and infant's respirations and breath sounds must be frequently checked. The chest should be transilluminated periodically to detect pneumothorax if this complication is likely. Equipment malfunction occasionally occurs and must be detected and corrected quickly. Although all the modern, highly developed equipment currently used in the NICU is a great asset, *the nurse is the most important and accurate monitor* of the infant's condition, and the tendency to rely on mechanical devices must be avoided.

Fluid therapy and feeding

The fluid requirements of the newborn are highly variable and depend on many factors. In the healthy full-term infant an intake of 75 to 90 ml/kg/24 hr is usually adequate during the first 24 to 48 hours of life, increasing to about 150 ml/kg/24 hr over the next few days. The premature infant, however, has increased insensible water losses and may normally require 140 to 160 ml/kg/24 hr. Water losses are also increased by tachypnea, abnormal gastrointestinal losses, administration of a concentrated solution (either orally or intravenously), and fever. The frequently used open radiant warmer bed further increases evaporative loss of water, as does the use of phototherapy for hyperbilirubinemia. Thus a small infant in whom several of these factors are operative may need an intake of 200 ml/kg/24 hr or even more. On the other hand, fluids should be restricted in some cases, depending on the infant's particular problems. The most important aspect of fluid therapy management is constant monitoring of the infant's state of hydration and appropriate readjustment of fluid intake. This is accomplished by following serial weights, intake and output, urine specific gravities (normal range 1.002 to 1.010), and serum electrolytes.

Caloric requirements are also somewhat variable and are higher in the low-birth-weight infant (120 to 150 cal/kg/24 hr) than in the full-term infant (110 to 130 cal/kg/24 hr). Increased metabolic rate, for any reason, increases caloric requirements. Various diseases, environmental temperature above or below the neutral thermal environment, and increased physical activity all increase the baby's needs.

Fluids are usually given intravenously to small, sick infants. Since volumes are relatively small and must be measured precisely, automatic infusion pumps with safety features to prevent accidental fluid overload are used. Fluids may be given through a peripheral vein, an umbilical arterial catheter (if one is needed for blood gas sampling), or a central venous line.

Tube feedings are begun on stable infants who are unable to take the bottle or breast orally, usually because of prematurity or respiratory or neurologic difficulty. Orogastric or nasogastric tubes can be used for either intermittent or continuous feeding. Longer tubes can be passed through the stomach into the small intestine for continuous infusions, so-called transpyloric or naso-duodenal feeding. Initially small amounts of diluted formula or breast milk are given. If these early feedings are well tolerated, the concentration and volumes are gradually advanced. Excessive feeding may cause regurgitation and aspiration or intestinal complications. Feeding intolerance must therefore be watched for by aspirating the stomach contents before giving feedings or periodically when feedings are continuous and by observing carefully for changes in abdominal girth, bowel sounds, and stooling patterns.

Nipple feedings may be attempted in the vigorous infant with intact gag and suck reflexes. The breast-feeding mother is encouraged to begin nursing as soon as the baby's condition permits. Until then, she may express milk manually or with a breast pump, freeze it, and bring it to the nursery, where it is stored to give to the baby at a later time.

Infants in whom intestinal feeding must be delayed for long periods are begun on parenteral (intravenous) hyperalimentation, which provides carbohydrate, fat, protein, vitamins, and minerals. Central venous catheters may be inserted for this purpose, or peripheral veins can be used. Complications may occur including sepsis (with central catheters), metabolic imbalance, and liver toxicity. Successful management requires a team effort involving the physician, nurse, and pharmacist.

Airway maintenance

Infants requiring ventilatory support are unable to clear secretions from their lungs and airways by normal mechanisms. Endotracheal tubes must therefore be suctioned to prevent airway occlusion and atelectasis and to minimize the risk of respiratory infections. The frequency of this suctioning depends on the disease process, primarily the amount and type of secretions present, ranging from every 2 hours in those with copious secretions to every 6 to 8 hours in patients with scant secretions.

Suction of the endotracheal tube should be performed with sterile technique, and the length of the suction catheter inserted should be no greater than the length of the endotracheal tube to minimize trauma to the tracheobronchial epithelium. The suctioning should be as gentle as possible and continued for no longer than 5 to 10 seconds, after which the catheter should be withdrawn and the baby ventilated briefly to allow for recovery before continuing suction. Small amounts (0.5 to 1 ml) of saline may be injected into the endotracheal tube to thin secretions if necessary. The infant should, of course, be monitored carefully during the suctioning procedure, ideally with a continuous transcutaneous blood gas reading or oximeter.

Infants with excessive secretions, such as those with pneumonia or meconium aspiration, may benefit from chest physiotherapy (CPT) before airway suctioning. Percussion or vibration should be done for 1 to 2 minutes either manually or with a specially adapted electric toothbrush or small portable vibrator. CPT should not be done on small premature infants with respiratory distress syndrome in the first few days of life because it may increase the risk of intracranial hemorrhage. Fortunately these patients do not usually have a significant amount of secretions.

Infants with respiratory disease or neurologic impairment should not be maintained in a flat supine position for extended periods of time. Their position should be alternated every few hours to prevent pooling of secretions in any one area of the lungs. A specific position may be indicated in cases of one-sided atelectasis or other localized problems.

Care of the umbilical catheter

Umbilical arterial catheters (UACs) are frequently used in the NICU, usually for monitoring arterial blood gases and aortic blood pressure in critically ill patients requiring ventilatory support. Umbilical *venous* catheters are used for exchange transfusions, emergency administration of fluids, medications, or blood, or occasionally for monitoring of central venous pressure. Either type of catheter may lead to serious complications if proper precautions are not observed. Hypovolemic shock or death may result from sudden blood loss if the catheter is accidentally removed or if loose connections at the stopcock or extension tubing allow leakage. Infection or emboli may be introduced with careless withdrawal of blood samples, administration of medications, or changing of tubing. Finally, clot formation in the aorta or other major arteries may lead to infarction of the kidneys, intestines, or lower extremities.

Most NICUs have written policies and procedures re-garding the use and care of UACs. These provide details, such as how to draw blood samples, how to connect and calibrate blood pressure monitoring equipment, and how to infuse various fluids and medications. Vasoconstrictive drugs, such as epinephrine, should never be given via the UAC, and hypertonic substances should be diluted or infused very slowly. Difficulty drawing blood, changes in the blood pressure tracing, and discoloration, coolness, or loss of pulses in the legs may indicate serious UAC complications, and immediate removal may be necessary.

COMMON PROBLEMS ENCOUNTERED IN THE NICU
Respiratory distress syndrome

Respiratory distress syndrome (RDS), or hyaline membrane disease, is the most common problem in the NICU and, before recent advances in ventilator management, was the leading cause of neonatal mortality (Fig. 15-3). It is most frequently seen in infants of less than 36 weeks' gestation, although occasionally a near-term baby is affected.

The onset of symptoms often occurs in the delivery room where the baby has low Apgar scores and requires assistance in establishing respirations. In other cases the infant may appear normal initially but begin to have expiratory grunting and nasal flaring in the first few hours

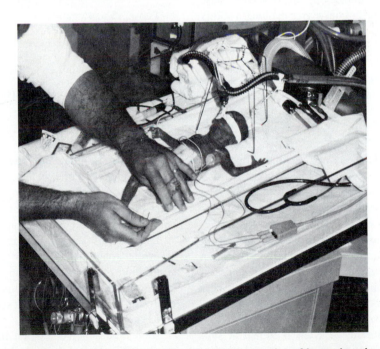

FIG 15-3 Another blood gas determination for a small representative of humanity who has respiratory distress syndrome. *(Courtesy Louis Gluck, MD, University of California—San Diego Medical Center.)*

of life (usually less than 6 hours). Respiratory distress becomes increasingly obvious in room air with progressive tachypnea, retractions, and cyanosis. A chest radiograph is diagnostic, revealing characteristic granular density, air bronchograms, and diminished lung volume. Arterial blood gases show hypoxia and usually a combined metabolic and respiratory acidosis.

Etiologic factors. The cause of RDS is somewhat controversial, but it is definitely a developmental disease (related to natural maturational changes) with many contributing factors. Biochemical lung maturity marked by the appearance of adequate amounts of surface-active phospholipid compounds in alveoli is important in preventing RDS.

These surface-active compounds, collectively referred to as surfactant, begin to appear in the fetal lung early in development but are not usually fully mature until about 36 to 37 weeks' gestation. Surfactant opposes the natural tendency of alveoli to collapse completely at the end of each expiration and thereby keeps the lung partially expanded at all times.

Infants in whom surfactant is deficient must completely reexpand their lungs with each breath, greatly increasing the work of breathing. Extreme stiffness of the lungs (decreased compliance) and progressive atelectasis (collapse of alveoli) result, leading to hypoxia, fatigue, and decreased ventilation, all of which cause acidosis. The acidosis further decreases the lung's ability to synthesize surfactant and also decreases pulmonary blood flow, thus worsening the RDS and creating a vicious cycle.

The amount of surfactant in the lungs normally increases significantly at approximately 33 to 34 weeks' gestation. Certain factors, such as chronic placental abruption, prolonged rupture of membranes, maternal hypertension, and possibly maternal narcotic drug use, induce earlier surfactant appearance and therefore protect the infant from RDS. On the other hand, maternal diabetes and erythroblastosis fetalis appear to delay lung maturation, and perinatal asphyxia worsens RDS.

Treatment. Treatment with various types of surfactant preparations has proven helpful in reducing signs of respiratory distress. Known as surfactant replacement therapy, this technique is currently in the final stages of clinical investigation and will be available in the near future. This major breakthrough promises to reduce significantly the incidence and severity of RDS.

Meanwhile the treatment of RDS is aimed at supporting the infant by assisting oxygenation and ventilation until the baby's lungs produce adequate surfactant

Blood gas analysis

Indications
To monitor oxygenation, ventilation, and acid-base balance

Methods of obtaining
1. Umbilical arterial or other indwelling arterial catheter
2. Arterial puncture (radial, temporal, or other)
3. Arterialized capillary blood sample drawn from heel, ulnar aspect of hand, or digit (extremity is first warmed for 5 to 10 minutes)

   Blood gas analysis can be performed on as little as 0.1 ml of blood drawn into a heparinized capillary tube, depending on the particular blood gas analyzer used. Care must be taken not to allow air bubbles or blood clots to enter the sample; sample should be placed on ice unless it is analyzed immediately.
4. Transcutaneous Po_2/Pco_2 monitor
5. Pulse oximeter (measures oxygen saturation only)

Normal values for arterial blood of newborns in room air
(Normal values in the first hours after birth are different)
pH   7.35 to 7.45
Po_2 70 to 100 mm Hg
         (40 to 50 mm Hg for capillary sample)
Pco_2 35 to 45 mm Hg

(usually within 2 or 3 days). The measures used depend on the severity of the disease. Mild to moderate cases are treated with increased concentrations of environmental oxygen, usually given by hood. More severely affected infants require continuous positive airway pressure (CPAP) to prevent the atelectasis that occurs at the end of expiration. This in turn improves oxygenation. This pressure is usually applied through nasal prongs or an endotracheal tube.

If the infant develops hypoxia, respiratory failure, or recurrent apnea despite CPAP and oxygen, mechanical ventilation is instituted with an infant respirator. Appropriate adjustments must be made for respiratory rate, expiratory and inspiratory pressures, and concentration of oxygen.

It must be remembered that all of these forms of treatment carry certain risks to the baby. High concentrations of inspired oxygen and ventilator pressures are known to be damaging to the lungs. High arterial P_{O_2} (exact critical levels are unknown) in the retinal arteries can cause blindness in premature infants. Infants receiving increased pressure therapy (CPAP or mechanical ventilation) are at risk for pneumothorax and cardiovascular disturbances. Endotracheal intubation predisposes the infant to infection, or the tube itself may become occluded with secretions. Because of these potential complications, the infant with RDS must be carefully evaluated, and the risks of therapy balanced against the benefits.

General supportive measures, such as proper regulation of fluids, acid-base status, and thermal environment, are of great importance in the infant with RDS. An umbilical artery catheter is often used for frequent arterial blood gas sampling and blood pressure monitoring as well as administration of parenteral fluids and medications. Antibiotics are not effective against the disease itself but are often used as a prophylactic measure. Transfusions are often necessary to replace blood drawn for testing.

Complications. Aside from the risks of therapy just mentioned, the complications of RDS include intracranial hemorrhage, patent ductus arteriosus (PDA), hypoglycemia, hypocalcemia, and hyperbilirubinemia. Intracranial hemorrhage is more common in infants of less than 32 weeks' gestation and is a major cause of death and disability. The onset of symptoms resulting from PDA usually coincides with the recovery phase of RDS. Typical congestive heart failure may occur with an enlarged heart and tachycardia. More often, however, an infant who has been improving clinically simply stops making progress and becomes dependent on oxygen, CPAP, or the ventilator. Fluid restriction and diuretics may be beneficial and often the PDA closes spontaneously, but some require surgical ligation or pharmacologic closure with indomethacin.

Prevention of RDS. Prenatal assessment of lung surfactant maturity can be done by performing an amniocentesis and analyzing surfactant in the amniotic fluid. The now-familiar L/S ratio compares the content of lecithin, an important surfactant, to sphingomyelin, an inactive phospholipid. An L/S ratio of 2.0 usually indicates lung maturity, as does the presence of another important compound, phosphatidyl glycerol (PG). Elective delivery (cesarean section or induction) should be delayed until the studies indicate lung maturity to minimize the risk of RDS. In some cases the administration of glucocorticoids to the mother 48 to 72 hours before delivery may stimulate fetal lung maturity and therefore decrease the risk of RDS.

Meconium aspiration

Staining of the amniotic fluid with meconium, the stool of the fetus, occurs in approximately 10% to 15% of all births. It may indicate intrauterine distress, and in some instances the infant may make gasping respiratory efforts before the head is delivered and thus aspirate the meconium into the lungs. Although normal amniotic fluid is usually harmless to the lungs, the particles of meconium produce obstruction of the airways and cause respiratory difficulty. The infant may be vigorous and breathing easily, but if significant intrauterine asphyxia has occurred, he will be depressed and require assistance in establishing respirations. In the latter case, intubation and direct tracheal suction are performed to remove as much meconium as possible before the use of positive pressure ventilation. Ideally this prevents forcing meconium from the airway into the lungs and reduces the severity of the disease. Suctioning of the baby's oropharynx after delivery of the head but before delivery of the shoulders and chest also minimizes the inhalation of meconium. Respiratory distress occurs in about 15% of meconium-stained infants and varies from mild to severe. In most cases distress resolves within 48 hours, but occasionally ventilatory assistance must be continued for longer periods. Treatment consists of oxygen, CPT and suction, and generally supportive measures. Antibiotics may be used, and mechanical ventilation is sometimes necessary for severe cases. Pneumothorax is a common complication.

Pneumothorax

Many newborns (possibly 1% of all babies) develop pneumothorax (free air in the pleural space), but the majority of them remain asymptomatic and the condition resolves without treatment. Pneumothorax usually occurs spontaneously as a result of the high intrathoracic pressures that infants generate when expanding their lungs with the first few breaths. Other cases may be caused by positive pressure ventilation or aspiration of meconium or blood. Premature infants are more susceptible to pneumothorax than full-term infants. Clinical signs include tachypnea, tachycardia, cyanosis, shifting of the cardiac impulse, decreased blood pressure, and irritability. Transillumination of the chest is significantly increased by a tension pneumothorax. The diagnosis is confirmed by chest radiograph.

Treatment of the infant with pneumothorax depends on the severity of the symptoms. The infant with mild or no signs needs only careful observation. If severe distress is present, the pneumothorax should be aspirated by needle and a chest tube inserted into the pleural space. The chest tube is usually connected to suction with a water seal. Follow-up radiographs are indicated to determine the position of the chest tube and reexpansion of the lung. Patency of the tube must be maintained by preventing kinking, clotting, and looping. The chest tube can usually be removed within a few days as the respiratory status improves.

Hyperbilirubinemia

Hyperbilirubinemia occurs to some degree in normal newborns and is often exaggerated in the premature or sick neonate. Bilirubin, most of which is formed from the breakdown of hemoglobin, is taken up by liver cells, where it is modified and excreted through the bile ducts into the intestine. This process is delayed in newborns, leading to so-called physiologic hyperbilirubinemia.

Hyperbilirubinemia is considered to be pathologic if the serum bilirubin level exceeds 12 mg/100 ml or if obvious jaundice appears in the first 24 hours. The most common cause is hemolytic disease (for example, Rh or ABO blood group incompatibility of the fetus and mother). Other causes sometimes encountered are polycythemia, excessive bruising, hemolytic anemias, sepsis, intrauterine viral infection, and metabolic disorders.

Hyperbilirubinemia is treated with phototherapy and, in severe cases, exchange transfusions. Phototherapy breaks down bilirubin in the skin. Infants receiving this treatment usually wear only an abbreviated diaper and eye shields. The babies must be periodically turned to ensure proper skin exposure, and they should be given more liquid to compensate for evaporative fluid loss associated with the treatment.

In an exchange transfusion, the infant's blood is replaced, ideally removing much of the excess bilirubin. The objective of the treatment is the prevention of kernicterus, a neurologic condition caused by deposit of bilirubin into the basal ganglia of the brain. Hearing loss may result from bilirubin toxicity to the auditory nerve. The exact serum bilirubin level at which damage occurs varies widely, depending on the maturity and clinical condition of the infant.

Neonatal sepsis

The newborn infant has incompletely developed immunologic responses and therefore has increased susceptibility to infection—bacterial, viral, and other types. Once an infection is acquired, it may quickly invade the bloodstream (neonatal sepsis or septicemia) and lead to meningitis, pneumonia, urinary tract infection, osteomyelitis, or other complications. Certain factors predispose infants to infection, including prematurity, prolonged rupture of membranes, maternal infection, difficult labor with fetal distress, and special procedures, such as resuscitation, intubation, and umbilical or central vein catheterization. Presenting signs are respiratory distress with grunting and tachypnea, poor feeding, vomiting, lethargy, temperature instability, jaundice, and apnea.

Group B streptococcal infections have been most often identified in the past years, but many other bacteria may cause sepsis, including other streptococci, *Staphylococcus, Listeria,* and Gram-negative organisms. In long-term NICU patients *Staphylococcus epidermidis* has become the most common pathogen, but less common bacteria such as *Citrobacter, Serratia, Pseudomonas,* or viruses may be encountered. Fungal infections, usually *Candida albicans,* have become more commonly seen in the past few years.

Early treatment is of extreme importance in obtaining a favorable outcome. Once infection is suspected, cultures should be taken promptly of blood, urine, spinal fluid, stool, tracheal aspirate, and additional sites as indicated. Broad-spectrum therapy, usually a combination of two antibiotics such as ampicillin and gentamicin, should be started immediately. Therapy may be changed later, when the results of cultures are obtained and sensitivities of the particular organism(s) are known.

Intrauterine infection

Although the fetus is protected by the mother from many infectious diseases, some microorganisms have the ability to cross the placenta and may cause significant damage. If a pregnant woman becomes infected at a time when her fetus is susceptible, intrauterine infection may result. These infections are commonly referred to as the TORCHES (*TO*xoplasmosis, *R*ubella, *C*ytomegalovirus, *HE*rpes, and *S*yphilis), although other agents are now known to cause fetal infection.

Rubella (German measles) is probably the best-known and most feared intrauterine infection. Rubella infection occurs in up to 50% of fetuses of mothers who acquire the disease during the first 8 weeks of pregnancy. The fetal infection rate then declines and is very low after the first trimester. Affected infants have demonstrated a variety of manifestations from the most severe congenital rubella syndrome (intrauterine growth retardation, cardiac defects, cataracts, deafness, anemia, jaundice, and mental retardation) to the apparently normal newborn with only mild hearing loss. Diagnosis can be confirmed by viral cultures of the infant's pharynx, urine, or stool and by antibody titers on the mother and infant. Immunization programs to prevent infection of pregnant women are of utmost importance, since no specific treatment exists.

Cytomegalovirus (CMV) is the most common intrauterine infection and, like rubella, may have a variety of effects in the infant. Most infants are asymptomatic, but others may have microcephaly, growth retardation, hepatitis, low platelet count, seizures, and pneumonia. Diagnosis is confirmed by cultures and by antibody studies.

Toxoplasmosis, a protozoan disease that may be contracted by the ingestion of raw meat or food contaminated with cat feces, is relatively uncommon in the United States. It may be entirely asymptomatic in the infected mother. It primarily affects the fetal central nervous system and may cause mental retardation, blindness, deafness, convulsions, and hydrocephalus. These infants should be treated with sulfadiazine and pyrimethamine, although much of the damage is probably irreversible.

Congenital syphilis is more likely if maternal infection occurs in the latter part of pregnancy, or infection may be acquired during the birth process. Infected infants usually appear normal in the immediate postpartum period, although prematurity and stillbirths sometimes result. Most cases of congenital syphilis exhibit a typical rash, profuse nasal discharge, radiographic defects of the long bones, and hepatitis in early infancy. Congenital syphilis is most often detected by screening for maternal disease with routine serologic testing on all pregnant women. Treatment with penicillin eradicates the disease, although mental retardation and other sequelae may not be totally prevented. (See also pp. 172-174.)

Recently identified as an important sexually transmitted bacterium, *Chlamydia trachomatis* is also acquired by the infant during birth. Conjunctivitis or pneumonitis can result during the first few weeks of life. Other organisms known to infect fetuses include hepatitis B virus and HIV, the virus that causes AIDS (acquired immune deficiency syndrome). Infants with these illnesses do not usually become symptomatic in the neonatal period. Herpes simplex virus may be transmitted from maternal genital infections to the infant during birth and cause a rapidly fatal illness (p. 174). As screening techniques and virology studies become more sensitive and widespread, knowledge of these fetal infections will increase, as will their relative importance in NICU patients.

Perinatal substance abuse

The increasing use of cocaine, especially "crack," by pregnant women has elevated the number of fetal deaths and premature deliveries. Such mothers may have placental detachment (abruption), causing significant maternal bleeding and hypoxia in the infant. Infants of these mothers may die or suffer brain damage. Others are exposed to the risks associated with premature birth.

Infants whose mothers are addicted to heroin, barbiturates, amphetamines, or other drugs inherit the drug dependence. These babies usually appear normal at birth but begin to show signs of withdrawal after 8 to 12 hours. Extreme irritability, constant crying, jitteriness, poor feeding, emesis, diarrhea, respiratory distress, and seizures may occur. Signs are alleviated by administration of paregoric, phenobarbital, or tranquilizers (chlorpromazine, diazepam) and by keeping the infant well wrapped in a quiet, dimly lit environment. Intravenous fluids may be necessary to prevent dehydration or hypoglycemia. Medication is gradually decreased and discontinued over several days.

Fetal alcohol syndrome

The fetal alcohol syndrome has been well documented in infants born to mothers with excessive alcohol intake during pregnancy. These infants may exhibit intrauterine growth retardation, microcephaly, mental deficiency, cardiac defects, and characteristic anomalies of the face and extremities. Lesser effects may occur in babies born to moderate drinkers and may be difficult to recognize, although intellectual impairment may result. These infants may experience withdrawal symptoms similar to those of infants of drug-addicted mothers.

Infants born to diabetic mothers

Infants born to diabetic mothers (IDMs) are predisposed to a number of neonatal disorders. Late intrauterine fetal deaths occur more commonly in diabetic mothers, so their pregnancies must be monitored carefully by the physician. Maternal blood glucose should be controlled as closely as possible, and the fetus should be evaluated frequently for abnormalities of growth and signs of distress. IDMs are at increased risk for RDS, especially if delivered prematurely. Amniocentesis is therefore usually performed to assess fetal lung maturity and help determine the optimum time for delivery.

When maternal diabetes is poorly controlled, the infants may be very large (10 or more pounds) and have a higher incidence of hypoglycemia. Blood glucose should be checked frequently in these infants and in any infant judged to be large for gestational age. Mild maternal diabetes may have gone undetected. Early institution of feedings may prevent hypoglycemia, or intravenous glucose water may be necessary. IDMs are also susceptible to hypocalcemia, hyperbilirubinemia, polycythemia, congenital anomalies, and renal vein thrombosis, especially if the mother's diabetes is not well controlled.

Infants born to mothers with severe or long-standing diabetes suffer intrauterine growth retardation and are usually small rather than large for their gestational age. Their lungs appear to mature early, and they may be protected from having RDS. The severity and duration of the mother's diabetes and her control during pregnancy are the most important factors influencing the infant's problems. (See also p. 169.)

Necrotizing enterocolitis

Necrotizing enterocolitis is an acute, sometimes lethal, intestinal disorder in the newborn and is most commonly seen in the small premature infant. Clinical signs include abdominal distention, vomiting, diarrhea with blood in the stool, apnea, lethargy, hypothermia, and shock. Positive diagnosis is established by abdominal radiographic examination, which may show air in the intestinal wall or free air in the peritoneal cavity.

Initial treatment consists of nasogastric suction, intravenous fluids, antibiotics, and transfusions. Serial abdominal radiographs are performed at frequent intervals to detect progression of the disease or perforation of the bowel, either of which is an indication for surgery. During surgery the areas of necrotic bowel are resected, and a colostomy is usually performed. Anastomosis of the intestine is then done as an elective procedure after the infant has recovered.

The cause of necrotizing enterocolitis is unknown, but inadequate blood flow to the gut is probably important. Such ischemia may damage the intestine and increase susceptibility to infection and possible harmful effects of digestive enzymes.

Postmaturity

Postmature infants are those who are born after 42 or more weeks' gestation. They have dry, parchmentlike skin, long fingernails, and a wide-eyed, alert expression. Meconium staining of the skin is common, and meconium aspiration occurs more frequently than with normal-term infants. Mortality of the postmature infant is nearly twice as high as that of the full-term infant. Postmature infants have diminished glycogen stores and are therefore susceptible to hypoglycemia. They should be fed early and have periodic blood glucose determinations.

• • •

It is important to remember that the material presented here represents only some of the highlights of neonatal intensive care nursing. The student interested in this area should refer to one of the many books currently available on the subject.

Key Concepts

1. The main objective of the NICU is to provide the earliest and maximum degree of medical and nursing care for the infant at risk so that each infant attains the best possible outcome.

2. Newborns may be admitted to the NICU with the following problems: prematurity and its various complications, birth defects, infection, jaundice, hypoglycemia, or perinatal asphyxia.

3. The comprehensive regional perinatal center provides an obstetric-perinatal service for outpatient and inpatient care of high-risk mothers and their fetuses, often operates a newborn transport system, supervises continuing education for health professionals in the region, provides long-term follow-up of infants treated in the NICU, and is responsible for ongoing research in perinatal-neonatal medicine.

4. Health care personnel can reduce the anxiety of parents whose infants are transferred to a regional NICU by restricting visiting only when absolutely necessary, encouraging them to touch and hold their infant, and involving them as much as possible in daily routines such as feeding and bathing. Parents should be kept informed of their child's progress and counseled appropriately.

5. An increased incidence of neonatal disease is seen in infants whose mothers have any of the following risk factors: lack of prenatal care, poor nutrition, or other socioeconomic problems; previous history of obstetric complications; and medical illnesses. Complications in labor and delivery that may signal potential neonatal problems include premature labor, premature rupture of membranes, abnormal presentation or fetal size, multiple births, meconium-stained amniotic fluid, and inappropriate maternal analgesia or anesthesia.

6. Small premature infants have difficulty maintaining

body temperature because they have thin skin that is not insulated by the subcutaneous fat characteristic of full-term infants, increased proportion of body surface area to body mass, and immature central nervous system temperature regulators.

7. The infant's intake and output must be carefully measured and charted. Output includes urine, stool, and blood withdrawn for diagnostic tests. Urine can be measured using disposable diapers or plastic collection bags, and is tested for blood, glucose, protein, pH, and specific gravity. Stools should be described and checked for occult blood.

8. When caring for an infant receiving oxygen-enriched ventilatory support, the nurse should frequently monitor the oxygen content of the air-oxygen, mixture, ventilator settings, endotracheal tube position, and the infant's respirations and breath sounds.

9. The premature or low-birth-weight infant experiences increased water losses as a result of tachypnea, abnormal gastrointestinal losses, administration of a concentrated solution, fever, the use of an open radiant warmer bed, and phototherapy. The infant's state of hydration is monitored by following serial weights, intake and output, urine specific gravities, and serum electrolytes.

10. Overfeeding a premature infant may cause regurgitation and aspiration or intestinal complications. Feeding intolerance can be evaluated by aspirating the stomach contents before giving feedings or periodically when feedings are continuous, and by observing for changes in abdominal girth, bowel sounds, and stooling patterns.

11. Nourishment can be provided to newborns through nipple feeding, orogastric or nasogastric tubes, transpyloric or nasoduodenal feedings, or parenteral hyperalimentation.

12. The patency of the airway of infants receiving ventilatory support can be maintained by suctioning endotracheal tubes, injecting small amounts of saline into the tube to thin secretions, and by administering chest physiotherapy before airway suctioning.

13. Infants with respiratory disease or neurologic impairment should not be maintained in a flat supine position for extended periods of time, but should be repositioned every few hours to prevent pooling of secretions.

14. If proper precautions are not observed, umbilical catheters may result in hypovolemic shock or death from sudden blood loss, infection or emboli, or clot formation leading to infarction of the kidneys, intestines, or lower extremities. Indications of possible complications include difficulty in drawing blood, changes in the blood pressure tracing, and discoloration, coolness, or loss of pulses in the legs.

15. Infants with RDS lack biochemical lung maturity marked by the appearance of adequate amounts of surface-active phospholipid compounds in alveoli. Prenatal assessment of lung surfactant maturity can be done by performing an amniocentesis and analyzing surfactant in the amniotic fluid.

16. Respiratory distress occurs in about 15% of meconium-stained infants and varies from mild to severe. Distress usually resolves within 48 hours.

17. Clinical signs of pneumothorax include tachypnea, tachycardia, cyanosis, shifting of the cardiac impulse, decreased blood pressure, and irritability. The diagnosis is confirmed by chest radiograph.

18. Hyperbilirubinemia is treated with phototherapy and, in severe cases, exchange transfusions. Infants receiving phototherapy usually wear only an abbreviated diaper and eye shields. They must be periodically turned to ensure proper skin exposure and should be given additional liquid to compensate for evaporative fluid loss.

19. Certain factors predispose infants to infection, such as prematurity, prolonged rupture of membranes, maternal infection, fetal distress during labor, and certain special procedures.

20. If a pregnant woman becomes infected with certain microorganisms, its possible for them to cross the placenta and infect the fetus. These infections are known as the TORCHES (*TO*xoplasmosis, *R*ubella, *C*ytomegalovirus, *HE*rpes, and *S*yphilis), and may cause a variety of effects in the infant.

21. An infant who has inherited the mother's drug dependence usually begin to show signs of withdrawal after 8 to 12 hours. Treatment includes the administration of paregoric, phenobarbitol, or tranquilizers, and keeping the infant well wrapped in a quiet, dimly lit environment.

22. An infant born to a mother with excessive alcohol intake during pregnancy may exhibit intrauterine growth retardation, microcephaly, mental deficiency, cardiac defects, and characteristic anomalies of the face and extremities.

23. The severity and duration of the mother's diabetes and her control during pregnancy are the most important factors influencing problems in the infant.

Problems may include RDS, hypoglycemia, hypocalcemia, hyperbilirubinemia, polycythemia, congenital anomalies, and renal vein thrombosis.

24. Necrotizing enterocolitis is an acute, sometimes lethal, intestinal disorder most commonly seen in the small premature infant.

25. Infants born after 42 or more weeks' gestation are considered postmature and have nearly twice the mortality rate as that of the full-term infant.

Discussion Questions

1. Neonatal intensive care units are usually located in large cities and are part of a major medical center. What plan of care is recommended if a high-risk birth is anticipated? What if there is no warning and birth occurs at a location some distance from the nearest NICU?

2. Why is respiratory distress syndrome a major concern in the premature infant? What observations indicate respiratory distress? What diagnostic tests? What is the typical treatment of an infant with RDS? Are there any risks involved in this treatment?

3. Infections acquired before or after birth place the neonate at increased risk. Identify those infections most likely to be contracted before birth. What can be done to reduce this risk? Identify those infections most likely to be contracted at or after birth. What can be done to reduce this risk?

4. Fetal problems related to life habits/addictions of the mother such as alcohol or drug abuse are becoming increasingly common. The newborn becomes the victim of the mother's problem. What do you think should be done in these situations? How could you recognize fetal alcohol syndrome or drug withdrawal in the newborn? What special care will the infant need? What about the mother? Does she require special care? Should other social service agencies be included in the plan of care?

UNIT
V

SUGGESTED SELECTED READINGS AND REFERENCES

General

American Academy of Pediatrics and American College of Obstetricians and Gynecologists: Guidelines for perinatal care, ed 2, Elk Grove Village, Ill, 1988, The Academy.

Anderson GC: Pacifiers: the positive side, MCN 11(2):122, 1986.

Booth CL, Johnson-Crowley N, and Barnard KE: Infant massage and exercise: worth the effort? MCN 10(3):184, 1985.

Brazelton TB: Neonatal behavioral assessment scale, ed 2, Philadelphia, 1984, JB Lippincott Co.

Buckner EB: Use of Brazelton neonatal behavior assessment in planning care for patients and newborns, J Obstet Gynecol Neonatal Nurs 12(1):26, 1983.

Coody D: Congenital hypothyroidism, Pediatr Nurs 10(5):342, 1984.

D'Apolito K: The neonate's response to pain, MCN 9(4):256, 1984.

Foley KL: Caring for the parents of newborn twins, MCN 4(4):221, 1979.

Furrh CB and Copley R: One precious moment: what you can offer when a newborn infant dies, Nursing 89 19(9):52, 1989.

Gino C: SIDS research that causes pain, Am J Nurs 88(10):1353, 1988.

Harrison LL: Teaching stimulation strategies to parents of infants at high risk, MCN 14(2):125, 1989.

Holaday B: Changing views of infant care, 1914-1980, Pediatr Nurs 7(1):21, 1981.

Horn M and Manion J: Creative grandparenting: bonding the generations, J Obstet Gynecol Neonatal Nurs 15(3):233, 1985.

Judd JM: Assessing the newborn from head to toe, Nursing '85 15(12):34, 1985.

Klaus MH and Kennell JH: Bonding: the beginnings of parent to infant attachment, St Louis, 1983, The CV Mosby Co.

Lohnes RC: Reading the fine print, Am J Nurs 86(9):1029, 1986.

Loring C: Newborns: first feeding, first breath, Nursing '89 19(1):109, 1989.

Ludington-Hoe SM: What can newborns really see? Am J Nurs 83(9):1286, 1983.

Marecki M and others: Early sibling attachment, J Obstet Gynecol Neonatal Nurs 14(5):418, 1985.

Mitchell K and Mills NM: Is the sensitive period in parent-infant bonding overrated? Pediatr Nurs 9(2):91, 1983.

Nugent JK: The Brazelton neonatal behavioral assessment scale: implications for intervention, Pediatr Nurs 7(3):18, 1981.

O'Doherty N: Atlas of the newborn, ed 2, Hingham, Mass, 1985, Kluwer Academic Publishers.

Page GG: How well do we evaluate and control infants' pain? Am J Nurs 89(3):317, 1989.

Sherwen LN, Smith DW, and Cueman MA: Common concerns of adoptive mothers, Pediatr Nurs 10(2):127, 1984.

Smith J: Big differences in little people, Am J Nurs 88(4):458, 1988.

Wagner TJ and Hindi-Alexander M: Hazards of baby powder? Pediatr Nurs 10(2):124, 1984.

Watters NE: Combined mother-infant nursing care, J Obstet Gynecol Neonatal Nurs 14(6):478, 1985.

Woolsey SF: Support after sudden infant death, Am J Nurs 88(10):1348, 1988.

Circumcision

Anderson GF: Circumcision, Pediatr Ann 18(3):205, 1989.

Engel NS: Lidocaine dorsal penile nerve block for circumcision, MCN 14(5):311, 1989.

Gibbons MB: Circumcision: the controversy continues, Pediatr Nurs 10(2):103, 1984.

Lincoln GA: Neonatal circumcision: is it needed? J Obstet Gynecol Neonatal Nurs 15(6):463, 1986.

Nesrallah PF: Circumcision: pros and cons, Prim Care 12(12):593, 1985.

Pelosi MA and Apuzzio J: Making circumcision safe and painless, Contemp OB/GYN 24(1):42, 1984.

Wayland JR and Higgins PC: Newborn circumcision: father's involvement, Pediatr Nurs 9(1):41, 1983.

Feeding

Anderson GH: Human milk feeding, Pediatr Clin North Am 32(2):335, 1985.

Barger J and Bull P: A comparison of the bacterial composition of breast milk stored at room temperature and stored in the refrigerator, Int J Childbirth Educ 2(3):29, 1987.

Beckholt AP: Breast milk for infants who cannot breastfeed, J Obstet Gynecol Neonatal Nurs 19(3):216, 1990.

Broussard AB: Anticipatory guidance: adding solids to the infant's diet, J Obstet Gynecol Neonatal Nurs 13(4):239, 1984.

Charles D and Larsen B: How colostrum and milk protect the newborn, Contemp OB/GYN 24(1):143, 1984.

Coreil J and Murphy JE: Maternal commitment lactation practices and breast-feeding duration, J Obstet Gynecol Neonatal Nurs 17(4):273, 1988.

Costa KM: A comparison of colony counts of breast milk using two methods of breast cleansing, J Obstet Gynecol Neonatal Nurs 18(3):231, 1989.

Edgehouse L and Radzyminski SG: A device for supplementing breast-feeding, MCN 15(1):34, 1990.

Gaull GE and others: Current issues in feeding the normal infant, Pediatrics 75(suppl):135, 1985.

Gulick EE: Infant health and breast-feeding, Pediatr Nurs 9(5):359, 1983.

Kahn A and others: Insomnia and cow's milk allergy in infants, Pediatrics 76(6):880, 1985.

Kelts D and Jones E, editors: Manual of pediatric nutrition, Boston, 1984, Little, Brown & Co, Inc.

La Leche League International: The womanly art of breast-feeding, ed 4, New York, 1987, New American Library.

Marmet C and Shell E: Training neonates to suck correctly, MCN 9(6):401, 1984.

Meier P and Wilks S: The bacteria in expressed mother's milk, MCN 12(6):420, 1987.

Nice FJ: Can a breast-feeding mother take medication without harming her infant? MCN 14(1):17, 1989.

Pipes PL: Nutrition in infancy and childhood, ed 4, St Louis, 1989, Times Mirror/Mosby College Publishing.

Reiff MI and Essock-Vitale SM: Hospital influences on early infant-feeding practices, Pediatrics 76(6):872, 1985.

Reifsnider E and Myers ST: Employed mothers can breast-feed, too! MCN 10(4):256, 1985.

Shrago L and Bocar D: The infant's contribution to breastfeeding, J Obstet Gynecol Neonatal Nurs 19(3):209, 1990.

Stahl MD and Guida DA: Slow weight gain in the breast-fed infant: management options, Pediatr Nurs 10(2):117, 1984.

Tiedje LB and Collins C: Combining employment and motherhood, MCN 14(1):23, 1989.

Walker M and Driscoll JW: Sore nipples: the new mother's nemesis, MCN 14(4):260, 1989.

Williams KM and Morse JM: Weaning patterns of first time mothers, MCN 14(3):188, 1989.

Wink DM: Getting through the maze of infant formulas, Am J Nurs 85(4):388, 1985.

Wishon PM and Kinnick VG: Helping infants overcome the problem of obesity, MCN 11(2):118, 1986.

Temperature maintenance

Britton GR: Early mother-infant contact and infant temperature stabilization, J Obstet Gynecol Neonatal Nurs 7(2):84, 1980.

Capobianco JA: How to safeguard the infant against life-threatening heat loss, Nursing '80 10(5):64, 1980.

Davis V: The structure and function of brown adipose tissue in the neonate, J Obstet Gynecol Neonatal Nurs 9(6):368, 1980.

Gardner S: The mother as incubator—after delivery, J Obstet Gynecol Neonatal Nurs 8(3):174, 1979.

Greer PS: Head coverings for newborns under radiant warmers, J Obstet Gynecol Neonatal Nurs 17(4):265, 1988.

Holzman IR: A method to maintain infant temperature, Am J Dis Child 139(4):390, 1985.

Noerr B: Nursing care to maintain neonatal thermoregulation, Crit Care Nurs 4(2):102, 1984.

Why not wrap the baby? Am J Nurs 86(11):1220, 1986.

Wong D: From sites to sensors: taking infants' temperatures, Am J Nurs 89(3):321, 1989.

Prematurity

Anderson GC, Marks EA, and Wahlberg V: Kangaroo care for premature infants, Am J Nurs 86(7):807, 1986.

Budreau G: The perceived attractiveness of preterm infants with cranial molding, J Obstet Gynecol Neonatal Nurs 18(1):38, 1989.

Felton GH and Martin B: The high cost of preterm labor, RN 48(8):47, 1985.

Gennaro S: Maternal anxiety, problem-solving ability, and adaptation to the premature infant, Pediatr Nurs 11(5):343, 1985.

George DS and others: The latest on retinopathy of prematurity, MCN 13(4):254, 1988.

Jenkins RL and Tock MKS: Helping parents to bond to their premature infant, MCN 11(1):32, 1986.

McCormick A: Special considerations in the nursing care of the very low birth weight infant, J Obstet Gynecol Neonatal Nurs 13(6):357, 1984.

Meier P and Anderson GC: Responses of small preterm infants to bottle and breast feeding, MCN 12(2):97, 1987.

Rice BR and Feeg VD: First year developmental outcomes for multiple-risk premature infants, Pediatr Nurs 11(1):30, 1985.

Sammons WAH and Levsi JM: Premature infants: a different beginning, St Louis, 1985, The CV Mosby Co.

Wink DM: Better breast milk for preemies, Am J Nurs 89(1):48, 1989.

Wong D: Simple soothers for LBW infants, Am J Nurs 88(9):1170, 1988.

Infections and infection control

American Academy of Pediatrics/American College of Obstetricians and Gynecologists: Guidelines for perinatal care, ed 2, Elk Grove Village, Ill, 1988, The Academy.

Andrich MP and Golden SM: Umbilical cord care: a study of bacitracin ointment vs. triple dye, Clin Pediatr 23(6):342, 1984.

Becker L and Lagomarsino W: Isolation guidelines for perinatal patients: creating a new protocol, MCN 12(6):400, 1987.

Bond GB: Serratia: an endemic hospital resident, Am J Nurs 81(12):2183, 1981.

Bourcier KM and others: Chlamydia and condylomata acuminata: an update for the nurse practitioner, J Obstet Gynecol Neonatal Nurs 16(1):17, 1987.

Campbell VG: Covergowns for newborn infection control? MCN 12(1):54, 1987.

Crow S: Calling in sick: how to decide, Nursing '90 20(3):63, 1990.

Hammerschlag MR and others: Efficacy of neonatal ocular prophylaxis for prevention of chlamydial and gonorrheal conjunctivitis, N Engl J Med 320(12):769, 1989.

Jackson MM: Infection prevention and control for HIV and other infectious agents in obstetric and gynecologic and neonatal settings, NAACOG Clinical Issues 1(1):115, 1990.

Larson E: Handwashing: it's essential—even when you use gloves, Am J Nurs 89(7):934, 1989.

Larson E: Trends in neonatal infections, J Obstet Gynecol Neonatal Nurs 16(6):404, 1987.

Lynch P and others: Implementing and evaluating a system of generic infection precautions: body substance isolation, Am J Infect Control 18(1):1, 1990.

Solheim K and Spellacy C: Sibling visitation: effects on newborn infection rates, J Obstet Gynecol Neonatal Nurs 17(1):43, 1988.

Wiley K and Grohar J: Human immunodeficiency virus and precautions for obstetric, gynecologic and neonatal nurses, J Obstet Gynecol Neonatal Nurs 17(3):165, 1988.

Neonatal intensive care unit

Bethea SW: Primary nursing in the infant special care unit, J Obstet Gynecol Neonatal Nurs 14(3):202, 1985.

Cagan J: Weaning parents from intensive care unit care, MCN 13(4):275, 1988.

Frank LS: A national survey of pain and agitation in the neonatal intensive care unit, J Obstet Gynecol Neonatal Nurs 16(6):387, 1987.

Gordin PC: Assessing and managing agitation in a critically ill infant, MCN 15(1):26, 1990.

Hawkins-Walsh E: Diminishing anxiety in parents of sick newborns, MCN 5(1):30, 1980.

Ioli J and Richardson M: Giving surfactant to premature infants, Am J Nurs 90(3):59, 1990.

Klaus, MH and Fanaroff AA: Care of the high-risk neonate, Philadelphia, 1986, WB Saunders Co.

Korones SB and Lancaster J: High-risk newborn infants: the basis for intensive nursing care, ed 4, St Louis, 1986, The CV Mosby Co.

Merenstein GB and Gardner SL: Handbook of neonatal intensive care, St Louis, 1989, The CV Mosby Co.

Perkin RM and Anas NG: Resuscitation and stabilization of the child with respiratory disease, Pediatr Ann 15(1):43, 1986.

Sande D: Preventing burnout in intensive care nurseries, Pediatr Nurs 9(5):368, 1983.

Schraeder BD: Attachment and parenting despite lengthy intensive care, MCN 5(1):37, 1980.

Thomas KA: How the NICU environment sounds to a preterm infant, MCN 14(4):249, 1989.

Troy P and others: Sibling visiting in the NICU, Am J Nurs 88(1):68, 1988.

Weibley TT: Inside the incubator, MCN 14(2):96, 1989.

Wooten B: Death of an infant, MCN 6(4):257, 1981.

Abnormalities of the newborn

Avery ME and Taeusch HW: Diseases of the newborn, ed 5, Philadelphia, 1984, WB Saunders Co.

Bartlett D and Davis A: Recognizing fetal alcohol syndrome in the nursery, J Obstet Gynecol Neonatal Nurs 9(4):223, 1980.

Bernardo ML: Craniosynostosis: the child's care from detection through correction (pictorial), MCN 4(4):234, 1979.

Burnett J: Congenital adrenocortical hyperplasia, Am J Nurs 80(7):1304, 1980.

Campbell JR: Inguinal and scrotal problems in infants and children, Pediatr Ann 18(3):189, 1989.

Carmen S: Neonatal hypoglycemia in response to maternal glucose infusion before delivery, J Obstet Gynecol Neonatal Nurs 15(4):319, 1986.

Crocker AC: The causes of mental retardation, Pediatr Ann 18(10):623, 1989.

Fisher C: The abnormal infant: protecting yourself against blame, RN 53(4):69, 1990.

Gantt L and Thompson C: Short gut syndrome in the infant, Am J Nurs 85(11):1263, 1985.

Greenwald JL: Hyperbilirubinemia, in otherwise healthy infants, Am Fam Physician 38(6):151, 1988.

Jackson PL: Primary care needs of children with hydrocephalus, J Pediatr Health Care 4(2):59, 1990.

Martin LW and others: Esophageal atresia, Surg Clin North Am 65(3):1099, 1985.

Merker L, Higgins P, and Kinnard E: Assessing narcotic addiction in neonates, Pediatr Nurs 11(3):177, 1985.

Messer SS: PKU: a mother's perspective, Pediatr Nurs 11(2):121, 1985.

Miller G: Myopathies of infant and childhood, Pediatr Ann 18(7):439, 1989.

Rubin IL: Mental retardation—the perinatal period: antecedents and sequelae, 18(10):653, 1989.

Schaming D and others: When babies are born with orthopedic problems, RN 53(4):62, 1990.

Smith JE and Deitch KB: Cocaine: A maternal, fetal, and neonatal risk, J Pediatr Health Care 1(3):120, 1987.

Stephens CJ: The fetal alcohol syndrome: cause for concern, MCN 6(4):251, 1981.

Wilkerson NN: Treating hyperbilirubinemia, MCN 14(1):32, 1989.

Growth, Development, and Health Supervision

16

Structural, Functional, and Psychologic Changes in the Child

CHAPTER OBJECTIVES

After studying this chapter, the student should be able to perform the following:

1 Define the following terms: growth, development, maturation, genes, chromosomes, karyotype, pedigree, consanguinity, and heterozygous and homozygous inheritance.

2 State five principles of growth and development.

3 Identify the periods of greatest physical growth during an individual's life span.

4 Explain the mechanism of autosomal dominant inheritance, give one example, and construct a "probability box."

5 Explain the mechanism of autosomal recessive inheritance, give one example, and construct a "probability box."

6 Explain why X-linked recessive disorders are usually expressed only by the male child; cite one example.

7 Discuss the role of the genetic counselor and the techniques that are available to this professional for assisting families.

8 Discuss the purpose of the U.S. Human Genome Project.

9 Discuss two diagnostic methods that are commonly employed for genetic screening during the first trimester of pregnancy.

10 List five examples of environmental influences on a child.

11 Demonstrate the use of the measurement called "percentile rank" on the NCHS growth charts and state what it indicates.

12 Explain different methods of evaluating growth and indicate which of them is considered the best for assessing a child's general growth progress.

13 Trace the average growth in height in children from birth through the first year, second year, preschool period, and from 6 to 10 years.

14 Indicate the intervals at which the birth weight of a child usually doubles and triples.

15 Identify centers of ossification that can be evaluated in children for bone-age studies.

16 Discuss the normal progress of dentition in children, stating which teeth usually appear first and second and the age at which the eruption of all 20 primary teeth is customarily complete.

17 Explain what is meant by cephalocaudal and proximodistal development.

18 State the normal sequence of prehension and the typical timetable cited for these accomplishments.

19 Trace the normal locomotion sequence starting with head and chest elevation and ending with walking alone.

20 Describe the process of habituation and its posssible role as a predictor of intelligence.

21 Describe the three main styles of parenting. Can more than one style be used by a parent?

22 P.E.T. has been helpful to many parents. What is meant by active listening? What are the three elements of an I-message?

23 List six techniques used to shape behavior and moral values. Which would you prefer to use? Why?

CONCEPTS OF GROWTH AND DEVELOPMENT

As children grow up they are constantly changing physically and functionally. This is the main distinction between the child and the adult. Growth is exhibited by all healthy children, although it may be impaired by malnutrition and disease. Child growth and development are the features that characterize pediatrics as a specialty.

Every nurse interested in the care of children should have a basic understanding of the stages of human growth and development. Such an understanding is of great help in evaluating the physical, intellectual, emotional, and social behavior of the dynamic child patient (Table 16-1).

Terminology

The terms "growth" and "development" are closely bound together and sometimes used interchangeably. Increases in structure (growth) are accompanied by increases in function (development). As children grow in size, they mature mentally, emotionally, and socially. Differences in the way a child thinks, feels, and acts are just as real as changes in size.

As growth and development proceed, various levels of maturity are observable. *Maturation* is the process in which inherited tendencies begin to unfold, independent of any special practice or training. All children have their own built-in growth patterns. Some children have patterns that allow them to mature rapidly; other children are very slow physically, mentally, and emotionally, and are called late maturers. A wide range can exist in the growth and development rates of normal children. Whereas one child enjoys walking at 12 months of age, another may be 15 months old when he takes his first steps. Each child advances physiologically toward maturity at his own rate.

Because children, learning methods, and child-rearing practices are similar in many different cultures, some generalizations can be made concerning growth and development. Although these generalizations are not applicable in every case, they do provide valuable points of departure in understanding and dealing with groups. This discussion of growth and development follows the child through an orderly sequence beginning with the prenatal phase and continuing through infancy, childhood, and adolescence.

Principles

The normal growth and development of a child through the prenatal period, infancy, childhood, and adolescence are guided by certain basic principles, five of which are described below. Growth and development (1) occur in an orderly sequence; (2) are, though continuous, characterized by spurts of growth and periods of relative rest; (3) progress at highly individualized rates from child to child; (4) vary at different ages for specific structures; and (5) represent a total process involving the whole child.

Orderly sequence. Growth and development occur in an orderly sequence and are continuous. The sequence of development is the same for all children, even though some children do things earlier than others. Children generally creep before they stand and stand alone before they walk. *Average* children talk before they read and usually read before they can write. One child reads at 4 years of age, and another reads at 6 years of age. What happens at one stage influences what happens in the next stage; each stage in the development of the individual is an outgrowth of an earlier stage. During the first year, babies babble; as they grow, they begin to say simple

Table 16-1 Progressive stages of development

Stages of life	Divisions of life stages	Chronologic age
Prenatal		
Conception to birth	Germinal	Conception to 10 days' gestation
	Embryonic	10 days to 2 months' gestation
	Fetal	2 months' gestation to birth
Infancy		
Birth to 1 year	Newborn (neonate)	Birth to 1 month
	Infancy	1 month to 1 year
Childhood		
1 to 12 years	Toddler	1 to 3 years
	Preschool	3 to 6 years
	School	6 to 10 years
	Preadolescence (puberty)	10 to 12 years
Adolescence		
12 to 19 years	Early adolescence	12 to 16 years
	Late adolescence	16 to 19 years

words. The toddler uses words in phrases, and the preschooler uses words in short sentences. No child speaks clearly before babbling, and each stage in the sequence of development can be anticipated.

Continuity. Growth and development continue from the moment of conception until the individual reaches maturity, but at no time is growth even and regular. Spurts and rest periods occur within the development of a child, even though no real interruptions occur until growth is completed. Growth is greatest during the prenatal period and is still rapid during infancy and early childhood. The rate is slow but constant in middle childhood. It shows a spurt during early puberty and then tapers off in the latter part of puberty.

Differences in growth rates. All children have their own unique growth timetables. A child who develops rapidly during the early years of life will continue to do so. Whereas one child may sit unaided at 6 months of age and walk alone at 9 months of age, his sibling may sit unaided at 8 months and walk alone at 15 months. Even in the same family, no two children grow at the same rate.

Variation of growth rates for different body structures. Not all parts of the body mature at the same time. The brain attains its adult size when the child is about 6 or 7 years of age, but it certainly does not complete maturation until many years later. Different phases of physical and mental growth occur at their own individual rates, and maturity is reached at different times.

Growth and development as a total process. The child does not grow physically one day and mentally the next but grows physically, mentally, socially, and emotionally at the same time. The child develops as a whole being. Changes in interest and mental growth are closely related to development in walking and talking. Growth is a total process involving the whole child, not just the body, mind, and emotions. Each child passes slowly and almost imperceptibly from stage to stage, preserving a patterned integration of behavior throughout life.

GENETIC AND ENVIRONMENTAL INFLUENCES AND LIMITATIONS

Every child's growth and development (pattern, rate, rhythm, and extent) are governed by genetic and environmental forces. Within the broad categories of genetic and environmental influences are many overlapping and diverse factors, such as sex differences, endocrine gland function, racial ancestry, cellular mutations, and other inherited strengths and weaknesses; psychologic and cultural milieu, nutritional and physical advantages or disadvantages; and intercurrent malformation or disease. For many years controversy raged regarding the respective importance of genetics and environment, or "nature versus nurture." Since then this interest has been somewhat tempered, and most writers in the field contend that both are important and try to determine ways that both can be improved to enhance the individual and society.

Genetic influences

A child's cellular inheritance and early embryonic growth may be a lifetime asset or a continuing liability. About one fourth of all hospitalized children have diseases or defects with genetic components. The science of genetics is based on principles of inheritance first described in the mid-1880s by the Augustinian monk scientist, Gregor Mendel. Mendel's law explains certain aspects of gene activity in humans during the formation of gametes (eggs and sperm) and during fertilization (the union of an egg and spermatazoon).

Genes, the hereditary elements, are defined lengths of deoxyribonucleic acid (DNA) located on structures called chromosomes, which are found in every cell's nucleus. DNA consists of pairs of four nucleotide bases: adenine (A), guanine (G), cytosine (C), and thymine (T) found in a double helix formation. DNA directs the assembly of amino acids into proteins essential for normal functioning. When cells divide, the DNA duplicates itself and passes on its genetic code to the next generation of cells. Twenty-three chromosomes from each parent, combining to make a total of 46, endow the offspring at fertilization. Each of 22 chromosomes donated by one parent has a microscopically similar counterpart that is donated by the other parent. These chromosomic counterparts can be paired whether the developing individual is a boy or a girl. They are called *autosomes*. Each pair of autosomal chromosomes is different in its genetic content and appearance. Two other, different chromosomes, labeled X and Y, determine sex. They are called *sex chromosomes*. Each parent donates only one. The mother is able to contribute only an X chromosome, while the father may give to his child either an X or a Y chromosome. Babies having an XX inheritance are girls; those with XY are boys.

There are three known general pathways involved in the etiology of genetic disease: (1) Mendelian patterns of inheritance involving only one or two defective genes; (2) multifactorial disorders related to multiple gene defects and environmental factors; and (3) gross genetic imbalances caused by chromosomal abnormalities. Defects in chromosomal structure or numbers can be considered *packaging defects*. The chromosomes are the "packages" that carry the genes from generation to generation. Defects in individual genes—the *contents* of these packages—are not evident on inspection of the chromosomes themselves but are revealed by disease and abnormalities in the affected person.

A brief discussion of the various modes of inheritance will provide the student with an understanding of the basic characteristics associated with each inheritance pattern.

The Mendelian disorders may be subdivided into four distinct patterns of inheritance. Each involves one or two defective genes. To observe the distribution pattern of a specific trait in a family, it is essential to have detailed background information of the child's relatives. The construction of a chart that utilizes standard symbols to designate family members, their relationships, and other pertinent information is called a pedigree or family tree. Pedigrees are valuable in demonstrating the various modes of inheritance for a given disorder in a particular family. For disorders with more than one mode of transmission, reviews of genetic pedigrees may establish the specific type of transmission. For example, a disorder called retinitis pigmentosa may be recessive, au-

tosomal dominant, or sex-linked. A pedigree is most helpful in determining the type of inheritance patterns present.

Two terms often used to describe an individual's gene inheritance are *heterozygous* and *homozygous*. When a specific gene that controls a certain characteristic is contributed by one parent and a nonmatching gene for that characteristic is donated by the other parent, the inheritance for that trait is said to be heterozygous. If both parents donate matching genes, it is said to be homozygous.

Autosomal dominant inheritance. An autosomal dominant genetic disorder expresses itself even though the defect is limited to a single gene on one of two paired autosomal chromosomes. Usually one parent has a single gene defect that dominates its normal gene partner (heterozygous dominant inheritance). As the parent may give either the normal or abnormal gene to the offspring, each of that parent's children has a 50% chance of being affected. Males and females are affected equally. If the offspring does not inherit the dominant gene, that person will not transmit the trait or disorder. Usually the first affected individual in a family represents a new mutation. This genetic change, depending on the individual's re-

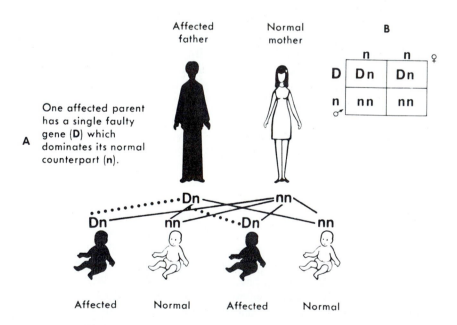

Affected father

Normal mother

B

	n	n	♀
D	**Dn**	**Dn**	
n	**nn**	**nn**	

♂

A One affected parent has a single faulty gene (**D**) which dominates its normal counterpart (**n**).

Dn .... nn

Dn — nn — Dn — nn

Affected   Normal   Affected   Normal

Each child's chances of inheriting either the **D** or the **n** from the affected parent are 50%.

FIG 16-1 **A,** Dominant inheritance. **B,** Different method of expressing probability of dominant inheritance exemplified in **A.** (*A, Courtesy The National Foundation–March of Dimes.*)

productivity either may be transmitted to the next generation or ends with the original person affected (Fig. 16-1).

Autosomal recessive inheritance. Autosomal recessive disorders are expressed only when the individual has two affected paired genes for the particular disorder (homozygous inheritance). Since both parents contribute one gene for each trait, these disorders are inherited from both parents. Most often, the parents are carriers of one abnormal gene that is dominated by its normal paired gene. The parents have an essentially normal appearance and, as a result, are unaware of the gene's presence until an offspring inherits both genes and is affected. It should be emphasized that the probability of having a child with an autosomal recessive disorder increases when the parents share a common ancestor and thus share a common gene pool. This is referred to as *consanguinity*. Males and females are affected with equal frequency. Each child has a 25% chance of being affected, a 50% chance of being a carrier, and a 25% chance of not inheriting the gene from either parent. Affected children whose mates

do not carry this gene will have unaffected children who will all be carriers of the gene (Fig. 16-2).

X-linked inheritance. Each individual has two sex chromosomes that differ from the autosomal chromosomes in that they are not alike in both sexes (males = XY, females = XX). A female may be homozygous for genes located on the two X chromosomes, but a male can only be heterozygous because he carries only one X chromosome.

X-linked recessive inheritance. X-linked recessive inheritance involves genes located on the X chromosome. The defective X-linked gene of an affected male must come from his mother, who is a carrier, because fathers give male offspring only a Y chromosome. A recessive X-linked gene in a female usually is matched by a normal dominant gene on the paired X chromosomes, and the disorder is not expressed. However, a male who inherits a recessive X-linked gene on his one X chromosome is always affected, because there is never a matching gene on the Y. Females affected with an X-linked recessive disorder are rare because they must carry affected genes

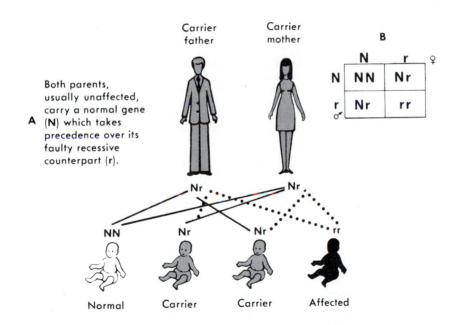

The odds for each child are:
1. A 25% risk of inheriting a "double dose" of r genes which may cause a serious birth defect
2. A 25% chance of inheriting two Ns, thus being unaffected
3. A 50% chance of being a carrier as both parents are

FIG 16-2 A, Recessive inheritance. **B,** Different method of expressing probability of rece
inheritance exemplified in **A.** (**A,** *Courtesy The National Foundation—The March of Din*

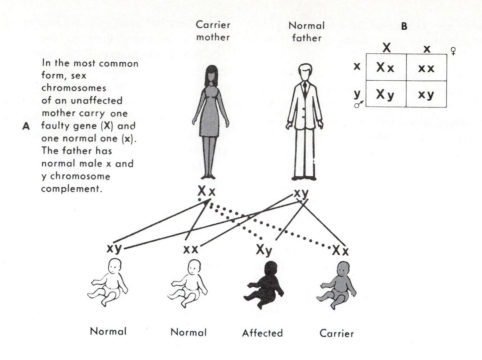

FIG 16-3 A, X-linked inheritance. **B,** Different method of expressing most common form of X-linked inheritance exemplified in **A.** (*A, Courtesy The National Foundation—The March of Dimes.*)

on both their X chromosomes. Each male child of a female carrier has a 50% chance of being affected; each female offspring has a 50% chance of being a carrier. No male-to-male transmission occurs, but the female offspring of an affected male all will be carriers, because they inherit the father's only X chromosome with the defective recessive gene. Transmission occurs from one generation to the next with only males affected in the majority of families; a generation may be skipped if only females inherit the recessive gene and the males are unaffected (Fig. 16-3).

X-linked dominant inheritance. In X-linked dominant disorders, females are affected if they carry a single abnormal gene on one of the X chromosomes. The inheritance pattern of an X-linked dominant trait resembles autosomal dominant inheritance with one exception—

the trait is transmitted from an affected male to all his daughters, but not to his sons. An affected female's offspring has a 50% chance of being affected whether male or female. In X-linked dominant disorders, usually twice as many females as males are affected.

Multifactorial inheritance. Multifactorial disorders result from an interaction between multiple defective genes and environmental influences. A thorough analysis of the family pedigree does not reveal a distinctive mode of inheritance as with mendelian patterns of inheritance. However, the increased incidence rate for such disorders in relatives of affected persons, especially in identical twins, yields evidence of a genetic factor. The recurrence risk for the disorder depends on the number of affected persons within a family, how closely related they are to the person seeking genetic counseling, and the sex of the

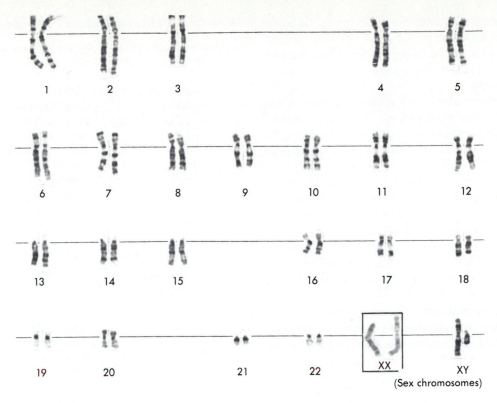

FIG 16-4 High-resolution G-banded human karyotype (male). *Insert shows XX pair from normal female. (Courtesy C. Bradshaw, UCSD Medical Genetics, La Jolla, Calif.)*

affected persons. It has been established that certain multifactorial disorders are more likely to occur in one sex than in the other. A pedigree demonstrates which people within a family are affected so that the recurrence risk can be established.

Chromosomal abnormalities. Recent developments permit accurate identification of each chromosome by using a special straining technique that produces a characteristic banding pattern for each chromosomal pair. The standard systematized arrangement of chromosomes is called a *karyotype*. It is an orderly arrangement of an individual's autosomal and sex chromosomes, according to size, shape, and banding pattern, as they appear in cutouts of photographic enlargements (Fig. 16-4). Chromosomal disorders can be diagnosed in a cytogenetics laboratory by examining the chromosomal pattern of cells derived by a culture of any of several body tissues. A leukocyte culture obtained from a blood sample is most often used. Syndromes are now being identified that are associated with specific chromosomal abnormalities. Chromosomal abnormalities result from various failures

in the production of ova and sperm within the two gonads (meiosis) and from abnormal segregation of chromosomes during the first several mitotic divisions of body cells (mitosis). This latter cause results in cells with different chromosomal numbers within one individual, a condition called *mosaicism*.

One kind of chromosomal change that may be inherited involves the transfer of material between two chromosomes, called a *translocation*. In a balanced translocation, all the chromosomal material is present in the cell, though not located in its normal position; an unbalanced translocation occurs when a portion of the chromosomal material has been lost or additional material has been gained. This unbalanced condition usually is associated with serious defects in the individual. A parent carrying a balanced translocation, though normal, is at risk of having offspring with an unbalanced translocation. The pedigree may be used to help identify those persons at risk for carrying a balanced translocation. It is recommended that such persons undergo a chromosome analysis (karyotype). Should they carry the translocation, each pregnancy may be monitored by means of amniocentesis (see discussion on p. 52). The parents then have the option of either continuing or terminating the pregnancy if the fetus is found to have an unbalanced chromosomal pattern.

Another chromosomal abnormality is related to *nondisjunction* of the chromosomes. This occurs when a chromosomal pair does not separate normally during formation of the sex cells in the ovary or testes (meiosis) or when the body cells divide (mitosis). If the gamete carrying the extra chromosome was fertilized, the offspring would then have a total chromosomal count of 47 rather than 46 per cell. This phenomenon is often related to advanced maternal age. The most common disorder resulting from this process is one type of Down syndrome (trisomy 21). An extra chromosome at the number 21 position produces mental retardation and other physical deviations (see p. 280).

The most common chromosome abnormality is simply a change in the total chromosome number. In general, a reduction of the total number of autosomal chromosomes is incompatible with life. An increase in the total number of autosomes results in multiple physical abnormalities, mental retardation, and often a limited life span. Numeric disorders of the sex chromosomes may also be present. One condition, characterized by a complete chromosome loss (45 instead of 46), that is compatible with life is Turner's syndrome, coded as 45 XO, indicating that one X chromosome is missing (Table 16-2).

The human genome

The U.S. Human Genome Project has been initiated with the purpose of creating a complete map and sequence of all 3 billion base pairs of DNA that make up the human genetic complement.

There are an estimated 50,000 to 100,000 genes. About 1,500 genes have been mapped to specific chromosomes and chromosome regions; 600 or more genes have had the DNA sequenced. The ultimate goal of this project is to provide information to help understand genetic disease in general. Initially, single gene disorders will be evaluated but as more information accumulates, multifactorial diseases will be better understood and hopefully treated. Predictive and preventative medicine based on the identification of susceptibility to disease should also be forthcoming as a result of this project.

Prenatal diagnosis

Genetic screening is now available for certain defects to determine the parental carrier status. Simple blood

Table 16-2 Patterns of inheritance and common disorders

Autosomal dominant inheritance	Achondroplastic dwarfism
	Huntington's chorea
	Neurofibromatosis
Autosomal recessive inheritance	Albinism
	Cystic fibrosis
	Phenylketonuria
	Sickle cell disease
	Tay-Sachs disease
X-linked recessive inheritance	Duchenne's muscular dystrophy
	Hemophilia
	Hurler's syndrome
X-linked dominant inheritance	Vitamin D-resistant rickets
Multifactorial inheritance	Cleft lip, cleft palate
	Clubfoot
	Congenital heart disease
	Dislocated hip
	Pyloric stenosis
	Spina bifida
	Anencephaly
Chromosomal abnormalities	Klinefelter's syndrome (XXY)
	Trisomy 13
	Trisomy 18
	Trisomy 21 (Down syndrome)
	Turner's syndrome (XO)

studies can reveal whether one or both parents carry a defective gene, such as sickle cell trait. It can then be predicted that if both parents carry the sickle cell trait, their unborn child has a 25% chance of having sickle cell disease. Such carrier testing is available for other genetic diseases such as Tay-Sachs and thalassemia.

Parents often wish to know prenatally whether a fetus is affected or not. Some disorders such as neural tube defects, which involve incomplete development of the brain or exposed spinal cord, can be screened by measuring the amount of alphafetoprotein (AFP) in the mother's blood. If the AFP is elevated, the client is referred for diagnostic testing, which may include ultrasound and amniocentesis.

Amniocentesis is usually performed at 16 weeks, although prenatal diagnosis centers now offer early amniocentesis between 10 and 14 weeks. Another technique, chorionic villi sampling, provides an alternative approach to prenatal diagnosis. At the 10th to 11th week of pregnancy, a transcervical or transabdominal approach is used to obtain extra-embryonic, placental tissue, which is genetically identical with the fetus. Chromosome or DNA analysis can then be performed on this tissue or on amniotic cells obtained through amniocentesis.

Direct DNA analysis or the utilization of specific genetic markers found in DNA material is now available for the prenatal diagnosis of such disorders as cystic fibrosis, Duchennes muscular dystrophy, Huntington's chorea, sickle cell anemia, and other genetic diseases. Health care providers now have an obligation to inform couples with at-risk pregnancies that genetic prenatal diagnosis for certain conditions is available.

Genetic counseling

Although individual birth defects may seem relatively rare (4% to 5% of all births), the total number of families affected is well into the millions. About 250,000 American babies are born each year with mild to severe physical or mental defects. With each passing year more disorders are identified as genetic problems, thereby increasing the known incidence of hereditary disease.

A genetic counselor is a health professional who is capable of communicating to the parents the magnitude of, the implications of, and the alternatives for dealing with the risk of hereditary disorders occurring within a family. Unfortunately, most genetic counseling is occasioned by the birth of a defective child. Much care, sympathy, understanding, and insight into human nature are necessary to communicate effectively all the implications and possible options relating to the genetic disorder.

Using pedigree studies, modern laboratory detection techniques (such as blood tests, enzyme assays, amniocentesis, chorionic villi sampling, and chromosome analysis), and knowledge of basic laws of heredity and incidence statistics, a genetic counselor can often predict the probability of the recurrence of a given abnormality in a family. The primary aim is to prevent genetic defects or, when that is impossible, to reduce their damaging effects to a minimum. Genetic counseling is a form of preventive medicine. It involves the delivery of genetic information: diagnosis, prognosis, presentation of odds for recurrence, and the effect of genetic diseases on the family. It is a field with its own body of knowledge and requiring its own expertise. Because a wide range of laboratory resources and consultative skills are frequently required, genetic counseling is most often available in large medical centers. A list of genetic counseling centers throughout the United States is sent to physicians or to the general public, free on request, from the Professional Educational Department of the National Foundation—March of Dimes (see also p. 229).

Environmental influences

Although the impact of a child's genetic background is great, another modifying force also exerts an important influence on growth and development—environment. Examples of environmental factors include: the family composition, interrelationships, culture and lifestyles; the degree and type of accessibility and stimulation offered by the primary care givers to the inquisitive infant and young child; health habits, nutrition, and the presence of malformation or disease. A child not only interprets his environment in terms of inherited tendencies and mental ability but also in terms of health and emotional balance. A strong, happy child makes the best use of his environment and is most able to deal with obstacles or defects in his surroundings.

Home and family. To develop naturally and wholesomely, a child needs devoted care and a family setting that is loving, accepting, and understanding. Such a home ideally supplies the growing child with more than just the physical necessities. It provides positive, helpful, broad maternal and paternal role models. It fosters respect for the individual not on the basis of beauty or intelligence (over which the child may have little control) but according to the child's attitudes, behavior, and willingness to accept and complete appropriate responsibilities. It increases the sense of personal esteem in ways that allow the child to seek experiences and enjoy new opportunities and challenges. The psychologic nurture given in the home is as important as physical support. Lack of real affection alone can result in, among other things, little or no smiling, loss of appetite, poor sleep, failure to gain weight, and persistent respiratory tract infections. Numerous studies indicate that children deprived of love and the kindly stimulation of the home fail to thrive. For an additional consideration of the impact of the family and parenting practices on the development of the child, turn to p. 337.

Nutrition. The growing child is vulnerable to many nutritional inadequacies. Disturbed patterns of skeletal development caused by the lack or overabundance of one nutrient exemplify the need for balance. Lack of protein during the prenatal period and early infancy may limit the number and size of brain cells. A well-balanced diet is essential for the development of bones and teeth, good skin, resistance to disease caused by dietary deficiency and infections, and general physical well-being. Clarification of the nutritional needs of children and the general abundance of high-quality foods have simplified the feeding of infants and children. Despite this, nutritional inadequacies may occur in the midst of plenty through faulty dietary habits, food fads, or psychic tensions centering around mealtime and the feeding situation.

Overnutrition seems to present more problems in the United States than does undernutrition. However, a severe form of protein deprivation, kwashiorkor, is common in underdeveloped countries of South America and Africa. Kwashiorkor is found among children under 4 years of age. It typically manifests itself after the child is weaned because of the birth of a younger sibling. Characteristically these children lag in growth and skeletal development. (For more information regarding nutritional needs see p. 385.)

Disease. Illness is both a physical and a psychologic hazard for the young child. Arrested growth is the obvious effect of fever and anorexia. Prolonged illness causes a definite decrease in the rate of growth and height and decreased ability to function. Any disease that interferes with physical activity and metabolic processes over a long period deters normal progress. Although some growth loss may occur during a minor illness, a subsequent growth spurt compensates for the temporary setback.

Uncontrolled diabetes always results in retarded growth in both height and weight. Chronic heart disability associated with hypoxia hampers growth, as do malabsorption syndromes such as cystic fibrosis and celiac disease.

Growth and development depend on each other and represent a continuous process of interactions between genetic potential on one hand and environment on the other. The kind of environment children live in determines whether or not they can realize all their inborn capacities for physical, social, mental, and emotional growth. Although nothing can make children do more than their inborn capacities permit, they must have a favorable environment to develop and learn as fast as their growth patterns allow.

PHYSICAL GROWTH

Although all phases of growth are continuous and take place concurrently, for convenience and clarity discussions of the main aspects of growth and development are presented here separately. Since physical growth is most obvious, it is discussed first.

Physical growth may be divided into four well-defined periods:

1. The period of very rapid growth during infancy

2. The period of slow, steady growth during childhood years
3. The period of the growth spurt during puberty
4. The period of decreasing growth and attainment of maximum height during adolescence

The greatest increase in extrauterine growth occurs during the early part of infancy. Small, steady gains continue during the slow periods. This general pattern of growth is characteristic of all the body systems with two exceptions. The nervous system grows rapidly during infancy, then decelerates, and after puberty ceases growing; the reproductive organs, however, grow very slowly until sexual maturation, which occurs during the pubertal growth spurt.

Tables of average height and weight are commonly used to show what a boy or girl of a particular age should approximate. In the course of development, observable trends in height and weight imply that one can draw certain conclusions regarding these aspects of growth. Growth norms can be successfully determined for a group of children and may serve as a point of reference for making comparisons. However, any table of averages should be interpreted with caution. Although these tables may accurately state averages, they do not necessarily state what is desirable for individuals. Growth charts for infants and children in the United States have been constructed to show weight, length, weight for various lengths, and head circumference. (For the full set of growth charts see Appendix B.) Clinical use of the charts can immediately show how the growth of any child ranks in comparison with the rest of the United States' child population of the same age and sex. The primary use of these charts is to detect nutritional and growth disturbances clinically.

The best method of evaluating a child's general growth progress is by comparing the child with himself from time to time. A large number of observations and measurements recorded periodically demonstrates the individuality of the child's own progress.

Height

Infants average about 20 inches in length at birth. During the first year of life the child grows about 10 inches. Five inches are added during the second year, and the child grows 3 inches a year during the preschool period. From the sixth to the tenth year of life the annual gain is reduced to approximately 2 inches. The maximum growth in height occurs during the pubertal period at the approximate time of sexual maturity. Growth in height reaches a peak for boys at about 14 years of age and a year or so earlier for girls. It ceases sometime before the twenties.

Puberty occurs at widely different ages. An early pubertal growth spurt is associated with an early cessation of growth. Individuals who mature late tend to grow for a longer period of time and ultimately become tall adults.

Weight

At birth the infant weighs about 7½ pounds. This weight doubles by the end of the fifth month of life, and by 1 year the birth weight has approximately tripled. A sharp drop in the rate of gain occurs after the first year. The child characteristically appears lanky and even

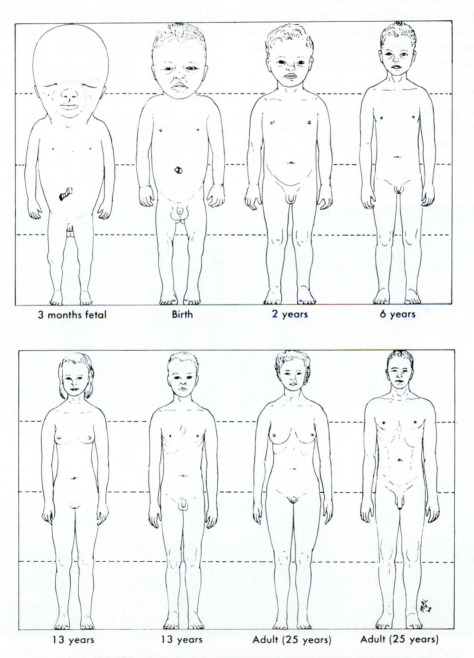

3 months fetal	Birth	2 years	6 years

13 years	13 years	Adult (25 years)	Adult (25 years)

FIG 16-5 Changes in body proportions, fetus to maturity.

skinny. During the preschool years the weight rises slowly, averaging about 5 pounds each year.

During the school years the weight gain is slightly increased. Weight varies more than height, since it is readily susceptible to external factors, such as dietary intake.

Generally boys are taller and heavier than girls, except in the years preceding puberty. A rapid gain in weight usually occurs in both sexes during puberty, corresponding closely with the gain in height. Girls begin their preadolescent growth spurt at about 10 to 12 years of age, 2 years earlier than boys. In addition, girls typically reach their adult proportions sooner than boys.

Body proportions (Fig. 16-5)

Distinct changes in body proportions occur between birth and maturity. The small child not only differs from the adult in size but also in body form. At birth the head is relatively large, about one fourth of the total body length, whereas in the adult it is about one eighth to one tenth of the body length. An infant's arms and legs are relatively short. During infancy the trunk is longer than the extremities. The midpoint of the total length of the infant is at the umbilicus, whereas in the adult it is at the symphysis pubis.

During puberty, adult proportions are attained, and the characteristic mature body shape for each sex becomes differentiated. The straight leg lines of the young girl become curved by 15 years of age. Her hips grow wider, but her shoulders remain narrow. The boy's shoulders become broader, whereas his hips remain narrow.

Body proportion and build, or physique, is unique to the individual. Within the individual's own general pattern—slender, stocky, muscular—each child's growth seems to be constant.

Bone formation

During the early days of fetal development, bones begin as simple connective tissue. Later this tissue becomes cartilage. By the end of the fifth month of ges-

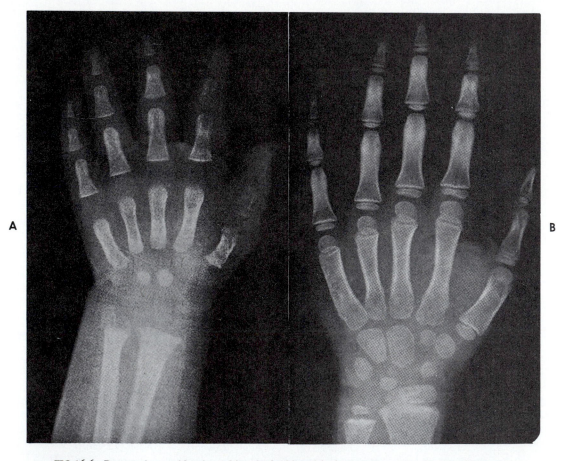

FIG 16-6 Progressive ossification of hand of white girl. **A,** Age 3 months. **B,** Age 6 years, 3 months. *(From Todd TW: Atlas of skeletal maturation, St Louis, 1937, The CV Mosby Co.)*

tation, certain mineral salts, especially calcium phosphate, are deposited in the cartilage, causing it to harden. Cartilage is gradually replaced by bone; this process is called *ossification*. During the early years of life, cartilage persists between the diaphysis (shaft) and epiphyses (ends) of long bones. Bones grow in length by a continual thickening of the epiphyseal cartilage.

As the child grows, changes occur in the texture, size, and shape of the "old" bones, and new bones appear. Bone development continues in an orderly sequence and is complete by the third decade of life.

Bone age can be determined by x-ray examination of certain joints. The information gained is compared with a standard. The x-ray films are studied to detect the following:

1. The appearance of new bones
2. Changes in the contour of the ends of bones
3. The union of the epiphyses with the bone shaft

Growth of the long bones is complete when the epiphyses and diaphyses are fused.

Bone development of the hand and wrist is a good index of the individual's progress in skeletal growth. Since boys lag behind girls in bone development at all ages, separate standards are used.

At birth the ends of the arm bones (epiphyses) are not developed, and the carpal bones are not present (Fig. 16-6). Shortly after, the carpal bones and epiphyses gradually appear, and changes in the size and contour of the ends of bones continue through the school years. Bone development of the wrist and hand is complete at the seventeenth year of life for girls and 2 years later for boys.

Tooth formation (Fig. 16-7)

The foundation of a child's tooth structure is formed early in fetal life. At birth all the primary (deciduous, baby) teeth and the first permanent teeth (6-year molars) are developing in the child's jaw. Dentition is widely varied.

It is not always possible to predict exactly when the first tooth will erupt, but it is possible to predict with

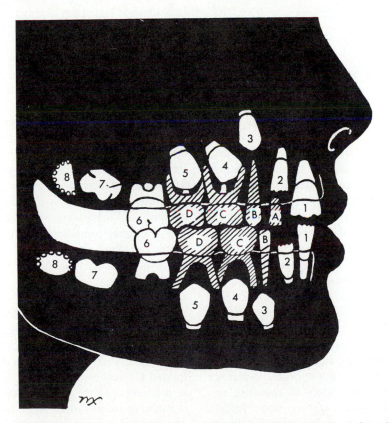

FIG 16-7 Illustration of 7-year-old child with good occlusion. Primary teeth: *A,* lateral incisors; *B,* cuspids; *C,* first molars; *D,* second molars. Permanent teeth: *1,* central incisors; *2,* lateral incisors; *3,* cuspids; *4,* first bicuspids; *5,* second bicuspids; *6,* first molars; *7,* second molars; *8,* site of wisdom teeth.

Table 16-3   Typical pattern of dentition

Teeth	Lower (mandibular) appear at age	Upper (maxillary) appear at age
Primary		
Central incisors	5 to 7 months	6 to 8 months
Lateral incisors	12 to 15 months	8 to 11 months
Cuspids (canines)	16 to 20 months	16 to 20 months
First molars	10 to 16 months	10 to 16 months
Second molars	20 to 30 months	20 to 30 months
Total per jaw—10		
Total—20		
Permanent		
Central incisors	6 to 7 years	6 to 7 years
Lateral incisors	7 to 9 years	8 to 9 years
Cuspids (canines)	8 to 11 years	11 to 12 years
First bicuspids	10 to 12 years	10 to 11 years
Second bicuspids	11 to 13 years	10 to 12 years
First molars (6-year molars)	6 to 7 years	6 to 7 years
Second molars (12-year molars)	12 to 13 years	12 to 13 years
Third molars (wisdom teeth)	17 to 22 years	17 to 22 years
Total set—32		

some accuracy which teeth will erupt first (Table 16-3). The two lower central incisors usually appear first, between 5 and 7 months of age. The upper central incisors appear next. Most children have 6 teeth at 1 year of age and all 20 primary teeth by 2½ years of age.

Wide variation occurs in the pattern of tooth shedding and permanent tooth eruption. Before the appearance of the first molars (6-year molars), all the permanent teeth are growing and maturing. During this time the roots of the primary teeth are disappearing by the process of resorption. Only the crown of the primary tooth is left when the permanent tooth below is ready to erupt. The loose crown then drops out. The care and preservation of the primary teeth are important. Unless they are beyond repair, primary teeth should not be pulled out. They contribute in large measure to proper alignment and good health of the permanent teeth.

Tetracycline antibiotics have an adverse effect on newly formed bones. The drug stains developing teeth with a yellow-brown material. Tetracyclines also cross the placenta. After the fourth month of gestation, the primary teeth of the developing fetus are also affected. Such discoloration of the teeth may be prevented by *not using* the drugs during pregnancy and the first 8 years of life.

MOTOR DEVELOPMENT

As their bodies grow children acquire the ability to function in increasingly complex ways. Motor changes accompany physical growth. Motor abilities involve various types of body movements that result from the coordinated activity of nerves and muscles. Maturation of the nervous system and learning are interrelated in the acquisition of motor abilities.

Motor development is the process of learning, controlling, and integrating muscular responses. Great advances in body control and locomotion are accomplished during the first 2 years of life. At first an uncoordinated, helpless infant, the child is soon able to sit, stand, walk, reach, and grasp.

Like other phases of growth, motor development unfolds in an orderly sequence that is closely related to the maturation of the nervous system. It follows a definite sequence. Characteristically, motor development begins in the head region of the individual and moves down toward the feet (cephalocaudal). Development also tends to proceed from the center of the body toward the extremities (proximodistal). At first motor response to stimulation (such as an ice cube touching the foot) is diffuse, involving the whole body. As maturation proceeds, the response becomes more specific and may involve only the withdrawal of the foot. The sequence of motor development is similar for all children, but the rate at which the development progresses varies with each child.

Prehension and locomotion provide examples of the usual sequences in the course of motor development.

Prehension

The development of the ability to oppose the thumb to the fingers in picking up an object is preceded by reaching, grasping, and raking movements. Early attempts in reaching also involve eye-hand coordination.

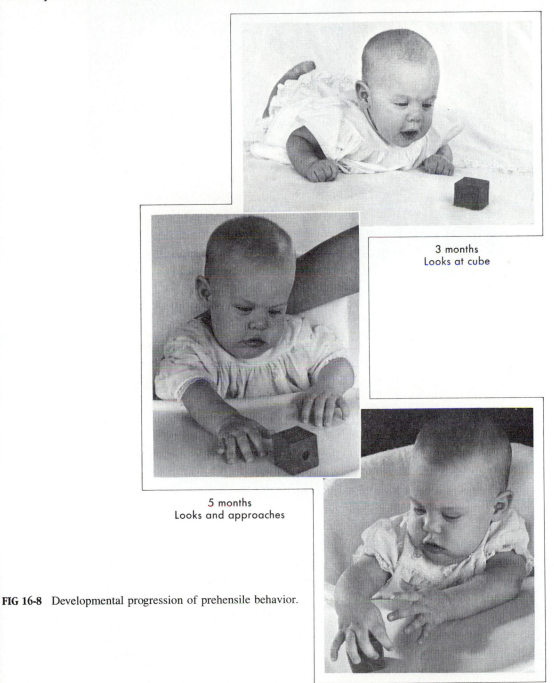

3 months
Looks at cube

5 months
Looks and approaches

6 months
Looks and crudely grasps with whole hand

FIG 16-8 Developmental progression of prehensile behavior.

Continued.

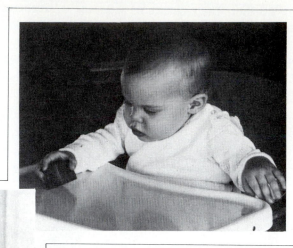

9 months
Looks and deftly
grasps with fingers

12 months
Looks, grasps with
forefinger and thumb,
and deftly releases

15 months
Looks, grasps, and releases,
to build a tower of two blocks

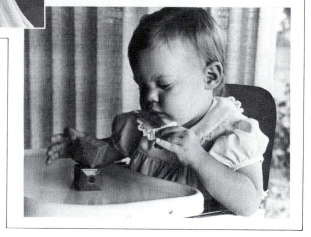

FIG 16-8, cont'd   Developmental progression of prehensile behavior.

Effective use of the hands for picking up small objects or for grasping is called *prehension*. The developmental sequence proceeds from eye-hand coordination in grasping to reaching without looking, from large muscle activity of the arms and shoulders to fine muscle activity of the fingers, and from a crude pawing closure to a closure of the fingertips that is accomplished in a refined fashion.

Gesell tested prehension by placing little red cubes before babies. He described the grasping sequence as follows (Fig. 16-8).

Development progression in grasping

12 weeks	Looks at cube
20 weeks	Looks and approaches
24 weeks	Looks and crudely grasps with whole hand
36 weeks	Looks and deftly grasps with fingers
52 weeks	Looks, grasps with forefinger and thumb, and deftly releases
15 months	Looks, grasps, and releases to build a tower of two cubes*

*From Gesell A and Ilg LB: The child from five to ten, New York, 1946, Harper & Row, Publishers.

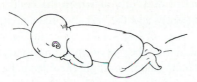

Birth
Keeps his legs tucked up under him and bears his weight on his knees, abdomen, chest, and head.

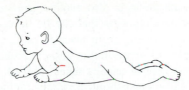

2-3 months
Extends his legs and lifts his chest and head to look around.

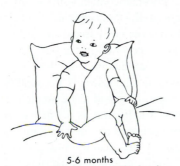

5-6 months
Can sit up with support, hold his head up, and is alert to surroundings.

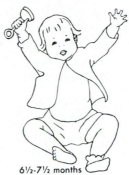

6½-7½ months
Sits up alone and steadily without support. Legs are bowed to help balance.

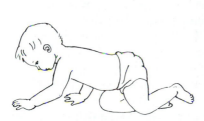

8-9 months
Creeping; the trunk is carried free from floor. With practice, rhythm appears and only one limb moves at a time.

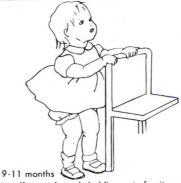

9-11 months
Pulls himself up and stands holding onto furniture. Feet far apart, head and upper trunk carried forward.

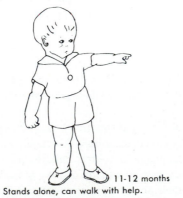

11-12 months
Stands alone, can walk with help.

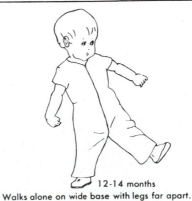

12-14 months
Walks alone on wide base with legs far apart.

FIG 16-9 Guideposts in motor development, emphasizing average child.

Locomotion

The ability to walk alone is also attained gradually after a sequence of developments that can be traced to the first days of life. Moving from place to place and walking are examples of gross motor skills. Complete establishment of this control usually takes most of the first year for early walkers and about 15 months for those who mature later.

The walking sequence begins when the baby is able to hold his head up, and it is half accomplished when the baby can sit alone. When an infant is able to change from a prone to a sitting position, he tends to begin to creep. The infant usually creeps to an object or person and pulls up to a standing position. Gradually the baby stands alone and finally walks independently.

The motor sequence (Fig. 16-9)

½ to 1	month	Lifts head
2 to 3	months	Raises chest
3 to 4	months	Turns from side to back
5 to 6	months	Sits with support
6 to 7	months	Rolls from back to abdomen
6½ to 7½	months	Sits alone
8 to 9	months	Creeps
9 to 11	months	Pulls self up
11 to 12	months	Walks with help
12 to 14	months	Walks alone

Prehension and locomotion develop independent of any teaching. Knowledge of these motor abilities "just comes." Each skill follows an orderly sequential course the rate of which may be affected by environmental factors.

As each skill develops, opportunity to use and practice it is necessary. This means that the child needs plenty of space for walking and objects to pick up and handle; most of all the child needs health, vigor, freedom, and encouragement to venture. The nurse who understands the development of motor skills does not restrict the child to his crib but encourages the child's full capacity for motor growth.

INTELLECTUAL DEVELOPMENT

Of all the factors influencing the overall development of the child, intelligence seems to be the most important. Superior intelligence is associated with superior development, whereas inferior intelligence is associated with retarded development.

Intelligence, defined as the ability to solve problems or achieve a goal, affects the child's observation, thought, and understanding. It strongly influences the level of difficulty at which the child is able to function efficiently and the scope of his activities.

Many changes take place in the intellectual life of children as they develop from infancy to adulthood. At birth the centers of higher intellectual activity in the brain are not fully developed. Furthermore, the sensory acuity necessary for these higher intellectual functions is likewise immature. The mental world of the newborn infant seems to consist primarily of experiences arising through direct physical contact with the environment and through the sensations that originate within the child's own body. New experiences expand the individual's mental world and are interpreted in the light of previous learning. Although "habituation," or the length of time of certain behavioral responses, is not readily detected by casual observers, it is said to be predictive of an infant's intelligence. Habituation is defined as the period of time that elapses between the infant's initial response to a repeated stimuli and the cessation of that response. The duration of a child's response is measured by skin electrode and an assessment of motor activity. The shorter the habituation, the higher the intellectual potential. No one knows whether infants who demonstrate rapid habituation investigate more. Watching intently is an important primary skill.

Beginning very early, children exhibit the ability to imagine and to engage in make-believe activities, which aid children in exploring the real world, organizing experiences, and solving problems. Through make-believe, children are able to participate in a wider range of experiences and to partially overcome their own limitations. Such fantasies are a necessary and normal part of learning.

As growth proceeds, the ability to concentrate develops. Children's attention spans are likely to be longer during activities that they have chosen or that are at least related to their own desires.

The development of a child's ability to reason is gradual and continuous. Young children are concerned with events related to their own immediate experience and well-being. As they grow, they become increasingly able to occupy themselves with more remote issues and to deal with abstractions. Such changes can be noted in the enlarged meanings associated with various terms in the language individual children use, in the interest and ability they eventually display in facing social issues, and in their ability to relate to events in the world beyond their immediate experience.

EMOTIONAL GROWTH

Every infant, child, and adult possesses the drive to express himself in some way. The reaction that accompanies either the satisfaction or frustration of a basic need may be termed an "emotion." Another way of describing an emotional response is to define it as a psychologic reaction caused by internal or external stimuli. Although emotions are not identical to basic drives, they are related. The basic drives can be physical, social, intellectual, or personal. Emotional experience includes feelings, impulses, and physiologic reactions. For example, if a baby's needs are fulfilled, he is happy, joyful, contented, or loving; if a baby's drives are frustrated, he is anxious, fretful, frightened, or angry. Physiologic changes initiated by emotions may stimulate a person to violent action.

All emotions cause a physical response. But just as no two persons think or act alike, no two react to the same emotion in the same way. For example, in response to fear one person may feel belligerent, another anxious, and still another depressed. As soon as one begins to experience emotion, physiologic changes take place. Manifestations of these changes include facial expressions, laughter, and crying.

Emotions appear early in life. Even during the first days of life the infant's need to satisfy his physical needs is accompanied by emotional response. The infant usually reacts by crying or kicking. Soon the baby finds a given stimulation pleasant or unpleasant. When the infant is hungry or uncomfortable, an unpleasant state results, and he reacts by crying or restlessness. When the infant's wants are satisfied, a pleasant state of well-being ensues, which is expressed by cooing, gurgling, or sleep. Thus the emotional responses of the infant are initially stimulated by physiologic needs. A baby's pleasant responses to attention reward the care giver. Ideally both infant and mother satisfy their needs through these encounters and bonding is strengthened.

Through a combination of maturation and learning, more specialized responses soon occur. By the end of the first year, emotions of fear, rage, excitement, anger, and joy become recognizable, and facial expression, vocalization, and body movement become part of the child's emotional equipment. Changes in the expression of the emotions continue progressively throughout the childhood years.

Love. Love is the most important of all the emotions, because it is the foundation on which all positive relationships are built. Children's first love is centered on their mothers, since she usually is the one who initially loves and serves them. The child's capacity for affection and love develops gradually from this early association. During the normal course of development children transfer a part of their affection to others who share their pleasures and achievements. Eventually this love will grow to form the nucleus of another family—the child's own. A child who receives loving and considerate care is prepared to give as well as receive love. For such children security is not simply a passive thing but a safe feeling that allows them to be venturesome in the belief that people will be good to them.

Fear. Fear is aroused naturally when infants experience any startling, sudden occurrence such as a loud noise, an unexpected jar, or a fall. They characteristically respond to these threats to their security with crying and general body distress. The young child acquires other fears that are associated with objects and persons in the immediate environment. As children become older, fearful responses become increasingly specific, and they are expressed by withdrawal from the fearful situation. Later, children learn to avoid situations that cause anxiety.

Once a child becomes afraid in a certain situation, repetition of the same or similar situation usually reproduces fear. However, if the boy or girl learns that the situation is not truly hazardous, the fear diminishes or disappears. Parents and other adults should not laugh at or ridicule a child's fears—identified or unnamed as they may be—but should help the child to understand the situation or thing that is frightening. Reasonable fear is a valuable safeguard against many dangers. Fear acts as a check on behavior. A person may be driven to action by anger, hate, or jealousy, but his conduct is held within reasonable bounds through the fear of consequences. In other words, fear may act as a negative guide to more orderly behavior.

Anger. Anger denotes a variety of emotional states that range from turbulent rage to milder forms of resentment. In infancy, anger arises primarily through interference with body movement or gratification of basic needs such as feeding. Crying, screaming, biting, hitting, and kicking are expressions of anger. In early childhood anger may take the form of numerous acts of disobedience and resistance. When children learn to talk they gain command of new ways to express their anger. Children may find outbursts of anger useful for attracting attention to themselves and for obtaining a desired end. Children are even more likely to give vent to anger when suffering from lack of sleep, hunger, or fatigue.

Approaches to help shape social behavior and moral values

Personal health maintenance (involves both parents and children)

    Provide regular health supervision: health examinations

    Monitor nutrition, sleep, exercise, immunization, drug abuse, and safety education

    Afford opportunities to increase understanding and skills and promote self-esteem

Modifications of environment

    Provide convenient age-appropriate areas for both energetic and quiet play involving both large and small muscles and activities such as music, picture stories, and reading

    Promote safety and include adequate supervision

    Encourage the gradual development of independent, responsible self-care as the child becomes capable (e.g., personal hygiene, dressing, and the completion of assigned household tasks)

Clarification of relationships, methods of communication, and expectations

    Define rules and responsibilities

    Respect the contributions and interests of the individual (provision of quality times with parents)

    Recognize the accomplishments of the family working as a team

    Lead to an understanding and appreciation of one's role and potential in the family and community

Selected techniques to shape behavior

    Model: teach by example

    Use P.E.T. techniques: active listening, I-messages, and negotiated conflict resolution to influence behavior

    Teach the "reality principle": make the child appropriately accountable for results of choices; a selective experience of logical consequences

    Practice distractions or substitution for troublesome toddler activities

    Employ "time-out" (for preschool and young school-age children): withdraw a child from activity for 5- to 10-minute intervals. Older children may be isolated (sent to their room) for about 1 hour or grounded (excluded from certain events).

    Introduce positive practices as part of the response to a difficulty: sincere apology; efforts to repair the damage or right the wrong

    Utilize point systems based on behaviors: reward appropriate expected activity and reduce rewards for failure to achieve or negative behavior

    Administer limited corporal (physical) punishment accompanied by explanations for its use and assurances of love. This technique is sometimes reserved only for "willful disobedience or disrespect for parental authority."

Anger may be controlled in small children by guarding the child's general health and physical condition and by providing regular meals, sleep, and time with mother and father for pleasurable experiences. Feelings of anger may be frightening. Young children need to be reassured that these feelings are very common. However, they also need to be guided toward more appropriate means for expressing anger. They are likely to feel more secure when behavior such as "acting out," hitting, and biting are firmly limited by adults. Parents can also aid by maintaining poise and self-control, refusing to be manipulated by theatrical displays of emotion (temper tantrums). This is usually best accomplished by leaving the child and the scene of the display, if possible. Following through with a clearly defined "time-out" period as soon as practical may be helpful. See the box above.

Jealousy. Jealousy is an emotional response compounded of anger, fear, and love. It is an emotion that, in general, seems to arise when persons or objects threaten to take away something, share something, or interfere with that which is felt to belong to oneself. In the young child, jealousy tends to develop when the child is threatened by possible loss of love, for instance, as a result of the presence of a newborn brother or sister initiating *sibling rivalry*. Because of the mother's preoccupation with the infant, the older child may equate loss of time and attention with loss of love. This child may see the younger sibling as an unwanted competitor and become jealous. The reaction of the child may be active and result in either aggression toward or competition with the new baby. Thus the jealous child may resort to hitting the baby or may turn to infantile habits to gain the desired attention. A negative reaction may consist in withdrawal from competition or repression. For example, a child may sulk or refuse meals. The expression of jealousy varies with age. Behavior caused by such personal envy gradually becomes less direct and less openly violent; it is more subtle but no less real.

The factors precipitating emotions and the reaction patterns they initiate have typical stages of development and can be traced just like the other stages of growth and development. Emotional responses not only vary in form and intensity from person to person but also from age to age. The emotions identified and the reactions they stimulate are closely related to the person's maturity and life experience. Emotions always find an outlet; if the most desired expression is blocked, another perhaps less desirable emotion is substituted. This observation has many practical applications and is basic to the understanding of many behavior problems and the concept of psychosomatic illness. Talking out problems and learning to communicate rather than "acting out" feelings or burying them in the subconscious, where they can cause physical and emotional problems, is extremely important.

SOCIAL BEHAVIOR AND MORAL VALUES

The immediate environment of children as provided by their parents or significant caretakers is of immense importance to their physical, intellectual, and emotional well-being. It is a potent ingredient in the formation of their personal sense of worth, behaviors, and moral values.

Functions of the family

In all cultures, the principal provider of nurturing to the child has been the family. However, the makeup of the unit that constitutes a family has varied and does vary greatly among different groups, locations, and socioeconomic conditions. In the mid-20th century, the typical American family was most likely to be described as "nuclear," that is, consisting of a mother, father, and children. At times, other members such as grandparents, aunts and uncles, and others may have joined the household to extend the scope of that family concept. Family roles were less flexible. Many middle-class mothers did not work outside the home and were the main caregivers for young children, whereas the male parent usually worked in the community and was more often the source of family income.

Today, the form of the typical American family unit is more difficult to describe. Much more diversity is apparent and roles and responsibilities reveal wide possibilities not present previously. The nuclear family is much less common. When both parents are present, they often work outside the home. Male or female single parent families are increasing, as are blended or adoptive

families. Members of some family structures find it more difficult to provide or obtain the appropriate skills or assistance needed to function adequately.

The family may be functionally defined as a special grouping, usually of biologically related persons bound by strong ties of intimacy and caring whose commitments usually have included provisions for the following:

1. Physical safety, growth and development
2. Emotional and social support and family life skill practice
3. Teaching of ethical and spiritual concepts, community responsibilities, and world views
4. Assistance with role definition, career exploration, development of independence, separate residence, and self-realization

Through the years as society has changed, the expectations and functions of families have changed. As more basic needs of survival and education are met or provided by society, less critical but important considerations are often emphasized. On the other hand, if basic needs are not being met by the family or community resources, family dysfunction and societal strain sooner or later become apparent.

An assessment by the nurse of the structure of the family, its composition, and its ability to meet health-related physical or psychologic needs can be of special importance. The nurse may not be able to provide the assistance personally but perceptions of need may be shared with other health professionals for validation and care.

The responsibility of parenting

Although most adults have learned something about parenting through the role modeling of mothers and fathers, requests for help in learning to parent are fairly common. Through parenting a child in a family is introduced to the requirements and rituals of social groups and is assisted in becoming a productive member in these groups. It is an early part of the "civilizing experience." Parenting, by no means an exact science, does include a number of skills that can be learned for the benefit of all. Classes and books specifically about parenting or homemaking are readily available in most communities, but many people are unaware of the types of help they provide. Numerous abilities may be enhanced or learned that may aid the parent directly or indirectly. Classes may include learning how to plan and prepare relatively inexpensive nutritious meals, design a balanced budget, anticipate changes in growth and development, use com-

Table 16-4 Three main styles of parenting

Style	Description
Authoritarian/Autocratic Emphasizes obedience and respect of parental role	Characterized by rather rigid, clearly defined rules. Negative reinforcement is more frequently applied for noncompliance than rewards granted for compliance.
Permissive/Laissez-faire Emphasizes relative freedom from parental restraint and direction	Characterized by lack of or few defined limits. Parent is more likely to use reasoning to guide child, and few punitive measures are applied. Child may learn consequence of action the hard way, and may have difficulty fitting into structured environment of school, etc.
Authoritative/Democratic Emphasizes rational issue-related guidance	Characterized by input from both parent and child for problem solving. Rules tend to be flexible depending on situation. This style encourages development of analysis and responsibility.

munity resources, and relate to one's children in beneficial, happy ways.

Much has been written about styles of parenting. Usually three main styles are identified: authoritarian/autocratic; permissive/laissez-faire and authoritative/democratic (Table 16-4). Most parents mix styles of parenting depending on the situation involved. The style (unless carried to an extreme) does not seem as important as whether the parents are able to provide adequate care and whether their expectations of a child's behavior and their reactions to it are basically consistent and child-appropriate, benefiting the family as a whole. ("Consistent" in this context means predictable and/or equitable, for example, knowledge of dependable follow-through

by the parent regarding behavior and expected consequences rather than blanket uniformity in the treatment of all children or lack of recognition of extenuating circumstances.) Some parents use a certain parenting pattern, even if it is ineffective or abusive, because it is all they know. It was "modeled" to them (taught by example) by their parents.

An authoritative/democratic parenting style is generally considered to be ultimately the most effective because it seeks input from both the child and the parent in problem solving and encourages analysis and self-discipline. The methods endorsed are initially more time-consuming but are usually deemed more productive in the long run. Thomas Gordon has explored and refined this style in his Parent Effectiveness Training (P.E.T.) programs. His training has promoted the use of certain techniques that assist communication and conflict resolution that have been valuable in shaping interactions within the family membership. Some of these techniques will be noted briefly later in this section.

One of the tasks of parenting has been described as moving the child's focus from the *pleasure principle* to the *reality principle*. In other words, as he grows, he is taught that immediate gratification of desires is not always wise or possible and that everyone from time to time is forced to wait for certain experiences or rewards. Children (and adults) should realize that everyone needs to develop self-control and an awareness of the kinds of situations that interrupt plans or make it impossible to do just what one wants to do at the time one wants to do it. It should also be observed that certain preparations may be necessary to be able to enjoy pleasurable outcomes.

Undoubtedly, part of the reality principle that will also be discovered in this process is that parents are not "all-knowing" or without flaw. Therefore, mothers and fathers should feel free to indicate that they too are still learning and growing. (It is a relief to not be expected to be perfect!) The role of parents is sufficiently demanding and dynamic.

Communication techniques and concerns

Communication is necessary for any relationship to endure. It is critical to the proper functioning of the family and the creation of the close attachments important to mothers, fathers, and their offspring. Communication need not always be verbal. Think of examples of nonverbal communication: a caress, a smile, a hummed lullaby, a nodding head. However, even these behaviors may be ambiguous. Those interested in communication are concerned about their ability to say what they mean. They are even more concerned about the greater need to listen attentively to what is being said in order to determine the meanings of others.

Parents are advised, if at all possible, to listen intently, empathetically, without verbalizing questions, comments, interpretations, or evaluations while children are sharing their perceptions and explanations. Interruptions may sidetrack children, causing them to stop a discussion, prematurely closing off communication and stifling what could be an important and gratifying trust-building experience for both parent and child.

In Parent Effectiveness Training sessions, Thomas Gordon lists four basic listening skills which may be used when a significant problem is suspected:

1. Passive listening—silence
2. Use of acknowledgment responses—for example, oh!, uh-huh
3. Door openers—for example, "Would you like to talk about it?"
4. Active listening—the most useful tool when used appropriately (when a conversation is not forced, privacy is respected, sufficient time is available, and the technique is not overused)

Active listening is a supportive communication technique that reflects the child's feelings back to him. It is used to indicate acceptance of a child with a problem; it allows emotional release and sharing and may help the child discover an effective answer to his problem and allow the parent a view of the difficulty and the dynamics of the solution. By feeding back the information that the child shares, the parent's perceptions are verified and this helps the child express and organize his thoughts.

Here is an example of an active listening dialogue:

Tom: (an angry high school freshman arriving home): I never want to go back to Mr. Blake's English class again!
Parent: You're upset about Mr. Blake's English class!
Tom: Yes, I tried real hard on that theme last week, I spent a lot of time. I got a C−. Jerry wrote his in 45 minutes (only 1½ pages) and got an "A".
Parent: You're frustrated because you spent more time and effort than Jerry and didn't get as good a grade as he did.
Tom: You got it! I don't understand why—guess I'll ask Mr. Blake.

For the parent who is having a problem with the behavior of a child, P.E.T. recommends "I-messages." I-messages include three elements: (a) the parent's feelings regarding the behavior, (b) a nonblameful description of the specific behavior, and (c) the tangible (concrete) effect of the behavior on the parent. Because they share feelings and consequences without depreciating or "putting down" the child, I-messages may achieve results without producing negative confrontations. They give the child data instead of blame. I-messages do *not* spell out which specific solution should be used to avoid the described consequences. The solutions are generated by the child and may be very creative and quite acceptable. An example of a problem-identifying I-message would be, "I get upset when I can't hear my friend on the telephone because there is so much commotion and noise in the room; trying to hear her this way wastes my time and energy."

I-messages may also be used to express positive feelings regarding a child's activities and are superior to ordinary praise, which may be experienced as manipulative. Such an I-message would be, "When you come in and hug me after school, it feels so good—the rest of my housework seems easier!"

If a problem is not solved through active listening or I-messages, then conflict-resolution is advocated. This is a method of cooperative problem solving, which is designed to meet the needs of both parties in a no-lose or win-win result.

Child-appropriate parental expectations and reactions

If parents are to be successful in teaching family life skills and social values, communications with their children should be child-appropriate. This means, in part, that parents should be acquainted with the typical patterns of growth and development represented by various ages and stages and the need for anticipatory guidance (see Chapter 17). However, not all children grow at the same rate or respond in the same way to the same stimuli. So, in addition to a child's calendar age, his abilities and previous experiences will also affect communication. Usually parents are sensitive to differences in a child's skills, temperament, and personality as well as to his interests and dislikes—even as children are alert to differences in their caregivers.

Indeed, although consistency in dealing with children is many times held up as an ideal, it is difficult and perhaps unrealistic to try to maintain completely because of the many personal and situational variables that may complicate the family portrait. Parents who identify considerable differences in behavior tolerances, for example, should support one another in such a way that the child will not find it profitable to play one parent against the other and thus precipitate a power struggle. Nor must the child be caught in the middle of such differences.

Parents must work them out so that they do not become a source of confusion to the child.

Role modeling

The day-by-day life example (model) presented by the parent is probably the most effective communication technique known. "Do as I say, not as I do" is *not* effective modeling! A thoughtful, courteous parent is much more likely to produce a thoughtful, patient child, willing to talk about and resolve problems rather than act out frustrations with damaging behavior.

In some families no adult male (or female) may be present to serve as a positive role model for the children. In this case, special efforts should be made to ensure that boys and girls have healthy relationships with adults who demonstrate the qualities desired. Role modeling is one of the goals of such organizations as Big Sisters/Big Brothers and various youth associations sponsored by churches, synagogues, and other community groups.

Through the years, many approaches have been advocated to promote constructive behavior and instill worthy moral values in each developing generation of society. Even a brief perusal of the current literature will reveal a wide range of sometimes conflicting suggestions regarding the best way to guide and prepare our children for their tomorrows. See the box on p. 336 for a list of some of these recommendations. They involve personal health maintenance, environmental modifications, clarification of parent/child communications and mutual expectations, and, finally, possible techniques of control or negotiation to achieve the goals desired.

This last category regarding techniques of negotiation is particularly controversial. For example, some parents feel that negotiations may be inappropriate and/or too time-consuming and that reward systems are too complex and difficult to maintain and border on bribery. Others conclude that listening techniques and the mutual search for solutions may take longer but result in superior self-discipline compliance and teach problem-solving skills. Some mothers and fathers are satisfied with a system of rewards for specific behaviors. If they use money for the reward (a variable allowance), they may believe that the technique is very helpful in teaching how to use money and habits of charity and thrift. The final technique listed—that of applying limited physical punishment—causes the most comment and objections. Such activity may show that the most effective way to control is through physical confrontation, a belief that has not been proved. Also, the possible impulsive escalation of such techniques may and do result in injurious abuse. Surely the attitude of the administrator, explanation of desired behaviors, and assurance of the parents' continuing love are extremely important if this technique is employed. It is estimated that about 85% of parents in the United States have used some type of physical punishment during their child care experiences.

It is largely in the home that the child's basic moral and spiritual concepts are developed. Community agencies, school, and church make significant contributions, but they seldom occupy the primary position in the child's esteem. It is the parents' behavior and not their words that influences the child. To reword an old saying, "What they are speaks so loud that the child does not hear what they say."

Physical growth, psychologic development, social ability, and moral sensitivity should not proceed independently of one another. They are like branches of the same tree, which, when mature, provide strength, protection, meaning, and beauty to both the individual and the community.

Key Concepts

1. A child's normal growth and development are guided by certain basic principles. Growth and development 1) occur in an orderly sequence; 2) are, although continuous, characterized by spurts of growth and periods of relative rest; 3) progress at highly individualized rates; 4) vary at different ages for specific structures; and 5) represent a total process involving the whole child.

2. Every child's growth and development are governed by genetic and environmental forces. A child's cellular inheritance and early embryonic growth will affect the pattern of growth and development.

3. Genetic problems are of three major types: 1) Men-

delian patterns of inheritance involving only one or two defective genes; 2) multifactorial disorders related to multiple gene defects and environmental factors; and 3) gross genetic imbalances caused by chromosomal abnormalities.

4. The genetic counselor uses various genetic information to determine the probability of the occurrence of a given abnormality in a family. The goal of genetic counseling is to prevent genetic defects or reduce their damaging effects to a minimum.

5. Environmental factors that influence a child's growth and development include the following: family composition and interrelationships, culture and life-

styles, stimulation, health habits, nutrition, and malformation or disease.

6. Physical growth may be divided into four periods: 1) rapid growth during infancy; 2) slow, steady growth during childhood; 3) the growth spurt during puberty; and 4) decreasing growth and attainment of maximum height.

7. Growth norms serve as a point of reference for evaluating the growth of an individual child. Since these averages do not necessarily reflect what is desirable for each individual, a child's general progress should be evaluated by comparing the child with himself from time to time.

8. Growth can be measured by the level of bone formation. Bone development continues in an orderly sequence and bone age can be determined by x-ray examination of certain joints.

9. Dentition is widely varied. Patterns of tooth shedding and permanent tooth eruption also vary. Most children have six teeth at 1 year of age and all 20 primary teeth by 2½ years of age.

10. Motor development proceeds in an orderly sequence, but the rate varies with each individual child. Prehension and locomotion provide examples of the usual sequences in the course of motor development.

11. Of all the factors influencing the overall development of the child, intelligence seems to be the most important. It strongly influences the level of difficulty at which the child is able to function efficiently and the scope of his activities. Many changes take place in the intellectual lives of children in their development from infancy to adulthood.

12. The factors precipitating emotions and the reaction patterns they initiate have typical stages of development and can be traced just as the other stages of growth and development can. Emotional responses vary in form and intensity from person to person and from age to age. Significant emotions include love, fear, anger, and jealousy.

13. The immediate environment of children provided by their parents or caretakers is of immense importance to their physical, intellectual, and emotional well-being. It is important for the nurse to assess the structure of the family, its composition, and its ability to meet health related physical or psychologic needs.

14. Three main styles of parenting have been identified: 1) authoritarian/autocratic; 2) permissive/laissez-faire; and 3) authoritative/democratic. Most parents mix these styles depending on the type of situation encountered.

15. Communication is critical to the proper functioning of the family and to the creation of close attachments between family members. P.E.T. indicates that active listening is the most useful tool for parents dealing with their children.

16. "I-messages" are recommended for parents having a problem with a child's behavior. I-messages include the parent's feelings regarding the behavior, a non-blameful description of the behavior, and the tangible effect of the behavior on the parent.

17. Many approaches have been advocated to promote constructive behavior and instill worthy moral values. Techniques include personal health maintenance, modifications of environment, clarification of parent-child communications and mutual expectations, and techniques of control or negotiation to achieve desired goals.

Discussion Questions

1. Discuss the principles of growth and development as described in this chapter. What impact does this have on your nursing care?
2. Carrier testing is available for which autosomal recessive conditions?
3. Discuss a situation in which genetic testing is advisable. What is the role of the genetic counselor?
4. Environment plays a significant role in the growth and development of an infant. Identify and discuss those factors in the home environment which you feel will have a major impact. As a nurse what can you do to promote a healthy environment?
5. If physical, motor, intellectual, and emotional growth and development all unfold in an orderly sequence, why is each child so different?

17

Ages and Stages of Childhood and Youth

CHAPTER OBJECTIVES

After studying this chapter, the student should be able to perform the following:

1 Indicate the average daily weight gain of an infant during the first 6 months and his growth in height during the first year.
2 List five subjects of anticipatory guidance for parents of children of the following ages: 2 weeks, 2 months, 5 months, 10 months, 16 months, 30 months, 3 years, 4 years, and 5 years.
3 Describe the psychosocial challenges as identified by Erik Erikson for the following age groups: infant, toddler, preschooler, school-aged child, early adolescent, and older adolescent.
4 Explain the significance of the following words or phrases and the age group(s) that they describe: separation anxiety, crawling, creeping, parallel play, ritualism, imaginary friend, hero worship, and peer pressure.

5 Identify the average ages for these infant behaviors: raises head, disappearance of Moro and rooting reflexes, sleeps 8 to 10 hours through the night, rolls from abdomen to back, sits with support, rolls from back to abdomen, says "ma-ma."
6 State where and when the first primary tooth usually erupts and when a complete set of baby teeth is obtained.
7 Indicate when the following skills usually appear: kicks ball, throws ball overhand, bowel training established, brushes teeth, buttons and unbuttons clothes, uses one foot per step when going downstairs.
8 Describe the main purpose of the DENVER II Screening Test.
9 Identify four basic tasks of adolescence.

In caring for children, one must have an awareness of the approximate ages at which the child is capable of various activities and functions and the different types of behavior that are likely to emerge at each stage of development. This information assists the nurse in fostering the child's growth and development while caring for him in illness and in health. Many books have been written to describe the physical, motor, and psychologic changes that take place as an individual goes through the process called "growing up." Table 17-1 is designed to assist the student in rapidly identifying the outstanding characteristics of certain ages, as well as in associating those characteristics with the basic challenges of psychosocial stages of development identified by the psychoanalyst Erik Erikson. It also offers anticipatory guidance for the various stages of growth to help provide for the needs of the child and the development of parenting skills by the mother and father. The nurse must remember as she observes and teaches that a child's understanding is influenced by his or her previous experiences and intellectual and educational levels. The performance times noted are averages only, and allowance must always be made for individual differences. The reader is referred to pp. 380-390 for more detailed nutritional expectations.

This chapter also includes a discussion of the DENVER II Developmental Screening Test and the Prescreening Developmental questionnaire, both of which are often used with young children.

THE DENVER II (DEVELOPMENTAL SCREENING TEST)*

The Denver Developmental Screening Test (DDST), a device for detecting developmental delays in infancy and preschool years, evaluates the child's achievement in four major areas of development: gross motor, fine motor adaptive, language, and personal-social. It was originally standardized on a large cross section of the Denver population in 1967 and has undergone two revisions since its original form. The latest and a major revision is the DENVER II which differs from the DDST by including many more language items, and a reduction in the total amount of report items. A pool of 336 items was analyzed and a final selection of 125 items was made on the basis of eight criteria. The items are displayed on the test form which has an age scale corresponding to the American Academy of Pediatrics recommended

health maintenance visits (see Fig. 17-32, A). For other differences review the DENVER II Screening Manual. The test is administered with ease and speed and lends itself to serial evaluations on the same test sheet. The directions for administration of the DENVER II are on the back side of the test sheet (see Fig. 17-32, B).

A simpler related preliminary screening instrument designed to identify those children who require screening with the Denver II is the Revised Denver Prescreening Developmental Questionnaire (R-PDQ) 1986. It facilitates periodic development screening of all children. The R-PDQ is a parent-answered prescreening test which consists of 105 questions arranged in chronologic order, ranging from 3 months to 6 years. Parents respond to age-appropriate questions to be answered with "yes" or "no" on the appropriate form, (orange: 0 to 9 months; purple: 9 to 24 months; gold: 2 to 4 years; white: 4 to 6 years). Children who have no age-appropriate delays are considered to be developing normally. Children who have one delay should be rescheduled for screening in 1 month. If on rescreening the child has one or more delays he should be screened with the DENVER II as soon as possible. Also, children having two or more delays on their first R-PDQ should be screened with the Denver II as soon as possible. Since development is a dynamic process that may be retarded at various ages, developmental screening should be repeated periodically for every child.

Test materials for the DENVER II

The screening manual is designed to teach those performing the screening test the step by step procedures in administration and interpretation of the test. The manual also contains data on the ages at which 25%, 50%, 75%, and 90% of children performed the various items.

The DENVER II test kit contains a skein of red wool, a box of raisins, a rattle with a narrow handle, a small glass bottle with ⅝-inch opening, a bell, a tennis ball, the test form, a pencil, eight 1-inch cubical counting blocks, a doll, a feeding bottle and a cup.

In addition to the materials necessary to administer the DENVER II a technical manual is available that contains step by step instructions for teaching the administration of the test and a test of proficiency to determine if the student is able to properly administer and interpret the test. There is also a videotape available to give students an overview of how to administer and interpret the test properly. It is suggested that this videotape be viewed before studying the Denver II Screening Manual.

*Prepared by WK Frankenburg and others, University of Colorado, reprinted with permission of the authors.

Table 17-1   Ages and stages of maturation

Infancy (0 to 1 yr)—newborn (birth to 1 mo)

Physical growth	Motor development	Language development	Anticipatory guidance	Basic psychosocial challenges
Average weight 7½ lb (3.4 kg)	Readily assumes fetal position		Development	In each stage of child development a central problem has to be solved, temporarily at least, if child is to proceed with vigor and confidence to next stage; each type of challenge appears in its purest form at a particular stage of child development
Gains 1 oz/day (5 to 7 oz weekly for first 6 mo)	Rooting, sucking, tonic neck, grasp, plantar, and Moro reflex present		Early evening crying	
Average height 20 inches (grows 10 inches during first yr)	Raises head but not stable		Sneezing normal	
Head circumference 13 to 14 in (33 to 35.5 cm)	Turns head from side to side		Sleeps 20 hr/day	
Head measures one fourth total length			Regards faces	
Pulse 110 to 150 beats/min			Will eat every 2½ to 4 hr	
Respiration 30 to 50 breaths/min			Breast-fed infants may eat more often	Trust vs mistrust: As infants grow older, they acquire increasing awareness of themselves as individuals who can be happy and satisfied or frustrated and anxious; when they sense they are loved (i.e., needs are gratified), they are happy, content; they begin to develop a basic sense of trust, which is fostered by a warm and loving mother-child and father-child relationship; discontinuities in care bring frustration and pain; child may then develop basic mistrust that may last throughout life
			Safety	
			Burp well	
			Prevent suffocation in crib	
			Car safety restraint	
			Stimulation	
			Colorful hanging toys	
			Talk to infant	
			Use of touch	
			Feeding practices	
			Hold while feeding	
			Diaper care	
			Avoiding diarrhea or constipation	
			Bathing	Significant person: mother

Table 17-1 Ages and stages of maturation—cont'd

Infancy (0 to 1 yr)—newborn (birth to 1 mo)

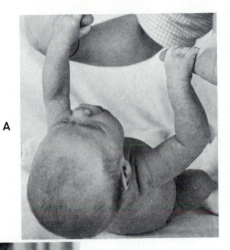

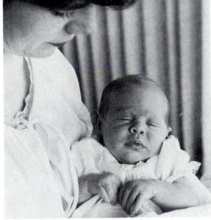

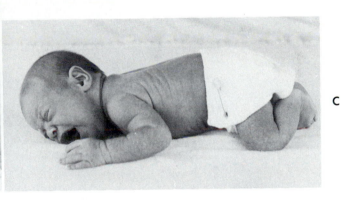

FIG 17-1 Newborn infant. **A,** Grasp reflex is strong. **B,** Sleeps 20 hours a day. **C,** Readily assumes fetal position.

Continued.

Table 17-1   Ages and stages of maturation—cont'd

Infancy (0 to 1 yr)—1 to 3 mo

Physical growth	Motor development	Language development	Anticipatory guidance	Basic psychosocial challenges

Posterior fontanel closes at 1½ to 3 mo
Grows in height about 1 inch/mo
Head circumference increases ⅓ to ¾ in (1 or 2 cm)/mo
	Activity diffuse and random
	Specific reflex activities
	May initiate facial expressions
	Cries with tears 2 mo—can hold rattle; coos, laughs, squeals
	Raises head 45 degrees
	3 mo—raises head 90 degrees
	Will attempt to roll over
		Cooing	Development
			  Head control increasing, alert, likes to look around
			  Follows objects 180 degrees
			5 wk—may sleep 6 to 8 hr through night
			Safety
			  See Newborn
			  Prevent falls
			  Car safety restraint
			  Pacifier
			Stimulation
			  Infant seat
			  Mobile
			  Talk to and touch infant
			  Musical toys
			Feeding practices
			  May "spit up" approximately 1 tbsp
			Other
			  Thumbsucking
			  Immunizations
			  Fever instructions	

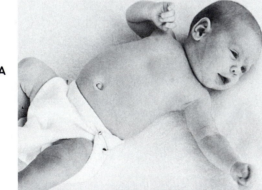
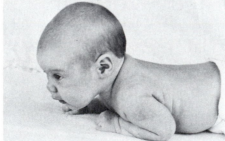
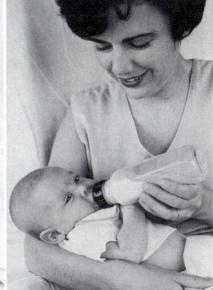

FIG 17-2 Infant at 1 month. **A,** Tonic neck posture readily assumed. **B,** Lifts and turns head when prone. **C,** Held while feeding.

Table 17-1 Ages and stages of maturation—cont'd

Infancy (0 to 1 yr)—1 to 3 mo

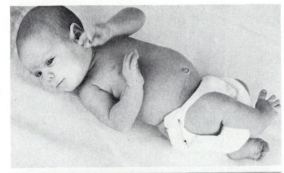

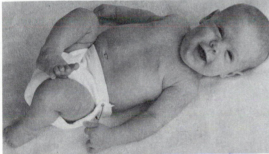

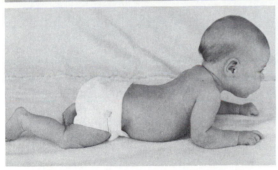

FIG 17-3 Infant at 2 months. **A,** Activity diffuse and random. **B,** Sociable smile appears. **C,** Raises head 45 degrees. **D,** Eyes follow objects.

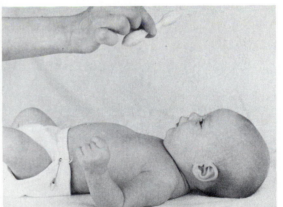

Continued.

Table 17-1   Ages and stages of maturation—cont'd

Infancy (0 to 1 yr)—3 to 6 mo

Physical growth	Motor development	Language development	Anticipatory guidance	Basic psychosocial challenges

Birth weight doubled by 5 mo
Head circumference increases 1/3 in (1 cm)/mo until age 12 mo
	3 to 4 mo—purposefully turns from back to side
	Reaches out at objects
	4 mo—rooting and Moro reflex absent
	5 mo—asymmetric tonic neck reflex absent
	5 mo—rolls from abdomen to back
	6 mo—sits with support
	Palmar grasp absent
		Sociable smile, squeals, coos
		Imitates several tones
		5 mo—understands name and babbles vowel-like sounds
		Responds to human sound more definitively
			Sleeps 8 to 10 hr through night
			Development
			  Spitting up
			  Teething
			Safety
			  Prevent falls and burns
			  Car safety restraint
			Stimulation
			  Play-yard observation
			  Vocal interaction
			  Games
			  Toys to mouth, grab and touch
			Feeding practices
			  Introduce cereal and cup at 5 to 6 mo (see Table 18-1)
			Immunization	

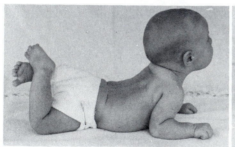 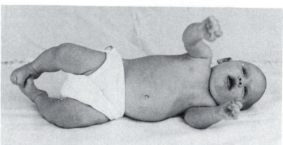

FIG 17-4   Infant at 3 months. **A,** Raises head when prone, supports self on forearms. **B,** Turns from back to side.

Table 17-1 Ages and stages of maturation—cont'd

Infancy (0 to 1 yr)—3 to 6 mo

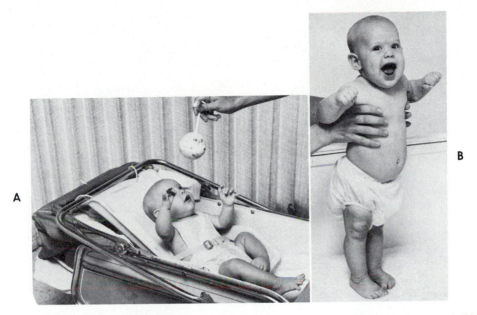

FIG 17-5 Infant at 4 months. **A,** Reaches and grasps at objects. **B,** Pushes with feet when held erect.

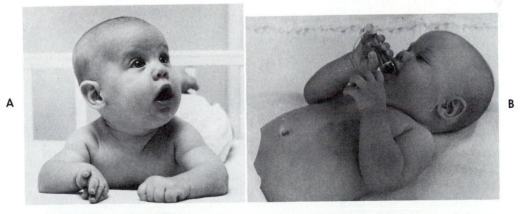

FIG 17-6 Infant at 5 months. **A,** Understands name and babbles. **B,** Manipulates and chews small objects.

Continued.

Table 17-1 Ages and stages of maturation—cont'd

Infancy (0 to 1 yr)—6 to 11 mo

Physical growth	Motor development	Language development	Anticipatory guidance	Basic psychosocial challenges
First primary teeth appear 6 mo—lower central incisors 7½ mo—upper central incisors 10 mo—upper lateral incisors Pulse 110 to 120 beats/min Respirations 30 to 40 breaths/min Blood pressure 90/60 mm Hg	6 mo—rolls from back to abdomen 6½ to 7½ mo—sits alone 9 mo—creeps 10 mo—pulls self to stand Crude pincer grasp, picks up small object using thumb and finger in opposition 9 to 12 mo—may begin cruising, walking Rejects confinement or restraint	Can grunt, growl, and gurgle; says "da-da" or "ma-ma"	Development Puts everything in mouth 7 to 9 mo—fear of strangers Special blanket or toy Dentition and dental care Safety Discipline—begin setting limits Prevent burns, poisoning, ingestion of small objects, falls, drowning Child-proof home Car safety restraint Stimulation Motion, nesting, and cuddle type of toys Peek-a-boo; pat-a-cake Kitchen utensils Feeding practices Finger foods, cup 9 mo—wean from bottle, no bottles in bed, breast-feeding ad lib	

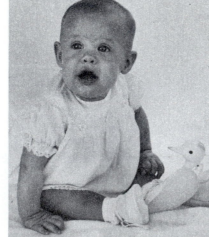
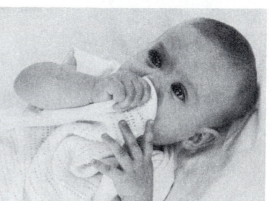

FIG 17-7 Infant at 6 months. **A,** Sits alone, leaning forward on one hand. **B,** Sleeps with favorite blanket and thumb in mouth.

Table 17-1 Ages and stages of maturation—cont'd

Infancy (0 to 1 yr)—6 to 11 mo

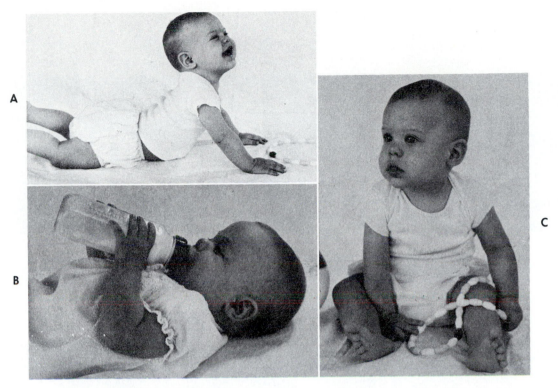

FIG 17-8 Infant at 7 months. **A,** Propels self forward on abdomen (crawling). **B,** Can hold bottle. **C,** Sits alone without support.

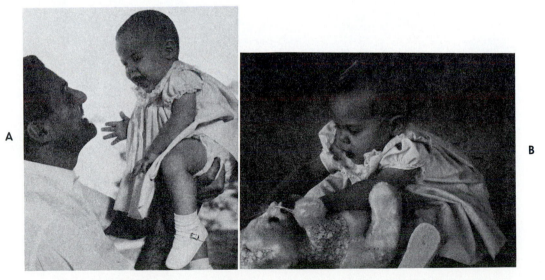

FIG 17-9 Infant at 8 months. **A,** Bubbles, gurgles, loves to play with adults. **B,** Can lean forward and straighten up.

Continued.

Table 17-1   Ages and stages of maturation—cont'd

Infancy (0 to 1 yr)—6 to 11 mo

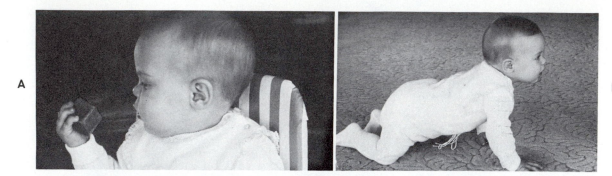

FIG 17-10   Infant at 9 months. **A,** Grasps small objects. **B,** Propels self forward on all fours, trunk above and parallel with floor (creeping).

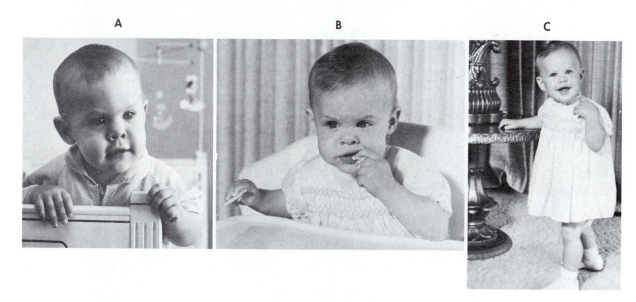

FIG 17-11   Infant at 10 to 11 months. **A,** Can pull self to standing position. **B,** Enjoys finger foods, using thumb and finger in opposition. **C,** Cruises around, holding on to furniture.

Table 17-1 Ages and stages of maturation—cont'd

Infancy (0 to 1 yr)—12 mo

Physical growth	Motor development	Language development	Anticipatory guidance	Basic psychosocial challenges

Birth weight tripled; height 29 to 30 in
6 teeth
Pulse 100 to 110 beats/min
Respirations 20 to 34 breaths/min
Blood pressure 96/66 mm Hg
	Walks alone with wide stance and short steps
	Picks up small objects with forefinger and thumb
	Drinks from cup with ease
		Says "ma-ma" and "da-da" plus two other small words such as "no-no" and "bye-bye"	Development
			  Negativism begins
			  Likes to explore
			  Plays spontaneously
			  1 nap/day
			  Cooperates in dressing
			  Gives a kiss
			Safety
			  See precautions for 6 to 11 mo
			Stimulation
			  Push and pull toys
			  Read to child
			Feeding practices
			  3 meals/day
				Trust, cornerstone of a healthy personality, usually established by end of first year

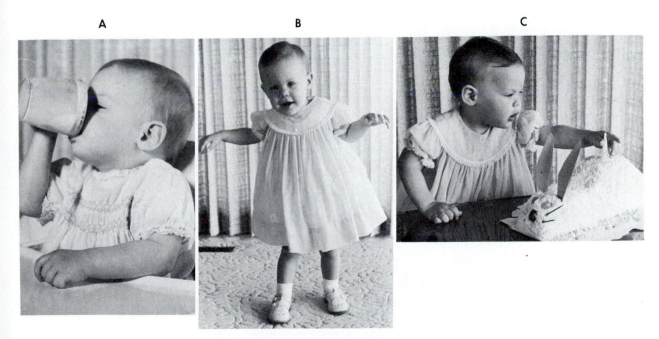

FIG 17-12 Infant at 12 months. **A,** Drinks from cup with ease. **B,** Walks alone with wide stance and short steps. **C,** Has good finger-thumb opposition.

Continued.

Table 17-1   Ages and stages of maturation—cont'd

Toddler (1 to 3 yr)—15 to 18 mo

Physical growth	Motor development	Language development	Anticipatory guidance	Basic psychosocial challenges

Growth rate slows
Abdomen protrudes
8 to 12 teeth
Anterior fontanel closed
	Walks well without support
	Builds a tower of two blocks
	Uses spoon but spills
	Can throw object
	Ceaseless activity
	Walks upstairs holding on
	Need for active mastery of newfound motor skills
		Vocabulary of 6 to 10 words; follows simple commands
		Uses jargon that will develop into sentences
			Development
			  Toilet training— may show signs of readiness
			  May be assertive and independent
			  Anger and temper tantrums
			  Ritualistic behavior
			  Takes off shoes and socks
			  Can climb into everything
			Safety
			  Lock medications
			Toddler immunizations
			Stimulation
			  Enjoys coloring, spontaneous scribbling
			  Moves from solitary to parallel play (playing beside but not with other children)
			  Turns pages of book
			Feeding practices
			  Small servings
			  Decrease in appetite
				Self-esteem (autonomy) vs shame and doubt: Children's energies centered around asserting that they are individuals with their own minds and wills; they must have right to choose; they want to do more and more for themselves; feelings of self-esteem, pride, and independence develop; with guidance from parents and others, they learn to make decisions and to become more self-reliant; those who guide growing children wisely will be firm, will avoid shaming them and causing them to doubt their sense of worth
				Significant persons: parents

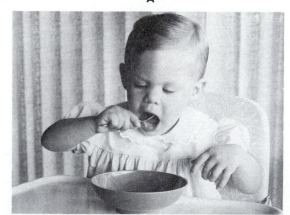

A

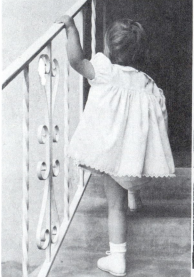

B

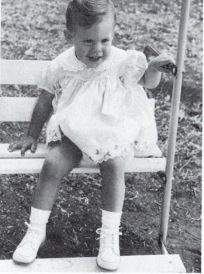

C

FIG 17-13   Toddler at 15 months. **A,** Uses spoon but spills. **B,** Walks upstairs holding on. **C,** Plays outside.

Table 17-1 Ages and stages of maturation—cont'd

Toddler (1 to 3 yr)—15 to 18 mo

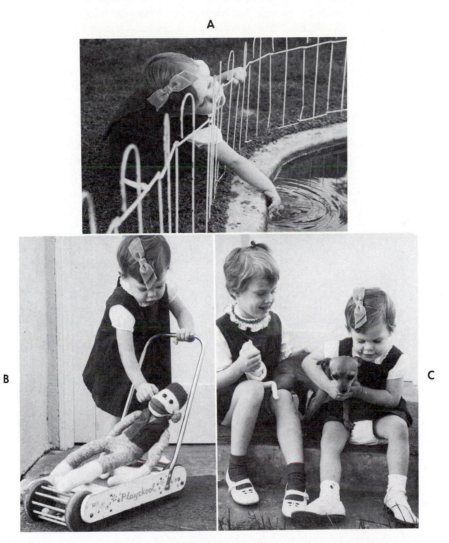

FIG 17-14 Toddler at 18 months. **A,** Needs independence but supervision too. **B,** Loves to push and pull toys. **C,** Moves from solitary to parallel play.

Continued.

Table 17-1   Ages and stages of maturation—cont'd

Toddler (1 to 3 yr)—24 mo

Physical growth	Motor development	Language development	Anticipatory guidance	Basic psychosocial challenges

Grows 3 to 5 in in second year
Gains 5 lb in second year
Weighs 26 to 28 lb
16 teeth
Pulse 90 to 120 beats/min
Respirations 20 to 35 breaths/min
	Walks up and down stairs alone
	Runs without falling
	Opens door
	Kicks ball
	Throws ball overhand
	Overestimates own capabilities
		Names familiar objects; says simple phrases; has vocabulary of 300 words; "me" and "mine" dominate	Development
			  Bowel control usually achieved
			  Has difficulty sharing
			  Dressing ability increases
			  Thumbsucking and temper tantrums decrease
			  Bedtime rituals important
			  Discipline—limits must be set; define unacceptable behavior
			Safety
			  Set limits
			  See previous precautions
			  Continue to childproof
			  Avoid foods that may be aspirated
			Stimulation
			  Will advance to cooperative play in next 12 mo
			  Picture books, stories
			  Begins to imitate doing household tasks
			Feeding practices
			  Dexterity increases
			  Appetite fluctuates
			  Feeds self	

Table 17-1   Ages and stages of maturation—cont'd

Toddler (1 to 3 yr)—24 mo

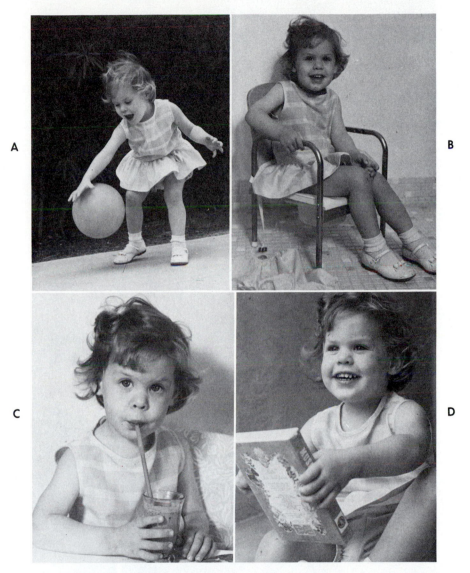

FIG 17-15   Toddler at 24 months. **A,** Muscular coordination greatly advanced. **B,** Verbalizes toilet needs. **C,** Drinks from straw. **D,** Enjoys picture books.   *Continued.*

Table 17-1   Ages and stages of maturation—cont'd

Toddler (1 to 3 yr)—30 mo

Physical growth	Motor development	Language development	Anticipatory guidance	Basic psychosocial challenges

Complete set of 20 primary teeth	Builds tower of 8 blocks
	Jumps with both feet
	Walks on tiptoes
	Undresses self easily
		Says full name; sings
		Begins to express needs
			Development
			  Loves routine
			  Magical thinking
			  Bladder training improves
			  Washes and dries hands
			  Make first dental appointment
			Safety
			  Prevent burns, falls, drownings, ingestions
			  Provide stimulation in car seat to help keep content, secure
			Stimulation
			  Exposure to other children
			  Coloring, finger-painting, games, cooking group
			  Short attention span
			Feeding practices
			  Definite likes and dislikes
			Sexual curiosity continues	

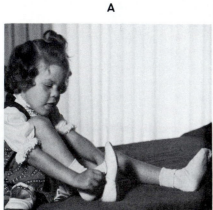
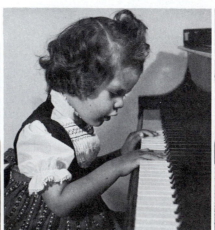
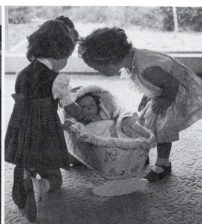

FIG 17-16   Toddler at 30 months. **A,** Can put shoes on. **B,** Attempts to sing simple songs. **C,** Enjoys playing with others.

Table 17-1 Ages and stages of maturation—cont'd

Preschool (3 to 6 yr)—3 yr

Physical growth	Motor development	Language development	Anticipatory guidance	Basic psychosocial challenges

Relatively slow growth; gains about 5 lb; height increases average of 3 in/yr	Uses stairs with alternate feet
	Strings large beads
	Hops on 1 foot
	Rides tricycle
		Has vocabulary of 900 words or more
		Knows 2 colors
		May talk with imaginary playmate
			Development
			  Can brush teeth
			  May display sibling rivalry
			  Bladder control usually achieved
			  Interest in sexuality
			  Needs 12 hr sleep a day
			  Allow independence within limits of safety
			Safety
			  Child overestimates capabilities—set limits
			Stimulation
			  Will soon enjoy cooperative play
			  Desires constant activity
			  Resents interference with play or possessions
			  Climbing activities essential
			  Wagons, kiddie cars, tricycles, and boats enjoyed
			Feeding habits
			  Food "jags" common; may not like "mixtures," i.e., casseroles
			  Regularity of mealtime important
				Initiative vs guilt: Knowing that they are persons in their own right, preschool children want to find out what kind of persons they can be; they imagine what it is like to be grown up; little girls want to be like "mama" and boys like "daddy"; they imitate parents and yearn to share in their activities; by this age, conscience has developed; an age of avid curiosity and consuming fantasies, which lead to feeings of guilt and anxiety; initiative must be fostered and care taken that young children do not feel guilty because they dared to dream
				Significant persons: basic family

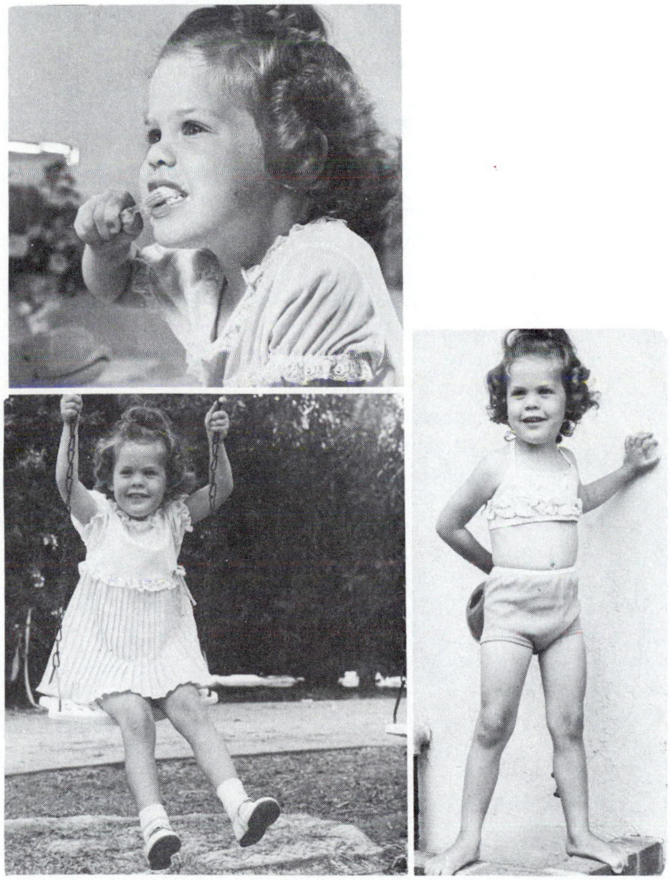

FIG 17-17 Preschooler at 3 years. **A,** Can brush teeth and wash hands. **B,** Can pump swing with legs. **C,** Knows own age and sex and has good balance.

Continued.

Table 17-1 Ages and stages of maturation—cont'd

Preschool (3 to 6 yr)—4 yr

Physical growth	Motor development	Language development	Anticipatory guidance	Basic psychosocial challenges
Height 39 to 41 in Weight 35 to 37 lb Continued relatively slow growth at rate of 3-year-old Pulse 100 beats/min Respirations 20 to 25 breaths/min Blood pressure 100/68 mm Hg	Uses 1 foot per step when going down stairs Climbs and jumps well Increasing finger dexterity Buttons and unbuttons clothes	Vocabulary of 1,500 words Can explain own drawing; knows several colors; repeats rhymes and songs Asks many questions	Development Magical thinking Sexual curiosity Continues becoming more self-sufficient Knows own age Safety May use seatbelt when weight reaches 40 to 50 lbs Teach safety precautions, i.e., cross streets on signals Avoid hot radiator and stove Preschool immunization Stimulation Moves from cooperative play with one child to small group play—plan projects accordingly Prepare for school Feeding practices Avoid between-meal snacks	

Table 17-1   Ages and stages of maturation—cont'd

Preschool (3 to 6 yr)—4 yr

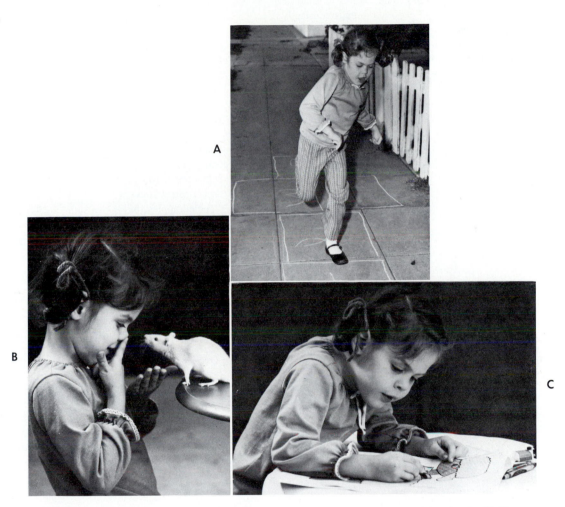

FIG 17-18 Preschooler at 4 years. **A,** Hops on one leg. **B,** Enjoys playing with animals. **C,** Has increasing finger dexterity with crayons.

Continued.

Table 17-1 Ages and stages of maturation—cont'd

Preschool (3 to 6 yr)—5 yr

Physical growth	Motor development	Language development	Anticipatory guidance	Basic psychosocial challenges

Height 43 to 44 in
Weight 40 lbs
May lose lower central incisors
Pulse 100 beats/min
Respirations 20 to 25 breaths/min
Blood pressure 94/55 mm Hg
	Good muscular coordination; can hop, skip, run, and catch ball
	Climbs on jungle gym
	Handles tricycle well
	Needs rest periods
		Names all primary colors and coins
		Talks in sentences; talks constantly
			Development
			  Prints
			  Dresses and undresses without assistance
			  Sensitive to praise
			Safety
			  Reinforce safety precautions
			Stimulation
			  Enjoys group activities, conformity, rules
			Feeding practices
			  Likes finger foods, i.e., carrot sticks, peeled apples, bananas
			  Teach importance of preventing caries	

Table 17-1   Ages and stages of maturation—cont'd

Preschool (3 to 6 yr)—5 yr

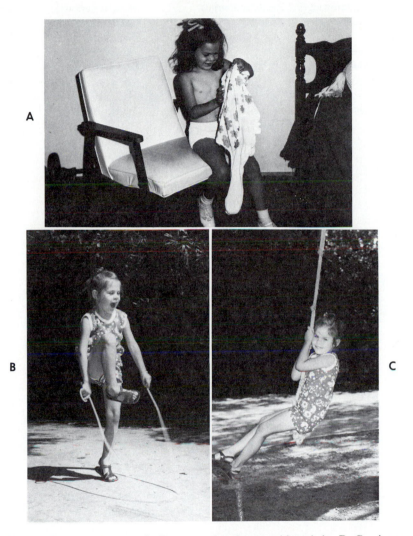

FIG 17-19   Preschooler at 5 years. **A,** Dresses and undresses without help. **B,** Can jump rope. **C,** Has good muscular coordination.

Continued.

Table 17-1 Ages and stages of maturation—cont'd

School age (6 to 10 yr)—6 and 7 yr

Physical growth	Motor development	Language development	Anticipatory guidance	Basic psychosocial challenges
6 yr molars; first permanent teeth	Good balance	Vocabulary of 2,500 words	Development	Industry vs inferiority: Preoccupation with fan-
Annual growth of 2 in	Increased dexterity	Reads and writes	Can bathe self	tasy subsides; children
Height 47 to 48 in	Advanced throwing	Counts	Modest; curious	want to be engaged in real
Weight 50 to 51 lb	Roller skates	May tell time	Conscious of rules	tasks that they can carry
Loses upper inci-	Swims		Household chores	through; in learning to ac-
sors	Ties shoes		important	cept instruction and win
	Enjoys outdoor		Begins to write	recognition by producing
	sports; can ride bi-		Allow independence	"things," they develop
	cycle, swim, jump		Safety	sense of adequacy and ac-
	rope, walk straight		Clubs, gangs, hero	complishment; when chil-
	line		worship pro-	dren do not receive recog-
			nounced—may	nition for their efforts,
			cause problems	they develop sense of in-
				adequacy and inferiority
				Significant persons: school
				and neighborhood friends

Table 17-1   Ages and stages of maturation—cont'd

School age (6 to 10 yr)—6 and 7 yr

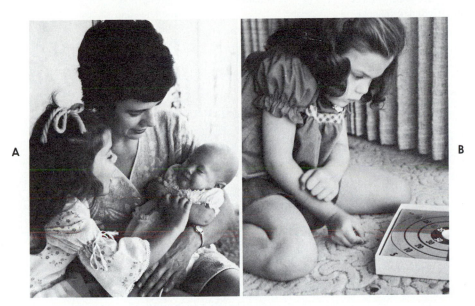

FIG 17-20   School age—6 years. **A,** Helps with younger children. **B,** Has increased interest in games.

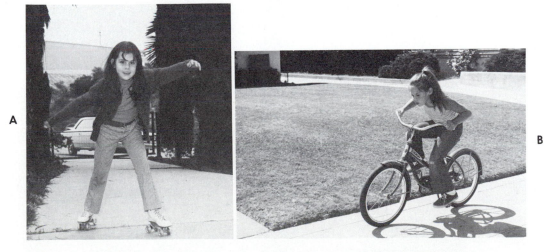

FIG 17-21   School age—7 years. **A,** Can roller skate. **B,** Can ride bicycle.   *Continued.*

Table 17-1   Ages and stages of maturation—cont'd

School age (6 to 10 yr)—8 and 9 yr

Physical growth	Motor development	Language development	Anticipatory guidance	Basic psychosocial challenges

Gradual increase in size—steady growth
Pulse 90 beats/min
Respirations 16 to 20 breaths/min
Blood pressure 106/56 mm Hg
	Movements more graceful; able to accomplish more
	Complex manual skills
		8 yr—tells days of week
		9 yr—tells months of year
		Enjoys puns, jokes, stories
		Reading, a useful tool, and may be enjoyable pastime
			Stimulation
			  Enjoys solitary and group play
			  Bicycles and skates are enjoyed
			  Competitive sports valued
			  Prefers own sex; peer group important
			  Favorite television shows
			  Continues to enjoy stories
			  May enjoy collections
			Feeding practices
			  Desires afternoon snacks
			  Teach importance of good nutrition; allow time for adequate breakfast
			  May have problems with manners and mealtime punctuality
			Good eaters from 8 yr on	

Table 17-1   Ages and stages of maturation—cont'd

School age (6 to 10 yr)—8 and 9 yr

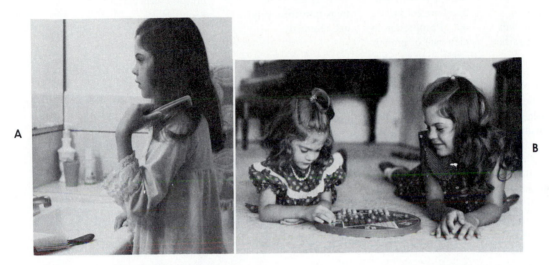

FIG 17-22   School age—8 years. **A,** Personal hygiene important. **B,** Satisfaction gained helping younger sister to learn.

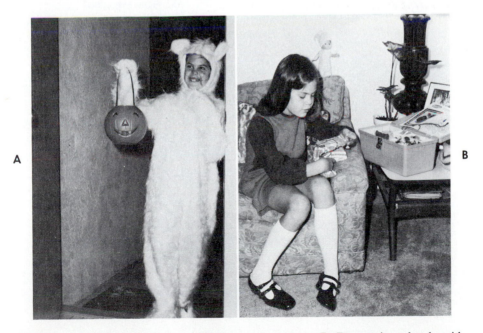

FIG 17-23   School age—9 years. **A,** Halloween—enjoys puns. **B,** Engages in real task, with recognition important.

Continued.

Table 17-1   Ages and stages of maturation—cont'd

Preadolescence (10 to 12 yr)

Physical growth	Motor development	Language development	Anticipatory guidance	Basic psychosocial challenges
Appearance and development of secondary sexual characteristics Pubescent growth spurt; 2 yr earlier for girls Girls may show widening of hips, budding breasts, pubic hair, and occasionally menses Boys ahead of girls in physical strength and endurance; boys increase in muscle mass and bone size especially shoulder girdle and ribs; penis and scrotum enlarge	Poor control will ensue if body framework and muscular development are out of proportion in their rate of growth Posture may be poor	Vocabulary increases; language reflects increasing ability to think introspectively and abstractly	Development Four basic tasks of preadolescence and adolescence: 1. Emancipation from parents and other adults 2. Development of healthy self-concept 3. Beginning acquisition of skills for future 4. Understanding psychosexual differences Possible problems 1. Obesity caused by inactivity and ravenous appetite 2. Poor nutrition (fad diets); need for increased protein 3. Acne associated with hormonal changes 4. Poor self-image (changing body image) 5. Peer pressure; ambivalence toward parents and other adults 6. Lack of sexual identity 7. Adolescent pregnancy 8. Venereal disease 9. Accidents	

Table 17-1   Ages and stages of maturation—cont'd

Preadolescence (10 to 12 yr)

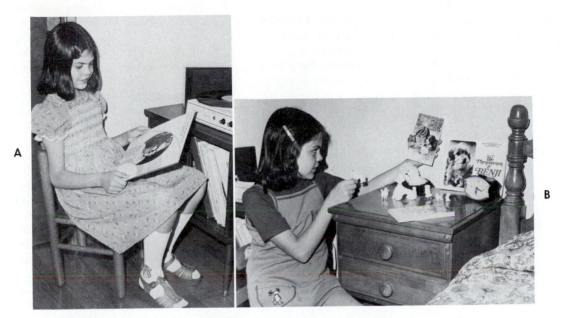

FIG 17-24   Preadolescence—10 years. **A,** Listening to music common pastime. **B,** Has many collections.

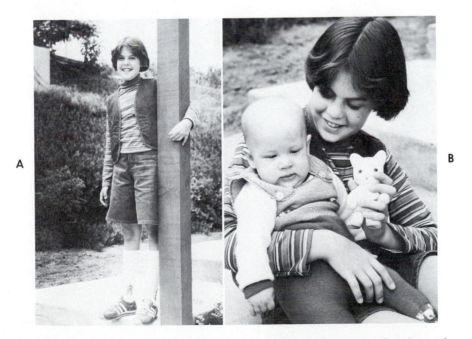

FIG 17-25   Preadolescence—11 years. **A,** Growing up fast. **B,** Baby-sitting favorite pastime.   *Continued.*

Table 17-1   Ages and stages of maturation—cont'd

Adolescence (12 to 19 yr)—early adolescence (12 through 15 yr)

Physical growth	Motor development	Language development	Anticipatory guidance	Basic psychosocial challenges

Wide individual variability as to onset and rate of growth
 	
Girls: growth spurt between 10 and 14 yr, gain 2 to 8 in (5 to 20 cm) in height, 15 to 55 lb (7 to 25 kg) in weight; menarche occurs 2 yr after pubescent changes
 	
Boys: growth spurt at 12 to 16 yr, gain 4 to 12 in (10 to 30 cm) in height and 15 to 65 lb (7 to 30 kg) in weight
 	
Growth of pubic, axillary, and upper lip hair; facial hair appears 2 yr after pubic hair
	Wide individual variability
	
	Hands and feet out of proportion; self-conscious, awkward
		Increased vocabulary influenced by attainment of intellectual maturity
		
		Talkative but not communicative; giggly
			Development
			  See preadolescent section
			  Needs parental respect and acceptance
			  Preparing for difficult decisions of late adolescence, i.e., continuing education, work, military service, dating, marriage plans, financial responsibilities, political and religious affiliations
				Identity vs diffusion: Adolescents seek to establish a sense of identity; if a good foundation has been laid (including building blocks of trust, autonomy, sexual identification, initiative, and learning), they will be able to integrate childhood identifications, basic biologic drives, native endowment, and opportunities offered in social roles to feel secure regarding their part in society; self-diffusion or lack of a feeling of identity may be temporarily unavoidable because of physiologic changes and psychologic upheavals in this period
				
				Significant persons: peer group

Table 17-1   Ages and stages of maturation—cont'd

Adolescence (12 to 19 yr)—early adolescence (12 through 15 yr)

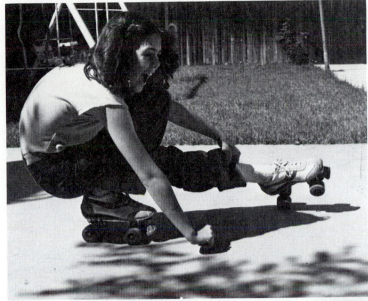

A

FIG 17-26   Early adolescence—12 to 15 years. **A,** Good coordination.

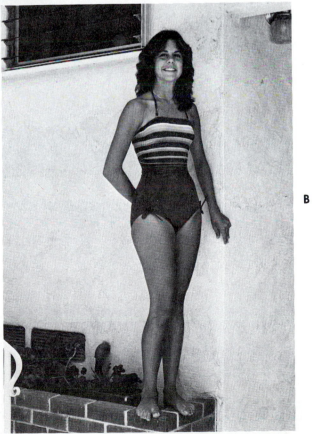

B

FIG 17-26, cont'd   **B,** Moving toward maturity—13 years. (See Fig. 17-17, *C,* for same pose 10 years earlier.)

Continued.

Table 17-1   Ages and stages of maturation—cont'd

Adolescence (12 to 19 yr)—early adolescence (12 through 15 yr)

A   B

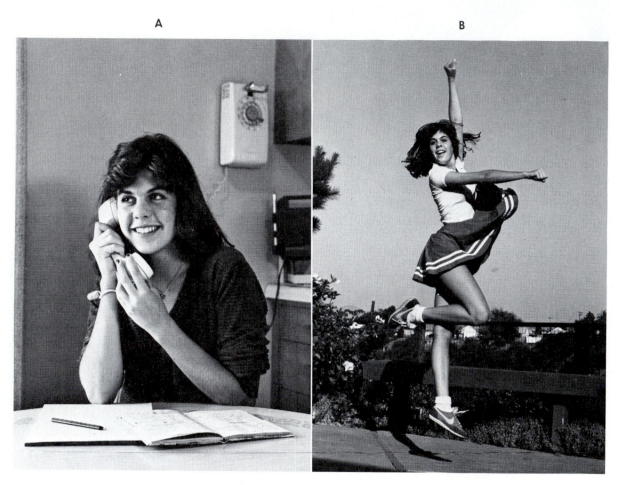

FIG 17-27   Adolescence—14 years. **A,** Talkative—many hours spent on telephone. **B,** Athletic ability highly prized.

Table 17-1 Ages and stages of maturation—cont'd

Adolescence (12 to 19 yr)—early adolescence (12 through 15 yr)

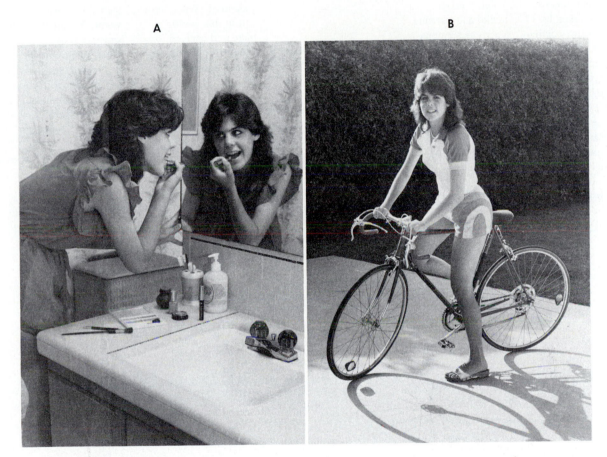

A   B

FIG 17-28 Early adolescence—15 years. **A,** Different-colored make-up for every occasion.
B, Exercise—a must for the figure.

Continued.

Table 17-1   Ages and stages of maturation—cont'd

Late adolescence (16 to 19 yr)

Physical growth	Motor development	Language development	Anticipatory guidance	Basic psychosocial challenges
Adult size and proportion usually attained Spermatogenesis established by 17 yr; slow, continuous growth in height ceases at 18 to 20 yr in boys and at 16 to 17 yr in girls Pulse 70 to 86 beats/min Respirations 14 to 16 breaths/min Blood presure 118/60 mm Hg	Improvement in coordination; strength and athletic ability highly prized Social and sporting activities emphasized		Dominant developmental thrust Establishment of ego identity: "Where do I fit in this world?" Increased concern for philosophic and religious questions	Intimacy vs isolation: When young persons feel secure in their identity, they are then able to establish warm, meaningful, constructive relationships with others and eventually a love-based, mutually satisfying sexual relationship; when they are unable to relate to others, they may develop a deep sense of isolation Significant person: opposite sex partner

Table 17-1 Ages and stages of maturation—cont'd

Late adolescence (16 to 19 yr)

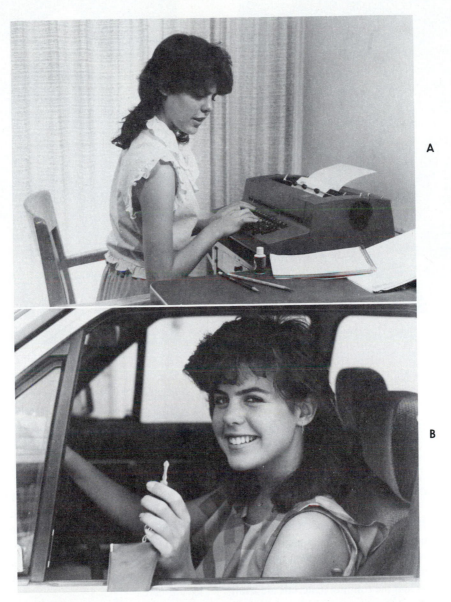

FIG 17-29 Late adolescence—16 years. **A,** Homework every night, except weekends. **B,** Wheels at last—another gray hair for mother!

Continued.

Table 17-1 Ages and stages of maturation—cont'd

Late adolescence (16 to 19 yr)

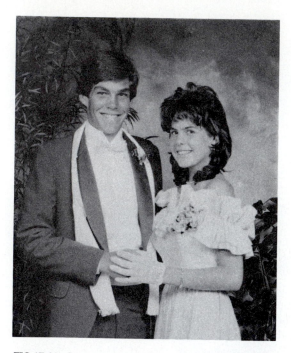

FIG 17-30 Late adolescence—17 years. Junior prom.

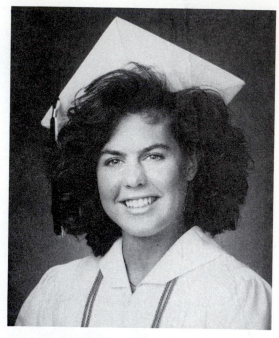

FIG 17-31 Late adolescence—18 years. Graduation.

CAUTION

1. Fig. 17-32 is an overview of the test and is not complete.
2. The DENVER II is not an intelligence test. It is intended as a screening instrument for use in clinical practice to note whether the development of a particular child is within the normal range.
3. The test materials and the training materials are available through Denver Developmental Materials, Inc., P.O. Box 6919, Denver, Colorado 80206-0919, (303) 355-4729.

Nurses should counsel parents that they cannot prevent or hurry growth, nor can they "do the growing" for their children. Adults can provide a healthy and happy environment in which children can grow, develop, and reach their optimum potential. Adults can provide the right equipment, abundant space, encouragement, and tender loving care.

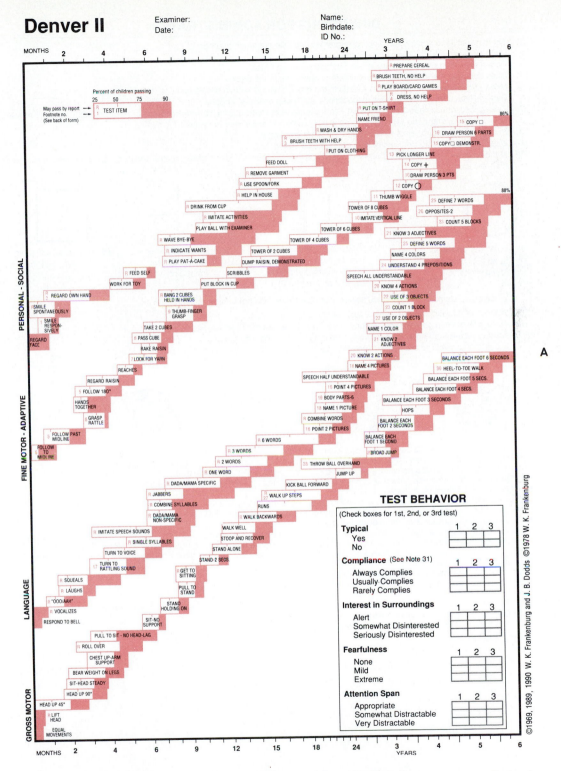

FIG 17-32 **A,** Denver Developmental Screening Test sheet. *Continued.*

DIRECTIONS FOR ADMINISTRATION

1. Try to get child to smile by smiling, talking or waving. Do not touch him/her.
2. Child must stare at hand several seconds.
3. Parent may help guide toothbrush and put toothpaste on brush.
4. Child does not have to be able to tie shoes or button/zip in the back.
5. Move yarn slowly in an arc from one side to the other, about 8" above child's face.
6. Pass if child grasps rattle when it is touched to the backs or tips of fingers.
7. Pass if child tries to see where yarn went. Yarn should be dropped quickly from sight from tester's hand without arm movement.
8. Child must transfer cube from hand to hand without help of body, mouth, or table.
9. Pass if child picks up raisin with any part of thumb and finger.
10. Line can vary only 30 degrees or less from tester's line.
11. Make a fist with thumb pointing upward and wiggle only the thumb. Pass if child imitates and does not move any fingers other than the thumb.

12. Pass any enclosed form. Fail continuous round motions.
13. Which line is longer? (Not bigger.) Turn paper upside down and repeat. (pass 3 of 3 or 5 of 6)
14. Pass any lines crossing near midpoint.
15. Have child copy first. If failed, demonstrate.

When giving items 12, 14, and 15, do not name the forms. Do not demonstrate 12 and 14.

16. When scoring, each pair (2 arms, 2 legs, etc.) counts as one part.
17. Place one cube in cup and shake gently near child's ear, but out of sight. Repeat for other ear.
18. Point to picture and have child name it. (No credit is given for sounds only.)
   If less than 4 pictures are named correctly, have child point to picture as each is named by tester.

B

 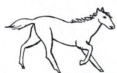   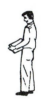

19. Using doll, tell child: Show me the nose, eyes, ears, mouth, hands, feet, tummy, hair. Pass 6 of 8.
20. Using pictures, ask child: Which one flies?... says meow?... talks?... barks?... gallops? Pass 2 of 5, 4 of 5.
21. Ask child: What do you do when you are cold?... tired?... hungry? Pass 2 of 3, 3 of 3.
22. Ask child: What do you do with a cup? What is a chair used for? What is a pencil used for? Action words must be included in answers.
23. Pass if child correctly places and says how many blocks are on paper. (1, 5).
24. Tell child: Put block **on** table; **under** table; **in front of** me, **behind** me. Pass 4 of 4. (Do not help child by pointing, moving head or eyes.)
25. Ask child: What is a ball?... lake?... desk?... house?... banana?... curtain?... fence?... ceiling? Pass if defined in terms of use, shape, what it is made of, or general category (such as banana is fruit, not just yellow). Pass 5 of 8, 7 of 8.
26. Ask child: If a horse is big, a mouse is __? If fire is hot, ice is __? If the sun shines during the day, the moon shines during the __? Pass 2 of 3.
27. Child may use wall or rail only, not person. May not crawl.
28. Child must throw ball overhand 3 feet to within arm's reach of tester.
29. Child must perform standing broad jump over width of test sheet (8 1/2 inches).
30. Tell child to walk forward, ⚬⚬⚬⚬⚬⚬➤ heel within 1 inch of toe. Tester may demonstrate. Child must walk 4 consecutive steps.
31. In the second year, half of normal children are non-compliant.

OBSERVATIONS:

FIG 17-32, cont'd   B, Reverse side of test sheet.

Key Concepts

1. Development at a given age may be measured by physical growth, motor development, and language development. Each stage presents basic psychosocial challenges. Anticipatory guidance identifies the needs of the child at each stage and assists in the development of parenting skills.

2. During infancy (birth to 1 year) the child grows and develops rapidly. By 1 year of age the child has six teeth and his birth weight has tripled. He can usually walk alone, pick up small objects, drink from a cup, and say several simple words. The basic psychosocial challenge is the development of trust versus mistrust. Anticipatory guidance includes development, safety, stimulation, feeding practices, bathing, and immunizations.

3. The growth rate slows during toddler years (1 to 3 years). By the age of 3 the child can run and climb stairs, string large beads, throw a ball, and ride a tricycle. He has a vocabulary of 900 words, knows his full name, and begins to express his needs. His basic psychosocial challenge is self-esteem versus shame and doubt. Anticipatory guidance includes development, safety, stimulation, feeding practices, immunizations, and sexual curiosity.

4. The average preschooler (3 to 6 years) weighs 40 pounds and is 43 to 44 inches tall by the age of 5. He has increasing finger dexterity and good muscle coordination. He uses his 1,500-word vocabulary in sentences, talking constantly and asking numerous questions. His basic psychosocial challenge is initiative versus guilt. Anticipatory guidance includes development, safety, immunizations, stimulation, and feeding practices.

5. Steady growth is seen in the school-aged child (6 to 10 years). Balance, dexterity, and manual skills are well developed. He can count, read, and write, and has a 2,500-word vocabulary. His basic psychosocial challenge is industry versus inferiority. Anticipatory guidance includes development, safety, stimulation, and feeding practices.

6. Preadolescence usually occurs between 10 to 12 years of age and involves a growth spurt and the appearance and development of secondary sexual characteristics. Poor motor control may ensue if body framework and muscular development are out of proportion in their rate of growth. Anticipatory guidance includes developmental challenges and possible future problems.

7. During adolescence (12 to 19 years) adult size and proportion are usually attained. Motor development varies widely and coordination improves. Intellectual maturity is attained. Basic psychosocial challenges include identification versus diffusion, followed by intimacy versus isolation. Anticipatory guidance includes immunization, nutrition, exercise, and vocational guidance as well as those which were first introduced during preadolescence.

8. The DENVER II Developmental Screening Test evaluates the child's achievement in four major areas of development: gross motor, fine motor adaptive, language, and personal-social.

Discussion Questions

1. The DENVER II Developmental Screening Test is helpful in estimating a child's level of development. Discuss the precautions to take when administering the test.

2. Discuss the anticipatory guidance that the nurse should provide to parents at their child's 6-month check-up.

3. Discuss Erikson's psychosocial challenges. Observe a toddler and compare your observations with the stage of development described.

4. Safety is an area of concern throughout life. The safety concerns related to children change greatly as the child moves from one stage to another. Discuss the major safety concerns of the preadolescent and the teaching required.

18

Preventive Pediatrics

CHAPTER OBJECTIVES

After studying this chapter, the student should be able to perform the following:

1 Indicate recommended feeding practices for formula-fed infants—type and amount of fluid intake, typical hunger patterns, need for vitamins, and use of skim and whole milk.
2 Discuss neuromuscular indicators for the introduction of semisolids and the typical sequential development of skills that lead to successful self-feeding.
3 Review Fig. 18-3, and explain the main reason why an infant needs more calories per kilogram than an older child.
4 Discuss the important roles of the minerals, iron, calcium, and fluoride in the growth of a child.
5 Outline the recommended active immunization schedule for normal infants and children from 2 months to

16 years of age, including protection against eight different infectious diseases.
6 Describe the impact of injuries on the pediatric population, and state three principles advocated for reducing the incidence of accidental death and injury.
7 List six different safeguards that, if followed, can reduce the occurrence of accidental poisonings.
8 Discuss the use of syrup of ipecac, when it should not be used to produce vomiting, how it is given, and the dose usually recommended for children over 1 year of age.
9 Identify six possible clues of nonaccidental injury, and discuss the legal obligation of physicians and nurses to report suspicious findings.

The valuable "ounce of prevention" that everyone has heard mentioned so often is frequently measured in milliliters, drops, or minutes spent with the physician and nurse for regular health supervision. Maintenance of an individual's optimum physical and mental health is a major goal of the physician and nurse.

Child health supervision is an extension of the prenatal care received by the mother and the developing fetus. Such supervision is designed to detect the presence of deformity or disease, to provide help in interpreting nutritional requirements and assuring proper food intake,

to protect against certain preventable infectious diseases, and to offer appropriate counseling in child-rearing practices and commonly encountered child behavior patterns. Records of the child's individual health history are maintained, and height, weight, and blood pressure are plotted in graph form. Health supervision may be carried on by the private physician, nurse practitioner, a public facility, or a child health conference.

Infants are usually scheduled to visit the physician monthly for the first 6 months and then every other month until their first birthday. Two to four visits should be made during the second year, and visits should be at least yearly thereafter. Special attention should be directed toward detection of any hearing impairment, visual defect, or orthopedic difficulty. Professional dental supervision should be started before any real problem is apparent, before the child's third birthday. Dental care at home should begin when dentition occurs.

School-age children in United States society, because of their multiple community contacts and the activities of the school nurse or public health nurses in some schools, usually receive more consistent health supervision than do preschool children. Even so, school-age children should have annual physical examinations and appropriate help and counseling as their growth and development levels require.

The following topics of study are fundamental to the consideration of preventive pediatrics. It is hoped that these introductory discussions of basic nutrition, immunization, and child safety will encourage the student to continue an investigation of the positive approach to health with increasing interest and reward.

SELF-FEEDING AND BASIC NUTRITION

Feeding and eating can be very natural. One should remember that a number of studies have indicated that infants and children select food of the right type at the right time and in the right amounts if it is available to them from the beginning of the self-feeding process. Babies accept solid foods and feed themselves when their neuromuscular progress permits them to do so.

Physiologic guides

Hunger vs. appetite. Infants have a rhythmic pattern of hunger contractions characterized by discomfort, restlessness, and crying. The rhythm of hunger contractions differs in each baby, but they usually reappear every 3 to 4 hours and more frequently in breast-fed babies. Babies should be fed according to their hunger rhythms, because rigidly prescribed feeding schedules ignore these hunger patterns. The normal infant's nutritional needs can be met for the first 6 months by breast-feeding or iron/vitamin fortified formula plus flouride. The Committee on Nutrition of the American Academy of Pediatrics urges that "all bottle-fed infants be given an iron fortified formula for at least the first 12 months of life." The amount of breast milk or formula consumed varies from day to day, but in general most infants take 2.5 ounces of formula per pound of body weight, distributed over a 24-hour period. After solid foods are introduced when the infant is about 5 to 6 months of age, this amount

decreases. When sucking stops and the healthy infant falls asleep, the hunger-appetite mechanism has been satisfied. The infant should not be coaxed or forced to take more milk, regardless of the amount remaining in the bottle.

During infancy, hunger prompted by physiologic needs chiefly controls food intake. Before 6 months of age an infant takes almost any liquid consistently. However, in the latter half of the first year, preferences related to taste, appearance, and culture (that is, appetite) become important. Parental diet, likes, and dislikes begin to condition the child's eating habits. By 1 year the baby shows definite preferences and dislikes. If the conditioning process has not been adverse, appetite may be trusted as a physiologic index of the infant's nutritional needs. It is believed that if babies refuse an essential food item, they should not be forced to take it, since they will accept it later when they need it.

Breast or formula feeding should be continued through the first year of life. Whole milk may be introduced in the second year of life. Skim milk should be avoided until after the second birthday, unless prescribed by the pediatrician, as skim milk is not nutritionally sound for infants. It provides an inadequate intake of fat, fatty acids, and calories, and protein in excess of four times the estimated requirements.

Developmental guides

Protrusion reflex. The protrusion reflex manifests itself when the infant pushes out solid food placed on the anterior third of the tongue. This response, common during the first 9 weeks, disappears by the fourth month of life. It does not interfere with the baby's bottle- or breast-feeding, because any nipple empties into the back of the mouth. However, it makes early feeding of solid foods difficult. The disappearance of the protrusion reflex and the development of the ability to sit with minimal support are the neuromuscular indications for the introduction of semisolid food. There appears to be no advantage in introducing solids (baby foods) during the first 6 months of life.

Getting the baby to accept the spoon willingly is an important learning process that proceeds slowly. Usually new food should be offered first while the baby is hungry. However, *very* hungry babies may refuse new foods because of their urgent desire for milk and their low frustration tolerance. (See Table 18-1.)

Self-feeding. Hand-to-mouth self-feeding begins before the infant is 1 year of age. If an infant is prevented from feeding himself when neuromuscularly ready, the

Table 18-1   Feeding for the first 12 months of life

					Month						
1	2	3	4	5	6	7	8	9	10	11	12

Breast milk: Nutritionally sound, believed to provide immunity, facilitates a close mother-baby relationship, decreases allergies, decreases incidence of dental caries and malocclusion

Formula: 24-32 oz/24 hr: well tolerated when breast milk is not available

Iron fortified rice cereal: source of calories, iron and fiber; avoid wheat products first 12 months of life.

Strained vegetables: source of calories, fiber, iron, Vitamins A and B, and minerals. Introduce yellow vegetables before green.

Strained fruits: source of calories, iron, fiber, Vitamin C, and minerals. Will offset constipating effect of cereals.

Plain lowfat yogurt: excellent source of calcium, phosphorus, Vitamin B, and protein

Meats: source of protein, calories, iron, and vitamins

Finger foods: assists in teething and fine motor coordination

acquisition of this skill may be delayed for weeks or months. A 6-month-old child can usually put his hands around a supported bottle and guide it to his lips. By 6 months of age, it is a good idea to begin offering juice, formula, or breast milk from a cup, regardless of whether the mother is still nursing or bottle-feeding. If permitted, a 7-month-old may hold the formula bottle himself. At 8 months a baby can feed himself crackers. Chewing motions appear at about 8 or 9 months and are the neuromuscular indications that lumpy foods can be introduced whether the teeth are present or not. Chopped foods should be introduced gradually. If undigested food appears in the stool, one should wait a week and try again. By 6 to 8 months an empty plastic or metal cup may be placed on the baby's tray for practice. At 10 months of age the baby can begin to practice with a spoon. Shortly after 12 months he can use a cup well, and by 18 months he can use a spoon skillfully. Self-feeding is usually accomplished between 12 and 18 months and combines feeding skills using the spoon, hand, or cup. Several foods are not recommended for children 12 to 24 months of age because of possible aspiration or poor digestibility. These include corn, leafy vegetables, cucumbers, chocolate, olives, peanut butter, uncooked onions, baked beans, grapes, and hot dogs. Nuts and popcorn should be avoided until age 4 years.

Nursing bottle caries. "Nursing bottle caries," or "nursing bottle syndrome," refers to the rampant decay of the upper anterior primary teeth resulting from bottle feeding of high carbohydrate fluids beyond 12 months (Fig. 18-1). This devastating condition, which may occur as early as 9 to 10 months, is attributed to bottle propping at night and at naptimes. When the fluid-filled nipple with a sugar-sweetened beverage remains in the child's mouth, the flow of saliva is minimized and therefore cannot neutralize juice acidity or the acidity developed in the bacteria-laden plaque, both of which promote decalcification of tooth enamel. The result is painful, unattractive, and severely damaged carious teeth. Any child with caries of the anterior teeth, especially the maxillary anterior teeth, should be referred immediately for pediatric dental evaluation and treatment (Figs. 18-1 and 18-2).

Nursing bottle caries can be prevented. Well-baby assessments should include appropriate counseling regarding adverse effects of using the bottle at naptime or night time beyond the age of 9 to 12 months. Proper techniques of tooth brushing, restricting intake of sucrose-containing

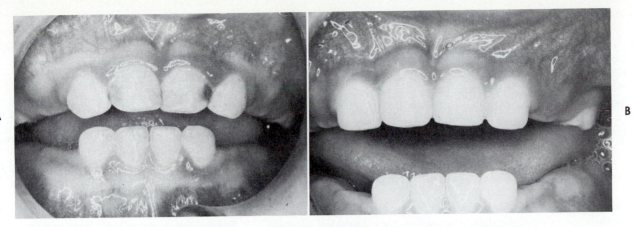

FIG 18-1 A, Decayed teeth. Nursing bottle caries evidenced at 9 months of age. **B,** Teeth returned to normal health and function through aesthetic restoration. *(Courtesy Barry H. Gruer, DDS, MS, San Diego, Calif.)*

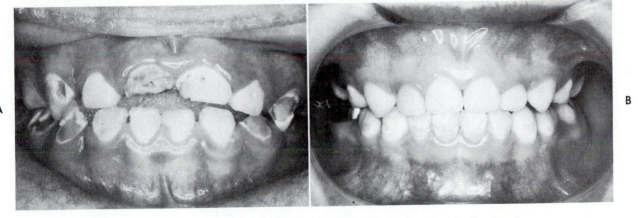

FIG 18-2 A, Extreme rampant caries that began with overretention of bottle. **B,** Complete restoration of primary teeth, providing child a means for mastication, speech, and improved aesthetic appearance. *(Courtesy Barry H. Gruer, DDS, MS San Diego, Calif.)*

carbohydrates, especially between meals, and maintaining desirable fluoride intakes should be encouraged.

Basic nutrition concepts (Table 18-2)

A happy healthy child reflects good eating habits. Good nutrition is like a good insurance policy. During the course of a lifetime it pays dividends in the form of a well-developed baby with good muscles, smooth skin, glossy hair, and clear bright eyes. What children eat and how they eat is established in their earliest years. Studies have shown that obesity may be associated with an in-

crease in adipose fat cell number (hyperplasia) and in cell size (hypertrophy) or with only an increase in the size of the cell. The number of adipose cells in children who became obese in the first year of life is higher than in those who became obese in later childhood. Dieting in later life can reduce cell size but not the cell number that was laid down in childhood. Thus early feeding practices are of utmost importance.

All systems and tissues in the body depend on proper nourishment for their existence and maintenance; this nourishment is obtained from the foods each person eats

Table 18-2   Clinical signs of nutritional status

	Good	Poor
General appearance	Alert, responsive	Listless, apathetic, cachexic
Hair	Shiny, lustrous; healthy scalp	Stringy, dull, brittle, dry, depigmented
Neck (glands)	No enlargement	Thyroid enlargement
Skin (face and neck)	Smooth, slightly moist; good color, reddish pink mucous membranes	Greasy, discolored, scaly
Eyes	Bright, clear, no fatigue circles beneath	Dryness, signs of infection, increased vascularity, glassiness, thickened conjunctiva
Lips	Good color, moist	Dry, scaly, swollen, angular lesions (stomatitis)
Tongue	Good pink color, surface papillae present, no lesions	Papillary atrophy, smooth appearance; swollen, red, beefy (glossitis)
Gums	Good pink color; no swelling or bleeding, firm	Marginal redness or swelling, receding, spongy
Teeth	Straight, no crowding, well-shaped jaw, clean, no discoloration	Unfilled caries, absent teeth, worn surfaces, mottled, malpositioned
Skin (general)	Smooth, slightly moist, good color	Rough, dry, scaly, pale, pigmented, irritated, petechiae, bruises
Abdomen	Flat	Swollen
Legs, feet	No tenderness, weakness or swelling; good color	Edema, tender calf, tingling, weakness
Skeleton	No malformation	Bowlegs, knock-knees, chest deformity at diaphragm, beaded ribs, prominent scapulae
Weight	Normal for height, age, body build	Overweight or underweight
Posture	Erect, arms and legs straight, abdomen in, chest out	Sagging shoulders, sunken chest, humped back
Muscles	Well developed, firm	Flaccid, poor tone; undeveloped, tender
Nervous control	Good attention span for age, does not cry easily, not irritable or restless	Inattentive, irritable
Gastrointestinal function	Good appetite and digestion; normal, regular elimination	Anorexia, indigestion, constipation or diarrhea
General vitality	Good endurance, energetic, sleeps well at night, vigorous	Easily fatigued, no energy, falls asleep in school, looks tired, apathetic

From Williams SR: Nutrition and diet therapy, ed 5, St Louis, 1981; The CV Mosby Co, p. 494.

and drinks. Food must perform three functions within the body:

1. Provide heat and energy
2. Build and repair body tissues
3. Regulate body processes

Substances essential to perform these vital functions are the following:

1. Oxygen
2. Water
3. Carbohydrates
4. Proteins
5. Fats
6. Minerals
7. Vitamins
8. Fiber

Oxygen. Oxygen is so vital to the activity of the body cells that without it life would cease immediately. The natural source of oxygen is fresh air. Through the activity of the respiratory system, oxygen enters the circulating blood, which carries it to every living cell. An abundance of fresh air is desirable at all ages.

Water. Second only to oxygen, water is necessary for life. Without water, death ensues in just a few days. The body of the infant contains proportionately more water (75% to 80%) than the adult (60% to 65%). The adult value is reached at about 12 years of age.

Water is a basic constituent of all cells and is a major component in blood, lymph, spinal fluid, and the various body excretions such as urine and sweat. In infancy considerable water is lost through the kidneys and skin. To keep pace with normal fluid losses, the infant must receive an equal fluid intake. The infant is subject to conditions causing water loss, notably fever, vomiting, and diarrhea. Unless water intake is increased during these abnormal states, symptoms of dehydration and its consequences appear rapidly. (See pp. 472-473.)

Carbohydrates. Carbohydrates serve as the body's primary source of heat and energy. Examples of carbohydrate-rich foods include grains, fruits, vegetables, and sweets. (Pure sugar is 100% carbohydrate.) Carbohydrates not used for heat and energy are stored in many of the body's organs (especially in the liver and muscles as glycogen), or they are converted in the liver to glucose when carbohydrate is not available in the food consumed. Since immediate heat and energy requirements have priority over tissue growth and repair, the body is also capable of using tissue fat and protein to furnish its energy needs. It is therefore important to have sufficient carbohydrates in the diet to meet these needs adequately, thus sparing protein for its primary use of building and maintaining tissues. The waste products of carbohydrate metabolism are excreted from the body in the form of carbon dioxide and water.

Protein. Protein requirements are greatest during infancy. Every living cell and almost all body fluids contain protein. Protein is necessary for the growth, repair, and maintenance of all body tissues. Immune bodies, which help the body resist infection, contain protein. Enzymes and hormones also include protein in their composition.

The end products of protein digestion are amino acids—small units, which, when properly reassembled, form the needed body protein. Of the many amino acids known, nine are essential for normal growth and body maintenance. Amino acids are found in varying amounts in various forms in foods.

Proteins are divided into three groups: complete, partially complete, and incomplete. The complete proteins contain all nine essential amino acids. A dietary supply of these amino acids is necessary because they cannot be synthesized by the body. Proteins from animal sources such as meats, poultry, fresh eggs, milk, and cheese provide the essential amino acids. Gelatin is 100% protein from an animal source but is not a complete protein.

Partially complete proteins are found in cereal products and vegetables. They contain many amino acids but not all the essential ones. When protein intake is insufficient, the result is a slow rate of growth and increased susceptibility to bacterial infections.

Incomplete proteins such as corn and gelatin can neither maintain nor support life. When an incomplete protein is the only source of protein, malnutrition, or marasmus, results.

Children receive adequate amounts of protein in meat, milk, and eggs. The overall protein value may be improved when both animal and vegetable protein are eaten together. Since no amino acids are stored in the body, it is essential that food contain sufficient amounts. Amino acids not needed by the body tissues are returned to the liver where approximately half are converted into urea, a waste product excreted by the kidney, and half are changed into glycogen or fatty tissue and stored to meet future energy requirements.

Finally, it is important to note that all nine essential amino acids work together. New tissue cannot be formed unless all the essential amino acids are present in the bloodstream simultaneously. Therefore it is imperative that some form of complete protein be included at each meal.

Human milk is believed to contain an ideal pattern of amino acids and is thus of high biologic value. In addition to those essential amino acids required by the adult, the infant requires histidine. The premature infant also requires tyrosine, cystine, and taurine.

Fats. Certain fatty acids found in dietary fats are necessary to maintain good nutrition. These essential fatty acids permit normal growth and the health and maintenance of normal skin. Fat also provides the vehicle of absorption of the fat-soluble vitamins, A, D, E, and K. Unless dissolved in fats, these vitamins cannot be retained in the body in adequate amounts.

Fats are found in both animal and vegetable foods. Fat contributes about 40% of the calories in human milk. Egg yolks, butter, meat, soybean oil, cottonseed oil, corn oil, and olive oil are good sources of the essential fatty acids. One of these sources must be included in the daily diet, since the essential fatty acids cannot be synthesized from other fats. The waste products of fat metabolism, like those of carbohydrate metabolism, are carbon dioxide and water.

If fat intake is inadequate, the child may not receive the essential fatty acids required to prevent the formation of certain types of skin lesions or to promote optimum myelinization of the brain. Brain cells reach adult numbers by approximately 8 months of age. Brain size by cell enlargement is completed by 2 years of age. Skimmed milk is an inappropriate food source during the first 2 years of life. (See p. 381.)

Energy requirements. Whenever work is to be performed by the body, energy is needed. The body must be supplied with fuel in the form of food in sufficient amounts to meet the energy requirements of that person. To determine how much food a child needs, it is necessary to know the child's metabolic rate, or rate of heat production. The unit of heat in metabolism is called a *kilogram calorie*. (It may be defined as the amount of

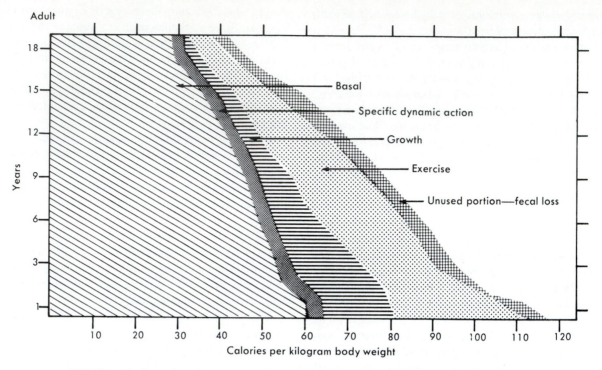

FIG 18-3 To determine total caloric requirements of child, multiply weight in kilograms by number of calories for age.

heat needed to raise the temperature of 1 kilogram of water 1° C.) A person's *basal metabolic rate* (BMR) is described as the minimum amount of heat produced by body cells when the body is at rest with only vital processes, such as circulation and respiration, functioning. Several factors—size, age, sex, hormonal levels, and body temperature—influence the BMR. The *total metabolic rate* of a person represents the total amount of heat produced by the body in a given time (usually 24 hours) under normal conditions. The total metabolic rate of a child represents the amount of food the body must burn not only to keep alive and awake but also to continue physical activity, to support growth, to supply specific dynamic action (ingestion and assimilation of food), and to replace calories lost (Fig. 18-3).

Total energy expended determines the need for calories. The fuel values of energy-producing foods are as follows:

Carbohydrates	4 cal/g
Protein	4 cal/g
Fats	9 cal/g

The average distribution of calories in a well-balanced diet is as follows:

	Infant	Child
Carbohydrates	29% to 58%	50%
Protein	7% to 16%	15%
Fat	35% to 55%	35% (or less)

If the number of grams of carbohydrate, protein, and fat in a food is known, the caloric value can be determined by multiplying each by the appropriate fuel value.

When food is not available, the body's nutritional reserves and tissues are used to meet its need for caloric energy. Carbohydrates stored as glycogen in different body organs are used first; fat deposits are next. Usually, fat in the extremities is used before fat located in the trunk. Fat in the cheek pads disappears last. Recessed cheeks in young children usually indicate severe malnutrition.

Minerals

Calcium	Copper	Molybdenum
Magnesium	Zinc	Selenium
Sodium	Phosphorus	Fluoride
Potassium	Manganese	Arsenic
Iron	Chloride	Cobalt
Iodine		

The preceding list indicates minerals that are essential to many body structures and functions. The action of minerals are interrelated in the body, and often one mineral is combined with another to complete the reaction. (For example, in the bones, calcium and phosphorus function together, and sufficient vitamin D is necessary for the proper use of calcium.) Most of these minerals are readily obtained from a well-balanced diet. Calcium and iron require special attention. Deficits of the other minerals do not ordinarily arise from inadequate intake. However, large amounts of minerals may be lost through vomiting and diarrhea. There is also concern now that excess intake of sodium, which may result from the addition of salt to baby foods in the home, predisposes some infants to hypertension in later life.

Fluoride. Fluoride is an essential mineral found in minute quantities in many foods. The main role of fluoride in the body lies in its ability to reduce the incidence of dental caries. Public water fluoridation is the most economical and effective preventive measure against dental caries. Fluorides act to inhibit the demineralization of tooth enamel and its ultimate carious destruction. Fluoridated drinking water, which contains one part per million (1 ppm), reduces caries by 50% to 60%. The additional use of topical fluoride can contribute to a further decline by 20% to 30%. Since municipal water fluoridation is not available to all, various dietary alternatives are suggested. Tablets, lozenges, or drops should be prescribed when drinking water contains less than 0.8 ppm fluoride (Table 18-3). If community water is not sufficiently fluoridated naturally, fluoridated water or supplemental fluoride should be prescribed and given on a daily basis from birth until eruption of all permanent teeth. Precaution should be taken to prevent an excessive intake of fluoride, which produces mottling of tooth enamel (dental fluorosis). Continuous, systemic concentrations of fluoride greater than 2 ppm may produce a brown stain on teeth, which is of aesthetic concern, although the strength of the teeth is not diminished.

Iron. One of the most vital elements in the body is iron. It is a component of hemoglobin, the oxygen-bearing element in the blood. Iron is required for growth, and the need for iron varies with the rapidity of growth at different periods of infancy and childhood.

In the United States, 30% of children between the ages of 6 and 30 months from lower socioeconomic backgrounds and 5% from upper middle-class families of the same age group suffer from iron-deficiency anemia. Iron deficiency leads to the development of anemia, or insufficient hemoglobin for the needs of the body. Anemia causes few deaths but contributes seriously to the weakness, ill health, and substandard performance of many children throughout the world. The greatest incidence of iron-deficiency anemia ocurrs in infants and young children. Cow's milk does not contain sufficient iron. When the stores present at birth become depleted (at 4 to 7 months of age), iron-deficiency anemia develops unless a supplement is given. Iron-fortified formula and supplementation of iron-fortified cereal after 6 months help ensure an adequate iron status in both breast-fed and bottle-fed infants. Foods rich in iron are liver, meat, dark-green leafy vegetables, and egg yolk.

Calcium. Relatively large amounts of calcium are required for many vital functions in the body. Calcium is essential for normal heart action and is an important element in the blood-clotting mechanism. Calcium builds bones and teeth and is necessary for normal musculoskeletal action. When the diet is calcium-deficient, the blood uses the calcium in the bones to maintain its normal composition. Bowed legs and rickets may result. Hypocalcemia may cause neonatal tetany, crying, muscle twitching, and convulsions. Unrelieved, it may end in death. Milk products are good calcium sources. Lactose-free products are available for those children who are lactose-intolerant.

Table 18-3 Current fluoride dosage recommendations

Fluoride content of drinking water (ppm)	Daily dosage (F ion)		
	Birth to age 2 (mg)	Age 2-3 (mg)	Age 3-14 (mg)
Less than 0.3	0.25	0.50	1.00
0.3 to 0.7	0	0.25	0.50
Over 0.7	Fluoride dietary supplements unnecessary		

Approved by the Council on Dental Therapeutics of the American Dental Association.

Vitamins

Fat-Soluble	Water-Soluble
A	C
D	B Complex
E	Thiamin (B_1)
K	Riboflavin (B_2)
	Niacin
	Folic acid
	Pyridoxine (B_6)
	Biotin
	Pantothenic acid
	Cyanocobalamin (B_{12})

Vitamins are organic compounds found in minute quantities of foods. They participate as catalysts in almost all metabolic processes and are vital to growth and good health. Vitamins A and D are the only two vitamins stored in the body. Excessive intake of these two vitamins results in toxic manifestations such as skin lesions, liver enlargement, and bone spurs. Any vitamin may be lacking, causing disturbances in the pattern of growth, metabolism, and development of the child.

The best sources of vitamins are found in the natural foods. A well-balanced diet containing the basic four food groups (see Fig. 5-2) ensures an adequate supply of vitamins. There are six vitamins that merit special consideration (Tables 18-4 and 18-5). The foods that supply these vitamins also supply all other known vitamin needs.

Prevention of atherosclerosis and coronary heart disease

Many researchers believe that atherosclerosis, which leads to coronary heart disease, has its origins in childhood. The Committee on Nutrition of the American Academy of Pediatrics (AAP), the American Heart Association, and the National Institutes of Health Consensus Conference on lowering blood cholesterol to prevent heart disease have recommended a "prudent" diet for children who are older than 2 years of age. Unfortunately, there is no consensus on what defines a prudent

Table 18-4   Significant vitamins

Vitamin	Function	Effects of deficiency
A	Promotes good eyesight	Nightblindness
	Aids in maintaining resistance to infections	Frequent infections
	Maintains skin integrity	Dry, rough skin, papular eruptions
	Helps form and maintain mucous membrane	Burning, itching eyes
	Helps in formation of bones and teeth	Retarded growth; thin and defective tooth enamel
B complex		
B_1 (thiamin)	Aids in maintenance and function of nervous system	Beriberi
	Regulates appetite, normal digestion	Listlessness, fatigue, and irritability
	Promotes feeling of general well-being	Anorexia, vomiting, and diarrhea
		Generalized weakness; gross symptoms of neuromuscular, digestive, and cardiovascular impairment
B_2 (riboflavin)	Aids in eye adaptation to light	Photophobia; impairment of visual acuity; cataracts
	Provides essentials for metabolism of carbohydrate, fat, and protein	Impaired formation of blood cells
	Necessary for normal growth	Anemia
Niacin (nicotinic acid)	Essential for normal function of digestive tract and nervous system	General poor health
		Gastrointestinal changes—loss of appetite, nausea, vomiting, abdominal pain, red tongue, ulcers and fissures of tongue
		Dermatitis
		Nervous system manifestations—headaches and dizziness, impairment of memory, and neurotic symptoms
C (ascorbic acid)	Important role in formation, maintenance, and repair of teeth, bones, and blood vessels	Scurvy
	Facilitates absorption of dietary iron	Loose teeth; faulty bones; slow growth
	Maintenance of normal blood hemoglobin levels	Weakness and irritability
		Delayed healing of wounds
		Cutaneous hemorrhages
D	Enhances absorption of calcium and phosphorus	Rickets
	Plays a vital role in formation of normal bone	Retarded growth and lack of vigor
		Variety of bone deformities—large head, pigeon chest, kyphosis, and curved long bones
	Promotes tooth development	Teeth erupt late and decay early

diet for children. The wisest general recommendations at present emphasize substituting polyunsaturated and monosaturated fat for saturated fats, moderately reducing total fat, dietary cholesterol and salt, and avoiding obesity.

The long-term effects of breast-feeding on cholesterol metabolism are not likely due to the differences in cholesterol intake between formula-fed and breast-fed infants. Rather, researchers believe that the fatty acid composition, immunoglobulins, and hormones in breast milk may have a long-term beneficial effect on cholesterol homeostasis.

Many proponents of early cholesterol screening recommend that the screening should be universal, beginning between age 2 and 5 years. Others recommend testing only those children whose first-degree (parents or siblings) or second-degree relatives (grandparents, aunts, uncles) have a history of stroke or atherosclerosis/coronary heart disease under 65 years of age or a positive family history of elevated cholesterol.

Most researchers agree that a total lifestyle approach is optimal and that anticipatory guidance, related to all risk factors, must begin in childhood. Recommendations are advocating smoking prevention/cessation; regular monitoring of blood pressure beginning at age 3; promoting regular physical activity to increase high density lipoproteins (HDLs) thought to be protective against coronary artery disease; and, finally, ongoing counseling on

Table 18-5 Recommended daily menu patterns based on the four food groups*

Food groups featuring leader nutrient equivalents		Servings per day			Food groups featuring leader nutrient equivalents		Servings per day		
		Child	Teenager	Adult			Child	Teenager	Adult
Milk group {	Calcium Riboflavin B₂ Protein	3	4	2	Fruit-vegetable group {	Vitamins A and C	4	4	4
1 cup milk, yogurt, or *calcium equivalent* 1½ slices (1½ oz) cheddar cheese 2 cups cottage cheese† 1¾ cups ice cream 1 cup pudding (foods made from milk contain part of nutrients obtained by a serving of milk)					Dark-green leafy or yellow vegetables 3-4 times weekly—citrus fruit daily ½ cooked or juice 1 cup raw Usually 1 average-sized fruit				
					Grain group {	Carbohydrate Thiamin B₁ Iron Niacin	4	4	4
					Whole-grain, fortified, or enriched products				
Meat group {	Protein Niacin Iron Thiamin B₁	2	2	2	Other foods {	Carbohydrates Fats	As needed to meet caloric needs (adult servings of four groups only supply approximately 1,200 calories)		
2 oz cooked lean meat, fish, poultry, or *protein equivalent* 2 eggs 2 slices (2 oz) cheddar cheese† ½ cup cottage cheese† 1 cup dried beans, peas 4 tbsp peanut butter					Butter, margarine, mayonnaise, oils (1 tbsp = 100 calories) Approximately 100-calorie servings: 2-3 inch cookies 1⅓ oz pie 2 tbsp sugar, jam, honey ⅓ cup ice cream				

*Adapted from the *Guide to good eating—a recommended daily pattern,* courtesy National Dairy Council.

†Count cheese as serving of milk or meat, not both simultaneously.

Table 18-6 Food and Nutrition Board, National Academy of Sciences—National Research Council recommended dietary allowances,[a] revised 1989

(Designed for the maintenance of good nutrition of practically all healthy people in the United States)

| | | Weight[b] | | Height[b] | | Protein | Fat-soluble vitamins | | | |
| | | | | | | | Vita-min A | Vita-min D | Vita-min E | Vita-min K |
Category	Age (years)	kg	lb	cm	in	(g)	(μg RE)[c]	(μg)[d]	(mg α-TE)[e]	(μg)
Infants	0.0-0.5	6	13	60	24	13	375	7.5	3	5
	0.5-1.0	9	20	71	28	14	375	10	4	10
Children	1-3	13	29	90	35	16	400	10	6	15
	4-6	20	44	112	44	24	500	10	7	20
	7-10	28	62	132	52	28	700	10	7	30
Males	11-14	45	99	157	62	45	1,000	10	10	45
	15-18	66	145	176	69	59	1,000	10	10	65
	19-24	72	160	177	70	58	1,000	10	10	70
Females	11-14	46	101	157	62	46	800	10	8	45
	15-18	55	120	163	64	44	800	10	8	55
	19-24	58	128	164	65	46	800	10	8	60

[a]The allowances, expressed as average daily intakes over time, are intended to provide for individual variations among most normal persons as they live in the United States under usual environmental stresses. Diets should be based on a variety of common foods in order to provide other nutrients for which human requirements have been less well defined.

[b]Weights and heights of Reference Adults are actual medians for the U.S. population of the designated age, as reported by NHANES II. The median weights and heights of those under 19 years of age were taken from Hamill et al. (1979). The use of these figures does not imply that the height-to-weight ratios are ideal.

the importance of maintaining an ideal body weight. The nurse in a variety of health care settings has a unique opportunity to assess family history, provide anticipatory guidance and education, and encourage lifestyle changes, thus reducing the incidence of coronary artery disease.

Summary

Digestion refers to those processes that prepare food for assimilation into the bloodstream or lymphatics of the body, whereas metabolism refers to all the changes that occur in the use of those nutrients by the cells and the generation of heat and energy. Amino acids, essential fatty acids, vitamins, and minerals are used primarily for cell growth and repair. They are also used in the formation of enzymes, hormones, and other body substances. Carbohydrates and fats are used primarily for caloric energy (that is, to supply fuel to keep the body warm) and mechanical energy for performing the body's work. When caloric needs are not met by fats and carbohydrates, protein is then used for energy. Adequate intake of carbohydrates and fats spares protein for cell growth. Thus the diet must contain a balance of all six substances—carbohydrates, fats, proteins, vitamins, minerals, and water; each one plays a vital role in the processes of growth and development (Table 18-6).

Much research is currently underway in an effort to determine any diet modifications that will help decrease the incidence of high blood pressure, heart disease, and other health problems later in life.

IMMUNIZATION

The brilliant success achieved in conquering the classic contagious diseases of childhood is attributed to immunization through which a person is able to build up defenses against certain infectious diseases. When individuals can resist a certain disease, they are said to be immune. They are immune because antibodies are present that injure or destroy the disease-producing agent or neutralize its toxins. Active immunization (artificial) is achieved when certain substances called *antigens* are injected into the body to stimulate the production of antibodies. Immunization is the best and cheapest method of preventing illness. In fact, it is the most routine procedure in preventive pediatrics.

Because the mechanisms for developing immunity are immature in infants, they are highly susceptible to some infections. The protection they have against infection is obtained from the mother, if she is immune. Any passive immunity acquired from the mother lasts about 4 to 6 months and may protect the child against diphtheria,

Water-soluble vitamins							Minerals						
Vita-min C (mg)	Thia-min (mg)	Ribo-flavin (mg)	Niacin (mg NE)[f]	Vita-min B$_6$ (mg)	Fo-late (µg)	Vitamin B$_{12}$ (µg)	Cal-cium (mg)	Phos-phorus (mg)	Mag-nesium (mg)	Iron (mg)	Zinc (mg)	Iodine (µg)	Sele-nium (µg)
30	0.3	0.4	5	0.3	25	0.3	400	300	40	6	5	40	10
35	0.4	0.5	6	0.6	35	0.5	600	500	60	10	5	50	15
40	0.7	0.8	9	1.0	50	0.7	800	800	80	10	10	70	20
45	0.9	1.1	12	1.1	75	1.0	800	800	120	10	10	90	20
45	1.0	1.2	13	1.4	100	1.4	800	800	170	10	10	120	30
50	1.3	1.5	17	1.7	150	2.0	1,200	1,200	270	12	15	150	40
60	1.5	1.8	20	2.0	200	2.0	1,200	1,200	400	12	15	150	50
60	1.5	1.7	19	2.0	200	2.0	1,200	1,200	350	10	15	150	70
50	1.1	1.3	15	1.4	150	2.0	1,200	1,200	280	15	12	150	45
60	1.1	1.3	15	1.5	180	2.0	1,200	1,200	300	15	12	150	50
60	1.1	1.3	15	1.6	180	2.0	1,200	1,200	280	15	12	150	55

[c] Retinol equivalents. 1 retinol equivalent = 1 µg retinol or 6 µg β-carotene.

[d] As cholecalciferol. 10 µg cholecalciferol = 400 IU of vitamin D.

[e] α-Tocopherol equivalents. 1 mg d-α tocopherol = 1 α-TE.

[f] 1 NE (niacin equivalent) is equal to 1 mg of niacin or 60 mg of dietary tryptophan.

tetanus, measles, and poliomyelitis. Because such passive protection varies greatly among infants and no passive immunity exists against pertussis (whooping cough), immunization should be initiated as early as possible. Combined antigens reduce the number of injections, enhance the action of each, and establish a desired immunity within the first 6 months of life.

Current practice begins immunization when the infant is between 8 and 12 weeks of age (Tables 18-7 to 18-10). A "triple toxoid" of diphtheria, tetanus, and pertussis antigens in one injection and a concurrent feeding of oral polio vaccine are given. The "triple toxoid" DTP is given three times, not less than 1 month apart. The necessity of preventing the high mortality from pertussis (whooping cough) in infancy is the main reason for the early start in basic DTP immunization. However, pertussis vaccine is not considered to be as satisfactory as diphtheria and tetanus toxoids because it does not provide absolute protection.

After the initial series of immunizations, recall or booster doses are given to stimulate high antibody levels and maintain maximum immunity. Children who have received three doses of triple toxoid (DTP) and two or three doses of oral polio vaccine (OPV) should be given a booster dose at 18 months of age. Subsequent booster doses are recommended between 4 and 7 years of age. Active, up-to-date immunization produces a degree of resistance in children comparable to that which follows the natural infection.

Precautions

1. A separate sterile needle and syringe, preferably disposable, should be used for each injection.
2. Preferred sites for subcutaneous and intramuscular injections include the anterolateral aspect of the upper thigh and the deltoid muscle of the upper arm. Each injection should be given at a different site.
3. A 1-inch needle (22-gauge) is the preferred length for intramuscular injections.
4. The infant/child should be adequately restrained before an injection.
5. Toxoids and vaccines (antigens) containing alum are given intramuscularly, preferably into the midlateral/anterolateral thigh or deltoid muscles.
6. The package insert should be read before administration of the immunization.
7. Patients and parents should be informed of any possible side effect or adverse reaction. They should be counseled in relation to the benefits of the vaccine and the risks of the disease.

Table 18-7   Recommended schedule for active immunization of normal infants and children[a]

Recommended age[b]	Vaccine(s)[c]	Comments
2 mo	DTP#1,[d] OPV#1[e]	OPV and DTP can be given earlier in areas of high endemicity
4 mo	DTP#2, OPV#2	6-wk to 2-mo interval desired between OPV doses
6 mo	DTP#3	An additional dose of OPV at this time is optional in areas with a high risk of poliovirus exposure
15 mo[f]	MMR,[g] DTP#4, OPV#3	Completion of primary series of DTP and OPV
18 mo	HbCV[h]	Conjugate preferred over polysaccharide vaccine[i]
4-6 yr	DTP#5,[j] OPV#4	At or before school entry
14-16 yr	Td[k]	Repeat every 10 yr throughout life

From Immunization Practices Advisory Committee (ACIP), Centers for Disease Control, MMWR 38:210, 1989.

[a]See Table 18-8 for the recommended immunization schedules for infants and children up to their seventh birthday not immunized at the recommended times.

[b]These recommended ages should not be construed as absolute, e.g., 2 months can be 6-10 weeks. However, MMR should not be given to children <12 months of age. If exposure to measles disease is considered likely, then children 6 through 11 months old may be immunized with single-antigen measles vaccine. These children should be reimmunized with MMR when they are approximately 15 months of age.

[c]For all products used, consult the manufacturers' package enclosures for instructions regarding storage, handling, dosage, and administration. Immunobiologics prepared by different manufacturers can vary, and those of the same manufacturer can change from time to time. The package inserts are useful references for specific products, but they may not always be consistent with current ACIP and American Academy of Pediatrics immunization schedules.

[d]DTP, diphtheria and tetanus toxoids and pertussis vaccine, adsorbed. DTP may be used up to the seventh birthday. The first dose can be given at 6 weeks of age and the second and third doses given 4-8 weeks after the preceding dose.

[e]OPV, poliovirus vaccine live oral, trivalent: contains poliovirus types 1, 2, and 3.

[f]Provided at least 6 months have elapsed since DTP#3 or, if fewer than 3 doses of DTP have been received, at least 6 weeks since the last previous dose of DTP or OPV. MMR vaccine should not be delayed to allow simultaneous administration with DTP and OPV. Administering MMR at 15 months and DTP#4 and OPV#3 at 18 months continues to be an acceptable alternative.

[g]MMR, measles, mumps, and rubella virus vaccine, live. Counties that report ≥5 cases of measles among preschool children during each of the last 5 years should implement a routine 2-dose measles vaccination schedule for preschoolers. The first dose should be administered at 9 months or the first health-care contact thereafter. Infants vaccinated before their first birthday should receive a second dose at about 15 months of age. Single-antigen measles vaccine should be used for children aged <1 year and MMR for children after their first birthday. If resources do not allow a routine 2-dose schedule, an acceptable alternative is to lower the routine age for MMR vaccination to 12 months.

[h]HbCV, vaccine composed of *Haemophilus influenzae* b polysaccharide antigen conjugated to a protein carrier. Children <5 years of age previously vaccinated with polysaccharide vaccine between the ages of 18 and 23 months should be revaccinated with a single dose of conjugate vaccine if at least 2 months have elapsed since the receipt of the polysaccharide vaccine.

[i]If HbCV is not available, an acceptable alternative is to give *Haemophilus influenzae* b polysaccharide vaccine (HbPV) at age ≥24 months. Children at high risk for *Haemophilus influenzae* type b disease where conjugate vaccine is not available may be vaccinated with HbPV at 18 months of age and revaccinated at 24 months.

[j]Up to the seventh birthday.

[k]Td, tetanus and diphtheria toxoids, adsorbed (for use in persons aged ≥7 years): contains the same amount of tetanus toxoid as DTP or DT but a reduced dose of diphtheria toxoid.

8. Systemic reactions such as fever, rashes, and arthralgia subside within 48 hours and are controlled by symptomatic measures and antipyretics.

9. Aspirin or Tylenol, 1 grain per year of age (up to 5 grains), may be given 2 hours after the injection. This dosage may be repeated as needed *not more than five times at 4-hour intervals* without medical consultation.

Contraindications*

1. Acute febrile illness; *minor infections* not associated with fever (such as the common cold) are *not* contraindications. Interruption of the recommended schedule, with a delay between doses, does not interfere with the final immunity achieved.

2. Pertussis immunization should not be repeated if a history of fever of 105° F (40.5° C) or over, severe screaming episodes, collapse, symptoms of central nervous system disorders, or platelet destruction (such as petechiae or bruising) has been noted after a DTP injection (Table 18-11). DT should be used instead.

3. Nonprogressive neurologic disorders *do not* constitute a valid reason for deferring or withholding routine immunization. However, if the child has an evolving neuropathic process, it may be necessary to avoid all immunizations.

*For a more detailed discussion refer to the Red Book (1988), pp 19 to 28.

Table 18-8   Recommended immunization schedule for infants and children up to the seventh birthday not immunized at the recommended time in early infancy[a]

Timing	Vaccine(s)	Comments
First visit	DTP#1,[b] OPV#1,[c] MMR[d] if child is aged ≥15 mo and HbCV[e] if child is aged ≥18 mo	DTP, OPV, and MMR should be administered simultaneously to children aged ≥15 mo, if appropriate. DTP, OPV, MMR, and HbCV may be given simultaneously to children aged 18 mo-5 yr
2 mo after DTP#1, OPV#1	DTP#2,[f] OPV#2	
2 mo after DTP#2	DTP#3[f]	An additional dose of OPV at this time is optional in areas with a high risk of poliovirus exposure
6-12 mo after DTP#3	DTP#4, OPV#3	
Preschool[g] (4-6 yr)	DTP#5, OPV#4	Preferably at or before school entry
14-16 yr	Td[h]	Repeat every 10 yr throughout life

From Immunization Practices Advisory Committee (ACIP) Centers for Disease Control, MMWR 38:211, 1989.

[a]If initiated in the first year of life, give DTP#1, 2, and 3 and OPV#1 and 2 according to this schedule; give MMR when the child becomes 15 months old.

[b]DTP, diphtheria and tetanus toxoids and pertussis vaccine, adsorbed. DTP can be used up to the seventh birthday.

[c]OPV, poliovirus vaccine live oral, trivalent: contains poliovirus types 1, 2, and 3.

[d]MMR, measles, mumps, and rubella virus vaccine, live.

[e]HbCV, vaccine composed of *Haemophilus influenzae* b polysaccharide antigen conjugated to a protein carrier. If HbCV is not available, an acceptable alternative is to give *Haemophilus influenzae* b polysaccharide vaccine (HbPV) at 24 months of age. If HbCV is unavailable and if the child is at high risk for *Haemophilus influenzae* type b disease, HbPV may be given at 18 months of age with a second dose at 24 months. Children aged <5 years who were previously vaccinated with HbPV between 18 and 23 months of age should be revaccinated with a single dose of HbCV at least 2 months after the initial dose of HbPV. Either HbCV or HbPV can be administered up to the fifth birthday. However, they are not generally recommended for persons ≥5 years of age.

[f]The second and third doses of DTP can be given 4-8 weeks after the preceding dose.

[g]The preschool doses are not necessary if the fourth dose of DTP and third dose of OPV are administered after the fourth birthday.

[h]Td, tetanus and diphtheria toxoids, adsorbed (for use in persons aged ≥7 years): contains the same dose of tetanus toxoid as DTP or DT and a reduced dose of diphtheria toxoid.

4. Immunization procedures are deferred during the administration of steroids, irradiation, and anticancer drug therapy because antibody response is depressed or abnormal. Immunizations should also be deferred if the child has recently received (within 12 weeks) immune globulin, plasma, or blood.

5. Infants, children, and other household contacts of individuals with an immunologic deficiency should not receive oral poliovirus vaccine, because the polio viruses are transmissible to the immunocompromised individual.

6. Live virus vaccines against measles, rubella, and mumps are *not* given to pregnant women or patients with generalized malignancy.

7. If allergic reactions were experienced after immunization, the same or related vaccine should be avoided.

German measles (rubella) vaccine

The principal objective of rubella (German measles) control is to prevent congenital rubella infection (CRI) (Fig. 18-4), which can result in miscarriage, abortion, stillbirth, and CRS (mild to severe multiple organ congenital anomalies such as heart defects, hearing loss, and cataracts) in infants.

This can best be achieved by eliminating the transmission of the virus among children, who are the primary sources of infection for susceptible pregnant women. All children between 15 months of age and puberty should receive the live rubella virus vaccine. It is not recommended for younger infants because of possible interference in active antibody formation by persisting maternal rubella antibody. Children of pregant women may be given rubella vaccine, since the vaccine virus is not communicable. However, immunization with live virus vaccine during pregnancy should be avoided because of possible risk to the fetus.

Mumps virus vaccine

The principal objective of the mumps vaccine is prevention of mumps in preadolescent males and young male adults. Live attenuated mumps virus vaccine is recommended for all susceptible children over 15 months of age and especially for preadolescent males and men who have not had the disease. MMR is the vaccine of choice

Table 18-9 Recommended immunization schedule for persons ≥7 years of age not immunized at the recommended time in early infancy

Timing	Vaccine(s)	Comments
First visit	Td#1,* OPV#1,† and MMR‡	OPV not routinely recommended for persons aged ≥18 yr
2 mo after Td#1, OPV#1	Td#2, OPV#2	OPV may be given as soon as 6 wk after OPV#1
6-12 mo after Td#2, OPV#2	Td#3, OPV#3	OPV#3 may be given as soon as 6 wk after OPV#2
10 yr after Td#3	Td	Repeat every 10 yr throughout life

From Immunization Practices Advisory Committee (ACIP) Centers for Disease Control, MMWR 38:212, 1989.

*Td, tetanus and diphtheria toxoids, adsorbed (for adult use) (for use after the seventh birthday). The DTP doses given to children <7 years who remain incompletely immunized at age ≥7 years should be counted as prior exposure to tetanus and diphtheria toxoids (e.g., a child who previously received 2 doses of DTP needs only 1 dose of Td to complete a primary series for tetanus and diphtheria).

†OPV, poliovirus vaccine live oral, trivalent: contains poliovirus types 1, 2, and 3. When polio vaccine is to be given to persons ≥18 years, poliovirus vaccine inactivated (IPV) is preferred.

‡MMR, measles, mumps, and rubella virus vaccine, live. Persons born before 1957 can generally be considered immune to measles and mumps and need not be immunized. Since medical personnel are at higher risk for acquiring measles than the general population, medical facilities may wish to consider requiring proof of measles immunity for employees born before 1957. Rubella vaccine can be given to persons of any age, particularly to nonpregnant women of childbearing age. MMR can be used since administration of vaccine to persons already immune is not deleterious.

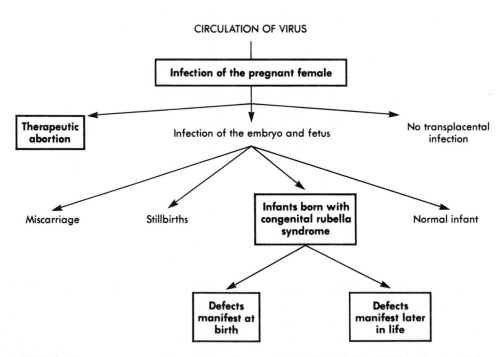

FIG 18-4 The occurrence and monitoring of congenital rubella infection (CRI) and congenital rubella syndrome (CRS). *(Modified from Centers for Disease Control, MMWR 33 [3SS]:1SS, 1984.)*

Table 18-10 Summary of Immunization Practices Advisory Committee Recommendations for tetanus prophylaxis in routine wound management

History of adsorbed tetanus toxoid (doses)	Clean minor wounds		All other wounds*	
	Td†	TIG	Td†	TIG
Unknown or <3 doses	Yes	No	Yes	Yes
≥3 doses‡	No§	No	No¶	No

From MMWR 39:39, 1990.

*Such as, but not limited to, wounds contaminated with dirt, feces, soil, or saliva; puncture wounds; avulsions; and wounds resulting from missiles, crushing, burns, or frostbite.

†For children <7 years of age, DTP (DT if pertussis vaccine is contraindicated). For persons ≥7 years of age, Td is preferred to tetanus toxoid alone.

‡If only three doses of *fluid* toxoid have been received, a fourth dose of toxoid, preferably an adsorbed toxoid, should be given.

§Yes, if >10 years since last dose.

¶Yes, if >5 years since last dose.

Table 18-11 Adverse events occurring within 48 hours of DTP immunizations

Event	Frequency*
Local	
Redness	⅓ doses
Swelling	⅖ doses
Pain	½ doses
Mild/moderate systemic	
Fever 38° C (100.4° F)	½ doses
Drowsiness	⅓ doses
Fretfulness	½ doses
Vomiting	¹⁄₁₅ doses
Anorexia	⅕ doses
More serious systemic	
Persistent, inconsolable crying— duration, 3 hours	¹⁄₁₀₀ doses
High-pitched, unusual cry	¹⁄₉₀₀ doses
Fever 40.5° C (105° F)	¹⁄₃₃₀ doses
Collapse (hypotonic-hyporespon- sive episode)	¹⁄₁,₇₅₀ doses
Convulsions (with or without fever)	¹⁄₁,₇₅₀ doses
Acute encephalopathy†	¹⁄₁,₁₁₀,₀₀₀ doses
Permanent neurologic deficit†	¹⁄₁,₃₁₀,₀₀₀ doses

From MMWR 34:411, 1985.

*Number of adverse events per total number of doses regardless of dose number in DTP series.

†Occurring within 7 days of DTP immunizations.

for persons likely to be susceptible to mumps (as well as measles and rubella). The vaccine should not be given to pregnant women.

Measles (rubeola) vaccine

Measles (rubeola) is often a serious disease. It is frequently complicated by middle ear infection or bronchopneumonia. Encephalitis occurs in about 1 of every 1,000 reported cases; survivors of this complication often have permanent brain damage and mental retardation. Death associated with complications occurs in 1 of every 1,000 cases, and the risk of death is greater in infants and young children. Because of recent outbreaks a routine two-dose measles vaccination schedule is now recommended. See schedule, Table 18-12. Revaccination is recommended for persons who received measles vaccine before 1980. Measles antibodies develop in at least 95% of susceptible children vaccinated at 15 or more months. Measles vaccine produces an inapparent or mild, noncommunicable infection. Because measles is often a severe disease with frequent complications, live measles vaccine may be given as early as 6 to 9 months of age if exposure of the infant is probable. A second dose must be given at about 15 months of age.

School-entrance laws require documentation of measles immunity at the time of entry into kindergarten or first grade. The existence of these regulations that require immunity to measles to be documented before children are allowed to enter kindergarten or first grade has been shown to correlate with reduced incidence of measles.

Smallpox vaccine

Global eradication of smallpox was declared in 1980 by the World Health Organization (WHO). Smallpox vaccine is currently indicated only for laboratory workers directly involved with smallpox viruses.

Haemophilus influenzae b conjugate vaccine

Haemophilus influenzae type b is one of the major causes of serious systemic disease among infants and young children, especially those younger than 18 months. It is the leading cause of bacterial meningitis, and the *Haemophilus* species is the most common cause of invasive infections including septicemia, pneumonia, epiglottitis, cellulitis, arthritis, osteomyelitis, and pericarditis. The mortality rate from *H. influenzae* b meningitis is 5% to 10%, and even when antibiotic treatment is

Table 18-12   1989 recommendations for measles vaccination

Routine childhood schedule, United States	
Most areas	Two doses*† -first dose at 15 months -second dose at 4-6 years (entry to kindergarten or first grade)‡
High-risk areas§	Two doses*† -first dose at 12 months -second dose at 4-6 years (entry to kindergarten or first grade)‡
Colleges and other educational institutions post-high school	Documentation of receipt of two doses of measles vaccine after the first birthday† or other evidence of measles immunity.¶
Medical personnel beginning employment	Documentation of receipt of two doses of measles vaccine after the first birthday† or other evidence of measles immunity.¶

From MMWR 38:4, 1989.

*Both doses should preferably be given as combined measles, mumps, rubella vaccine (MMR).

†No less than 1 month apart. If no documentation of any dose of vaccine, vaccine should be given at the time of school entry or employment and no less than 1 month later.

‡Some areas may elect to administer the second dose at an older age or to multiple age groups.

§A county with more than five cases among preschool-aged children during each of the last 5 years, a county with a recent outbreak among unvaccinated preschool-aged children, or a county with a large inner-city urban population. These recommendations may be applied to an entire county or to identified risk areas within a county.

¶Prior physician-diagnosed measles disease, laboratory evidence of measles immunity, or birth before 1957.

provided, neurologic sequelae are observed in at least 25% to 35% of survivors.

Haemophilus type b conjugate vaccine is licensed and is now routinely recommended for all children at 15 months of age instead of 18 months.* Children who attend day-care facilities and children with certain chronic conditions, such as sickle cell disease and antibody deficiency disease, are at increased risk of *H. influenzae* infections.

*Immunization Practices Advisory Committee (ACIP), Centers for Disease Control, MMWR 39:232, 1990.

Passive immunity

Immune globulin (human) (IG), formerly called immune serum globulin or gamma globulin, is an antibody-rich fraction of pooled plasma from normal donors. It confers temporary immunity that is attained in approximately 2 days and lasts from 1 to 6 weeks. The large, viscous dose should be divided and given intramuscularly in two different sites with an 18- or 20-gauge needle. IG is limited in supply and has been clearly documented to be helpful in prevention or modification of measles and viral hepatitis A (HAV) and in the treatment of certain antibody deficiencies. IG does not transmit hepatitis B virus, human immunodeficiency virus (HIV), or other infectious diseases.

Specific immune globulins (human)

Special preparations of specific immune globulin are obtained from a preselected human donor pool and include hepatitis B immune globulin (HBIG), varicella zoster immune globulin (VZIG), rabies immune globulin (RIG), and tetanus immune globulin (TIG).

Immune globulin intravenous (human)

Immune globulin intravenous (IGIV) is derived from a similar pool to that of the IG pool but is prepared to be suitable for intravenous use. Indications for use include replacement therapy in antibody deficiency disorders, idiopathic thrombocytopenic purpura, Kawasaki disease, premature infants, and AIDS. IGIV should be used only when its efficacy has been established, and the instructions given in the package insert should be followed.

Patient education and nursing responsibilities

Parents should be educated about the benefits and risks of each immunization their child is to receive. The physician is responsible for informing the parents regarding the nature, prevalence, and risks of the infection or disease that is being prevented or modified. Verbal statements should be reinforced by written documents.

Every child should be immunized against the preventable contagious diseases. The office nurse can do a great deal by her efficient, yet kindly manner to help parents realize the importance of continuing the immunization program. She should be sure that the parents have been informed about the immunization the child is receiving. She should be aware of any allergies that the child has demonstrated and learn whether there have been any noteworthy reactions to previous immunizations.

The nurse's good-humored recognition that the med-

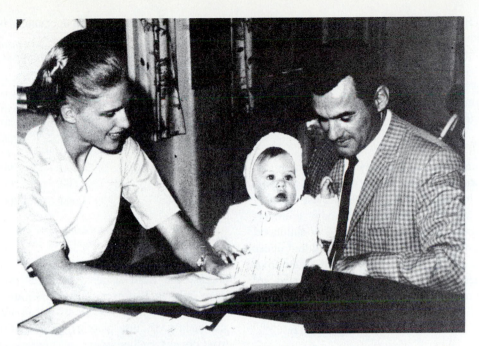

FIG 18-5 Immunizations should not be given without follow-up instructions to parents. This nurse is explaining the World Health Organization immunization record and what to do if certain signs and symptoms develop after Mary Ann's inoculation. *(Courtesy Naval Hospital, San Diego, Calif.)*

icine does sting a bit and that a sincere "ouch" is not out of place may help wary youngsters. A matter-of-fact, positive attitude rather than an overly solicitous manner seems to offer some support to the parent and child.

Record keeping

A continuous written record should be given to the parents. The date and time of the next appointment should be clearly understood (Fig. 18-5). The following information regarding the vaccine/immunization should be entered into the patient's medical record as well as his retained record.

1. Date: month, day, and year
2. Name of the vaccine/immunization
3. Manufacturer, lot number, and expiration date
4. Site and route of administration
5. Name, address, and title of nurse administering the vaccine

The National Childhood Vaccine Injury Act (1988) requires that the information listed above and any events occurring after the vaccine be recorded on the patient's permanent medical record. The law stipulates that chil-

dren who are inadvertently injured must go through a compensation system before attempting to sue either the manufacturer or the person who gave the vaccine. The system is designed to ensure fair compensation to children and to provide protection from liability for vaccine manufacturers and providers. (For details, see p. 22 in *Report of the Committee on Infectious Diseases,* ed. 21, American Academy of Pediatrics, 1988.)

It is also important to record all immunizations received on the patient's WHO immunization record, clinic folder, and hospital record, if one exists. Immunization status is reviewed at the time of each health assessment, illness, or injury.

It is equally worthwhile to inquire about the current status of the parents' immunizations. The proverbial daily apple really is not too successful in preventing illness, but regular immunization is a proved and necessary protection for both young and old.

• • •

Immunization is so important that information about the procedure should be given in prenatal classes. New parents are very concerned about "doing what is right" for their child. Before going home from the hospital, the mother and father should be reminded again about the immunization program. Although immunizations are usually given by the private practitioner or the nurse as part of the baby's regular health checkups, parents should be told of community resources where free immunization services are available.

CHILD SAFETY

Successful prevention and treatment of infectious diseases and nutritional disorders have resulted in a significant decrease in child mortality. The greatest threat to the health and well-being of the child today is injury. Injuries are responsible for more than 50% of childhood fatalities. An estimated 8,000 to 12,000 children under 15 years of age die annually in the United States from injuries. Injuries kill more children than the next six leading causes of childhood death combined.

	Death rates* (ages 1 to 14)
Accidents	14.6
Cancer	3.5
Congenital anomalities	2.8
Homicide	1.5
Heart disease	1.3
Human immunodeficiency disease	0.2
Suicide	0.5
Pneumonia and influenza	0.6

The magnitude of the injury problem is further stressed by the fact that 19 million children suffer nonfatal injuries every year. Many of these children are crippled or permanently disabled for life. In 1984 over 550,000 children were treated in hospital emergency rooms for toy-related injuries (Table 18-11). Of course, not all childhood injuries are brought to the attention of medical personnel. Perhaps an additional 25% of children up to 14 years of age have significant but unreported injuries. Thus the conservative figure of 19 million childhood injuries indicates that a serious national problem exists.

Accidental injury

Few people know what injury really means except that injury represents the leading cause of death in the United States before age 55, the largest cause of years of potential life lost, and a cost of over $100 billion annually. Injury is a term not yet widely understood, probably

*Rates per 100,000 population 1987. Advance Report of Final Mortality Statistics, 1987. From National Center for Health Statistics, Monthly Vital Statistics Report (suppl) 38, September 26, 1989.

Table 18-13 Accidental death in children, 1988*

Type of accident	0 to 4 years	5 to 14 years	Total
Motor vehicle	1,200	2,500	3,700
Drowning	800	500	1,300
Fires, burns	850	450	1,300
Ingestion of objects	260	40	300
Firearms	20	230	250
Poisoning	110	90	200
Falls	160	90	250
Other	500	500	1,000
TOTAL	3,900	4,400	8,300

Data from the National Safety Council: Accident facts, 1989, pp 6-7.
*Deaths per 100,000 population in each age group.

because the word accident has been used to describe many injuries. However, most injuries are *not* accidental.

The most common accidents that injure children consist mainly of cuts, piercings with instruments, blows from objects, animal bites, and injuries related to motor vehicles. Motor vehicles are the major cause of death from injury. Also ranked among the leading causes of fatal injuries are drownings, fires, and ingestion of objects (Table 18-13).

Certain factors seem to be influential in causing childhood injuries: (1) approximately one half of all fatalities occur in children under 5 years of age; (2) boys at all ages have more accidents than girls; (3) the nonwhite population has a considerably higher incidence of accidents than does the white population; (4) most injuries occur during the spring and summer months; (5) a higher percentage of injuries occurs in the home, especially during the preschool period; (6) the child between 1 and 2 years of age is most vulnerable to injuries of all sorts; and (7) some children are accident-prone. Combinations of certain personality characteristics and environmental influences predispose a child toward repetitive injuries.

Prevention. Good safety habits could eliminate many of the causes of injury. Gains in safeguarding the lives of children depend on injury prevention (Figs. 18-6 to 18-12).

Continued emphasis has been placed on two particular approaches to injury prevention: (1) elimination of specific environmental hazards peculiar to different age groups and (2) supervision of small children by adults, to be gradually replaced by training for safety. A glance at the data of the past years shows a continued increase in the actual number of injuries.

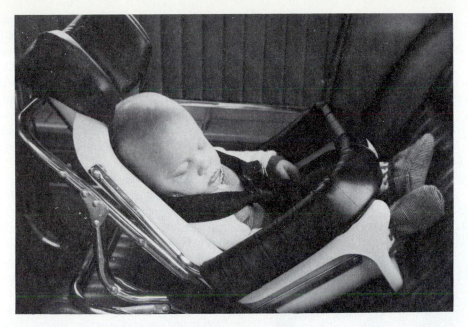

FIG 18-6 Correct use of infant car carrier. Children weighing less than 40 to 50 pounds (18.8 to 22.7 kg) need special safety restraints designed to distribute crash forces over large body area. All car occupants should ride restrained. Infants and young children should be restrained in the back seat. Purchasing and properly using crash-safe automotive restraints are keys to prevention or reduction of severe injuries. *(For information and evaluation of restraints, contact Physicians for Automotive Safety, 50 Union Avenue, Irvington, NJ, 07111.)*

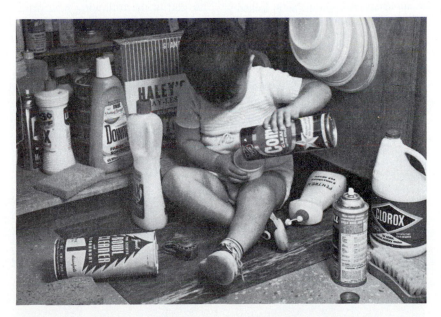

FIG 18-7 Young children may eat and drink anything regardless of taste. Keep household poisons in *locked* cupboard.

Vital statistics in the United States indicate the number of children injured and the kinds of situations causing the injuries. However, they do not provide sufficient detail about each individual case to describe fully the complete situation of each accident. This prevents making valid conclusions concerning injury causation and prevention in childhood. Often vital information is not recorded. This is undoubtedly why specific recommendations for the prevention of certain injuries have not always been effective.

To date no single approach to injury prevention has been formulated. The widespread misinterpretation that injuries happen by chance is reflected in the use of the unscientific term *accident*. Accident implies that the event was unpredictable. However most "accidents" are predictable and preventable.

Injuries are the result of a large number of complex mechanisms. Like other illnesses they can be conquered only through systematic investigation. To understand the nature and cause of injuries, several factors must be considered simultaneously: the host (the child who is affected), the agent (the object that is the direct cause), and the environment (the situation in which the injury takes place). This is the epidemiologic approach to the study of injuries.

Although a great deal remains to be learned about the interaction of these major factors, the existing knowledge has led to the following new principles aimed at injury prevention:

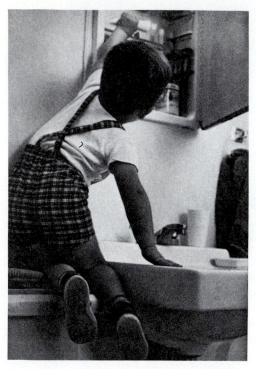

FIG 18-8 Pink pills are *not* candy. Keep medicine in locked cabinet.

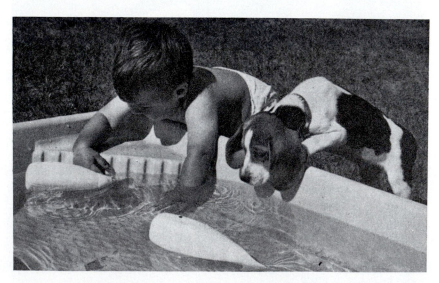

FIG 18-9 Even shallow water is dangerous for an unattended child.

1. Control of the agent whenever possible (for example, use of child-protective caps on medicine-bottles and household products)
2. Recognition and protection of a vulnerable host (young, inquisitive children, especially those with a history of injuries)
3. Control of the environment or milieu by offering consistent love and discipline.

Control of each factor can lead to control of the injury itself.

Alerting and instructing parents. All parents should be made aware of the dangers confronting children at each stage of their development, particularly the toddler and the preschooler (Table 18-14). Parents need to realize fully that normal children search for adventure and are ignorant of consequences. Parents should know that fatigue, hunger, family discord, and anxiety increase the likelihood of an injury. A wise and loving parent knows that discipline is a fundamental prerequisite for injury prevention. This discipline of obedience rapidly becomes the only reliable method for ensuring protection of the school-age child.

All children and families should be instructed in safety. Community educational efforts aimed at injury prevention should include information on fire and burn prevention, including flame-retardant clothing, smoke detectors, fire escapes and drills; water and play safety; approved automobile restraint devices; and use and

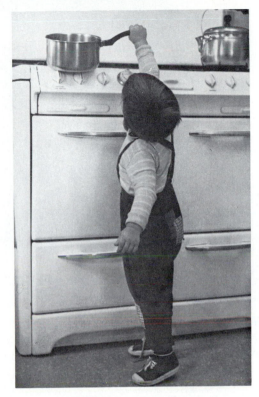

FIG 18-10 Always turn handles of pots and pans to back of stove.

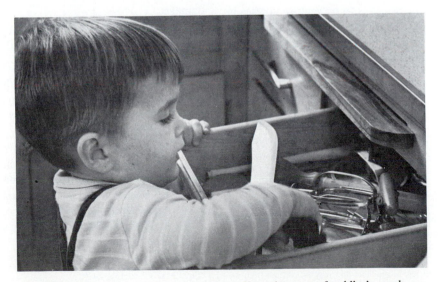

FIG 18-11 Knives are always dangerous. Keep them out of toddler's reach.

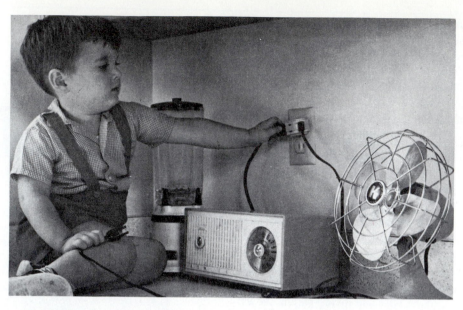

FIG 18-12   Disconnect appliances not in use. Plug outlets and prevent hurts and burns.

proper storage of potentially toxic household chemicals, medicines, cosmetics, tools, and equipment. Individual responsibility and alertness multiplied to ensure intelligent community involvement are needed.

The Injury Prevention Program (TIPP)*

Anticipatory guidance for injury prevention should be an integral part of child health care. Recently the American Academy of Pediatrics initiated The Injury Prevention Program (TIPP) which is considered one of the most useful and practical approaches to preventing injuries in children. TIPP consists of a series of easy-to-use patient information handouts and questionnaires designed for parents and for children through age 4 years. It provides the practitioner with printed, approved guidelines to injury prevention, organized according to the child's age and stage of development. TIPP is now considered a significant part of anticipatory guidance, which is recognized as being as much a part of routine health supervision as the history and physical examination.

Poison ingestion

Many different kinds of toxic substances have been known to be swallowed by children (Fig. 18-7). The most common poisons are found in the medicine cabinet and under the kitchen sink. Often parental negligence is

directly responsible for the loss of a child's life. Most accidental poisonings in childhood are preventable.

Each year several hundred children die as the result of accidental poisoning, and an estimated 500,000 to 2 million children are involved in poisoning incidents. A large number of accidental poisonings occur in children under 4 years of age, the "age of curiosity." These children are not selective about what they ingest. A number of nonfatal poisoning victims are left with permanent disabilities such as esophageal stricture or hepatic or renal damage.

Precautions to reduce the risk.* The following recommendations must be repeated until parents learn them.

1. Household products and medicines should be kept out of reach and sight of children, preferably in a locked cabinet or closet. When one leaves the room even briefly, containers of such products should be moved to a safe place.
2. Medicines should be stored separately from other household products and kept in their original containers—never in cups or soda bottles.
3. All products should be properly labeled, and the label should be read before use.
4. A light should be turned on when one gives or takes medicine.

*Information or the TIPP Kit is available and may be ordered from the Academy of Pediatrics, (800) 433-1096.

*From MMWR 35:151, 1986.

Table 18-14 Injuries common at various stages of development

Typical behavior	Type of accident	Precaution and safety education
Infant		
Sleeps most of time	Suffocation	Use a firm mattress, no pillow; destroy plastic covers and filmy bags
Wiggles and rolls	Falls	Never leave child unattended on a surface such as a table or sofa; keep crib bars up
Helpless in water	Drowning	Never leave alone in bathtub or near pools
Sucks on objects	Choking; ingestion of foreign objects	Keep small objects out of reach, especially pins or other sharp objects; buy toys too large to swallow
	Poisoning	Keep medicines and poisons in a locked cabinet
Toddler		
Roams all over house	Falls	Use gates on stairways; keep windows and doors locked; fence yard
Climbs into things		
Takes things apart	Cuts	Provide large, sturdy toys without sharp edges or small removable parts; keep sharp instruments and knives out of reach
Curious about everything	Burns	Needs constant supervision; never leave hot coffeepot or running water unattended; turn pot handles inward; keep matches locked up; treat flimsy clothing with fire-retardant (7 oz borax, 3 oz boric acid, 2 qt hot water)
Pokes and probes with fingers	Electric shock	Keep electrical appliances out of reach; cap unused light sockets with safety plugs
Chews everything	Poisoning	Keep medicines, cosmetics, and household poisons out of reach
	Ingestion of foreign objects and aspiration	Keep small objects such as coins, beans, needles, pins, jewelry, and doll's eyes out of reach
Enjoys playing in water	Drowning	Keep away from unattended pools and ponds; stay with child while in bathtub; fence in bodies of water
Rides tricycle	Motor vehicle accidents	Be firm and instruct child to keep clear of driveways and out of streets
Likes to ride in car and wants to go everywhere with mother		Instruct child in proper car safety; keep car doors locked and use safety belts or other approved restraints; never allow child to sit or stand in front seat of a car or allow child to put hands or head out of window
Preschooler		
Ventures into neighborhood		Teach child safety rules and demonstrate principles by good example; enforce obedience
		Do not overprotect—preschoolers can begin to protect themselves, and overprotection deprives them of experience they need in growing up and learning independence
Inquisitive	Burns	Teach children danger of open flames and hot objects
Rides bicycle	Motor vehicle accidents	Instruct them in proper traffic safety rules—look both ways before crossing street, walk, never run across street, go with traffic light and walk in crosswalk, and never dart into street to go after a ball
Plays ball		
Climbs trees and fences	Falls	Teach them good footing and proper handholds when climbing
Enjoys playing in water	Drowning	Begin swimming instruction; never let child play around unsupervised pools
Plays rough; runs up and down stairs	Blows; cuts	Check play areas for hazards
		Store dangerous tools and equipment in a locked cupboard

Continued.

Table 18-14   Injuries common at various stages of development—cont'd

Typical behavior	Type of accident	Precaution and safety education
Preschooler—cont'd	Poisoning	Teach child not to taste unidentified foods, especially berries
		Lock up poisons; store in labeled bottles
		Discard old medicines down drain before putting containers in trash
Early school age, 6 to 9 yr		
Adventurous	Motor vehicle accidents	Needs intensive instruction in safety rules
Will try anything	Drowning	Encourage swimming safety
Loyal to friends	Falls	Point out importance of fun and not getting hurt
		Needs to know consequences for failing to follow rules
	Burns	Teach child to avoid smoldering fires; bottles and cans may explode and cause fatal injuries
		Teach child danger of matches and fires
		Teach proper use of chemistry sets
	Firearms	Point out serious consequences of playing with dry ice, fireworks, and other hazardous materials
Late school age, 10 to 14 yr		
Rides bicycle constantly	Motor vehicle accidents	Enforce safety rules; explain reasons for them
Plays away from home, often in hazardous places	Drowning; burns; explosions	Know where child is at all times
Has lots of energy and enjoys strenuous play	Sprains; concussions	Point out importance of safe play
Enjoys working with power tools	Lacerations	Show children how to work around house safely (they should not use power tools unless tools are in good condition and they have knowledge of their use and safety); use proper equipment and keep it in good condition
Curious about firearms	Gunshot wounds	Lock up firearms and ammunition in separate locations

5. Since children tend to imitate adults, adults should avoid taking medications in their presence. Medicine should not be drunk from the bottle.

6. Medicines should be referred to by their correct names.

7. Medicine cabinets should be cleaned out periodically. One should discard old medicines by flushing them down the drain, rinsing the container with water, and discarding it.

8. Household substances in child-resistant packaging should be used. Prescription medicines should be contained in safety packaging. Safety features should be carefully resecured after use.

Emergency supportive treatment. All poisonings in childhood are treated as an urgent emergency. Supportive and symptomatic treatment should be initiated immediately, even though the specific poisonous substance may

not be known. Check the child's breathing immediately. Ensure that there is a clear airway and fresh air. CPR or mouth-to-mouth resuscitation may be lifesaving. Initiate immediate irrigation and dilution of highly corrosive substances associated with dermal or ocular exposure. In the event of caustic ingestion, immediate administration of water or milk to irrigate or dilute the poison has been advised. After first aid has been administered, call the physician or Poison Control Center immediately and bring the child and the poisonous substance to a hospital emergency room. (See section on poison control centers.)

Immediate management. The following immediate action should be taken in the case of poisoning:

1. Identify and remove the poison.
2. Administer the antidote.
3. Administer other supportive treatment.

Removal of poison. In most cases the immediate necessity is to empty the child's stomach, even if hours have passed since the ingestion. If not contraindicated, emesis should be induced if possible. Removal (after prevention) is the most important aspect of poison management. However, emesis should *not* be induced in the event of ingestion of corrosives (lye or strong acids), strychnine, or hydrocarbons (kerosene, gasoline, fuel oil, paint thinner, and cleaning fluid). Emesis also should not be initiated if the child exhibits a decreased level of consciousness or is convulsing.

1. Administration of 15 ml of *syrup of ipecac* followed by 1 cup of water is the most effective way to induce emesis in a child over 12 months of age. The dose may be repeated once in 20 minutes if vomiting has not occurred. The child's head and shoulders should be lowered to prevent aspiration of the vomitus. A subcutaneous injection of apomorphine is sometimes used in the hospital in lieu of syrup of ipecac. An antidote such as naloxone (Narcan) must be given after vomiting has occurred to counteract the depressant effects of the apomorphine. Packaged in 1 fluid ounce containers, syrup of ipecac may be sold without a prescription. Parents should be carefully counseled at the 1-year, well-child visit concerning poison prevention. Information regarding syrup of ipecac should be emphasized so that parents may have it available for use if necessary.

2. Gastric lavage is usually reserved for use when emesis is contraindicated or for the child who has not vomited after two doses of syrup of ipecac. A gastric tube with a large lumen is inserted, and the stomach contents are aspirated first and then irrigated with copious amounts of physiologic saline. Because of the time lapse in getting to the hospital and because the stomach normally traps material inaccessible to the lumen of the tube, chemical emesis is favored over gastric lavage.

Specific measures can be instituted as soon as the particular poison is identified. In most cases of acute poisoning, the physician can identify the agent by a quick history of the incident or by the label on the container. The poison container should always be brought to the hospital with the child.

Poison control centers. Information about poisons and emergency treatment of poison ingestion may be obtained immediately by telephoning the nearest Poison Control Center. More than 250,000 toxic or potentially toxic trade name products are on the consumer market.

Federal law requires that the ingredients of drugs, pesticides, and caustic products be clearly stated on labels. However, many household products frequently involved in accidental ingestions are not required to be so labeled. To assist physicians with their very grave problem of identification, Poison Control Centers have been established in key areas of the United States. These centers are usually associated with medical schools or large hospitals equipped with laboratories, library, house staff, and faculty. They are available to dispense information 24 hours a day. They also serve as treatment centers and are actively engaged in programs of public education to prevent accidental poisoning. In some areas the Poison Control Centers give information to physicians only. However, parents should be instructed to keep the Poison Control Center number on their telephone. Other callers receive first-aid instruction and are advised to call the physician at once.

Administration of antidotes. Antidotes should be given immediately after emesis or lavage to render any remaining poison inert or prevent its absorption. Specific antidotes are not available for all poisons. Among the few available antidotes is dimercaprol (BAL, British antilewisite), which is a good antidote for arsenic, mercury, antimony, and lead poisoning.

Activated charcoal, an old remedy, is a powerful physical antidote that adsorbs most poisons to itself. It effectively reduces the absorption of most substances. It should not be used with other substances, such as syrup of ipecac, that may interfere with its adsorptive capacity or with which it may interfere. Large doses of adsorbent should be used. Optimal adsorption occurs when charcoal is administered in doses 5 to 10 times the amount of the ingested substance. Activated charcoal is usually administered in water and is available in 6 to 8 oz containers to which water can be added.

The antidote should be put in the Levin tube before the tube is removed from the stomach. The specific antidote is given if one is available.

Overtreatment by emetics, sedatives, and stimulants is dangerous and should be avoided. Overtreatment may result in more harm than does the ingestion of the poison. Keep the patient comfortable, warm, and dry.

Acute salicylate (aspirin) poisoning. Until recently, salicylate intoxication was the most common cause of accidental poisoning in children. The decreased incidence of salicylate poisoning is attributed to safety packaging of aspirin (including a limited number of 36 baby aspirins per bottle) and increased public awareness of the dangers of aspirin. Currently about 50% of all hospital-

izations for salicylate poisonings are caused by therapeutic misuse of aspirin, usually by a poorly informed
parent.

The widespread use and availability of salicylates are
prime factors in overdosage. The use of salicylates is so
commonplace that parents and sometimes physicians
underestimate the toxicity of the drug. Salicylates act
rapidly but are excreted slowly. A small dose repeated
frequently may accumulate to cause a severe state of
salicylate poisoning.

Candy-flavored aspirin was invented to obtain an accurate, small dosage and improve the taste, but children
should never be told that medicine is candy; flavored
aspirin should *never* be left within a child's reach (see
Fig. 18-8).

A common but grave error occurs when the parent
mistakenly gives the child a teaspoon of oil of wintergreen instead of cough medicine. One teaspoon of oil of
wintergreen contains as much salicylate as 60 grains of
aspirin. It represents a lethal dose in most cases.

Ingestion of acetaminophen, birth control pills, iron,
and cosmetics is on the rise.

Clinical signs. There are many clinical signs of salicylate poisoning in children. In acute poisoning the first
manifestation is hyperpnea with an increase in respiration
depth. Severe acidosis, electrolyte imbalance, and dehydration follow. Other common symptoms include restlessness, extreme thirst, high temperature (usually 103°
F or higher), profuse sweating, oliguria, tinnitus, tremors, delirium, convulsions, and coma. Cerebral hemorrhage may occur.

Treatment. The treatment for acute salicylate poisoning is always immediate emesis. Parents should attempt
to induce vomiting as soon as the discovery is made. The
physician or nearest Poison Control Center should be
called for emergency instructions. The child is usually
ordered to the hospital. The parents are requested to bring
with the child any implicated container, loose pills, and
sometimes the material vomited.

Emesis may be induced with syrup of ipecac in the
emergency room. After evacuation of the stomach, activated charcoal is administered. A blood specimen is
ordered immediately to determine the level of salicylate
intoxication (30 mg/100 ml invariably is associated with
symptoms). Peak levels are usually reached about 90
minutes after ingestion. Treatment of salicylate intoxication is aimed at correcting electrolyte imbalance. Measures are instituted to promote the rapid excretion of
salicylates in the urine. Parenteral fluids are given both
to combat dehydration and to facilitate prompt excretion
of salicylates from the body.

Nursing care. Nursing care for salicylate poisoning is
supportive. Fever may be reduced by cool sponges,
hourly urinary output is recorded, and pH of the urine
is tested with Nitrazine paper. Accurate hourly output
notations help determine amounts of parenteral fluids
necessary. Temperature, pulse, and respiration are
checked every 15 minutes until stable; oxygen is given
as necessary. Exchange transfusions or dialysis may be
considered in severe, life-threatening intoxication.

Misuse of drugs

Abuse of drugs by youth in society is a major and
growing social and personal problem in the United States.
The average age level of drug users is dropping steadily.
Many junior high and grade school children are frequent
offenders.

The word "drug" is used widely to mean a substance
taken for pleasurable purposes, usually with the implications of illicitness and danger. The term drug
dependence includes *addiction* (which implies tissue dependence, tolerance, and withdrawal symptoms) and *habituation* (which specifies the continuing nature of the
drug-taking and implies psychologic rather than physiologic dependence). One may become addicted to heroin
and other opium derivatives (narcotics), habituated to
barbiturates, or dependent on any of these or on psy-
chedelic drugs (for example, lysergic acid diethylamide
[LSD] or mescaline), amphetamines, alcohol, or marijuana.

The subject of drug abuse cannot be treated in any
detail in this text, but students must acquire adequate
knowledge and insight into treatment of this problem.
Because of the severity and widespread nature of the
difficulty, it is likely that pediatric nurses will encounter
a variety of different situations related to drug abuse.

Drug reactions vary. A heroin overdose produces a
severe depression, whereas an amphetamine overdose
results in hyperactivity and overstimulation. Violent psychologic reactions, varying from hallucinations to severe
psychoses (paranoia) may result from LSD use.

In the last decade the use of LSD (acid) has declined.
Unfortunately, phencyclidine (PCP or angel dust) abuse
became more common for a time. Now, the greatest
threat is concentrated cocaine ("crack"). The severe impact of cocaine abuse today may be noted in pediatrics,
with the birth of babies to addicted mothers or with the
sequelae of abuse and neglect flowing inevitably from
the parent's addiction.

Nurses should be alert for any unusual behavior not
typical of the individual or age group. Such signs include
abnormal dilation of the pupils, excitability, talkative-

ness, profuse perspiration, staggering, mental confusion, disturbances in perception, and general personality changes. The nurse can best assist these patients initially by a calm, supportive manner and a quiet atmosphere, carefully attempting through conversation to make the patient aware of reality.

Sincere concern by the nurse for the substance abuser can in some cases help build a communication bridge to society that helps rehabilitate the individual. Unfortunately, such successes have been less common than the failures. Care of the parent-child unit may mandate that the addict parent obtain treatment; otherwise the risk of loss or permanent major injury to the child exists.

Child abuse (nonaccidental injury)

The term "child abuse" includes many types of physical, sexual, mental, and emotional molestation, injury, and neglect. Hundreds of children are killed annually, and thousands of others are permanently harmed at the hands of adults, usually their parents.

Affected children commonly manifest abrasions, lacerations, burns, skull fractures, intracranial bleeding, and multiple long bone fractures in various stages of healing, as well as personality disturbances and mental impairment. One type of child abuse in which the victim is characterized by severe physical injury and neglect was in the past called the *battered child syndrome*. Neglected, nonaccidentally injured children brought to the hospital are typically under 3 years of age, frequently boys. Many times they are born out of wedlock, unwanted, mentally retarded, or physically malformed. The children are often too young or too afraid to talk.

Parents of such children are described as emotionally immature and unready to accept the responsibilities of parenthood. Child abuse occurs in all socioeconomic levels, but often the parents are burdened by adverse social conditions, financial strain, social isolation, and personal frustration. Some have reversed roles with their children, expecting them to provide love, gratification, and fulfillment to meet their own needs. Many of these parents were abused themselves. They are repeating familiar parental behavior experienced in childhood and have not learned different coping mechanisms. Repeat abuse occurs in over 70% of abuse cases. Prompt and early recognition of child abuse may break the vicious cycle before permanent injury or death of not only the involved child but also his siblings results.

Recognition. When first admitted to the hospital, neglected and nonaccidentally injured children typically shut their eyes, turn their heads away, and cry irritably, in contrast to well-nurtured children who characteristi-

cally cry loudly and reach out for their parents. The skillful observer may recognize the difficulty when parents offer no reasonable explanation regarding the character, circumstances, or nature of the trauma sustained.

Protection. As part of public comprehensive child welfare services, most communities have established "protective services" for neglected and abused children. The purpose of a protective service is not only to provide care and protection for the child but also to help parents who "want to be good" but for some reason are unable to assume their role. Why else do parents bring their neglected and battered children to the hospital? They always run the risk of punishment. Could an abused or neglected child be their way of actually asking for help? The emergence of self-help parent groups such as Parents Anonymous, as well as "hot lines" nationwide, are a direct outgrowth of parents' need for help and anonymity.

Management of this serious problem may range from professional counseling and the introduction and explanation of various community services involved in child care—for example, crisis nurseries and lay therapists (parent aides who may serve as role models and friends)—to criminal court action. Juvenile courts have power over "neglected children" but do not employ criminal sanctions against the parents. However, when the case is reported, prosecuting agencies may institute criminal charges. According to recent studies, criminal prosecution is a poor means of preventing child abuse. Usually, criminal proceedings divide the family and cause parents to hate their children. Legal action is advisable only when all other means of protection and prevention have failed.

Perinatal nurses are in an ideal position for identifying potential child abusers.

One 2½-year-old boy entered the hospital to have his leg checked. He weighed 19 pounds, one front tooth was missing, a fingernail was pulled off, his head and face were covered with skin lesions, and his right femur was broken (see Fig. 31-3). The only information offered by his mother was, "He was very clumsy and stumbled in the yard." Two weeks passed before he would turn to look at anyone. His parents visited once in a period of 2 months. Suspicion should always be aroused when any of the following are noted: abnormal uncleanliness, malnutrition, multiple soft tissue injuries or burns in various stages of healing, and illness obviously caused by lack of medical attention. Often the behavior of the child indicates that he has no real expectation of being comforted or helped.

Reporting. Because parental neglect and abuse are difficult to understand, they may go unrecognized. Children may recover from their injuries and go home, only to be battered again. The alert nurse is usually the first to suspect that a child has been abused. She should carefully chart what she observes and *report* the situation to the physician at once! Every state requires that nurses and physicians report suspicions to the police department or to the appropriate child protection service in the community. After a written report has been submitted, the case is carefully investigated. The person participating in good faith in making a report is immune from civil or criminal liability. Willful refusal to report child neglect or abuse is a violation of the law.

Key Concepts

1. The normal infant's nutritional needs can be adequately met for the first 6 months by breast-feeding or iron-fortified formula plus vitamins. Cereal, fruits, vegetables, yogurt, meats, and finger foods are added gradually between 5 and 12 months of age.

2. Self-feeding is usually accomplished between 12 and 18 months.

3. All systems and tissues in the body depend on proper nourishment for their existence and maintenance. Food must perform three functions within the body: 1) provide heat and energy; 2) build and repair body tissues; and 3) regulate body processes. The following substances are essential to perform these functions: oxygen, water, carbohydrates, proteins, fats, minerals, vitamins, and fiber.

4. To determine how much food a child needs to meet energy requirements, it is necessary to know the child's metabolic rate.

5. The main role of fluoride is its ability to reduce the incidence of dental caries. If community water is not fluoridated, fluoridated water or supplemental fluoride should be given daily from birth until the eruption of all permanent teeth.

6. Iron is one of the most vital elements in the body and is required for growth.

7. Relatively large amounts of calcium are required for many vital functions in the body.

8. Vitamins act as catalysts in almost all metabolic processes and are vital to growth and good health.

9. Many researchers believe that atherosclerosis, which leads to coronary heart disease, has its origins in childhood. A total life-style approach for prevention is optimal.

10. According to current practice, immunizations begin when the infant is between 8 and 12 weeks old. Active, up-to-date immunization produces a degree of resistance in children comparable to that which follows a natural infection.

11. All children between 15 months of age and puberty should receive the live rubella virus vaccine. Live attenuated mumps virus vaccine is recommended for all susceptible children over 15 months of age, especially preadolescent males and men who have not had the disease.

12. A routine two-dose measles (rubeola) vaccination schedule is now recommended. Live measles vaccine may be given as early as 6 to 9 months of age if exposure of the infant is probable. A second dose must be given at about 15 months of age.

13. *Haemophilus influenza* type b conjugate vaccine is now routinely recommended for all children at 15 months of age.

14. Human immune globulin has been clearly documented to be helpful in prevention or modification of measles and viral hepatitis A and in the treatment of certain antibody deficiencies.

15. The greatest threat to the health and well-being of the child today is accidental injury. Continued emphasis has been placed on two particular approaches to injury prevention: 1) elimination of specific environmental hazards peculiar to different age groups; and 2) supervision of small children by adults, gradually to be replaced by training for safety.

16. Anticipatory guidance for injury prevention should be an integral part of child health care.

17. The majority of accidental poisonings in childhood are preventable. Parents should be informed of precautions to reduce the risk of accidental poisoning.

18. All childhood poisonings are treated as an urgent emergency. Supportive and symptomatic treatment should be initiated immediately. The Poison Control Center or physician should be notified and specific measures instituted as soon as the particular poison is identified.

19. Until recently, salicylate (aspirin) intoxication was the most frequent cause of accidental poisoning in children. The treatment of acute salicylate poisoning is always immediate emesis. Nursing care is supportive.

20. Abuse of drugs by youth is a major and growing problem in the United States. Nurses should be alert for any unusual behavior not typical of the individual or age group.

21. Prompt and early recognition of child abuse is essential to prevent permanent injury or death. Management of this serious problem may range from professional counseling and referral to various community services to criminal court action.

22. Every state requires that nurses and physicians report suspicions of child abuse to the police department or to the appropriate child protection serve in the community.

Discussion Questions

1. Discuss the different areas that are considered when performing a nutritional assessment.

2. The mother of a 6-month-old is attempting to start solid food. Discuss the order in which solids foods should be introduced, and some of the concerns related to introduction of solids such as protrusion reflex, aspiration, allergies, nutritional adequacy, and so on. How would you explain all of this to the mother?

3. What immunizations are recommended for infants and children? How often are boosters required for tetanus? Where are immunizations available in your community?

4. Accidents are the leading cause of injury and death in children. Discuss the major types of injuries that occur at different ages. What can be done by the nurse to reduce their occurrence?

5. You are working in a public school as part of a health screening team. You observe that one of the children has several bruises visible on his arms and face. What would you do?

UNIT
VI

SUGGESTED SELECTED READINGS AND REFERENCES

Growth and development—general

Barker-Stotts K: Action stat! Strangulation, Nursing '89 19(3):33, 1989.

Bearinger L and Gephart J: Priorities for adolescent health: recommendations of a national conference, MCN 12(3):161, 1987.

Bydlon-Brown B and Billman RR: Nobody cares if I live or die! Will somebody please help me, Am J Nurs 88(10):1358, 1988.

Gemma PB: Coping with suicidal behavior, MCN 14(2):101, 1989.

Johnsen D and Nowjack-Raymer R: Baby bottle tooth decay (BBTD): issues, assessment, and an opportunity for the nutritionist, J Am Diet Assoc 89(8):1112, 1989.

Lamb JM: The suicidal adolescent: how you can help, Nursing '90 20(5):72, 1990.

Palmer CA: Diet and nutrition crucial factors in the dental health of children, World Rev Nutr Diet 58:131, 1989.

Reynolds EA and Ramenofsky ML: The emotional impact of trauma on toddlers, MCN 13(2):106, 1988.

Rhyme MC and others: Children at risk for depression, Am J Nurs 86(12):1379, 1986.

Ross B and Cobb KL: Family nursing: a nursing process approach, Redwood City, Calif, 1988, Addison-Wesley Nursing.

Substance abuse

Barbour BG: Is fetal alcohol syndrome completely irreversible? MCN 14(1):44, 1989.

Burpo RH: A step beyond "Just say no," MCN 13(6):428, 1988.

Centers for Disease Control: Progress toward achieving the 1990 national objectives for the misuse of alcohol and drugs, MMWR 39(15):256, 1990.

House MA: Cocaine, Am J Nurs 90(4):41, 1990.

Lewis KDS, Bennett B, and Schmeder NH: The care of infants menaced by cocaine abuse, MCN 15(5):324, 1989.

Lindmark B: Maternal use of alcohol and breast-fed infants, N Engl J Med 322(5):338, 1990.

Little RE and others: Maternal alcohol use during breast-feeding and infant mental and motor development at one year, N Engl J Med 321(7):425, 1989.

McNaull FW: Lung cancer: Tobaccoism: what keeps Americans hooked, Am J Nurs 87(11):1430, 1987.

Methadone maintenance has a tragic price. Am J Nurs 88(12):1630, 1988.

Miller NS, Gold MS, and Millman R: PCP: a dangerous drug, Am Fam Physician 38(3):215, 1988.

Povenmire KI and House MA: Recognizing the cocaine addict, Nursing '90 20(5):46, 1990.

Powell AH and Minick MP: Alcohol withdrawal syndrome, Am J Nurs 88(3):312, 1988.

Rich J: Action stat! Acute alcohol intoxication, Nursing '89 19(9):33, 1989.

Smith J: The dangers of prenatal cocaine use, MCN 13(3):174, 1988.

US Preventative Services Task Force (Washington DC): Screening for alcohol and other drug abuse, Am Fam Physician 40(1):137, 1989.

Vandegear F: Cocaine—the deadliest addiction, Nursing '89 19(2):72, 1989.

Nutrition and problem diets

Akridge K: Anorexia nervosa, J Obstet Gynecol Neonatal Nurs 18(1):25, 1989.

American Academy of Pediatrics Committee on Nutrition: Follow-up or weaning formulas, Pediatrics 83(6):1067, 1989.

Dorf A: Tube feeding the young child: current practices and concerns of pediatric nutritionists, J Am Diet Assoc 89(11):1658, 1989.

Fahey PJ, Boltri JM, and Monk JS: Key issues in nutrition during childhood and adolescence, Postgrad Med 81(4):301, 1987.

Flood M: Addictive eating disorders, Nurs Clin North Am 24(1):45, 1989.

Frank GC, Vaden A, and Martin J: School health promotion: child nutrition programs, J School Health 57(10):451, 1987.

Heird WC: Advances in infant nutrition over the past quarter century, J Am Coll Nutr 8(suppl):225, 1989.

Hine RJ and others: Early nutrition intervention services for children with special health care needs, J Am Diet Assoc 89(11):1636, 1989.

Jacobs C and Dwyer JT: Vegetarian children: appropriate diets, Am J Clin Nutr 48(3 suppl):811, 1988.

Kemm JR: Eating patterns in childhood and adult health, Nutr Health 4(4):205, 1987.

Kurinig N and others: Does maternal employment affect breast-feeding? Am J Public Health 79(9):1247, 1989.

Research on improving infant feeding practices to prevent diarrhea or reduce its severity, Bull WHO 67(1):27, 1989.

Taras HL and others: Early childhood diet: recommendations of pediatric health care providers, J Am Diet Assoc 88(11):1417, 1988.

Winick M, editor: Nutrition, Pediatr Ann 19(4):(entire issue), 1990.

Parenting

Allaire S: How a chronically ill mother manages, Am J Nurs 88(1):46, 1988.

Beebe BM: Tips for toddlers, New York, 1983, Dell Publishing Co.

Brazelton TB: Families, crisis and caring, New York, 1989, Addison-Wesley Publishing Co.

Brazelton TB: Working and caring, Menlo Park, Calif, 1985, Addison-Wesley Publishing Co.

Castiglia PT and Petrini MA: Selecting a developmental screening tool, Pediatr Nurs 11(1):8, 1985.

Crocker AC: Mental retardation, Pediatr Ann 18(10):(entire issue), 1989.

Dobson D: Dare to discipline, Wheaton, Ill, 1970, Tyndale House Publishers.

Dormire SL, Strauss SS, and Clarke BA: Social support and adaptation to the parent role in first-time adolescent mothers, J Obstet Gynecol Neonatal Nurs 18(4):327, 1989.

Elkind D: The hurried child-growing up too fast, too soon, Menlo Park, Calif, 1988, Addison-Wesley Publishing Co.

Freiberg KL: Human development: a lifespan approach, ed 3, Boston, 1987, Jones and Bartlett Publishers.

Gilliss CL and others: A health-education program for day-care centers, MCN 14(4):266, 1989.

Ginott HG: Between parent and child, New York, 1961, Macmillan Publishing Co.

Gordon T: P.E.T. in action, New York, 1978, Bantam Books.

Gordon T: Teaching children self-discipline at home and at school, New York, 1989, Times Books–Random House.

Greenspan S and Greenspan NT: The essential partnership, New York, 1989, Viking Penguin Inc.

Hammer D and Drabman RS: Child discipline: what we know and what we can recommend, Pediatr Nurs 7(5):31, 1981.

Howe J: Parenting and functions of the family. In Scipien GM and others, editors: Pediatric nursing care, St Louis, 1990, The CV Mosby Co.

Koch M: Baby exercise has low impact on development, Am J Nurs 89(1):11, 1989.

Lombardino LJ, Stapell JB, and Gerhardt KJ: Evaluating communicative behaviors in infancy, J Pediatr Health Care 1(5):241, 1987.

Mitchell K: Parenting: In Mott SR, Fazekas NF, and James SR, editors: Nursing care of children and families, Menlo Park, Calif, 1985, Addison-Wesley Publishing Co.

National Commission on Working Women: Who cares for the kids? Washington DC, The Commission, 1985.

Nugent KE: Routine care: promoting development in hospitalized infants, MCN 14(5):319, 1989.

Shaw HSW: Telephone audiotapes for parenting education: do they really help? MCN 11(2):108, 1986.

Spock B: Dr. Spock on parenting, New York, 1988, Simon & Schuster.

Starr RM and Gravitz RF: Pit and fissure sealants in the prevention of tooth decay, Pediatr Nurs 11(4):289, 1985.

Taylor MO: Teaching parents about their impaired adolescent's sexuality, MCN 14(3):109, 1989.

Valente S: The suicidal teenager, Nursing '85 15(12):47, 1985.

Abuse and neglect

Aiken MM: Documenting sexual abuse in prepubertal girls, MCN 15(3):176, 1990.

Bruce DA and Zimmerman RA: Shaken impact syndrome, Pediatr Ann 18(8):482, 1989.

Bullock LF and McFarlane J: The birth weight/battering connections, Am J Nurs 89(9):1153, 1989.

Chadwick D: Color atlas of child sexual abuse, St Louis, 1989, Mosby—Year Book.

Kessler DB and New MI: Emerging trends in child abuse and neglect, Pediatr Ann 18(8):471, 1989.

Mittleman RE, Mittleman HS, and Wetli CV: What child abuse really looks like, Am J Nurs 87(9):1185, 1987.

Nelms BC: Violence: the epidemic is growing, J Pediatr Health Care 3(4):173, 1989.

Rhodes AM: The nurses' legal obligations for reporting child abuse, MCN 12(5):313, 1987.

Soditus C and Mock D: Interrupting the cycle of child abuse, MCN 13(3):196, 1988.

Switzer JV: Reporting child abuse, Am J Nurs 86(6):663, 1986.

The sad state of childrens' health includes a rise in abuse, Am J Nurs 89(9):1115, 1989.

Tittle K: When the parents couldn't care less, Nursing '88 18(11):68, 1988.

Wissow LS and Wilson MN: The use of consumer injury registry data to evaluate physical abuse, Child Abuse Negl 12(1):25, 1988.

Zdanuk JM, Harris CC, and Wisian NL: Adolescent pregnancy and incest: the nurse's role as counselor, J Obstet Gynecol Neonatal Nurs 16(2):99, 1987.

Safety/injuries

Bass JL and others: Educating parents about injury prevention, Pediatr Clin North Am 32(1):233, 1985.

Dyment PG, (guest editor): Adolescent injuries, Pediatr Ann 17(2): (entire issue) 1988.

Edwards KS and Forsyth BW: Lead screening at pediatric teaching programs, Am J Dis Child 143(12):1455, 1989.

Gallagher SS, Hunter P, and Guyer B: A home prevention program for children, Pediatr Clin North Am 32(1):95, 1985.

Guidelines for health supervision, Elk Grove Village, Ill, 1985, American Academy of Pediatrics.

Gunnip A and others: Car seats helping parents do it right! J Pediatr Health Care 1(4):190, 1987.

Guyer B and Gallagher SS: An approach to the epidemiology of childhood injuries, Pediatr Clin North Am 32(1):5, 1985.

Hepler B, Sutheimer C, and Sunshine I: Role of the toxicology laboratory in suspected ingestions, Pediatr Clin North Am 33(2):245, 1986.

Kidwell-Udin P, Jacobson D, and Jensen R: It's never too soon to teach car safety, MCN 12(5):344, 1987.

Killam P and Smith K: Getting kids into car seats, MCN 13(2):124, 1988.

Lawson D, Sleet DA, and Amoni M: Priorities for motor vehicle occupant protection among children and youth, J Health Educ 15(5):27, 1984.

Lewander WJ and Lacouture PG: Office management of acute pediatric poisonings, Pediatr Emerg Care 5(4):262, 1989.

Micik S and Miclette M: Injury prevention in the community: a systems approach, Pediatr Clin North Am 32(1):251, 1985.

Molly PJ: Childhood injuries, Public Health Curr 27(4):23, 1987.

Needleman HL: The persistent threat of lead: medical and sociological issues, Curr Probl Pediatr 18(12):697, 1988.

Rick J: Action stat; electric window strangulation, Nursing '88 18(3):33, 1988.

Rivara FP, Bergman AB, and Drake C: Parental attitudes and practices toward children as pedestrians, Pediatrics 84(6):1017, 1989.

Robitaille Y and others: Evaluation of an infant car seat program in a low-income community, Am J Dis Child 144(1):74, 1990.

Shovin JT and others: Near drowning: neurological evaluation is your guide to managing the near-drowning victims, Am J Nurs 89(5):680, 1989.

Skolnick A: Health and safety standards being developed for child-care programs, JAMA 262(24):3387, 1989.

Spyker DA: Submersion injury: epidemiology, prevention and management, Pediatr Clin North Am 32(1):113, 1985.

Steinhart CM and Pearson-Shaver AL: Poisoning, Crit Care Clin 4(4):845, 1988.

Tenenbein M: Pediatric toxicology: current controversies and recent advances, Curr Probl Pediatr 16(4):185, 1986.

Testing child safety seats for preemies, Am J Nurs 89(12):1605, 1989.

Thomson R: Helping to prevent accidents in the home, Nurs Stand 4(16):28, 1990.

Wintemute GJ and Wright MA: Swimming pool owners' opinions of strategies for prevention of drowning, Pediatrics 85(1):63, 1990.

Wong DL: Dispelling some myths about Ipecac, Am J Nurs 88(7):952, 1988.

Wyatt DM: Are you prepared for a hospital fire? Nursing '85 (2):15, 1985.

Zuckerman B and Duby J: Developmental approach to injury prevention, Pediatr Clin North Am 32(1):17, 1985.

Immunization

Centers for Disease Control: General recommendations on immunization, MMWR 38(13):205, 1989.

Centers for Disease Control: Measles prevention, MMWR 38(S-9):1, 1989.

Centers for Disease Control: National childhood vaccine injury act: requirements for permanent vaccination records and for reporting of selected events after vaccination, MMWR 37(13):197, 1988.

Centers for Disease Control: Progress toward achieving the national 1990 objectives for immunization, MMWR 37(40):613, 1988.

Centers for Disease Control: Protection against viral hepatitis (ACIP), MMWR 39(RR-2):1, 1990.

Centers for Disease Control: Rubella and congenital rubella syndrome—United States 1985-1988, MMWR 38(11):173, 1989.

Centers for Disease Control: Tetanus 1987-1988, MMWR 39(3):37, 1990.

Centers for Disease Control: Update: tuberculosis elimination—United States, MMWR 39(10):153, 1990.

Current status of varicella vaccine: Pediatrics 78(4): entire issue, 1986.

Hepatitis B prenatal/postnatal care, US Preventative Services Task Force, Washington DC: screening for hepatitis B, Am Fam Physician 40(1):131, 1989.

Kick JF and others: Optimum needle length for DTP inoculation of infants, Pediatrics 84(1):136, 1989.

Klein JO and Gerety RJ (editors): Current status of haemophilus influenzae type b vaccines, Pediatrics 85(4):entire issue, 1990.

Koblin B and others: Response of preterm infants to diphtheria-tetanus-pertussis vaccine, Pediatr Infect Dis J 7(10):704, 1988.

Salerno MC and Jackson MM: What does the "national childhood vaccine injury act" require of nurses? Am J Nurs 88(7):1019, 1988.

Takenberg JA, editor: Avoiding the threat of hepatitis, Nursing '89 19(10):32C, 1989.

The Child, the Family, and the Hospital Setting

19

Hospitalization of the Child

CHAPTER OBJECTIVES

After studying this chapter, the student should be able to perform the following:

1 Relate three kinds of information about a child that will guide a parent or nurse in preparing him for hospitalization, a nursing procedure, or other interruption in routine.
2 List six ways in which pediatric units and caregivers have tried to reduce stress on a child and his family when medical or surgical care is needed.

3 Explain the three classic phases of separation anxiety as they are typically manifested by the 1- to 4-year-old child.
4 Discuss three nursing principles that help children cope with hospitalization and explain how they may be implemented.

For most persons, regardless of age, hospitalization is a necessary but not a particularly welcome interlude in their lives. Often a stay in the hospital is not planned, and suddenly one enters a rather strange world with many of one's normal social defenses changed, such as family and community role, privacy—even clothes. This turn of events is disruptive for the adult, but it is potentially more disruptive for the dependent toddler, the impressionable young child, and the insecure adolescent.

PREPARATION FOR HOSPITALIZATION

Not many years ago the preparation of children and their parents for the experience of hospitalization was not considered. Emphasis was placed on the child's disease rather than the fact that this was a person with certain capabilities and needs who happened to be ill. Typically the parents brought their child to the pediatric ward, signed some papers, and said a hasty and usually tearful good-bye. Perhaps the child was placed in a special semi-isolation admission area to be observed for 24 to 48 hours for the possible onset of contagious disease before being transferred to the main pediatric ward. Little was done to prepare the child or his parents for this sudden change in their pattern of living.

Today, although a great deal remains to be learned about children's needs and family relationships, health providers recognize that the old approach and many of the old methods were incomplete and unnecessarily traumatic for all concerned. Attempts have been made to shorten hospitalization, use special care-by-parent units, or avoid admission altogether by relying on outpatient departments and surgi-centers designed for minor operations and recovery requiring less than a day. The modern nurse recognizes that the family may have a great deal to offer the hospitalized child. When properly prepared and supported, the parents will be able to help the child during a difficult but potentially constructive period in the child's life.

COPING WITH HOSPITALIZATION

While hospitalized, little patients should continue to grow physically, emotionally, intellectually, and socially in spite of illness. Three principles for nursing children may be suggested to encourage their growth.

Maintain a basic sense of trust

Whether a child is well or sick, he needs to feel secure. Maintaining a sense of trust is crucial. Experiences associated with the fulfillment of basic needs are prime sources for development and support. Parents are best able to fulfill their child's basic needs and give a quality of care that enhances trust and a feeling of security.

A sense of trust should be established between the nurse and the parent and child during the admission process. When admitting the child to the hospital, the nurse routinely checks his pulse, respiration, and temperature. During this procedure she explains to the child what is being done and she answers the parents' questions. Parents judge the nurse's ability to care for their child at this time.

When parents perceive the nurse as a confident (in her knowledge), warm, and gentle person, a trusting relationship develops. Fears of their child's hospitalization subside, and they begin to trust and have faith in the nurse. Parents become relaxed and may even talk about their many difficulties. Worries about an operation, the cost of surgery, and uncertainty of the child's recovery are some of the problems they face. Although it is not always possible to remove all anxieties, the nurse can assist parents step-by-step to solve the concrete problems they face each day. Taking time to listen to them and to answer their questions often relieves many fears. Frequent rounds, easy availability, and a willingness to help and explain make parents more comfortable. The parents' feelings of confidence and trust carry over to the child.

Gradually, as the child's body becomes more dependable, he seeks within his environment ways of gaining active exercise and a greater range of sensory experiences. He investigates, listens, touches, and even tastes in these efforts. Most important is not the fulfillment of these needs but the manner in which they are fulfilled.

Protect from fear, frustration, and pain

Children often are afraid of hospitals and fear what nurses and doctors might do to them. Parental threats of sending the child to the doctor as punishment confuse the child and help develop the idea that illness may be a punishment. The necessary diagnostic measures and treatment procedures may cause great apprehension and physical discomfort. The nurse can readily see from the responses of many children that illness imposes difficult emotional adjustments to unpleasant and painful experiences.

Unpleasant experiences can be minimized by giving the child every opportunity to talk about his fears. His questions should be answered truthfully, simply, and patiently. Preparing the child emotionally for a procedure is very helpful. However, a child should not be told of unpleasant procedures too far in advance so that fantasies and fears may not be activated.

Because a child is interested only in that which will affect him, information about a treatment must be focused on how he will feel and what he may do during the procedure. A painful procedure should be explained just before it is done. Telling the child that the injection will hurt does not necessarily result in acceptance, but the fact that the nurse has been truthful shows him that she understands his reactions. Honest explanations lessen a child's fears and strengthen his trust and confidence in the nurse.

Protection against pain and feelings of distress promote constructive uses of hospital experience. Friendly, comforting hands, answering a child's cry, not forcing him to eat nor waking him from sleep all are sound nursing decisions that enable the child to use his inner strengths to get well.

Facilitate social contacts and communication with the outside world

A common danger for a child who is hospitalized for a long period of time is that he may begin to feel dependent. His stay in the hospital may lessen his initiative because he gets so much satisfaction from being nursed. Physical restoration from illness is not enough. Adverse effects of extended hospitalization must be offset by educational opportunities in the hospital that provide experiences for growth and development. Often a child is socially immature because he has come from a protective hospital environment. In order to combat the isolation illness may inflict, the child needs to be provided with experiences that are as comparable as possible to those he would be experiencing if he were not hospitalized—his world of home, schoolwork, and recreation. This includes activities suitable to his physical condition, which bring him the companionship of children his own age. A well-rounded program of guidance, instruction, and recreation will develop self-respect, encourage initiative, and help fulfill the needs of the whole child.

Guidance. Guidance, that is, training or teaching the child how to live and care for himself may be very productive. It is often easier for the nurse to go ahead and provide the care needed; however, by careful planning and suggestion, a more constructive program may be devised with the child working along with the nurse. For example, during the early morning period, which is a busy time in the hospital, many boys and girls can be taught to take care of their personal belongings and attend to their personal hygiene. Success is a strong incentive to every boy and girl, and the child who feels he has succeeded in accomplishing something worthwhile develops more self-esteem and self-confidence.

Each morning while observing the child, the nurse is confronted with questions about his illness, body, and medical procedures. One essential aspect of a constructive hospital experience is to create a balanced, emotional climate in which it is possible to learn by asking questions. The nurse is uniquely qualified to educate the child about his body and his illness. Talking with the child and answering questions may calm specific fears and contribute to his long-range education and development.

Instruction. The public school system is responsible for providing education for all children, including children in the hospital for extended periods. Pediatric hospitals should supply adequate space for educational facilities. The schoolroom should be large enough to accommodate a group of children in beds, wheelchairs, or carts. The nurse should arrange routine procedures and treatments in order to allow adequate time for a consistent educational program.

Recreation. Play periods are included daily as an integral part of the educational program. In the hospital a supervised play program provides a warm, friendly atmosphere that will help the child develop normally while his body mends. A place to play, suitable materials, and other youngsters to play with are what children need. Because play is a child's way of learning, toys, materials, and equipment are learning tools. Paints, modeling clay, dolls, blocks, games, books, and toys are some of the materials with which children rebuild the world to their size—a world they bring with them of people, things, and feelings. Children play wherever they are. A child's play is his occupation just as surely as teaching may be his father's occupation.

A play program should be designed to help protect children from the effects of separation from family, of isolation, and of harmful experiences such as intrusive procedures. Play offers healing for hurts and sadness. Children who fear treatments are helped to release their pent-up feelings in their use of dolls and other toys. Janie, age 5 years and confined to the hospital for chemotherapy, picked up her doll one day and said, "Don't cry Janie. It isn't your fault. Mommy is going to come every day to take care of you." The attitudes and feelings that children reveal in their play are full of meaning. Every opportunity should be afforded the sick child to release his feelings so that any bad feelings from his experiences in the hospital don't linger as he grows into adulthood. Unless the deep-lying impulses satisfied by play are allowed to express themselves in childhood, adult life may suffer. (See also p. 428.)

The parents

The heart of the problem in preparing children for hospitalization lies in the preparation of their parents, who are best able to help their children. It is imperative that parents receive sufficient knowledge of the child's illness so that they readily understand the need for hospitalization. It is also necessary for parents to have some understanding of the tests and treatments given to their child and the risk and discomfort involved.

A child's morale will inevitably reflect the parents' outlook. When parents are inadequately prepared, they cannot adequately prepare their child. It is extremely important that the parents have sound information about the child's illness, confidence in their physician's recommendations, and the devoted interest of warm, intelligent, and understanding nurses.

The siblings

In addition to the ill child becoming fully informed about the need for hospitalization, siblings should also be included in the explanation so that they too can understand what is happening. Siblings are often affected by the illness of a brother or sister. Fears and imaginations of the brothers and sisters can be worse than the fears of the ill child. Siblings may use fantasy to substitute for a lack of knowledge about hospitalization. However, what a child makes up to substitute for reality can often be more frightening than the truth. When reality is explained in a way that is developmentally appropriate, children can usually understand and cope with potentially serious situations. Open communication and education of all family members help to minimize the well siblings' misconceptions and fantasies about the ill child.

A child's hospitalization is a stressful experience for the entire family. Sibling rivalry may be intensified because of the shift of family attention. When parents spend most of their time with the ill child as they often do, the well siblings begin to develop feelings of rejection, abandonment, anger, and jealousy. Siblings should be allowed to discuss their feelings with parents and how they feel toward the ill child. Sibling visitation is an excellent way to decrease sibling rivalry and should be permitted and encouraged. Because most young children learn best through direct experience they benefit by seeing the ill child in the hospital setting.

The child

According to their level of understanding, children should be told why it is necessary for them to go to the hospital. The truth is less frightening to youngsters than the ideas their imaginations invent. Children who are not given the true reason for hospitalization often believe that they have been punished or sent away because they have been naughty. Of course, if the truth is to be supportive, children must have confidence in their parents and other authority figures based on previous experience of their trustworthiness. Such an attitude cannot be established in a day. Its foundation is laid during the first year and perpetuated through each stage of life.

Telling children about surgery is a highly individual matter and depends on the child's age, level of understanding, and emotional makeup. Usually a brief, simple explanation of what is wrong and what must be done to change it or make it better helps the child develop a sound and healthy attitude. A detailed explanation of the operation is not necessary; the child needs the truth but not always the whole truth. The belief that an event has been explained relieves tension.

Pediatric units in hospitals throughout the United States have developed methods to prepare parents and children for hospitalization. Colorful booklets and pamphlets, telephone calls, hospital tours, preadmission or orientation parties including movies and puppet shows, and the use of television sets all have lessened the trauma of admission to the hospital. Advising parents of procedures and inviting children and their parents to visit the hospital before admission help children to know what to expect (Fig. 19-1). Allowing the child to share in planning for a hospital stay or helping to pack a suitcase is sometimes rewarding.

Children should know in advance what the hospital is like. They should be told simply and in a matter-of-fact manner about such things as the differences between hospital beds and beds at home, use of the bedpan and urinals, baths in bed, special schooling, the playroom, and the food service. If a young child knows in advance about the big, wiggly scale that he must stand on to see how heavy he is and some of the other things that happen

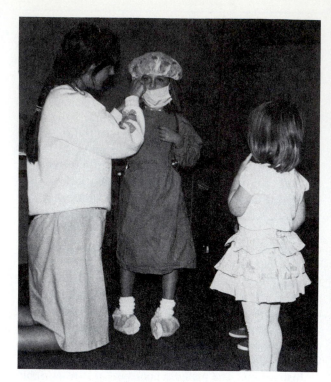

FIG 19-1 Inviting children and their parents to visit the hospital before admission helps them to know what to expect.

at the hospital, he is less shocked when he faces them directly (Fig. 19-2).

It is not always possible, necessary, or desirable for children to know everything that will happen. All they need to know is enough to assure them that what happens is according to plan and that their parents will be at their side whenever possible. When they cannot be there, kind friends, physicians, and nurses will help care for them until they can go home again.

Printed information sheets completed by parents, ideally before admission, are helpful. They request brief background material regarding the health history, habits, skills, likes, dislikes, fears, and family composition of the young patient; this information assists the staff in individualizing care.

Liberal visiting hours that include sibling visitation, rooming-in facilities, and appropriate parent participation in care make it much easier for the mother and father to continue their supportive role and help counteract any sense of isolation or desertion the child may feel. However, no matter how well children are prepared for hospitalization, they may still cry at the prospect of treatment, needles, and pain. The nurse should explain to the parents that this is a natural reaction and encourage them

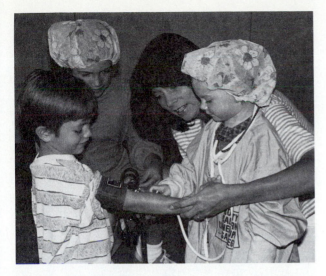

FIG 19-2 If the child knows in advance what will happen, he is less likely to be shocked when he faces the situation directly. (*Courtesy Children's Hospital and Health Center, San Diego, Calif.*)

to stay with their child, since they are best able to comfort the youngster with the thought of feeling better when it is over. Usually the parents' presence helps the child to weather each difficulty as it comes and greatly reduce the risk of emotional trauma.

AGE AND DEVELOPMENTAL NEEDS

The age of the child and his stage of development at the time of his illness or hospitalization are prime factors in understanding its significance in his life. In addition children come to the hospital with their own unique personalities, past experiences, and methods of dealing with anxiety. The nurse can encourage emotional growth by accepting these children as they are and by assisting them to continue in their present stage of development. For example, often young children are expected to conform to hospital rules by staying in cribs when, in essence, they have had the run of the whole house before hospitalization. Unless acutely ill, a child may refuse to stay in bed. The nurse should not arbitrarily urge the child to "stay there." She should be aware of the dangers of restricting children to cribs when they otherwise could be ambulatory. For the toddler, sustained restriction of movement may lead to a severe state of anxiety and hostility. Whenever the basic motor urge is thwarted, the child becomes frustrated and angry and may regress. This drive is constructively handled by the wise nurse who devises ways to allow the child freedom to move about safely.

In general, when a child must be hospitalized, flexible and adaptive arrangements become necessary both to help maintain the family unity and to respect the needs of both the child patient and other members of the family. The nurse must try to provide both the physical and social environment appropriate for the child's continuing development.

The infant

During the first year of life, infants develop trust by having their needs met in a consistent, satisfying manner. Rooming-in accommodations are most desirable for the hospitalized infant, and his parent, too. The repetition of the same feeding routine, basic physical care by the mother or the same person in the same way provides a sense of security or trust that is vital to his development. Since the very young infant does not know or recognize his mother, he is likely to be content in the hospital, provided that these needs are adequately fulfilled by the nurse. However, by the time the child has reached the second half of his first year, he becomes increasingly aware of mother as a specific source of gratification.

When parents of a young child are unable to come to the hospital for prolonged periods, the hospitalized child is exposed to additional traumatic factors resulting in frustration of those inborn needs that are normally met in a family environment. Hospitalization interrupts the mother-child relationship and arouses the fear of desertion. As a result, the child may fail to thrive physically, socially, and psychologically. In extreme situations, maternal deprivation may be manifested as a general marasmus or wasting away.

The toddler

Considerable evidence has shown that under certain circumstances children may view hospitalization as desertion by their parents and thus may be profoundly affected by their hospital experience.

Studies have pointed out that children between 1 and 4 years of age are most likely to suffer when parent-child separation occurs. *Separation anxiety* tapers off beyond 5 years of age but never disappears entirely during childhood. Separation anxiety is characteristic of all young children who have established a healthy parent-child relationship. The phenomenon of "settling in," or adjustment to hospitalization and separation, is deceptive. Robertson* found that children under 4 years of age expe-

*Robertson J: Young children in hospitals, New York, 1958, Basic Books, Inc.

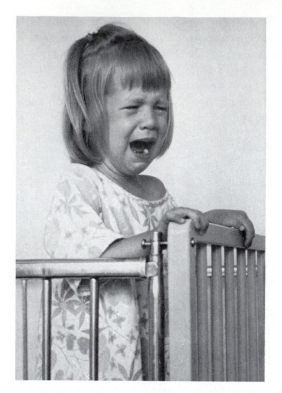

FIG 19-3   Phase I: protest. First day after admission, child (2½ years old) cries aloud for "Mama," shakes the crib, and is alert for signs of her mother's return. *(Courtesy Children's Hospital and Health Center, San Diego, Calif.)*

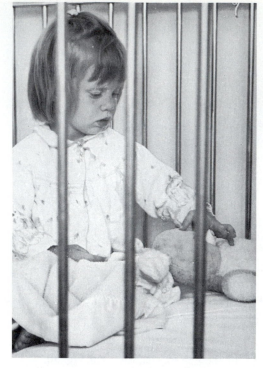

FIG 19-4   Phase II: despair. Four days after admission, child has become apathetic and withdrawn. She does not understand why her mother has left her or why she is in the hospital. *(Courtesy Children's Hospital and Health Center, San Diego, Calif.)*

rience three phases in the process of settling into the hospital: protest, despair, and denial. These emotional phases may not be as severe when pediatric policies are more enlightened, but they are probably still there.

At first young children *protest* the separation (Fig. 19-3). They cry aloud for "Mama," shake the crib, throw themselves around, and are alert for any signs of mother's return. The nurse may pick up the child and try to quiet him, but this is to no avail. Telling children to stop crying only conveys to them that they are not understood and adds to their feelings of helplessness. This phase may last for a few days or even up to 1 week.

During the phase of *despair* the child becomes apathetic and withdrawn, signs often mistaken for acceptance (Fig. 19-4). Instead of crying loudly, the child sobs. The hope of mother's return fades, but the wish for her return remains. During this quiet stage, distress seemingly has lessened, and the nurse presumes that the child is "settling in." When the parents arrive, the child may turn away and cry aloud. These children do not understand why they are in the hospital. They reject their

parents in the same way that their parents seem to have rejected them. Parents spend most of the visiting time trying to get the child to respond to them more normally, and just as the child brightens up, the parents must leave again. Children's piteous cries on the parents' arrival and departure lead the nurse to mistakenly think that the youngsters are better off without their parents. The nurse, understanding the reason for this behavior, can be of great help to parents who dread coming back because they anticipate their child's distress. The parents need to realize how much their child needs them, and they should be encouraged to come often. When they leave, they should be sure to tell the child when they will come back. It is unfair for parents to tell their child that they are going for a cup of coffee when they are actually leaving. Children have lain awake all night waiting for parents to return.

Gradually the stage of *denial* follows despair. Children begin to show more interest in the surroundings, are more responsive to nursing attention, and actually deny the need for their parents. When their mothers come, they

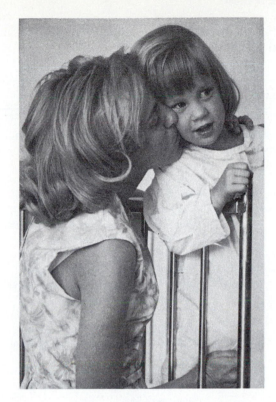

FIG 19-5   Phase III: denial. Eight days after admission, child cannot tolerate intensity of distress so she represses need for mother. When her mother comes, she seems hardly to know her and is happy and cheerful. *(Courtesy Children's Hospital and Health Center, San Diego, Calif.)*

may seem to hardly know them, may be happy and cheerful throughout the visit, and may even wave good-bye (Fig. 19-5). Psychologists have explained this phenomenon as the inability of young children to tolerate the intensity of distress, which causes them to repress the need for their mothers. However, after these young children return home, they often demonstrate their disturbed feelings by regressive, babylike behavior and by clinging to their mothers. This only confirms that the complacency they exhibited in the hospital was a façade.

The preschool child

The preschool child demonstrates separation anxiety to a lesser degree than does the toddler. His focus has changed from earlier separation fears and loss of love to his physical integrity. He believes that his illness is punishment for wrongdoing, and he fears he will be medically punished by mutilation. The preschool child is particularly sensitive to surgical procedures and bodily intrusion such as rectal temperatures, injections, and blood tests. If he is immobilized or confined, feelings of frus-

tration and despair occur, which are often manifested by social withdrawal.

Preschool children struggle to understand and to assimilate the illness experience. Routine hospital procedures can be overwhelming to him. The medicine tastes bitter, shots hurt, and the x-ray machines and other hospital equipment are frightening. At times, his mother is the only acceptable buffer between him and the frightening hospital. The only really effective way to prevent psychologic distress is to provide overnight facilities for parents so that Mom or Dad can be with the sick child as often as possible. Without his mother, even if he has been prepared, the preschooler finds hospitalization to be a terrifying experience.

The school-age child

School-age children worry about having to give up their independence. It seems to them that doctors and nurses can do whatever they please to their bodies, that is, draw blood, enforce medication, operate. School-age children seem more bothered by the disease process and its treatment. The school-age child is very aware that he is different and that uncontrollable things are happening to his body through illness or surgery. He blames himself for his illness and often experiences treatments and procedures as punishment. Imagination persists strongly throughout the school-age years. Like the preschooler, he often fantasizes. Fears of mutilation influence his degree of emotional reaction. Kind nurses who encourage free expression and demonstrate understanding are most welcomed by these children.

School-age children can cope fairly well if their illnesses are short and if they have meaningful adults to support their coping. To some extent these children have learned to rely on adults and other children when away from home. They can understand that hospitalization is a temporary situation and that their parents come only at certain times.

The adolescent

Adolescents are particularly affected by the confinement and dependency inherent in hospitalization. The typical adolescent needs for independence, copious quantities of food, physical activity, and a peer group are hard to supply in a hospital setting. The adolescent is most vulnerable in those illnesses or accidents that make him different from his peers. He may be afraid that his illness or surgery will have a permanently crippling effect, which will interfere with his future participation in school, sports, social activities, and even marriage.

Illness and hospitalization at a time when the indi-

The Hospitalized Child

Selected nursing diagnoses	Expected outcomes	Interventions
A. Anxiety related to separation from mother (or primary caregiver). Clinical manifestations: Prolonged crying during separation, disinterest in play, lack of response to comfort measures of familiar nurse, parental report of being unable to stay with child for extended periods.	Child tolerates necessary absence of mother or primary caregiver without severe distress or prolonged anxiety. Child demonstrates positive coping behaviors throughout hospital stay.	Develop sense of familiarity and eventual trust between child and nurse. Attempt consistency in nurse-patient assignments. Facilitate presence of security objects and items associated with home. Learn child's normal home routines and follow these when possible. Visit child frequently during parent's absence, even if for short periods. Offer physical contact—holding, rocking, etc.,—when possible. Utilize play and playroom as often as possible. Create a social and active environment for child when possible. Provide positive reinforcement for participation in ADLs, treatments and unit activities. Ensure mother's understanding of separation anxiety. Make parent comfortable and welcome to stay with child as much as possible. Encourage parent's presence during traumatic procedures if feasible. Keep child's bed/room area "safe"; perform painful procedures in treatment room. Offer assistance in preventing separation if possible: e.g., helping to secure transportation or child care for parents and siblings. Show understanding and acceptance of necessary separation and assure parent of close supervision during her absence. Encourage visits from other relatives and friends. Emphasize importance of being honest with child at all times.
B. Fear related to painful and/or invasive procedures.	Child verbalizes fear and maintains some control during traumatic procedures.	Encourage child to verbalize feelings, both before and after procedure. Facilitate presence of parent, if desired by parent and child.

Selected nursing diagnoses	Expected outcomes	Interventions
Clinical manifestations: Expression of distress, anticipatory crying, withdrawal, repeated questions, verbalized fear.		Keep child's bed/room area "safe"; perform potentially painful procedures in treament room if possible. Explain reason for procedure to child and parent. Anticipate sequence of events and sensations with child. Answer child's questions as simply as possible, with consideration of the child's level of understanding. Choose terminology to ensure understanding and avoid frightening associations. Utilize visual aids, doll, or stuffed animal to enhance understanding and acceptance of explanation. Discuss how child can behave during procedure to maximize control and minimize discomfort. Include child in decision making when appropriate. Teach parent how to help during procedure. Use distractions and/or relaxation techniques during procedure if appropriate. Enable procedure to be performed as quickly as possible. Allow role playing and directed play as indicated before or after procedure. Give positive feedback when possible.

vidual is dealing with major developmental tasks regarding independence, sexual identity, peer relations, and future job and career goals add extra stress to an already critical period. Although hospitalization may impede the accomplishment of developmental tasks, it may in some instances aid in their accomplishment. Whether hospitalization is ultimately a positive or negative experience for the adolescent depends to a large degree on the understanding, interest, and sensitive care given by nurses.

PROLONGED HOSPITALIZATION

Long-term hospitalization imposes numerous anxieties on children of all ages. During a serious illness even older children have a great need for their parents and can tolerate their absence only for short periods. They need to know that their parents will be there when they need them most and that they are loved and missed. (See Chapters 20 and 21.)

• • •

This discussion has highlighted the psychologic risk of hospitalization. However, it is comforting to note that children usually are able to survive the event of hospitalization without significant emotional scars. It is largely the nurse's function to see that the original trauma is slight and the scars minimal.

Key Concepts

1. Three principles for nursing sick children are suggested to encourage their growth: (1) maintain a basic sense of trust; (2) protect them from fear, frustration, and pain; and (3) facilitate social contacts and communication with the outside world.

2. A well-rounded program of guidance, instruction, and recreation develops self-respect, encourages initiative, and helps fulfill the needs of the whole child.

3. It is imperative that parents are prepared for their child's hospitalization because they are best able to help prepare the child.

4. Siblings should be provided explanations about the hospitalization, should be allowed to communicate their feelings, and should be encouraged to visit their brother or sister.

5. In preparation for hospitalization, children should be provided with truthful explanations in keeping with their level of understanding, should be allowed to visit the hospital, and should be involved with planning for their stay.

6. The age of the child and his stage of development at the time of hospitalization are prime factors in understanding its significance in his life.

7. Children between 1 and 4 years of age are most likely to suffer when parent-child separation occurs. There are three phases of separation anxiety: protest, despair, and denial.

Discussion Questions

1. Refer to the ages and stages of development. What fears are most likely to occur if a child in each of these stages is hospitalized?

2. What techniques would you choose to help you explain the hospital and hospital procedures to children in each of these stages?

3. How could you help reduce a parent's anxiety regarding the need to hospitalize a child?

4. Separation of parent and child is difficult, particularly if the child is ill. What are hospitals in your area doing to reduce this trauma for both parents and children?

5. Many young children who have been toilet-trained become incontinent when they enter the hospital. What is this called? How would you explain this behavior to a parent?

20

Rehabilitation of the Long-Term Pediatric Patient

CHAPTER OBJECTIVES

After studying this chapter, the student should be able to perform the following:

1 Define rehabilitation and state how it differs from habilitation.

2 Discuss three recommendations related to psychologic support, noted in the text, which are thought to be especially appropriate when nursing children and young people with long-term illnesses or disabilities.

3 Explain why the staffing pattern in a rehab unit usually needs to be 30% to 60% above typical medical-surgical ratios.

4 Indicate signs and symptoms of autonomic dysreflexia and the emergency treatment advised.

5 Explain the use of the Levels of Cognitive Functioning Scale developed at Rancho Los Amigos Hospital in Downey, California.

6 Point out six hazards of long-term bed rest.

7 Present a suggested schedule for a skin tolerance check.

8 List three ways that urinary control may be achieved by persons with neurogenic bladders.

9 Describe how a 10-year-old girl may safely perform a clean self-catheterization in the bathroom at home. What equipment will she need?

10 Identify three problems associated with the use of Foley catheters and state how their incidence may be reduced.

11 Emphasize five factors that influence bowel patterns, making regularity difficult.

12 Describe the process of behavior modification based on stimulus-response techniques, including the terms *intermittent reinforcement, shaping,* and *trapping.*

For most children the period of hospitalization is brief—a day or two, perhaps a week. Increasingly, the trend is to shorten the treatment period away from home whenever possible; a shorter stay in the hospital has psychologic, social, and financial advantages for the child and the family. However, for a few patients, hospitalization is still prolonged. The severely ill child who has a long, complicated convalescence, the child undergoing elaborate orthopedic corrections, and the teenager with a damaged spinal cord who is struggling to recapture skills once considered automatic and to adjust to new expectations and goals all are examples of relatively long-term pediatric patients. The following is a brief discussion of the needs of boys and girls who stay in the hospital for extended periods; it emphasizes the nursing perspectives, challenges, and skills of a relatively new specialty within a specialty—that of pediatric rehabilitation.

The term *habilitation* refers to the ability to perform

those daily activities that are characteristic of the normal functions for one's age and culture. Some children for various reasons never become completely habilitated.

In a general sense the definition of rehabilitation is "to restore to a functional state." The families of those patients who have suffered devastating physical disabilities characteristically need a coordinated multidisciplinary team that considers not only the physical but the sociologic, emotional, vocational, and spiritual aspects of the patient's total situation. The rehabilitation of children is made more complex by their continuing need for normal growth and development in the face of disability.

Pediatric rehabilitation is based on at least two concepts: first, that each person is unique and has individual basic worth, and second, that the task involves a committed group of people working together as a team with a common goal. The overall goal of pediatric rehabilitation is to foster maximal growth, development, independence, and personal fulfillment within the limitations of the handicap. Many allied health professionals form the core rehabilitation team: physicians, nurses, physical and occupational therapists, speech and hearing pathologists, medical social service workers, dietitians, financial counselors, recreational therapists (Child Life representatives), teachers, and educational consultants. Representatives of other specialty areas, such as psychology, psychiatry, psychometric testing, and vocational counseling, as well as community agencies, are available as needed. Team physicians represent each specialty, and the community physician, public health nurse, and teacher are invited to be part of the team for their patient. Each team member evaluates the patient, makes recommendations in writing, and participates in patient planning conferences. The patient and family are prime members of the team and are included appropriately in conferences where current status and progress are discussed and new goals are set.

The needs of the area served by the rehabilitation center dictate the types of patients seen. Patients with various diagnoses who have functional, mobility, and cognitive problems usually make up the patient population.

Generally speaking, any patient with a devastating injury or illness that produces lasting or permanent physical disabilities can and should be treated by the rehabilitation team. Nursing principles of rehabilitation must be initiated at the onset of illness or injury to prevent complications and further loss of function. Realistically, many of these children initially require specialized lifesaving care, which can be delivered more effectively in intensive care or medical-surgical units. Ideally the principles of both acute and long-term care will be delivered simultaneously. When the patient's condition has stabilized and the youngster is no longer "ill" as such, it is time to consider transfer to the rehabilitation unit.

In the best circumstances a rehabilitation program provides an inpatient unit, an outpatient clinic, and supportive community agency relationships. They all help the patient and the family progress more smoothly from onset of illness or injury back to home and community as a functioning, worthwhile part of society. Some patients may continue to return to a rehabilitation program periodically as they grow older and their needs change or their abilities alter.

Throughout the patients' progression from the initial care facility back to the home and community, there must be no surprises. The transition of the patient to units, wards, agencies, and levels of any program must be done smoothly without breaks in continuity. The patient, family, and team members must be kept informed of the patient's status, program, and goals. Continuity in care during and after transfer to the rehabilitation unit takes the coordinated effort and skills of all the persons involved. One person must coordinate the process of admission. Frequently this is the responsibility of the nurse.

Staffing of a rehabilitation unit needs to be 30% to 60% above the typical medical-surgical ratios. Fastidious nursing care, continual teaching, and reinforcement are required. Independence comes with patience, repetition, and allowing the patient or family member to "do" rather than the traditional "doing for." The program is expensive, and the cost must be passed on to the patient, insurance companies, and government agencies, but the independence gained may in the end reduce the total financial outlay. Needless to say, the patient, family, and rehabilitation team must expend great amounts of emotional and physical energy, as well as monetary resources.

Before contributing to the formation of an individualized care plan, each team member must assess the patient's current status. A logical, systematic approach will ensure the inclusion of all important facts in the nursing assessment. (See the box on p. 427 for a suggested initial assessment outline.)

Using this evaluation of the patient's current status and pertinent history, one can formulate nursing interventions for existing and potential problems and identify teaching needs. Successful teaching also includes assessment of the cultural values, lifestyle, and learning capabilities of the child and the parents. Teaching needs and nursing intervention must always be discussed with

Initial nursing assessment outline

Introduction	Name, age, chief complaint or problem, circumstances of present injury or illness, referring physician
History	Past injuries, illnesses, hospitalizations
Vital signs	Temperature, pulse, respiration, blood pressure
Allergies	Reactions to drugs, food, airborne particles, contact agents
System check*	
Neurosensory	Level of consciousness, orientation, neurologic checks, intellectual level, balance, coordination, sensory abnormalities, emotional stability
Integumentary (skin and mucous membranes)	Turgor, general condition, complete description of lesions, condition of mouth
Musculoskeletal	Muscle strength, range of motion, motor abnormalities, amputations (follow-up evaluation by PT), current therapy
Respiratory	Pattern and sound of respirations, URI? cough? Pulmonary function studies (follow-up evaluation by PT and RT)
Urinary	Vocabulary? Normal voiding or ostomy? (Continence? Urinary draining devices, catheter size, catheterization program)
Gastrointestinal	Vocabulary? Schedule: time, frequency, bowel movement consistency, normal movement or ostomy? Effect of diet?
Diet	Type, likes and dislikes, time and amount; method: bottle, oral gavage, gastrostomy etc.
Health supervision	Dates of last dental, eye, and hearing examinations; performed by? Immunizations? Safety problems?
Growth and development (activities of daily living; motor skills)	Independent, with assistance; dependent: feeding, turning, transfer, bathing, dressing, toileting, standing, walking, grooming, dental hygiene (follow-up evaluation by OT and PT)
Equipment brought	Cane, crutches, walker, wheelchair, braces, appliances, scooterboards
Current medications and treatments	Medication: dosage, time, route, effects? Treatments: time, duration, specifics
Family composition	Parents, marital status, age, siblings, extended family, resources (follow-up evaluation by MSS)
Social and educational interests	Level of education, special friends, hobbies, security items, community contacts
Understanding of injury or illness	By patient, by family
Specialized care needs	

PT, physical therapy; OT, occupational therapy; RT, respiratory therapy; MSS, medical social service.
*In making this assessment, ascertain the status of the patient before his injury or illness.

the patient—in a manner appropriate to the child's age—and with the parents to determine the family's readiness to learn. Mutual strategies, goals, and target dates can then be incorporated into a written plan. Visual materials and demonstrations giving clear explanations of the treatment rationale and its importance to the patient enhance learning.

When the patient's progress is sufficient, as shown on the unit and during progressive home passes, discharge plans are finalized. Discharge should also be coordinated by one person. There should be a home visit by a member of the rehab team before discharge to help plan for program needs or physical changes within the home. These will be evaluated during progressive pass experiences. Before discharge, arrangements for the following may need to be made: community public health nurse follow-up, admission to a regular or special school, methods of obtaining supplies and medications, return appointments to community physicians, and the sharing of phone numbers of team members with the family.

After discharge, regular visits to a rehabilitation clinic enable the team to reevaluate each patient with feedback from the school, public health nurse, and other outside agencies.

Because of improved medical care during the last 25 years, increasing numbers of people with various disabilities have been absorbed into society. As a cohesive group, they are beginning to represent a political force. Through consumer awareness and pressure, legislation for the disabled has brought about improved wheelchair accessibility in many public buildings and businesses, leading to improved educational and employment opportunities. Additionally, the courts have begun to attack discrimination in the job market, making job performance the sole criterion for employment.

PSYCHOLOGIC SUPPORT OF LONG-TERM PATIENTS AND THEIR FAMILIES

The character and severity of an injury or disease may be sources of considerable stress, but prolonged isolation from normal surroundings, the strange environment of the hospital, and frequent encounters with the many different people involved in patient care make hospitalization particularly difficult. The limited experience and development of the child increase the potential for emotional trauma at this time.

The three principles of nursing care described as appropriate for all hospitalized children in Chapter 19—(1) maintain a basic sense of trust, (2) protect from fear, frustration, and pain, and (3) facilitate social contacts

and communication with the outside world—are particularly applicable to the long-term patient.

A sense of trust is best fostered in children when their parents trust the people working in the facility. This trust is gradually developed as the parents and child learn that the staff, demonstrating forethought, accessibility, and reliability as well as technical skills, cares about them. It may be strengthened through the primary nursing concept or at least the consistent assignment of one or two nurses for each child's care. Trust also increases as the staff helps the family with their grief for the child who is injured or has been impaired by disease. The grief experienced by the parents, family, and friends of these patients has some similarity to that encountered by those who mourn the death of a loved one.

Often the three-stage pattern of shock and denial, developing awareness, and restitution or resolution can be identified. The response of shock and disbelief is often still present on arrival at the rehabilitation unit. Statements such as "When will my child walk again?" and "When she is better, things will be like they were before," demonstrate the denial. Each statement does not require refuting but should not be reinforced. The counseling nurse should reinforce reality through an understanding but factual discussion of the patient's status, problems, and required nursing care. Involving the family in this care helps them feel useful, important, and needed.

The second stage of mourning is demonstrated by increasing awareness and feelings of guilt and anger. Laments of "Why me?" "It's all my fault," "If only I'd looked sooner," or "I shouldn't have let him go," poignantly demonstrate guilt. Anger is often directed toward the child for being careless or disobedient. One parent may accuse the other of being at fault. Often anger is directed at the hospital staff, since this outlet is "safer" than accusing a family member. Criticism of nursing care, the physician, or staff personalities is the most common manifestation. Understanding the causes of these feelings enables the staff to support the family. Reassurance that the accident was unpreventable (if, indeed, it was) will help. Giving the parents information about their child's condition and involving the family in care-giving and decision-making are essential. Nonjudgmental listening and prompt attention to problems help to smooth the way toward the third stage of grieving: restitution or resolution.

The last stage of grieving involves the sharing of grief with others and, it is hoped, the support of relatives and friends. When a loved one dies, a funeral may help a family to accept their loss. In the case of disability, the family frequently substitutes ritualistic behavior such as an exact time for visitation, weekly visits to a special physician, or daily trips to church. Some families seem to adjust to the changes imposed by disability better than others. Unfortunately, the stresses are great, and family dissolution all too often results. Trust helps ease these stresses. Trust through open communication helps the family work through the problems.

The parents and team must realize that as children become aware of their disabilities and limitations, they too go through a grieving process. They may verbalize anger, quietly withdraw, or become overly cooperative. At times these children may show little motivation or may refuse to learn new skills. The goal during this period should be to assist the child to adjust to a new body image and activities of daily living rather than acceptance of the disability. Psychosocial support can help the child, parents, and team work through this normal process.

It is impossible and probably undesirable to protect a patient completely from fear, pain, or even frustration. However, these unpleasant feelings may be reduced. Since young children need to do little to prepare themselves in advance for most procedures, the knowledge that a certain procedure will be done usually need not be shared until just before its actual performance. Then these children should be told in simple, truthful terms how the test or nursing activity will affect them and what they can do to help. Later, opportunities to verbalize and to express themselves through drawings, play acting, story telling, or music should be made available. Feelings that cannot be put into words need to find an outlet before they, in turn, become symptoms. (See p. 416.)

The need for emotional release ties in with the need to facilitate social interaction and contact with the community. Maintaining friendships is sometimes difficult for a child with flagging energy and extended illness. Yet the knowledge that one still has such relationships encourages stability and incentive and usually makes return to the neighborhood after hospitalization less traumatic. Short, chaperoned trips to recreational areas, to cultural centers, or just to visit friends can also be a method of maintaining one's place in the world outside. These passes should begin as soon as the family has been given necessary instructions and has demonstrated competence in the child's care. Much support and encouragement are often needed, since the hospital often provides a safe, accepting environment of the child's disability, and this acceptance may not exist in the community. The child and parents must be prepared to respond to stares, handle avoidance, and answer questions.

The addition of a Child Life Specialist to the staff of many hospitals is a welcome event. This specially prepared professional helps patients participate in a wide range of constructive activities either in groups or as individuals. A monthly newspaper planned by the patients, hobby fairs, and picnics on nearby lawns are sample activities.

Whether in a rehabilitation unit or regular hospital area, convalescing long-term patients should be given the opportunity and responsibility of continuing their education. Ideally a classroom for ambulatory patients will be available and provision made for tutors from the public school system. Telephone or TV tutoring is also available in some areas. It is possible in some cases to maintain contact with the class and school attended before hospitalization and to work on assignments in the rehab unit. Education is extremely important to those capable young people whose vocational choices may be somewhat narrowed.

CONDITIONS COMMONLY ENCOUNTERED

Common diagnoses found in rehabilitation units include spinal cord injuries, anomalies or diseases of the central nervous system, and brain injury caused by trauma, tumor, or disease. Since students working on the rehabilitation unit frequently meet patients with these problems, they are discussed briefly below.

Spinal cord injury

Children suffer spinal cord injury less frequently than adults do. Spinal cord trauma in teenagers and children occurs most often as a result of automobile or, less frequently, diving accidents and gunshot wounds. Although the spinal cord is partially protected by bone, shearing or torsion forces can destroy or severely damage the cord. The affected portion of the body is determined by the level of spinal injury. The higher the cord injury, the greater will be the resulting disability. Paraplegic patients (persons whose paralysis or functional loss involves lower extremities), even though they may experience loss of bowel and bladder control and perineal sensation, can be totally independent; quadriplegic patients (persons whose paralysis or functional loss involves all four extremities) may need supervision or assistance. The more hand function available, the more independent the patient will be. With improved emergency care and quicker retrieval, increased numbers of patients with high spinal cord injuries (C1, C2, and C3 levels) are surviving. These patients have no function below shoulder level. Their basic care remains the same as that required by other quadriplegic patients, but the nurse must become familiar with ventilatory equipment and be prepared for more intense psychologic and adjustment problems. Eventual resocialization requires sophisticated electronic equipment such as electric wheelchairs with tongue switches, as well as environmental control systems to operate a television, radio, telephone, or intercom.

The application of lifesaving measures is of initial importance in the management of the patient with spinal cord injury. Immobilization and stabilization of the spine are paramount. These are often accomplished with a "halo" apparatus that may be worn for a period of 10 to 12 weeks until the spine is stabilized. This apparatus consists of a halo ring to immobilize the head and metal bars that attach the ring to a vest that encompasses the chest and supports the apparatus weight. Plastic vests are often used, but a plaster vest may be needed for the irregularly shaped chest or back. The halo apparatus allows the child to have extra mobility to sit, stand, or lie prone, usually causing respiratory, circulatory, and muscular problems to improve.

Orders for the child in a halo apparatus include administration of a mild analgesic for initial discomfort. The nurse should report swallowing problems, difficulty in opening the mouth, and loosened pins. The pins holding the halo barely penetrate the skull. Therefore these pin sites must be meticulously cleaned twice a day. Half-strength peroxide is often employed. The use of povidone-iodine (Betadine) solution is currently discouraged for routine pin care because of reports of possible allergic reactions and potential pin deterioration. Separate sterile applicators should be used for each pin. Some serosanguineous drainage is expected initially, but one must check for any change or increase in drainage, redness, swelling, or pain that would indicate development of infection. Although the vests have a protective inner lining, pressure sores may develop over the scapulae and shoulders. These sores may be prevented with proper body positioning and frequent changes in position. The vest's resistance tends to inhibit respiratory function; therefore, deep breathing and coughing exercises must be encouraged. Observation for spinal cord trauma by performance of daily upper extremity neurologic assessments is required. Any changes should be reported immediately to the physician. Finally, the nurse must teach the child some general safety rules to prevent falls that may inflict greater damage. During the time of bony healing the complications of bed rest must be prevented. The patient needs meticulous skin care, periodic range-of-motion exercises, adequate fluid intake, venous-support stockings (TED hose), bowel and bladder programs,

and special respiratory care. The patient with injury at midtrunk level or above requires more than position changes and coughing. Because the respiratory muscles have been affected, incentive spirometers are valuable. An upper respiratory tract infection is a serious threat to this patient.

The higher the level of the cord injury, the less tolerance the patient displays for an upright position. The application of elastic hose from toes to groin or of a snug-fitting corset before the patient sits helps prevent pooling of blood in the lower extremities. Gradually (over a period of days), increasing the angle of the wheelchair back and lowering the legs help prevent dizziness, perspiration, fainting, and other signs of hypotension. When these symptoms occur, tipping the wheelchair back to lower the patient's head relieves the symptoms.

Below the level of injury, temperature regulation is affected in these patients, since skin nerve endings that combine with the central nervous system are not functioning to control temperature. The skin does not perspire to aid cooling, nor do the muscles shiver to produce heat. Therefore the skin may be injured by extremes of heat or cold that the patient cannot perceive, and the patient must be made aware of this possibility. In addition, the patient's response to an inflammatory process may register a higher body temperature than is typical for that type of problem. Control is usually obtained by uncovering the patient or using acetaminophen (Tylenol).

In the patient with an injury above midtrunk, or T6, a complication known as *autonomic dysreflexia* or *hyperreflexia* may arise. This is a very serious rise in the blood pressure that can lead to a cerebrovascular accident (CVA) or seizures. Signs and symptoms include flushing, headache, sweating, feelings of nasal stuffiness, goose bumps, bradycardia, and a rapid increase in blood pressure. These result from sympathetic nervous system activity and are usually related to physical stimuli such as bladder and bowel distention, severe pressure sores, and urinary tract infection. Less frequently, external stimuli may trigger autonomic dysreflexia. It should be treated by elevating the patient's head and removing the stimulus. A distended bladder is drained. If the patient does not improve, hydralazine hydrochloride can be given. Patients who are subject to such episodes and their family members should be fully instructed in self-care before discharge.

Brain injury

A result of the fast-paced and highly technologic society in which we live is an increase in accidents and traumatic injuries. Those children who survive severe

Table 20-1 Levels of cognitive functioning

Level	Patient behavior	Nursing intervention
I. No response	Patient appears to be in deep sleep and is unresponsive to visual, auditory, or painful stimuli.	Be calm and soothing in manner of speech and physical manipulation of the patient.
II. Generalized response	Patient reacts inconsistently and nonpurposefully to stimuli in a nonspecific manner. Responses may be physiologic changes, gross body movements, and vocalization.	Do not talk with others when working with the patient. Assume that the patient can understand what is being said.
III. Localized response	Patient reacts specifically but inconsistently to stimuli. He can track and focus on objects and turn toward or away from auditory stimuli. The patient may withdraw from painful stimuli. Simple commands may be followed in an inconsistent or delayed manner. The patient may show vague awareness of self and body by responding to discomfort by pulling at a nasogastric tube or restraints.	Talk to the patient about things he is doing or about family members and friends. Do not overwhelm the patient with talking. Control environmental stimuli. Activation of patient's behavioral responses at these levels is dependent upon external stimuli; too much can suppress movement toward awareness of the environment. Encourage the family to follow the same pattern of care.
IV. Confused-agitated	Patient is in a heightened state of activity with severely decreased ability to process information. The patient may scream, cry, pull at tubes, verbalize inappropriately, confabulate, or become euphoric or hostile. Inability to discriminate among persons or objects is common. Patients at this level are often unable to cooperate with treatment efforts.	Be calm and soothing when working with the patient. Describe what you are going to do with the patient before beginning the activity. Talk in a slow soft voice. Loudness may be startling. Multiple stimuli within the environment may be more than the patient can handle. If the patient becomes upset, allow him time to adjust or remove the patient from the situation.
V. Confused inappropriate, nonagitated	Patient appears alert and is able to follow simple commands. More complex commands produce responses that are nonpurposeful or fragmented. The patient may show some agitated behavior but at this level, only in response to external stimuli. The patient is highly distractible, verbalizes inappropriately, and demonstrates severe memory impairment. Self-care activities and feeding can be managed with assistance. Mobile patients often wander randomly.	Create an environment for the patient that can produce purposeful and appropriate responses to internal and external stimuli with greater frequency and duration. Present only one task at a time and allow the patient to complete the task or a great portion of it before presenting another task. Tell the patient what you are going to do several minutes before you begin. Explain again just before working with the patient. Demonstrate instructions or use gestures whenever possible.
VI. Confused-appropriate	Patient shows goal-directed behavior but is dependent on input for direction; is able to relearn old skills such as self-care but requires maximum assistance with learning new skills. Selective attention to difficult tasks may be impaired; has increased awareness of self and family members.	Maintain a structured quiet environment for the patient. Describe the daily routine to him on a daily basis. Keep him metally challenged by reading and playing games with him.

Continued.

Table 20-1   Levels of cognitive functioning—cont'd

	Level	Patient behavior	Nursing intervention
VII.	Automatic-appropriate	Patient appears appropriate and oriented. He goes through daily routine in an automatic, robotlike fashion; has recall of activites and increased awareness of self and family. There is superficial awareness of, but lack of insight into, his condition. He has decreased judgment and problem-solving abilities and a lack of realistic planning. At this level the patient demonstrates poor safety awareness.	Provide structure through the use of an orientation board or a daily schedule. Place a clock and a large calendar in the patient's room. Instruction should be used only for those activities or times when he becomes confused. Have the patient keep a written daily log of his activities to assist in orientation.
VIII.	Purposeful and appropriate	Patient is alert and oriented and is able to recall and integrate past and recent events. Carryover for new learning is now evident. Patient needs no supervision once activities are learned; is independent at home but has difficulty in abstract reasoning and stress intolerance may persist.	

Adapted from Hagen C, Malkmus D, and Durham P: Levels of cognitive functioning. In Rehabilitation of the head injured adult: comprehensive physical management, Downey, Calif, 1979, Staff Association of Rancho Los Amigos Medical Center, Inc.

head trauma resulting from automobile or bicycle accidents, falls, or nonaccidental trauma caused by shaking, all are potential candidates for rehabilitation. Initial lifesaving management seeks to prevent complications; consequently, tracheostomy and ventilator care become important aspects of the rehabilitation care plan. Children who have suffered cerebral vascular accidents, brain tumors, and anoxic insults caused by meningitis, near drowning, and status epilepticus may also benefit from rehabilitation services.

The physical needs of all these children may be considerable and in many ways not unlike those of the patient with spinal cord injury. The progress of the child varies according to the severity of the injury and the areas of the brain affected. The minimally injured child may completely recover or have a limp, speech defect such as dysarthria (difficulty pronouncing words) or a cognitive disorder (difficulty with sequencing thought) or a shortened attention span. These areas, however, must be addressed because they will affect the child's resocialization and academic progress. Another patient may suffer severe brain injury and may be left with multiple deficits or may be totally nonfunctional.

The brain-injured patient typically regains awareness and orientation slowly. Eight helpful levels of cognitive function and behavioral response (developed at Rancho Los Amigos Medical Center, Downey, California) have been identified in the recovery process. Table 20-1 describes these eight Levels of Cognitive Functioning and corresponding strategies for nursing intervention. Stimuli should be presented in a manner that matches the patient's present functioning level yet offers a challenge of advancement to the next level.

Sensory stimulation must be carefully planned by the team and introduced slowly. The physical and occupational therapists work with the patient in developing both fine and gross motor coordination. Though strong, such patients may be unable to feed or dress themselves. Activities of daily living (ADLs) are introduced early in the rehabilitation program so that, ideally, the patient can begin to achieve some degree of independence. Speech, intellect and emotional stability are typically affected. Since the healing process of the brain is measured in months to years in these children, ongoing psychologic testing and educational counseling are helpful. The more severely affected children usually attend special schools but are mainstreamed whenever possible.

A child with an impaired intellect and a functional body may ultimately be happy and satisfied. A child with a reasonable intellect and severe physical dysfunction, such as aphasia (loss of normal speech) or ataxia (lack of coordination of voluntary muscles producing a characteristic abnormal staggering gait and/or uncontrolled upper extremity movement) understands his condition and frequently has a great deal of difficulty adjusting.

At puberty the brain-injured person also has awakened sexual interest. If the brain injury occurs during this time, the patient may be difficult to manage in the rehabilitation unit, since the individual has little or no control over his inhibitions. Parents must be cautioned that the child may be overly friendly and invite unwanted sexual encounters.

PHYSICAL ASPECTS OF REHABILITATION

The complications of prolonged bed rest and immobility represent the greatest dangers to the life of the long-term patient (Fig. 20-1). Examples of such complications are as follows:

1. Motor and sensory loss involving superficial nerves, skin ulcers, and skeletal deformities
2. Muscle wasting and shortening (contractures), bone calcium loss, ankylosis of joints, edema, venous stasis, and thrombosis from disuse atrophy
3. Urinary tract infection, stones, constipation, and fecal impaction related to poor fluid intake and lack of mobility
4. Hypostatic pneumonia from pooling of secretions in the lungs
5. Depression and psychologic disorders resulting from isolation and interference in normal activities
6. Disturbance in normal growth and development

The meticulous application of a few basic nursing principles can prevent many of these complications from occurring. These principles are discussed in the following sections.

Routine skin care

An adequate blood supply keeps the skin functioning and in repair. A lack of blood to an area will cause deprived cells to die. The small vessels in the skin form a network that supplies the skin from many directions. Any pressure, such as that from sitting, standing, lying, braces, shoes, or appliances, causes compression of these small vessels and does not allow blood to the cells. Where bony prominences (such as hips, sacrum, and knees) are close to the surface, there is no muscle tissue to pad or distribute the pressure evenly, and considerable pressure develops, which can cause great damage to the skin. The sequence of events leading to skin breakdown and the sores or lesions that result are described in Fig. 20-2.

When red marks are seen, the child must not bear pressure on that area until the skin has returned to normal. Any surface that comes into contact with the skin must be suspect. Soft, moldable surfaces distribute pressure over a larger area, and any one spot receives less pressure, with less damage resulting. If you recall the difference between sitting on a concrete step and a well-

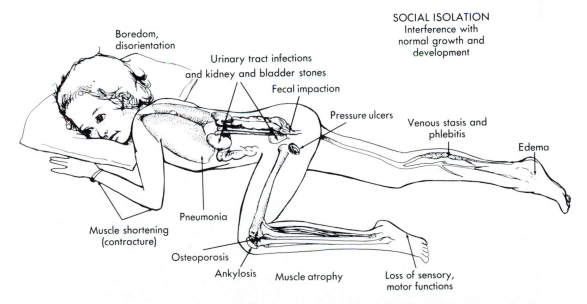

FIG 20-1 Complications of prolonged bed rest. All these complications may not be seen in every patient!

Response to pressure: the sequence of events	What you see
Caution signs	
1. Area pinkness, leaving area in a few minutes.*	
2. Discrete darker reddish spot persisting up to 1 hour.*	
3. Discrete darker reddish spot persisting over 1 hour to several days. The more time needed for the area to regain color after a finger blanching test, the more time needed for return to normal.	
Pressure sores or decubitus ulcers	
4. An unbroken or open blister, sometimes with no color change. May be confused with burn; takes days to heal.	
5. A partial-thickness ulcer, damaging part of epidermis; heals from bottom and edges; takes days to heal.	
6. A full-thickness ulcer, damaging full depth of epidermis; heals only from edges; takes days to weeks.	
7. A penetrating ulcer, involving bone and connective tissue; takes perhaps months to heal.	
*Best time to treat to prevent sequence. Practice prevention: total body inspections twice daily; pressure point inspections with each position change.	

FIG 20-2 Skin signals.

Suggested schedule for skin tolerance check

Trial periods

1. Beginning periods—15 minutes
   Increase by 15-minute periods according to tolerance until 2-hour level is reached

2. After 2-hour level is reached, trial periods may be increased to 30 minutes

Observations of pressure areas (red marks)

Clearing in 15 minutes or no pressure area seen, increase trial period by 15 minutes
Clearing in 30 minutes, repeat trial period
Clearing in 45 minutes, reduce trial by 15 minutes
Persists 60 minutes or more, keep patient off area
Use same clearing time evaluation, but substitute 30-minute trial periods

NOTE: Any interruption in the use of a brace, appliance, or position may require a reevaluation period. Prolonged intervals between their use may mean starting again at the beginning of the schedule. When any pressure area is detected, check methods of positioning. Cocoa butter or lotion applied daily to bony prominences helps keep skin supple.

upholstered chair, you will appreciate why items such as foam rubber mattresses, wheelchair cushions, and soft leather shoes are encouraged.

For the patient who is wheelchair bound and who lacks sensation over the buttocks area, it is imperative that pressure be relieved over the bony ischial prominences. The method for relieving pressure is called a "chair raise." For the paraplegic patient it consists of lifting the buttocks by using the arms of the wheelchair to raise oneself or alternately shifting from side to side. Recommended frequency for the paraplegic patient is every 20 or 30 minutes for 30 seconds. This activity should soon become automatic so that the paraplegic does it without having to think about it. The quadriplegic patient must have assistance to relieve this ischial pressure.

The use of new braces, shoes, or different positions or postures must always be instituted gradually and evaluated frequently. (See box on p. 434 for suggested schedule.)

In addition to pressure-caused skin problems, one must be aware of the danger of burns, bumps, scratches, and even pimples. Burns can be caused by hot car upholstery, electric blankets, sunburn, hot sand at the beach, spilled hot drinks, and other accidents. Although they may appear to be minor, these can be very serious and must be seen by the physician. Any abrasion or scratch that involves a pressure-bearing surface must be completely healed before pressure bearing is resumed. Diaper rashes and irritations that do not quickly respond to the application of Desitin ointment or zinc oxide paste should be examined immediately before a severe problem results. Pimples or abrasions on weight-bearing surfaces should be cleaned gently with mild soap and water and observed closely for increasing size and severity. Because of poor blood supply to scar tissue, healed sores may leave scars that are susceptible to future breakdown and may interfere with a child's ability to live a normal life and hold a job as he grows into a responsible adult. A small amount of time spent daily in prevention will save a great deal of time, trouble, and money later. Remember the following: (1) never permit any pressure on reddened areas, blisters, or sores; (2) increase positioning times according to the guidelines; and (3) regularly check total body skin, using mirrors as necessary. Teach the child and the family these precautions. By the age of 10 or 11 years a child, with supervision, should be assuming responsibility for his own skin care.

If a patient with an existing pressure sore is admitted, some treatment must be undertaken. Many theories exist regarding what to put on a pressure sore. The fact is that one can almost say, "Put anything on it but the patient!" No weight bearing should be allowed. It may be possible to avoid the one position that causes pressure; however, if there are ulcers in several different places, the nurse may have no alternative but to position the patient carefully on an affected side. If this must be done, pressure must be relieved from the ulcer by bridging either side of the ulcer with foam rubber pads or pillows, thus freeing the lesion itself from pressure. Circular or doughnut-shaped supports are not recommended.

Pressure sores must be kept clean. Whatever agent is used, cleaning must be done gently to preserve the new delicate epithelium being formed. Physiologic saline or half-strength hydrogen peroxide on applicator sticks have been used to clean away drainage. If the ulcer is infected, a topical enzyme, such as Travase or Elase, and hydrotherapy will debride the sore. A small pressure sore may be left open to the air to dry. Covered sores should be taped loosely to allow air circulation. Op-Site is effective in areas where incontinence is a problem because it prevents moisture from entering the wound but allows passage of air and gases. Debrisan (hydrophilic wound-cleaning beads) absorbs excess drainage from clean sores. However, it should not be used in tracts.

Large ulcers are better managed by moist dressings. A sterile, fine-mesh gauze pad, such as any eye pad, is cut the exact size of the crater and moistened with physiologic saline solution. This should be covered with a dry dressing taped down with paper tape to prevent drying. The dressing is changed every 4 to 6 hours, depending on the drainage present and how long it stays moist. If it is allowed to dry, the gauze should be soaked off to preserve the new epithelium. As the ulcer heals, the gauze is reduced in size until finally one can leave the shrunken ulcer open to the air.

Positioning

In the discussion of skin care we have underlined the importance of relieving pressure by turning and changing position. Proper anatomic positioning can help prevent skeletal deformities, muscle shortening (contractures), and venous stasis. Six basic positions may be used: back (supine), abdominal (prone), lying on either side, sitting, or standing. These all can be modified to a certain degree. Positioning problems vary according to the diagnosis and individual needs of the patient. Fig. 20-3 illustrates good prone positioning to prevent pressure areas and contractures and to protect catheter drainage when necessary.

Another positioning device is the splint. "Resting splints" are designed to maintain the position of an ex-

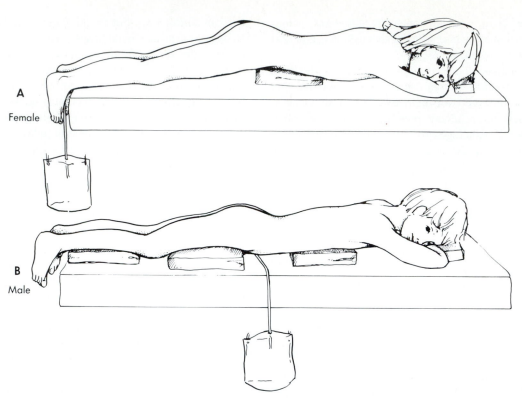

FIG 20-3 A, Prone position with pillow below breast level and small foam rubber support under forehead. Note position of Foley catheter between legs. **B,** Prone position with pillows under chest, thighs, and shins to leave hips, knees, and feet free from pressure. Note position of Foley catheter.

tremity. There are also splints designed to improve alignment or support the extremity so that improved mobility can be achieved.

Venous pooling and the danger of thrombosis can be decreased by thigh-high, closed-toe support stockings to help collapse the superficial leg veins. To further prevent venous stasis, as well as muscle shortening and contractures, a full range of motion should be carried out. The nurse is responsible for ranging joints *without* stretching muscles. The bywords are gentleness and patience. The hands and fingers are exceptionally delicate, and specific instructions about appropriate range should be obtained from the physician or the physical or occupational therapist. Overzealous range of the fingers can make the hand less functional later.

Position changes also lessen stasis of fluid in the lungs. With regular deep breathing, an incentive spirometer, and coughing, pneumonia may be prevented. Changing position and forcing fluids will also help prevent urinary stones and constipation.

Naturally, as soon as patients are physically able to tolerate a wheelchair, they should be placed in a more normal sitting position, even if they are still comatose. These wheelchairs have special supports and/or belts to facilitate a more upright position while maintaining safe body alignment. This maneuver adds a position to the patient's repertoire and lets them see people and their environment from the more customary vertical perspective, which helps to prevent disorientation.

Another technique is use of a tilt table designed to bring the supine patient to a more upright position. Here, the patient is safely restrained with belts placed at chest, hips, and knees. The position of the tilt table is gradually elevated; the child usually "tilts" for about 30 minutes, for a total of 2 to 3 times per day (see Fig. 31-16).

Depression, disorientation, and hallucinations can result from prolonged horizontal positioning and social isolation of the normal individual. This, added to the physical and emotional trauma of an injury, is a tremendous problem. Anything that stimulates and orients the mind—people, predictable routines, a clock or calendar—is helpful. Frequent visits by the nurse (just to say hello) help. Conversation with the patient while in the room or delivering care is essential. The presence of parents and siblings and the friendship of another patient who has experienced a similar injury and made progress helps tremendously.

Interference with growth and development, manifested by disrupted bone growth, delay in reaching skill or functional milestones, or inability to play normally, occurs too frequently in young disabled children. They must have the chance to explore and move about the floor and, if possible, achieve the vertical position. Their environment should be as "homey" as possible and include measured amounts of supervised responsibility and freedom appropriate for their age, abilities, and general condition.

Urinary bladder care

Neurogenic bladder disease (NGB) refers to bladder dysfunction resulting from lesions of the central or peripheral nervous system. The goals are (1) preservation of normal urinary tract anatomy and renal function, (2) prevention of significant urinary infection, and (3) attainment of urinary continence.

The lower urinary tract (bladder and urethra) has two basic functions—the storage and evacuation of urine. The bladder is capable of expanding in response to increasing intravesical volumes without a significant rise in intravesical pressure. When a person with normal bladder control desires to void, intravesical pressure is raised as bladder outlet resistance falls. When intravesical pressure is higher than outlet resistance, urine flows.

Urination is a highly complex, coordinated activity under the control of the parasympathetic and sympathetic nervous systems. The parasympathetic system promotes bladder emptying; the sympathetic system promotes storage. A balance between these two systems provides for reliable low pressure storage and controllable emptying. Disorders of the central or peripheral nervous systems can lead to an imbalance, resulting in inability to store urine reliably, or in the storage of urine at high intravesical pressures, or the inability to empty the bladder effectively. High intravesical pressures can lead to upper tract dilatation, infection, and renal damage. Loss of storage ability leads to incontinence and danger of skin inflammation.

NGB can occur from injury to or disease in the brain, spinal cord, or peripheral nerves. Historically NGB has been classified according to the level of the lesion, as patterns of dysfunction vary with the level.

The *uninhibited neurologic bladder* results from damage to the brain center that controls voluntary voiding. A typical patient is one who has suffered a stroke. They recognize that the bladder is about to contract and empty, but are unable to inhibit this activity. Voiding commences in a low pressure, coordinated fashion, but without voluntary control. This pattern is normal in infants and young children before they are toilet trained.

The *reflex neurologic bladder* is the result of spinal cord injury or disease that occurs above the voiding reflex arc located in the lower cord. Traumatic spinal cord injury is the most common cause. The bladder works automatically, without the patient's awareness or controllability. The relaxation of the bladder outlet may not be coordinated with bladder contractions. Bladder contractions against contracted sphincters cause intermittent high intravesical pressures and renal damage is likely. Since reflex voiding is not controllable the patient is not reliably dry. Occasionally a *balanced bladder* can be attained by reflex emptying elicited by stimulation of the pubic genital area with massaging or stroking, This prompts voiding at controllable intervals. Unfortunately, reflex bladder contractions may occur in response to other motions (chair transfers, coughing, etc.) with resultant incontinence.

An *autonomic neurogenic bladder* results from injury to the voiding reflex arc in the area of the sacral spine (S2-4) or to the peripheral sensory or motor nerves that lead to and from this area. In these patients the bladder is relatively atonic and does not contract. Urine leaks out of the bladder in an overflow fashion. If the sensory nerves are the only ones involved (as in diabetes), the patient may be able to void voluntarily, but never has the urge to void and the bladder is gradually enlarged and damaged. If the motor nerves only are involved (as in a herniated disc), the sensation of a need to void and even pain from overdistention may occur, but the patient is not able to generate a bladder contraction.

The most common cause of neurogenic bladder in a child is spina bifida (myelomeningocele), in which the posterior elements of the spine fail to close during development leaving the underlying spinal cord exposed. The classification of neurogenic bladder above does not apply to this disorder because unpredictable, mixed abnormalities of bladder and sphincter dysfunction occur. These children are best classified by the abnormality of function they exhibit, that is, as failure to store or as failure to empty.

Clean intermittent catheterization (CIC). In patients with failure to empty problems programs of clean intermittent catheterization (CIC) have been very beneficial (Fig. 20-4). Every bladder has a point at which passive filling causes intravesical pressure to be higher than outlet resistance. If the bladder is emptied by catheterization before this point is reached, an individual can theoretically remain dry between catheterizations. In addition to providing a means of continence, CIC offers a method of keeping intravesical pressure at a lower level, thus protecting the kidneys.

Catheterization is generally performed every 4 hours during the day, using a clean rather than a sterile technique. The parent or patient is advised to lubricate the catheter with a water-soluble lubricant, and cleanse the perineal area with soap and water. Infants are generally catheterized in the supine position whereas older children may catheterize while sitting on a toilet. Females are taught to separate the labia with the index and ring finger of their nondominant hand while inserting the catheter with the opposite hand. Males hold the penis erect, taking care not to pinch off the urethra. The parent/patient is instructed to insert the catheter until a stream of urine is obtained, then advance the catheter about 1 inch farther. It is sometimes helpful to slowly rotate the catheter while applying gentle pressure as the catheter passes through the external sphincter and prostatic urethra. A slight "give" may be encountered as the catheter passes through the sphincter area in males. The catheter is held in place until the stream of urine stops at which time the catheter is slowly withdrawn. The patient stops withdrawal any time that a stream is again encountered.

After the catheter has been removed, it is washed with soap and water, dried with a clean paper towel and stored in a clean plastic bag or container until the next use. At the initiation of the CIC program the parent is instructed to keep accurate records of the child's intake and output and to note whether the child remains dry between catheterizations.

There are times when CIC may not be possible or appropriate. CIC is unsatisfactory for patients with intermittent reflex bladder contractions, poor stretchability of their bladder muscle, or incompetent bladder outlets. Urodynamic studies better define these problems for more specific management. Anticholinergic drug's (probanthine, ditropan, etc.) are used to control or lessen reflex contractions. Adrengenic drugs (ephedrine, propadrine, etc.) improve bladder neck competence. Surgical enlargement of the bladder using segments of intestine (augmentation enterocystoplasty) is useful in treating poor

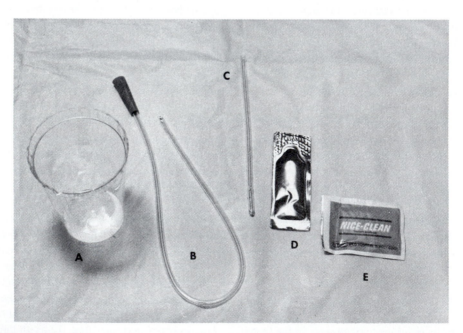

FIG 20-4 Supplies for clean catheterization technique: **A,** calibrated plastic container; **B,** catheter for male; **C,** catheter for female; **D,** lubricant; and **E,** cleansing wipe.

compliance or low capacity bladders. Surgical reconstruction or compression procedures can improve incompetent bladder necks, not controlled by adrenergic drugs. If the above pharmacologic and/or surgical measures are successful in converting storage or control problems to a failure to empty status, then CIC can be initiated.

Children who develop upper urinary tract damage because of high intravesical pressures either from uncoordinated reflex bladder contractions occurring against a closed bladder outlet or from poor bladder compliance are managed in a similar way to the failure to empty group of children. However, close medical management of all children with spina bifida together with early urodynamic evaluation in infancy identifies those children at risk for upper urinary tract deterioration and allows for preventive rather than salvage therapy.

Children who are on a program of CIC often have asymptomatic positive urine cultures. These are generally not a matter of concern and are not treated unless symptoms develop or the child has associated vesicoureteral reflux. Unexplained fevers or the sudden onset of wetting between catheterizations in a previously dry child, are symptoms of a significant urinary tract infection.

External urinary collection devices. For the child who does not use intermittent catheterization an external device may be desirable. Many collection devices are available for boys. Some new female external collection devices are now on the market for adolescents and adults, but no successful device exists for young girls. Regular diapers are frequently used for young children and as the child grows, custom-fitted diapers may be purchased or made from patterns. Since urine may contribute to skin breakdown, a protecting ointment should be applied with each diaper change. Meticulous skin observation and care are needed to protect the vulnerable perineal areas.

Catheter care. In the past indwelling urinary catheters were used fairly frequently in rehab areas. Now with the increased utilization of clean intermittent catheterization and various triggering mechanisms to stimulate planned voiding, Foley catheters are seldom, if ever encountered. However, in certain situations a child or youth may not meet the criteria for a successful CIC program. In this event, indwelling catheters still occasionally may be employed.

Proper catheter care can help prevent abscesses and periurethral fistulas and can reduce infections. The male patient with a Foley catheter usually has more problems. The smaller catheter that will drain without clogging is desired. The catheter should be taped to the abdomen so that the penis and catheter are directed toward the upper body. This helps prevent the catheter from being accidentally pulled, causing damage to the sphincter or urethra. It also eliminates the constant movement of the catheter and penis and irritation and destruction of urethral mucosa. This position prevents excessive pressure against the urethra by the elimination of the normal S-curve from the penis to the bladder. Foley catheters in girls should be taped to the thigh. The patient should be taught the importance of maintaining straight gravity drainage. Maintaining a sterile closed system, and forcing fluids is important. The use of Foley catheters is associated with infection, stone formation, and periuretheral abscesses and fistulas.

Bowel care

Neurogenic bowel may be classified in the same way as neurogenic bladder. Uninhibited neurogenic bowel results in defecation without volitional control when the rectum fills. The reflex, or spastic, bowel exhibits above-normal rectal sphincter tone. When the rectum fills, frequent automatic, partial emptying results. In autonomous neurogenic bowel the rectal sphincter is flaccid and frequent small stools may result.

When the patient has lost normal control, a bowel program should be established early. This helps protect already vulnerable skin from rashes and breakdown. Then, too, the socialization of the older child can be drastically affected by soiling, obnoxious odors, and diapers.

An adequate program consists in (1) keeping the stool normal or slightly firmer than normal (soiling is more likely to occur if it is soft or liquid) and (2) scheduling evacuation time. All children are individuals, and their programs must be tailored precisely to their needs. Therefore one child's program may not be identical with that of another child with a similar problem.

Many factors influence bowel patterns. Diet has a very great effect; disruption of eating patterns—skipping meals, eating extra meals, or changing meal times, amounts, or types of food eaten—may disturb the program by causing constipation or diarrhea. By trial and error one learns exactly what foods constipate or loosen the stool for each patient. Generally, citrus juices, prune juice, and bulk (or roughage) items, such as raw vegetables and nuts, tend to loosen the stool. Inadequate fluid intake and foods such as bananas and cheese constipate. Gas-forming items, such as beans and cabbage, may cause diarrhea. Most of these foods are not a problem unless eaten in larger than normal quantities. A normal, stable diet with sufficient fluid intake usually keeps the stool as desired. If possible, any changes in factors affecting bowel habits should be added singly so that the effect of each change will be known.

Bowel patterns are also affected by physical activity. Inactivity usually constipates, whereas great increases of activity may speed the movement of food through the digestive system and cause accidents. Aging, a change of climate or community, altered living patterns, anxiety, and stress may all have their effect.

A number of reflexes, techniques, and agents can be employed to assist in establishing a sound bowel program free of accidents. These include the gastrocolic reflex, digital stimulation, abdominal straining, stool softeners, and bisacodyl (Dulcolax) suppositories.

The gastrocolic reflex is an increase in the peristaltic muscle activity of the large bowel after the stomach has distended from ingestion of food or warm liquids. Therefore about 30 minutes after a meal is a logical time to carry out a bowel program. If the stool is too hard in spite of fluid and dietary measures, stool softeners, such as dioctyl calcium sulfosuccinate (Colace) or dioctyl sodium sulfosuccinate (Surfak), which retain water in the stool, may be used.

Bisacodyl is a safe means of chemically inducing peristaltic movement of the large bowel. It is more predictable and safer than irritating laxatives or mineral oils that could decrease vitamin absorption. An appropriately sized bisacodyl suppository is inserted high up in the rectum, against the side of the bowel wall so that it will dissolve and be absorbed easily. Bisacodyl usually dissolves in 10 to 15 minutes, reaching peak action in another 10 or 15 minutes. Bisacodyl small-volume enemas may be effective for the paraplegic or meningomyelocele patient.

Digital stimulation does not refer to the digital removal of stool from the rectum. It is a gentle circular motion made by the gloved finger inserted ½ inch (1.25 cm) against the rectal sphincter muscle. The patient may be positioned on the left side or may sit on a raised toilet seat. This gentle motion both relaxes and dilates the rectal sphincter and causes peristaltic muscle contractions of the large bowel. The procedure should be continued for 10 to 15 minutes. It can be used in conjunction with suppositories or by itself. As evacuation occurs, one should gently pull the rectum to one side and allow the stool to be eliminated.

Although any number and combination of these techniques and agents may be used in the child's bowel training, the program should start with the least and the simplest. The time of day for evacuation should be chosen with regard to previous bowel habits, daily schedules, time limitations, and personal preferences. A reasonable time seems to be about 30 minutes after the morning or evening meal. Once a time is selected, it must remain consistent within 30 minutes.

For a child with a spinal cord injury, one possible routine might be as follows: (1) Immediately after breakfast, insert one half of a Dulcolax suppository as high as possible into the rectum. (The amount depends on age and size of the child. Too much causes abdominal cramping; too little, no action.) (2) Wait 10 to 15 minutes, continuing personal care. (3) Place the child on a "potty chair" or toilet with the feet touching the floor so that the hips are flexed into the squat position. (4) Have the child lean forward against the thighs (to increase intraabdominal pressure), and massage the abdominal muscles. Encourage the child to strain at the same time. (Have children who do not understand this blow on a toy balloon.) If diarrhea should occur, it is wise to check for impaction because liquid feces can seep around impaction, resulting in false diarrhea.

Consistency in the program is essential. Some young children may require the program twice a day. A bowel program takes time, patience, and attention to detail but in most instances is very rewarding.

BEHAVIORAL ASPECTS OF REHABILITATION

Many problems that are encountered in rehabilitation, though based on physiologic disability, are psychologic in content. If undesirable behavior can be changed, the long-term outlook for the patient improves. One method of behavioral change, based on the work of B.F. Skinner and his stimulus response (S-R) techniques, is called *behavioral modification*. A behavior is an action—something a person does. It may be desirable or undesirable. To be changed, using this technique, it must be observable, describable, and measurable.

An action can be made to occur more often by following it with a favorable consequence—a *positive reinforcer*. A behavior may be reduced or eliminated by withdrawing its reinforcer or influenced less effectively by punishment.

While recovering from head trauma, 4-year-old Joseph became incontinent of urine. By positive reinforcement of an observable, describable target behavior that can be counted, he again learned to void in the toilet.

After recording the number and frequency of his voidings, his primary nurse established a toileting schedule. The nurses explained what behavior was expected, then remained with him quietly. When Joseph voided into the toilet, he was immediately reinforced with praise, a smile, and a few minutes of attention. In a short time Joseph was voiding in the toilet, and as his physical and mental condition improved, by further reinforcement he was able to summon the nurse for assistance to the bathroom. In examining Joseph's problem, his nurse discovered that busy staff members had nagged and cajoled him when he voided incontinently. Because Joseph had valued their attention, their actions had reinforced incontinent voiding. During the modification program, if he voided incontinently, his nurse would change him in a matter-of-fact manner, withholding both positive and negative attention.

A reinforcer must affect the frequency of the behavior. If the rate of behavior does not change, no reinforcement has taken place and a true reinforcer must be found. For Joseph praise was appropriate, although a toy or food might have been successful in another situation. A reinforcer must be delivered promptly only when the target behavior occurs. Joseph was reinforced with praise immediately on voiding in the toilet; otherwise, he was matter-of-factly returned to bed. Early in a program, reinforcement may occur after each desired behavior (continuous). Later it may be intermittent—a more effective and efficient technique.

At times it is inconvenient to deliver reinforcers at the time of target behavior. In this instance a token may be delivered after each desired behavior to be exchanged later for a desired reinforcer. This makes it possible to use a variety of reinforcers for single or multiple behaviors. Adults use this system when they work for money.

As Joseph progressed, he learned to dress himself. Each time he completed a dressing behavior he was praised and a poker chip was placed in a glass by his bed. Each chip was worth 5 minutes of evening television time. When establishing a token trade rate, one should aim for a high rate of success. As the patient progresses, trade rates should be revised to require increased performance for a given amount of reinforcement.

A large task achieved through a series of small, planned successes is called *shaping*. When Joseph learned to dress himself, he began with putting on his socks. In the beginning he was reinforced when he picked up his socks to prepare to put them on. Later he received reinforcement only when he placed his socks over his toes. Finally, his reward was given only after he pulled his socks over his heels.

Generalization occurs when a behavior learned in one situation occurs in another environment or time, or as a broadened scope of behavior (for example, patients who learn to walk in the hospital, then return home where they walk, dress, and brush their hair). They have generalized in all three aspects. This can be accomplished by direct methods using a trained family member or visiting nurse to reinforce the behavior. An indirect approach is called *trapping*, which ties the desired behavior to a naturally occurring reinforcer. Assuming that the previous patient enjoyed the socialization of school, attendance would involve dressing, grooming, and walking. These target behaviors are reinforced by attending school. Trapping increases the chance that the behavior will continue.

In behavioral terms, punishment is either the withdrawal of a reinforcer or application of an aversive stimulus. We believe that the latter method is rarely appropriate for the health professional. In some instances isolation or loss of privileges may apply; however, aversive stimuli are more often used to reinforce the adult's feelings of power and control. The effect of punishment is relatively temporary and produces reactions of fear, anxiety, frustration, and hostility. Alternative approaches are (1) changing the circumstances that evoke undesirable behavior, (2) reinforcing an incompatible behavior, (3) permitting the behavior in a safe place until the desire is satiated, and (4) extinguishing the behavior through lack of reinforcement. Family and staff attention is perhaps the strongest reinforcer of behavior.

• • •

The broad goal of pediatric rehabilitation—to foster growth and development, to improve function, independence, and personal fulfillment—represents a tremendous challenge. It requires all the support of the family, patient, and rehabilitation team. Its rewards may be delayed but are definite, nonetheless.

Key Concepts

1. Pediatric rehabilitation is based on at least two concepts: (1) each person is unique and has individual basic worth and (2) the task involves a committed group of people working together as a team with a common goal. The overall goal is to foster maximal growth, development, independence, and personal fulfillment within the limitations of the handicap.

2. A rehabilitation unit requires 30% to 60% more staff than the typical medical-surgical unit to provide fastidious nursing care, continual teaching, and reinforcement.

3. Three principles of nursing care that are particularly applicable to the long-term patient are (1) maintain a basic sense of trust; (2) protect from fear, frustration, and pain; and (3) facilitate social contacts and communication with the outside world.

4. The child who is injured or has been impaired by disease, as well as his family and friends, experiences grief similar to that encountered by those mourning the death of a loved one. A three-stage pattern of shock and denial, developing awareness, and restitution or resolution can often be identified.

5. Psychosocial support of these children includes providing opportunities to express their feelings, facilitating social contact and interaction, and assisting them to continue their education.

6. Common diagnoses found in rehabilitation units include spinal cord injuries, anomalies, or diseases of the central nervous system, and brain injury caused by trauma, tumor, or disease.

7. In the patient with an injury above midtrunk, autonomic dysreflexia may arise. Symptoms include flushing, headache, sweating, feelings of nasal stuffiness, goose bumps, bradycardia, and a rapid increase in blood pressure. Treatment includes elevating the patient's head and removing the stimulus.

8. The brain-injured patient typically regains awareness and orientation slowly. Eight helpful levels of cognitive function and behavioral response have been identified in the recovery process.

9. The complications of prolonged bed rest and immobility represent the greatest dangers to the life of the long-term patient. Such complications include motor and sensory loss, contractures, edema, thrombosis, urinary tract infection, fecal impaction, hypostatic pneumonia, psychologic disorders, and disturbances in normal growth and development.

10. Routine skin care should include the following: prevent pressure on reddened areas, blisters, or sores; increase positioning times according to the guidelines; and regularly check total body skin.

11. Proper anatomic positioning can help prevent skeletal deformities, muscle shortening, and venous stasis.

12. The primary goals of management of the pediatric neurogenic bladder are preservation of normal urinary tract anatomy and renal function, prevention of significant urinary infection, and attainment of social urinary continence.

13. Clean intermittent catheterization provides a means of continence and offers a method of keeping intravesical pressure at a lower level, protecting the kidneys.

14. Factors that influence bowel patterns include diet, physical activity, aging, change of climate or community, altered living patterns, anxiety, and stress.

15. Behavior modification can be accomplished by positively reinforcing desirable actions. A behavior may be reduced or eliminated by withdrawing its reinforcer or, less effectively, by punishment.

Discussion Questions

1. In childhood rehabilitation the team includes teachers and educational consultants. Why are these team members especially important for the child?

2. Nursing in rehabilitation focuses on teaching the parents and child to "do" as much as possible. Why is this better than "doing for" the family and child? How would you respond if the mother says, "You can do it so much better than I can?"

3. Severe illness or injury causes stress in the family. What indications might you observe that indicates high stress level? What can you as the nurse do to help reduce this stress?

4. Identify specific injuries and illnesses that require specialized long-term rehabilitative care. In what setting would individuals with these problems receive the best care?

5. With the trend toward care in the home whenever possible, what teaching regarding physical care should be provided to the parents? What do you think about parents performing "nursing skills" such as catheterization and suctioning in the home?

21

The Dying Child, the Family, and the Nurse

CHAPTER OBJECTIVES

After studying this chapter, the student should be able to perform the following:

1 Identify the kinds of understandings that help the nurse provide the sensitive support that a family needs when facing a life-threatening illness of a child.
2 State four factors that contribute to a child's concept of death.
3 Describe the typical progression in the growth of a child's understanding of the nature of death, based on age at less than 3 years; 5 to 6 years; 7 years; 10 to 11 years.
4 List four ways in which children who are unable to verbalize their fears may express themselves.
5 Discuss the need for usual behavioral expectations

and discipline for the child who has a life-threatening condition.
6 Discuss the concerns for appropriate communication, careful listening, honesty, and hope when interacting with an ill child and his family.
7 Explain three main stresses that all hospitalized children may encounter but that may be particularly difficult for the potentially fatally ill child and his family.
8 Indicate the four phases of mourning described by Bowlby, and explain how knowledge of them may be helpful to the nurse.

Few nursing assignments are more challenging than helping a family with a child who is afflicted with an illness that is often fatal. Since the nurse cannot change the reality of the tragic situation, she frequently feels sorrowful. Probably no human experience cuts so deeply into the center of one's heart as the loss of a child.

THE CHALLENGE OF UNCERTAINTY

Although this chapter deals with the dying child, concern for the physical and psychologic support of the child during the chronic phase of a terminal illness cannot be overlooked.

Today, because of great medical and technologic ad-

vances, children with fatal illnesses typically live longer than ever before. Helping such a child reach his developmental potential, physically, intellectually, psychologically, and socially, has become a multidisciplinary challenge. Frequently the short-term or long-term prognosis may be uncertain. The burden of such uncertainty calls for much time and energy from those who provide the child's care.

The chronicity of terminal illness requires much understanding. One must not only have a working knowledge of the ongoing medical treatment but, more important, its psychosocial implications for the child. Psychologic strength is very important if the necessary adaptability is to be sustained during this period of prolonged instability. The nurse can promote this quality by honesty, knowledge, and understanding care.

It is extremely important that the child be prepared for living as long as any possibility of life remains. Communicating this concept to the child's family, teachers, and other significant persons is essential! For example, the school-age child with a life-threatening illness frequently experiences scholastic difficulties because of absences, psychologic problems and fears, and "differentness" caused by amputation, chemotherapy, and other treatment or disease sequelae. These problems must be recognized and addressed as vigorously as possible to maintain the child's own psychologic well-being and rapport with his peer group.

To face the almost overwhelming demands of a long-term, life-threatening illness, the child, parents, and hospital personnel need to recognize and use many supportive measures.

Understanding the child's reactions (influenced by his developmental level and possible concept of death), typical parental reactions, and one's personal feelings and philosophy concerning death helps the nurse to provide the sensitive support the family needs.

REACTIONS OF THE CHILD
Child's concept of death

A child's concept of death depends to a considerable extent on his age, intellect, life experience, and cultural background. Children under the age of 3 years have no awareness or understanding of death. They fear being separated from people who are an integral part of their lives, such as parents or other consistent caregivers. If these significant people detach themselves physically or emotionally from the dying child, the child senses this and becomes fearful at first, then extremely withdrawn. Young children typically do not perceive death as final or terminal. For children 3 to 5 years of age, death is denied; it is only a change of some kind and is not permanent. Children 5 to 6 years of age recognize death but cannot conceive of it as resulting from chance or a natural happening. Causation is personified. Death to them is like part of a game of cowboys and Indians. Everybody kills each other, and then they resurrect themselves and play another game. Hence, when someone dies, in the child's mind the event is usually thought of not only as a deprivation but also as a personal abandonment. It may be considered a hostile act on the part of the person who died.

From approximately 6 years of age and onward, children seem gradually to be accommodating themselves to the proposition that death is final. Many 6- and 7-year-olds suspect that their parents will die someday and that they too may die, but they are comforted by the thought that the death of their parents (and their own death) is still a long time away.

Children 9 to 10 years of age and older achieve a realistic concept of death as a permanent biologic process. A child over 10 years of age is capable of integrating the concept of "not being" if the parents can do so. As children approach adolescence, they are equipped with the intellectual tools necessary to comprehend time, space, life, and death in a logical manner. At about 10 or 11 years of age, children can understand the universality and permanence of death.

In spite of the common depiction of violence in the newspapers and on television, children in the United States are often shielded from any real involvement with or explanation of death. Dying is not typically viewed as a normal part of the life cycle. Yet studies have indicated that children often fear—usually in terms of separation and loss of security—their own deaths or those of their loved ones. Since life includes death, deliberate, thoughtful education about death in the observation of nature and daily life is appropriate.

Children who are terminally ill rarely manifest an *overt* concern about death, probably because they attempt to repress their anxiety concerning it. Nevertheless, children should be allowed to express their fears verbally if they are capable or through play media (drawing pictures; relating to puppets; playing with dollhouse or paper doll families; and handling, pounding, and shaping clay) if they are not. Highly susceptible to the attitudes of their parents, terminally ill children will likely sense the gravity of the situation and will need to ventilate their feelings. They pick up many cues from their families and surroundings that something has changed, that something different, important, and probably bad is happening or will occur. These cues may include a change in expectations, less emphasis on discipline, unnatural silences or forced chatter, and unusual gifts. These children should not be deprived of the security of usual behavioral expectations, and they should be allowed to participate in their normal activities as much as medical assessment considers possible. Often the children should be reassured that their illness is not their fault and is not a punishment for anything they did.

What to tell the child

If a child with a life-threatening illness asks about dying, a statement such as, "You have a serious illness, but no illness is without hope," is likely to be believed and reassuring. To deprive a person of hope even when the outcome is clouded is unrealistic and unkind. One must also individualize responses according to the child's understanding and circumstances. If the child sees or asks about the death of another child, you might say, "Johnny was very sick and died." Answer questions simply and always truthfully. Keep in mind the child's level of comprehension. Opportunities to talk should be given. Many times older children select one staff member who appears open and accepting of what they say for sharing their fears and concerns. Most important is the maintenance of an atmosphere that allows patients to ask as much or as little as they wish. Nurses, social workers, psychiatrists, or ministers may be used effectively in this role as well.

The majority of parents say they believe that when the terminally ill child asks, he needs to be told honestly that he is dying. To hold out false hope or to deny the imminence of death is very confusing to the child who senses the gravity of his illness. The child knows from the behavior of those close to him that he is going to die. Being honest with the child allows him to express his fears and concerns and ask questions about what happens when a person dies and what will await him after death; this can be answered in terms of the family's religious beliefs. Many children take comfort in knowing that relatives or friends who have died will be "waiting" for them.

It is important to talk with families about giving their child "permission to die." They can reassure the child that he has worked hard, fought his disease as best he could, and now it is permissible to stop fighting. It helps for parents to let their child know that he will be missed greatly and never forgotten, but that they and any brothers and sisters will be all right and will be able to go on with their lives.

Three stresses of terminal illness

In addition to having illnesses that cause considerable distress, children suffering from terminal illnesses are subjected to three stresses common to other hospitalized children: separation from parents, traumatic procedures, and isolation. Modification of hospital routine and procedure must be considered.

Separation from parents. Depriving parents and children of each other when permanent separation will soon take place would be particularly unfortunate. Children want their parents. Nurses should encourage parents to touch the child. The warmth of physical contact is the most primitive and basic nonverbal comforting technique humans possess. It can communicate a solace or comfort to the frightened child that words can never produce.

Traumatic procedures. When parents understand the reasons why tubes are inserted, intravenous feedings are ordered, blood is withdrawn, and other treatments are initiated, they feel more satisfied. Parents are usually best able to console and protect their children from fear. Similarly the nurse is best able to help children allay their fears through their parents. By helping parents to understand, you will have helped the child. Also, allowing the child as much control as possible over the necessary procedures and routines is vitally important. Let him make choices among appropriate alternatives and participate in decisions relative to his care. In essence, encourage and allow independence.

You can also help older children by transferring their attention and concern from their incurable illness to curable problems or symptoms they may be experiencing. Listen with interest and attention to all their complaints, particularly ones related to intercurrent infections, such as rashes, which can be eliminated. Children can receive enormous reassurance and relief if these complaints are treated intensively. They are not being deserted. Wahl calls this method of relieving anxiety "trading up."

Isolation. The most dreaded possibility does not seem to be that of dying but of dying alone. Children feel secure with other children, and they know nothing too terrible can happen when Mom and Dad are there.

In the hospital setting. Do not isolate the dying child from his siblings, friends, other relatives, or staff. Usually you cannot conceal a child's death from other children in the unit. Encourage parents and relatives to say when they will come back. It implies a promise: "I will see you again, and you will have nothing to fear in the interim." Although relatives and staff are encouraged not to isolate the child, the nurse should not permit constant or unduly prolonged visits that the child may interpret as a "death watch." Parents also need respite to attend to other responsibilities, to rest, and to reorganize. They should not be encouraged to stay continually. Arrangements can usually be made for someone to stay with the child, allowing parents periods of change.

It has been found that most children are very concerned about their special possessions and what will happen to them when they are gone. Many children, even in the younger age groups, find it comforting to make a "will" in which they designate who is to have their favorite toys or treasured books. Older children, particularly those who have spent much time in the hospital, frequently want to be sure they are not forgotten and may take comfort in planning for the donation in their memory of a plaque, a TV, video game, or toys to the hospital.

NURSING CARE PLAN

The Terminally Ill Child

Selected nursing diagnoses	Expected outcomes	Interventions
A. Alteration in comfort related to terminal process. Clinical manifestations: Verbal complaints of discomfort, crying, guarding, refusing to move, increased respiration and heart rate, blood pressure, restlessness.	Child exhibits behaviors indicating a state of psychologic/physiologic comfort.	Limit physical care to essentials. Maintain pleasant environment (privacy, dimmed lights, quiet room for closeness of loved ones). Allow any items of importance to child (toys, clothing). Assist family members with comforting measures. See Nursing Care Plan on the Child in Pain on p. 525.
B. Self-care deficit related to terminal process. Clinical manifestations: Decreased LOC, fatigue, pain, loss of bowel and bladder control.	Child maintains independence with ADLs when possible.	Encourage participation with ADL's and assist when needed. Limit physical care to essentials. Maintain skin integrity (bathing, repositioning). Encourage oral intake when possible. Encourage family members to assist with care of child, and be sensitive to their personal needs. Discuss options for home respite care and hospice.
C. Anticipatory grieving related to impending death. Clinical manifestations: Parent/child crying, withdrawal, expressed feelings of guilt, anger, hopelessness.	Child/family verbalizes feelings and desires. Child/parent may grieve at their own pace. Child/parent/nurse interact effectively throughout terminal period.	Assess child/family's understanding of physical state. Encourage child/family to discuss feelings and behaviors in nonjudgmental manner. Maintain a "normal" atmosphere to provide sense of security. Assist child to express feelings (verbal expression, art, play therapy). Keep family informed of changes in child's status. Arrange support from other disciplines (social service, psychologist, spiritual counselor). Assist child/family through grieving process.

One patient donated a Serojet (device used for numbing the site prior to bone marrow aspiration or lumbar puncture). He said he wanted to be sure one was always available to other children having these procedures done. Another child wanted a refrigerator donated to "his" room so that other children could have their favorite foods close at hand.

Dying at home

A fairly recent innovation has been the practice of allowing terminally ill children, when the parents agree and cooperate, to spend their last weeks or months at home. Nursing care in these situations must be adapted to the family and to the facilities available. Although home care for the terminally ill is a change from recent methods, it has been the norm during most of human history. With the advent of specialized diagnostic and emergency services available only in hospitals, this significant event was often moved outside the home. Yet for many sick children who can no longer benefit from the sophisticated facilities offered in a hospital, the home may be the place of most comfort and security if the family is willing and able to provide the care needed.

Impetus for this type of terminal care has come particularly from the work of Ida Marie Martinson and the experiences of nursing and medical personnel and parents who participated in the Home Care for the Dying Child Project, first developed as a research study at the University of Minnesota.* The nurse should refer to Martinson, Spinetta, and others for more detailed perspectives.

Another recent trend has been the organization of volunteer nurses who reside near the affected family and can more easily provide the on-call support essential to the family. Decreased costs associated with this type of support are an important factor. The consulting home care nurse should be prepared to refer the family to financial and other community resources as part of the total care plan. One should bear in mind that financial disaster for the family added to the loss of the dying child can destroy the entire family unit. Follow-up by the nurse after death is extremely important in aiding family adjustment.

Many families have found the home care method very fulfilling. It helps decrease the parents' feelings of helplessness, although the final result may be unchanged. Researchers report that the child's emotional well-being and comfort are much enhanced by the familiar surroundings and association with family members. Even if a medical emergency requires rehospitalization, the survivors have expressed great satisfaction in the home experience that was possible.

Specialized centers for the care of the dying (hospices), first developed in Europe, are a relatively new development in the United States. Centers devoted to pediatric patients are even more recent. The team care that is ideally offered in these settings seems to hold much promise.

PARENTAL REACTIONS

One of the nurse's most important roles in the management of the child with a terminal illness is helping the grieving parents. Integrating the tragic event of death into their life experience is most difficult. The parents' reactions to the prospective death of the child may be likened to the mechanism of separation anxiety. However, it has much deeper meaning than most separation anxieties that parents and children face.

The mourning process

In recent years much has been written regarding the reactions of patients who face a terminal illness and of the behaviors of parents and close family members or friends when they mourn the impending death of a child. The descriptions and analyses offered are not to be construed as undeviating or as applicable to all persons and situations, but they may form guidelines for the interpretation and anticipation of events that will be helpful to all concerned.

John Bowlby* was one of the earliest writers in the field to describe the mourning process. He identified four phases in the natural mourning process: (1) numbness, (2) yearning and searching, (3) despair and disorganization, and (4) hope and rebuilding. Bowlby's work covers the phases of mourning in the period following death. However, anticipatory mourning often begins before death occurs, and Bowlby's phases have been helpful in describing parental reactions before the death of the child.

Mourning is the process of healing that helps people face and recover from loss. The normal healing process takes a year or more. The clearest evidence of recovery is the ability to remember comfortably and realistically both the pleasures and disappointments of the lost relationship.

Most persons progress through the basic phases de-

*Martinson IM: Home care for the dying child: professional and family perspectives, New York, 1976, Appleton-Century-Crofts.

*Bowlby J: Attachment and loss: loss sadness and depression, vol 4, New York 1980, Basic Books Inc, Publishers.

scribed below, whether the child's death occurs before, after, or during the process. But it is very important for nurses to be aware of and sensitive to the different interactions that may occur among family members and nurses themselves, depending on the phase of the mourning process individually experienced when death occurs.

Numbness. The first phase is characterized by a state of shock at the news of the loss or of the impending loss. Denial also occurs during this phase. For some parents their denial may be a positive response allowing them time to adapt to the loss. Denial may range from extreme to slight and will come and go throughout all of the stages. The overriding need of this phase is for protection from the pain of the loss, and this need is met by refusal to recognize the diagnosis or loss.

Yearning and searching. The second phase involves an intense desire to find the lost loved one. Many strong emotions are brought into play—anxiety, yearning, anger, and guilt. Parents cannot believe that this could happen to their child. Often a parent's attitude is one of suspicion, hostility, and constant criticism. Hope for the child is stressed but in a nonspecific way. Parents tell themselves, "Something will be discovered." They want to try anything that might offer hope for a cure no matter how irrational it may seem.

Anxiety is manifested by an intense need to weep, an empty feeling in the abdomen, loss of appetite, and other body complaints. With anxiety there is yearning, longing for a sign that a cure will be found and that the child will get well. Guilt feelings are constantly expressed in tears: "If only I had done this or that, if only I had notified the physician sooner." It is natural and necessary to cry, to be angry, and to feel guilty. These are all healthy signs of normal grief. It is a stage in the gradual process of accepting a great loss.

Involvement of parents when possible in the physical care of the child is extremely important in facilitating parental adaptation. But although parental participation in the care of the sick child is desirable, it should not be at the expense of the emotional and physical well-being of the rest of the family. Mothers and fathers usually want to be with their sick child and need to feel that they personally have done everything possible for the child. Feelings of guilt are somewhat relieved by the expenditure of personal effort in the care of the child. Parents are encouraged to participate realistically in the physical care of their children by bathing, feeding, or entertaining them and escorting them to the laboratory and x-ray departments. Thus parents become integrated into the hos-

pital routine, and communication with personnel is enhanced.

During the initial period in the hospital, parents physically cling to their children. They are involved solely in their care. After a while parents want to help with the care of other children. Assisting children to the playroom and reading to a group rather than just their own child are examples of this desire. Manifestations of the capacity to help other children mark a turning point in parental adjustment that reflects acceptance of the child's illness and ultimate death.

Actually, the second phase of the mourning process as described by Bowlby is very similar to the stages noted by Elizabeth Kübler-Ross in which she describes the ill patient's reaction as "No, not me!" (shock and denial) and "Why me? Why now?" (anger, rage, and envy). The parent's mourning, however, also typically includes a destructive guilt factor.

Despair and disorganization. The third phase in Bowlby's mourning process also finds a parallel in the observations of Kübler-Ross. It is similar to her "Yes, me, but . . ." (bargaining) and "Yes, me" (depression) stages.

Facing and accepting the reality of the fatal illness, parents feel helpless. Life is stripped of meaning. Active, realistic efforts to prolong life typify the early part of this phase.

Usually, the mother is the parent who spends the most time ministering to the needs of the sick child. During this time the nurse must be aware that her attempts to cope with the situation may fluctuate from gentle, assured bedside care to inappropriate, exhausting activity. At one moment she may express exaggerated gratitude to the nurses and medical staff; in the next she is overly critical. Her emotions may range from philosophic resignation to sentimentality. She is emotionally fragile and inconsistent.

The reality of the fatal illness and its meaning begins more and more to penetrate the mother's consciousness. Her denial of the character of the illness may disappear, but hope of a cure persists. Her hope is more specific now, often related to particular scientific efforts. Mothers begin to cling less to their children and encourage them to participate in hospital activities. Parents should be encouraged to express their feelings of depression and defeat during moments away from the child. This helps them move beyond the initial shock and recognize some of the specific things they still have to offer their child. Every attempt must be made to enable parents to see the continuing value of their function as parents, despite their feelings of despair and helplessness in the face of death.

As the child's physical energy begins to diminish, preoccupation with measures that involve treatment of the disease begins to subside, and parents are interested in relieving the child's discomfort and pain. Although they continue to hope that their efforts will save the child, the intensity of the expectation is gradually reduced. They are separating themselves emotionally from the child.

Hope and rebuilding. The fourth phase is characterized by a calm acceptance of the child's impending death. Separation from the child is no longer an adaptive problem for the parents. The mother or father remains with the child whenever possible but with adequate consideration for the remainder of the family. For the first time the parents express a wish that the child could die so that the suffering would end.

Many parents never reach this fourth phase of mourning during their child's illness. It may not be until after the child dies that this phase begins. With the loss acknowledged and the depth of pain plumbed, new people, relationships, and activities become meaningful. Some parents take interest in organizations such as the Cancer Society and the Cystic Fibrosis Association. By so doing, the mourner is able to reduce preoccupation with self and the dead child. This allows the parents to reinvest feelings in other love objects—spouse, remaining children, or close relatives. Again, the last stage of "yes" (described by Kübler Ross as acceptance or resignation) appears appropriate.

SIBLING REACTIONS

Brothers and sisters are often disturbed by the continuing illness and may require considerable parental support. Parents should be encouraged to divide their time among the various members of the family as the situation warrants. The importance of communication with siblings must always be borne in mind by the parents and all others in contact with the family during this period. They need the same type of communication and support that the parents require. However, their needs and understanding depend on their ages. Nursing care for the family should include the siblings.

Martinson reports that home care for dying children does not have an adverse effect on siblings, even when they actually witness the death. In fact, the experience of participating in terminal care seems to remove many of the false anxieties and fantasies experienced by siblings who could not participate in the hospital experience.

THE NURSE'S REACTIONS
Personal concepts of death

Awareness of one's feelings about death is essential to giving comprehensive nursing care to dying children and their parents. Information about children's concepts of death and their parents' fears is not enough. To give sensitive and supportive care to the dying child, the nurse needs help in understanding her own fears about death. The nurse may find her role particularly frustrating if she feels herself a failure because she cannot cure or rehabilitate the child. Her concept of nursing must be changed to include helping the family "cope"—an extremely valid and worthy goal.

Fear of death is the most inescapable and realistic of human fears. Fear and anxiety lead to convictions of immortality on a conscious or unconscious level that are universal to all humans. Each individual recognizes that other people must die but feels an inward assurance that it need never happen to him or her.

Every person feels or reacts differently to the death experience. If this reality (death) is so painful that one handles it by either immersing oneself in it or utterly denying it, it will be difficult to fulfill one's role as a nurse. Nurses ought to let themselves recognize, at least to a limited degree, the awe and fear that everyone experiences in the face of death. Fear of death is handled in several ways: (1) by a religious belief in immortality, (2) by a denial of the awe felt for death, (3) by withdrawal from the dying child, and (4) by the formation of various phobias or compulsions. Nurses are involuntarily influenced by illogical but protective defenses in the presence of impending death. However, if they are to help parents who are experiencing deep grief and distress, nurses must not ridicule parents or isolate themselves from them. Nurses are not to punish parents. Instead, they must become aware of their own feelings. They must try to understand better how they themselves feel about death and about nursing a young human being who will probably experience death soon.

The entire bedside staff should be given aid by the formation of support groups, appropriate patient conferences, and access to information regarding helpful techniques and approaches. Nurses who care for dying children frequently find it difficult to admit to themselves or to others that they need support. Ongoing open communication among staff members can be encouraged by the provision of regularly scheduled meetings that give permission to staff to avail themselves of informal support from other staff members. To cope successfully with the loss of a child, nurses must recognize that although the outcome (death of the child) was inevitable, the professional care and support they provided for the patient and family were the very best possible. They have given comfort to those who need it most and, in turn, can take comfort in this knowledge.

Nursing the dying child requires courage. The nurse must remember that courage is not the absence of fear but the willingness and ability to function in its presence. Nurses who care for dying children and counsel their parents must preserve a sympathy and empathy and yet be free enough of emotional involvement to do their work well. Nurses should not become so personally involved with the dying child that they neglect the other children who have an equal need for nursing care.

PARENT/STAFF SUPPORT GROUPS

There has been a trend in university centers to set aside special times for the staff to meet with the parents of children with life-threatening diseases. Common problems are shared in these small mutual support groups. Discussions have centered around the nature of the disease and its treatment, as well as the emotional problems faced by parents, siblings, friends, and staff. Most of the groups intermittently include physicians, nurses, a social worker, and a psychiatrist. As a result parents and staff have shared increased understanding of each other's problems. The meetings provide opportunities for parents to meet unit physicians and nurses in a more relaxed setting and with ample time for discussion. Specific benefits from these meetings include mutual support during times of stress and uncertainty, the realization that discipline of the child is still desirable, and the possibility for sharing feelings about death and dying. But perhaps the most important benefit is the opportunity for parents to share and identify with one another on a level common to each.

Sudden infant death syndrome

The sudden death of a child from unknown causes is particularly tragic. Statistically, sudden infant death syndrome (SIDS) is the *second leading cause* of infant mortality in the United States. SIDS, defined as the unexpected death of a previously healthy infant between 1 month and 1 year of age, is usually a diagnosis of exclusion, dependent on a complete autopsy examination. The etiology of SIDS is unclear, although several risk factors are known. Siblings of SIDS victims have a tenfold increased risk of SIDS. Black and Native Americans have a rate of SIDS two to three times that of whites.

Preterm and low birth weight infants, as well as infants of multiple gestations, are thought to be at increased risk. Significant research over the past decade has increased our understanding of the factors associated with the sudden, unexpected deaths of infants, but the cause remains elusive. Although, of course, these infants are not hospitalized, the nurse may encounter a family who has lost a child under these circumstances. She must not underestimate the intensity or duration of mourning felt and must be a compassionate listener and provider of information. The National Sudden Infant Death Syndrome Foundation and the SIDS Information and Counseling Centers have been established by Public Law 92-270 and are excellent resources for parents and family members.

Basic concepts of religion

The comfort the nurse can give to the parents of the dying child is important. Knowing their religious beliefs concerning death may be a great help. Often the nurse observes that parents with deep faith in God find real comfort in their religious beliefs. For Catholics and Protestants who believe in personal immortality great solace and comfort can be found in the conviction that they will one day rejoin their loved ones.

In the Jewish faith the concept of immortality is not clearly defined. Judaism teaches that perhaps there is a life after death, but the only immortality of which man is certain is the immortality he may achieve while he is still alive or through his descendants.

Knowing the basic concepts of the various religious faiths concerning death may be of great assistance to the nurse. The nurse is not expected to be a theologian nor should she attempt to share her religious beliefs concerning death unless she is asked, but the nurse can help the child and the parents by supplying physical and emotional support and the comfort of spiritual counsel by contacting any clergyman the parents desire. This spiritual advisor, especially one who has added skills in personal counseling to his religious training, can well be the one to whom a parent may turn. He can communicate comfort to parents when friends and relatives are helpless.

• • •

Death is inevitable but no less difficult because of its inevitability. Just as it may be the nurse's privilege to help parents and their infant at the event of birth, it may also be her privilege to ease and comfort a mother and father and a small human being who has come to life's last hours. May she do so with gentleness, reverence, and skill.

Key Concepts

1. When dealing with the family of a terminally ill child, the nurse must have both a working knowledge of the ongoing medical treatment and an understanding of its psychosocial implications for the child and family.

2. A child's concept of death is influenced by his age, intellect, life experiences, and cultural background.

3. Children who are terminally ill rarely manifest an overt concern about death. They should, however, be allowed to express their fears verbally or through play media.

4. When dealing with the terminally ill child, the nurse should answer questions simply and truthfully, keeping in mind the child's level of comprehension.

5. Children suffering from terminal illnesses are subjected to three stresses common to other hospitalized children: separation from parents, traumatic procedures, and isolation.

6. For many terminally ill children who can no longer benefit from hospital facilities, the home may be the most comfortable and secure place to spend their final weeks or months. Nursing care must be adapted to the family and to the facilities available.

7. Bowlby identified four phases in the natural mourning process: (1) numbness, (2) yearning and searching, (3) despair and disorganization, and (4) hope and rebuilding. Although these phases are not to be construed as undeviating or applicable to all persons and situations, they provide guidelines for interpretation and anticipation of events.

8. The importance of communication with siblings must be remembered by the parents and all others in contact with the family of a dying child.

9. To give sensitive and supportive care to the dying child and his family, the nurse must come to terms with her own feelings about death.

10. Knowing the basic concepts of the various religious faiths concerning death may be of great assistance to the nurse caring for the family of a dying child.

Discussion Questions

1. How does a child's concept of death change at various ages? How can the nurse help a child express his feelings regarding death?

2. Children are very sensitive to the attitudes and emotions of the adults around them. How do adults respond to death and dying? What impact does or should this have on the parents and health care providers?

3. Terminal illness is stressful to the child, the parents, and the health care providers. What are the greatest stressors? What can be done to reduce these?

4. Do you think that the death of a child is more difficult to cope with than the death of an adult? If so, why? If not, why not? What can be done to help parents through the grieving process?

5. Sudden infant death syndrome (SIDS) can result in the death of an apparently normal infant. What feelings might the parents experience in this situation? What resources are available in your community for families who experienced SIDS?

SUGGESTED SELECTED READINGS AND REFERENCES

Hospitalization

Azarnoff P: Preparing well children for possible hospitalization, Pediatr Nurs 11(1):53, 1985.

Campbell IR, Scaife JM, and Johnstone JM: Psychological effects of day care surgery compared with inpatient surgery, J Arch Dis Child 63(4):415, 1988.

Caty S, Ellerton ML, and Ritchie JA: Coping in hospitalized children: an analysis of published care studies, Nurs Res 33(5):277, 1984.

Coucouvanis JA and Solomons HC: Handling complicated visitation problems of hospitalized children, MCN 8(2):131, 1983.

Craft MF and Waytt N: Effect of visitation upon siblings of hospitalized children, Matern Child Nurs J 15(1):47, 1986.

Dorn LD: Children's concepts of illness: clinical applications, Pediatr Nurs 10(5):325, 1984.

Flint NS and Walsh M: Visiting policies in pediatrics: parents perceptions and preferences, J Pediatr Nurs 3(4):237, 1988.

Fore CV and Holmes SS: A care-by-parent unit revisited, MCN 8(12):408, 1983.

Hodapp RM: Effects of hospitalization on young children: implications of two theories, Child Health Care 10(4):83, 1982.

Huth MM: Guidelines for conducting hospital tours of early school-age children, Pediatr Nurs 9(6):414, 1983.

Knafl KA, Deatrick JA, and Kodakek S: How parents manage jobs and a child's hospitalization, MCN 7(2):125, 1982.

Koss T and Teter M: Welcoming a family when a child is hospitalized, MCN 5(1):51, 1980.

Lamb JM and Rodgers DR: Assisting the hostile, hospitalized child, MCN 8(5):336, 1983.

La Montagne LL: Three coping strategies used by school-age children, Pediatr Nurs 10(1):25, 1984.

Licamele WL and Goldberg RL: Childhood reactions to illness and hospitalization, Am Fam Physician, 36(3):227, 1987.

Marchant R: Caring for hospitalized inner-city children: Pediatr Nurs 11(2):129, 1985.

McCain GC and Bies DC: Television viewing and the hospitalized child, Pediatr Nurs 9(1):33, 1983.

Nelms BC: Stress during childhood: long lasting effects? Pediatr Nurs 11(2):95, 1985.

Pazola KJ and Gerberg AK: Teen groups: a forum for the hospitalized adolescent, MCN 10(4):265, 1985.

Perrin J and others: Hospitalization for children requiring surgery, Pediatrics 77(4):587, 1986.

Robertson J: Young children in hospitals, New York, 1958, Basic Books Inc Publishers.

Schum TR: Effects of hospitalization derived from a family diary, Clin Pediatr 28(8):366, 1989.

Stevens KR: Humanistic nursing care for critically ill children, Nurs Clin North Am 16(4):611, 1981.

Temmerman RR: Preoperative fears of older children, AORN J 38(11):827, 1983.

Teyber EC and Littlehales DE: Coping with feelings: seriously ill children, their families and hospital staff, Child Health Care 10(3):58, 1981.

Vipperman JF and Rages PM: Childhood coping: how nurses can help, Pediatr Nurs 6(2):11, 1980.

Whaley LF and Wong DL: Effective communication strategies for pediatric practice, Pediatr Nurs 11(6):429, 1985.

Wood SP: School-aged children's perception of the causes of illness, Pediatr Nurs 9(2):101, 1983.

Zurlinden JK: Minimizing the impact of hospitalization for children and their families, MCN 10(3):178, 1985.

Zweig CD: Reducing stress when a child is admitted to the hospital, MCN 11(1):24, 1986.

Rehabilitation/long-term illness

Acute care rehab shortens stays for patients with brain injuries, Am J Nurs 89(6):795, 1989.

Altshuler A, Meyer J and Butz M: Even children can learn to do clean self-catheterization, Am J Nurs 77(1):97, 1977.

Bakke K: Ethical dilemmas: institutionalizing a severely disabled child, Pediatr Nurs 7(6):27, 1981.

Brady MH: Longlife care of the child with Duchenne muscular dystrophy, MCN 4(4):227, 1979.

Brewster AB: Chronically ill hospitalized children's concepts of their illness, Pediatrics 69(3):355, 1982.

Brock W and others: Intermittent catheterization in the management of neurogenic vesical dysfunction in children, J Urol 125(3):391, 1981.

Burkett KW: Trends in pediatric rehabilitation, Nurs Clin North Am 24(1):239, 1989.

Carlson CE: Psychosocial aspects of neurologic disability, Nurs Clin North Am 15(2):209, 1980.

Conti MT and Eutropius L: Preventing UTIs: what works? AM J Nurs 87(3):307, 1987.

Davis JH: Children and pets: a therapeutic connection, Pediatr Nurs 11(5):377, 1985.

Dittmar S: Rehabilitation nursing: process and application, St Louis, 1989, The CV Mosby Co.

Does continuous passive motion help knees, Am J Nurs 87(8):1012, 1987.

Downey JA and Low NL, editors: The child with disabling illness: principles of rehabilitation, ed 2, New York, 1982, Raven Press.

Elsea SB: Professionally speaking, ethics in maternal-child nursing, MCN 10(5):303, 1985.

Finnie N: Handling the young cerebral palsied child at home, ed 2, New York, 1975, EP Dutton, Inc.

Gaspard NJ: Care of the adolescent male with traumatic head injury, J Rehabil 51(2):58, 1985.

Horner MM, Rawlins P, and Giles K: How parents of children with chronic conditions perceive their own needs, MCN 12(1):40, 1987.

Huddleston K and others: MIC or Foley: comparing gastrostomy tubes, MCN 14(1):20, 1987.

Johnson MP: Support groups for parents of chronically ill children, Pediatr Nurs 8(3):160, 1982.

Killam PE and others: Behavioral pediatric weight rehabilitation for children with myelomeningocele, MCN 8(4):280, 1983.

Lazure LL: Defusing the dangers of autonomic dysreflexia, Nursing '80 10(9):52, 1980.

Loughrey L: Avoiding the pit-falls of rehabilitation at home, Nursing '89 19(10):63, 1989.

Martin N, Holt N and Hicks D: Comprehensive rehabilitation nursing, New York, 1981, McGraw-Hill Book Co, Inc.

McKeever PT: Fathering the chronically ill child, MCN 6(2):124, 1981.

McNichol J: When eating doesn't come naturally, MCN 14(1):23, 1989.

Miller RA and Evans WE: Immediate postop prosthesis, 87(3):310, 1987.

Monsen R: Phases in the caring relationship: from adversary to ally to coordinator, MCN 11(5):316, 1986.

Norris RM: Commonplace tips for working with blind patients, Am J Nurs 89(3):360, 1989.

Olson E and others: Hazards of immobility: effects on cardio-vascular function; effects on respiratory function (reissue of April 1967 article), Am J Nurs 90(3):43, 1990.

Pierce PM and Giovineo G: REACH: self-care for the chronically ill child, Pediatr Nurs 9(1):37, 1983.

Retik A: Urinary tract disorders in children: new approaches, Hosp Pract 19(8):121, 1984.

Robinson CA: Double blind: a dilemma for parents of chronically ill children, Pediatr Nurs 11(2):112, 1985.

Rodgers BM and others: Depression in the chronically ill or handicapped school-age child, MCN 6(4):266, 1981.

Rose MH and Thomas RB, editors: Children with chronic conditions: nursing in a family and community context, Orlando, Fla, 1987, Grune & Stratton.

Rubin M: The physiology of bed rest, Am J Nurs 88(1):50, 1988.

Schaefer RS and Proffer DS: Sports medicine for wheelchair athletes, Am Fam Physician 39(5):239, 1989.

Shanks S, editor: Nursing and the management of pediatric communication disorders, San Diego, Calif, 1983, College Hill Press, Inc.

Stax TE, editor: Selected issues in pediatric rehabilitation, Pediatr Ann 17(12):(entire issue), 1988.

Vigliarolo D: Managing bowel incontinence in children with meningomyelocele, Am J Nurs 80(1):105, 1980.

Wilde MH: Living with a foley, Am J Nurs 86(10):1121, 1986.

Willey T: High-tech beds and mattress overlays: a decision guide, Am J Nurs, 89(9):1142, 1989.

Death and dying

Adams DW and Deveau EJ: Coping with childhood cancer, Reston Va, 1984, Reston Publishing Co, Inc.

Adams FE: Six very good reasons why we react differently to various dying patients, Nursing '84 14(6):41, 1984.

Archer DN and Smith AC: Sorrow has many faces, Nursing '88 18(5):43, 1988.

Carr D and Knupp CSF: Grief and perinatal loss: a community hospital approach to support, J Obstet Gynecol Neonatal Nurs 14(2):130, 1985.

Chee CM: Professionally speaking, a child's right to die, MCN 7(2):81, 1982.

Chitwood L: A lesson in living, Nursing '84 14(1):54, 1984.

Clements DB: Reminiscence: a tool for aiding families under stress, MCN 11(2):114, 1986.

Corcoran DK: Helping patients who've had near death experiences, Nursing '88 18(11):34, 1988.

D'Addio D: Reach out and touch, Am J Nurs 79(6):1081, 1979.

Davenport J: Common questions about withdrawal of life support, Am Fam Physician 39(1):201, 1989.

Dettmore D: Spiritual care: remembering your patient's forgotten needs, Nursing '84 14(10):46, 1984.

Ferszt GG and Taylor PB: When your patient needs spiritual comfort, Nursing '88 18(4):48, 1988.

Gray E: The emotional and play needs of the dying child, Issues Comprehensive Pediatr Nurs 12(2-3):207, 1989.

Herring JE: "How can you do that?" Nursing '88 18(12):65, 1988.

Hoffman Y: Surviving a child's suicide, Am J Nurs 87(7):955, 1987.

Holloway N: Dysfunctional grieving; when the hurt doesn't go away, Nursing '88 18(8):32C, 1988.

Jackson PL: When the baby isn't perfect, Am J Nurs 85(4):396, 1985.

Johnson S: Giving emotional support to families after a patient dies, Nurs Life 3(1):34, 1983.

Johnson SH: Ten ways to help the family of a critically ill patient, Nursing '86, 16(1):50 1986.

Kotsubo CZ: Helping families survive SIDS, Nursing '83 13(5):94, 1983.

Martinson IM: Caring for the dying child, Nurs Clin North Am 14(3):467, 1979.

McBride MM: Children's literature on death and dying, Pediatr Nurs 5(3):31, 1979.

Mina CF: A program for helping grieving parents, MCN 10(2):118, 1985.

Null S: Nursing care to ease parents' grief, MCN 14(2):84, 1989.

Ragonese R: Darlene's legacy—my most unforgettable patient, Nursing '89 19(1):61, 1989.

Ryan J: The neglected crisis, Am J Nurs 84(10):1257, 1984.

Sanders CM: Grief: the mourning after, Somerset, NJ, 1989, John Wiley & Sons, Inc.

Spinetta JJ and Deasy-Spinetta P, editors: Living with childhood cancer, St Louis, 1981, The CV Mosby Co.

Stevens CA: Helping Peter face the dark, Nursing '85 15(11):96, 1985.

Stoll RI: Guidelines for spiritual assessment, Am J Nurs 79(8):1574, 1979.

Thomas NT and Cordell AS: The dying infant: aiding the parents in the detachment process, Pediatr Nurs 9(5):355, 1983.

Vogel LJ: Helping a child understand death, Philadelphia, 1975, Fortress Press.

Pediatric Procedures

22

Hospital Admission and Discharge

CHAPTER OBJECTIVES

After studying this chapter, the student should be able to perform the following:

1 Describe the role of the pediatric nurse, and discuss qualifications necessary or desirable for this position.
2 Make a pediatric admission checklist that could be used to record background information, observational data, and routine examination results.
3 State how a blood pressure cuff size is properly selected.

4 Explain three ways in which an infant's blood pressure may be obtained.
5 Determine whether a pulse, respiratory rate, or BP is within normal limits for a certain age group (using Table 22-1 or Fig. 22-2).
6 Describe how to obtain a urine specimen from an infant or toddler.

First impressions are important, especially when parents and their child are involved. At times hospitalization of a child may be planned, and a previsit to the pediatric department may be possible to reassure parents and patient, but for many families hospitalization comes as an abrupt, unscheduled and frightening experience. A cordial, smooth introduction to hospital life, extended by a nurse who is sincerely interested in the family involved, does much to ease the anxiety inherent in the situation. All good nurses minister to more than the hospitalized patient's needs. They are alert to the needs, expressed or unspoken, of all family members. However, perhaps nowhere more than in the care of the child is the nurse's response to the entire family so crucial. If the trust of the parent or guardian can be secured initially, the nurse has obtained vital cooperation, a less tense, more relaxed mother and father, and a calmer child. A few more minutes spent at the time of admission may save hours of time later on (Fig. 22-1).

If first impressions are important, so are last contacts. The dismissal may be a most helpful period for the parent, or it may be a confusing "getaway." The following discussion is intended to help the nurse function well in these two eventful situations.

ADMISSION
Identification

The admitting nurse should be introduced or should introduce herself to both the new patient and the parents. In many hospitals identification of the patient is accomplished through use of a bracelet, which should be checked for accuracy. The parent's surname may be different from the child's. This should be clearly and discreetly noted to understand the situation better and prevent embarrassing incidents. To help the staff know their small patients better, many pediatric departments send out questionnaires to the parents of prospective patients requesting helpful information regarding the abilities,

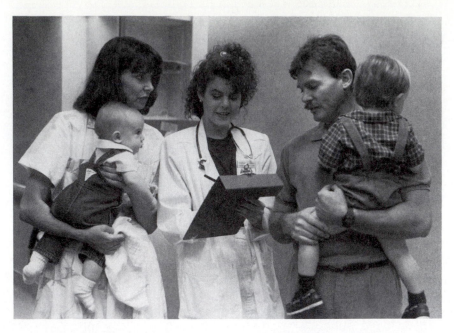

FIG 22-1 For most people coming to the hospital is a special and not too pleasant experience. This time baby brother will be having day surgery, and Mom and Dad express considerable concern.

habits, likes, and dislikes of the child. Nicknames and special vocabulary used by the child are also investigated. It is good to know that 3-year-old Edmund Atherton Barnstow III responds to "Barney" and loves grape-flavored popsicles.

Qualifications of a pediatric nurse

The pediatric nurse should feel friendly toward and comfortable with children. She should gain great satisfaction in helping children to become better equipped to meet the demands of life. Her loving concern for children should be expressed through a warm not "gushy" approach. Children can readily detect people who genuinely care about them. Nurses who find it difficult to work with children because of inexperience with or isolation from this age group need not feel that they will never function successfully in a pediatric area. But they must really want to learn to know children and think of them as persons and not as *problems*. If nurses are willing to be patient, if they are alert, adaptable, and imaginative, and if they are knowledgeable, kind, and understanding, they possess the potential assets for pediatric nursing.

Nurses frequently find the pediatric area emotionally taxing. It is sad indeed to see a tender, innocent child suffer or a young boy or girl whose life had been bright with promise suddenly struck down by disease or death.

Health professionals do not know all the answers to the philosophic questions created by such circumstances, but they do know that these children and young people and their parents need help. There must be those who are willing to try to help them and who are especially prepared to do so.

The nature of a pediatric nurse's responsibilities dictates that she possess an ample portion of both fortitude and *discretion*. She must think at least twice before she speaks. Detailed or crucial information about a patient must come from an authoritative source, such as the *head nurse, nursing supervisor,* or *attending physician,* and should be given only to those directly involved, usually attending personnel or parents. Well-meaning but curious casual inquirers should not be given diagnoses or progress reports. Finally, the nurse must develop the capacity for benevolent self-criticism and evaluation of her own actions so that she can constantly improve her ability to meet her patient's needs.

Nurse-parent role

Newer concepts of pediatric care do not picture the pediatric nurse as an authoritarian dispenser of knowledge and skill who alone has the ability to meet any need of the small patient. She is not a substitute mother, usurping the biologic or legal mother's position. However, she is a practitioner who has the advantage of special practical and theoretic education and training not available to most mothers, and she is a person who cares about children, sick or well. The aims of the pediatric nurse and the child's parents should be the same—to help develop each child's potential to the optimum level and to produce a creative, contributing member of society who finds high purpose in life and a role worth pursuing. The family learns from the nurse, and the wise nurse learns from the family.

The amount of parental participation in the care of the hospitalized child depends on the condition of the child and the response and abilities of the parents. To say that they should be allowed to do nothing when they have probably had total responsibility for their child until he was admitted to the hospital is unrealistic and even unkind. On the other hand, if parents give baths to their child, feed him, and complete his routine hygienic care alone, much valuable observation of the child is lost by nursing personnel, and much potential mutual teaching between child, nurse, and parent never takes place. At times, extended unrelieved participation at the bedside may produce an exhausted, worried mother or father instead of more relaxed, cooperative parents.

Perhaps, when the parent and child seem to gain much from parental participation in hospital care, it is best to carry out such care with the nurse helping the parents and vice versa. Then learning is enhanced, observation and reporting are more accurate, and any legal complications of parental care are prevented or minimized.

Some parents are unable to share constructively in the care of their hospitalized children. Others do not wish to participate. Occasionally children may be more relaxed when the mother and father do not participate. Parent anxiety caused by possible feelings of guilt, inadequacy, or frustration may be sensed by children and cause them, in turn, to be anxious. In certain cases the child may be confused about the role of the parent when the mother or father is at the bedside and the nurse must minister to the small child. In this situation, asking the parents to take a brief rest period until the procedure is completed may benefit both parent and child. For the most part, however, the presence of the parents is a real asset to the child. The mother and father, depending on the condition of the child, can help and be helped by sharing in the admission of the child. They may aid by undressing the child, positioning him for temperature readings, helping with feedings, and providing comfort by their presence. However, no parent should be made to feel that unless he or she is at the bedside the child will not receive complete and loving nursing care. This would cause many anxieties. Parents should not be made to think that they are neglecting their duty to the child unless they are at the bedside almost constantly. The liberal visiting privileges currently extended to parents in pediatric hospitals are designed to ease tensions, not create them. An excellent rule to follow is found in many nursing texts: "The modern pediatric nurse is mother and father's friend and helper—not their substitute."

Orientation

If the circumstances of hospital admission and the patient's age and condition permit, the child and parents should be oriented to the unit and introduced to other children. The parents should be introduced to key personnel and shown where such conveniences as the public telephone, rest rooms, public dining area, and waiting rooms are located. Many children receive a simple toy such as a hand puppet or coloring book at the time of admission, which helps to entertain and to pass the difficult periods of waiting for examination or surgery. The nurse should be sure the child has something appropriate at the bedside for diversion. A specially beloved toy or blanket may be brought from home. The nurse should make sure that any personal toys or clothing kept at the hospital are carefully labeled. In most cases the use of the child's own clothes, with the exception of bathrobes and slippers, is discouraged because of the high incidence of loss in the hospital laundry, despite attempts by the staff to avoid such confusion.

When the nurse is speaking to children, it is psychologically good technique to either bend or crouch down to their eye level for special introductions, serious talks, or mutual enjoyment. No one likes to talk to knees or to stretch to look up all the time.

NURSING PROCEDURES

Patients are usually admitted directly to their own units. During the admission, it is customary to secure the following:

1. Pertinent information regarding the child's family structure, habits, vocabulary, possible allergies, normal diet, history of childhood illnesses, current immunization status, and recent exposure to contagious diseases (especially chickenpox). A brief description of current health problems, any ongoing treatment or medication schedules, and the child's preparation for hospitalization should be included. This type of information may be obtained on a form filled out by the parent while the admission is in progress if it was not secured before the actual hospitalization.
2. Height, weight, and age
   a. Babies are routinely weighed without clothes.

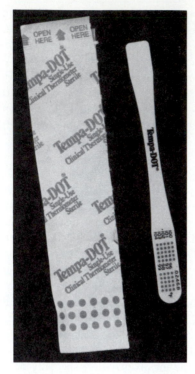

FIG 22-2 The Tempa-Dot single-use sterile clinical thermometer properly used provides a reliable quick oral or axillary reading. The temperature end (dots) is placed under the tongue as far back as possible into either heat pocket. The patient should press his tongue down on the thermometer and close his mouth for 1 minute. After removing the thermometer, the nurse should wait 10 seconds for dots to stabilize. The last blue dot indicates the correct temperature.

    b. Be sure that the scale is covered with a diaper or technique paper and is balanced before weighing.

    c. Many hospitals record the weight in both pounds/ounces and metric measurements.

    d. This information is used to

      (1) Determine dosages of medications and anesthesia

      (2) Determine general condition and progress

      (3) *Note:* All children with diarrhea and vomiting or intake-output problems are routinely weighed every morning before breakfast.

3. Temperature

    a. Glass or electronic (rectal, axillary, or oral) thermometers or Tempa-Dots may be employed, depending on the policy of the hospital and the desire of the physician. The method may be altered, depending on the child's age, diagnosis, condition, and tolerance of the method.

    b. Never leave a child alone with a thermometer in place (oral, rectal, or axillary). When rectal temperatures are

secured, always have one hand on the thermometer and another on the child to ensure safety and accuracy.

    c. A glass thermometer should not be used for an oral temperature if the following occurs:

      (1) The child has seizures or poor muscular control. (There is danger that the child may bite the thermometer, causing self-injury.)

      (2) The child has difficulty keeping the mouth closed because of oral surgery, general condition, or breathing difficulties. (Mouth surgery itself may contraindicate oral temperatures.)

    d. In current references the following temperatures are usually defined as fever:

      (1) Oral and axillary temperatures above 100° F (37.8° C)

      (2) Rectal temperatures above 100.4° F (38° C)

Temperature elevations should be reported promptly according to hospital policy to the charge nurse or team leader as soon as determined. Children with abnormal temperatures should have temperature checks more frequently (see p. 578).

    e. Rectal temperatures are now generally not recommended for children under 6 years old and are contraindicated in young infants, and persons with cancer, diarrhea, or rectal pathology.

    f. Being consistent, minimizing trauma to the patient, and maximizing accuracy all should be considered when deciding on the best route for each patient.

4. Pulse

    a. For infants an apical pulse rate is secured by placing a stethoscope between the left nipple and sternum. It is too difficult to secure an accurate radial pulse rate using standard methods.

    b. Other pulse points may be used with the older child (the temple, the neck) if keeping the wrist still is difficult.

    c. Pulse determinations can usually be made by timing for 30 seconds and multiplying by 2 on the very young child.

    d. Irregularity, quality, and rate should be noted.

    e. The activity of the child should be taken into account. (For example, the pulse of a sleeping child should be so labeled.)

    f. For rate ranges see Table 22-1.

Table 22-1 Approximate pulse and respiration rates at rest based on age*

Age	Pulse	Respiration
Birth-1 mo	110-150	30-45
1 mo-1 yr	100-140	26-34
1-2 yr	90-120	20-30
2-6 yr	90-110	20-30
6-10 yr	80-100	18-26
Over 10 yr	76-90	16-24

*Pulse and respiration rates become slower with age.

5. Respirations
   a. The rate and character of respirations are important. The nurse should detect and describe wheezing and other respiratory abnormalities, such as sternal retractions.
   b. For rate ranges see Table 22-1.
6. Blood pressure
   a. The correct size of cuff is very important. The cuff bladder should be 20% (one-fifth) wider than the diameter of the extremity or cover two thirds of the upper arm measured from the shoulder to the elbow. Some authorities have recommended a cuff even larger for infants and young children.* The same cuff should be used consecutively if possible.
   b. It is sometimes difficult to determine the BP of an infant.
      (1) Infants should be supine.
      (2) If regular auscultation is not helpful, the systolic pressure can be secured by *palpation* of the brachial pulse as the cuff is gradually deflated. This systolic

*Steinfeld L and others: Sphygmomanometry in the pediatric patient, J Pediatr 92:934, 1978.

reading is usually recorded over P (for example, 86/P).
      (3) In some areas a Doppler or arterial pressure transducer apparatus is used. It provides both systolic and diastolic readings but is a relatively expensive unit.
      (4) The "flush method" may be used with fair-skinned children. The distal portion of an upper or lower limb is made pale by the application of wrappings or manual pressure. The blood is prevented from entering the blanched hand or foot by an inflated cuff. The cuff is slowly deflated and the reading recorded when a flush, indicating the passage of blood beyond the cuff into the exposed hand or foot, is noted. Usually two people are needed to observe the flush and manometer reading concurrently. The number obtained represents an approximate average of the systolic and diastolic pressures and is recorded over F (for example, 50/F).
   c. Any unusual activity of the child just before or during the blood pressure determination must be noted. Try to obtain a BP while the child is quiet.

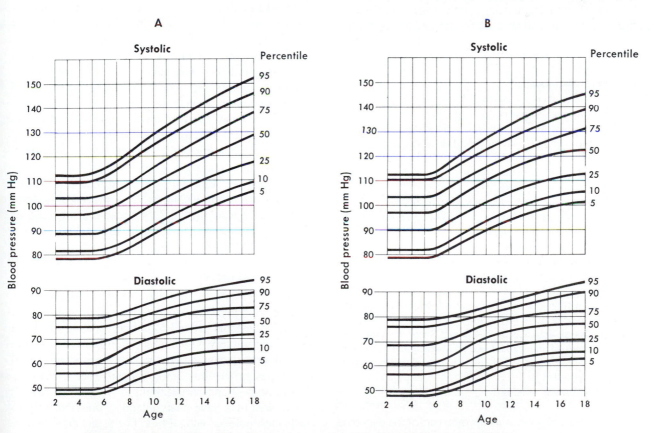

FIG 22-3 A, Percentiles of blood pressure measurement in boys (right arm, seated).
B, Percentiles of blood pressure measurement in girls (right arm, seated). *(From Blumenthal S and others: Pediatrics 59(suppl):803, 1977; News and Comment 29:8-13, 1978. Copyright American Academy of Pediatrics, 1977 and 1978.)*

   d. The average blood pressure at birth is 80/46. For percentile readings for boys and girls ages 2 to 18 years of age, see Fig. 22-3. Most children's blood pressures vary considerably. These charts may be used to evaluate the blood pressure readings obtained, although their real function is to serve as a device for plotting blood pressure over a period of time. Blood pressure measurements should be obtained and plotted at least once yearly.

7. General appearance and behavior as evaluated through observation

   a. Overall clinical *appearance*
      (1) In no acute distress
      (2) Mildly ill
      (3) Severely ill

   b. Growth and development
      (1) Appropriate for age and sex of child
      (2) Special physical considerations, such as orthopedic problems, imperfect vision, deafness, speech or language barriers, malnutrition, obesity, cosmetic defects, prostheses (dentures, glasses, contact lenses, artificial eyes, limbs), surgically created stomas, history of seizures, and general vigor
      (3) Cultural, intellectual, and emotional considerations, such as cultural heritage (for example, Hispanic-American), mentally retarded or gifted, parent-child-nurse interaction, and initial response to hospitalization

   c. Skin manifestations
      (1) Unusual color—flushed, pale cyanotic, or jaundiced
      (2) Unusual birthmarks or scars
      (3) Rashes, bruises, possible boils, blisters, or possible infestations (body or head lice or scabies)
      (4) State of cleanliness

   d. Nervous system manifestations
      (1) Level of consciousness
      (2) Abnormally or unequally dilated pupils
      (3) Tremor, twitching, or periods of blank staring
      (4) Limp, flaccid extremities
      (5) Bulging fontanels
      (6) One-sided or lower-extremity weakness or paralysis

   e. Other signs and symptoms important to note on admission
      (1) Diarrhea, nausea, vomiting, or abdominal distention (type of stool or emesis)
      (2) Nasal drainage or coughing (Signs of respiratory tract infection noted in a child scheduled for surgery should be reported immediately. Surgery may be cancelled.)
      (3) Difficulty voiding

All of these observations become part of the data base that makes up the admission assessment of the child. Emphasis should be placed on learning the reason for hospital admission and carefully observing the body systems involved.

Collection of specimens

In addition to the preceding measurements and observations, the patient is routinely scheduled for urinalysis and blood examinations.

Urine specimens. The collection of a urine specimen in a child over 2½ years is seldom difficult. The collection of a specimen from an infant or young toddler poses real problems. Various methods have been recommended. Most pediatric nurses, after careful cleansing of the perineal area, position small sterile adhesive-backed plastic bags over the urethra that adhere to the perineal region or base of the penis (Fig. 22-4 and p. 507). These are usually satisfactory except when the child has a rash or perineal excoriations. The bag must be checked frequently to prevent losing the urine collection. When a prolonged urine collection is needed, a 24-hour pediatric urine specimen bag with an attached drainage tube may be used, or a small feeding tube may be specially inserted into the top of the routine collection bag and the bag periodically emptied with a syringe.

Blood samples. A blood specimen is usually not secured by the nurse, but she may help restrain the child as the physician or laboratory technician obtains the specimen. It may be obtained from a toe, heel, ear, or finger prick, an arterial puncture of the arm, or a venous puncture in the arm or neck. If children must be restrained and if they are old enough to understand, they should be told that the hands, sheets, or other appliances that may be employed are used to help them hold still so that the physician can help them get well. They should not think of the restraints as a means of punishment. Various types of restraints are used during a child's hospitalization. These are discussed in Chapter 23. Common procedures or diagnostic tests that may be ordered at the time of admission (spinal puncture, sweat test, and so on) are discussed in Chapter 24.

Diet and fluid orders

The diet of a newly admitted child depends, of course, on the reason for the hospitalization and the child's age, food allergies, and general condition. Patients scheduled for pending surgery might not be allowed anything to eat or drink or may have orders for a certain amount of fluid until a designated time before surgery later in the day. Be sure to post appropriate signs near or on the child.

Children may have many allergies, often not only to medicines, pollens, animal furs, fibers, and dust but also to common foods. Chocolate, milk, wheat products, tomatoes, oranges, and strawberries are among the frequent offenders. Nurses should be alerted to these problems and the allergic manifestations they usually

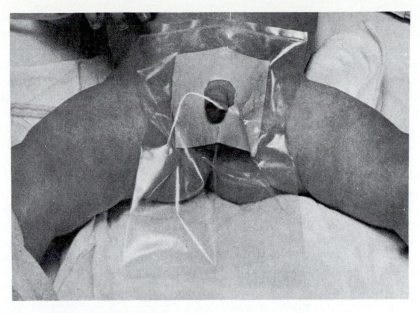

FIG 22-4 Application of one type of adhesive-backed plastic bag for collection of urine specimen. Be sure it is not upside down!

cause. The cultural patterns of some patients may cause feeding problems and poor acceptance of the routine hospital diet.

Admission responsibility

The member of the nursing team who has the responsibility of admitting a patient depends on the condition and needs of the child. In certain situations the admission may be made in its entirety by a registered nurse. At other times it may be a joint or delegated responsibility carried out by both the registered nurse and the licensed vocational nurse.

As a result of the admission interview, observations, and examinations, a plan for nursing care should be formulated based on the patient's needs and individual characteristics.

DISCHARGE
Plans for dismissal

The discharge day is usually extremely busy for parents. Arrangements must be made for transportation (for example, a child in a hip spica cast won't fit in every car). Maybe the child's father or mother has to take time off from work to provide transportation. Perhaps special child care arrangements need to be found. The child usually must be dismissed in the morning to avoid a hospital charge for an additional day. If possible, the nurse should write out any instructions for home care

concerning observations to be made or medications and procedures prescribed rather than rely on oral instructions to the parents. The arrangements for the next follow-up visit to the physician should be clear.

Preparation for home care

Extended needs after discharge. When home care after discharge involves special skills, continued procedures, or particular stress, preparations for discharge may need to begin days before the actual departure of the child. Some hospitals currently employ a special discharge or "continuity of care" nurse who helps the parents or child caregivers to plan for continued home care, teaching them necessary skills while the child is still hospitalized (for example, instructions on gavage, dressing changes, stoma care, or IV observation). Ideally, more than one member of the family and, if appropriate, the patient himself should be taught the skills that will be necessary for care.

The discharge nurse may also go to the home to assess needs and check patient progress. The location of the sleeping quarters of the child may need to be changed to save steps and provide greater opportunity for observation. Special equipment or supplies may need to be improvised, borrowed, rented, or purchased. The services of a visiting nurse may be required. Patients are being discharged from hospital settings much earlier than ever before. They need special support.

Possible behavior changes. Parents should be cautioned that hospitalization affects children differently. Occasionally, children have a period of difficulty readjusting to life at home. They may regress developmentally, and activities that they had already mastered before their illness may not be attempted. Irritability and wetting by a previously toilet-trained child are common.

Actual leave-taking

At the time of discharge, every attempt should be made to send all of the child's belongings home with the parent. Return trips to the hospital to pick up articles left behind are annoying. Bedside stands, closets, cupboards, bedclothes, and flooring must be carefully scrutinized.

Before actually leaving the hospital premises, the parent (or responsible adult) must sign a form indicating who is taking the child. Great care must be taken that the person who is given responsibility for the child at the time of discharge has the legal right to assume that responsibility. At this time a final check is made regarding any medications to be taken home or special instructions to be given.

If at all possible, the child should be taken to the point of actual transfer (usually to a car) in a wheelchair, a rolling bassinette, or on a gurney. The child must always be accompanied by a nurse or hospital employee.

• • •

Admissions and discharges are part of the everyday pattern of hospital routine. The nurse must remember that they are far from routine for most of the patients and parents who find themselves within the sound of her voice and the influence of her actions.

Key Concepts
---

1. Potential assets for pediatric nursing include patience, alertness, adaptability, imagination, knowledgeability, kindness, and understanding.

2. The amount of parental participation in the care of the hospitalized child depends on the condition of the child and the response and abilities of the parents. Parents should not be totally excluded from providing care, nor should they be given excessive responsibility.

3. During the admission assessment, the following information becomes part of the data base: patient's history; height, weight, and age; temperature; pulse; respirations; blood pressure; and general appearance and behavior.

4. The patient is routinely scheduled for urinalysis and blood examinations. The nurse is usually responsible for securing the urine specimen and assisting the physician or laboratory technician in obtaining a blood specimen.

5. The diet of a newly admitted child depends on the reason for hospitalization and the child's age, food allergies, and general condition.

6. Discharge preparation should include written instructions for home care and arrangements for follow-up visits to the physician. Parents need specific instructions on how to care for their child at home, especially with today's trend of early discharge.

Discussion Questions
---

1. Pediatrics is viewed as a specialized area of nursing. Discuss the special skills and attitudes required of a nurse working in pediatrics. Are all well-educated nurses capable of being pediatric nurses?

2. How can the pediatric nurse best establish a trusting relationship with the child? With the parents? What can the nurse do to maintain this trust?

3. How does assessing vital signs (temperature, pulse, respirations, blood pressure) of a child differ from adult assessment? What particular safety precautions should be taken?

4. Subjective data can be obtained from both the parents and from the child. How would you attempt to get this type of information from the child? How would you vary your history taking technique based on the age of the child?

5. What modifications and special nursing techniques are used when attempting to collect blood and urine specimens from a young child?

Basic Patient Needs and Daily Planning

Every patient has individual needs that are personal and special because of their unique combination or background. At the same time, these needs may be said to represent the needs of all people, because they usually fall into broader, more basic categories of care. For this presentation the patient's needs have been grouped to form seven areas of discussion.

BASIC PATIENT NEEDS

The nursing staff is responsible for helping to provide the following:
1. Safety
2. Observation and assessment
3. Diagnostic procedures
4. Supportive procedures

a. Aiding respiration and oxygenation
b. Regulating body temperature
c. Positioning and appropriate activity
d. Adequate nourishment and fluid balance
e. Cleanliness
f. Rest
g. Diversion, self-expression, coping mechanisms, and acceptance

5. Medications and special treatments
6. Rehabilitation
7. Recording of events

Safety

Safety is a constant problem in any hospital. In a pediatric hospital it seems to be both constant and compounded. The environment must be continually evaluated to prevent accidents because the patients are often too small to regulate their own surroundings, and they lack the judgment to evaluate their own environments properly. Unrestrained or unattended children in high beds or cribs should always have the bed or crib sides securely raised. No nurse should turn her back on an unrestrained child in a crib with the side lowered. Young children who have climbing urges should be placed in special protective beds unless supervision is constant (Fig. 23-1). Beds of inquisitive boys and girls should be at a "no touch" distance from wall electricity, suction, and oxygen outlets. No antiseptics or other supplies, which may be ingested by the curious child, should be left at the bedside. Toys should be checked for sharp edges, points, or other potential dangers. Plastic bags should not be used for storage of toys or playthings. Notices of the child's known allergies should be clearly posted in his unit. All equipment should be in good working order and used properly. Special precautions should be observed when administering oxygen. When a child is transported in a wheelchair, in most instances a waist or jacket restraint should be used to prevent the child's tipping forward or sliding down. Unnecessary traffic and congestion in the halls should be avoided.

An important component of safety is firm but kind discipline. Explaining the reason for some rules to the child who is old enough to understand often works wonders. Good discipline also means realistic expectations and prompt follow-through by the nurse responsible for supervising behavior. It means that nurses must not give choices when no alternatives are possible. It also means offering a choice when the opportunity to choose would bring pleasure, importance, and a sense of self-direction or achievement to the child. Promises kept, a "yes" that

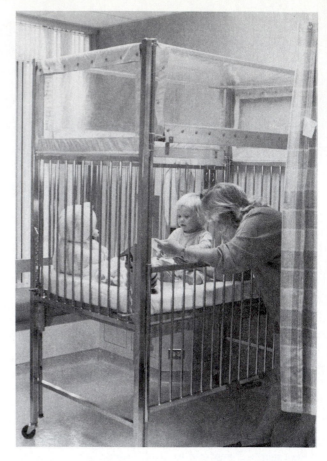

FIG 23-1 High top cribs are designed to protect ambitious climbers. *(Courtesy Children's Hospital and Health Center, San Diego, Calif.)*

means yes and a "no" that means no, and a loving regard for the ultimate welfare of the child are extremely significant in maintaining good discipline.

Sometimes children must be restrained during treatment to protect them from themselves. Such restraint should never be presented as a punishment but as one way to help children hold themselves still for a little while. An example of such a restraint is the "mummy wrap" (Fig. 23-2). A commercial mummy restraint used in many emergency rooms is the Olympic papoose board shown in Fig. 23-3. Another type of control used to prevent children from touching their faces or pulling on gavage tubes is elbow restraints, which are usually fastened to the hospital gown (Fig. 23-4, *A*). However, elbow restraints are not effective if the child can reach his face with a toy or an implement without bending his

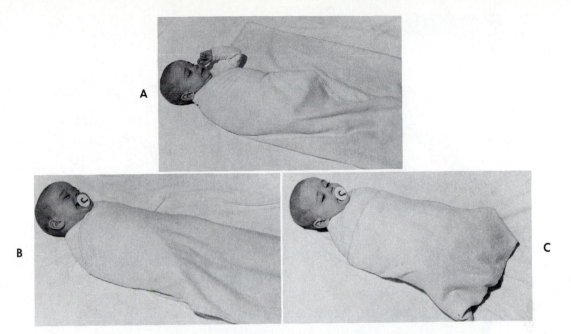

FIG 23-2 Covered chest mummy wrap. **A,** Center baby's head at edge of "short side" of open baby blanket or sheet. Place one arm at his side and pull blanket snugly over his shoulder, arm, and chest and tuck the blanket under the baby. **B,** Position opposite arm similarly and pull opposite corner over and around baby. **C,** Open out loose end of blanket and bring it up and around baby snugly. (We do not generally advocate pacifiers but believe they have a place in certain situations.)

arms. To control leg and arm motion, specially constructed ankle and wrist restraints (Fig. 23-4, *B*) or the time-proven clove hitch tie (Fig. 23-5) may be used. A pediatric Posey belt may be employed to allow some movement in bed while preventing the patient from rising. A jacket restraint is pictured in Fig. 23-6.

Most restraints must be removed about every 2 hours to check circulation and exercise the body part involved. Restraints should be constructed so that they do not become tighter with increased tension, impairing circulation or endangering the child's respiration.

Observation and assessment

Observation is crucial to the welfare of the patient. To plan and pursue the care of a patient intelligently, enlightened systematic assessment must take place. Observational study of the pediatric patient is particularly important and complex because many small children cannot express themselves and because many variables are associated with different stages of growth and development. Observation of the patient should be made, especially in light of the patient's medical and nursing diagnosis. For example, if his medical diagnosis is pneu-

monia, the fact that the child is pale and has a frequent, loose cough producing thick, white mucus is significant. Sometimes negative observations are important to make. It is important to record that a child admitted because of convulsions has had no seizures for a certain period. The observation that a child hospitalized for vomiting and diarrhea retained a feeding and had no stools for a specific interval may be significant. When observing the whole patient and recording appearance, activity, and treatment, refer to his diagnosis. What is especially important for the physician or supervising nurse to know? A change in the bed placement is sometimes needed for closer observation of the child.

Diagnostic procedures

The diagnostic procedures ordered must be understood so that adequate preparation, execution, and follow-up can be provided. It is impossible to describe within this brief text all the diagnostic procedures encountered by the nurse in a pediatric setting. But for some of the more common tests and a description of specimen collection, consult Chapter 24 and the hospital procedure manual. It should be remembered that many diagnostic studies

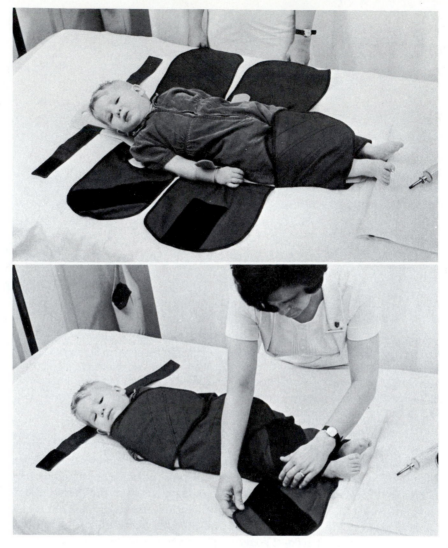

FIG 23-3 Preparing to restrain child for gastric lavage using Olympic papoose board. Various wraps are possible with Velcro-lined restraining folds. *(Courtesy Olympic-Surgical Co, Inc, Seattle.)*

require the parent's or guardian's informed written consent.

In the morning the nurse must be careful to determine whether any of her patients should not receive anything to eat or drink and whether they are listed as NPO. Many laboratory tests do not limit water intake. After a test is complete for which a patient has been fasting, the nurse must be sure to inquire if the patient may resume his diet. If so, the prescribed foods or liquids must be secured.

Supportive procedures

Various types of supportive procedures and techniques are used to maintain or improve the physical and emotional resources of the patient. These may include special provisions for aiding respiration or oxygenation, regulating body temperature, positioning and encouraging appropriate activity, maintaining fluid balance or nutrition, relieving pain, or improving body function. They also include the interest and love expressed by parents, family, friends, and nurses and the physical and spiritual

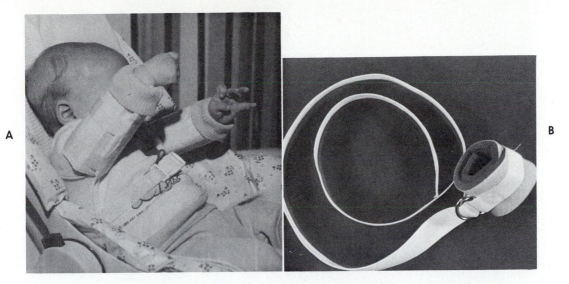

FIG 23-4 A, Baby cannot touch his cleft lip repair but can move his arms, an advantage of elbow restraints. **B,** Extremity restraint incorporating Velcro fastener.

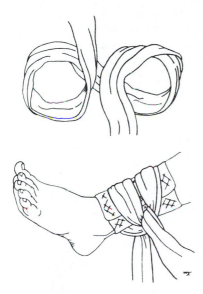

FIG 23-5 Application of clove hitch restraint. Formed loops are placed one on top of other and body part put through opening. Body part should always be previously padded.

serenity promoted by the development of trust. The use of oxygen and humidification equipment is discussed in a separate chapter, as are the methods of regulating body temperature. Positioning of the child in bed is described in the following paragraphs.

Supervision of position and activity. Even children who are ambulatory and active need to be supervised so that they do not develop poor posture habits that will interfere with the optimum function of their bodies and cause them to feel less than their best. Children in bed, particularly if they must remain fairly quiet for long periods, must maintain good alignment, functional positions, range of motion, and tissue health for all body parts. (Read also the section on skin care and positioning, pp. 433-434.) Barring special treatments involving traction, casting, or specifically ordered body placement, the child in bed, whether supine (on back) or prone (on abdomen) must maintain a posture that would be considered well aligned if the child were standing. This is important for those who are not able to change their position easily. Included in this section are some illustrations showing examples of proper positioning.

If patients remain in bed for extended periods without adequate foot support or with tight covers pressing down on their feet, they will develop tightening of the Achilles tendon, or heel cord, causing *footdrop,* which makes walking difficult. One leg may fall outward toward the side *(external rotation)* causing deformity or it may remain in a common flexed position, which if not changed often, can result in fixation and *contracture* in a relatively short period. Arms positioned on top of the chest and a partially flexed head position decrease respiratory capacity. Flexed arm and hand positions (very typical of the arthritic patient), if maintained, cause flexion con-

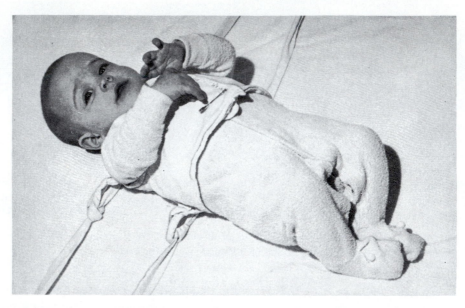

FIG 23-6 Restraining jacket. Ties are fastened to bedspring frame, and pins are placed in front, on top, or underneath, depending on child's age. It is best, if possible, to elevate head of bed to avoid problems with aspiration. Ties may be modified to allow some toddlers to sit up in bed. It may also be used as wheelchair restraint for small children.

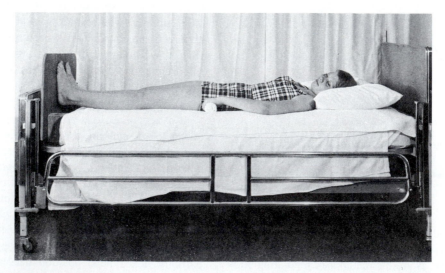

FIG 23-7 Good body alignment in supine position. *(Courtesy Children's Hospital and Health Center, San Diego, Calif.)*

tractures of the shoulder and elbow and *wristdrop*, with loss of function in the hand.

Fig. 23-7 illustrates how good alignment may be achieved with the help of a footboard, pillows, and hand rolls. Incapacitated teenage patients usually need considerable help. It should be noted that a type of foot support is being employed. (However, partially paralyzed patients who exhibit considerable muscle spasticity may be unable to tolerate a hard footboard without tissue damage occurring. They may need a soft boot type support.) The knees are straight up, rotated neither to the inside nor outside. Sometimes this correct position is maintained in part by a rectangularly folded blanket that has been partially slipped under the buttocks of the patient. The long protruding end is then rolled under tightly toward the thigh to stabilize the leg in a neutral position. This is a *trochanter roll*. Some patients appreciate a small pillow placed in the small of the back. The arms are alternately rotated for comfort. Soft hand rolls help maintain functional finger-thumb relationships.

When the patient is in the prone or abdominal position (Fig. 23-8) the toes should be either over the end of the mattress pointing down between the foot of the bed and the mattress or over the edge of a pillow. A thin pillow support under the abdomen takes pressure off the chest and reduces the lumbar curve. The arms are usually comfortable if abducted and flexed. A pillow may not be required under the head.

The side-lying position is often preferred. The main problem with this position is the strain placed on the hip joint and lower back by the upper leg if it is allowed to fall forward. For a patient who has no back or hip problems and is able to move freely, this is no great difficulty. However, if these problems or conditions exist, the side-lying position should be properly maintained by the addition of one or two pillows supporting the upper leg, as in Fig. 23-9. Sometimes a pillow tucked lengthwise against the back is comforting. A support for the upper hand relieves the chest.

Good positioning and frequent turning (every 2 hours or less) does much to comfort the patient, prevent respiratory, circulatory, and urinary complications, reduce deformity, and speed rehabilitation. Infants and toddlers do not require such elaborate supports to maintain alignment and prevent deformity, but they do need to be frequently turned and positioned if they do not move themselves. Older infants or young toddlers often sleep with their heads and chests on the mattress, faces turned to the side, while their knees are pulled under their abdomens to make their buttocks form the highest point of their sleeping silhouettes. This is a perfectly normal and characteristic posture for this age. A young infant should not be left unattended flat on his back because of the danger of aspiration. A rolled blanket should be placed at the infant's back to maintain a side position.

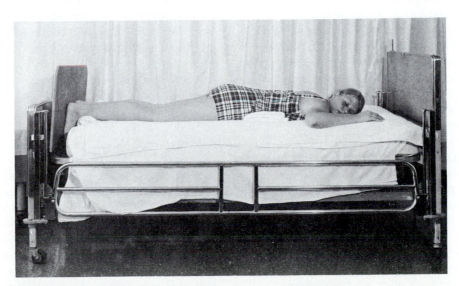

FIG 23-8 Good body alignment in prone position. *(Courtesy Children's Hospital and Health Center, San Diego, Calif.)*

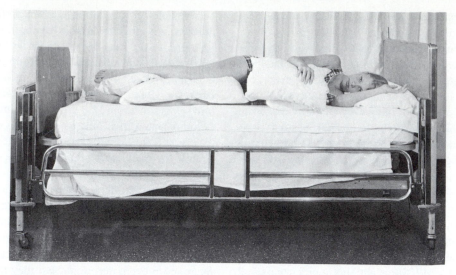

FIG 23-9 Good body alignment in side-lying position. *(Courtesy Children's Hospital and Health Center, San Diego, Calif.)*

Nourishment and fluid balance

Diet. The diet of a patient does not consist of the diet order that the physician writes on the patient's chart. It is not that easy. The diet consists of what a patient eats, drinks, and retains of the food and drink sent from the kitchen or prepared by the nursing staff in response to the physician's order. Some diets look beautiful on paper but, unfortunately, are never eaten.

Before a tray is served to a patient, it should be carefully checked to see that it is compatible with his diet order, food allergies, abilities, and cultural or religious background. Nuts, raw carrots, and celery should not be served to toddlers who can aspirate such chunky foods. Common diets served in the pediatric area are clear liquid, full liquid, soft, high protein, high carbohydrate, low residue, diabetic, and salt- or sodium-restricted. Nursing students should review these diets in a diet manual.

A child must often be helped at mealtime. A nurse cannot simply put a tray on a bed or crib table and expect even an older child to eat automatically. The utensils should be appropriate. The food must be easily available and attractive. Some young children prefer trying to feed themselves, but very young children enjoy being held during meals. Bibs and nurse's feeding gowns ease laundry problems. Encourage parents to visit at mealtime if possible. Their presence often increases intake.

Infants often drink better if they have a breathing space between the time they finish their solids and are offered their formula. Infants and toddlers who need a greater fluid intake may be offered fluids before solid foods, when appetites are sharpest, to encourage fluid acceptance. Plastic bottles should be used with older infants who enjoy holding their own bottle.

Whether it is necessary to record every bit of food eaten by a child depends on the diagnosis and the child's condition. A diabetic child requires close observation and recording of food intake. The true diet of a patient with any metabolic, growth and development, digestive, or feeding problems should be carefully recorded. A calorie count or written record of the amount of each food item eaten is often kept at the bedside.

Intakes for patients with stabilized conditions can be described as "ate well," "ate fairly well," or "ate poorly." *All* pediatric patients are routinely on a regimen of measured fluid intake, expressed in cubic centimeters (cc) or milliliters (ml). Most are on a measured fluid output regimen.

Hydration. Fluid intake is of greater immediate importance than solid feeding. The hydration of a child is extremely important. A young child may become dehydrated more rapidly than an adult. An infant is especially vulnerable, having a greater surface area and higher metabolic rate per unit of weight than an adult. Maintaining an adequate fluid intake is one of the very important responsibilities of the bedside nurse. The amount of fluid that is urged depends on the size and condition of the child. Nursing students are reminded that patients who are immobilized in casts or traction apparatus and all those with indwelling urinary catheters must have special attention to ensure abundant fluid intake.

Encouragement. Ensuring oral intake often calls for a nurse's ingenuity, patience, and persistence. Small amounts taken frequently are tolerated better by the ill child than copious amounts taken rapidly, no matter how willingly. Fluids taken rapidly are often not retained by children who are ill, upset, or excited.

The kinds of fluids offered to children depend on their diet orders and any allergies they have. Clear fluids include any liquid through which one can see the bottom of the container—water, bouillon, strained fruit juices, popsicles, gelatin, and soft drinks. A full liquid diet includes unstrained fruit juices and milk products such as ice cream, sherbet, milkshakes, and creamed soups.

Learning which fluids the child has accepted well in the past may save time. Offering a choice is often helpful. Sometimes the manner in which fluids are offered is significant. Some older babies seem insulted by a bottle and drink well from a cup. Others regress and take fluids only from a bottle with a certain kind of nipple. (Remember that propping a bottle is not a safe practice.) Some small children are accustomed to warm milk; others like it cold. Older children often reject milk unless it is ice cold. A nurse who is able to sit down with the child beside her or in her lap and offer fluid as part of good companionship is more likely to be successful than the nurse who expresses her frustration in constant verbal harassment. In some cases the use of straws, doll tea-party dishes, colored ice cubes, or a paper star on the fluid intake record may help. Popsicles are usually very acceptable. Plain water should not be forgotten in the search for fluids. With older children, the factual knowledge that other steps (intravenous feedings) will be necessary to ensure hydration if oral fluid intake is too low may encourage drinking. For most children a carton of milk and a glass of fruit juice at breakfast, a glass of some other fluid or dish of ice cream or gelatin equaling approximately 200 ml during midmorning, soup and beverage at lunch, and a midafternoon liquid snack fulfill the dietary responsibilities of the day nursing shift.

Restriction. Children with renal disease, central nervous system disease, including meningitis, or heart disease may require restricted fluid intake. Patients scheduled for operative procedures are usually not allowed any oral intake for several hours before their surgeries. After the procedures the amount and types of fluids offered may be restricted. For instance, in some cases, after heart surgery oral liquid intake may be limited and offered only in small quantities for an extended period. Some postsurgical patients are allowed nothing by mouth for a considerable period after their procedures, receiving their fluids parenterally (by other routes than oral, such as by vein) until the physician believes that oral administration can be attempted. The child who has had stomach or intestinal surgery is initially offered very small amounts at a time to ascertain tolerance and to decrease stress on the surgical site. Infants with severe cases of diarrhea and vomiting are usually not allowed anything by mouth or are placed on a limited oral intake to rest the gastrointestinal tract. Fluids for these patients are also administered *parenterally.*

Fluid and electrolyte balance. It has become increasingly apparent in recent years that the content and volume of the body fluid is a key consideration in the maintenance of cellular health and therefore the health of the total individual. The body organs and systems function to maintain the proper internal and external cellular environment and enable the survival of the person. The following brief, simplified discussion of fluid and electrolyte balance is included because an understanding of this area of biology has become more and more necessary for the general public and the bedside nurse.

The body functions in sensitive equilibrium. One of the most delicate balances maintained by the body is demonstrated by the composition of body fluid. Major ingredients of this fluid are water and certain chemicals termed *electrolytes*. Electrolytes develop electric charges when they are dissolved in water. Some electrolytes carry a positive charge and are called *cations*. Negatively charged electrolytes are called *anions*. In either case the electrolytes are referred to as *ions*. A small number of chemical compounds that do not ionize or carry electrical charges are also found in body fluid. Organic compounds such as glucose and urea are the main nonelectrolytes of body fluid. (See Table 23-1.)

Body fluid occupies three permeable compartments (Fig. 23-10): blood vessels, tissue spaces (interstitial areas outside of tissue cells), and the areas inside the cells. *Extracellular fluid* (ECF) is located within the blood vessels and between the tissue cells, and *intracellular fluid* (ICF) lies inside the tissue cells.

Every tissue cell is surrounded by a semipermeable membrane that permits selective passage of certain substances and free passage of water molecules in both directions. Water passes from the side containing the least amount of electrolytes and other dissolved compounds to the side that contains more dissolved compounds. This water movement is called osmosis. In health a dynamic

Table 23-1   Major electrolytes and imbalances

Electrolyte	Deficit	Excess

Sodium (Na⁺)—normal value 136-143 mEq/L*	*Hyponatremia*
	Associated with dehydration; sodium losses from the body in excess of water losses; Na⁺ below 130 mEq/L
	  Muscular weakness; abdominal cramps; clammy skin; weak, rapid pulse; hypotension; drowsiness; confusion; coma
	Predisposing factors—excessive sweating and water intake; gastrointestinal suction and excessive oral water intake; glucose water infusion without sodium; diarrhea; renal disease; cystic fibrosis; central nervous system disease
		Hypernatremia
		Associated with dehydration; water losses from the body in excess of sodium losses; Na⁺ above 150 mEq/L
		  Thirst; dry skin; loss of skin elasticity ("doughy" tissue turgor); fever; weight loss; scanty urine formation; confusion; stupor; seizures; circulatory embarrassment
		
		Predisposing factors—sodium chloride infusion; inadequate water intake; water diarrhea; renal concentrating disease; anorexia; nausea; vomiting; high fever
		Additional feeding factors—infant feedings of undiluted cow's milk; boiled skim milk; powdered electrolyte mixtures: salt and sugar mixtures; bouillon soup, and so forth

Potassium (K⁺)—normal value 4.1-5.6 mEq/L	*Hypokalemia†* K⁺ below 3.5 mEq/L Weak pulse; hypotension; muscular weakness; diminished reflexes; loss of peristalsis, cardiac arrest Predisposing factors—diuretics; diarrhea; vomiting; gastric suctioning	*Hyperkalemia* K⁺ above 5.7 mEq/L Nausea; apprehension; muscular weakness; confusion; hypotension; cardiac arrest Predisposing factors—burns, excessive tissue damage; excessive infusion of potassium; kidney disease; severe dehydration with scanty urine formation; adrenal insufficiency
Calcium (Ca⁺⁺)—normal value 10-12 mg/100 ml (5-6 mEq/L)	*Hypocalcemia* Ca⁺⁺ below 9 mg/100 ml Tetany; tingling around mouth and fingers; muscular cramps; convulsions Predisposing factors—hypoactive parathyroid; malabsorption syndromes; chronic renal disease; distressed newborns	*Hypercalcemia (rare)* Ca⁺⁺ above 12 mg/100 ml Vomiting; constipation; polyuria; abdominal pains; headache Predisposing factors—prolonged bed rest; overactive parathyroid; overdose of vitamin D
Bicarbonate (HCO₃)⁻ normal value 19-26 mEq/L	*Metabolic acidosis* HCO₃ below 12 mEq/L Apathy, drowsiness or lethargy; deep rapid breathing (Kussmaul type) disorientation; stupor; weakness; coma Predisposing factors—diabetes mellitus; starvation; kidney insufficiency; excessive parenteral NaCl; severe diarrhea; salicylate intoxication; respiratory alkalosis	*Metabolic alkalosis* HCO₃⁻ above 30 mEq/L Depressed, shallow respirations; hypertonic muscles; tetany; disorientation Predisposing factors—vomiting (pyloric stenosis); ingestion of alkali; chloride-deficient diets or formulas; gastric suction; diuretics; respiratory insufficiency

*Milliequivalents per liter (mEq/L).

†Potassium may be given intravenously only after urinary output is well established.

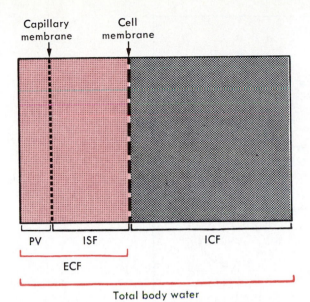

FIG 23-10 Body fluid compartments. *PV*, Plasma volume; *ISF*, interstitial fluid; *ECF*, extracellular fluid; *ICF*, intracellular fluid.

equilibrium of electrolytes and water is maintained between the two areas. Therefore, although each of the fluid compartments of the body contains electrolytes, the concentration and composition of electrolytes in the water of each compartment vary. The electrolytes found in the fluid inside the cells differ greatly in amount from those found in the fluid outside the cells. Interstitial fluid in the tissue spaces is similar to plasma (the fluid portion of the blood), except that it contains very little protein. In interstitial fluid the principal cation is sodium, and the main anions are chlorides and bicarbonates. Intracellular cations are mostly potassium and magnesium, whereas the anions are chiefly phosphates and bicarbonates. Thus chemical differences exist between the extracellular and the intracellular fluids.

Water equalizes quickly in all body compartments. Therefore rapid water intake does not result in edema but causes swelling of the body's cells and expands and dilutes both the intracellular and extracellular compartments. Salt- and protein-containing solutions remain primarily in the extracellular compartments. Excessive salt intake may lead to edema and visible swelling.

Acid-base balance. The acidity or alkalinity of a solution depends on the concentration of hydrogen, or the H ions present. An acid may be simply defined as a compound that has enough H ions to give some away.

A base or alkali is a compound possessing few H ions. An increase in H ions makes a solution more acid, and a decrease makes a solution more alkaline. The concentration of hydrogen ions is expressed by pH. A neutral fluid has a pH of 7.0 (a lower pH means higher hydrogen ion concentration). An acid solution has a pH value below 7; an alkaline solution has a pH value above 7. The acid-base balance of the blood is maintained in an extremely narrow pH range, normally 7.35 to 7.45. Any slight deviation from this range causes pronounced changes in the cellular functions. This in turn may threaten life. Blood is normally slightly alkaline (pH 7.4). The acid-base balance is maintained by the action of the lungs, kidneys, and buffer systems. The lungs assist in maintaining this equilibrium by varying the rate at which carbon dioxide is blown off, retaining it in acidic form when blood plasma is getting too alkaline or increasing the respiratory rate when the plasma is becoming too acid. When disturbances in blood pH are primarily the result of disease or abnormalities of the respiratory system, the problems resulting are termed either *respiratory alkalosis* or *respiratory acidosis*. The kidneys assist in maintaining the normal pH of blood by regulating the rates of excretion of acids and bases in the urine. Excessive retention of base or loss of acids through diseases of body systems other than the respiratory apparatus results in *metabolic alkalosis;* likewise, excessive retention of acids or loss of base produces *metabolic acidosis*.

Chemical buffer systems protect the acid-base balance of solution by rapidly offsetting changes in its ionized H concentration. Buffer systems defend and maintain the pH of body fluids by protecting against added acid or base.

Fluid volume. The volume of blood plasma, interstitial fluid, and intracellular fluid normally remains relatively constant. Any blood plasma changes that take place during illness usually reflect changes in all body fluids. Since plasma is relatively easy to obtain from the body and the other fluids are not, it is the chosen fluid for analysis.

Maintenance therapy. Fluid therapy aimed at replacing the patient's daily loss of water, electrolytes, and calories is termed *maintenance therapy*. The purpose of maintenance fluid is to keep the body in neutral balance for water, sodium, potassium, and chloride. Water and electrolyte requirements for normal maintenance depend on the child's metabolic rate (calories metabolized), which changes with maturation (Fig. 23-11). Pediatric caloric expenditure can be easily calculated by using the formula in the box.

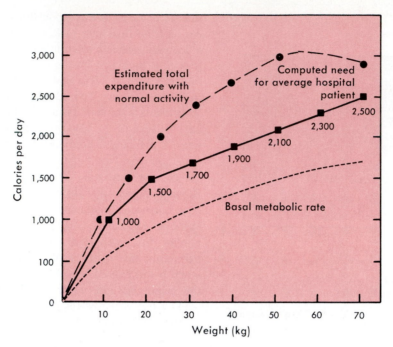

FIG 23-11 Comparison of energy expenditure in basal and ideal state. *(Modified from Holliday MA and Segar WE: Pediatrics 19:824, 1957.)*

The store of fluid in the body comes from ingested liquid and food. A cardinal principle of fluid balance is that fluid intake must equal fluid output. Under normal conditions the requirement for water is usually derived from the need to replace water lost across the skin and lungs (insensible water losses), which maintain body temperature and dissipate the body's metabolic heat and water lost through urine and stool (see boxes on p. 477).

Fluid requirements may be increased in children with increased insensible losses associated with fever, burns, hyperthyroidism, increased respirations, or increased urine production (diabetes insipidus). Less fluid is required when insensible losses are reduced (for example, when children are in croup tents, are on respirators with increased humidity, or have abnormal decreased urine output as in renal failure). Any condition that interferes with an adequate intake of fluid or produces excessive fluid loss threatens the life of the young child.

When fluids are administered parenterally, maintenance electrolytes are necessary to replace urinary, stool, and skin losses of sodium, chloride, and potassium. A child usually needs 3 mEq of sodium, 2 mEq of chloride, and 2 mEq of potassium per 100 kcal expended to meet his maintenance requirements. These electrolyte requirements usually do not need to be altered when maintenance

water requirements are varied. It is important to note, however, that sodium is not given to patients in heart or renal failure. Potassium is excreted almost exclusively by the kidneys; therefore replacement of potassium is withheld until the child has demonstrated adequate renal function. Potassium is omitted if the child is oliguric.

To prevent acidosis and ketosis, reduce protein breakdown, and provide calories, glucose must also be added to most parenteral fluids. Although full caloric replacement is difficult to accomplish, about 5 g/100 kcal/24 hr of glucose should be given. Fluid maintenance and electrolyte requirements should be administered over the greater part of the 24-hour period for which they were intended.

Fluid compartments. Fig. 23-12 illustrates that plasma is the only portion of body water in contact with the external environment. It is the first fluid storage supply to be tapped in gastrointestinal disturbances (vomiting or diarrhea) rapid respirations, or deficient fluid intake. Interstitial fluid is the reservoir that responds most easily to the shifting fluid conditions present in disease (for example, overhydration may cause edema, and dehydration causes the skin to lose its turgor and become wrinkled). The intracellular compartment represents the largest reservoir and is the least accessible. Here water is

Caloric expenditure for average hospitalized child for 24 hours

Body weight (kg)	Caloric expenditure
0 to 10	100 kcal/kg
10 to 20	1,000 kcal + 50 kcal for each kg over 10 kg
Over 20	1,500 kcal + 20 kcal for each kg over 20 kg

Maintenance fluid requirements are proportional to caloric expenditure and can be readily calculated when the caloric requirements have been determined as discussed below. The need for water can be estimated to be 100 ml/100 kcal or 1 ml/kcal. Therefore the milliliters of water required are equal to the calories as ascertained by the previous method (for example, a 12 kg child would require 1,000 + (2 × 50) = 1,100 cal and 1,100 ml of water).

Maintenance water requirements*

Output per 100 ml intake	
Urine	60 ml
Insensible water loss†	
Skin	30 ml
Lungs	15 ml
Sweat	0 to 25 ml
Stool water	5 to 10 ml
Hidden intake	
Water of oxidation	Approximately 10 ml (subtract from output)
	100 ml/100 kcal

*Daily water requirements will approximate 100 ml/100 kcal metabolized.
†Water losses associated with diarrhea or with heavy sweating must be treated as abnormal. Replacement requirements must be computed separately.

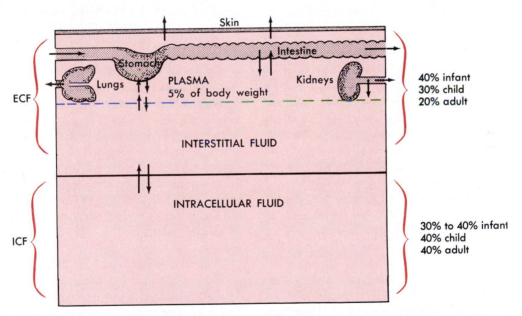

FIG 23-12 Relative fluid balance in children and adults expressed in percentage of total body weight.

lost or gained over a period of days. Without water a well infant in a temperate environment can live 3 days or more, and an adult can survive about 10 days.

Several differences between body fluid compartments in the infant and older child must be considered. A newborn infant's weight is approximately 80% water, the older child's is 70% water, and the adult's is 60% water. This percentage varies with the amount of fat. Since fat is essentially water-free, a lean individual has a greater proportion of water to total body weight. The proportion of intracellular fluid to body weight remains comparatively constant at all ages. Extracellular fluid constitutes

NURSING CARE PLAN

The Child with a Fluid Volume Deficit

Selected nursing diagnoses	Expected outcomes	Interventions
A. Fluid volume deficit related to active losses from vomiting or diarrhea. Clinical manifestations: Thirst, lethargy, irritability, sunken fontanel, dry mucous membranes, absence of tears, soft and sunken eyes, poor skin turgor, decreased urinary output, weight loss, increased pulse, temperature, and respiration rate, decreased BP, poor peripheral circulation.	Child maintains adequate hydration.	Assess child for signs of dehydration; see opposite column for clinical manifestations. Make NPO. Monitor IV fluids as ordered. Maintain strict I&O. Obtain daily weight (same time and scale). Check urine, specific gravity of void. Monitor IV fluids as ordered. Utilize creative methods for drinking (colorful straws and cups, drinking from syringe) when allowed until symptoms subside. Offer child's favorite fluids as appropriate.

about 40% of the infant's weight as compared with 20% of the adult's body weight. An infant, then, may approach a fluid loss of 10% of body weight before a severe fluid deficit occurs, whereas a weight loss of 5% represents a severe fluid volume deficit in the adult. However, one should remember that 10% of a baby's body weight is not very much.

Although the infant's body has a relatively greater fluid content per pound, a baby is *more vulnerable* to fluid volume deficit than the adult. There are several reasons why infants lose a proportionately larger volume of water daily. The baby's body surface in relation to body weight is three times that of the older child. Therefore infants lose a relatively greater amount of fluid through the skin and gastrointestinal tract. Their high metabolic rate produces more waste products, which must be diluted for excretion. Their immature kidneys are less able to concentrate urine, thus adding to the volume of urine. Accumulation of acidic wastes (because of the high metabolic rate and immature kidneys) stimulates respiration, causing greater evaporation through the lungs. Infants may react to infections with higher temperatures, which also result in a higher water loss from evaporation. As the nurse reviews these facts about

the infant's body fluid balance, she can more readily understand why the infant, at one-twentieth the adult's weight, requires one third as much water.

Dehydration. Inadequate fluid intake or excessive fluid loss causes dehydration. It is almost always associated with fever, burns, vomiting, diarrhea, hyperventilation, or hemorrhage. Dehydration seldom denotes water loss alone but rather loss of fluid volume, electrolytes, and water. During periods of dehydration, plasma volume is usually maintained at the expense of interstitial volume.

Clinically, dehydration is described as the percentage of body weight that has been lost as water. The most accurate method to assess the child's degree of dehydration is by noting changes in body weight.

Mild	5%
Moderate	7% to 10%
Severe	10% to 15%

Since accurate recorded weight before the child's episode of dehydration is seldom available, clinical signs of dehydration have been defined.

Early signs of dehydration in a patient are dry lips and mucous membranes, diminished urinary output, reduced weight, and lethargy. Moderate dehydration is further characterized by depressed fontanels, sunken eyeballs, loss of skin turgor, and oliguria. As dehydration increases, the child becomes acutely ill, and the circulation may fail. The skin is grayish; the pulse is rapid and weak. Temperature elevation and low blood pressure are characteristic. Recorded output is scant, and weight loss is obvious—10% or higher. Apathy, restlessness, and even convulsions may occur. An infant's condition may require the use of preweighed diapers to determine output. Each gram increase in the weight of a urine-wet diaper is counted as 1 ml of output. Obviously, diapers must be changed and weighed promptly. The blanket under the infant may need to be preweighed as well. It should be next to a waterproof pad.

Intravenous therapy. Because it is often difficult to perform and maintain a conventional intravenous infusion for prolonged periods in the small child, a *cutdown* may be performed (Fig. 23-13). This is a minor but important surgical procedure that is usually completed in the treatment room. The physician "cuts down" to a vein, directly exposing it. Small plastic tubing is inserted into a minute nick in the vein and sutured in place. This tubing is then joined to the intravenous tubing. The increased

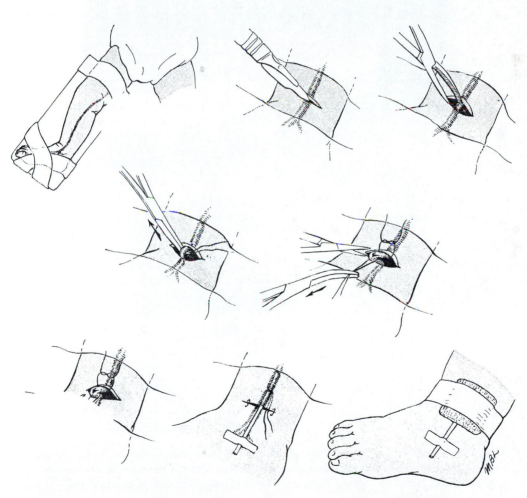

FIG 23-13 Cutdown procedure. Great care is necessary in immobilizing leg to prevent impairment of circulation and pressure areas. Cutdown may be used for a number of days to help maintain fluid balance or administer medication. It is used when vein access is difficult or precarious.

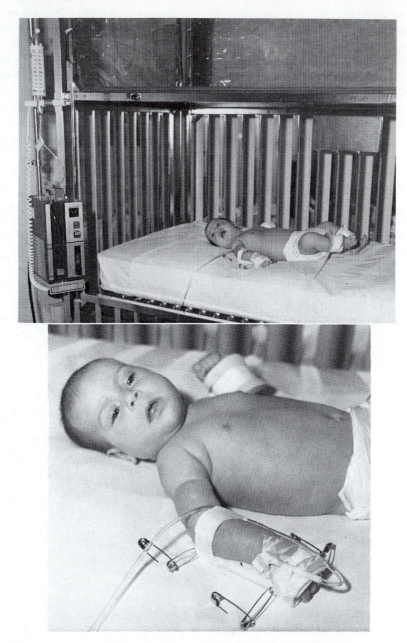

FIG 23-14 Intravenous fluid with IVAC gravity flow infusion controller can be set for specific amount of fluid delivery and is able to detect infiltration. Side rail down for illustration only. Arm board is pinned to bedding. Close-up shows arm immobilization. *(Courtesy Naval Hospital, San Diego.)*

use of small angiocatheters, which are threaded through a needle puncture into a vein, has reduced the need for cutdowns.

Whether fluids are administered through a cutdown or a needle puncture through the skin into a vein of the scalp or extremity, it is important that the amount of fluid given to the child is gauged very carefully to prevent overloading the circulatory system. The rate of flow ordered should be known, marked on the bottle, and meticulously observed. Special pediatric intravenous counting chambers simplify calculation. The typical drop size is 1/60 ml or 60 drops/ml. Although a number of semi-automatic infusion sets have added a special margin of safety to administering fluids, the nurse must continue to keep a close watch on the flow rate, the infusion site, and the child's response to the fluid therapy. The infant and small child must be appropriately restrained to prevent dislodging the infusion. The nurse should be aware that changes in the child's position may slow or speed the infusion, and the nurse should frequently observe the rate of flow in the drip chamber (Fig. 23-14). Extreme care should be exercised in moving the patient. The vocational nurse shares responsibility for observation of the intravenous apparatus with the supervising registered nurse. If the nurse observes an infusion running more rapidly than ordered, she should slow it to the known

rate, but she must immediately check the physician's orders to verify the desired drip rate. The area surrounding the IV needle must be checked frequently to detect infiltration or inflammation. Pain and swelling are signs of possible dislocation of the needle.

The responsibility for observation is even greater if the child is receiving blood. There is more danger of circulatory overload, tissue damage, and untoward reactions. Patients receiving blood should be carefully watched and, when necessary and possible, questioned regarding back or chest pain or chills. The temperature, pulse, and respiratory rate should be frequently determined and the skin observed for hives to detect any possible incompatibility.

Parenteral hyperalimentation. Some children who cannot tolerate oral or nasogastric feedings can survive by intravenous alimentation. Total parenteral hyperalimentation provides glucose; proteins, fats (lipids), minerals, vitamins, and fluid necessary for normal growth and weight gain. Two intravenous methods for total parenteral nutrition (TPN) are currently used: (1) a central venous line may be established by threading a silastic catheter through an incision on the side of the neck into a jugular to the superior vena cava (2) a multipurpose Hickman and or Broviac catheter may be installed by way of the jugular vein into the right atrium, exiting via

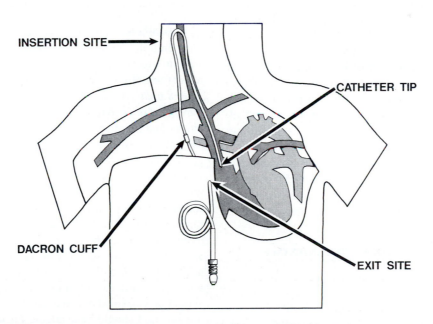

INSERTION SITE

CATHETER TIP

DACRON CUFF

EXIT SITE

FIG 23-15 The Hickman indwelling right atrial catheter provides long-term venous access for drawing blood and for giving total parenteral nutrition, medications, and blood products. *(Courtesy Virginia Shumate, BSN, Children's Hospital and Health Center, San Diego, Calif.)*

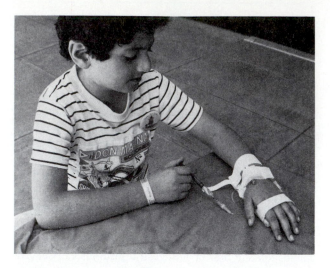

FIG 23-16 Young boy with hemophilia injecting heparin flush into his heparin lock.

a subcutaneous tunnel on the right thorax or sternum (Fig. 23-15). Peripheral or surface veins may be used as a temporary method for more diluted nutritional supplement, that is, peripheral hyperalimentation. The first two approaches may be preferable, since a concentrated life-sustaining solution can be given at a uniform rate into large veins where it will dilute rapidly and thereby prevent thrombosis and phlebitis. However, meticulous sterile technique is required to prevent infection. Hyperalimentation using peripheral veins runs the risk of severe tissue damage if infiltration should occur.

For short-term venous access the heparin lock is used for patients receiving intermittent medicines. It allows more mobility without the need for continuous intravenous fluids or frequent venipunctures. The heparin lock (Fig. 23-16) consists of a short flexible catheter or scalp vein needle attached to plastic tubing sealed by a rubber insert that is maintained in a manner ensuring patency and sterility. The following procedure is included to increase the licensed vocational nurse's understanding of the heparin lock technique, although state regulations may limit her function in this area.

HEPARIN LOCK INSTALLATION AND MAINTENANCE

EQUIPMENT

1. Tourniquet
2. Povidone-iodine solution sponges
3. Adhesive tape
4. 2 × 2 in sterile gauze pads
5. A special 22- or 24-gauge intravascular catheter (Quick-cath), or No. 23 or 25 gauge butterfly scalp vein needle

6. Heparin lock injection adaptor
7. Heparin lock flush (10 to 100 units/ml heparinized solution)
8. 3-ml syringe for heparin lock flush
9. 25-gauge 5/8-inch needle for subsequent clearing of tubing, Quick-cath, or needle with saline and/or heparin lock flush
10. Alcohol sponges
11. 3-ml syringe for normal saline

PROCEDURE (protocols vary in different agencies, and modifications may occur according to type of patient, equipment used and medication administered. Refer to agency procedure.)

1. Skin is cleansed; intravascular catheter or needle is inserted into arm vein and taped in position.
2. Heparin lock injection adaptor is attached.
3. Injection port is cleansed with alcohol before any injection or infusion is performed. Small needles (23- to 25-gauge) must be used to prevent large puncture holes in the injection port.
   a. Saline can be used to clear tubing of any blood or tubing can be flushed before a change in tubing solutions.
   b. Heparin lock flush is instilled last to maintain the patency of the line.
   c. A heparin lock should be checked for patency and flushed with saline or heparin lock flush 1.0 ml.
   d. Careful instructions and return demonstrations must accompany the outpatient use of this device.

Cleanliness. Satisfying the need for cleanliness is almost entirely the responsibility of the nursing staff. The way in which it is met depends on the condition of the patient and the facilities of the pediatric unit.

Bed bath. A bath is usually administered each day to prevent skin irritation and provide refreshment, stimulation, and comfort. It also serves as an excellent period for patient observation and evaluation. Bed baths are given routinely to patients who are quite ill, are especially susceptible to chilling and respiratory tract infections, have dressings or incisions to be protected, or are in traction or casts. Most children with elevated temperatures usually have bed baths, although occasionally a tepid tub bath may be ordered to reduce fever. Bed baths are carried out in essentially the same manner for children as for adults. A bath blanket or towel should be used for a covering, and except in the case of an infant, the area should be curtained or screened. Unless contraindicated, a good light should be available for the bath area to aid in the detection of any special changes in skin color, rashes, or other abnormalities.

Perineal care. Children should be helped with the care

of their genitalia if they are too young to cleanse the area properly. Any irritation of the penis or labia should be reported. If a little boy is uncircumcised, no extraordinary force should be exerted to retract the foreskin, nor once retracted should it remain so, but observation of the area for cleanliness and possible inflammation should be made. Occasionally, more formal perineal care using an irrigation technique is desirable to encourage cleanliness, especially in the case of older girls having their menses.

Nails. The nails of young children often need attention. Cleaning the nails when necessary should be part of the daily care. Usually, the nails of children may be cut or filed without an order except when the patient is diabetic or has peripheral circulatory, sensory, or bleeding disorders.

Oral hygiene. Oral hygiene should also be carried out routinely. However, remember that a child with a recent cleft lip, cleft palate, or dental repair usually is not allowed to have a brush or anything hard in his mouth. For those too young to have more than two or three teeth, oral hygiene may be a simple drink of water, but for older children the essentials of good care of the teeth should be taught. A small toothbrush that can easily fit into the mouth is needed. Massage of the gums and correct brushing and flossing of the teeth are important health habits and often make food and fluid intake more pleasant. Cracked or dry lips may be lubricated with petrolatum.

Bed patients are usually dressed in pajamas or gowns, but sometimes if the child is convalescent, a bright dress or shirt may be a big lift to the morale of the child and parents.

Unit care. Part of the daily care of the patients is the care of their units. The bath is not technically complete until the unit is clean and orderly. Whether a complete linen change is necessary depends on its condition. Most children's beds need frequent changes, but linen should not be used needlessly.

The patient's bedside stand should be neat (inside and out), and the unit furniture wiped down with a moist paper towel. The aim is not to have each bed "just so" with a neat and clean but unhappy occupant; instead, the intention is to cut down on confusion and reduce safety hazards. Children *need* their toys and a certain amount of freedom in their bed activities. But they are not aided by mounds of equipment taking over their beds or cribs. In some hospitals, special bags are available for toy storage. In addition, the patient's room should be comfortably warm and well ventilated but free from drafts.

Tub bath. When tub baths are allowed, the amount of supervision required depends on the age and condition of the child. Young children should never be left alone because of the danger of burning from the hot water faucet, drowning, or falling while trying to climb out. Teenagers usually resent observation in the tub room and many times need only a minimum of supervision. Unless a prolonged tub bath is ordered for treatment purposes, the bath should not be too extended. There is greater possibility of chilling, and others may be waiting in line. When facilities are available, there is a greater tendency than formerly to give hospitalized children tub baths. Use of bubble bath and shampoo in bath water have been found to cause urinary tract irritation in some children. Be sure to clean the tub well after each child is finished.

A prolonged tub bath lasts at least 20 minutes. It may be ordered to relax the muscles before physical therapy, to help remove dressings or crusts, or to apply a certain soothing medication to the skin, such as oatmeal or Alpha Keri. To help the patient relax in the bath and get the whole body in contact with the water, a pillow may be constructed from a rolled bath blanket to raise the head out of the water while the child lies flat in the tub. If a rubber headrest is available, it may be used for this purpose.

Infant tub bath. The infant receiving a tub bath is placed in a small basin for greater security and easier handling. The following procedure can be used for a newborn infant whose umbilicus has healed or, with modification, for an older infant. It can be carried out at the bedside, at a special table or counter, or at home in a clean sink. Wherever the bath is given, the principles are the same, although the organization and details of equipment may be different. The nurse may wish to place the tub on a bedside table and use the bed for drying and dressing the infant. Use of a technique or feeding gown by the nurse may help reduce cross-infection and protect her uniform. The older child who enjoys the bath and is able to sit steadily may be allowed more freedom in the tub.

INFANT TUB BATH

MATERIALS NEEDED

1. Baby bathtub, large basin, or bathinette
2. Suggested supplies on tray
   a. Mild soap
   b. Jar of cotton balls
   c. Jar of safety pins
   d. Bottle of baby lotion

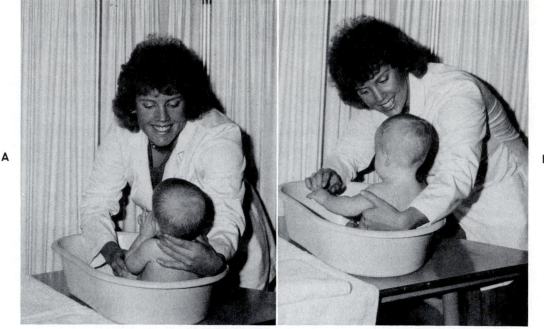

FIG 23-17 **A** and **B,** Two methods of supporting infant during tub bath.

e. Bottle of sterile water
f. Box of tissues
3. Large towel or mat used for drying and dressing area
4. Bag or hamper for discard of dirty clothes
5. Wastebasket to receive trash
6. One soft towel for drying
7. Two soft washcloths or paper mesh squares
8. Clean baby clothes stacked in order of use
   a. Diaper
   b. Shirt
   c. Kimono
   d. Receiving blanket
9. Apron or feeding gown

PRINCIPLES

1. Maintain infant warmth as much as possible
2. Wash, proceeding from clean to dirty areas
3. Support the infant appropriately, maintaining control of his head and guarding his safety (Fig. 23-17)
4. Use the bath time for careful observation and stimulation; enjoy the baby

PROCEDURE

1. Check the temperature of the room (should be 72° to 75° F [22° to 24° C] and free from drafts).
2. Wash hands thoroughly; put on apron.
3. Assemble equipment. (Never leave baby alone in tub, for instance, to seek supplies or answer the phone.)

4. Fill tub one third full of water that is at a temperature comfortable to your elbow.
5. Place the infant, still dressed to preserve body heat, on the mat.
   a. Inspect eyes, wash lids proceeding from the inner corner of the eye outward. A fresh washcloth surface or cotton dipped in clear water is appropriate.
   b. Inspect the ears; wash outer folds. Do not probe canals.
   c. Wash the face with the washcloth and clear water from the tub. Dry.
   d. Soap the scalp; support infant, using the football hold (see p. 256). The infant's head is held over the tub, his ears covered by the nurse's fingers. Rinse the scalp carefully. Dry. Check for "cradle cap."
6. Remove shirt and diaper. If the buttocks are grossly soiled with stool, discard the washcloth used for the cleanup and use another to continue the bath, or use tissues for initial cleanup.
7. The infant's body may be soaped either before being placed in the tub for rinsing or during the time he is in the tub, whichever way the nurse feels more secure.
8. Lift the child carefully into the tub, feet first, using appropriate holds.
9. After a relatively brief period, lift the infant out of the tub and place on a towel on the mat; pat infant dry.
10. Inspect and clean female genitalia with damp cotton balls or tissues as needed, wiping from front to back.

Retraction of the foreskin on male infants should not be forced. Many infants have adhesions in the area. Gently cleanse the glans.

11. Dry the infant carefully; dress in clean clothes and a receiving blanket.
12. Offer drinking water and inspect his mouth.

NOTE: The use of talcum powder is not necessary and has been associated with instances of aspiration. Baby oil has been thought to block pores and encourage infection.

Shampoo. The state of the patient's scalp, the patient's general condition, and the length of the hair determine the need for a shampoo.

Whether a shampoo for an older child must be ordered by the physician depends on hospital policy, the condition of the child, and the type of shampoo contemplated. Many children can easily have their hair shampooed by lying on a gurney with their heads extended over the end next to a sink or tub. A trough to guide the water may be constructed of plastic or rubber sheeting. If a wall spray hose is used, great care should be taken in regulating the temperature of the water before it touches the child.

If the child is bedfast, a simple head basin and trough can be constructed from two bath blankets rolled together lengthwise (like a snake) and curved into a horseshoe shape with the open end pointing toward the side of the bed. This form is draped by a plastic sheeting to make a waterproof basin that leads off the side of the bed into a large bath basin or baby tub. Some hospitals use inflated Kelly pads. A few have bed shampoo basins available, similar to those found in beauty salons. The hair must be rinsed of suds until squeaky clean. Some patients like a vinegar or lemon rinse. Hair should be dried quickly to prevent chilling the child.

Rest. Personal and environmental cleanliness and order should promote rest, but rest is not automatic. Nap times must be provided and promoted. Most children do best with a rest period after lunch, lasting at least 1 hour. Other nap times should be encouraged, depending on the needs of the child. Shades should be drawn, the television set turned off, the area straightened up, and the child covered comfortably. A reminder of something pleasant that can happen after a rest is often helpful in making the nap more acceptable.

Diversion, self-expression, coping mechanisms, and acceptance (Table 23-2). A convalescing child should not be expected to sit or lie quietly all day long without diversion and opportunities for self-expression. Although rest is very important, a child may rest better when allowed moderate activity during the day. To stay perfectly still is impossible, and the attempt may be fatiguing in itself. The nurse can help by supplying appropriate toys, providing suitable television programs, setting up controlled group play for patients in the same room when possible, playing with the child herself, or asking for the help of the "play lady" or auxiliary worker. She may enlist the aid of occupational or recreational therapists or Child Life workers if they are available. A hospital library may be a good resource.

Play is a learning activity that promotes physical, mental, emotional, and social growth. In play children develop new abilities, acquire knowledge about themselves, and explore the feel, look, and taste of the world around them. They use play to express what they are thinking and feeling and to relate and interact with others. Dramatic play is recognized as a form of emotional release.

The nurse can help children choose play materials that will be fun and satisfying. The following principles should be kept in mind when choosing toys: (1) suitability for a particular age, (2) safety, and (3) durability.

Choosing the right play materials at the right time is not an easy task. However, an understanding of the wide variety of play interests can often give helpful clues.

Every child needs a well-balanced toy selection for all-around development. The choice should be planned to stimulate (1) social play, (2) dramatic play, (3) creative play, (4) manipulation and constructive play, and (5) active physical play.

Play activity is as vital to growth as medicine, food, and sleep. What is the worth of a healed body if the mind is permanently limited from lack of opportunity to grow socially and emotionally?

Medication

The administration of medication to young children entails special skills and knowledge. It is a particularly heavy responsibility because dosages vary so greatly from child to child, as the result of weight, body area, and metabolic differences.

General principles. Pediatric dosages may be calculated in different ways. Age is still used occasionally as a basis for determination.

Young's rule:

Child's dose =

$$\frac{\text{Age of child in years}}{\text{Age of child in years} + 12} \times \text{Average adult dose}$$

Table 23-2 Play-and-get-well chart

Age	Interest	Toys	Books
Infant (Birth to 1 yr)	Toys that attract the eye, make little sounds, and tempt grasping hands	Bright hanging objects; large plastic rings; string of bright-colored rings; rubber toys that squeak; tinkling bells	None (enjoys a song or lullaby)
Toddler (1 to 3 yr)	Toys that enable parallel play, provide security and attention, and help development of muscle coordination	Nest of blocks; mallet and wooden pegs; trucks and cars; cuddly toy animals; large dolls; rocking horse; toy telephone; musical toys; kiddie car	Large linen picture books; nursery rhymes; ABC books; farm and zoo animal stories Likes the same story over and over again
Preschooler (3 to 6 yr)	Toys that stimulate child's imagination and develop creative abilities	Nurse and doctor sets; trains and trucks; Tinker Toys; cabin logs; magnets; toy army men; record player; hand puppets; crayons and color books; dolls and clothes; simple puzzles; modeling clay; scrapbooks; cuddly toy animals	Dr. Seuss books; Golden Books; once-upon-a-time stories Enjoys stories about airplanes, trains, and police and fire stations Likes to look at pictures while being read to
Early school age (6 to 10 yr)	Application of mental as well as physical skills Interest and enjoyment in playing with children of same sex Realistic toys that bring child into contact with world outside hospital	Craft sets; models; picture painting; stamp collection; string marionettes; spool knitting; beadwork Games such as Monopoly, checkers, and Clue Paper and pencil games; jigsaw puzzles; paper dolls; video games	Comic books; riddle books; crossword puzzles; fairy tales; adventure stories; simple science book; how and why books; who-when-where books; *Highlights*
Middle school age (10 to 12 yr)	Adaptable to group activities Combine companionship and challenge and coordinate work and play in teams	Card games; photoelectric football; science toys; chess; checkers Skill crafts such as sculpting and wood carving Walkie-talkie; telescope; transistor radio; camera; television; picture viewer	Comic books; school textbooks; biographies; adventure stories Junior classics such as *Heidi, Little Women, Treasure Island, Robin Hood, Alice in Wonderland, Andersen's Fairy Tales, Aesop's Tales*

Because the sizes of children who are the same age may differ, Clark's rule, which is based on weight, is the safer way to calculate dosage:

Clark's rule:

Child's dose =

$$\frac{\textbf{Weight of child in pounds}}{150} \times \textbf{Average adult dose}$$

Another concept used in computing pediatric dosage is based on the surface area of a child.*

*Campbell J: The BSA method of calculating pediatric drug dosage, Am J Matern Child Nurs 3:357, 1978.

With this method one must know the metric weight and height of the child to calculate the surface area in square meters. The average surface area of an adult is calculated to be 1.7 square meters. The final formula used is:

$$\frac{\textbf{Surface area of child (m}^2\textbf{)}}{1.7} \times \textbf{Average adult dose}$$

Some dosages must be individualized for the specific child by his physician.

Giving medication is sometimes difficult because the child often does not recognize the need for the medicine and may, despite the kindliest approach, resist its administration. However, although the licensed vocational nurse usually is not given major responsibility in the administration of medicines in the pediatric area, she should know the principles involved and receive practice in giving selected medications to children during her pediatric experience.

As with the administration of medication anytime, the following factors must be identified:

1. The right patient
2. The right medication in the right form
3. The right dosage
4. The right method of administration
5. The right time of administration

Before any medication is given, it should be identified on a medicine card or on the medication Kardex. In some hospitals, orders for certain medications must be renewed after a certain time. Common medications that are often automatically stopped unless reordered are broad-spectrum antibiotics and narcotics. Medications that are ordered on an "as necessary" or p.r.n. basis must be checked to see when they were last given to prevent too-frequent administration. It also must be determined whether the need for the medication truly exists. The nurse should look up any unfamiliar medication before assuming the responsibility for its administration. She should know its common usages, contraindications, side effects, common dosages, and peculiarities of administration.

Common measurements. Before giving medications, the nurse should review the common measurements used in the metric and apothecary systems and frequently used conversions. There should be an easily read table available for her reference. Some of the most common conversions follow:

1 dram (℥, dr)	= 4 ml
1 teaspoon (tsp)	= 5 ml
1 tablespoon (tbsp)	= 15 ml
1 ounce (℥, oz)	= 30 ml
15 or 16 minims (℥xv or ℥xvi)	= 1 ml
15 grains (gr xv)	= 1 g
1 grain (gr i)	= 0.06 g or 60 to 65 mg

Oral medication

Preparation. If possible, medications for children are prepared as solutions for greater ease in administration. Suspensions must always be shaken well before being poured. Most may be diluted, although it is not wise to dilute medicines more than a few milliliters to wash out

the measuring container. Children might not take the increased volume easily. Placing medication in a baby's formula is also precarious. If the baby refuses to take all the formula, how much of the medication has been taken? Was the medication evenly distributed throughout? These are difficult questions to answer.

Administration. Before giving any type of medication, the nurse must check the patient's identification. Very young children cannot identify themselves. It is imperative that the nurse check their identification bands.

Always place a bib on a small child before administering oral medications. Such a simple maneuver saves many extra changes and important minutes of the nurse's time, which is best used in other ways. Remember, if a child is given water or other fluid to wash down a pill, this liquid must be recorded on the intake record.

Fluid medications may be given fairly easily to infants when placed in a nipple fitted in a standard ring (used on ring-and-disc–type baby bottles). The baby sucks out the medication while the nurse supports the head to prevent aspiration. Small medication cups are also employed. Syringes may also be used to administer oral fluids, thus increasing the accuracy of the dose. The medicine is poured slowly with the baby in a sitting position or with his head elevated. Rubber-tipped medicine droppers may be helpful too. Pills and capsules usually must be crushed or opened for children under 5 years of age. Giving nonliquid medication to younger children may also increase the danger of aspiration. The medication may be placed in syrup, or jelly and given from a spoon. Many of these medications are bitter so that a good disguise must be used. However, children must never be told that they are receiving candy when they are being medicated.

The child who takes medicine well should be praised for being such a big boy or girl. If children find it difficult to take medicine, they should be made to feel that the nurse understands some of their distaste and fear and wants to help them during this brief but difficult period. Although a young child may be helped by gentle restraint in the administration of medicines (the nurse may hold the child on her lap with one of the child's hands wedged behind her and the other controlled by her encircling arm and hand) (Fig. 23-18), pouring medication down the throat of a struggling, crying youngster is an invitation to aspiration, early emesis of the medication, and subsequent trying periods when medicine time comes again. At times children respond much better if allowed to hold the cup and drink at their own rate. Many of the small, disposable medicine cups are safe play objects for suc-

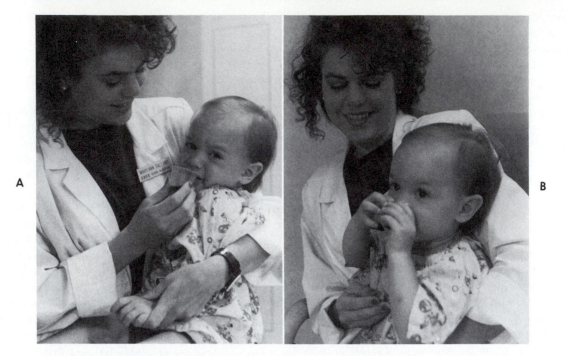

FIG 23-18 **A,** Medicine time—the nurse appropriately encircles Chris with her arm and holds his hand. His other arm is tucked behind her back. He will take the medicine in this position but he much prefers to hold the cup himself and take the medicine until "all gone" (**B**).

cessful medicine takers, who in turn pretend to medicate dolls and stuffed toys.

Intramuscular injections. When the nurse gives an intramuscular injection to a child, she usually needs a second person to help support, distract, restrain, or comfort the child. If the child is old enough to understand, the nurse should explain the procedure just before administering the injection. Resistant, tearful children might be told that the medicine will help them get better so that they can go home sooner. The infant or younger child needs to be restrained adequately to ensure safe and correct administration of the drug. For most infants and children an injection simply means "hurt" and may establish a lasting fear. To lessen a child's fear and to maintain a degree of trust, the nurse should always comfort him by holding him afterward. When dealing with an older child she should indicate that she understands why he reacts the way he does.

EQUIPMENT

1. Damp antiseptic sponge
2. 1 or 3 ml syringe
3. 22-gauge, 1-inch needle for infants and children
4. 23-gauge, ¾-inch needle for tiny infants
5. Band-Aid?

Because the gluteal muscle is not well developed in the infant or young child, and permanent sciatic nerve damage is possible, the buttocks are never used for an intramuscular injection. The most desirable sites for pediatric injections are the lateral and anterior aspects of the thighs, the deltoid areas, and the soft tissue inferior to the iliac crests (Fig. 23-19). The medicine and syringe should be completely prepared and ready for use before the nurse enters the child's room.

Method. The site is cleansed with the antiseptic damp sponge, using a circular motion. The skin is pulled taut. In young children who have minimal muscle, the needle is inserted at a slightly oblique angle; if the child is large and well developed, it is inserted perpendicularly. The plunger is pulled back to ensure that the needle is not in a blood vessel, and the medicine is injected slowly. The sponge is placed over the needle, the needle is quickly withdrawn, and the area is gently wiped with the sponge. A bandage is usually placed over the site. Many older children seem to be helped a great deal if they can grasp the crib sides with their hands and count during an injection. Some gain satisfaction in helping to put on a Band-Aid after the procedure. Afterward a child should be comforted by the nurse administering the injection, if possible. After all, she is not his enemy but a special

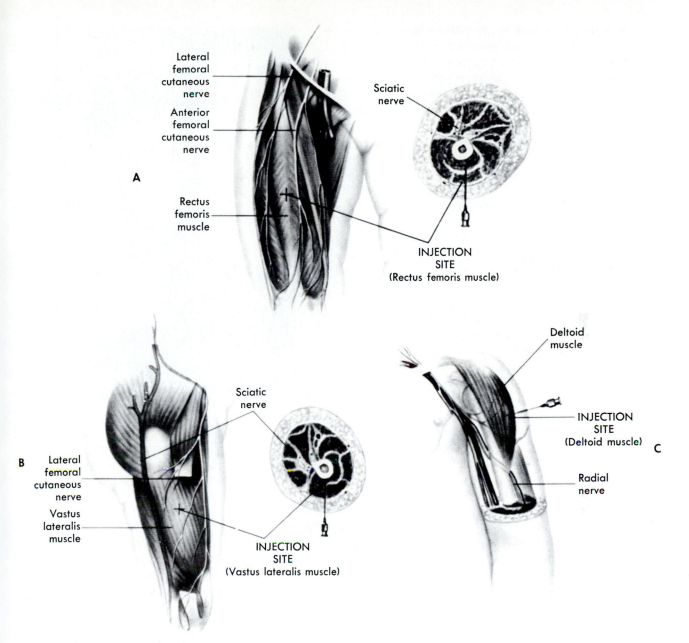

FIG 23-19 Site of injection chart. Most desirable sites for pediatric intramuscular injections are rectus femoris muscle (**A**); vastus lateralis muscle (**B**); deltoid muscle (**C**).

friend, and everything should be done to help the child recognize this.

Suppositories. Aspirin, sedative drugs, and bowel stimulants are often given to children in the form of rectal suppositories. Most of these suppositories can be lubricated with a jellylike material before insertion. Since they are often refrigerated to preserve their shape, warming them, unwrapped, in a clean hand for about a minute may be helpful. The nurse should wear a clean glove for the insertion of the suppository. The child should be asked to take a deep breath, if possible, and the medication should be pushed about 2 inches past the rectal sphincter. After insertion, pressure should be exerted on the buttocks, holding them together for more than a minute. Otherwise the suppository may be ejected and its effect lost.

Nose drops. Nose drops are ordered fairly often for infants and children. They are primarily used to combat nasal congestion and make breathing, eating, and drinking easier. In the case of an infant, nose drops may be ordered 20 minutes before meals to improve sucking and formula intake. If the nose is very congested, gentle suctioning of the nasal passageway may be indicated before the drops are administered. It does no good if the drops only roll in and out again or do not remain in the nose. Young children do not understand the reason for nose drops and may need to be gently restrained by a second person or by a modified mummy restraint. The child should be lying down with the head tilted back over a folded towel or small pillow. The dropper should be pointed slightly toward the top of the nasal cavity. The child should maintain this position for several seconds after the instillation. Oily nose drops should be avoided because of the possibility of aspiration and lipoid pneumonia.

Ear drops. Ear drops are still used occasionally in the pediatric area. They should not be cold but close to body temperature or warm. Cold ear drops are painful. The child's head should be resting comfortably on the bed, turned with the ear to be treated exposed. When ear drops are given to children under 3 years of age, the earlobe should be gently pulled down and back to straighten the canal. Older children and adults should have their earlobes pulled up and back for the same reason. After instillation, cotton should not be routinely inserted because it may interfere with drainage of discharge to the exterior or serve to soak up the recently instilled medication.

Eye drops. Eye drops, when ordered, should not be dropped on the cornea but instilled in the lower conjunctival sac while the child, lying flat, tries to look at the hair on top of his head. After instillation of the eye drops, his eyes should be lightly closed, not squeezed shut, since this may force out the medication. It is a good practice with some toxic medications such as atropine to put a little pressure at the inner angle of the eye after the drop has been placed to prevent drainage into the nose through the tear duct.

Topical medication. Ointments or creams may be applied to the skin with a finger cot or buttered on gauze with a sterile tongue blade if the area is to be covered with a sterile compress. Liniments and lotions are often applied with clean hands or cotton balls, depending on their contents and the condition of the area to be treated.

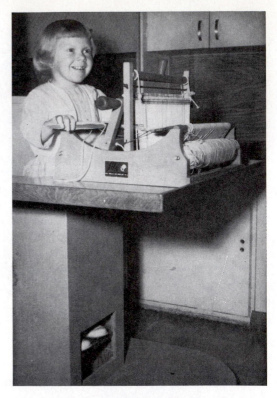

FIG 23-20 Susan enjoys her weaving in occupational therapy. Stand-up table with little gate at back helps her maintain balance. Finger exercise encourages joint movement that is so necessary for rheumatoid arthritis patients like Susan. *(Courtesy Children's Hospital and Health Center, San Diego, Calif.)*

Special treatments

Special treatments related to the particular physical problem that the child may be facing are discussed in separate chapters describing procedures involving the various body functions, systems, or diseases.

Provisions for rehabilitation

As convalescence progresses, provisions for rehabilitation may be necessary to recapture skills lost during illness. This usually begins during hospitalization and continues after discharge. In some cases the problem involved is not so much rehabilitation as *habilitation*, or the formation of skills not previously mastered. This is particularly true of patients suffering from neuromusculoskeletal problems. Emphasis is placed on the development of function with the least cosmetic defect and maximum appearance of normalcy. Priority is placed on skills needed for daily tasks. The hospital may have a special rehabilitation unit. (See discussion in Chapter 20.)

Physical therapy. Those engaged in the specialty of physical therapy concern themselves primarily with the treatment of disease and injury by physical agents such as heat, cold, electricity, and water. The most common techniques used involve therapeutic exercises in and out of water. These specially prescribed exercises are fundamental to the treatment of delayed motor development and respiratory, orthopedic, and neuromuscular disease. They are designed to prevent and correct deformities, increase muscle strength and function, and establish normal postural reflexes. The physical therapist institutes normal patterns of motion and teaches coordination, balance, walking, and stair-climbing (with and without orthopedic appliances), as well as other activities of daily living (ADL). Thus through the careful selection of techniques the physical therapist prevents deformity, relieves pain, and promotes functional capacity.

Occupational therapy. Occupational therapy is more often concerned with the maintenance or stimulation of small muscle control necessary for the accomplishment of more refined but equally important skills involving finger and wrist manipulation (Fig. 23-20). Occupational therapy uses many crafts to motivate and involve the patient in activities that strengthen muscles or are psychologically stimulating. Weaving, ceramics, shell jewelry manufacturing, woodworking, and painting are usually just means to an end—a better-functioning patient. Often the occupational therapy department can locate or fashion equipment to aid the patient in carrying out necessary ADLs: appliances that help malfunctioning hands to hold combs and toothbrushes, special cups, plate guards, angled spoons and forks to help with eating, and elastic shoelaces and long-handled gadget sticks to aid in dressing are just a few of many possibilities (see Fig. 31-17).

Other specialties. Speech therapists and hearing specialists often help to fit the child or youth for life by meeting the child's needs for communication and participation. A bedside teacher provided by the public school system may make the return transition from hospital to regular school less difficult. Greater provision for socialization, according to the developmental needs of the child, should be considered to provide for optimum personality development for children undergoing long-term hospitalization. A sense of individual worth, importance, and purposefulness should be fostered.

• • •

An appreciation of the importance of individuals and the contributions they make to their world should be part of the nursing perspective of the staff. If the child or youth is personally incapable of making a constructive contribution, society itself may become a source of growth and hope by channeling efforts toward rewarding research and increasing compassion and understanding. A nurse should have a faith that recognizes the tragic realities of life without destroying its sweetness, a philosophy that allows her to give without becoming empty and brittle, and an outlook that carefully measures minutes in the light of an eternity.

Recording

Although the recording of nursing observations and care may seem to be of minor importance when compared with the proper execution of these responsibilities, clear, concise, and appropriate record keeping is a nursing necessity. Nursing notes serve as a permanent record of the patient's treatments, medications, and changing condition. It is especially important to have a clear record of pediatric patients who often, because of their ages, lack communication skills. The nurse's notes may help influence therapy, may be important in research studies, or may become of specific legal importance.

The notes should be hand-printed in ink. Errors in charting should never be erased. Instead, a line should be drawn neatly through the error, so that the entry can still be read, and the portion labeled "error." All notes should be signed with the first initial, last name, and title of the person making them. In recording, one should always ask oneself, "What is the reason for this child's hospital entry? What signs and symptoms are significant to record? Is there any change in condition? Is the intake and output record accurate?" If the child has had any bowel movements, they should be described in terms of amount, consistency, and color. Of course, treatments and medications and patient reactions also form part of the record and are recorded after they are completed or administered. Special teaching and demonstrations of procedures to patients or parents should also be noted. The visits of physicians and parents and relatives are important too.

The nurse should not be too wordy, but she should give an accurate description of the condition of her patient. Good charting for most nurses is not automatic. If it develops, it is the result of concentrated effort and experience. Each hospital probably has a different form to use, but the principles of charting remain the same.

DAILY PLANNING FOR PATIENT CARE

After the basic needs of patients have been identified, planning nursing care to meet the needs of patients takes time, ingenuity, and experience. The student requires guidance in executing nursing care so that priorities are recognized and work progresses safely and efficiently, benefiting all the patients and staff.

When given her morning assignment and report, a student must plan her individual care to accomplish her goals in the best way possible. To do this, she must be aware of the organization of the nursing unit and the staff utilization pattern. The head nurse, team leader, or student instructor may assist in her planning.

Usually, the best beginning is a *quick* tour of all assigned patients to check on any immediate needs. The following things can be achieved during the tour:

1. Introduce the nurse to the child and the parent, when appropriate.
2. Check the general safety of the patient's environment.
   a. Restraints and siderails, crib nets
   b. Intravenous apparatus for rate of flow and possible infiltration and type of solution
   c. Humidification devices for function
   d. Oxygen equipment
   e. Inappropriate toys
3. Help set up and supervise breakfast, when appropriate, checking diet for accuracy (know whether any patients need to be weighed before eating).
4. Evaluate the need for supplies.
   a. Linen
   b. Sizes of underwear, dresses, trousers, shirts, hospital gowns, or pajamas
   c. Procedural supplies
      (1) Dressing supplies
      (2) Solutions—irrigating sets, and so on

After this brief "grand tour" the patient's needs must be evaluated again. In deciding which patient should receive basic care first, one must consider the following:

1. Any prior appointments that have been scheduled for the patients

a. X-ray examination or therapy
   b. Physical therapy
   c. Speech therapy
   d. Bedside tutoring
   e. Scheduled dressing changes
2. General condition of the patient
   a. As a general rule, the patient who is least comfortable has the priority.
   b. Presurgical patients who have had a preoperative medication are usually not disturbed.
   c. Patients who are sleeping and need the rest may, at the discretion of the supervising nurse, be left temporarily undisturbed. Sleep may be their most pressing need.
3. Types of treatment that are ordered and when they are to be given
   a. Enemas are ordinarily given before the bath and bed change.
   b. Shampoos are ordinarily given after the bath but before the bed change.
   c. A patient's care is preferably completed before a blood transfusion or other infusions are started.
   d. Ideally, sterile dressings are best changed when local movement, bed making, and mopping are at a minimum.
4. Hospital routine
   a. Taking the temperature, pulse, respiration, and blood pressure is routine for most patients; the time at which it is done depends on the hospital policy and the type of nursing organization pattern folowed.
   b. Meal schedules: Children usually need more supervision and aid than adults; babies are usually fed their ordered solids, bathed, and then given their fluids.

A good rule to follow, saving steps and time during the morning, is to never go anywhere empty-handed if possible. Usually something needs to be carried to or from a patient's unit.

An active mind, gentle skill, and good humor should accompany a nurse's many steps.

Key Concepts

1. The nursing staff is responsible for helping to provide the following: safety, observation and assessment, supportive procedures, medications and special treatments, rehabilitation, and recording of events.

2. The pediatric hospital unit must be continually evaluated to prevent accidents because the patients are often too small to regulate their own surroundings and they lack the judgment to properly evaluate their own environment.

3. Sometimes children must be restrained during treatment to protect themselves. Restraints should be constructed so that they do not become tighter with increased tension, impairing circulation or endangering respiration.

4. Observation and assessment of the pediatric patient are particularly important and complex because small children may be unable to express themselves and because many variables are associated with different stages of growth and development.

5. Diagnostic procedures must be understood so that adequate preparation, execution, and follow-up can be provided.

6. Various types of supportive procedures and techniques are used to maintain or improve the physical and emotional resources of the patient. These include supervision of position and activity, nourishment and fluid balance, cleanliness, rest and diversion, self-expression, coping mechanisms, and acceptance.

7. Children in bed, particularly if they must remain fairly quiet for long periods, must maintain good alignment, functional positions, range of motion, and tissue health for all body parts.

8. All pediatric patients are routinely on a regimen of measured fluid intake; most are on a measured fluid output regimen as well.

9. Hydration is extremely important because a young child may become dehydrated more rapidly than an adult. The amount of fluid that is urged depends on the child's size and condition. Ensuring adequate oral intake often requires ingenuity, patience, and persistence.

10. One of the most delicate balances maintained by the body is demonstrated by the composition of body fluid. Major ingredients of this fluid are water and electrolytes.

11. Body fluid occupies three permeable compartments: blood vessels, tissue spaces, and the areas inside the cells. Extracellular fluid is located within the blood vessels and between the tissue cells; intracellular fluid lies inside the tissue cells. Chemical differences exist between extracellular and intracellular fluids.

12. The four main electrolytes in the body are sodium, potassium, calcium, and bicarbonate. Deficits or excesses are called electrolyte imbalances and may require intervention.

13. Acid-base balance is maintained by the action of the lungs, kidneys, and buffer systems. Any slight deviation from the normal range causes pronounced changes in the cellular functions that may threaten life.

14. Fluid therapy aimed at replacing the patient's daily loss of water, electrolytes, and calories is termed maintenance therapy. The purpose of maintenance fluid is to keep the body in neutral balance for water, sodium, potassium, and chloride.

15. Infants are more vulnerable to fluid volume deficits than adults for the following reasons: their body surface in relation to body weight is greater, therefore they lose a relatively greater amount of fluid through the skin and gastrointestinal tract; their high metabolic rate produces more waste products, which must be diluted for excretion; their immature kidneys are less able to concentrate urine, resulting in greater urine volume; and accumulation of acidic wastes stimulates respiration, causing greater evaporation through the lungs.

16. Early signs of dehydration are dry lips and mucous membranes, diminished urinary output, reduced weight, and lethargy.

17. It is important that the amount of fluid administered intravenously to a child be gauged very carefully to prevent overloading the circulatory system. The nurse must keep a close watch on the flow rate, the infusion site, and the child's response to therapy.

18. Some children who cannot tolerate oral or nasogastric feedings can survive by intravenous alimentation. Total parenteral hyperalimentation provides glucose, proteins, fats, minerals, vitamins, and fluid necessary for normal growth and weight gain.

19. The heparin lock is used for patients receiving intermittent medication, and allows more mobility without the need for continuous IV fluids or frequent venipunctures.

20. Methods of meeting the patient's needs for cleanliness depend on the condition of the patient and the facilities available on the unit. Bed baths, tub baths, shampooing, and other hygiene measures are almost always the responsibility of the nursing staff.

21. Play is a learning activity that promotes physical, mental, emotional, and social growth. The following principles should be kept in mind when selecting toys for children: suitability for a particular age, safety, and durability.

22. The following factors must be identified before administering medication: the right patient, the right medication in the right form, the right dosage, the right method of administration, and the right time for administration.

23. Fluid medications may be fairly easily given to infants by placing the medication in a nipple fitted in a standard ring, a small medicine cup, a syringe, or a rubber-tipped medicine dropper.

24. The buttocks are never used for an intramuscular injection for an infant or young child. The most desirable injection sites are the lateral and anterior aspects of the thighs, the deltoid areas, and the soft tissue inferior to the iliac crests.

25. Nose drops are ordered fairly frequently for infants and children, primarily to combat nasal congestion and make breathing, eating, and drinking easier.

26. As convalescence progresses, provisions for rehabilitation may be necessary, including physical and occupational therapy. Physical therapy is designed to prevent deformity, relieve pain, and promote functional capacity. Occupational therapy is more often concerned with the maintenance or stimulation of small muscle control necessary for the skills involving finger and wrist manipulation.

27. Nursing notes serve as a permanent record of the patient's treatments, medications, and changing conditions. The nurse's notes may help influence therapy, may be important in research studies, or may become of specific legal importance.

Discussion Questions

1. Starting at birth, identify the developmental activities that increase the safety risks for children. How does this relate to the hospitalized child? How does it relate to home safety? (Each student could select a different age and present pertinent material.)

2. Discuss the reasons why careful monitoring and maintenance of fluids are of particular importance in children. How is fluid balance assessed? What special techniques are used for oral and IV intake? What special techniques may be used to measure output?

3. Pediatric medication dosage is calculated using specific rules or formulas. What are the accepted formulas?

4. When injections are given to infants and children, how do the sites and equipment differ from those used for adults?

5. Play is often called the work of childhood. How do departments such as occupational therapy and physical therapy incorporate "play activities" into treatment? How are certain toys and games determined to be appropriate for specific ages?

24

Common Diagnostic Tests Used in Evaluating Maternal and Child Health

CHAPTER OBJECTIVES

After studying this chapter, the student should be able to perform the following:

1 Cite the components of a typical complete blood count and urinalysis.
2 Identify what size needle should be used for routine blood draws, and state why smaller gauge needles should be avoided.
3 Repeat some of the advantages or disadvantages of the following equipment used to obtain venous blood specimens: winged infusion or scalp vein needles, eccentric tip blood-drawing syringes, and Vacutainer devices.
4 Identify special needs for capillary blood collection, the sites of choice, and the devices used.
5 Indicate which specimen tubes of blood must be in-

verted four to six times immediately following collection and which should be left undisturbed.
6 Describe how to collect a clean-catch or midstream urine specimen.
7 Explain how to assist the physician and help the infant undergoing a percutaneous bladder aspiration (bladder tap).
8 Describe how to initiate and collect timed urine or stool specimens.
9 Describe a correct method of holding a young child during a lumbar puncture.

A day does not pass in a busy hospital without many diagnostic tests being performed. The tests may entail the services of the clinical laboratory, the x-ray department, the operating room suite, or other specialized areas. They may be performed in the nursing unit. Although the nurse does not need to know the details of all these procedures, she should know the purpose of the test, whether patient preparation is necessary, the general procedure followed during the test, its effect on the patient, and the follow-up care needed.

For convenience the tests described in this chapter are

arranged in table form and are grouped as follows: tests of blood specimens, tests of urine specimens, tests of stool specimens, miscellaneous specialized tests, and x-ray tests. Only those tests commonly performed and of special interest in obstetric or pediatric areas are described. The details of each test frequently differ from hospital to hospital, even though automated laboratory techniques are often employed. The nurse is advised to consult the procedure manual of the institution where she is employed before participating in any test.

Text continued on p. 502.

Table 24-1 Tests of blood specimens

Test	Purpose and rationale	Preparation of patient and specimen	Special considerations	Normal value
Albumin, globulin, total protein, and A/G ratio (usually performed together)	To aid in diagnosis or evaluation of treatment of many diseases, including those of liver and kidney Blood may contain excessive globulin when albumin is abnormally displaced or lost, causing change in blood protein and A/G ratio	Fasting patient Specimen—minimum 3 ml clotted blood (red top tube); pediatric collection may be capillary blood in Microtainers		Adults: A/G ratio—1.5-2.5:1 Total protein 6-8 g/dl Newborn: lower levels
Antistreptolysin O titer (ASTO or ASO titer)	To aid in diagnosis of suspected rheumatic fever, although not specific for this disease Indicates antibodies formed from recent streptococcal infections	Nonfasting patient Specimen—minimum 3 ml clotted blood (red top tube)		50-166 Todd units
Arterial blood gases (ABGs)	To evaluate respiratory exchange and acid-base balance	Specimen—1 ml from arterial puncture or arterial line collected in heparinized syringe Blood gas evaluation may be performed by capillary collection in the nursery by use of special pipets Some facilities perform tests for venous blood gases as well	Place syringe (or capillary tube if from capillary draw) containing specimen in ice immediately and transport for analysis	P_{CO_2} 35-45 mm Hg P_{O_2} 75-100 mm Hg pH 7.35-7.45 Arterial, capillary, and venous blood have different normal values
Bleeding time "Simplate"—disposable, controlled device and modification of Ivy Bleeding Time	To determine time needed for constriction of small blood vessels To evaluate patient's status when excessive bleeding might be a problem; frequent "T and A" screen To assist in diagnosis of bleeding disorders	Blood pressure cuff is applied and 40 mm Hg is maintained by placing a hemostat between bulb and cuff Incision device is placed laterally about 4 inches below antecubital area and triggered; stop watch is set Drops of blood are removed by allowing filter paper be-	Exact procedure necessary or results invalid Bleeding time is interval between triggering of device until bleeding ceases	Usually up to 10 minutes; may be continued 30 minutes to evaluate bleeding potential

Test	Purpose	Specimen/Procedure	Observations	Normal values
Blood counts Differential; "diff"—part of complete blood count (CBC)	Counts kinds of white blood cells (WBCs) present expressed as percentage with 100 WBC counted Evaluates types, and abnormalities of WBCs, red blood cells (RBCs), and platelets (thrombocytes)	Nonfasting patient Uniform, thin smear made from capillary blood test Some smears made from anticoagulant tube (purple top) may show cell distortion	Morphology of WBCs, RBCs, and platelets is noted (size, shape, abnormalities)	Percentage patterns vary with age Adult: Neutrophils—50%-65%, increased during infections; eosinophils—1%-6%, increased in allergic conditions and parasitic infections; basophils—0%-1%, increased in some blood disorders; lymphocytes—25%-40%, increased in some viral and bacterial infections; monocytes—0%-5%, increased during some infections Children: varied normal patterns according to age and maturity of child Infant: percentages of lymphocytes and neutrophils reversed
Hematocrit (Hct) or packed cell volume (PCV)—part of CBC	To determine relative percentage of RBCs in plasma Reliable screening test for certain anemias, hemorrhage, dehydration	Nonfasting patient Specimen—3 ml minimum venous blood; anticoagulant tube (purple top) may be performed by nurse, rather than in laboratory "Crit" centrifuge used with red top (heparinized) capillary tubes to collect capillary blood Height of RBC column is read on special graph and recorded as percent of total		Adult: Male—40%-50% Female—35%-45% Child (2-6 months of age): may be as low as 35% Newborn: 45%-65%
Hemoglobin (HgB or Hb)—part of the CBC	To determine amount of hemoglobin in RBCs available for transport in oxygen—carbon dioxide exchange Hemoglobin levels are proportional to red color in blood	Nonfasting patient Specimen—3 ml venous blood anticoagulant tube (purple top) Capillary collection by use of Microtainer		Adult: Male—14-17 g/dl Female—11.5-15 g/dl Infants: Higher normal levels than older children or adult (14-19 g/dl; low of 11 g/dl may be seen at 3-4 months of age)

Continued.

Table 24-1 Tests of blood specimens—cont'd

Test	Purpose and rationale	Preparation of patient and specimen	Special considerations	Normal value
Platelet count (thrombocyte)—not part of CBC	Platelets necessary for proper clotting To aid in diagnosis of diseases of clotting and bleeding To determine bleeding potential before surgery	Nonfasting patient Specimens—may be from 3 ml minimum anticoagulant (purple top); special capillary blood collection in infants usual; not done from blood smear		Methods and thus normal values may differ Usually 250,000-450,000/mm^3
Red blood cell count (erythrocyte or RBC)—part of CBC	To aid diagnosis of anemia type or effects of disease on blood cells RBCs carry O_2 to tissues and CO_2 from tissues Elevated counts indicate dehydration, cardiopulmonary problems, specific disease processes (e.g., polycythemia vera); low counts indicate anemias (cause usually needs more study)	Nonfasting patient Specimen—3 ml minimum venous blood; anticoagulant tube (purple top); special capillary collection by Microtainers		Adult: Male—4.5-5.5 million/mm^3 Female—4-4.5 million/mm^3 Child: usually 4-5.6 million/mm^3 Newborn: has higher RBC count than adult
White blood cell count (leukocytes or WBCs)—part of CBC	WBCs combat infectious organisms Blood levels usually elevated in bacterial infections and some viral infections High in most leukemias	Nonfasting patient Specimen—3 ml minimum venous blood; anticoagulant tube (purple top) Special capillary collection by Microtainers		Adult: range usually 5,000-10,000/mm^3 Newborn: WBC averages 20,000/mm^3 at birth with counts as high as 38,000/mm^3 considered normal Infants: count usually falls with age and approaches adult values by age 3 years
Blood culture	To identify microorganisms that may be circulating in bloodstream Antibiotic sensitivity tests may be done if organism present Special media available emitting low-level radioactivity if organisms present; saves time in diagnosis	Nonfasting patient Specimen—special venous blood culture media; often performed when temperature spikes present Drawn under strict aseptic conditions before administration of antibiotics Requires laboratory incubation at 37° C (98.6° F) for organisms to grow	Area of collection must be cleansed with iodine prep using careful aseptic technique Preliminary reports may be available in 36 hours Specimen may be collected aerobically or anaerobically (with or without air)—check with hospital procedure manual	Negative culture

glucose)	normal glucose metabolism; hyperglycemia or hypoglycemia caused by diabetes mellitus or insulin treatment as well as other diseases	specimens depending on patient's needs and diagnosis Timed postprandial (after eating) tests are common Specimen—3 ml minimum venous blood; anticoagulant tube (gray top tube) Capillary collection may be done by Microtainer or even "crit" tubes if performed 'stat'	ing special strips increasingly employed by patients and staff Usually capillary blood and dipstick for Glucometers and Dextrometers	toluidine method) but normals depend on timing
Blood grouping (ABO grouping)	To determine blood group for possible transfusion or maternal-newborn studies and ABO incompatibilities	Nonfasting patient Exercise extreme care in specimen/patient identification and collection Specimen—most often minimum 5 ml in clot tube (red top tube); rarely, additive tube, (purple top) is requested		Four main blood types found in US population: A—38% B—12% AB—5% O—45%
Rh factor (Rh_0 or RhD)	To determine blood type for possible transfusion and for maternal-newborn studies; identify high-risk mothers at beginning of prenatal care Although other Rh subgroups are potential problems, the most common source of difficulty is RhD (Rh_0)	Nonfasting patient Extreme care exercised in patient/specimen collection and ID Most often 5 ml clotted blood (red top tube) Rarely an additive tube (purple top tube) requested Usually performed concurrently with blood grouping		85% of Americans Rh+ (positive); 15% of Americans Rh− (negative)
Blood urea nitrogen (BUN)	To determine kidney disease or urinary obstruction Urea, a waste product of protein metabolism, normally excreted by kidney; if urinary system fails, blood urea levels will be elevated	Fasting patient Specimen—3 ml minimum clotted venous blood in clot tube (red top) Capillary blood may be collected in Microtainer		7-20 mg/dl (depending on method)

Continued.

Table 24·1 Tests of blood specimens—cont'd

Test	Purpose and rationale	Preparation of patient and specimen	Special considerations	Normal value
Coombs' test	To monitor level of antibody formation in Rh-negative mother initiated by Rh factor from fetus entering mother's blood To help determine Rh status of unborn infant To determine need for prophylactic administration of RhoGAM to mother before delivery To assess need for treatment of newborn including blood replacement transfusion	Nonfasting patient Specimen—usually 5 ml clotted blood (red top tube) obtained from mother by venipuncture May be obtained from newborn as cord blood, by arterial line, or by venipuncture	Direct or indirect Coombs' test may be ordered, depending on purpose Mother's blood before childbirth—indirect Infant cord blood—direct	If direct Coombs' test negative and baby Rh_0 (RhD) positive or D^u positive and mother is negative, mother is immune globulin candidate
C-reactive protein (CRP)	To aid detection of inflammation and tissue breakdown Nonspecific test, often for diagnosis of rheumatic fever and infarctions	Serum from a red top vacuum tube or capillary blood in a Microtainer depending on specimen needs		Normally, no C-reactive protein present
Glucose tolerance test (GTT)	To aid in determination of abnormal glucose metabolism To plot a "metabolic curve" up to a period of 5 hours, using blood glucose and urine glucose over required time to diagnose specific diseases	Fasting patient (high CHO diet 1 day before for validity) Specific dose of glucose given orally after fasting; blood and urine specimens obtained Specimens obtained at exact intervals (usually ½ hr, 1 hr, 2 hr, 3 hr, etc) after administration of glucose Normal amounts of water given to ensure collection of urine specimens Specimens—3 ml minimum venous blood in anticoagulant tube (gray top) at precise times For children microtainers may	Adults: Prepared dose of either 75 or 100 g/dl water Commercial preparations made to resemble soft drinks Children: Dosage calculated according to body weight in lesser amounts of water Comparison with standard curves indicates various diseases Diabetes mellitus and liver and kidney diseases may be diagnosed	Peak of not more than 150 mg/dl blood and a return to below fasting level after 2 hours Glycosuria is abnormal

Test	Purpose	Specimen/Procedure	Special Considerations	Normal Values
		"crit" tubes (red top) are sometimes used when specimens are to be analyzed immediately		
PKU (test for phenylketonuria)	To identify early excessive amounts of phenylalanine in infant for prevention of mental retardation by use of restrictive diet. Metabolic disorder that requires adherence to restrictive diets throughout life	Capillary blood obtained 72 hr to 7 days after birth (should be after infant has ingested milk). Mothers birthing at home are urged to have baby tested at a specific time. Requires saturation of five "dime-sized" circles on special paper with capillary blood; blood must saturate both sides of paper before examiner proceeds to next circle	Many states mandate test performance. If tested before 24 hours or elevated result, repeat test before 3 weeks of age. Phenylalanine is not present in urine until third day in milk-fed babies	1.2-3.4 mg/dl phenylalanine level above 8 mg/dl blood diagnostic of PKU
Sedimentation rate (ESR, Sed rate)	To aid in detection of inflammation and tissue breakdown. Nonspecific test; if rate is elevated, may point to rheumatic fever activity, arthritis, infections, infarctions, and cancer. Usually elevated during pregnancy	Nonfasting patient. Specimen—3 ml minimum venous blood in anticoagulant tube (purple top). Blood placed in a calibrated thin tube and level of plasma separation from cells in exactly 1 hour is expressed in mm/hour	Some methods provide a "correction factor" for anemia patients	Adults: Male—0-10 mm/hour Female—0-20 mm/hour Children under 12 years; usually 0-20 mm/hour (Wintrobe)
Serology test for syphilis—STS (RPR, VDRL, TPI, ABS)	To aid in detection of syphilis. Legally required before marriage in most states; routine test in prenatal examinations. Performed on infants whose mothers show reactive result to test to detect congenital syphilis	Nonfasting patient. Specimen—serum from 5 ml clotted blood tube (red top)	Reactive results should be handled discreetly. Occasionally persons show reactive results throughout life when screening tests are performed, although not communicable after treatment	Nonreactive. Because occasional false positives may result from screening with RPR and VDRL tests, confirmatory tests are performed
T_4 (thyroxine) assay	Adult: to identify thyroid abnormalities. Infant: to identify congenital hypothyroidism and prevent mental retardation	Specimen—5 ml minimum venous blood in clot tube (red top). Infant: cord blood or capillary blood collected in two blue top "crit" tubes	All infants should be screened. T_4 levels of 4µg/dl or less are tested for thyroid-stimulating hormone (TSH). TSH levels greater than 25 µg/dl are diagnostic for congenital hypothyroidism	After 1 month 4-11 g/dl, 5 days—1 month 14-21 µg/dl, Birth—4 days 14-23 µg/dl, Cord blood 8-12 µg/dl

BLOOD SPECIMEN TESTS (Table 24-1)
General considerations

Many hospitals employ specialists—phlebotomists—who are usually considered a part of the laboratory department and whose skills include a variety of specialized techniques for all types of blood specimen collection. However, the nurse, the licensed technologist, and sometimes even the physician may collect specimens for testing purposes, depending on the special needs of the facility and the individual patient. For instance, in many outpatient clinics or convalescent facilities the nurse is responsible for collection of specimens to be sent to a reference laboratory. In some states, regulations require that nurses and other personnel obtain a "blood-drawing certificate" indicating successful completion of an educational program that includes both theory and clinical experience.

Some blood specimens for chemical analysis must be collected after a period of fasting. Nurses should be aware of the test procedures that require fasting before blood withdrawal and must take appropriate measures to ensure that such requirements are met. Orders for laboratory specimens to be drawn in the morning should not automatically trigger the withholding of food or fluids from the patient. Individual tests differ. Unless an extraordinary condition exists, water may be allowed in normal amounts for fasting patients for laboratory procedures.

Blood specimens used for determining therapeutic drug levels are sometimes drawn at specific times following the administration of a drug (for instance, gentamicin or tobramycin). Often two specimens—a "peak" and a "trough"—are collected to determine drug levels in the blood. It is extremely important for the nurse to indicate exactly when the drug was administered so that testing is accurate. The following blood specimens are frequently obtained.

Venous blood
Sites

Adults. Most blood specimens are obtained by venipuncture because of the relative ease of collecting large amounts of blood. The amount of blood to be drawn and the sites for collection may differ depending on the laboratory requirements and hospital policies. The most common site is the antecubital space, but the back of the hand and the veins on the lower arm may be considered as alternative sites if problems exist in the individual patient. Evaluation of the type of procedure to be used in collection depends on the expertise of the health professional in obtaining such specimens.

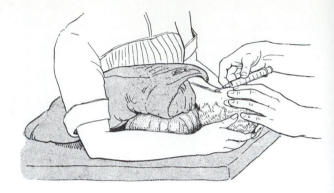

FIG 24-1 Suggested restraint and positioning for puncture of jugular vein.

Children—2 years or older. A venipuncture is usually performed if capillary puncture is impractical or unfeasible because of the minimum amount of blood needed or the patient's status. Most often the antecubital area is used for the procedure, since the veins tend to be larger and closer to the surface, although sometimes the nurse may use veins in the ankle or the top of the foot. Policies and procedures of the individual facility should be used as guidelines.

Infants and children under 2 years. The physician may use jugular veins if large amounts of blood must be obtained in emergencies or cannot be obtained elsewhere. Often the placement of an intravenous (IV) device is a consideration, and the IV procedure may be coupled with blood collection at the time of the device's insertion. The nurse must be acquainted with the minimum amounts needed for specific tests and the proper use of the color-coded tubes for specimen collection (Fig. 24-1).

Equipment. Equipment varies with procedures selected and the patient's condition (Fig. 24-2).

Tourniquet. Penrose surgical drains or disposable rubber tourniquets are recommended for most drawing procedures, since the amount of tension may be quickly and easily regulated. The wider Velcro type tourniquet is more difficult to adjust and is costly (and therefore less disposable) but is occasionally used by some personnel. Blood pressure cuffs are often used for difficult draws from young children and infants to reduce discomfort and trauma, as well as to better distend the veins.

Antiseptic sponges. Current methods recommend presterilized, individually packaged alcohol preps rather than non-sterile cotton balls doused with alcohol. Alcohol is a washing, degreasing, and dehydrating antiseptic frequently used; however, when sterile collection of a *specimen* is important (as for blood cultures), preparations containing povidone-iodine (Betadine) or chlorhexidine gluconate (Hibiclens) are often recommended. The nurse should inquire regarding allergies to iodine before applying povidone-iodine.

Needles. Needle size is important to obtain the best possible specimens with minimum trauma to the patient. Since blood-drawing procedures depend on specific patient and specimen needs, the choice must be carefully evaluated. Only 20- to 22-gauge needles should be used for most testing requirements. A needle smaller than 22 gauge should not be used, with the exception of the 23 gauge TW (thin wall) obtainable only in the winged infusion device. Even if veins seem small and a preliminary evaluation might indicate a need for smaller needles, reduced sizes should be avoided. The specimen will yield erroneous results because of undesirable hemolysis of red blood cells or small clots in the specimen itself. Also, the proper amount of blood may not be obtained because the system tends to "clot off."

Hypodermic needles. Hypodermic needles are used in conjunction with the eccentric tip syringe to make an effective unit, especially for difficult draws. Usually a 1-inch, regular bevel is desirable, since penetration of ½ inch into the vein is necessary to prevent hematoma formation.

Winged infusion devices. Winged infusion devices (Butterflies or scalp-vein needles) are especially useful in drawing blood from pediatric patients, as well as adults with small or "difficult" veins. Most often a ¾-inch long, 23-gauge TW (thin wall) needle is used because it has the interior capacity of a 22-gauge. Its design includes two plastic wings that, when squeezed together, allow a flat-as-possible penetration. Attached to the needle is a plastic tube supplied with an adaptor where a syringe may be connected to provide suction. It is particularly helpful in properly filling pediatric-sized vacuum tubes (pedi-tubes).

A syringe is attached to the adaptor at the end of the tubing and after entry into the vein, the syringe plunger is pulled to begin the fill. Only 10- to 12-ml syringes may be used. Smaller syringes do not provide enough suction, whereas larger ones fill too slowly, allowing the blood to clot before completion or cause the vein to collapse as a result of excessive suction. After obtaining the desired amount, the Butterfly needle is removed from the vein and inserted through the rubber top of a pedi-tube. The vacuum within the pedi-tube pulls the specimen

from the syringe into the tube. (When larger tubes of blood are necessary, a 20-gauge needle should be placed on the syringe after removing the Butterfly adaptor so that the greater suction will not hemolyze the blood as it passes through the needle into the tube.) By intermittently relaxing the pull on the syringe plunger during the draw, the vein does not collapse and sufficient amounts of blood are secured.

The flat entry of the butterfly needle causes less pain when hand veins or other superficial or small veins must be used. Children find this device less painful and threatening. It doesn't look as if they are getting a "shot", and, once placed, it is stable and needs no taping or support for blood collection. (However, the butterfly is taped if it is to be used for IV administration after the blood collection is completed.) A helper is almost always needed to comfort and assist the child to maintain position or remain still during the procedure.

Vacutainer-type needles. Vacutainer-type multidraw needles are used for most adult blood collection. The procedure should be limited to adults and should be used only in the antecubital area and where no identifiable patient problem exists. Other procedures are better choices for collection from the back of the hand and the lower arm.

Children find Vacutainer needles intimidating, because the insertion and removal of tubes cause stress and sometimes pain. A special gasket on the portion of the needle entering the collection tube prevents regurgitation of the blood into the needle holder when the tubes are changed. This permits collection of sequential color-coded tubes without contamination of the reusable needle holder. However, some limitations do exist with Vacutainer needles: (1) because the constant suction tends to cause small veins to collapse, it is undesirable for other locations (such as the hand, wrist, or foot); (2) because the angle of entry is greater than with other devices, more pain may result from draws where bony structures are close to the vein; (3) hematomas may occur more frequently because the greater angle of entry may also be associated with accidental transection of the vein.

Vacutainer needle holders (shields). Plastic Vacutainer needle holders or shields allow the use of a two-way needle, which is screwed into the shield. When the vacuum tube is inserted into the shield after the venipuncture, the stopper is penetrated and the blood flows into the tube. The shield (needle holder) does not become contaminated and can be used again, although at some clinical facilities the custom is to discard the needle holder after completion along with the needle.

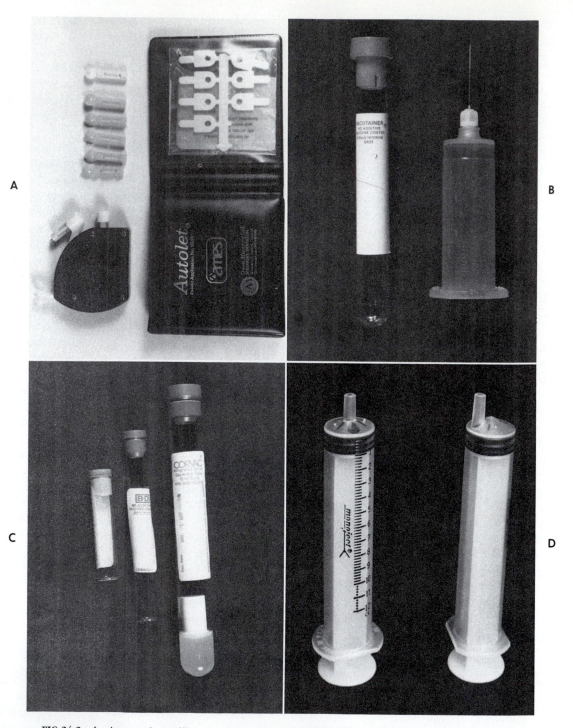

FIG 24-2 **A**, Automatic capillary puncture device (Autolet) used frequently by diabetic patients and nurses to secure relatively small amounts of blood. Presterilized disposable blades encased in plastic are inserted before triggering. **B**, *Left to right*: 7-ml vacuum tube; Vacutainer needle holder (shield) with multidraw needle in place. After penetration of vein, vacuum tube is pushed against needle within holder, causing rapid flow of blood specimen into tube. **C**, Three of several sizes of vacuum tubes used for blood collection. *Left to right*: 2- and 4-ml (used for pediatric specimens) and 15-ml tube containing serum separation material. **D**, *Left to right*: Center tip syringe; eccentric tip blood-drawing syringe, which permits angle of entry at 0 to 10 degrees.

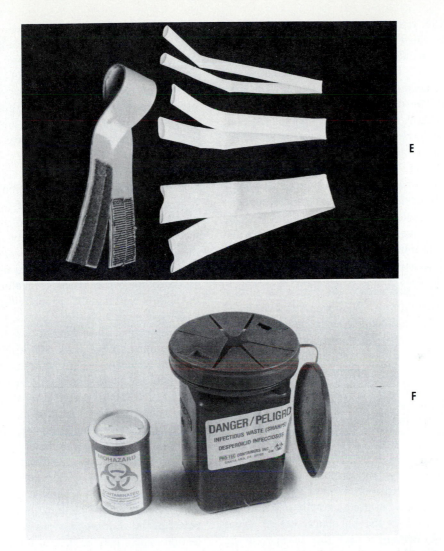

FIG 24-2, cont'd **E**, Various tourniquets used to restrict venous blood return in preparation for venipuncture; three sizes of Penrose drains and one Velcro type. **F**, Containers commonly used for disposal of "sharps" (needles, syringes, Butterflies, lancets, razors) before autoclaving and discarding. Note symbol for biologic hazard.

Syringes. True blood-drawing syringes have an eccentric tip, permitting a flat angle of entry into the vein. They also have a very tight barrel-to-plunger fit, producing more efficient suction and specimen collection. Although a 20-ml size is available, the 12-ml size syringe tip is the most versatile and is compatible with pediatric-sized collection tubes.

Vacuum tubes. All manufacturers of vacuum tubes abide by uniform color coding of the stoppers. The colors indicate the presence or absence of certain additives in the tubes. Since it is extremely important to choose the correct size and color for any given testing procedure, a collection manual should be constantly checked. The necessity of knowing the type of specimen to be collected (serum, plasma, or whole blood) and the specific color to be used cannot be overemphasized. The size of the tubes are 2, 3, and 4 ml in the pedi-tube sizes and 5, 7, 10, and 15 ml in regular sizes. Selecting the proper size tube and filling it adequately is necessary for accurate testing. Partially filling tubes is to be avoided, because results of tests are often erroneous. A much better procedure is to select a smaller tube and fill to the vacuum rather than put a small amount of blood in a larger tube.

Aftercare. After removal of the needle, the puncture site should be elevated while firm digital pressure is applied for about 2 minutes to avoid hematoma formation. A Band-Aid or 2- × 2-inch sterile gauze square is usually recommended to keep the puncture site clean. The latter is often wrapped by the stretch material that sticks to itself, avoiding allergy to tape and skin injury at removal.

Disposal containers for "sharps" and other materials. Extreme care is needed in handling materials contaminated with blood. Needles are dangerous if not handled and disposed of properly. A needle cutter should not be used. Although most guidelines do not recommend the recapping of needles, there are times when a needle must be covered promptly to provide safety when a disposal unit is not in immediate reach. The following is a suggested safe alternative to leaving the needle bare.

> *Place* the proper size needle cover on a flat surface open end toward you. With your dominant hand holding the venipuncture device and your *other hand behind your back* . . .
>
> *Insert* the needle into the cover, raising your hand to "scoop up" the cap. Holding the covered device in an upright position . . .
>
> *Use* your nondominant hand to grasp the needle cover from the sides *(not over the tip)* to pull down the cap tightly.

In blood drawing areas, on phlebotomy trays, and the like, rigid puncture-resistant disposal containers for sharps are mandatory. An entire syringe and needle set-up or Butterfly device is inserted carefully into the container. In many facilities the Vacutainer needle holder (shield) is reused, making it necessary to unscrew the needle and dispose of it separately. The tight fit of the contaminated needle and its location make it too dangerous to remove with one's fingers. Some health facilities use special "sharps" disposal containers equipped with plastic grippers to hold the needle while the shield is twisted off. At other facilities employees use hemostats or small forceps to unscrew the needle. Some use the safe one-handed capping method, which allows the needle to be safely unscrewed with its cap tightly in place. Other materials contaminated with blood are placed in a special plastic bag labeled "biologically contaminated." See the symbol for biologic hazard (Fig. 24-2, *F*). All these items are then autoclaved before disposal.

Application of universal precautions. The application of the concept of "universal precautions" is growing, owing to the dangers of blood-borne diseases and frequent exposure of health care personnel to potentially contaminated body fluids. This concept assumes that every patient is potentially infected. Appropriate protective measures should be used while performing procedures involving possible exposure. In some facilities, special signs appear in the rooms of all patients indicating what measures should be used. Certain situations involve use of gloves, masks, gowns, or goggles. Using gloves for phlebotomy in some instances may be optional. Many technicians state that gloves increase injuries.

Capillary blood

Sites. In adults and older children, the tip of the finger is frequently selected as the site for drawing capillary blood. In normal-sized children of 6 months to 3 years, the tip of the great toe should be considered. In infants the inner and outer sides of the plantar surface of the heel is the area of choice. The midplantar surface is avoided, since scar tissue formation may later impede the child's walking. Occasionally the earlobe is used for small specimen collection.

Equipment. The "Autolet" or other trigger devices are sometimes used when only a few drops of blood is needed. However, a sterile lancet is often employed and is overall the most satisfactory means of collecting capillary blood. It has a deeper predetermined depth of puncture. These "stickers" must be placed promptly into the special waste receptacle. Allowing them to become covered with paper tissues or bedding in cribs or Isolettes is dangerous. If a second "stick" is needed, a fresh lancet should be used.

Collection devices include capillary tubes, Microtainers, and particular solutions for dilution of blood samples. Special slide preparations and certain specimen collection papers may be needed for specific tests.

Cord blood

Cord blood is obtained from the placenta at birth or from the umbilical cord vessels (artery or vein) of the newborn by means of an umbilical catheter. It is useful in detecting Rh or other antibodies in the newborn. It may be used for cross-matching in preparation for blood exchange procedures.

Arterial blood

Arterial blood specimens are primarily used for arterial blood gas determinations (ABGs) and are taken from either the brachial or the radial arteries. The angle of entry is 45 to 90 degrees. The procedure is very different from venipuncture. A 22-gauge needle is fastened to a heparinized blood gas syringe. On completion of the collection, the syringe and needle are immediately immersed in a cup of ice and taken at once to be analyzed.

Blood gas analysis is not limited to arterial sources. In special care nurseries, capillary collection may be appropriate. Venous blood gas analysis is still performed in many facilities, although arterial collection dominates. Special certification is required for arterial blood collection.

Nursing considerations

Nursing care during specimen collection may consist simply of explaining the procedure to the young child and helping to support and restrain him. However, the qualified nurse may be responsible for the actual collection, depending on the certification needed and the hospital policy.

Blood specimens must be collected, labeled, transported, and checked into the laboratory properly.

When actually drawing specimens, the nurse must immediately invert those tubes containing anticoagulants four times to ensure mixture with the anticoagulant—the nurse should *never shake specimens*. Those tubes containing no anticoagulant (red top tubes) are allowed to clot, undisturbed, for ½ hour at room temperature. Labeling of the specimen is the responsibility of the person actually collecting it. This may be done by using the plastic "charge card" type of arrangement and pre-gummed labels. Many outpatient facilities may require only a clearly printed, hand-prepared label. Labeling must be done in the prescribed manner before the specimen is removed from the patient's presence. Date, time of specimen collection, and phlebotomist's initials should also be on the label.

Written requisitions must accompany every laboratory specimen. It is imperative to check the patients's ID number with that on the requisition and on the labels made for the collection tube. In outpatient facilities the patient, if possible, is asked to spell his name to ensure correct identification.

URINE SPECIMEN TESTS (Table 24-2)
General considerations

Urine specimens, except for bladder taps, are secured by the nurse. They may be obtained in various ways, depending on the physician's orders. Specimens may be ordered regulating the preparation of the patient or the timing of the specimen collection.

For a routine voided specimen, no special preparation is usually needed. The patient is asked to void into a clean container. Since children and some adults do not understand the word "void," terminology in accord with the age and education of the patient should be selected. Little children may say "pee-pee," "tinkle," "number 1,"

"pass water," or "urinate." The patient should be told not to put toilet paper in with the specimen. If the patient is menstruating, a routine voided specimen will be of only limited value. A "clean catch" may be ordered or the test deferred until later.

For a voided "clean-catch midstream specimen," special preparations are made before the specimen is collected. Necessary equipment may include the following:

1. Six or more sterile cotton balls or sterile wash packets, gauze compresses, or four povidone-iodine prep packets if patient is not allergic to iodine
2. Povidone-iodine solution in squeeze bottle or bowl if sterile wash packet is not used (or four povidone-iodine prep packets), other antiseptic or soap solution
3. Water for rinse of area
4. Paper bag or other waste receptacle
5. Sterile collecting container with tight-fitting lid
6. Clean gloves

For female patients the perineum is carefully cleansed with an appropriate product. The labia are retracted, and each cotton ball compress or prep is used only once, moving from front to back. Following cleansing with the antiseptic, the area is rinsed with sterile water using compresses, cotton balls, or an irrigation technique. The labia are kept retracted if possible. After the urinary stream begins, the collecting bottle is positioned to collect an adequate specimen and removed before the stream slows. Older patients may be able to carry out the procedure alone if properly instructed. Gloves are omitted if the patient collects the specimen. Younger patients may find it difficult to void when directed. Little girls may be washed off and placed directly on a sterile bedpan if unable to void with the labia retracted. Infants and toddlers must be "taped" for a specimen using a sterile plastic bag that adheres to the perineum with adhesive and tape. If the patient is well hydrated, the request for a specimen is more easily fulfilled. A midstream collection kit includes everything necessary for the collection of sterile specimens. For male patients the glans penis is carefully washed with antiseptic solution, and the foreskin, if present, is retracted to ensure proper cleansing (unless the infant is under 5 months of age). When the patient begins to void, the container is positioned to collect an adequate specimen and removed before the stream dwindles. Older boys and young men often carry out this procedure alone or with the assistance of an orderly.

To obtain a "three-glass specimen" (male patients), the glans penis is cleansed. Three sterile urine specimen

Table 24-2   Tests of urine specimens

Test	Purpose and rationale	Preparation of patient and specimen	Special considerations	Normal value
Routine urinalysis Acetone* (to detect ketonuria)	To determine presence of ketones in urine, a possible sign of developing acidosis found as a result of diabetes mellitus, starvation, vomiting and diarrhea, or prolonged protein diet	One drop of urine placed on Acetest tablet, and after 30 sec color change compared with scale; or dipstick analysis (Diastix) may be performed	Though uncommon, urine specimens of diabetics may be free from sugar but containing acetone. This is usually the result of other concurrent problems	No acetone present normally
Albumin* (to detect albuminuria)	To detect loss of plasma albumin through kidney. May indicate kidney disease, heart failure, drug poisoning, or toxemia of pregnancy	Dipstick analysis	Often done in conjunction with urine glucose test in prenatal checkups	Usually no albumin present; however, orthostatic or postural albuminuria sometimes occurs in absence of disease Albuminuria is common finding in newborn infant
Blood, occult*	To determine presence of free hemoglobin (hemolyzed cells) or intact RBCs	Dipstick analysis	Infections, injury, neoplasms, calculi—usual causes; hemolytic diseases also may cause presence	Normally none present
Glucose*	To detect presence and/ or amount of glucose in urine, caused by diabetes mellitus; liver and kidney disease	Clinitest—follow directions issued with Clinitest tablets *carefully*; the 5 drop and/or 2 drop method may be ordered depending on patient's condition; not specific for glucose, since other "reducing sugars" may give false-positive results Dipstick is specific for glucose—thus avoids false-positive results. May be used qualitatively for screening and positive color change noted without specific timing; precise timing must be done on second evaluation as a quantitative	When performing Clinitest, observe reaction—rapid passage through green, tan, orange, and finally to dark shade of greenish brown indicates amount of glucose is over 2% in 5 drop method; continue testing with 2 drop method, which indicates up to 5% glucose Do not touch tablets; store away from heat and sun; keep in dry place; replace lid tightly and immediately. Watch for "blue color and stickiness" in the tablet, invalidating results	No glucose present Clinitest sensitive to other simple sugars (lactose, pentose); confirmation test done by dipstick if Clinitest positive

Test			
Gross appearance (color, clarity, odor)	...to aid in estimation of degree of hydration and ability of kidneys to concentrate or dilute urine	...cate pathology; confirmation of cause of turbidity by microscopic examination	...of hydration or medication given—may change greatly from one time interval to next. Smoky urine may indicate hematuria
Cells (microscopic analysis)	Red blood cells and white blood cells found in urinary tract disease in large amounts	Need 12-15-ml specimen of urine; sediment examined microscopically after centrifugation	Presence of a few RBCs or WBCs in voided specimen of mature female has little significance, since these results may be caused by vaginal contamination. Recheck by clean-catch if large numbers present	Occasional red blood cell. A few white blood cells (0-5) in female; 0-2 in male. A moderate number of epithelial cells is inconsequential for females
Casts (microscopic analysis)	Casts usually represent abnormal sediment in urine; may be formed of several substances passing relatively slowly through tubules; presence usually indicates kidney disease	Specimen of urine sediment examined microscopically after centrifugation	Several types of casts; meaning differs with each type	Rare hyaline cast may be present; other types indicate pathologic conditions
Bacteria (microscopic analysis)	If large number present in fresh or refrigerated voided specimen, midstream clean-catch specimen may be ordered for culture	Specimen should be observed soon after collection or stored in refrigerator	Freshly voided specimens should be refrigerated within minutes to avoid bacterial growth	A few bacteria in voided specimen insignificant, especially in female patient. No bacteria in catheterized or midstream clean-catch specimen
Specific gravity (sp gr)	To measure density of urine as compared with distilled water. High specific gravity may occur in albuminuria, glycosuria, and dehydration. Low specific gravity may reflect kidney's inability to concentrate urine or overhydration	Tested with a urinometer (calibrated float) or refractometer (TS meter or total solid meter) that needs only 2 drops and is more accurate than urinometer (Fig. 24-3). Be sure to clean and dry urine chamber of refractometer immediately after use; dipstick now also available	Detects presence of many dissolved substances, but does not identify them. Also indicates patient's ability to concentrate or dilute urine when monitored with fluid intake/output records	Adult: 1.003-1.030. Newborn (after ingestion of milk): 1.002-1.010

*The dipstick analysis has become the routine screening procedure for the tests indicated. These strips also provide other essential information to the clinician not detailed here.

Continued.

Table 24-2   Tests of urine specimens—cont'd

Test	Purpose and rationale	Preparation of patient and specimen	Special considerations	Normal value
pH	To determine acidity or alkalinity of urine To differentiate acid urine from alkaline amniotic fluid to detect ruptured bag of waters	Strip of Nitrazine paper is dipped into urine, placed in a baby's diaper, or dampened by vaginal drainage; color change compared with scale Other dipsticks available Result <7 = acid Result >7 = alkaline (7 = neutral pH)	pH should be measured quickly because urine becomes alkaline on standing Sometimes alkaline urine is needed to keep excreted substances soluble (during sulfadiazine therapy or blood or tissue destruction), and therapy is directed to this end Acid pH is encouraged (medication or diet ordered to alter pH to kill bacteria requiring alkaline environment)	4.5-7.5 (urine is usually acid, but pH may vary, depending on diet, patient's condition, and age of specimen)
Vanillylmandelic acid (VMA—not a routine urine test)	To aid diagnosis of neuroblastoma and follow the response of therapy Urine measurements of vanillylmandelic acid (VMA)	24-hour urine specimen collected in refrigerated brown bottle with preservative hydrochloric acid; 2 days before collection diet restricted by elimination of bananas, ice cream, foods containing vanilla flavoring, and so on; no vigorous exercise on day before collection	Certain drugs interfere with test Discontinue 2 days before test Check hospital manual	0.5-7.0 mg/24 hr

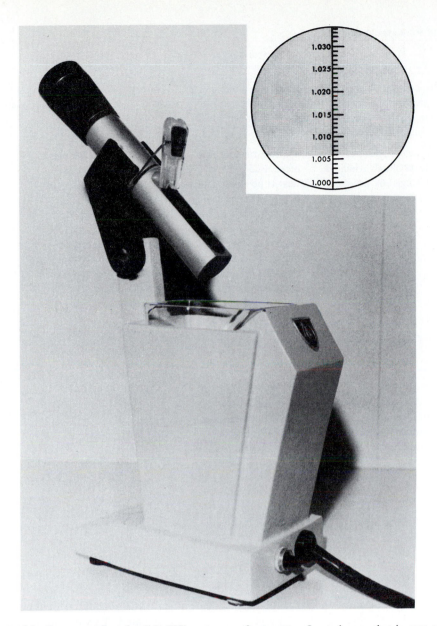

FIG 24-3 One type of total solids (TS) meter or refractometer. Inset shows what is seen on specific gravity scale with specific gravity of 1.006.

bottles are labeled No. 1, No. 2, and No. 3. The patient begins the urine stream, voiding approximately 20 ml in bottle No. 1. Without interrupting the urine stream he voids about 100 ml into bottle No. 2. Without interruption he continues to collect the specimen in No. 3 until his bladder is empty. The assistance of the orderly or a male nurse may be needed.

Catheterized specimen collection is used much less frequently because of danger of infection. Male cathe-

terizations usually are performed by a male nurse or orderly; female catheterization technique is described in Chapter 10. The urethra of the female infant curves downward; therefore the catheter should be inserted in a slightly downward direction.

A percutaneous bladder aspiration (bladder tap) specimen is obtained by a physician. If possible, the patient is given some fluid about 20 minutes before the tap. The patient is placed in a supine position on a firm surface.

Table 24-3   Tests of stool specimens

Test	Purpose and rationale	Preparation of patient and specimen	Special considerations	Normal value
Fat determination	To confirm diagnosis of steatorrhea (excess fat in stools), signs of celiac syndrome	Patient on normal diet 2 or 3 days before test Timed specimen usually ordered		Between 15% and 25% of weight of fecal sample
Occult blood	To detect presence of fecal blood, which is changed by process of digestion	Usually 3 random specimens used If test is positive, patient is placed on meat-free diet for 3 days and another specimen obtained. Positive findings may inidicate presence of an ulceration/neoplasm in gastrointestinal tract; further testing procedures may be indicated	Diet containing meat may sometimes cause positive result, depending on method used Hematest tablets or Hemoccult prepared packets with developer are available Various amounts are reported as trace, 1^+, 2^+, 3^+, and 4^+	No occult blood
Ova and parasites (see p. 516)				
Timed stool specimen	To determine amount of certain substances excreted in feces in given time	Patient should not void or place tissues in bedpan with stool Determine date and approximate time of previous defecations; this will be start of test collection; refrigerate total specimen until complete and then take to laboratory		

The abdominal area is cleansed with antiseptic. The puncture is made above the pubis with a 22-gauge (1-inch) or 21-gauge (1½-inch) needle with a 5- or 10-ml syringe attached to aspirate a specimen in a sterile manner. With female infants the labia are tightly closed, or pressure may be placed on the urethra to prevent voiding before the aspiration. The procedure should be delayed if the infant voids just before it is scheduled. Afterward, pressure is applied digitally with a gauze sponge over the tap site, and the site is covered with an adhesive bandage.

Timed specimens (most common is a 24-hour collection) usually consist of voided urine, although it may involve drainage from a urinary catheter. To begin the specimen collection, the patient empties his bladder and the time is noted. This first urine specimen is discarded. A large collection bottle of the type approved by the laboratory is labeled with the patient's name, his physician's name, and the time the discarded urine specimen was voided. This is the start of the test. All voided specimens for the ordered period are collected in this single large collection bottle. Even if a special preservative is used, the bottle is usually kept in a refrigerator or in a basin of ice unless instructed otherwise by the laboratory. At the exact end of the timed period the patient empties his bladder again and this specimen is added to the total collection. The total specimen is then sent to the laboratory. Since this represents the total urine output of a

Table 24-4 Miscellaneous specialized tests

Test	Purpose and rationale	Preparation of patient and specimen	Special considerations
Amniocentesis (see p. 52)			
Electrocardiogram (ECG or EKG)	To aid in determination of irregularities in electrical impulses controlling heart action and to help diagnose certain types of heart damage	Usually no special preparation except simple explanation; no pain involved Leads positioned on limbs and chest by technician	ECG on infant or child uses tiny electrodes often in place over long periods
Electroencephalogram (EEG)	To aid in determination of abnormalities in brain waves Useful in diagnosing convulsive disorders, brain tumors; estimating cerebral activity	Simple explanation Young children need to be sedated before test Testing takes about 1 hour; no pain involved Electrodes placed on scalp with adhesive substance by special technician in quiet atmosphere May need shampoo before and after test	
Fetal lung maturity Foam stability test (Shake test); positive result usually indicative of fetal lung maturity L/S (lecithin/sphingomyelin) ratio; 2:1, or 2, usually indicative of fetal lung maturity	To detect presence of surfactants denoting fetal lung maturity or possibility of respiratory distress syndrome	Amniocentesis necessary to secure sample of amniotic fluid for analysis	Used to best advantage to determine time of elective cesarean procedures
Lumbar puncture	To obtain cerebrospinal fluid specimens for cell count, protein and sugar content, culture, or Gram stain Spinal fluid glucose lowered in cases of meningitis Spinal fluid protein elevated in meningitis or subarachnoid hemorrhage White blood cell count moderately increased in encephalitis; greatly elevated in most cases of meningitis	Inform child just before procedure Positioning: place child on side with knees drawn up sufficiently to arch back, or in sitting position with spine curled forward to increase the space between vertebrae for needle insertion (Fig. 24-4) Child must be supported and maintained in position throughout procedure	Three specimens properly labeled, transported, and checked into the laboratory immediately Normal value in children: Pressure 70-200 mm of water Cell count 0-8 WBCs (under 5 yr) and 0-5 WBCs (over 5 yr), 0 RBCs Protein total 15-40 mg/dl Glucose 50-90 mg/dl
Nonstress test (NST)	Purpose same as OCT below but does not employ oxytocin Based on knowledge that FHR accelerates with fetal movement and baseline shows variability in "healthy" *reactive* fetus Effects of any contractions may also be evaluated	Semi-Fowler's position with external fetal and contraction monitors obtain baseline FHR and vital signs Run 20- to 40-min monitor strip; have mother confirm fetal movement Observe for accelerations with fetal movement and baseline FHR variability	Test done after 28 weeks' gestation; test shorter, less expensive, noninvasive vs OCT Reactive tests usually indicate fetal health Fetus may demonstrate rest-activity cycle of approximately 40 min, necessitating 40-min strip to observe FHR changes

Continued.

Table 24-4 Miscellaneous specialized tests—cont'd

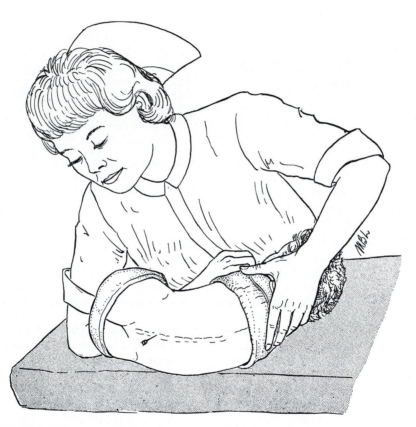

FIG 24-4 Restraining a small child or infant for lumbar puncture. When an older child (2 to 3 years of age) is positioned, child's head may be tucked under elbow, and nurse may have to lean over her charge in a gentle but firm fashion to maintain positioning.

Table 24-4 Miscellaneous specialized tests—cont'd

Test	Purpose and rationale	Preparation of patient and specimen	Special considerations
Nonstress test (NST)—cont'd			False nonreactive tests may occur as result of maternal sedative May be used in conjunction with OCT if test nonreactive
Nipple stimulation contraction stress test (NS-CST)	Purpose same as for OCT (below) but does not employ oxytocin Nipple stimulation causes release of oxytocin from posterior pituitary producing uterine contractions allowing evaluation of FHR response	One-to-one nursing advocated—private room Semi-Fowler's or left lateral position; external fetal and contraction monitors in place Obtain baseline FHR and vital signs If 3 interpretable contractions/10 min at least 40 sec long, NS-CST not necessary because that is goal of procedure Nipple stimulation should be intermittent and stop when contraction in progress Blood pressure monitored every 10 min	Check hospital procedure—methods of nipple stimulation vary Warm moist breast compresses appear to have no advantage Brushing across nipple with hand through clothing; tugging or rolling nipple under clothing Time periods vary, one or both breasts involved Hyperstimulation of uterus possible (contractions >90 sec or 5 or more/10 min) A negative test: no late deceleration with adequate contractions
Oxytocin challenge test (OCT) or Contraction stress test (CST)	To determine circulatory-respiratory reserve of utero-placento fetal unit before labor and evaluate ability of a *high-risk* fetus to withstand the stress of labor by recording the effect of oxytocin-induced contractions on his heart rate	Semi-Fowler's position with external fetal and contraction monitors Obtain a baseline FHR pattern and vital signs If 3 interpretable contractions with FHR present in 10 min, no oxytocin necessary If insufficient contractions, dilute oxytocin infusion begun Dosage increased to produce three contractions/10 min at not less than 2-min intervals lasting less than 1 min	Test done after 28 weeks' gestation Negative test: no late decelerations with adequate contractions Take blood pressure every 10 min to detect "supine hypotension" Tests may also be *equivocal* (inconsistent results) or unsatisfactory (failure to obtain adequate contraction or monitoring records) Contractions present in 80% of patients by 38 weeks Infusion pump required Average time for test approximately 90 min Avoid overstimulation of uterus Frequency of false-positive tests high False-negative tests infrequent

Continued.

Table 24-4 Miscellaneous specialized tests—cont'd

Test	Purpose and rationale	Preparation of patient and specimen	Special considerations
Sweat test	To help detect cystic fibrosis Abnormal amount of sodium chloride present in perspiration of affected persons Positive sweat chloride 60 mEq/L or higher Positive sweat sodium usually 10 mEq/L higher than sweat chloride	Pilocarpine iontophoresis: an electric current via attached electrodes drives pilocarpine into skin of forearm, stimulating local sweat production in about 5 min; a specimen of perspiration is then absorbed into gauze or filter paper; typical time for sweat collection is 30 min; sample is weighed and analyzed	
Magnetic resonance imaging (MRI)—No x-rays used; no risks of ionizing radiation	A combination of a strong magnetic field and radio frequency waves plus computer technology produce diagnostic images The interior of certain body parts can be studied from many angles with excellent imagery MRI is used most frequently for discovery or evaluation of CNS abnormality	Ask patient to void before Patient placed in tunnel-like body scanner with a special call button No movement allowed during scan Restless or claustrophobic patients may be sedated All metal objects (hairpins, belt buckles, snaps, zippers, coins, credit cards, jewelry, etc.) should be removed if possible; those that cannot be must be evaluated by radiologist before the scan Infusion pumps cannot be used in scanning room	Noninvasive technique; no known side effects Contrast media (if used) does not contain iodine Adverse reactions rare—consist of headache Objects containing iron may be affected by the magnet; patients with pace makers, Holter monitors, shrapnel, etc., are not candidates for test Machine makes loud knocking sound; ear plugs may be offered

patient within a known period, the collection *must* begin with an empty bladder. Twenty-four-hour urine specimens are notoriously difficult to obtain in pediatrics, especially from little girls.

Routine urine specimens should be properly collected, free of fecal material, labeled, transported, and checked into the laboratory with proper requisitions. Urine specimens should be sent promptly to the laboratory unless protected from deterioration by refrigeration or a preservative.

Urine for culture may be obtained by midstream clean-catch or catheterization. Replace the lid immediately after collection and ensure that the inner sides of the container are not touched. This type of specimen should *not* be refrigerated but should be sent immediately to the laboratory.

STOOL SPECIMEN TESTS (Table 24-3)
General considerations

Stool specimens are obtained by the nurse. They may be obtained by collection from a bedpan or diaper (for limited tests) or, occasionally, by rectal swabs, but specific needs should be verified by contacting the laboratory.

The stool specimen should be placed, with tongue blades, in a properly labeled, clean, disposable, wide-mouthed container with a tight-fitting lid. No stool material is permitted to be, or to have been, on the outside of the carton. The specimen must *not* be contaminated with urine. The specific test desired must be clearly indicated on the requisition, since many tests may be performed on the specimen. The entire specimen need not be sent to the laboratory unless a timed specimen is

Table 24-5 X-ray tests

Test	Purpose and rationale	Preparation of patient and specimen	Special considerations
Barium enema* (BE)	To aid in diagnosis of lower bowel pathology by outlining colon with radiopaque material May be part of treatment for intussusception	Cathartics and cleansing enemas may be ordered on previous day or morning of test Clear liquid diet may be given 1 day before test until test completion Barium enema given in x-ray department when patient is under fluoroscope; examination takes 1 to 2 hr Enema or cathartic may be ordered after radiographs completed to remove contrast media	Note and record patient's bowel movements after procedure
Brain scanning Computed tomography (CT scan)*	To provide a visual display of abnormal tissue within skull; useful in diagnosing brain tumors	Possible IV injection of radioactive isotope	If isotope used, patient should be NPO Allergy to iodine may alter technique used
Cystogram*	To aid in diagnosis of urinary obstruction or other abnormality by visualization of bladder, ureter, and urethra with radiopaque material during filling and emptying of bladder	Urethral catheter inserted prior to procedure Bladder emptied Radiopaque material injected into bladder and radiograph taken Catheter removed	
Voiding cystourethrogram*		Radiographs taken during voiding process	
Ciné cystourethrogram	To determine whether reflux appears or increases at voiding pressure	Continuous fluoroscopic pictures taken during voiding process	
Gastrointestinal series (GI series)*	To aid in diagnosis of stomach and small bowel disease by outlining areas with radiopaque material	Night before test, patient may have light supper No food, fluids, or medications after midnight until 6-hour radiographs X-ray department gives oral barium under fluoroscope Patient remains NPO until x-ray department gives release after 6-hour follow-up studies If 24-hr studies ordered, no enema or cathartic given until studies completed Check for enema or cathartic orders when test completed	

*If the nurse is holding or positioning the child during the x-ray procedure, she should wear a lead apron.

Continued.

Table 24-5 X-ray tests—cont'd

Test	Purpose and rationale	Preparation of patient and specimen	Special considerations
Intravenous pyelogram (IVP)*	To detect kidney or urinary disease by intravenous dye injection followed by abdominal radiographs	Cathartic or enema ordered on day before test Patient may eat light dinner with little fluid Fluids, food, and medications withheld after midnight Radiographs of abdomen taken before and after intravenous injection of dye by physician Fluids usually forced after completion of test to rid patient of residual contrast media	Allergy to iodine is contraindication to routine technique

*If the nurse is holding or positioning the child during the x-ray procedure, she should wear a lead apron.

ordered or the reason for the stool collection is the detection of a tapeworm head (scolex). Specimens for ova and parasites should be sent to the laboratory soon after collection. If transport will be delayed, about 2 ml of stool specimen should be placed in polyvinyl alcohol (PVA) solution and the container sealed tightly. The balance of the specimen can go in a carton to the refrigerator to be sent to the laboratory when possible.

TESTS OF SPUTUM
General considerations

Occasionally sputum specimens are requested for culture and sensitivity studies, cell analysis ("Pap" smear),

Gram stain, or wet mounts. They are usually difficult to obtain from young children. However, even older children and adults may find it difficult to produce material originating in the bronchial tree. Specimens are best secured from cooperating patients after undergoing IPPB treatment or chest therapy (cupping, vibration, and postural drainage).

For those who cannot cooperate, the use of a sterile specimen trap connected to a suction apparatus has been helpful. Avoid saliva if possible. It is better to obtain scant material from lower areas than more volume with saliva.

=========================== **Key Concepts** ===========================

1. Although nurses need not know the details of all diagnostic procedures, they should know the purpose of each test, what patient preparation is necessary, the general procedure followed during the test, its effect on the patient, and the follow-up care needed.
2. Components of a typical complete blood count (CBC) include a hematocrit (Hct), hemoglobin (Hgb), white blood cell count (WBC), red blood cell count (RBC), and differential blood smears (Diff).
3. The following types of blood specimens are frequently obtained: venous, capillary, cord, and arterial. Most blood specimens are obtained by venipuncture.
4. Sites for venipuncture vary according to the patient's age and the amount of blood to be drawn. Equipment

also varies, but usually includes a tourniquet, antiseptic sponges, needles, syringes, and vacuum tubes.
5. Needle size is important to obtain the best possible specimens with minimum trauma to the patient. Only 20- to 22-gauge needles should be used for most blood draws. Smaller needles may result in a specimen that yields erroneous results because of unwanted hemolysis of red blood cells or small clots in the specimen itself. Also, the proper amount of blood may not be obtained because the system tends to "clot off."
6. Winged infusion devices (Butterflies or scalp-vein needles) are especially useful in drawing blood from pediatric patients because the flat entry causes less

pain, children feel less threatened because the device does not resemble a "shot," and, once placed, no taping or support is needed for blood collection.

7. Vacutainer-type needles, which are used for most adult specimens, should not be used for pediatric patients.

8. True blood-drawing syringes have an eccentric tip, permitting a flat angle of entry into the vein, and a tight barrel-to-plunger fit, producing more efficient suction and specimen collection.

9. It is extremely important to select the correct size vacuum tube with the appropriate color-coded stopper for any given testing procedure.

10. Extreme care should be used when handling materials contaminated with blood. Needles are especially dangerous if not handled and disposed of properly. Universal precautions should be observed.

11. The tip of the finger or great toe is frequently selected as the site for drawing capillary blood in children depending on their age. In infants the inner and outer sides of the plantar surface of the heel are the areas of choice. A sterile lancet is the most satisfactory means of collection.

12. Cord blood is useful in detecting Rh or other antibodies in the newborn and may be used for cross-matching in preparation for blood exchange procedures.

13. Arterial blood specimens are primarily used for arterial blood gas determinations. The procedure is very different from venipuncture and requires special certification.

14. Blood specimens must be collected, handled, labeled, transported, and checked into the laboratory properly.

15. Specimens containing anticoagulants must be immediately inverted four times to ensure mixture. Those containing no coagulant are allowed to clot undisturbed for ½ hour at room temperature.

16. Routine urinalysis includes acetone, albumin, occult blood, glucose, gross appearance, cells, casts, bacteria, specific gravity, and pH.

17. Urine specimens may be obtained in various ways; orders may regulate the preparation of the patient or the timing of the specimen collection.

18. For a routine voided urine specimen the patient simply voids into a clean container. For a clean-catch midstream specimen the perineal area or glans penis is first carefully cleansed. The specimen is then collected after the urinary stream begins, with the specimen container being removed before the stream slows.

19. A percutaneous bladder aspiration (bladder tap) specimen is obtained by a physician. In preparation, the patient is placed in a supine position on a firm surface and the abdominal area is cleansed with antiseptic. After the procedure, pressure is applied digitally with a gauze sponge over the tap site, and the site is covered with an adhesive bandage.

20. Timed specimens must begin with an empty bladder, therefore the first specimen is discarded. All voided specimens for the ordered period are then collected in a single large collection bottle, which is usually kept in a refrigerator or a basin of ice.

21. Tests of stool specimens include fat determination, occult blood, ova and parasites, and timed stool specimen.

22. Sputum specimens are occasionally requested for culture and sensitivity studies, cell analysis, Gram stain, or wet mounts. These specimens are usually difficult to obtain from young children.

23. Other specialized tests include amniocentesis, electrocardiogram, fetal lung maturity, lumbar puncture, nonstress test, oxytocin challenge test, nipple stimulation contraction stress test, sweat test, and magnetic resonance imagery (MRI).

24. X-ray tests include barium enema, brain scanning, voiding cystourethrogram, ciné cystourethrogram, gastrointestinal series, and intravenous pyelogram.

Discussion Questions

1. Collection of blood samples from children requires various techniques. Which sites are used for venipuncture? Why are these sites recommended? What unique precautions must be taken when drawing blood from an infant or child?

2. How does the preparation of a pediatric patient for diagnostic tests differ from the preparation of an adult? Are the normal values for blood-based tests the same as they are for adults or do they differ?

3. Obtaining a urine specimen from an infant or child can present a significant challenge. What equipment is used to obtain urine specimens? What are the special challenges involved in collection of a 24-hour specimen?

4. What special considerations and precautions are involved in a lumbar puncture of an infant or child? How is the child positioned and restrained for this procedure?

5. X-ray diagnostic tests can be frightening and confusing to a child and to the parents. How would you describe and explain three of the most common tests?

25

The Child Surgical Patient

CHAPTER OBJECTIVES

After studying this chapter, the student should be able to perform the following:

1 Discuss ways infants and young children differ from adults regarding:
   a. Metabolic rate
   b. Reserve physical resources
   c. Healing ability
   d. Time orientation
2 State at least five factors that should influence how a child is prepared for the experience of surgery.
3 List five teaching methods that might prepare a pediatric patient for a surgical procedure.
4 Identify four behaviors a child unable to verbalize may exhibit that help the nurse detect that he is experiencing pain.
5 Discuss three types of scales or measurements that may

be used by a child to help reveal the extent of pain or relief he feels. What kind of considerations influence his perception and reaction to pain?
6 Indicate six different ways (other than the administration of analgesics) that a parent, nurse, or child may ease pain.
7 Express the reasons and basic pediatric modifications for the following common hospital procedures:
   a. Skin preparation for surgery
   b. Cleansing enema
   c. Sterile dressing change
   d. Gavage feeding
   e. Gastrostomy feeding
   f. Nasogastric or intestinal tube irrigation

Anatomic relationships, physiologic activity, and psychologic responses are greatly influenced by the phenomena of normal growth and development.

This chapter discusses some of the differences that set the child apart from the adult and reviews routines and procedures encountered when nursing the pediatric surgical patient.

CHILD-ADULT DISTINCTIONS

The following list of child-adult distinctions is not complete, but may prove helpful in the evaluation of the needs of children.

1. The metabolic rate of infants and young children is much greater proportionately than that of adults. Children need to be fed more frequently and cannot go as long preoperatively without some form of fluid intake.
2. Abnormal fluid loss is more serious in the infant and young child than in the adult. Fluid intake and output must be calculated carefully, including fluid loss from diaphoresis or wound drainage. A 7-pound (3.2 kg) infant who sustains a blood loss of 1 ounce (30 ml) is comparable to a 150-pound

(68 kg) man who has lost 20 ounces (600 ml) of blood.

3. The child lacks the physical reserves that are available to the adult. The child's general condition may change rapidly, almost without warning.
4. The body tissues of the child heal quickly because of the rapid rate of metabolism and growth.
5. The young child lives more in the present than an adult does. This is both to the child's advantage and disadvantage. "Now" is understood and very important, but "later" is difficult to grasp. On the other hand, children seldom become upset by anticipating unpleasant future problems or prospects or worrying about finances or loss of a job.

PREPARATION FOR SURGERY

When simple surgery is contemplated, the trend is toward 1-day hospitalization or the performance of operative procedures at outpatient surgi-centers. However, many youngsters are still formally admitted to a hospital, even for minor surgery.

Preparing a child for the experience of surgery must be based on the following factors: age and developmental level; the child's perception of hospitalization and the upcoming surgery; the surgical procedure to be performed; postoperative care; previous hospitalization experience; expected length of hospitalization; and parental attitudes. (See Chapter 19.)

Psychologic preparation

The method of preparation must be geared to the actual developmental level of the child or the regressed level, not merely to chronologic age. Many nurses use role play, imagery, puppets, dolls, drawings, films, and selected visitation to special areas of the hospital in conjunction with group and individual discussions as methods of preoperative preparation. Research has demonstrated that children who receive systematic psychologic preparation and continued supportive care demonstrate less disturbed behavior and more cooperation in the postoperative period. Parents are also less anxious and more satisfied with the information and care received.

The nurse should remember that in all contacts with patients, regardless of age, explanations and emotional support should be adapted to the individual's ability to understand and to personal needs. She should also remember that as parents are reassured, the confidence they gain in turn helps support the child. The presence of parents at the bedside immediately before and after surgical and diagnostic procedures is usually beneficial.

Some hospitals admit parents to the recovery room area as well.

Physical preparation

Patients admitted for surgery should be especially assessed for the presence of respiratory infection and signs of malnutrition. Occasionally surgery may be delayed until the child's general condition improves. Basic evaluative blood and urine tests are performed usually within 24 hours of the surgery. Other diagnostic studies may have been previously performed.

Except in emergency situations physical preparation for surgery usually begins the night before the procedure. Although some children may be admitted to the hospital early in the morning of the day of minor surgery, many come into the hospital the previous afternoon.

If orthopedic surgery is planned, the child is usually given a povidone-iodine (Betadine) bath in the evening as ordered. The body part involved in the surgery is carefully washed and inspected. The fingernails or toenails of any extremity involved are cleansed and trimmed. Frequently any ordered shave of the operative area is delayed until the morning of surgery. If a shave prep is requested, it often is done in the operating room suite just before the procedure to reduce the possibility of infection. For some types of surgery, preparatory enemas may be ordered.

Food, fluids, and oral medications are withheld as ordered, depending on the type of surgery planned, the age of the child, and the time of the procedure. The fact that the child must not receive anything by mouth should be conspicuously posted. Children should be told of this so that they do not think that they have been forgotten when the breakfast trays are passed. Any loose or missing teeth should be noted and recorded on the chart. (It may be easier with babies to record the number of teeth present.)

Preoperative sedatives and analgesics may be ordered before certain procedures for various reasons, for example, to eliminate preoperative pain, to supplement and reduce anesthetic requirements, to lessen anxiety and body movement, to facilitate the induction of anesthesia, and to decrease airway secretions. However, there has been a trend to reduce the use of preoperative medication because of possible complications and patient distress at the time of administration when weighed against the benefits obtained. Each child is assessed individually, considering the procedure to be performed. If such medication is given, every effort should be made to see that the young child is allowed to rest, whether in the parent's arms or in the crib with the side rails secure until surgery. More prospective controlled studies of sedation and analgesia in infants and children are necessary to discover the optimal preoperative medication for various situations.

Children may be taken to surgery in their cribs or on carts, or they may walk or have to be carried. Many take a well-labeled security item such as a stuffed animal or special blanket. Eyeglasses and hearing aids are important for communication and must be considered for this trip as well. Unless scheduled to go to an intensive care unit, the child's unit is prepared for his return. The bed, if present, is made up according to the child's postoperative needs, and any special equipment is placed conveniently. An orthopedic patient may need a special mattress, overbed frame and trapeze, and extra-firm pillows. Additional equipment that may be required, depending on the individual, includes a suction machine, intravenous standard, oxygen apparatus, and properly sized restraints.

POSTOPERATIVE CARE
Immediate observation

When patients return to the nursing unit from the recovery room, their general condition must be noted. Periodically pulse, respirations, and blood pressure are determined and recorded. Until patients are responsive and alert, they should be kept on their abdomen or side unless the surgery performed contraindicates these positions. The nurse should note the condition and placement of any dressing and describe any apparent drainage. The presence of a plaster cast or mold should be recorded. Arms or legs in casts should be elevated, and frequent checks for circulatory disturbances should be made. Intravenous infusions should be checked for possible infiltration and correct rate of flow. Children should be protected from harming themselves (pulling out needles or tubes or tampering with suture lines) by the use of appropriate restraints, as necessary. If a child is immobilized with restraints for an extended period of time, it is imperative that appropriate range of motion be included in the plan of care and that explanation be given to the child and family. Urinary catheters should be connected to dependent drainage and stabilized properly. The type and amount of urinary drainage should be observed. The patient's skin color and temperature are checked. The nurse must always watch for and quickly report signs of shock: low blood pressure; cold, moist, pale, or cyanotic skin; rapid pulse; dilated pupils; and restlessness.

Diet

Whether oral fluids are allowed after the child is responsive depends on the physician's orders and the child's general condition. Sometimes surgical patients are not allowed oral fluids for a considerable period of time; instead, they are fed intravenously. When oral feedings are introduced, they are begun gradually, and the patient's tolerance is observed. The routine postsurgical diet follows this sequence with modifications for different age groups—clear liquid, full liquid, soft and regular foods. Rich, spicy, highly seasoned, or gas-forming foods should be avoided by the patient. Because of the confusion that may result, oral surgery patients are not served red gelatin products!

Ambulation

Early progressive ambulation for the general surgery patient is the rule in the modern care of patients. In only a few situations does the physician delay ambulation beyond the first postoperative day. The general surgery patient usually has orders to stand at the bedside and take a few steps the day after surgery. The nurse should be sure to follow these orders because judicious ambulation strengthens the patient, aids in the restoration of gastrointestinal function, and helps prevent complications such as pneumonia and the formation of blood clots and pressure areas.

When the patient's condition or young age makes it impossible or inadvisable to get out of bed, the nurse must be sure that the child is turned frequently, receives good skin care, and breathes deeply at intervals. The physician may order the use of incentive spirometers or intermittent positive-pressure treatments to aid lung expansion.

After surgery, toddlers and preschoolers usually move about spontaneously in their cribs or beds; ambulation presents few problems for them. However, older children may express the same timidity and fear of pain that most adult patients exhibit when asked to move or get up and may need a great deal of initial support and encouragement from their parents and the nursing staff.

Usually it is not long before these same youngsters are enjoying the freedom of the playroom. Most recover quickly, gather together their little hoard of treasures, and say their "goodbyes" in a few days. At times some possessions are overlooked; one nursing staff fondly remembers Bobby, who left his turtle in the linen closet!

Methods of preventing pain and promoting comfort

Although the following discussion of pain prevention has been placed in the context of the child surgical patient, it is readily understood that pain is experienced in many settings. The following considerations should benefit surgical, medical, emergency, and long-term patients of all ages in numerous places.

One of the major goals in patient care is to prevent pain and maintain optimum comfort. The assessment and management of pain in children, therefore, is of critical importance. In 1977 J.M. Eland initially drew attention to the fact that serious undertreatment of pain in children was widespread. Since then much attention and many research studies have been directed toward pain management in children, identifying sound assessment techniques, disproving long-standing misconceptions, and testing the effectiveness of a wide variety of methods for alleviating pain. Much has been learned, and each year our ability to detect and manage pain in children continues to improve.

The physiology of how pain occurs requires an understanding of many different aspects of both the central and peripheral nervous systems. Emotional and psychologic components also contribute significantly to the individual's response to pain. Pain, therefore, is extremely complex and difficult to assess objectively and reliably. It is also difficult to determine the best treatment, especially in the young child whose verbal skills and level of understanding are distinctly limited. The importance and challenge of accurate pain assessment cannot be overestimated.

Assessment of pain in children must include their physiologic and behavioral responses and shared perceptions. Although the infant and toddler are too young to reveal much about their perception of the pain they are experiencing, consultation with their parents may offer some of this missing data. Physiologically, the body responds to a painful stimulus by activating the autonomic nervous system. This causes an increase in the heart rate, pulse, blood pressure, sweating, muscle tension, and gastrointestinal motility. Although these signs and symptoms can be due to other causes as well, they should always be assessed when determining whether pain exists.

Behavioral clues are especially important when assessing the infant and toddler because these children are unable to use verbal means of describing their pain. Four multidimensional behaviors have been researched and suggested as useful in improving the nurse's assessment of the infant believed to be experiencing pain. These four dimensions are vocalization or cry, facial expression or grimacing, body movements involving all four extremities, and the autonomic nervous system responses described above. The assessment process is greatly enhanced by using an organized and consistent approach. The toddler often responds to pain through aggressive behavior such as biting, hitting, temper tantrums, and even verbal hostility. He may also exhibit ritualistic behaviors such as thumb-sucking, rocking, and teeth clenching, or he may be silent and regressive in his response.

The preschool child can verbalize fears and discomfort better than the toddler, but may distort reality significantly because of his understandably self-centered perspective (egocentricity) and magical thinking. He cannot clearly separate himself from the cause of his illness or pain, and has a very limited understanding of body intactness, which can greatly enhance his fears in the hospital situation, and thus also increase his pain. School-age children can usually describe the cause, type, quality, and quantity of pain, especially if given some preparation beforehand, and are able to respond to any one of many possible scales or questionnaires developed specifically to assist with a more accurate and reliable measurement of pain in both children and adults.

From preschool age on, it is possible and highly desirable to elicit the child's own perception of his pain experience, since one of the most widely used definitions of pain is that of Margo McCaffery—that pain is whatever the person experiencing it says it is. A variety of scales are available for use, and a few are applicable to children as young as age 3. The "faces" scale, in the form of drawn faces with progressive gradations of unhappy expressions (Fig. 25-1), and the Oucher scale,

0	1	2	3	4	5

FIG 25-1 Faces pain rating scale. *(From Whaley LF and Wong DL: Essentials of pediatric nursing, ed 3, 1989, St Louis, The CV Mosby Co.)*

which shows photographs of a child in various stages of pain, are both applicable to the preschool child. The poker chips scale uses five white plastic chips to depict "pieces of hurt" and is recommended for use starting at age 4. The validity and reliability of all scales increase with age; again, it is important to remember that some preparation of the child before the painful event greatly enhances its usefulness. Additional scales are the thermometer, the color scale, and the visual analog scale (a horizontal line depicting pain intensity from 0 to 10) as well as a variety of questionnaires and body diagrams that encourage more specific description and localization of the pain. It is most important to select a scale and/or questionnaire that is appropriate to the patient's age, to introduce it at a nonthreatening and pain-free time, and then to use that same scale in a consistent manner at regular intervals as long as pain remains a problem. It is only with this three-dimensional measurement of pain—physiologic, behavioral, and perceptual information—that the nurse can reliably decide first how to manage the child's pain and then determine the effectiveness of that management.

At the same time that the nurse is attempting an accurate assessment of her patient's pain, she must also be aware of the multitude of influential factors at work in determining his reaction to the painful experience. Age, sex, culture, previous experience with pain, fear, the presence of parents, the amount of preparation, and the child's individual temperament and personality all play a role in determining how each child responds to a given situation. A clear understanding of these factors is necessary in order to help the patient manage the pain he is experiencing.

After an accurate pain assessment is achieved, the goal of pain management must be threefold: (1) to eliminate suffering to the greatest degree possible; (2) to enhance each child's ability to cope; and (3) to respond when possible to the underlying reason for the pain. For instance, if the pain is caused by swelling and the edematous extremity is below the level of the heart, elevation of the affected extremity should be the immediate initial intervention.

When all has been done that is possible to treat the cause of the pain, the possible use of medication becomes of primary consideration. Parenteral narcotics are usually the best means of relieving severe pain. However, they should never be used alone, without consideration of additional pain relief measures nor indiscriminately without an awareness of the respiratory depression and other side effects that may occur with their use. Under these circumstances parenteral narcotics not only reduce the pain and stress of hospitalization, but also maximize the effectiveness of additional nursing pain relief measures and can help in preventing postoperative complications as well. A young child cannot breathe deeply and will refuse to ambulate or even move at all if he is in a moderate to severe amount of pain.

Other types of medications such as nonsteroidal anti-inflammatory drugs, muscle relaxants, and antiemetics are often ordered on an as needed basis at the same time, and can provide additional relief of specific complaints that may be contributing to the overall discomfort of the patient. The nurse must consider safety and comfort together when making the all-important determination of the right medication for the individual patient. A sound knowledge of pharmacology will direct appropriate use of narcotics when severe pain exists, a liberal use of nonnarcotic analgesics as the pain is lessening, and conscientious follow-up assessment to detect side effects and determine ongoing pain management.

In addition to medication, the nurse has a multitude of comfort-enhancing interventions available. Probably the most important among these is a positive attitude toward the benefit of each pain-relieving measure proposed, and the development of trust between the nurse and the patient that enables him to relax and relate in a more honest and open manner. Including the parents whenever possible is also crucial because their anxiety clearly contributes to the child's pain; their assistance, when they are supported and informed enough to give it, can help immeasurably in alleviating the child's discomfort.

There are cognitive, behavioral, and physical ways in which to offer pain relief. Cognitive measures include a careful, age-appropriate, and well-timed preparation for hospitalization, surgery, and painful procedures, which is essential to allaying anxiety and fear of the unknown. The child's level of understanding and concept of time help determine how much preparation should be given, and when it should occur. For the younger child, the simpler, more concrete, visual explanation is the most desirable, and the closer its timing is to the actual event, the better.

Behavioral methods of assisting with pain relief include a variety of relaxation techniques such as rhythmic breathing, massage, rocking, therapeutic touch, and the soothing voice of a parent, close friend, or concerned nurse. Guided imagery and hypnosis can be effective, particularly with specially trained personnel, and the simple concept of distraction can work wonders when assisted by the right person in the right way. Play therapy, music, story telling, videos, reading, and various types of games all can be used not only for distraction, but also to help the child gain a degree of mastery and control over his environment. In most children, this greater sense of control helps to decrease pain intensity.

Physical measures of pain control consist of transcutaneous electrical nerve stimulation (TENS), assuring adequate rest, repositioning, application of heat or cold, and elevation of the injured body part, any or all of which may be appropriate depending on the circumstances.

No matter what method or methods of pain control

NURSING CARE PLAN

Care of the Child in Pain

Selected nursing diagnoses	Expected outcomes	Interventions
A. Alteration in comfort, pain related to surgical procedure, inflammation, pressure. Clinical manifestations: HR, RR, BP increase, diaphoresis, restlessness, crying, facial grimacing, verbal report of child and/or parent, pain scale rating of >2 (1-10).	Child remains comfortable throughout hospitalization.	Assess VS and behavioral manifestations of pain, with consideration of level of growth and development. Teach child over age 3 and/or parent how to use appropriate pain scale. Assess location and quality of pain. Evaluate cause of pain and treat if possible. Approach child with confidence of ability to decrease his discomfort. Ensure administration of appropriate analgesic medication as needed. Assess for untoward effects of narcotic analgesia, especially respiratory depression and oversedation. Support in position of comfort. Decrease anxiety by encouraging parental presence, utilizing security objects and keeping child well informed. Make age-appropriate use of nonpharmacologic measures of pain relief, e.g., distraction, relaxation techniques, cutaneous stimulation, guided imagery, etc. Prepare child and/or parent for any painful procedures ahead of time and offer some measure of control if possible. Assess parental anxiety; keep them well informed and encourage participation in care when appropriate. Reassess child to determine response to pain relieving measures.

NURSING CARE PLAN

The Child Undergoing Surgery

Selected nursing diagnoses	Expected outcomes	Interventions
A. Potential for infection related to surgical procedure and anesthesia. Clinical Manifestations: Increase in temperature, respiration and heart rate, and blood pressure, cough, rales and rhonchi, anorexia, purulent drainage at surgical site.	Child exhibits no evidence of wound or respiratory infection.	Monitor vital signs for signs of infection. Provide analgesia prior to respiratory hygiene, ambulation, and wound care. Encourage coughing, deep breathing—may need to splint wound with pillow. Assist child in use of incentive spirometer. Ambulate child as ordered. Maintain aseptic technique and provide wound care as ordered. Promote nutritious diet when child tolerates oral feedings.
B. Anxiety related to surgery, unfamiliar surroundings, discomfort. Clinical Manifestations: Verbalized fear and anxiety, questioning, withdrawal.	Child ventilates concerns and decreases anxiety level.	Familiarize child with items and terms relating to surgery (masks, gowns, gurneys, NPO status, breathing exercises). Allow parents to remain with child as much as possible. Encourage questions and be honest with responses. See Nursing Care Plan for The Hospitalized Child on p. 422.
C. Alteration in Comfort, related to surgical procedure, wound care (See Nursing Care Plan for The Child Experiencing Pain on p. 525)		
D. Potential Fluid Volume Deficit related to NPO status, anorexia, N/V. (See Nursing Care Plan for The Child with Fluid Volume Deficit on p. 478)		

are used, the fact that the nurse's judgment determines it is of crucial importance. This responsibility is challenging, exciting, and sobering all at once. In accepting the responsibility, the nurse needs to maintain a current knowledge base, understand the degree to which personal experience and values influence decision making, and communicate readily with other members of the health team, realizing that it is only with multidisciplinary collaboration that the goal of optimal pain relief will be accomplished.

When working with a patient with chronic, persistent, or unresolved pain, the use of a Pain Flow Sheet can be an invaluable asset. It necessitates frequent documentation of pain assessment parameters, the patient's rating of his pain, methods used to relieve the pain, and both beneficial and adverse effects of those relief measures. Whether or not a Pain Flow Sheet is used, however, the nurse must conscientiously document in the patient's record the reason for, use of, and effects from each pain-relieving measure she administers. By doing this and by constantly reassessing the patient's condition, the nurse can make reliable judgments for ongoing pain management and help fellow workers to do the same.

Many promising prospects for improved pain management are being carefully researched and more and more frequently used in pediatrics. One example is patient-controlled analgesia (PCA). PCA allows the child to determine for himself when he needs pain medication and to administer that medication by pushing a button that sends the narcotic into his bloodstream through an existing intravenous line. The total amount he is allowed to receive is kept within safe limits, and children as young as 9 years of age have learned to use this system successfully. It is extremely encouraging to see the increased attention and research now being directed toward pain relief in children. Hopefully this will stimulate all nurses to use the knowledge at their disposal and the concern for the child's well-being to meet more effectively the challenge of safe and effective pain management for children of all ages.

COMMON PROCEDURES

A few of the common procedures encountered when nursing pediatric surgical patients are described in the following pages. Some of these treatments may also involve medical patients. At times parents may be instructed regarding these techniques as they assume nursing responsibilities for their child at home. They include skin preparation for surgery, cleansing enema, dressing change, gavage feeding, gastrostomy feeding, and irrigation of nasogastric or intestinal tubes.

SKIN PREPARATION FOR SURGERY

PURPOSES: To cleanse the area of prospective surgery to help prevent infection, to provide a clearly visible operative field, and to carefully inspect the skin for possible pustules, lesions, or signs of poor circulation. Skin preps are now frequently performed in the operating room just before surgery. Many surgeons are omitting a shave-prep of the operative site.

MATERIALS:

1. Sharp, sterile razor (if shave-prep is ordered)
2. Clean bowl for warm water
3. Prescribed soap or antibacterial solution
4. Waterproof pad or sheeting
5. Towels (2)
6. Washcloth or gauze sponge
7. Clean cotton applicators, if the areas to prepare involve the umbilicus or toes
8. Nail clippers, if extremities are involved
9. Bath blanket or drawsheet
10. Gooseneck lamp or other good light

PROCEDURE:

1. Check the order, the operative permit, and the time preoperative medications will be given.
2. Identify the patient.
3. Explain the procedure to patients according to their level of understanding. Small children usually respond to the explanation, "We're going to wash your tummy to make it very clean." When you are ready, begin by doing just that. Explain as you work. As the child gains confidence, you may show the youngster the tiny hairs on the arm and talk about how adults shave. Run your finger along the child's skin to show how the razor feels. Suggest that it may tickle a little but that being very still will help.
4. Position the lamp and raise the bed to a convenient working level.
5. Wash your hands.
6. Place the waterproof pad and towel under the patient to protect the bed.
7. Prepare and place the warm water and any ordered antibacterial agent conveniently. (Some physicians may order a dry shave.)
8. Apply tension to the skin with a washcloth or gauze sponge if you shave. (If the feet or fingernails are very dirty, they may be soaking in a basin of warm water while the adjacent areas are being shaved.)
9. Crouch down frequently to look *across* the surface of the skin to check for remaining hairs.
10. Retain your "prep setup" until the skin preparation has been checked by the team leader, head nurse, or instructor.
11. Record the procedure. Any skin lesions (for example, pustules) must be reported. Pustules are *not* to be

opened. Razor nicks should be treated with direct pressure with a sterile sponge and should be reported. Great care must be used in shaving, especially in areas of old scars, insect bites, or bony prominences, where nicking may easily occur.

12. In some cases a povidone-iodine (Betadine) scrub of 10 minutes may be ordered after the shave is complete. The physician may order the prepared area wrapped in sterile towels until surgery.

CLEANSING ENEMA (FIG. 25-2)

PURPOSES: To cleanse the lower bowel before surgery or diagnostic procedures, to relieve constipation or flatulence, and to aid in the expulsion of parasites

MATERIALS:

1. Rectal catheter or tubing and clamps, appropriately sized
   a. For infants, size 12 to 16 French
   b. For young child, size 12 to 20 French
   c. For older child, size 16 to 22 French
2. Container of ordered solution
   a. At 105° F (40.5° C) when given
   b. Suggested total amounts
      (1) Infant—60 to 100 ml
      (2) Toddler to 5 years—250 ml
      (3) School age—250 to 750 ml
   c. An infant or young child should not be expected to retain a cleansing enema until the total amount of fluid is given. Small amounts should be instilled and

then allowed to return around the catheter. The amount expelled should be measured if possible.
3. Lubricant and wipes
4. Asepto syringe barrel or enema can or bag, depending on the amount of fluid to be given and the size of the child

NOTE: Disposable enema setups may be easily used for some patients depending on amount of solution needed. At times commercially prepared enemas may be ordered for children over 2 years simplifying the procedure (e.g., Fleet phosphate-type ready-to-use enema, as ordered by the physician).

PROCEDURE:

1. Check the order.
2. Identify the patient.
3. Explain to the child what will be done as you do it according to the level of understanding. In the case of the very young child, understanding will not be complete, of course, but the tone of voice and the socialization such explanation offers can be helpful. Telling a small child that you are "going to put a little water in to help you go to the bathroom" sometimes helps.
4. Screen the unit and position the child. A number of positions are advocated when giving an infant or toddler an enema.
   a. For most children the side position with the upper leg flexed seems to be the most comfortable. The left side is preferred because this placement puts the descending colon lowest. However, a left-sided

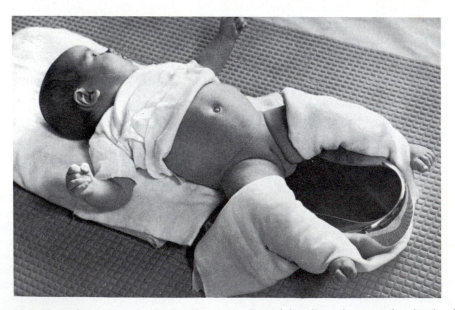

FIG 25-2 Example of infant positioning for enema. Restraining diaper is centered under tip of pan and then brought up and over infant's legs and pinned to itself.

position is not absolutely mandatory. In fact, some investigators question the supposed advantages of left-sided placement. Infants and small toddlers often do well if placed on a firm pillow, which has been draped with a lightweight plastic sheet and covered with an absorbent towel, with their hips pulled to the edge. The plastic extends over the side of the pillow into or beside a curved basin or small bedpan, which is placed snugly against the buttocks just below the rectum. For warmth, the child is covered by a bath blanket or towel.

b. If the infant is very active and a nurse has no one to help maintain the child in a side position, the infant may be gently restrained in supine position over a small bedpan. The back and head are supported by a small pillow or folded bath blanket. The buttocks are placed over the bedpan and the legs gently drawn to either side and secured by a diaper placed under the bedpan and drawn up and over the lower extremities and pinned to itself as illustrated in Fig. 25-2.

c. Older children with sphincter control are usually positioned on their sides and given enemas in basically the same way as any adult.

5. Place the ordered amount and type of solution in a can or Asepto barrel attached to a clamped rectal tube. Expel the air from the tube and lubricate the tip. Do not occlude the eyes of the catheter.

6. Gently insert the tubing approximately ½ to 3 inches (3.7 to 7.6 cm), depending on the size of the patient, into the rectum and observe the flow. Hold the container of solution no higher than 12 to 18 inches (30 to 46 cm) above the patient's hips.

7. Observe the patient closely during the procedure for an increase in respiratory and pulse rates and exhaustion.

8. As needed, put the child on a bedpan or potty chair, or allow the child to go to the bathroom.

9. Remove equipment and tidy up the area.

10. Record the procedure, the solution used, and the results obtained.

STERILE DRESSING CHANGE

PURPOSES: To protect the incision or wound from contamination by replacing soiled or wet dressings, to allow direct observation of the incision or wound to evaluate the healing process or measure wound drainage, to increase the cleanliness and comfort of the patient, and, in some instances, to apply local medications, carry out irrigations or debridement procedures (wet to dry dressings) that assist in treatment

MATERIALS: Materials vary according to the area to be dressed and whether sutures are to be removed or local debridement attempted, and according to the wishes of the physician. The following supplies may be needed, although not all the supplies listed are needed every time. Simple dressings may require only sterile compresses, handling forceps, adhesive tape, and a discard bag.

1. Dressing tray containing the following:
   a. Basic instrument kit with sterile instruments
      (1) Suture-remover scissors
      (2) Clip removers
      (3) Sharp-pointed suture scissors
      (4) Tissue forceps
      (5) Smooth forceps
      (6) Small hemostat
      (7) Probe
   b. Wrapped, sterile cotton applicators
   c. Wrapped, sterile dressings of various thicknesses and sizes
      (1) Thick, absorbent pads (ABD or composite pads)
      (2) 4×4-inch and 2×2-inch gauze squares (flats)
      (3) Nonadherent dressings (Telfa)
      (4) Soft gauze dressings that have been fluffed out (fluffs)
   d. Various sizes of gauze roller bandage, Kerlix, or Ace tensor bandage
   e. Various sizes and kinds of adhesive tape or Montgomery straps
2. Sterile gloves (used when the area to be dressed is large or difficult to manage)
3. Large paper or plastic bag to receive old dressings
4. Clean kidney basin for antiseptic pour-off overflow
5. Bandage scissors
6. Appropriate antiseptic, irrigating solution, or medication; sterile syringe and basin
7. Clean paper towels

PROCEDURE:

1. Check the order.
2. Select a time when there is little bedmaking or mopping activity in the area. These activities increase the bacteria count in the air.
3. Identify and screen the patient and explain the purpose of the dressing change according to the level of understanding. At times positioning assistance may be needed.
4. Drape the patient appropriately.
5. Adjust the lamp, if needed; position and open discard bag and kidney basin, if needed.
6. Wash your hands.
7. Open only those supplies needed.
8. Place sterile handling forceps on the edge of a sterile wrapper—points on the sterile surface, handles over the edge.
9. Remove bandages or adhesive tape (Always pull tape toward the incision or wound to prevent undue strain or pain.)

10. Lift off the top dressing, your hand protected by a clean, folded paper towel or clean plastic gloves. Contact only the side of the dressing that was exposed to the exterior. Drop dressing and towel or glove into open paper bag.

11. Lift off any remaining inner dressing with the sterile handling forceps or use sterile gloves. Be careful not to pull drains, if present. Dressings that stick to the skin usually may be moistened with a small amount of sterile saline solution to facilitate their removal. Always note the presence of a drain when recording the dressing change.

12. Cleanse the area gently of any old drainage present with mild antiseptic or solution as ordered, using sterile gauze sponges mounted on handling forceps or gloved hands. Pour the solution onto the sponge over the discard kidney basin or use a sterile basin. Dry the area with a sterile compress.

13. Place the new sterile dressing, appropriate for size of the incision and amount of drainage present, using handling forceps or sterile gloves. Remove gloves, if used, before handling tape.

14. Secure with adhesive tape, Elastoplast, or Montgomery tapes. If using adhesive tape, turn back the ends slightly "sticky side against sticky side" to make the tape easier to remove.

15. Discard used dressings, wash your hands, and tidy up the area.

16. Record the procedure and the condition of the wound or incision. Describe the type and amount of any drainage present and report any unusual odor. Note any skin irritation caused by adhesive. Note any drains present.

17. NOTE: If your patient is having the sterile dressings weighed to calculate the amount of wound drainage, you may:
    a. Weigh the total amount of dressings to be used in their sterile wrappers using a gram scale and mark their weight on the outside.
    b. Apply the dressings and save the wrappers carefully after marking the time and date of the dressing change next to the weight previously indicated.
    c. At the time of the next dressing change, discard the old dressings on the saved wrappers and weigh them again. The difference in weight expressed in grams will equal (for this purpose) the milliliters of drainage present.

GAVAGE FEEDING USING AN INDWELLING NASOGASTRIC TUBE OR ORAL FEEDING TUBE

PURPOSE: To avoid mouth and lip motion when it may endanger surgical repair, to nourish a child who is too weak to be fed orally in the normal fashion, and to supplement oral feeding when nutritional buildup is imperative and sufficient intake by normal means is impossible

(NOTE: When needed, feeding tubes for premature infants are now usually inserted orally before each feeding. Such an approach keeps the nose unobstructed and untraumatized, helps maintain a sucking reflex, and reduces incidence of bradycardia during insertion.)

MATERIALS:

1. Sterile Asepto or piston-type syringe (If the child is receiving sterilized formula, a sterile syringe will be secured for each feeding. If the child is not receiving sterilized formula, the nurse may wash and store the syringe in a clean manner for use next time.)
2. Container of formula (infants who receive sterilized formula will have the feeding tube sterilized)
3. Glass of water (bottle of sterile water for infants)
4. Towel or napkin
5. Possibly bib and infant seat
6. Appropriate tube and tape as needed
7. Stethoscope

PROCEDURE:

1. Check the order.
2. Identify the patient and explain the procedure according to his needs and level of understanding.
3. Briefly warm the formula, if necessary, so that it will be tepid at the time of the feeding. (Feeding cold formula, if not given by pump or slow drip, can be upsetting to the patient and may initiate vomiting.) Evaluate the consistency of the feeding: Is it too thick? Will it clog the tube? Many times you cannot dilute a feeding and administer the entire amount to maintain the caloric count ordered without overloading the stomach.
4. Unless contraindicated, raise the backrest of a child's bed or place a baby on his side, head elevated. An elevated position lets gravity aid the flow of the formula. Restrain as necessary.
5. Protect the area next to the tube opening with a towel.
6. If insertion of an oral tube is indicated:
    a. Measure the tube for insertion from the tip of the nose, to the lobe of the ear, to ½ inch below the xiphoid process; mark with tape.
    b. Gently pull down on the chin and advance the tube over the tongue to the tape marker.
    c. Observe the infant continually for color change, gagging, coughing, or respiratory distress. Withdraw the tube if any occurs.
    d. Secure the tube to the face with tape or hold it in place with one hand.
7. Test the position of the end of the tube by each of the following methods:
    a. Observe the length of the tube exposed.
    b. Inject approximately 1 to 5 ml of air (depending on patient) into the tube. Listen with a stethoscope just below the sternum for sound of air passage.

Withdraw the air and suction further for evidence of stomach contents, or, if ordered, measure entire aspirate to help determine digestion of previous feedings and current stomach capacity. Measured aspirate is usually returned to the stomach and the amount of the ordered feeding reduced by the amount of the aspirate.

   c. Ask the patient to hum, if possible. If the tube is in the trachea, the patient cannot hum.

8. Continue with the administration of the formula. In most instances allow the formula to flow by gravity. Exerting additional pressure may be dangerous. If the flow is sluggish, raise the barrel. If it is too fast, lower the barrel or pinch the tube. If the flow has stopped, change position of the patient slightly. If the flow still does not continue, *gentle* pressure with a syringe bulb or piston may *start* the flow. If no response is forthcoming, the tube must be removed and another inserted. If the infant is crying, flow will be slower than when the child is quiet.

9. Add more formula before the barrel is empty to avoid introducing additional air into the stomach. If the tube is to be left in place, when the formula is finished (just before the last few drops leave the barrel) add 5 to 15 ml of water to rinse the tube. (Failure to include this step will cause a clogged tube.) If the tube is to be removed, pinch it tightly before and during its quick removal to prevent drops of formula from entering the airway.

10. An infant must be burped after gavage just as he would be burped after routine oral feeding.

11. Record any aspirate obtained, the amount and type of feeding, and the tolerance of the patient.

GASTROSTOMY FEEDING

PURPOSE: To provide nourishment by way of a tube that has been surgically inserted through the abdominal wall into the stomach because of obstruction or surgical repair of the child's oroesophageal tract or to avoid the constant irritation of a nasogastric tube when oral feedings are not possible

MATERIALS:

1. Tray containing the following:
   a. Syringe barrel (sterile for small infants receiving sterilized formula)
   b. Container of formula (sterile for small infants)
   c. Container of water (sterile for small infants)
2. Towel or napkin

PROCEDURE:

1. Check the order.
2. Identify patient and explain the procedure according to his needs and level of understanding.
3. Evaluate the formula as for a gavage feeding. Position

the child either flat with his head raised or elevated in a semisitting position.

4. Attach the syringe barrel to the tube and fill with formula before unclamping the tube. (NOTE: There may be orders to aspirate the contents of the stomach into the barrel. The amount aspirated is noted, and it is allowed to return to the stomach. The feeding to be given is decreased accordingly to prevent overloading.)

5. Unclamp the tube and allow the fluid to flow slowly by gravity. Never use pressure of any kind to start the flow of formula into the gastrostomy tube. This may cause unwanted backflow into the esophagus.

6. Continue to add formula to the barrel before it completely empties to avoid introducing air into the stomach.

7. Finish the feeding by adding 15 to 30 ml of water to rinse the tube. Clamp off the tube before all the water leaves the barrel to avoid introducing air into the stomach. (NOTE: In some cases involving infants, the physician may order that the tube not be clamped but left opened with the barrel attached and elevated above the baby's body. The formula is allowed to return to the barrel as the child cries or changes position.)

8. Record the amount and type of feeding and the tolerance of the patient.

IRRIGATION OF A NASOGASTRIC OR INTESTINAL TUBE ATTACHED TO SUCTION

PURPOSES: To prevent the clogging and ensure the patency of an indwelling nasogastric or intestinal tube. The tube may have been inserted (1) to prevent vomiting or (2) to relieve postoperative abdominal distention, discomfort, and pressure on surgical repairs.

When the tube has been inserted for the reasons cited, it is attached to some type of suction or drainage device. Usually the suction ordered is intermittent; occasionally it may be continuous. High or low negative pressure may be prescribed. Sometimes only gravity drainage is ordered. Most children are placed on low intermittent suction. Irrigation is carried out only when the wishes of the physician concerning the individual case are known. Double-lumen or sump-type nasogastric tubes are frequently used. A small tube, or sump, which serves as an "airway," is incorporated into the larger suction tube. As the suction pulls out gastric contents, it also pulls in air via the airway; this helps prevent the end of the suction tube from "grabbing" the stomach mucosa and causing tissue damage.

MATERIALS: Unless the type of surgery makes it necessary to employ sterile technique, the materials used to irrigate a tube must be kept meticulously clean but need not be sterile. The type and amount of irrigating fluid to be used is ordered by the physician. Physiologic saline solution, often combined with a suspension of magnesium and aluminum hydroxides such as Maalox, is frequently requested. (The antacid helps to neutralize stomach acidity, thus preventing irritation and bleeding of gastric mucosa.) The amount used depends on the size of the child and the type of surgery performed.

A setup usually includes the following:

1. Syringe (10 to 30 ml, depending on amount to be used)
2. Basin or solution reservoir
3. Clamp
4. Towel and emesis basin
5. Ordered solution

PROCEDURE:

1. Identify the patient.
2. Explain the procedure to the child according to the level of understanding. For young children it is usually sufficient to say that you are putting a little "water" in the tube.
3. Draw up the amount and kind of solution ordered in the syringe.
4. Place a folded towel and emesis basin under the junction of the tube leading to the suction apparatus or gravity drainage.
5. Turn off any mechanical suction device.
6. Clamp the tubing that leads to the suction or drainage bag and disconnect the two parts of the tubing; wrap the end of the tubing that leads to the suction machine in a towel, cover it with cap, and hang it from a support on the machine or hold it between your last two fingers.
7. Fit the syringe of irrigating fluid into the patient's tube and gently instill the ordered amount. Whether the nurse will be allowed to withdraw any of the irrigating solution with the attached syringe will depend on the preferences of the physician. If a sump-type tube is being irrigated, the saline may be instilled in either the end of the sump or "airway" or the end of the suction tube. Regardless of the route used for irrigation after the instillation, approximately 10 cc of air should be injected into the sump to clear the tube. The sump tube outlet should never be clamped while the suction is in operation.
8. Detach the syringe and reconnect the tube either to the suction machine (removing the clamp and restarting the suction) or to the gravity drainage. (Recheck any suction setting.)
9. Remember, this patient is usually not allowed oral fluids except perhaps *small* amounts of ice chips. However, lubrication of the nares, renewal of the tape maintaining the tube's position, and oral hygiene are fairly common patient needs.
10. Record in the patient's output record the amount of irrigating fluid used. (NOTE: If a tube is not draining and resistance is encountered during an attempted ordered irrigation, the nurse should notify her supervisor immediately.)

One of the most satisfying aspects of the role of the pediatric nurse is watching children master their fears and anxieties about impending surgical procedures. A nurse truly fulfills the role of the helping person when she is able to assist children and their families to cope with a potentially traumatic situation.

Key Concepts

1. Child-adult distinctions that may help the nurse evaluate the needs of children include the following: the metabolic rate of infants and young children is proportionately much greater than that of adults; abnormal fluid loss is more serious in the infant and the young child than in the adult; the child lacks the physical reserves that are available to the adult; the body tissues of the child heal quickly; and the young child lives more in the present than an adult does.

2. Preparing a child for surgery must be based on the following factors: age and developmental level; the child's perception of hospitalization and the upcoming surgery; the surgical procedure to be performed; postoperative care; previous hospital experience; expected length of hospitalization; and parental attitudes.

3. Psychologic preparation must be geared to the child's developmental level, not merely to chronologic age. Parents should also be informed and reassured.

4. Postoperatively, pulse, respirations, and blood pressure are periodically assessed and recorded. The nurse must always watch for and quickly report any signs of shock.

5. The assessment and management of pain in children are of critical importance. The level of pain experienced is influenced by both physiologic and emotional factors; therefore, it is difficult to assess objectively and reliably.

6. Physical signs of pain include increases in heart rate, pulse, blood pressure, perspiration, muscle tension, and gastrointestinal motility.

7. In addition to the physical signs of pain, the nurse should assess an infant for vocalization or cry, facial expression or grimacing, and body movements involving all four extremities.

8. The toddler often responds to pain through aggressive or ritualistic behavior.

9. The preschool child can verbalize fears and discom-

fort better than the toddler, but may significantly distort reality.

10. School-age children can usually describe the cause, type, quality, and quantity of pain.

11. A variety of scales and questionnaires have been developed to assist with the measurement of pain. The validity and reliability of these tools increase with the child's age. Some preparation regarding these tools should be provided for the child before the painful experience.

12. The goal of pain management must be threefold: (1) to eliminate suffering to the greatest degree possible, (2) to enhance each child's ability to cope, and (3) to respond when possible to the underlying reason for the pain.

13. Narcotic and nonnarcotic medications may be used to relieve pain. Side effects and other pain relief measures must also be considered when determining the most appropriate medication for each patient.

14. In addition to medication, the nurse can offer pain relief in cognitive, behavioral, and physical ways.

15. Early progressive ambulation is usually ordered for the general surgery patient. When the child's condition or young age makes it impossible or inadvisable to get out of bed, the nurse must be sure that the child is turned frequently, receives good skin care, and breathes deeply at intervals.

16. Various procedures are encountered when caring for pediatric surgery patients, including skin preparation for surgery, cleansing enema, dressing change, gavage feeding, gastrostomy feeding, and irrigation of nasogastric or intestinal tubes. Parents may be instructed regarding these techniques if they are to care for their child at home.

Discussion Questions

1. What critical factors must be taken into consideration when preparing a child for surgery? Give some examples of how the preparation for surgery changes according to the child's age and developmental level.

2. More minor surgical procedures are being performed on a "day surgery" basis. How can proper preparation be done if the patient doesn't arrive until 1 or 2 hours before surgery?

3. With the trend toward early discharge, parents are becoming increasingly responsible for the nursing care of children having recently undergone surgery. What would you explain to the parents regarding diet, activity, care of the incision, and specific observations?

4. Identify the specific safety precautions that may be required to prevent a child from harm postoperatively. Why is it essential for the nurse to observe a child more often than an adult?

5. Do you think that children experience as much postoperative pain as adults do? Why? How would you assess a child for signs of pain or discomfort?

26

Aiding Respiration and Oxygenation

CHAPTER OBJECTIVES

After studying this chapter, the student should be able to perform the following:

1 Define respiration, PaO_2, SaO_2, hypoxemia.
2 List six signs of possible respiratory difficulty.
3 Give the normal values for arterial blood gases in children.
4 State the purpose of chest physiotherapy and identify four of its components.
5 Explain the purpose of the cuff on an endotracheal or tracheostomy tube.

6 Name three possible complications of suctioning endotracheal and tracheostomy tubes.
7 Cite four safety considerations associated with the administration of oxygen.
8 Give three reasons for placing patients on mechanical ventilation.

The process of respiration refers to gas exchange or the movement of oxygen from the atmosphere into the bloodstream and the movement of carbon dioxide from the bloodstream into the atmosphere. In some diseases ventilation of air into and out of the lungs, transfer of gases across the alveolar-capillary membrane, or blood flow is inhibited, thereby decreasing the amount of oxygen available for cellular function. To remedy this problem, various procedures, apparatuses, and medications have been developed for clearing the airway, enriching the oxygen content of inspired air, stimulating or maintaining adequate ventilatory effort, or achieving adequate circulation of blood.

Nurses can do a great deal to maintain and improve the respiratory function of their patients. They need to work closely with respiratory therapists to sustain optimal breathing and prevent respiratory dysfunction. In many

hospitals the responsibilities of respiratory therapists include supervision of gaseous and ventilator therapy, and performance of chest physiotherapy, and resuscitation measures.

HINDRANCES TO OXYGENATION OF THE BLOOD

To understand more clearly the types of problems encountered and the rationale of many of the treatments ordered, the student should review the structure and function of the respiratory system (Figs. 26-1 and 26-2). The passageways from the exterior of the body to the microscopic air sacs (alveoli), which make up the functional tissue of the lungs, must remain open to ensure proper oxygenation. Any obstruction, whether caused by the position of the tongue, aspiration of a foreign body, edema, a tumor, the presence of tenacious secretions in the laryngotracheobronchial "tree," or spasm of the bron-

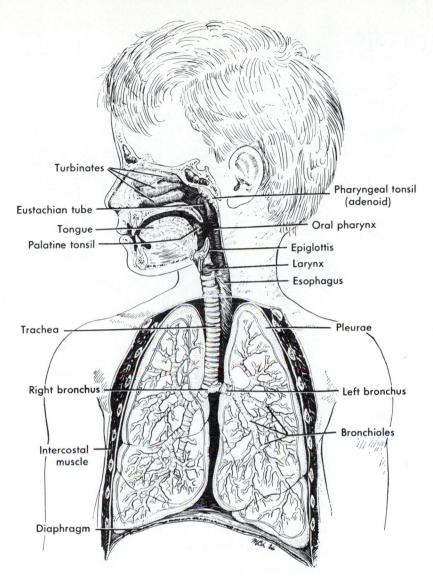

Turbinates

Eustachian tube

Tongue

Palatine tonsil

Pharyngeal tonsil
(adenoid)

Oral pharynx

Epiglottis

Larynx

Esophagus

Trachea

Pleurae

Right bronchus

Left bronchus

Bronchioles

Intercostal
muscle

Diaphragm

FIG 26-1 Normal respiratory tract.

chioles, will lead to respiratory difficulty. Conditions such as atelectasis, pneumonia, pulmonary edema, tuberculosis, and a malignancy that cause a depletion in the ability of the lung tissue to receive air and transfer oxygen and carbon dioxide may cause respiratory distress. Common pulmonary disorders in infants and children are respiratory distress syndrome (RDS), aspiration, pneumonia, bronchiolitis, croup, and asthma. Less common but most challenging is cystic fibrosis.

Any interruption in the mechanisms of breathing also affects respiration and therefore oxygenation. Of course,

in the final analysis the circulatory system must also be adequate to deliver oxygen to its final destination—the individual microscopic body cells.

CLINICAL SIGNS AND SYMPTOMS OF RESPIRATORY DIFFICULTY

A nurse should be thoroughly familiar with clinical signs of respiratory difficulty. Signs of respiratory difficulty include the following problems:

1. Depressed or elevated respiratory or cardiac rates

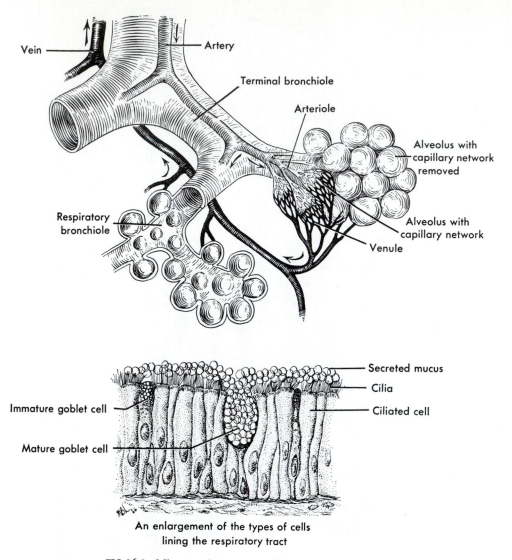

An enlargement of the types of cells
lining the respiratory tract

FIG 26-2   Microscopic anatomy of lower respiratory tract.

at rest for the age of the child considered (see p.
460 for a pulse and respiration table)
2. Any chest retractions, note kinds (Figs. 26-3 and
26-4 show types of retractions in infants)
3. Noisy, labored breathing, grunting, wheezing
4. Flaring nostrils and the use of facial and neck muscles in attempts to aid respirations
5. Pallor, cyanosis (gray to purple skin coloring),
which may be localized or generalized
6. Restlessness, apprehension, and disorientation
7. Inflamed respiratory tract with or without thick
nasal discharge and blockage of the nasal passageways

8. Frequent productive or nonproductive coughing
(however, the absence of coughing is not in itself
necessarily a sign of respiratory improvement)

The observation of any of the preceding signs and
symptoms deserves prompt report and evaluation. If a
child becomes cyanotic and a bedside oxygen unit is
available, it should first be determined that the child's
airway is open, then the oxygen should be started and
assistance sought for further evaluation of the patient.
The pulse rate and respirations should be counted. Many
children with circulatory and respiratory problems in
which fluid tends to collect in the chest or abdomen

CHEST MOVEMENT

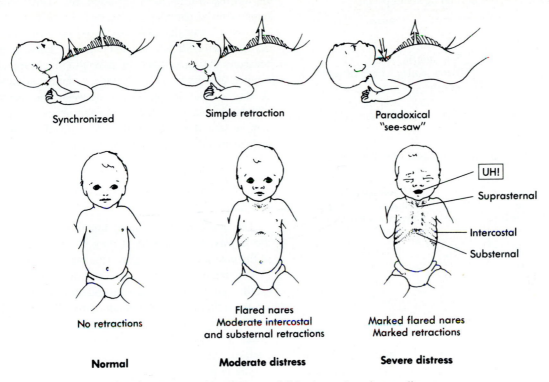

FIG 26-3 Types of respiration—visible signs of respiratory distress.

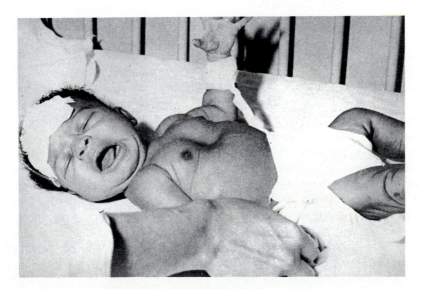

FIG 26-4 Deep substernal retractions caused by pneumonia (note hollow in chest area). The retractions lessened when the baby was placed upright in an infant chair. *(Courtesy Naval Hospital, San Diego, Calif.)*

Table 26-1 Normal ranges for arterial blood gases (ABGs) for infants and children beyond newborn period*

ABGs	Range
pH	7.35-7.45
$PaCO_2/PCO_2$	35-45 mmHg
PaO_2/PO_2	83-108 mmHg (Adult value 80-100 mmHg)

*Measurements at sea level—21% O_2. For newborn values see p. 304.

Table 26-2 Approximate relationships between PaO_2 and SaO_2 values*

Partial pressure of oxygen in arterial blood (PaO_2)	Percentage of hemoglobin saturated by oxygen in arterial blood (SaO_2)
100 mmHg	98%
60 mmHg	90%
45 mmHg	80%
30 mmHg	60%

*An SaO_2 of 90% or less signifies hypoxemia.

breathe more easily when propped in a semi-Fowler's position or supported in an infant seat. The most accurate way to determine the extent of oxygenation of a patient's blood is by chemical analysis of the oxygen and carbon dioxide levels in an arterial blood sample.

LABORATORY EVALUATION OF OXYGENATION

The term *hypoxemia* describes the presence of subnormal amounts of oxygen dissolved in arterial blood plasma. Tissue hypoxia occurs when a subnormal amount of oxygen is delivered to the body cells.

Clinical signs of tissue hypoxia may be identified. Tachycardia and tachypnea are common mechanisms triggered to correct the hypoxia. Other signs are hypertension, polycythemia, dysrhythmias, and low urine output. When more than one third of the body's hemoglobin is not oxygen-saturated, cyanosis may be present. A myriad of neurologic symptoms such as headache, anxiety, agitation, confusion, weakness, double vision, and drowsiness may be experienced. Eventually, coma may develop.

Although the clinical signs and symptoms of hypoxia are important manifestations, they are, nonspecific, and can relate to other organ dysfunction. Because tissue hypoxia cannot be directly measured, the most accurate way to determine the extent of oxygenation is through the measurement of the oxygen (PaO_2/PO_2) and carbon dioxide ($PaCO_2/PCO_2$) levels in an arterial blood sample. Indwelling arterial lines are often established when frequent arterial samples are needed. Pulse oximeters are also used clinically to measure oxygen saturation after comparison with arterial blood gases. Pulse oximeters measure the percentage of hemoglobin saturated with oxygen and have the advantage of being noninvasive. A direct relationship exists between the percentage of hemoglobin saturated by oxygen in an arterial blood sample (SaO_2) and the partial pressure of oxygen in an arterial blood sample (PaO_2/PO_2). See Tables 26-1 and 26-2.

SECURING AND MAINTAINING AN AIRWAY
Position

The first concern in aiding breathing always involves the airway. Occasionally it may be obstructed because of the position of the tongue. This may be especially true in the unconscious patient; the tongue is not actually swallowed, but falls backward and obstructs the pharynx. An open airway may be obtained by placing the patient on his back with his head in "sniffing" position and his lower jaw held up. This returns the tongue to normal position. At times the insertion of a plastic oropharyngeal airway is needed.

If the airway is obstructed by a foreign body or secretions, the emergency relief usually attempted *first* involves gravity drainage. However, in cases of choking, in which the patient is unable to speak or cough, several repeated, controlled, upward thrusts of the thumb-side of a fist just below the patient's rib cage are used (Heimlich maneuver). This causes the diaphragm to suddenly force air out through the airway, which may dislodge a foreign body. Further references and detailed instruction should be sought.* Occasionally the bronchi may need to be visualized for removal of a foreign body. A relatively small, flexible, fiberoptic bronchoscope is then employed.

To prevent aspiration, a child in danger of vomiting or regurgitating should be maintained on his side or abdomen. If this is impossible because of other more important considerations (such as the type of surgery or administration of an anesthetic), the head should be lowered and turned to the side during episodes of nausea and vomiting. Babies are sometimes placed upright in infant seats to help prevent vomiting.

*Nursing '85 Books: Nurse's reference library: Emergencies, Springhouse, Pa, 1985, Springhouse Corporation, pp 94-97. See also Fig. 26-5 and p. 549.

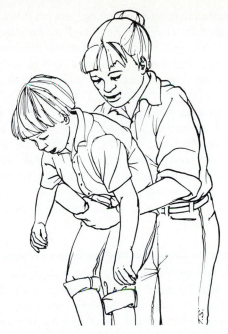

FIG 26-5 Heimlich maneuver. When a child is conscious, struggling to breathe, unable to speak or cough and sitting or standing, the rescuer wraps his or her arms around the child's waist. One hand grasps the opposite fist, which is positioned in the midline thumb side against the child's abdomen just above the navel and well below the xiphoid process. The rescuer's fist is pushed forcefully against the child's abdomen to produce a quick upward thrust. The thrusts are repeated until the foreign body is expelled or a series of 10 thrusts have been completed. *(Reproduced with permission. © Instructor's Manual for Basic Life Support, 1987. Copyright American Heart Association.)*

Nasopharyngeal suction

Suction of the naso-oropharyngeal passages may be necessary to clear the airway. Suction is accomplished by using a bulb syringe, or a catheter setup attached to wall or portable suction (see Fig. 13-1.) The following procedure points should be remembered when a catheter is used:

1. Catheter sizes vary with the size of the patient, usually as follows:
   a. Infants, size 5 to 8 French
   b. Children, size 8 to 10 French
   c. Youths and adults, size 12 to 14 French
2. An individual suction apparatus is used for each patient and is kept free from contamination. Although in some instances clean rather than sterile techniques would be acceptable for suctioning limited to the nose, mouth, and throat, trauma and hazards of infection are still possible. Therefore sterile precautions are used, especially when dealing with infants, young children, and patients who are particularly vulnerable to injury or sepsis. A two-glove technique (one sterile, one clean) is now encouraged to reduce the possibility of contamination and the danger of cross-infection.
3. At the outset, the drainage bottle should contain about 1 inch of disinfectant solution to make cleaning it easier and to reduce the number of organisms in the bottle.
4. Catheters should be lubricated with saline or water-soluble gel to ensure greater ease of insertion. Suctioning saline through the catheter before use will also verify that the suction is functioning properly.
5. During catheter insertion suction should be temporarily discontinued by pinching the catheter or uncovering the Y-tube or other thumb suction control opening. This will help prevent depletion of the patient's oxygen supply or injury to the mucous membranes. To suction the nose, the catheter should be guided along the floor of the nasal cavity, parallel with the roof of the mouth.
6. The lowest amount of suction necessary should be intermittently applied as the catheter is being rotated and withdrawn (see box below). Suction should not be prolonged (no more than 10 seconds). If administered too frequently, suction may aggravate rather than relieve congestion.
7. The catheter and connection tubing should be rinsed during and after use to prevent clogging.
8. The child usually needs to be restrained during the procedure.
9. The catheter should be discarded after each suctioning procedure.
10. Note should be taken of the type and relative amount of suctioned material obtained and the patient's tolerance of the procedure or relief obtained.

Suggested suction ranges

Neonate	60-80 mmHg
Child	80-100 mmHg
Teenager	100-120 mmHg

ENDOTRACHEAL AND TRACHEOSTOMY TUBE PLACEMENT AND SUCTION

Endotracheal intubation

When the patient's airway and oxygenation cannot be maintained using the previously mentioned treatments, an artificial airway or endotracheal tube must be inserted. Often the patient also needs to be supported on a mechanical ventilator at this time.

The indications for endotracheal intubation are generally of an emergency nature, such as need for airway maintenance, removal of secretions, prevention of aspiration in a compromised patient, respiratory insufficiency or failure, and/or the need to enhance oxygenation. An endotracheal tube is the most common artificial airway for short-term airway management, although it may be used for several weeks when prolonged ventilation is required.

Immediately after intubation, the adequacy of tube placement should be determined by observing symmetric chest movement, auscultating bilaterally equal breath sounds and absent breath sounds over the stomach. An x-ray should be taken to confirm its position. Occasionally an endotracheal tube can slip into the right mainstem bronchus, which is more nearly vertical to the trachea than the left. A reference mark should be made at the point of insertion into the mouth or nose in order to detect subsequent tube movement. Following intubation, the tube should be secured to the patient's face with benzoin and tape.

Tracheostomy

When it is anticipated that a child will need ventilatory support or airway maintenance for more than a few weeks, a tracheostomy is performed. A tracheostomy is an artificial surgical opening into the trachea, usually at the second through fourth tracheal rings, performed electively in the operating room. There is almost no such thing as an emergency tracheostomy anymore. A tracheostomy provides the best route for long-term airway maintenance because of easier secretion removal, increased patient acceptance and comfort, and the ability to eat and sometimes talk with the tube in place. (See p. 542.)

Types of artificial airways

Most tubes are made of plastic material and have an inflatable cuff attached (usually if the child is over 8 years old). This cuff or balloon is built into the end portion of an endotracheal or tracheostomy tube. When inflated, it creates a seal between the tube and the pa-

tient's trachea to prevent air leakage and provide a closed system, thereby enabling the patient to be adequately ventilated. The cuff should be of the low pressure, high volume type, and should be inflated with an intentional minimum air leak in order to prevent tracheal wall damage.

Tracheostomy tubes may be single lumen or double lumen. Single-lumen tubes consist of the tube and the cuff and an obturator, which is necessary during insertion. Double-lumen tubes have, in addition, an inner cannula that can be removed for cleaning. The obturator of the patient's indwelling (in situ) tube and another tube of the same size must be at the bedside in case of accidental removal.

Suctioning (endotracheal and tracheostomy tubes)

When the upper respiratory tract is bypassed, the defense system becomes impaired, and warming and humidification of gases must be done externally. Studies show contamination of the lower airways 24 hours after endotracheal intubation.*

The cough reflex is also compromised and tracheal suctioning must be performed through the artificial airway. The technique must be sterile to prevent infection.

Complications of tracheal suctioning via endotracheal tube or tracheostomy include hypoxemia and resulting cardiac arrythmias, and bronchospasm; airway irritation and possible infection caused by catheter; and atelectasis from applying too much suction. Suctioning should be performed only when necessary, that is, when secretions are audibly or visibly obstructing the artificial airway. Basically, the technique for endotracheal suctioning is as follows:

1. Oxygenate the patient. The patient should be given oxygen for several minutes prior to, during, and immediately after suctioning. (The concentration of O_2 used is usually 100% except in the case of newborns for whom lower oxygen concentrations are typically employed.)
2. Use a sterile disposable suction tray equipped with gloves, catheter, and saline solution. Rinse catheter in saline and test suction (Fig. 26-6).
3. Install 0.5 to 2 ml of sterile saline in trachea to help thin secretions during inspiration (an optional procedure; may initiate productive cough).
4. Insert the catheter applying *no* suction (finger off

---

*Heffner JE, Miller KS, and Sahn S: Tracheostomy in the intensive care unit: part II, Complications, Chest 90(3):430, 1987; Trout C: Artificial airways: tubes and trachs, Resp Care 21(6):513, 1976.

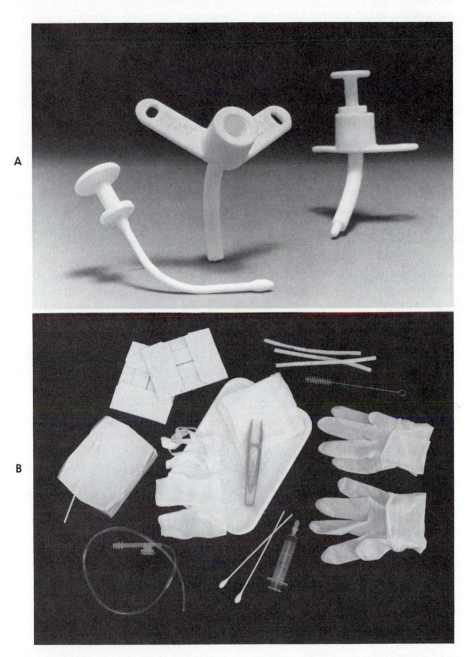

FIG 26-6 **A,** *Left to right*, Shiley pediatric tracheostomy tube obturator, pediatric tube, Shiley neonatal tracheostomy tube with obturator in place. **B,** Contents of tracheostomy suctioning and cleaning tray (Pharmaseal). *(A,* Courtesy Shiley, Inc.)

vent) during inspiration when the airways are open wider. The alert patient can be instructed to take a breath as the catheter is inserted.

5. Apply suction intermittently during expiration while rotating catheter in a circular motion.

6. Limit total time in which catheter is in trachea to 10 seconds.

Communication

Patients cannot talk with a patent endotracheal tube or a tracheostomy tube; therefore, they must rely on medical personnel to provide a means of communication. A young child who cannot yet write but cries for attention may be especially frightened. When appropriate, signal cords or handbells should always be available. Communication devices like magic slates, cards, talkboards, and a simple pen and pencil can be used for older children. When a tracheostomy tube can be plugged or a talking trach inserted, a patient with a tracheostomy is able to talk. Fortunately, body language usually can be easily interpreted. A nurse with a calm, reassuring manner is most helpful.

Medications

Medications are frequently ordered to aid in clearing the airway.

Nose drops. Nose drops, such as phenylephrine hydrochloride (Neo-Synephrine), may be ordered to shrink mucous membranes and ease nasal congestion.

Expectorants. Oral expectorants, which increase the bronchial secretions and may help thin mucus, are occasionally ordered. Common medications of this type are potassium iodide and guaifenesin syrup.

Aerosols. *Acetylcysteine* (Mucomyst) reduces the thickness and tenacity of mucus and is used primarily for patients with cystic fibrosis. It is, however, administered *with caution* because it has been known to cause bronchospasm and/or bleeding. Cephalosporin antibiotics are now being aerosolized to provide direct bactericidal effects in cystic fibrosis patients.

Cromolyn sodium (Intal) must be taken daily as prescribed for prophylaxis to prevent both allergy and exercise-induced asthma.

Albuterol (Proventil, Ventolin) and terbutaline sulfate (Brethine) are often used to relieve bronchospasm and dyspnea.

Metaproterenol sulfate (Alupent, Metaprel) is also given to provide bronchodilatation but has more cardiac side effects than albuterol or terbutaline.

Racemic epinephrine (Vaponefrin) has been success-

fully used to treat symptoms of laryngotracheobronchitis, also known as croup.

Injections. *Epinephrine hydrochloride* (Adrenalin) is indicated for the emergency treatment of anaphylactic allergic reactions to insect bites, foods, drugs, and other allergens as well as exercise-induced anaphylaxis. It can be given subcutaneously or intramuscularly. It is rapid-acting but may produce cardiac and neurologic side effects such as tachycardia, palpitations, hypertension, headache, and nervousness.

Aminophylline or *theophylline ethylenediamine* (Aminophyllin) may be given intravenously for acute bronchospasm associated with status asthmaticus. It may produce numerous side effects or adverse reactions (usually because of overdose) such as tachycardia, palpitations, flushing, **hypo**tension, and tachypnea, as well as epigastric pain, nausea and vomiting, headache, and irritability. Generalized convulsions may also occur. (See p. 713.)

Oral forms. *Theophylline* (Theo-Dur, Slo-bid, Slo-Phylline) is also available in different oral forms. Some types are immediate release; others are time-released to produce prolonged bronchodilatation for both preventing and treating asthma attacks.

This list is intended to provide only a basic survey of commonly used medications in pulmonary care.

Chest physiotherapy

Some respiratory diseases (for example, cystic fibrosis and bronchitis) produce such exaggerated amounts of tenacious secretions deep in the lungs that it may be difficult for the patient to expel them even with the aid of medications, humidification, and suction techniques. These secretions interfere with proper pulmonary ventilation and set the stage for frequent respiratory tract infections that further endanger the patient.

Chest physiotherapy is a therapeutic modality designed to improve pulmonary hygiene in patients with acute or chronic sputum production. It incorporates the use of breathing exercises, gravity-assisted positioning, percussion and vibration of the chest wall, followed by purposeful coughing and possible suctioning.

When respiratory therapists are available, they usually perform these maneuvers and instruct the family if continued treatment is necessary at home. If respiratory therapists are not available, nurses may be asked to learn the techniques. Anyone responsible for performing them should receive special instruction and be initially supervised in their use. The following brief explanation is not intended to take the place of such instruction.

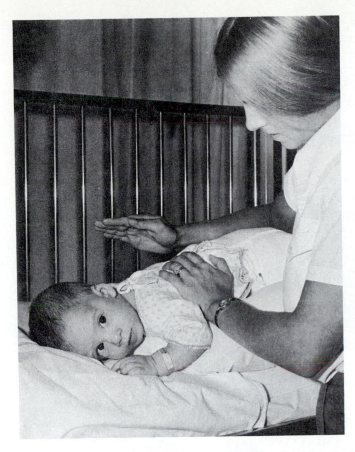

FIG 26-7 Respiratory therapist is performing early morning, before breakfast ritual on small patient with congenital structural weakness of bronchi. Scheduled percussion and vibrating have proved particularly helpful. *(Courtesy Children's Hospital and Health Center, San Diego, Calif.)*

The treatment is most effective when preceded by aerosol therapy and is enhanced by diaphragmatic breathing. It may be prescribed as a prophylactic as well as a therapeutic measure.

Various postures assumed by the patient help drain different parts of the lungs. Therefore the position or positions in which the patient is placed depends on the site of the congestion and the general aims of the therapeutic program. In general the placement of the patient enlists the forces of gravity and the sweeping action of the respiratory cilia in clearing the lungs. In infants the right upper lobe is frequently infected. In children bronchial secretions tend to collect in the lower lobes of the lung by gravity. Positions that drain the lower lobes utilize the Trendelenburg position. Any constrictive clothing should be removed. The patient's knees and hips should be flexed in the various positions necessary so

that relaxation will be promoted and less strain exerted on the abdominal muscles when coughing is encouraged. When a patient's chest must be lowered, usually all that is needed for an infant or young child is a well-positioned, firm pillow. (See Fig. 26-7.) Premature infants should *not* be placed in head-down positions because of the increased danger of intracranial hemorrhage. A baby or toddler may respond best when positioned on the nurse's or therapist's lap. An older child may assume a modified jack-knife position, lying over an elevated knee-gatch. The bed may be placed in Trendelenburg position for teenagers.

These assisted postural drainage techniques should be done before meals or at least 1 hour after eating. They are never initiated if the patient is hemorrhaging or in pain.

Two basic maneuvers are used: (1) percussion, also known as cupping or clapping and (2) vibrating. The first

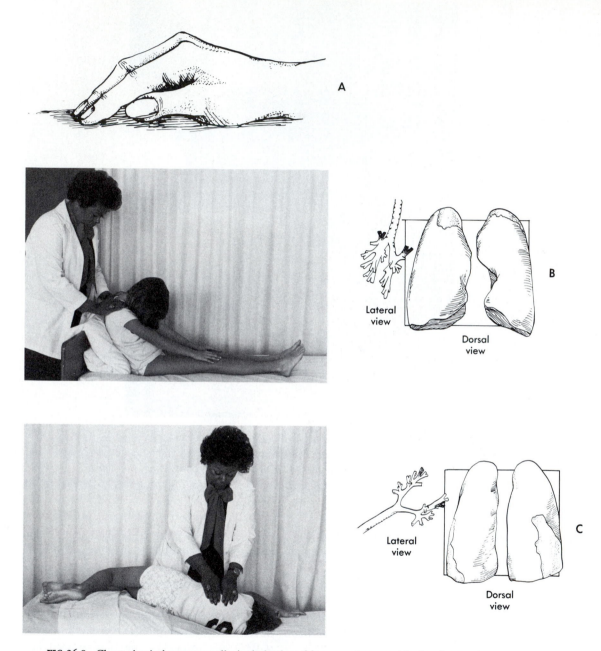

FIG 26-8 Chest physiotherapy usually includes breathing exercises, positioning (postural drainage), percussion, vibration, and effective coughing or suctioning to clear selected congested areas of the lung. Vibration is more difficult to perform, but is considered more effective than percussion. The entire range of possible positions is not illustrated. **A,** Percussion is accomplished by striking the cupped hand rhythmically against the chest wall, creating an air pocket between the therapist's hand and the chest wall. **B,** Position for drainage from upper lobes, apical segment. **C,** Position for drainage from lower lobes, lateral basal segments.

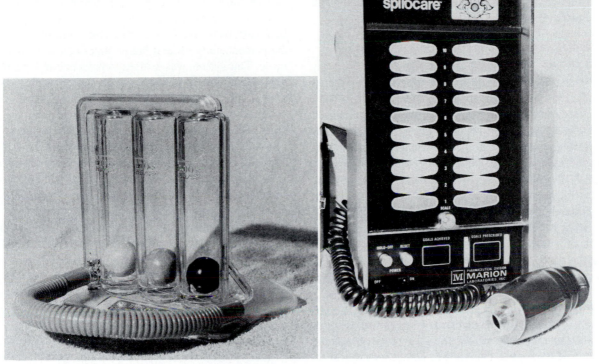

FIG 26-9 **A,** Triflo incentive spirometer; patient inhales and raises the balls. **B,** Spirocare
incentive breathing exercises; patient inhales, lighting up various colors as preset goals are
achieved. *(Photo by Bob Burgin, courtesy Children's Hospital and Health Center, San Diego,
Calif.)*

is performed with the palm of the hand raised, the fingers
and thumb forming the sides of a firm cup (Fig. 26-8,
A). When the cupped hands are gently but abruptly applied to the patient's chest wall, the wrist is alternately
flexed and extended. A characteristic hollow sound is
produced. The technique is continued for about 1 minute
over the affected area while the patient both inhales and
exhales. It is then followed by the vibrating motion, done
only while the patient is exhaling. This second maneuver
is accomplished by tensing the hands, arms, and shoulders and producing fine, gentle vibratory movements on
the chest wall for 5 or 6 exhalations. The two maneuvers
are then repeated several times, depending on the tolerance of the patient.

Soft percussion aids made from nipples or small face
masks may also be employed on infants and small children. Mechanical vibrators are very effective and less
tiring than manual vibration. Electric toothbrushes may

be used on infants and a G-5 apparatus on larger children.
Vibration is thought to be more effective than percussion.

Percussion techniques are performed on top of a light
shirt or diaper. Neither maneuver should be performed
directly over the spine, kidney area, abdomen, sternum,
or developed breast tissue. Coughing should be encouraged after each postural drainage position. If the patient
is unable to cough productively, suctioning should be
employed. The effectiveness of the treatment should be
evaluated by chest auscultation before and after the procedure.

Incentive spirometers, devices that indicate the approximate volume of inspiratory intake of patients during
breathing exercises, are found at the hospital bedsides of
persons of all ages. They help to encourage deep breathing for postoperative or relatively inactive patients to
avoid the onset of respiratory complications such as pneumonia. The patient is encouraged to practice voluntary

sustained inspiration. Deep breaths should be held for at least 2 seconds. Two types of incentive devices are pictured in Fig. 26-9. Many children enjoy the challenge these offer.

ADMINISTRATION OF OXYGEN/MIST
Safety factors

Various methods and devices are used to make inspired air richer in oxygen. The oxygen content of air in a well-ventilated room is about 21%. Therefore, any device used to increase the oxygen content must be capable of administering oxygen of a higher percentage. Although preterm infants may suffer eye damage and loss of sight as a result of retrolental fibroplasia caused by oxygen excesses in the blood, there are times when inspired air must contain more than 40% oxygen to meet their needs. The most accurate way of assessing the actual oxygen needs of these infants is by periodic blood gas determinations. The results of these tests are compared with the oxygen concentrations monitored by oxygen analyzers delivered in the hood or incubator.

When oxygen is being used, other safety factors involved must be clearly understood to avoid fire. Oxygen readily supports combustion, and all sources of possible ignition of flammable materials should be removed from the environment. If oxygen cylinders are used; they must be safely stored and maintained to avoid fire and explosion hazards.

Rules for oxygen administration. The following rules should be observed during oxygen administration:

1. No open flames, cigarettes, cigars, matches, cigarette lighters, or candles should be allowed in a room in which oxygen is being used. Signs that read OXYGEN IN USE—NO SMOKING should be clearly posted.
2. No electrical appliance is used unless it has been safety-checked. No device that is capable of producing a spark should be operated in the oxygen-enriched environment. Any electrical equipment used must be specially grounded to be safe.
3. All enclosed oxygen units (such as incubators or tents) should be "flushed" with oxygen before the patient is enclosed within them.
4. Because of the potential danger of excess carbon dioxide accumulation, all tents or enclosures should provide some method of ventilation or chemical control that will prevent this problem.

Methods of oxygen enrichment

Incubators with increased oxygen and/or mist. Incubators may be employed to provide both increased

oxygen and humidity to the infant, as well as a controlled environmental temperature. Incubator temperatures and oxygen concentrations (whenever supplementary oxygen is being used) should be recorded at least every 2 hours. Some incubators have oxygen delivery controls that limit the percentage to 40 and below unless an adjustment is made. This system was devised to prevent blindness from oxygen toxicity in prematures. However, some infants need to have concentrations above 40% to survive.

Head hoods for increased oxygen delivery for infants. Head hoods are often used for ill neonates receiving care under a warmer in intensive care units. Occasionally, they are placed within incubators to avoid wide variations in oxygen concentration, which may occur when the incubator is entered. The oxygen should be warmed and humidified. (Cold air blowing on an infant's face increases O_2 consumption.) Hourly oxygen concentration and temperature checks are recommended.

Oxygen and/or mist tents. A large oxygen tent may be ordered for an older child. Such a tent is usually a plastic canopy suspended from an overhead rod and attached to a cabinet containing a machine that, when properly adjusted, regulates the tent's ventilation and temperature and may also provide a control for increased humidity along with an opening for the appropriate oxy-

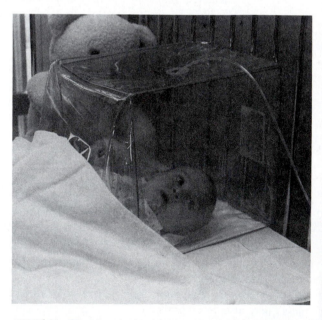

FIG 26-10 The view looking into a 12- × 12-inch pediatric oxygen tent or "Care-Cube." We wonder what Michael sees looking out. *(Courtesy Children's Hospital and Health Center, San Diego, Calif.)*

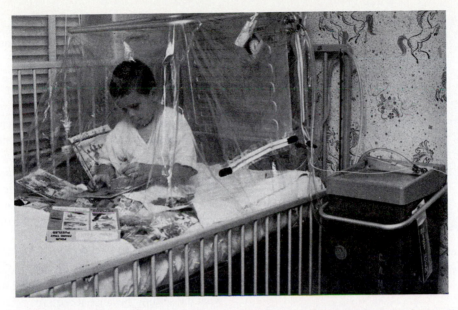

FIG 26-11 C.A.M. tent, used for oxygen or mist therapy, is cooled and ventilated electrically. Working apparatus is not near patient, and more room is available for activity. Side rail down for picture only. (*Courtesy Children's Hospital and Health Center, San Diego, Calif.*)

gen flow (Fig. 26-11). Such a tent may be set up in the following manner:

1. Place a bath blanket between the bed mattress and the bedspring to prevent snagging the plastic canopy, which can be easily torn.

2. Set the air circulation or ventilation control halfway between low and high. Set the temperature control at 70° F (21° C). In extremely hot weather the temperature setting should not be more than 10° to 15° F (5.5° to 8.3° C) below the room temperature to maintain the working efficiency of the tent. Arrange the ventilation deflectors so that the cool air entering the tent does not blow directly on the patient. Turn motor on, if so equipped.

3. Connect the oxygen inlet tube to the wall flow meter or oxygen cylinder regulator and start the flow at 15 L/min. Maintain this rate for 30 minutes and then analyze the oxygen concentration. The same concentration can be achieved by holding a flush valve open for at least 2 minutes after the tent has been placed around the patient. Always start oxygen or compressed air before closing a tent.

4. Many tents of this type seem drafty to patients. The amount of clothing necessary to protect the child from cold depends on the patient's own body temperature.

5. Mold the tent canopy around the child's body to prevent oxygen loss. If the tent is not tucked in properly, leakage will occur.

6. Plan nursing care so that the tent is opened as little as possible and many of the patient's needs are met during one interval.

Sometimes respiratory secretions are so thick that they are difficult to drain by gravity or remove by suction. Various procedures may be used to help thin out the mucus, such as simply increasing fluid intake, breathing cool moistened air provided by a convenient bedside humidifier, and, in the hospital setting, using a tent and humidification device to help relieve congestion. (Warm mist or steam tents are no longer used because of the danger of burns.) High humidity concentrations may be achieved with the addition of jet nebulizers to many types of tents (Fig. 26-9). Sterile distilled water alone or additional ordered medications may be used. Tents may often use compressed air rather than oxygen to achieve desired mist.

Patients placed in the cool, high humidity environments produced in such tents must be checked frequently to see whether their hair and clothing are damp. If the patients do not have excessively elevated temperatures, they should wear undershirts under their cotton gowns. Infants seem to do best when dressed in long-sleeved, footed sleepers.

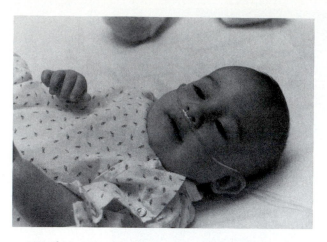

FIG 26-12 Infant receiving oxygen by nasal cannula. *(Courtesy Children's Hospital and Health Center, San Diego, Calif.)*

Nasal cannula. A common mode of delivering low concentrations of oxygen is by nasal cannula. One to six liters per minute will provide a fraction of inspired oxygen (FiO_2) concentration of 24% to 44%. The cannula is a lightweight, disposable soft plastic tube with two prongs that insert shallowly into each nostril. The cannula should not obstruct the nares, and the patient (if old enough) should be instructed to breathe through his nose. Oxygen administered by cannula should be passed through a humidifier to prevent uncomfortable drying of the mucous membranes.

Oxygen masks. Oxygen by mask is usually administered through a tube leading from the oxygen supply to a light, disposable, plastic face mask. Masks are capable of providing high oxygen concentrations quickly and are ideal for emergency use.

The simple mask is commonly used. This is an open-face mask that covers the nose and mouth, has vents for exhaled air, and can deliver oxygen concentrations of up to 60%. Oxygen flow rates of 5 to 6 L/min should be used to wash out the exhaled carbon dioxide that accumulates within the mask. One of the main uses of the simple mask is to deliver humidity or aerosol therapy.

A nonrebreathing mask is a mask with a reservoir bag system designed to deliver 90% to 100% oxygen when there is a tight seal over the face. Exhaled air is diverted to the atmosphere so that no carbon dioxide can be rebreathed.

Masks can be uncomfortable because they need to fit tightly on the face and because of the headstrap used to hold them in place. They must also be removed in order

for the patient to eat or cough. Nurses should be well acquainted with the particular oxygen equipment used in their setting.

STIMULATION AND MAINTENANCE OF RESPIRATORY EFFORT

If respiratory effort is absent or precarious, methods may be employed to stimulate or maintain respiration. They all presuppose an *adequate airway*.

In the delivery room or nursery, if a newborn is not breathing regularly, the nurse often stimulates more effective respirations by rubbing the infant's back, snapping the soles of the feet, or jarring the bed or incubator.

Mouth-to-mouth resuscitation

If respiration has actually ceased, mouth-to-mouth resuscitation is a practical, prompt source of aid, no matter what the setting, because it requires no additional equipment and can be instituted while other methods are being prepared for use. (Because of anxiety regarding possible exposure to infection during mouth-to-mouth ventilation, some nurses are carrying in their pockets airways or specially designed disposable patient "masks" wrapped and ready for use during emergency resuscitations.) The following is a description of mouth-to-mouth resuscitation, which can be used alone if cardiac function is adequate or with cardiac compression in the absence of heartbeat. (See Table 26-3.) Often children respond to mouth-to-mouth resuscitation alone.

If the child if found face down at the scene of a possible accident, the child must be rolled over in a manner that avoids twisting the neck or back and must be placed supine on a firm surface. If head or neck injury is suspected, the head tilt/chin lift maneuver is not used to open the airway. Instead, the jaw thrust maneuver is substituted. The caregiver positions herself behind the patient's head with her elbows on the supporting surface and reaches on each side of his head. She then places her middle and index fingers of each hand under his jaw while resting her thumbs near the corners of his mouth and lifts the jaw.

If head or spinal injury is not considered to be a problem, the standard head tilt/chin lift procedure is followed. The child's head is tipped slightly more than in the "sniffing" or neutral position used with infants. Only slight hyperextension is used with babies to avoid the possibility of collapsing the infant's trachea. The rescuer places his hand closest to the victim's head on the victim's forehead. Gently, the rescuer tilts the victim's head backward while using his other hand to raise the child's chin by placing his fingers against the bony jaw and lifting it upward. The head tilt-chin lift method clears the tongue and epiglottis from the airway and allows greater air exchange.

Obvious foreign material in the mouth should be removed. However, finger sweeps should be employed only if the victim of suspected airway obstruction is unconscious.

Two breaths of 1 to 1.5 seconds are performed (mouth-to-mouth with a child or youth, with the nose pinched; mouth-to-nose-and-mouth with an infant). Controlled breaths of air from the cheeks should be used with an infant, and gentle breaths just large enough to make the chest rise and fall with a child.

In children and adults continued foreign body airway obstruction may be relieved by the Heimlich maneuver. In the case of infants, abdominal thrusts (Heimlich maneuver) are not recommended because of possible injury to the abdominal organs, chiefly the liver. Instead a combination of four back blows and four chest thrusts is proposed. Chest thrusts in the infant are a succession of four external chest compressions similar to those performed during CPR.

After a clear airway is obtained, the circulatory status of the victim is evaluated. In infants it is now advised to feel for the brachial pulse instead of the apical pulse, because some infants may have good cardiac function but a heartbeat that is difficult to palpate. Although possibly less accessible in infants, the carotid pulse is sought in young children, as it is in adults.

If the pulse is present, rescue breathing is continued at a rate of 20 ventilations per minute for infants, 15 ventilations per minute for a child, and 12 to 15 per minute for children over 8 years of age and for adults.

Resuscitation of some kind is continued until the victim responds spontaneously or is pronounced dead or until the rescuer is physically unable to continue.

Cardiopulmonary resuscitation

1. See basic procedure on Table 26-3 and in following text.
2. External heart massage is not without danger. However, the danger of injury (broken ribs, traumatized liver) is probably less than the danger of circulatory collapse.
3. A precordial thump or blow on the chest is not recommended for children. It is used only on adults who display an arrest on a cardiac monitor.
4. CPR is usually not attempted in cases in which such dramatic efforts would delay a death that will take

place in minutes or hours after the treatment is terminated (for example, in a child dying of a malignancy).

A nurse should make use of every opportunity to secure practice and instruction regarding resuscitation measures during nonemergency situations. She should know where emergency resuscitation and oxygenation equipment is stored in the area in which she works. This includes knowledge of the location of the following items:

1. Resuscitation apparatus
2. Suction setup
3. Oxygen mask and cylinder
4. Emergency drug supply

Manual resuscitators

The use of manually controlled bag-valve-mask ventilation devices can be of great assistance in emergencies and for relatively short-term respiratory support. Use of such devices is much less fatiguing for the caregiver than mouth-to-mouth or mouth-to-airway resuscitation and also helps avoid the problem of possible disease transmission.

To be successful, one must be able to maintain an adequate airway using the typical techniques of head tilt and chin lift and/or oropharyngeal airway placement while also providing adequate support for the mask over the nose and mouth. The person providing ventilation may stand or sit behind the supine patient's head with the top of his head stabilized against her body. With one hand she holds the mask firmly against the patient's nose and mouth while maintaining his airway. With her other hand, she squeezes the air bag at a rate and depth compatible with the size and needs of the patient. Usually only enough bag pressure to achieve a rise and fall of the chest is recommended.

The typical rates are the same as those used for mouth-to-mouth resuscitation: infants, every 3 seconds; children 1 through 8 years (or size), every 4 seconds; and bigger persons, every 4 to 5 seconds. Too rapid, excited compression of the bag will cause greater respiratory distress. Time must be allowed for the patient to exhale adequately. When the patient makes an effort to breathe spontaneously, the treatment may be discontinued while the patient's respiratory attempts are evaluated.

There are two basic types of bag-valve-mask devices. Most commonly used are the self-inflating or automatic recoil bags (Ambu, Hope, Laerdal; and Penlon). Adult and pediatric size bags, masks, and oropharyngeal air-

Table 26-3 Emergency cardiopulmonary (CPR) reminders*

	Infants (less than 1 year)	Children (1 year through 8 years)	Older children and adults

CPR basic sequence

1. Identify problem
   a. Gasping or struggling for breath
   b. Lack of respiratory effort
   c. Cyanosis
   d. Limp extremities
2. Stimulate
   a. Shout, gently shake
   b. If unable to arouse, call out for help (if child unconscious and rescuer alone, perform CPR 1 minute before calling out for help)
3. Open airway (A)
   a. Head tilt, chin lift (if no neck injury suspected)
   b. Jaw thrust (without head tilt; safest when neck injury suspected)
   c. If airway remains obstructed, use Heimlich maneuver (abdominal thrusts) on children or adults
   d. Back blows, chest thrusts used for obstructed airway in infants (under 1 year)

4. Evaluate breathing (*B*)
   Look, listen, feel
5. Give two initial breaths
   a. 1 to 1.5 second each
   b. Only enough volume to make chest rise and fall
6. Evaluate circulation (*C*)
   a. Palpate for carotid pulse in children and adults
   b. Palpate infants brachial/femoral pulse
7. Use rescue breathing or CPR as needed

Consideration

Pressure point	Lower half of sternum (Locate the xiphoid process and measure up about two finger widths.)	Lower third of sternum	Midsternum—one finger breadth below the nipple line
Hands	Both	Heel of one hand	Tips of 2 fingers
Compression distance	1½ to 2 inches (4 to 5 cm)	1 to 1½ inches (2.5 to 3.8 cm)	½ to 1 inch (1.3 to 2.5 cm)
Compression/ventilation (CV)	Alone—15C/2V Two rescuers—5/1 (V = 1.5 seconds each)	5/1 (4-second cycle)	5/1 (3-second cycle)
C/V ratio	80-100C/12-15V/minute	80-100C/15V/minute	100C/20V/minute

*Victims should be supported on firm surface for best results. Breathing techniques now recommended make gastric distention and aspiration less likely. Effective CPR is accompanied by improvement in skin color and pupillary constriction. Check briefly for pulse after approximately 10 cycles or 1 minute of compression/ventilation and periodically thereafter. Each compression/relaxation phase should be of equal duration and performed in a smooth fashion. © Instructor's Manual for Basic Life Support, 1987. Copyright American Heart Association. (Illustrations reproduced with permission.)

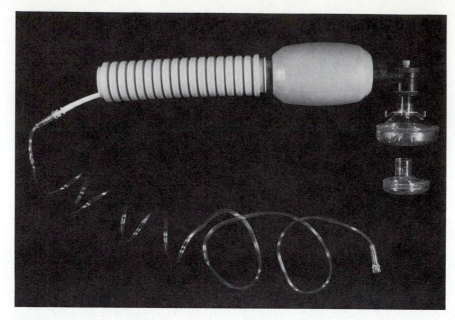

FIG 26-13 Puritan Bennett PMR II. A manual resuscitator that administers 40% oxygen unless equipped with an oxygen reservoir that provides a 100% oxygen concentration capability.

ways should be available. Concentrations of oxygen up to 40% may be obtained by attaching the green tubing from a standard cylinder wall source to the port at the base of the bag. However, a reservoir tubing can be adapted to most bag-breathing apparatuses to provide as much as 100% oxygen concentration. Some but not all self-inflating bags have pressure relief safety valves set at 35 to 40 cm H_2O, or they incorporate an intentional fixed leak to guard against the application of too much pressure and the danger of pneumothorax.

The second type of bag-valve-mask device is the thin rubber flow-inflating bag used commonly by anesthesiologists. During use they are constantly connected to a flow of gas, usually an oxygen/air mixture, but 100% oxygen concentrations can also be achieved. A manometer should be attached to the system to provide a visual indication of the applied pressure. Nurses should be knowledgeable regarding the equipment available.

Mechanical ventilators

If breathing needs to be supported for prolonged periods of time, mechanical ventilators are used. The most common indication for mechanical ventilation is impending or actual respiratory failure. Patients are placed on mechanical ventilators to treat hypoxemia and tissue hypoxia, to provide adequate ventilation for the patient who no longer can breathe on his own, to maintain positive pressure in the airways throughout the respiratory cycle, and to reduce the work of breathing.

Mechanical ventilators deliver air into the lungs through masks or endotracheal or tracheostomy tubes and administer any desired amount of oxygen from 21% to 100%. Positive pressure ventilators (PPV) are the most commonly used. They accomplish lung inflation by applying intermittent positive pressure ventilation (IPPV) or continuous positive pressure ventilation (CPPV) to the airway. Three different types of PP ventilators are volume-cycled; pressure-cycled; and time-cycled. Volume-cycled ventilators deliver a preset volume; pressure-cycled ventilators deliver gas until a preset pressure is achieved, and time-cycled ventilators deliver gas during a preset time interval.

High-frequency ventilation is a new type of PPV that delivers small tidal volumes at a high ventilatory rate in an effort to reduce barotrauma and cardiac complications associated with normal frequency mechanical ventilation.

Positive end-expiratory pressure (PEEP) is used to maintain an airway pressure greater than atmospheric pressure at the end of exhalation. Alveolar volume is thereby increased, hopefully decreasing hypoxemia and reducing the FiO_2 to less toxic levels. PEEP is often used in infant respiratory distress syndrome (IRDS).

For most of us breathing is so natural that we are often not aware of the process. An alert, knowledgeable nurse is in a strategic position to recognize alterations, abnormalities, and need for specific therapies. Skilled to meet patient needs, the nurse may be a vital link to life.

Key Concepts

1. Signs of respiratory difficulty are the following: altered resting respiratory or cardiac rates, chest retractions, labored breathing, flaring nostrils, pallor, cyanosis, restlessness, disorientation, inflamed respiratory tract, and frequent coughing.

2. Because the clinical signs and symptoms of hypoxia are nonspecific, laboratory evaluation of arterial blood is done to determine the extent of oxygenation. Pulse oximeters are also used clinically to measure oxygen saturation.

3. Methods for securing and maintaining an open airway include positioning, nasopharyngeal suctioning, endotracheal or tracheostomy tube placement and suctioning, medications, and chest physiotherapy.

4. An open airway may be maintained or established by positioning the patient so that obstructions are cleared and aspiration is prevented.

5. Suction of the naso-oropharyngeal passages is accomplished by using a bulb syringe or a catheter setup attached to mechanical suction.

6. When positioning and nasopharyngeal suctioning are insufficient to maintain the patient's airway and oxygenation, an artificial airway must be inserted. An endotracheal tube is most commonly used for short-term airway management; a tracheostomy provides the best route for long-term maintenance. Tracheal suctioning should be performed only when necessary.

7. Medications to aid in clearing the airway are nose drops, expectorants, aerosols, injections, and oral forms of medication.

8. Chest physiotherapy is designed to improve pulmonary hygiene in patients with acute or chronic sputum production. It incorporates breathing exercises, gravity-assisted positioning, percussion and vibration of the chest wall, followed by purposeful coughing and possible suctioning.

9. Rules for oxygen administration must be understood and carefully followed to avoid fire.

10. Methods of oxygen enrichment include incubators, head hoods, oxygen and mist tents, nasal cannula, and oxygen masks.

11. In the presence of an adequate airway, the following methods may be used to stimulate or maintain respiration: mouth-to-mouth resuscitation, cardiopulmonary resuscitation, manual resuscitators, and mechanical ventilators.

12. If respiration has ceased, mouth-to-mouth resuscitation is a practical, prompt source of aid.

13. The use of manually controlled bag-valve-mask ventilation devices is less fatiguing for the caregiver than mouth-to-mouth resuscitation and helps avoid possible disease transmission.

14. Patients are placed on mechanical ventilators to treat hypoxemia and tissue hypoxia, to provide adequate ventilation when the patient cannot do so, to maintain positive pressure in the airways throughout the respiratory cycle, and to reduce the work of breathing.

Discussion Questions

1. Identify various conditions that can result in airway obstruction. Which of these are most commonly seen in children?

2. What methods are used to relieve or reduce the airway obstruction?

3. A variety of medications are used to improve respiratory function. Identify the most common medications. For which therapeutic or adverse effects should the nurse be watching?

4. What techniques are used to facilitate drainage of fluids from the lungs? Why are many different positions necessary? What precautions should the nurse take when performing chest therapies?

5. What mechanical equipment is used to assist ventilation?

27

Traction, Casting, and Braces

CHAPTER OBJECTIVES

After studying this chapter, the student should be able to perform the following:

1 Define traction and enumerate four reasons for its use in orthopedics.
2 Contrast skin and skeletal traction in three different ways.
3 Identify three ways in which countertraction may be created to prevent the loss of traction.
4 Discuss four ways to help prevent pressure areas.
5 Describe four different traction setups noted in the chapter and the conditions for which they are usually prescribed.
6 Explain why casts are often "petaled" or lined and edged with stockinette.
7 List eight signs of possible neurovascular complications involving a casted or wrapped extremity.
8 Explain one method of measuring a supine patient for crutches.

This chapter presents for initial consideration or review basic nursing procedures and responsibilities involved in the care of patients receiving therapy in traction, casts, or braces. These patients may be hospitalized for various reasons; fractures, musculoskeletal diseases, and neurologic disorders account for most of their diagnoses. For more information regarding specific illnesses in this grouping, the student is referred to Chapter 31, which discusses in greater detail some of these problems and the nursing care they require. However, to prevent needless repetition, the orthopedic nursing entailed in the care of such patients is discussed separately in this section.

TRACTION

Traction, or methods of exerting pull, is discussed first because at times it must precede casting. Traction is used for the following reasons:

1. To bring a broken bone back into alignment (reduce a fracture) and provide immobilization for correct union
2. To secure a corrected position to treat a congenital or acquired deformity not involving a fracture (reduce a dislocated hip)
3. To prevent or treat contracture deformities
4. To relieve muscle spasm and pain (back injury)

Basic types

Traction may be exerted manually or by means of certain appliances. There are two main types of traction—skin and skeletal.

Skin traction. Skin traction indirectly helps position the bone by pulling on the skin and muscles. It is relatively simple to apply, involves no surgical operation, and may be accomplished in a home setting. However, only a limited amount of weight may be added with this type of traction, and occasionally the maximum amount

554

allowed is insufficient to produce the desired results. Also, the skin may show signs of irritation—allergic reactions, circulation difficulties, or friction—caused by the supportive wrapping. The weight is usually secured to the skin by running strips of adhesive material, cotton or perforated plastic-backed adhesive tape, or foam rubber up both sides of the extremity and securing the strips with a compression (Ace) bandage. The ends of the strips are then attached to a foot spreader, which in turn is connected to the desired weight.

Skeletal traction. Skeletal traction is secured by inserting a mechanical device directly into or through the bone and attaching the prescribed weight. The bone may be fixed with wires, pins, or tongs. Considerable weight may be attached to such devices, and no bulky or irritating skin wrappings are necessary. Nevertheless, skeletal traction, too, has its drawbacks. Since the bone is actually pierced, danger of infection is always present, and a surgical procedure is involved in both the insertion and the removal of the mechanical attachment. The areas where the holding devices are inserted through the skin must be frequently inspected for signs of inflammation, infection, and drainage. Special pin care may be ordered, usually involving the cleansing of the skin around the pin with hydrogen peroxide, followed by the application of a protective antimicrobial ointment.

Nursing considerations

The beginning student may express perplexity after viewing her first traction patient. Often there seems to be a surplus of weights, ropes, pulleys, and bars, and she wonders how they all fit in to produce a desired result. The mechanical apparatus used may seem complex, but the basic principles of traction that guide its use are neither numerous nor obscure.

Maintenance of proper traction. The maintenance of proper traction depends on the correct direction and amount of pull exerted through the use of ropes, pulleys, and weights and on the correct positioning or alignment of the patient. Therefore it is important that the nurse understand the orders concerning the care of each individual patient in traction and maintain the correct relationship of the various parts of the traction apparatus to the patient. The following points should be noted:

1. Pulleys increase the amount and change the direction of pull on a body part by a weight. A rope should ride smoothly on a pulley to exert the ordered weight.
2. Weights should not be added or subtracted by the nurse. Too much weight may cause the nonunion of a break; too little weight may cause unwanted overriding and an extremity of unequal length. Weights should always hang freely; they should be frequently observed so that they do not come to rest on a rung of the bed, a poorly placed chair, or the floor.
3. The amount of time that traction is applied should be clearly understood. Skin traction may occasionally be removed (but such removal always depends on the physician's order). Skeletal traction is continuous and should not be interrupted.
4. Ropes should be in good condition and frequently inspected for signs of wear. Knots should be taped for additional safety. Multiple weights attached to the same rope should be taped together so that they cannot easily fall or be removed. Some pediatric-orthopedic areas push the foot of a bed, over which weights hang, against the wall to discourage tampering by the small fingers of ambulatory patients.

Countertraction. Pull in one direction must be balanced by pull in the opposite direction for traction to remain effective. This opposing pull is called countertraction, not to be confused with *balanced traction* (p. 564).

Countertraction may be exerted in various ways. If the weights used to create the initial pull are not extremely heavy, it may only be necessary to keep the patient in a certain place in bed, checking periodically to see that the patient has not slipped. The patient's body provides the countertraction. The friction of the patient's body against the bedding may help prevent the child from slipping out of position.

If the pull is stronger, the end of the bed where the initial traction is applied may need to be elevated so that gravity increases the countertraction created by the patient's body weight. Elevation may be achieved through the use of grooved blocks under two legs of the bed, a mechanical bed lift, or special positioning of an electric bed.

If it is very difficult to maintain the child in proper position in bed, sometimes a restraint may be used (a restraining jacket or waist restraint). However, such devices may cause other problems—pressure areas, hypostatic pneumonia, and constipation. The use of restraints must be carefully evaluated.

Sometimes the treated body part is placed in a frame or splint that is lifted off the surface of the bed. When this arrangement is used, a counterweight may often be connected to the frame, exerting force in the opposing direction (see p. 563).

In review, countertraction is created in four basic ways:

1. Maintenance of body replacement in bed by constant observation and correction, if needed
2. Elevation of the part of the bed closest to the weights
3. Use of restraints
4. Application of a counterweight

The method employed depends on the desires of the physician and the responses of the patient. Failure to maintain correct placement in bed while the patient is in traction may (1) cause the weights, which are supposed to create initial pull, to rest on the floor or some other surface and temporarily stop traction altogether, in some cases allowing possible displacement, or (2) change the angle of pull and distort the result desired. Both situations are potentially harmful. When a nurse is told "Keep Susie's hips at the level of the tape markers on the bed," or "Be sure that Roger is kept pulled up in bed," it is to prevent these situations.

Activity and body position. The amount of movement and activity allowed for the patient in traction should be understood and promoted, and good body alignment and support should be maintained. Bedboards may be placed under the mattress to prevent sagging.

Some patients are allowed relatively little movement or position change because of their particular musculoskeletal problems or traction arrangements. If the nurse allows these patients to sit up or turn on their sides, the traction may be lost or altered so that treatment fails or perhaps even real damage may result. However, a patient who has a leg in a Thomas splint support, which is raised off the surface of the mattress, is allowed considerable movement because such a traction maintains proper alignment when the patient's trunk is raised. Even a slight amount of turning toward the splinted leg is usually possible. Such an arrangement is termed "balanced traction." When balanced, traction is used in conjunction with an overhead bar and trapeze, the patient enjoys considerable activity, and nursing care is greatly simplified (see pp. 562-563).

Although it is important that patients not be moved in a way that disrupts their traction, it is also important that they be moved to the extent permitted to encourage proper body function, elimination, respiration, and circulation and to avoid pressure areas. Exercise and correct positioning of the uninvolved extremities are very necessary to prevent other problems (stiffness or deformity) from occurring in some patients. As in all cases of prolonged immobilization, a high fluid intake should be encouraged. A diet well supplied with roughage and natural laxatives, such as prunes, helps prevent constipation. Special attention should be given to the prevention of footdrop or undesired internal or external rotation of the lower extremities.

Circulation and skin condition. The circulation and skin condition of a patient in traction or other immobilization devices such as casts should be frequently evaluated.

The skin of any patient who is bedfast for long periods and is permitted only limited movement must be meticulously observed and protected. Pressure areas are most likely to develop over bony prominences, such as the hips, sacrum, ankles, elbows, scapulae, and shoulders. Areas exposed to continuous friction are also likely spots for skin breakdown. If a Thomas splint is used, the skin area under the padded ring must be frequently inspected. The heels of both the affected and nonaffected leg should be carefully observed. Often the foot that is not being treated may develop a sore heel because the patient moves up in bed by digging the heel into the mattress to obtain leverage. To prevent unnecessary pressure, the linen must be kept smooth and tight, and crumbs and other irritating small objects must be eliminated from the bed. Skin traction wrappings may cause circulation and nerve interference similar to that occasionally encountered with the casted patient. Inability to dorsiflex the exposed big toe of a wrapped affected lower extremity should be reported to the physician promptly.

Pressure areas are much easier to prevent than to treat. Frequent inspection and cleansing of susceptible areas; use of an egg crate mattress; maintenance of wrinkle-free linen; continual elevation of the bed's head to an angle of less than 30 degrees; and encouragement of as much movement as is allowed, consistent with the patient's well-being, greatly reduces if not entirely eliminates pressure areas. Every complaint of skin tenderness, burning sensation, or aching should be investigated. It does not take long for a small red area to become an enlarged, open sore, particularly in areas where circulation may already be impaired. Any devices that lift a pressure area off a surface must be used with caution and frequently evaluated, since they may sometimes cause circulatory disturbances themselves. Patients who are paralyzed or suffer from sensory loss must receive special care and observation. A child in traction should routinely receive back and skin care during baths and at least twice more during the day. The use of an overhead bar and trapeze can greatly facilitate back and skin care

Table 27-1 Common types of traction

Name	Basic type	Most common indications	Major nursing considerations
Bryant's	Skin—to lower extremities	Fractured femur in child under 30 lb	Report immediately any signs of neurovascular problems
Buck's	Skin—to lower extremities	Hip or knee contractures or immobilization	Avoid skin breakdown around ankles and heels
Russell's	Skin (may incorporate skeletal)—to lower extremities	Hip contractures or immobilization for fractured femur	Maintain proper alignment with patient flat
90°–90°	Skeletal	Fractured femur—preschool- and school-age child	Avoid any movement of bed or traction setup

when such aids are feasible. If no such arrangement is possible, a nurse may press down on the mattress with one hand to allow her other hand to massage, or two nurses may work together to lift the child *slightly* to facilitate skin care, depending on the type of traction used.

Sometimes the use of imitation or genuine lamb's wool mats under the patient is helpful. Tincture of benzoin applications on closed areas of pressure or potential pressure are sometimes prescribed. The benzoin serves to toughen the areas of pressure. However, benzoin may stain the sheets.

Bed making. Some hospitals are supplied with special traction linen designed to fit under or around different traction appliances, such as the Thomas splint. A special "split" top sheet may be used on either side of the splint. More commonly a large sheet is simply pulled to one side over the uninvolved leg, and a light baby blanket is draped over the splinted leg at night. Another satisfactory and modest arrangement uses two blankets, each contained within a separate folded sheet. One such blanket-sheet combination is placed over the chest and abdomen of the patient, with open edges under the chin; the other is placed on top of the uninvolved leg and below the suspended leg, with open edges toward the foot of the bed where they are tucked in. The upper and lower blanket-sheet combinations are then pinned together around the thigh of the leg in traction. This makes a very neat bed. Traction patients may have special snap-on pajamas (tops and bottoms) to facilitate dressing, or perineal drapes or G-strings may be used.

Types of traction equipment

Traction equipment may vary depending on the individual needs of the patient (see Table 27-1).

External fixation. External fixation is a new adapta-

tion of an older method of treating complicated fractures and may be used instead of traction, casting, or internal fixation (Fig. 27-1). The external fixation device consists of pins inserted through the fractured bone and attached to a metal frame, which provides reduction and stabilization. Possible indications for its use are open comminuted fractures, fractures that occur with multiple injuries, or infected bone that fails to heal properly. The advantages of external fixation are an immediate and rigid stabilization of the fracture, an early mobilization of adjacent joints, and a shorter bed confinement. At the same time, it allows for complete visualization and treatment of an open wound. The major disadvantages lie in the cumbersome nature of the device and the sometimes frightening appearance of the open wound. In addition, the multiple pin sites present the possibility of infection. It thus becomes extremely important for the nurse to prepare the child ahead of time, to explain carefully the reason for its use to the child and his parents, and to provide meticulous pin site care to prevent infection of the pin tract. External fixation is less frequently seen in younger children because of their ability to heal rapidly, but it can offer earlier mobilization and rigid stabilization for the older child with a complicated fracture.

Bryant's traction. Bryant's traction is often used for the treatment of fractured femurs in young children (Fig. 27-2). Such patients must be carefully observed for developing circulation problems because the leg wrappings may interfere with the blood flow. Swollen, cool, or "blotchy" looking toes, slow blanching on pressure, or delayed return of skin color after pressure is released from a toenail bed all are signs that should be promptly reported. The pulse at the ankle may be checked to detect circulatory problems. Unexplained restlessness, crying, and complaints or indications of leg pain must be further evaluated immediately, and assessment for circulatory

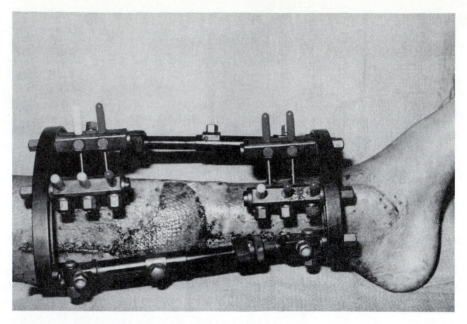

FIG 27-1 External fixation. Severe open fracture of tibia has been stabilized with Ace-Fisher external fixator. Skin defect has been closed with soleus muscle flap and covered with split-thickness skin graft. *(Courtesy F. Craig Swenson, MD, La Jolla, Calif.)*

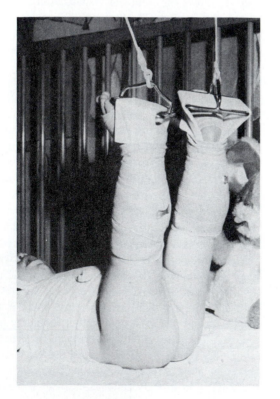

FIG 27-2 Bryant's or vertical traction may be used for infants or young children weighing less than 30 pounds. Pelvis is no longer lifted above mattress by traction, since this has been associated with circulatory problems in legs. Knees should be slightly flexed. Both legs are placed in traction even though only one may be fractured. Better alignment is maintained. *(Courtesy Children's Hospital and Health Center, San Diego, Calif.)*

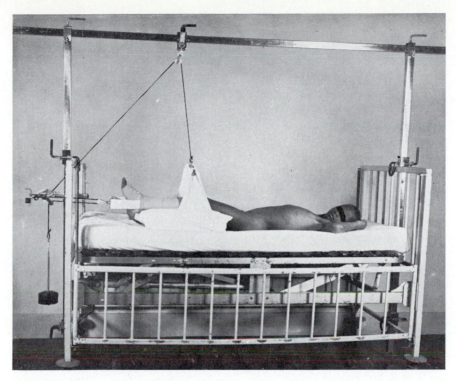

FIG 27-3 Russell's traction can be used to treat fractures in older children and adults. Split-Russell's traction makes use of two ropes, pulley, and weight setups for two directions of pull. Pillow under sling is not always present. *(From Brashear HR Jr and Raney RB: Shand's handbook of orthopaedic surgery, ed 9, St Louis, 1978, The CV Mosby Co.)*

impairment must be carried out on both the affected and unaffected extremity. This type of patient should be raised slightly during feedings to prevent aspiration. The jacket restraint can be loosened or removed if a responsible person is at the bedside, but it should be in place when the child is alone. If the nurse is rewrapping the Ace bandages, care must be taken to wrap them tightly enough to secure the traction but not so tightly as to impair circulation or prevent a slight degree of flexion in the knees. To make the bed, one nurse must lift the baby's body just enough to allow another nurse to slide the bed sheets under the hips and back. The weights should not be removed. Frequent back care and diaper changes are a necessity.

Russell's traction. Russell's traction, a skin traction using a sling and single rope arrangement attached to one weight supported by multiple pulleys, is used to treat undisplaced fractures and provide postoperative hip and knee immobilization in older children (Fig. 27-3). If the traction pull of the sling is separate and in the opposite direction, it is called split Russell traction. Because the extremity is suspended, more patient movement is allowed, and nursing care is considerably easier.

90°-90° Traction. 90°-90° traction is commonly used to reduce a fractured femur (Fig. 27-4). Both the hip and knee are placed in 90 degree flexion. A pin is inserted through the distal femur or proximal tibia, and traction is applied. A sling or cast on the lower leg is used for suspension.

Buck's extension. A rather simple, frequently used skin traction for treatment of hip synovitis or muscle spasm of the lower extremities or lower back is called Buck's extension (Fig. 27-5). Note the adhesive strips on the sides, the elastic bandage wrapping, the foot spreader (to prevent pressure of the adhesive strips against the ankle), the pulley, and the rope leading to the freely hanging weight. Some physicians order the placement of a small flattened pillow under the leg just above the Achilles tendon to protect the heel from pressure. In this picture the angle of the pull elevates the heel slightly off the bed.

Cervical traction. The patient in cervical traction may have a sling or halter arrangement around the chin and occiput (Fig. 27-6), or the patient may be placed in skeletal traction, which involves the placement of metal tongs into (but not through) the cranium (Fig. 27-7).

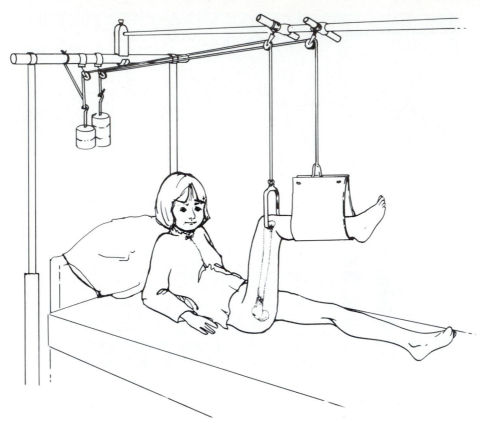

FIG 27-4 90°-90° traction through distal femur, commonly used for preschool- or school-age child.

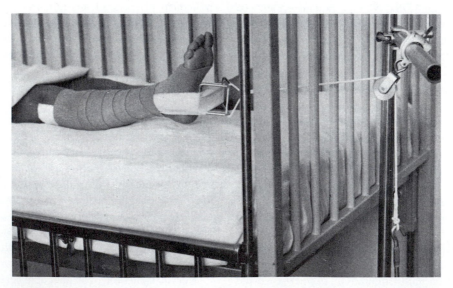

FIG 27-5 Buck's extension. Note that heel clears mattress. Some physicians use small flat pillow under leg to provide clearance. *(Courtesy Children's Hospital and Health Center, San Diego, Calif.)*

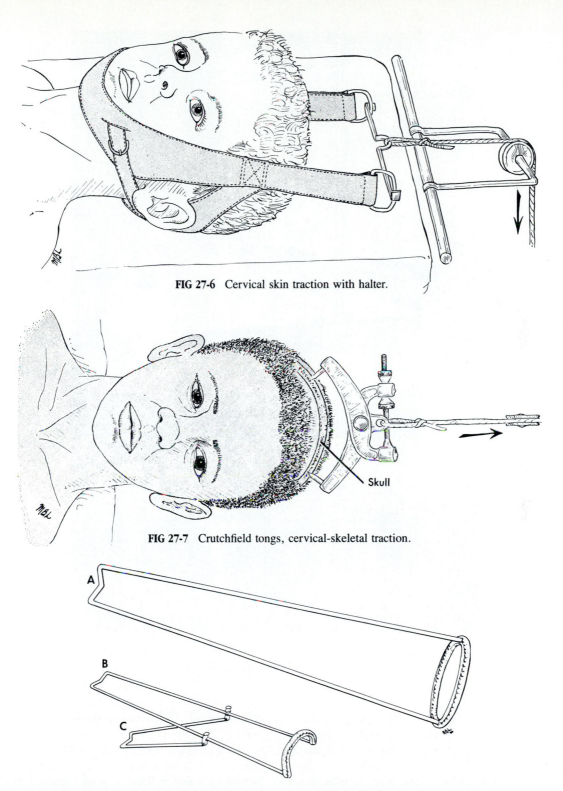

FIG 27-6 Cervical skin traction with halter.

FIG 27-7 Crutchfield tongs, cervical-skeletal traction.

FIG 27-8 **A,** Thomas splint with complete ring. **B,** Half-ring Thomas splint. **C,** Pearson attachment.

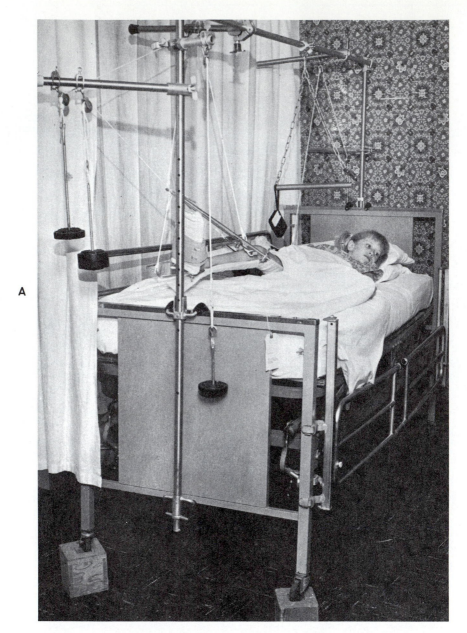

FIG 27-9 A, Patient in balanced traction. **B,** Explanatory drawing. **C,** Close-up view of leg.
(Courtesy Children's Hospital and Health Center, San Diego, Calif.)

Orders regarding the positioning of the patient, the movement allowed, and whether any elevation of the backrest
is permitted should be clearly understood. Patients in
skeletal-cervical traction are often positioned in slight
hyperextension, and flexion of the cervical spine is not
permitted. If cervical skin traction is used, foam rubber
padding may be necessary in the chin area to prevent

skin irritation. Gum chewing may relieve aching jaw
joints.

Pelvic traction. Occasionally pelvic traction may be
ordered to relieve lower back pain. Pelvic traction is
created by a pelvic band or girdle attached to a weight
or weights. Sometimes a thoracic belt may be used for
countertraction. Such an arrangement is designed to re-

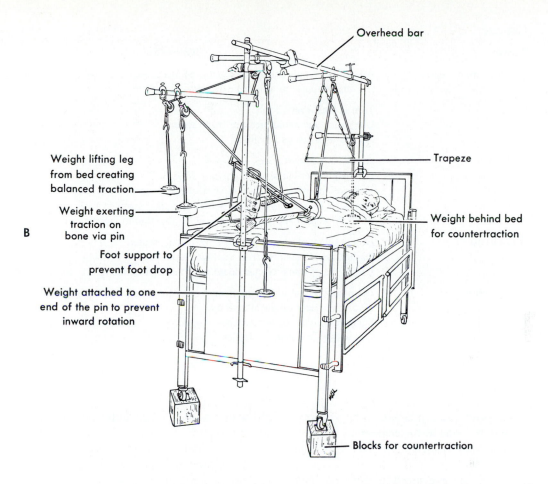

Overhead bar

Trapeze

Weight lifting leg from bed creating balanced traction

Weight exerting traction on bone via pin

Foot support to prevent foot drop

Weight attached to one end of the pin to prevent inward rotation

B

Weight behind bed for countertraction

Blocks for countertraction

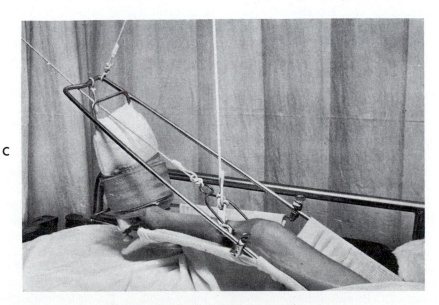

C

FIG 27-9, cont'd For legend see opposite page.

Table 27-2 Cast care

Objective	Intervention
Detect circulatory impairment early	Assess and report unexplained pain, edema, cool temperature, poor capillary refill, or loss of pulse in affected extremity.
Ensure even drying	Turn at least every 2 hr. Use palms and avoid pressure from fingers. Air dry as much as possible.
Prevent skin breakdown	Assess skin at cast edges every 4 hr. Use padding or cut away sharp cast edges. Turn patient often and support comfortably with pillows. Avoid use of sharp objects for scratching underneath cast. Keep skin clean and dry, giving special attention to perineal area.
Maintain integrity of cast	Do not allow plaster of paris cast to contact water. Do not use abduction bar to facilitate turning. Use of metal frame or cast board may facilitate toileting.
Promote maximum mobility	Facilitate optimal use of unaffected extremities, change environment often. Place child near center of activity. Support upright position whenever possible. Use wagon or adapted "stroller."

lieve muscle spasm and lessen pressure on nerve roots. Pelvic traction may be ordered for continuous or intermittent application. Many patients are given bathroom privileges.

Balanced traction. As previously mentioned, *balanced traction,* involving the suspension of the affected limb above the surface of the bed, provides the opportunity for more movement and activity by the patient. Patients may raise their hips, have their backrests elevated, or turn slightly toward the side of the splinted lower extremity. An overhead bar and trapeze greatly facilitate lifting. The suspension device takes up the slack created and maintains the line of traction. It is well to remember that no matter how much these patients want to stay up they should intermittently rest flat, without the elevation of the backrest, to prevent hip contractures.

Although suspended traction gives greater liberty of movement and effectively relieves heel pressure, the area where the ring of the Thomas splint rests must be frequently inspected for the development of skin problems. Each day the skin may be gently pulled up or down from under the ring and washed, dried and massaged. The ring, if leather, can be polished with saddle soap. Fig. 27-8 shows a Thomas splint with a complete ring and a Thomas half-ring splint with a Pearson attachment, which is used to support the extremity. Fig. 27-9 shows a young

girl with a balanced skeletal traction, including an extra support to prevent foot drop and an additional weight to correct a tendency toward internal rotation of the leg. Not long after this photograph was taken the girl was sent home in a long-leg plaster cast.

Neufeld's traction. More mobility is possible with this recent type of balanced traction setup that incorporates a skeletal pin into a plaster of Paris cast, ensuring both secure immobilization and substantial traction at the same time. An overhead pulley system enables maximum mobility, even to the point of the patient's moving to a bedside chair. It is used to treat a fractured femur in the older school-age child or adolescent who may be facing a prolonged period of time in traction.

CASTS (Table 27-2)

Casts are often applied subsequent to treatment by traction, supplying a form of external immobilization of a body part. Occasionally, a cast may be applied over a skeletal pin, thus continuing traction as well as contributing to immobilization. Such a procedure is called *plaster traction.* The ends of the protruding pins should be covered with plaster or some sort of protective device to prevent the snagging of clothing or bed coverings or injury to others. Plaster traction allows greater mobility for the patient (when feasible). In addition to immobilization and possible traction, casts may also be a means of aiding proper positioning or resting a body part.

The most common kind of cast consists of plaster of Paris—impregnated crinoline bandages that have been applied and molded while moist over some type of soft, protective layer and allowed to dry to a hard, resistant shell. Dry plaster of Paris is a form of calcium sulfate; when mixed with water, it forms the substance known as gypsum.

Plaster is most often used in the casting of the hospitalized child, but despite their greater expense, synthetic materials (fiberglass and plastic) are increasingly being used to form casts for ambulatory patients. They set rapidly and, depending on the substances and techniques used, may be ready for weight bearing 3 to 30 minutes after application. They are less bulky, light weight, and porous. When applied over special nonabsorbant linings, they may be immersed in water if the physician permits. If they do get wet for any reason, they must be carefully dried—a process that takes about an hour. Manufacturer's instructions must be consulted for details of application and care. Because they are more difficult to mold than plaster, synthetics are usually considered less effective for immobilizing severely displaced bones or unstable fractures until initial swelling has subsided. Parents and patients need to be aware that vigorous activity can misalign a fracture or even break a synthetic cast. The exterior of the cast is often rough and can snag clothing or scratch furniture or skin unless precautions are taken.

Application of the cast

Because of the "orderly disorder" that invariably accompanies plaster applications, it is preferable to schedule cast work in a room especially designed for such procedures—a room that is easily cleaned and contains all the equipment and supplies usually needed.

Commonly needed supplies are as follows:

1. Materials that protect the skin, to be wrapped around the body part before application of plaster or synthetics
   a. Sheet wadding (Webril)
   b. Tubular stockinette
2. Various widths of plaster of Paris bandages and strips (splints) or synthetic tapes
3. Materials to reinforce or protect areas of the cast or body that are under special pressure or strain
   a. Felt
   b. Yucca board

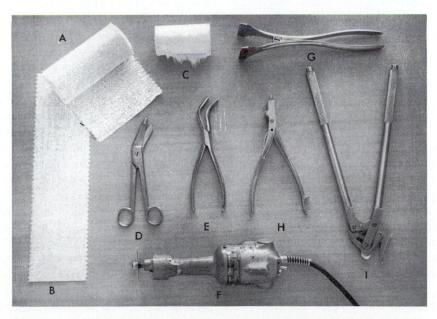

FIG 27-10 Instruments and materials used in preparing or removing plaster casts. **A,** Plaster roll; **B,** plaster strip or splint; **C,** Webril (sheet wadding); **D,** plaster shears (large bandage scissors); **E,** cast bender; **F,** cast cutter or saw (electric); **G** and **H,** cast spreaders; **I,** cast cutter (manual). *(Courtesy Children's Hospital and Health Center, San Diego, Calif.)*

c. Wire netting
d. Rubber heels (for leg casts of ambulatory patients)
4. Special tools (Fig. 27-10)
   a. Various types of cast knives
   b. Plaster shears
   c. Cast spreaders and cast benders
   d. Manual and electric cast cutters
   e. A bucket for water to moisten the cast materials (temperatures vary)
5. Other possible needs
   a. Cover gowns
   b. Gloves, caps, and masks
   c. Special lamps to cure certain synthetic casting materials (Lightcast II)

The furnishings of a cast room need not be elaborate. Usually an examining table, some benches, good lighting, an x-ray film view box, and a sink are sufficient. A sink with a plaster trap is convenient because the water used to soak the plaster of Paris rolls may be discarded into the drain without much danger of plugging the plumbing. If large body casts or scoliosis jackets are applied, additional supportive frames, tables, or slings are needed. Newspapers placed on the floor under the working area aid cleanup.

Preparation of the patient. Some patients undergoing casting procedures are anesthetized to aid muscle relaxation, relieve pain, and facilitate the entire procedure. Of course, patients who have open reductions of fractures or have had other operative procedures just before casting are always anesthetized. Small children are frequently anesthetized for closed reduction procedures. Such patients are given nothing by mouth for several hours before the procedure and usually receive preoperative sedation.

The nurse must make certain that the child and the parents have been informed of this procedure beforehand and know what to expect after the cast has been applied. Sometimes meeting another youngster with a cast or seeing a doll with a casted arm or leg is a helpful preparatory experience for the young boy or girl.

Duties of the nurse. The nurse helping the physician in the cast room is responsible for making available all the necessary equipment and supplies. When plaster of Paris is used, the desired width of plaster bandage is removed from its waxed paper wrapper and immersed on end in tepid water. When air bubbles no longer rise from the roll, the bandage is lifted from the water. The sides of the closed bandage are gently squeezed to remove water while retaining the plaster. The loose end of the bandage is unrolled slightly, and the roll is handed to the

physician for application. The bandage should not be dripping at the time of the transfer. The nurse may also assist by holding the extremity being casted. She may be asked to support part of the newly formed cast. If so, she should use only the palms of her hands in rendering such support to prevent the formation of pressure areas.

Cast changes and removal

Sometimes a patient must have one cast removed and another applied (Fig. 27-10). The frequency with which a child must have a cast changed depends on the child's rate of growth, the condition of the cast, and the progress of the desired correction. The plaster cast may be cut manually with a cast knife shaped like a short kitchen paring knife and a hand cast cutter. The cut is made along a line dampened by vinegar solution, hydrogen peroxide, or water from a syringe. A metal strip may be inserted just below the cutting line to protect the body part. An electric vibrating-blade cast cutter may be used instead. The electic saw makes a great deal of noise, which sometimes frightens the patient. When the cast has been carefully cut, the sections are separated by a cast spreader, and the padding underneath is released with large bandage scissors. The body part that was casted must be gently supported and handled and not forced into new, unfamiliar positions. Sudden lack of support or movement often causes considerable stress.

Professional opinion differs regarding the skin care of a patient who has been in a cast for a considerable time and who will almost immediately be enclosed in a cast again. Some physicians want their patients to have baths; others believe that the least amount of handling as possible is best. All wish to prevent trauma to the skin, which leads to trouble during the subsequent period of casting. If the use of a cast is discontinued permanently or for a considerable time, the physician may order a combination of gentle baths and the application of baby oil to help loosen the crust of old skin and sebaceous material that has collected on the body part that was under the cast. With patience and time this crust can be removed with no injury to the underlying epidermis.

Care of the newly casted patient and the cast

A newly casted patient may complain of the heat generated by the plaster as it undergoes physical reaction with the water. This heat of crystallization is transitory; however, in body casts it may cause considerable annoyance. Newly applied casts are soft, damp, and grayish white and have a slightly musty smell. They must be handled carefully.

Transfer of the patient. When transferring a newly

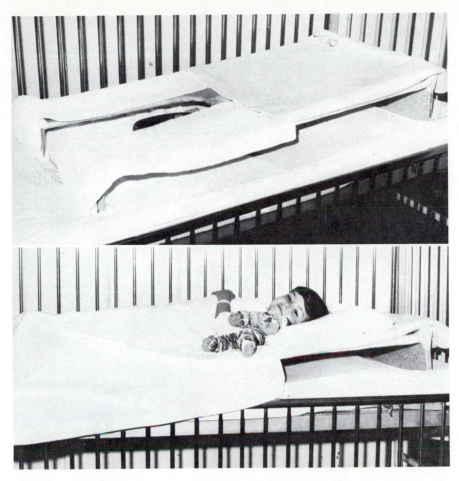

FIG 27-11 Cast board premeasured especially for patient. Note incline and positioned bedpan. *(Courtesy Children's Hospital and Health Center, San Diego, Calif.)*

casted patient, the nurse should lift the cast with the palms of the hands rather than grasp it by the fingers. Finger pressure may cause indentations, tissue injury, and disturbances in circulation. If the patient is in a body cast (hip spica) covering the trunk or hips and legs, many hands may be necessary to make an efficient, smooth transfer from cart to bed.

Preparation of the unit. The unit of a patient who is having a new body cast applied requires special preparation. Bed boards should be placed under the mattress to prevent sagging. Numerous firm pillows should be available to support the contours of the soft cast.

If the child is old enough and able to benefit from them, an overhead bar and trapeze should be attached to the bed. The room should be well ventilated to assist in the drying of the cast. Occasionally, special cast driers are available, or an undraped heat cradle may be used

to help speed drying. A new cast should be exposed to the air. However, for modesty's sake a G-string or diaper may be positioned over the perineal area. A fracture pan should be available in the bedside stand. In many hospitals infants and small children in body casts are measured for so-called cast boards or for a Bradford frame, which holds the child at a slight incline, elevated from the bed mattress (Fig. 27-11). A bedpan is kept positioned under the child at all times, and plastic strips, which are tucked into the perineal area of the cast, guide waste material into the pan below. Very young children who are incontinent can be "taped" with urine collection bags until the cast is dry enough to be protected against accidental soiling. If this is done before cast application, soiling can be more effectively prevented.

For patients with newly casted extremities, often all that is necessary for the nurse to have ready in the patient's unit is a supply of firm pillows to elevate the body part to help prevent swelling. Sometimes elevation is best maintained through the use of a gatch bed, placement of pillows under the end of the mattress, or suspension of the affected part from an intravenous pole. The cast should be left exposed to the air to facilitate drying, and the patient should be turned frequently. Most casts dry in approximately 24 hours.

Care of the cast. When the cast is dry, as indicated by a chalky white finish and a hard nonmoist surface, it should be protected against accidental wetting in the perineal region. This may be done in several ways. Various types of plastic material can be cut to fit under the perineal edge of the cast and to protect the curved band of the adjacent plaster. It can be held in place by pieces of water-repellent adhesive tape. Plastic adhesive tape can be cut into wedge-shaped pieces and positioned around and under the perineal rim and on the outer surface. Regardless of the method selected to protect the cast, the waterproof material should not be applied until the cast is dry because the adhesive usually does not stick until then.

When the cast is dry, all rough or potentially rough edges of the cast should be covered. This process is called

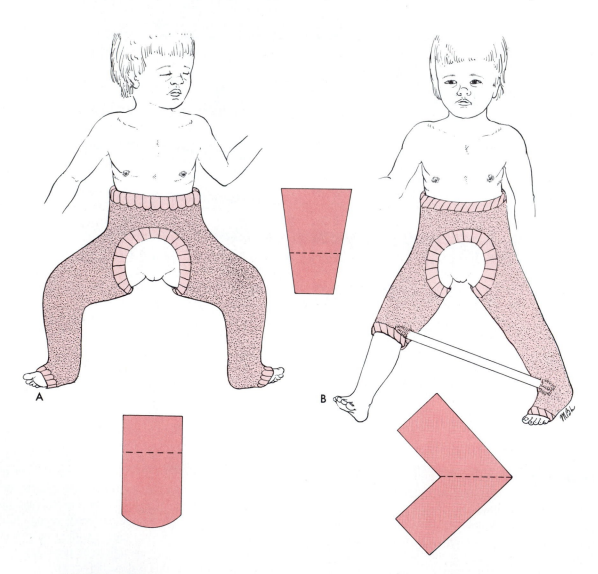

FIG 27-12 Different types of petaling. **A,** Bilateral hip spica cast. **B,** Unilateral hip spica cast with abductor bar.

Signs of neurovascular complications

Pain	Patient feels discomfort or burning sensation, especially when toes or fingers are passively stretched. Very small children are unable to verbalize subjective symptoms; they should be watched for unexplained "fussiness."
Puffiness	Toes or fingers are swollen.
Pallor	Toes or fingers are cold (they should be pink and warm). The nurse should compare them with uninvolved extremity if possible.
Purple tint	Toes or fingers are cyanotic or mottled.
Pressure response delay	Blanching sign is absent or delayed. Pressure is made on the nail beds to blanch the area. When the pressure is removed, the normal nail color should return immediately. If the area does not blanch, this is also significant because it indicates local congestion and lack of good circulation.
Pulselessness	A pulse in an extremity cannot be found (when the area to be palpated is accessible).
Paralysis	Toes or fingers cannot be moved properly by the child.
Paresthesia	Patient feels numbness and tingling.

"petaling" because the pieces of adhesive tape first used for this purpose were cut in the shape of flower petals. However, nurses currently use adhesive tape cut like chevrons, circles, or wedges, as well as the traditional "petal," to protect cast edges (Fig. 27-12). Petaling keeps small bits of plaster from the cast edges from falling into the cast, helps prevent skin irritation around the cast, and may waterproof and improve the appearance of the cast. If tubular stockinette is applied before the plaster bandage during the construction of the cast, it can be neatly trimmed, brought up over the cast edge, and secured with adhesive or plaster strips to make a smooth, attractive edging when the cast is dry.

Various methods have been employed to enhance the appearance of a cast and help protect it from damage and soil. Some physicians apply shellac, varnish, or plastic spray to a dry cast to increase its longevity and help keep it clean. It is best not to get a cast dirty or stained in the first place, but if it does become soiled, the nurse may clean the area with a damp, not wet, cloth and a small amount of white cleanser (such as Bon Ami) or fast-drying white shoe polish. Some dry, dirty areas may be covered by adhesive tape or additional plaster of Paris strips. Children should be cautioned against getting their casts damp. (Swimming is prohibited.)

Casts are a great help in correcting various musculoskeletal problems, but they may also cause or accentuate problems. The casted patient must be carefully observed to detect the development of any difficulties.

Observation for complications. A newly casted extremity may suffer impaired circulation. Sometimes cir-culatory problems compound themselves. Because of injury, operative procedure, or a tight cast application, there may be swelling under the cast. The increasingly tighter cast impedes circulation further, and tissue damage may take place. Certain signs and symptoms that indicate abnormal pressure and swelling should be reported to avoid significant tissue damage. Patients should be assessed frequently after casting and periodically thereafter (box above).

Excessive bleeding after surgery, as estimated by bloody drainage seeping through the cast layers, may be worrisome. The type of surgical procedure involved is a consideration. Physicians differ in opinion about marking the drainage stains and the time noted on a cast because it may alarm patients unduly.

When possible, the corresponding unaffected extremity should be compared with the casted arm or leg. Some people have cold hands most of the time, with or without casts. Any complaint of a burning sensation or pain should be promptly reported and investigated. Considerable damage can occur in a relatively short period. The body part may become numb and no additional complaints may be heard for some time, until tissue damage is significant.

A swelling casted extremity must be relieved promptly. A nurse should not hesitate to call a physician if circulation is impaired even though the hour is inconvenient. In the unusual situation in which no physician can be contacted, the nurse should be prepared to cut the cast herself. Certainly such a situation is extraordinary, but if no help is available for a considerable period, it is better to have a damaged cast than a gangrenous extremity. The usual emergency procedure involves cutting the cast in half and forming upper and lower, or anterior and posterior, shells. The inner wrappings should also be cut, since they may cause considerable pressure. The extremity may be maintained in the shell with the halves held loosely together by elastic bandage. Such a cast is said to be *bivalved*. Occasionally, physicians intentionally plan to bivalve casts; such casts provide support but also allow some movement and exposure and facilitate the skin care of an area. Bivalved casts are often used as splints in conjunction with elastic bandages.

Even when the cast is dry and relatively old, the daily care of the patient in a body cast or a hip spica cast should continue to include observation for disturbances in circulation and possible areas of pressure, skin breakdown, and infection. A peculiar, sweet, musty odor may indicate the presence of pus. The skin next to the cast edges must be carefully inspected and massaged. The heel and heel cord and the perineum especially should be watched for signs of irritation.

Turning the patient. The patient in a dry body cast is routinely turned at least every 2 or 3 hours in an attempt to prevent pressure sores and promote respiration and elimination. The number of people needed to turn a patient in a body cast depends on the size and general condition of the patient and the age of the cast. Remember the following when turning a patient in a large body cast:

1. If there is a choice, plan to turn the patient toward the nonoperative side.
2. Before turning the patient, pull or lift the child to the side of the bed, placing his "turning side" toward the center of the bed. Have the patient lift his hands above his head or, if this is not feasible, have them held against his sides with a towel or diaper placed between his hands and the cast just before turning to prevent injury. Do *not* use the abductor bar to turn the patient. It is held in place with only a few turns of plaster bandage. It helps support the cast, but it is not a handle.

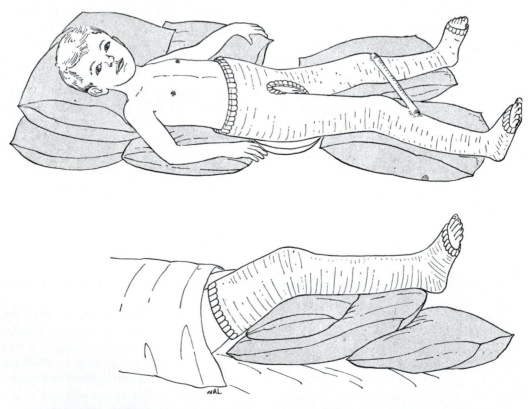

FIG 27-13 Methods of using pillows to support cast. Child shown at top is on bedpan.

3. If possible, place the protective pillows needed under the cast in the new position before the patient is turned.

   a. If the patient is placed *on his abdomen,* a flat pillow just below his chest area sometimes helps chest expansion and respiration. A small pillow for his head increases comfort. Legs should be supported to prevent his toes from digging into the bedding and the problem of footdrop. Curved up-and-down contours of the cast also should be protected from strain. The abdominal position is preferred for older children at mealtime to aid in swallowing and self-feeding.

   b. If the patient is *supine,* place a small pillow under his head. Curved up-and-down contours of the cast should be protected from strain, and the heels should be lifted from the mattress.

   c. Ensure that the edges of the cast do not press against the patient's skin. The patient should be made as comfortable as possible.

   d. A young child who is incontinent and does not have a cast board may be placed on a horseshoe-shaped pillow arrangement, and a small bedpan or large kidney-shaped basin may be positioned under the patient with a plastic strip tucked under the cast leading to the pan or basin (Fig. 27-13). Such a pillow support should elevate the child on a slight incline to prevent urine backflow into the cast.

Safety factors. Children in casts of any type must be carefully observed and taught not to put anything into the cast. Small objects, such as crayons and bobby pins, can cause pressure areas, pain, and infection. The nurse must also be vigilant regarding the use of so-called scratchers, employed to relieve itching. If scratchers are allowed at all, they must be relatively soft, such as a strip of gauze that has been strategically placed before the cast application is begun. Even pipe cleaners may cause excoriation and are not recommended for such purposes. Blowing air from a syringe—or from a hair dryer set on cool air—under the rim of the cast may be soothing. One must be sure that the child is not scratching a healing surgical incision.

General nursing considerations

Bathing. Parts of the body that might be overlooked during the daily bath are the fingers and the areas between the toes. Plaster crumbs may collect between the digits and cause pressure areas. Cotton-tipped applicators dipped in baby oil help clean these areas satisfactorily.

Diet and fluids. The child who is immobilized needs not only meticulous skin care but also special attention to diet and fluid intake to promote healing and prevent constipation and urinary stasis. A liberal fluid intake should be maintained, and a high-protein diet is often encouraged. At times prune juice or a mild laxative is indicated.

Support of a casted extremity. When a child with a casted extremity is allowed to be up in a chair, the cast should be elevated and not permitted to become dependent. The physician may order that a casted arm be supported in a sling. Several types of slings are available. The classic sling is formed from a triangular bandage. The fingers are exposed but the wrist is supported, and the hand is higher than the elbow. The knot should not rest over the cervical spine; this is uncomfortable and may cause a pressure area. Fig. 27-14 shows a com-

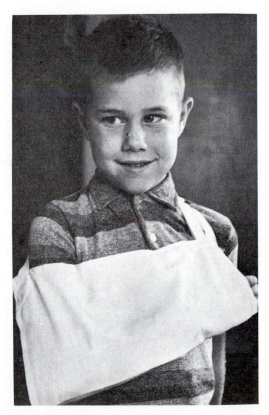

FIG 27-14 Commercial hammock-type sling. Note that arm enters sling from top, not from side.

NURSING CARE PLAN

The Child with Musculoskeletal Dysfunction

Selected nursing diagnoses	Expected outcomes	Interventions
A. Altered peripheral tissue perfusion, related to bleeding, edema, and increased pressure. Clinical manifestations: Progressive pain, positive passive stretch, weak or absent peripheral pulse, slow capillary refill, weakness or tingling in affected extremity.	Child maintains adequate peripheral circulation to affected extremity.	Assess for circulatory impairment every hour during first 24 hours following surgery or trauma, and every 4 hours thereafter. Notify physician if child has progressive pain in spite of analgesia and/or other signs of circulatory impairment. Compare affected extremity to unaffected, and note any changes from previous assessment. Elevate affected extremity at or above level of the heart. Ensure even drying of plaster of paris cast by turning child frequently and avoiding pressure on any one area. If rewrapping ace bandages, ensure secure but well distributed tension. Teach child and/or parent signs and symptoms to report that indicate circulatory impairment.
B. Impaired physical mobility related to cast or traction. Clinical manifestations: Mechanical restriction of normal movement, inability to move out of bed.	The child maintains maximum mobility within the limits of a cast or traction, and remains free of complications from decreased activity.	Explain limitations of movement necessitated by treatment plan, and rationale to child and/or parent. Discuss possible complications of restricted mobility and means of prevention. Encourage maximum movement possible while still maintaining optimal position of safety, function, and comfort. Assess joints, skin, abdomen, and lungs to ensure full function and absence of complications. Have child perform full ROM, active if possible, to all uninvolved extremities every shift. Help child minimize friction with movement and avoid prolonged pressure over bony prominences by changing position every 2 hours, use of trapeze, egg crate mattress, and back care every shift.

Selected nursing diagnoses	Expected outcomes	Interventions
		Monitor frequency and character of bowel movements; encourage diet with high fluid and fiber content; and secure order for stool softeners if needed. Maintain accurate I & O; offer bedpan to empty bladder at least every 4 hours; cleanse perineum well during bath and after each bowel movement. Encourage semi-Fowler's position or higher while awake, deep breathing every 4 hours; and use of incentive spirometer if indicated by unwillingness to deep breathe.
C. Diversional activity deficit related to restricted movement, unfamiliar surroundings, inability to participate in customary play activities. Clinical manifestations: Verbal and nonverbal expressions of boredom, disinterest in surroundings, flat emotional affect, restlessness.	Child participates actively in both structured and unstructured age appropriate play activities each day of hospitalization.	Learn of child's individual interests and favorite play things from child and parent. Schedule with child and parent each day to include times for both structured and unstructured play. Help decorate the bedside with objects of interest and reminders of home. Encourage frequent use of playroom and change child's environment often, if possible. Place child in room with peers, especially if school age or older, and foster interaction between roommates. Secure toys, games, and supplies for projects feasible for use in bed, and with consideration of child's individual age, interests, hobbies, and talents. Consider acquisition of tape recorder and/or radio and encourage its use for music, sports, and storytelling. Secure reading books appropriate to child's age and interests, and make time/effort to foster their use via nurse, parent, or volunteer. Facilitate contact with school teacher from home and plan time for help with assignments. Encourage contact by phone, letters, or visits with siblings and friends in addition to parents. Refer to Child Life Director if indicated. Allow use of TV occasionally, but only after participation in more productive activities.

mercially prepared hammock-type sling. It is available in several sizes.

When local swelling of an extremity is present or possible, some physicians order that the arm be elevated with pillows. If such elevation is to be effective, the child's wrist must be higher than the elbow, the elbow must be higher than the shoulder, and the entire extremity must be elevated above the level of the heart.

Diversion and intellectual stimulation. A person may be clean, free from pain, on the mend physically, but not particularly happy. The nurse who is interested in the total patient, not just the body in the cast, should help provide proper diversion, intellectual stimulation, and interpersonal contacts for her patients. During such a time older children can develop constructive hobbies and lasting interests.

Discharge. Many casted patients do not remain in the hospital for very long. Often the cast is applied, dried, protected, and petaled, and the patient's discharge is written within 48 hours or less. The family must be instructed in detail concerning skin care, observation for circulatory problems, cast protection, and cleansing if they are not already familiar with cast care. The need for maximum mobility within the child's limitations should be emphasized in order to enhance normal growth and development. Using proper body mechanics and seeking assistance when necessary may prevent injury to both parent and child. Appropriate transportation must be arranged. Patients in long-leg casts or hip spica casts cannot be comfortably placed in all automobiles. Discharging a patient with a cast should not be taken lightly, and sufficient time for teaching must be given to anticipate and answer the parents' questions. Videotapes and instruction handouts can be used to aid but not substitute for direct teaching.

BRACES

A removable, external support used to maintain position or provide strength to a body part is called a brace. A brace may be made of numerous kinds of material but characteristically is constructed of metal, leather, felt, and lacings. Braces are expensive but helpful pieces of equipment. They are individually fitted and produced, and they demand the respect of both patient and nurse. Braces furnish support by exerting pressure on at least three points of the body. There are many different types of braces. The Milwaukee brace for the treatment of scoliosis is one example of a body brace (Fig. 31-10). Short, below-the-knee braces for ankle or foot support or full-length leg braces for both knee and ankle stabilization are available.

Some patients (cerebral palsy victims) must have combined body and long leg braces because of extensive muscle involvement. Many braces include movable joints that can be locked with various mechanisms to provide greater stability for weight bearing.

Maintenance of the brace

The routine care of a brace includes protecting it from rust, carefully cleaning and oiling any hinges with a fine-grade oil, and removing any excess oil to prevent staining of leather supports or clothing. It also includes the care of any leather parts by the periodic application of saddle soap, followed by polishing. Cleaning fluids may be used on felt pads. Laces should be maintained intact and free from pressure-causing knots. Shoes incorporated in any leg brace should be frequently inspected for abnormal wear. Any missing parts (such as felt kneepads or screws) should be promptly reported because the loss may seriously jeopardize the brace's function.

Nursing responsibilities

The nurse and patient should be familiar with the purpose of each brace, the way in which it should be applied and positioned, when it should be worn, the length of time it should be worn, and its mechanism and maintenance. Patients wearing braces should be frequently inspected for bruises and pressure areas. Bony prominences can be protected beforehand by rubbing tincture of benzoin or a wet tea bag over the skin area. Trial periods should be gradually lengthened (p. 434). Those wearing leg braces should have well-fitted, "no-hole" stockings. A body brace is usually worn over a cotton shirt. It should be applied with the patient lying flat in bed. Back braces are buckled or laced from the bottom up, then adjusted as necessary with the patient in a standing position. A good orthotist (maker and fitter of braces) and a cooperative patient and family are essential to the successful use of a brace. In the event of the patient's persistent refusal to wear the brace, psychologic counseling may be advisable. A power struggle between parent and child must be prevented at all costs.

CRUTCHES

Often a patient is required to use crutches, with or without braces, to be ambulatory. The physical therapist is usually responsible for teaching crutch walking and the particular gait best suited to the individual patient. However, the nurse may be asked to measure patients for crutches and assist them in developing good habits involving their use.

One method of measuring a patient in the supine position for standard-type crutches is to measure the distance from the patient's axilla to a point 4 to 8 inches (10 to 20 cm) out from the patient's heel while the leg is extended and adducted. Ideally patients should wear the shoes that they will be using while walking. Another method involves subtracting 16 inches (41 cm) from the patient's height. Crutch length depends also on the condition of the patient and the gait selected.

The nurse should be sure that the rubber guards on the crutch ends are not worn smooth. The patient should not lean on the "armpit rests." The weight of the body should be borne by the hands. It is easier for a patient using crutches to rise from a firm rather than an overstuffed chair. When walking with a patient who is learning to use crutches, the nurse should walk behind her patient. In case of difficulty she may grasp the patient by the belt, trousers, or waist.

• • •

Orthopedic nursing can be extremely satisfying. It may take much skill, patience, determination, and time to achieve a straightened back or a corrected foot, but it is well worth the effort involved.

Key Concepts

1. Traction is used for the following reasons: to bring a broken bone back into alignment and provide immobilization for correct union, to secure a corrected position, to treat a congenital or acquired deformity not involving a fracture, to prevent or treat contracture deformities, and to relieve muscle spasm and pain.

2. The two main types of traction are skin and skeletal. Skin traction indirectly helps position the bone by pulling on the skin and muscles. Skeletal traction is secured by inserting a mechanical device directly into or through the bone and attaching the prescribed weight.

3. The maintenance of proper traction depends on the correct direction and amount of pull exerted through the use of ropes, pulleys, and weights and on the correct positioning or alignment of the patient.

4. Countertraction is created in four basic ways: maintenance of body placement in bed, elevation of the part of the bed closest to the weights, use of restraints, and application of a counterweight.

5. Although it is important that patients not be moved in a way that disrupts traction, it is also important that they be moved to the extent permitted to avoid pressure areas and encourage proper body function, elimination, respiration, and circulation.

6. The skin of a patient in traction must be meticulously observed and protected. Pressure areas may be reduced or eliminated by frequent inspection and cleansing of susceptible areas, use of an eggcrate mattress, maintenance of wrinkle-free linen, continual elevation of the bed's head to an angle of less than 30 degrees, and encouragement of as much movement as is allowed.

7. Some hospitals are supplied with special traction linen designed to fit under or around different traction appliances.

8. Traction equipment varies depending on the patient's individual needs. Common types are Bryant's, Buck's, Russell's, and 90°-90°.

9. External fixation may be used instead of traction, casting, or internal fixation. It is less frequently used for the younger child, but can offer earlier mobilization and rigid stabilization for the older child with a complicated fracture.

10. Bryant's traction is often used for the treatment of fractured femurs in young children. Such patients must be carefully observed for circulation problems because the traction may interfere with blood flow.

11. Russell's traction, a skin traction using a sling and single rope arrangement attached to one weight supported by multiple pulleys, is used to treat undisplaced fractures and provide postoperative hip and knee immobilization in older children.

12. In 90°-90° traction, both the hip and the knee are placed in 90 degree flexion. This type of traction is used to reduce a fractured femur.

13. Buck's extension is a rather simple, frequently used skin traction for treatment of the lower extremities or lower back.

14. Balanced traction, involving the suspension of the affected limb above the surface of the bed, provides the opportunity for more movement and activity by the patient.

15. In addition to immobilization and traction, casts may also be a means of aiding proper positioning or resting a body part. The nurse assisting the physician in applying a cast is responsible for making available all equipment and supplies. She may also be asked

to hold the extremity being casted or to support part of the newly formed cast.

16. Objectives of cast care include early detection of circulatory impairment, ensuring even drying, prevention of skin breakdown, maintenance of cast integrity, and promotion of maximum mobility.

17. Sometimes a patient must have one cast removed and another applied. The frequency with which a child must have a cast changed depends on his rate of growth, the condition of the cast, and the progress of the desired correction.

18. The unit of a patient with a newly applied body cast requires special preparation, including placement of bedboards under the mattress, numerous pillows, and a fracture pan or bedpan. Patients with newly casted extremities usually require only a supply of firm pillows to elevate the body part.

19. When the cast is dry, all rough or potentially rough edges are covered using a process called petaling. Petaling prevents small bits of plaster from the cast edges from falling into the cast, helps prevent skin irritation around the cast, and may waterproof and improve the appearance of the cast. Skin protection is also achieved by lining and edging the cast with a tubular stockinette.

20. Patients should be assessed frequently after casting and periodically thereafter. Signs of neurovascular complications are pain, puffiness, pallor, purple tint, pressure response delay, pulselessness, paralysis, and paresthesia.

21. The patient in a dry body cast is routinely turned at least every 2 to 3 hours to prevent pressure sores and promote respiration and elimination.

22. Nursing considerations for the casted patient include bathing, diet and fluids, support of the casted extremity, diversion and intellectual stimulation, and preparation for discharge.

23. Braces are individually fitted and produced, and various types are available. The nurse and patient should be familiar with the purpose of each brace, the way in which it should be applied and positioned, when and for how long it should be worn, and its mechanism and maintenance.

24. The nurse may be asked to measure patients for crutches and assist them in developing good habits involving their use. Crutch length can be measured in different ways and depends on the patient's condition and the gait selected.

Discussion Questions

1. What is meant by the terms traction, countertraction, and balanced traction? How do they differ?

2. What are the basic types of traction? Within these two basic types identify the specific forms of traction used for children?

3. Discuss the advantages of fiberglass casts.

4. What modifications are made regarding hygiene activities, bed making, and skin care when a pediatric patient is restricted by traction? By a cast?

5. What special nursing precautions are taken when a cast is newly applied? What special nursing observations are required when a cast is applied? Because many patients are discharged soon after cast application, the parent needs to be aware of how to care for the child. What would you explain about bathing, diapering, foreign objects, and circulation checks?

28

Methods of Temperature Control and Therapeutic Uses of Heat and Cold

CHAPTER OBJECTIVES

After studying this chapter, the student should be able to perform the following:

1 State the usual definition of fever taken by the oral, rectal, and axillary routes.

2 List four mechanisms by which the body produces heat and regulates its own temperature.

3 Indicate six methods that help a person maintain or increase body temperature.

4 What type of disorders are associated with an elevation in the body's temperature set-point, and what method of temperature control is commonly used for such problems?

5 Indicate six methods that help a person lower body temperature.

6 Define the terms evaporation, radiation, conduction, and convection as they relate to the regulation of body heat; cite an example of each.

7 Define "neutral thermal environment" as it relates to the body temperature maintenance of an infant.

8 Explain the meaning of the admission note "febrile seizure" on a chart.

9 Translate the following directions for water temperature into thermometer reading ranges: neutral or warm, hot, and very hot.

10 Discuss possible dangers involved in the local surface application of heat or cold.

11 Explain what is meant by reflex vasoconstriction or vasodilatation.

12 Describe an acceptable method of administering a tepid water sponge bath.

The regulation of body heat and the effects of localized temperature change on body parts are significant considerations in the medical and nursing care of many patients. Although the aims and methods of temperature control are not without controversy, the perceptive regulation of body temperature through the use of selective therapies not only may bring greater comfort to the patient but also may prevent complications that occur in the presence of high temperature or abnormal loss of body heat. Appropriate temperature maintenance may be particularly critical for small infants by conserving calories and preventing acidosis.

Occasionally extremes of body temperature have been induced for therapeutic reasons. Local hot and cold applications are commonly used for treatment. Both the regulation of general body temperature and local reac-

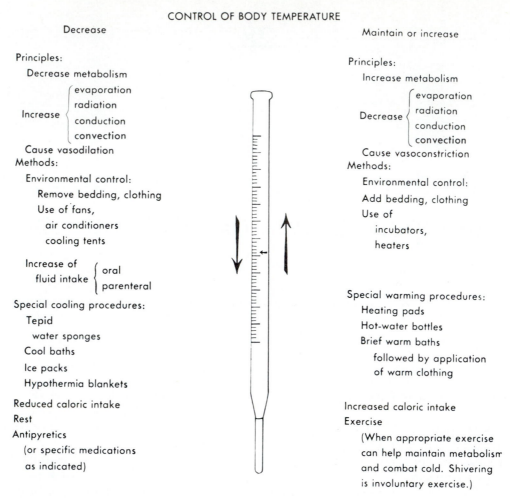

CONTROL OF BODY TEMPERATURE

Decrease

Principles:
  Decrease metabolism
  Increase { evaporation
             radiation
             conduction
             convection
  Cause vasodilation
Methods:
  Environmental control:
    Remove bedding, clothing
    Use of fans,
      air conditioners
      cooling tents
  Increase of { oral
  fluid intake { parenteral
  Special cooling procedures:
    Tepid
      water sponges
    Cool baths
    Ice packs
    Hypothermia blankets

  Reduced caloric intake
  Rest
  Antipyretics
    (or specific medications
    as indicated)

Maintain or increase

Principles:
  Increase metabolism
  Decrease { evaporation
             radiation
             conduction
             convection
  Cause vasoconstriction
Methods:
  Environmental control:
    Add bedding, clothing
    Use of
      incubators,
      heaters

  Special warming procedures:
    Heating pads
    Hot-water bottles
    Brief warm baths
      followed by application
      of warm clothing

  Increased caloric intake
  Exercise
    (When appropriate exercise
    can help maintain metabolism
    and combat cold. Shivering
    is involuntary exercise.)

FIG 28-1 In health, the body keeps its temperature within safe ranges. However, during unusual conditions or illness, normal temperature controls may be disturbed, and special regulating measures may be needed.

tions to temperature extremes are briefly discussed in the following paragraphs.

BODY TEMPERATURE

Regulation (Fig. 28-1)

Although the normal oral temperature is often cited as 98.6° F (37° C) (see Table 28-1), these figures indicate an average normal oral temperature. However, even the normal *range* of oral temperature is variously defined. Oral temperatures ranging from 97.6° to 99° F (36.4° to 37.2° C) are not considered abnormal, and some other published ranges of normal are more expansive. A number of authors consider an oral or axillary reading greater than 100° F (37.8° C) to be fever. Rectal temperatures higher than 100.4° F (38° C) normally indicate fever.

It has been taught that rectal temperatures are about 1° F higher than those taken orally and that axillary temperatures usually register about 1° F lower. This relationship has not been supported by careful investigation. Axillary temperatures are increasingly favored for infants and young children. They are less invasive and can be as meaningful.

Infants and young children have relatively high metabolic rates and usually higher normal temperatures than older persons. During a 24-hour period, people typically demonstrate a predictable change in body temperature. Readings taken between 4 and 8 PM usually are higher, whereas those taken during the usual sleep interval are characteristically lower. Environmental conditions, type of dress, and activities all influence a person's body tem-

Table 28-1 Approximate Celsius/Fahrenheit temperature conversions

	Celsius	Fahrenheit
Boiling point	100°	212°
Harmful fever*	41.7	107.0
	41.6	106.8
	41.4	106.5
	41.2	106.2
	41.1	106.0
	41.0	105.8
	40.8	105.4
	40.6	105.1
	40.5	105.0
	40.4	104.7
	40.2	104.4
	40.0	104.0
	39.8	103.6
	39.6	103.3
	39.4	103.0
	39.2	102.6
	39.0	102.2
	38.9	102.0
	38.8	101.8
	38.6	101.5
	38.4	101.1
	38.3	101.0
	38.2	100.8
	38.0	100.4
	37.8	100.0
	37.6	99.7
	37.4	99.3
	37.2	99.0
Average oral temperature	37.0	98.6
	36.8	98.2
	36.7	98.0
	36.6	97.9
	36.4	97.5
	36.2	97.2
	36.0	96.8
	35.8	96.4
Freezing point	0.0	32.0

*NOTE: Generally the appearance and behavior of a person is more significant than the degree of temperature recorded. The rapidity of the rise of a fever is also important. A rapid rise in temperature is often associated with seizures. Controversy continues regarding the definition of harmful fever 106° vs. 107° F [Schmitt BD: Pediatrics 74(5):929, 1984 Reeves-Swift R: MCN 15(2):82, 1990]. Temperature measured orally

Conversion Formulas: $°C \times \frac{9}{5} + 32 = °F$

$$°F - 32 \times \frac{5}{9} = °C$$

perature. Normal body temperature in a human being represents a balance between heat production and heat loss in the body. Most body heat is inadvertently created in the process of normal body functions. Production of body heat is the result of the activity of all cells, made possible by the oxidation or burning of foodstuffs within those cells. Blood, flowing through the various parts of the body, helps distribute heat, and although measured body temperature may differ depending on the method by which it is determined (oral, rectal, axillary, or skin probe), it is remarkable that these various measurements do not differ more than they do. Temperatures measured near arteries are often called core temperatures. Examples are oral, rectal and axillary readings in contrast to those measured by a skin probe.

Body heat is conserved by the involuntary constriction of the blood vessels of the skin, forcing more blood into the warm interior of the body and cutting it off from cooler areas near the skin's surface; it is also conserved by the automatic reduction of perspiration. Of course, the maintenance of body heat is also aided by the voluntary activity of the person. Adding a sweater or coat to provide better insulation or exercising to increase metabolism and circulation increases tolerance to cold. Much heat is produced through the activity of the skeletal muscles. When additional warmth is necessary, these muscles may even contract involuntarily to produce heat, a process called shivering. Conversely, removing insulation, increasing surface evaporation, and reducing muscular activity decrease body heat.

Body heat is lost primarily through the dilatation of the capillaries in the skin, the *evaporation* of increased perspiration on the skin's surface, and the process of warming inspired air, which is subsequently exhaled. Heat naturally moves from a warmer to a cooler area or surface. Heat transfer occurs even when objects of different temperatures do not touch. This heat loss, called *radiation,* is more rapid if a significant difference in the temperatures of neighboring objects exists. Placing a body part directly in contact with a surface cooler than itself causes heat loss by *conduction.* Some surfaces remove body heat much more rapidly than others. They are called "good conductors of heat." Cooler air flowing on the body, particularly the face, can be the source of considerable heat loss by *convection* (conduction to air). All of these mechanisms of heat transfer or loss may become operative, and the nurse trying to conserve a patient's body heat must understand them. For example, a wet, nude newborn may be in jeopardy if placed in a draft or in contact with rapidly flowing oxygen while lying on a cool surface near cool walls and supply tables.

The area of the body that ultimately controls the unconscious processes necessary for the regulation of heat production, heat maintenance, and heat loss is thought to be located deep in the brain. The part of the brain considered most responsible for heat regulation is the hypothalamus, often dubbed the "thermostat" of the body responsible for setting the systemic temperature. Through the action of the autonomic nervous system, it probably controls the processes of vasoconstriction and vasodilatation, the associated activity of the sweat glands, and the involuntary skeletal muscle motion. The hypothalamus influences various aspects of body temperature through hormonal stimulation and control.

In infants and young children temperature regulation is not perfected, and rather wide swings in body temperature occur readily. During the first days of life an infant is more likely to be influenced by the temperature of the environment; hence the frequent use of incubators. Toddlers and young school-age children may react to the common infectious diseases of childhood by running temperatures of 104° F (40° C) or more. A child may initiate a temperature elevation during a hard crying spell.

Causes and effects of elevated body temperature

Elevated body temperature may be caused by three basic processes:

1. Elevation of the body's temperature set-point or control located in the hypothalamus—associated with infection, allergy, malignancy, radiation and central nervous system disorders
2. Excessive heat production by the body not involving an elevation in temperature set-point—associated with aspirin overdose, hyperthyroidism, and "malignant hyperthermia" (a serious condition involving an inherited muscle disorder and the administration of anesthesia and neuroblocking agents)
3. Defective heat loss mechanism preventing the body from dissipating excess heat not involving an elevation in temperature set-point—associated with heat stroke, burns

Many of the instances of elevations in body temperature that the parent or nurse encounters are that of the resetting of the body's thermostat or set-point. An elevated systemic temperature, whether initiated by infectious processes, dehydration (inadequate intake, vomiting, or diarrhea), too many clothes or coverings, or other mechanisms, usually causes considerable discomfort and distress for pediatric patients and their parents. Young children may experience a rather rapid rise in temperature, especially in response to viral infections. In general, the rapidity of a rise in body temperature is more significant than the fact that a moderately high fever exists. However, patients may be ill without an abnormal rise in body heat.

About 4% of children with a fever may exhibit convulsions. These so-called *febrile seizures* may occur at temperatures that are not extremely elevated. Whether the temperature causes the seizures or some other factor is involved is not clear. Although a seizure is frightening and parents are especially fearful regarding the possibility of brain damage, research indicates that such damage does not occur from fever in itself until levels of 106° to 107° F (41.1° to 41.7° C) are reached (see p. 579).

The belief that certain fevers may represent a therapeutic response by the body which helps support the immune system and fight infection has been changing the management of some elevated temperatures. For example, routine orders such as "acetaminophen (Tylenol) to reduce fever of 101° F" are not as common. Efforts are concentrated on finding the cause of the fever and prescribing appropriate therapy to eliminate its initial cause. If acetaminophen is given, it is often administered for its analgesic as well as its antipyretic effects (p. 582).

To evaluate fever it is necessary to assess the patient's total condition and behavior and to monitor the temperature consistently. A rapid rise in temperature (especially spiking fevers) even in the "lower readings" can cause a seizure. A high fever of 105° F or more may *depress* the immune system. Some patients may have underlying cardiorespiratory problems that may cause the elevated metabolism and accompanying rising pulse and respiratory rates associated with fever to be detrimental to their conditions. Other problems such as neurologic disease may cause special concern. Thus, fever can become a complex consideration.

Causes and effects of depressed body temperature

A depressed body temperature may simply reflect inactivity. The early morning temperature reading may be low only because body processes are at a naturally low ebb. However, an abnormally low systemic temperature may also indicate circulatory collapse or the tiring of basic body processes before death.

For some patients undergoing cardiac and thoracic surgery it may be particularly desirable to slow down metabolism during surgery and postoperative care by cooling the body to extremely low temperatures to rest the heart and respiratory system. The narrowing of the blood vessels in the skin that results from surface cooling forces the blood into the interior of the body, increases viscosity (thickens the blood), slows the blood flow, and necessitates less oxygen intake. Uncompensated by muscle activity, the drop in temperature is of therapeutic importance. However, such a severe reduction in metabolism requires special equipment and personnel and cannot be safely maintained indefinitely.

A less dramatic reduction in body temperature may increase metabolism because of the body's continuing compensatory efforts to maintain a normal temperature. Such efforts may decrease blood glucose used for fuel and consume more oxygen. This is particularly important to remember when caring for the neonate. At-risk infants subjected to this type of continued cold stress rapidly become hypoglycemic and, in addition, are unable to increase their oxygen intake sufficiently to meet their metabolic needs. Cellular metabolism in the absence of adequate oxygen produces lactic acid, and acidosis results. Such a sequence of events is avoided by maintaining a neutral thermal environment in which an infant is able to maintain body temperature with the least expenditure of energy as measured by oxygen consumption. Adequate weight gain and proper acid-base balance is enhanced. A neutral thermal environment for a baby is usually achieved when the abdominal skin temperature registers between 97.7° F (36.5° C)* and 98.6° F (37° C).

Raising body temperature

At times it becomes the duty of the nurse to carry out techniques to maintain or raise body temperature. This may be done to provide comfort, regulate metabolism, or combat exposure. It may be accomplished most simply by increasing room temperatures, applying more blankets, adding clothing, and offering warm but not hot drinks. In the home situation, placing children who have been chilled in a *brief* warm bath, dressing them warmly, and tucking them in bed is a time-honored technique.

In an emergency situation in which no incubator is available, the warmest place for a newborn infant would be directly next to the mother, who could share her own body heat. However, an infant can be most easily warmed by an incubator, a cozy box supplied with a built-in heating unit, or one of the open, radiant-heat infant warmers.

Infant incubator. Incubators are often used to maintain or gradually increase the body temperature of newborn infants. They allow close observation of a nude or partially clad baby without jeopardizing body temperature. Incubators are plastic enclosures that also may provide additional humidity and oxygen for their small residents. Three basic designs are available: (1) those with hinged lids that are lifted up to expose the infant; (2) those that, in addition to hinged lids, provide special portholes or panels for access to the infant (Fig. 28-2); and (3) those that lift up from the side, creating an open, horizontal slitlike access to the infant (Fig. 28-3). Before opening any part of an incubator, the nurse should read the temperature of the air inside and record any oxygen concentration percentage. The baby's body temperature should be recorded with that of the ambient air temperature on the baby's graphic chart. How warm an incubator is kept to conserve the infant's energy depends on the baby's gestational age when born, his present age, weight, and condition.

In some models of incubators the temperature of the artificial environment may be automatically controlled by the baby's own skin temperature through the use of a heat-sensitive probe taped to the baby. This may be advantageous in maintaining body temperature. Such incubator controls are to achieve a neutral thermal environment. However, an early abnormal rise in an infant's temperature may be masked unless the simultaneous records of the temperature of the incubator and the skin of the infant are compared. This is because, as the infant's temperature rises, the heat source will not be activated and the incubator temperature will decrease. Conversely, if the probe becomes detached from the infant undetected, the unit may overheat. The temperature setting of incubators may also be adjusted manually, depending on the results of intermittent temperature readings.

The application of local heat is helpful in raising total body temperature. The use of hot-water bottles, various heating pads, and hypothermia blankets, which may be regulated to function like giant heating blankets, is discussed in detail on p. 584.

Reducing body temperature

Approximately six basic methods may reduce fever or lower body temperature.

Fluid intake. The first method of body temperature reduction typically involves encouraging fluid intake. It has already been noted that fever may result from dehydration. Frequently, if oral fluids are impractical because of the state of the gastrointestinal tract or ex-

---

*American Academy of Pediatrics and American College of Obstetricians and Gynecologists: Guidelines for perinatal care, ed 2, Elk Grove Village, Ill, 1988 the Acacemy.

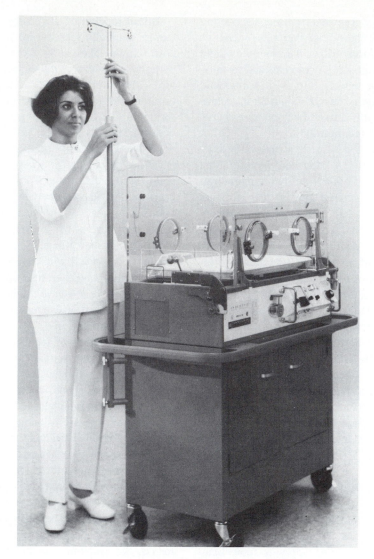

FIG 28-2 Isolette infant incubator, Model C-86. *(Courtesy Isolette—A Narco Medical Co, Warminster, Pa.)*

aggerated body need, fluids must be administered intravenously.

Environmental control. Body temperature may be lowered and the patient made more comfortable by altering the immediate environment. The removal of extra blankets and heavy clothing (unless the patient is complaining of chills and shivering) is often helpful. A well-ventilated, draft-free room may also be an aid. In warm weather well-placed fans that circulate the air without directly blowing on the patient may be used.

Medication. Medications called antipyretics may be ordered to help reduce fever. The most frequently prescribed medications have been acetylsalicylic acid, commonly known as aspirin, and the nonsalicylate acetaminophen (Tylenol or Tempra). Both are analgesics and antipyretics. They help reduce the elevated set-point of the hypothalamus.

These medications are not ordered as liberally for fever as in the past because low fevers, usually considered to be less than 102° F (38.8° C), are often thought to be helpful in combating infections. There is also a concern that a fever (a possible sign of a disease process) may

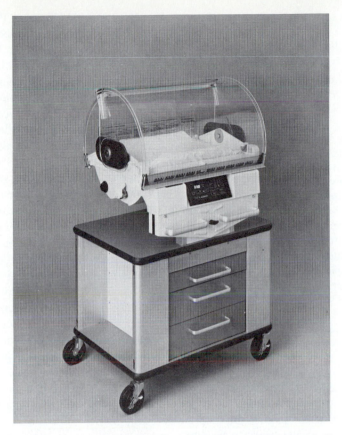

FIG 28-3   Intensive care incubator. *(Courtesy Ohio Medical Products, Madison, Wis.)*

be masked by their use, obscuring one indication of diagnosis or progress in treatment. There is still a lingering concern regarding the use of aspirin for the treatment of viral disease in children because of its suggested association with Reye syndrome.

TEPID TUB OR SPONGE BATHS

PURPOSES: Cooling by means of a tepid water tub bath or sponging techniques in the crib or bed have long been used in pediatrics in an effort to control elevated temperatures and relieve discomfort. Tepid tub or sponge baths are said to be most effective for the treatment of temperature elevations *not* caused by a rise in set-point (See p. 580, categories 2 and 3.)

PREPARATION: The procedure selected and the materials needed depend on the age, condition, and reaction of the individual child or young person.

The tepid tub bath: Best for infants or older children.

MATERIALS:

1. Wash cloths, towels
2. Convenient baby tub or standard bath tub
3. Floating toys, plastic headrest

4. Light gown or pajamas
5. Appropriate water supplies

PROCEDURE:

1. Explain procedure according to patient's understanding.
2. Place warm water about 98° F (36.6° C) in tub, only enough for a shallow bath.
3. Support child as necessary in tub—supine if possible. Never leave patient alone.
4. Place a moist washcloth on child's forehead, if appropriate.
5. Spray or pour warm water over child's body.
6. Gradually reduce temperature of bath water by adding cooler water if tolerated.
7. Observe carefully for onset of chilling or shivering. Discontinue if chilling is seen.
8. Continue bath for about 20 to 25 minutes.
9. Dry and dress in lightweight clothing.

Tepid sponge bath: Best for most toddlers.

MATERIALS:

1. Waterproof sheet

2. Absorbent bath blanket or towels, depending on the size of the child
3. Light bath blanket to place over patient
4. Basin of tepid water at about 85° to 90° F (29.4° to 32.2° C)
5. Four washcloths

PROCEDURE:

1. Explain the procedure to the child in simple terms.
2. Place the child on top of waterproof sheeting and absorbent blanket (unless this is already part of the base of the bed) fairly close to the side of the bed so that he may be easily reached. Remove pillows.
3. Undress the child and cover with the light bath blanket.
4. Rub the skin of the anterior trunk and extremities briefly with a dry washcloth to bring the blood to the surface to decrease the sensation of chilling and aid in heat reduction when the tepid moist washcloths are applied.
5. Place moist, not dripping, folded washcloths on the axilla and groin on the side of the child you will sponge last.
6. Wash the child's face and neck with the solution; place a wet washcloth on his forehead.
7. Expose only the area being sponged. Use firm, long strokes in sponging the upper extremity, thorax, abdomen, and lower extremity on the side farthest away. Place the washcloths on the groin and axilla of the opposite side. Continue sponging the patient—first the upper extremity, then the thorax, abdomen, and lower extremity.
8. Evaluate periodically the patient's reaction. How are the child's color, pulse, and respirations? (If the child seems to be chilled or shivering excessively or protests and becomes agitated or if other unfavorable reactions occur, stop the treatment, lightly cover the patient, and report to the supervising nurse.)
9. Turn the patient on his side. Rub and sponge the back firmly.
10. Gently rub the skin dry at the end of the sponge bath with a towel, and dress the child in a light gown. The procedure should take about 20 to 25 minutes.
11. Cover the child with a light sheet or blanket. Remove the bed protectors and encourage rest.

NOTE: An alternative to the tepid water sponge bath described above is wrapping with moist tepid towels instead of sponging with washcloths. These towels must be changed as soon as they become warm.

POSTPROCEDURE FOR ALL METHODS:

1. Check the patient's temperature, pulse, and respiration 30 minutes after the sponge bath; report to the supervising nurse.
2. Record the procedure, patient's reaction, and results.

Hypothermia blankets. Patients with temperature elevations that are exaggerated or fail to respond to other methods of treatment may be placed on so-called hypothermia blankets (resembling K-pads in reverse).

Several types of hypothermia blankets are manufactured. Although the operating instructions on each may differ, the principles involved are similar. Cold, distilled water or alcohol and distilled water (depending on the model) are circulated through tubes embedded in a plastic mat or mats. The water is cooled and circulated by a refrigeration pump unit to which the pads are attached. With some units, adjustment of the pad temperature is accomplished manually by the nurse, depending on the patient's temperature. With others, a rectal probe is inserted, facilitating continuous monitoring of the patient's temperature. The temperature of the patient, registered by the probe, may regulate the temperature of the pads automatically, according to predetermined temperature settings. Several pads of various sizes may be used both under and over the patient, according to need. A light bath blanket or sheet is always placed between the patient and the plastic pad. The pad should not be folded or creased, and no pins should be used to secure them. The temperature desired and the time it is to be used should be ordered by the attending physician.

LOCAL APPLICATION OF HEAT OR COLD
Local application of heat

Local application of heat and cold for the treatment of disease may be ancient therapy, but it is also a useful contemporary method. Local heat is frequently ordered to prevent chilling, relieve pain, hasten superficial abscess formation or the drainage of an infected wound, and relieve congestion in one body part by increasing blood supply to another.

Effects. The primary effect of locally applied heat is vasodilatation of the treated area (skin becomes warm and pink). Locally applied heat also speeds up metabolism, enhances associated muscle relaxation, increases the temperature of the underlying skin, subcutaneous tissue, and muscle, and even raises the skin temperature of remote body areas. Studies have shown that immersion of an arm in a hot soak raises the temperature of the big toe. Controversy exists regarding the degree of reflex vasodilatation achieved in *deep* tissues through the application of surface heat. When the effects of heat are desired in the deep-lying organs of the body, diathermy treatments, using high-frequency currents or ultrasound, are often ordered. These treatments are administered with special equipment and are seldom part of the nurse's responsibility. They more properly lie within the sphere of the physical therapist.

Dangers. The surface application of heat is not without danger. The nurse should never apply heat (other than in the form of extra blankets) without a physician's order.

When an internal abscess or localized infection is suspected (such as appendicitis), local heat should never be applied because of the danger of rupture, subsequent spread of infection, and peritonitis.

Skin temperatures over 110° F (43.3° C) cause tissue damage. However, compresses or soaks that are prepared with solutions above 110° F do not necessarily raise skin temperatures to 110° F. Skin temperatures depend on the extent of the exposure to heat—body area, time, method employed, and temperature of the solution.

Water temperatures have been placed by several authors in the following descriptive classifications:

Neutral (warm)	93° F (33.8° C) to 98° F (36.6° C)
Hot	98° F (36.6° C) to 105° F (40.5° C)
Very Hot	105° F (40.5° C) to 115° F (46.1° C)

The area receiving heat treatments should be observed frequently for signs of congestion and tissue damage. Nerve endings that detect the presence of heat and cold adjust to extreme temperatures and become less sensitive to variations. Temperatures may be inadvertently increased to an injurious level unless this loss of sensitivity is recognized. Fair-skinned persons are more likely to be burned than dark-pigmented persons and should be observed especially closely. Special precautions should be taken when the area to be treated reveals poor circulation or sensory loss. Patients may unknowingly sustain tissue damage from burning because of the lack of feeling in the area.

The time interval ordered for heat application should be carefully observed. If significant warmth is applied to a local area longer than about 1 hour (some say 30 to 45 minutes), a reflex vasoconstriction may reduce the blood supply to the area, and a reverse effect may occur.

Methods

Dry heat. Dry heat may be administered by an electric heating pad, a hot-water bottle, or a unit that circulates warm water through a plastic pad. An electric heating pad is rarely used in a hospital setting because of the danger of electrical malfunction, and the problems of maintenance and disinfection. Hot-water bottles are not recommended because many accidental burnings have resulted from their use. If hot-water bottles are employed for infants and young children, they should never contain water hotter than 115° F (46.1° C), although temperatures up to 120° F (48.8° C) are permitted for older children and adults. They should be emptied of excess air, tightly stoppered, and turned upside down to check for leaks. A dry, warm cloth cover should be placed on the bottle to provide proper insulation. Hot-water bottles should

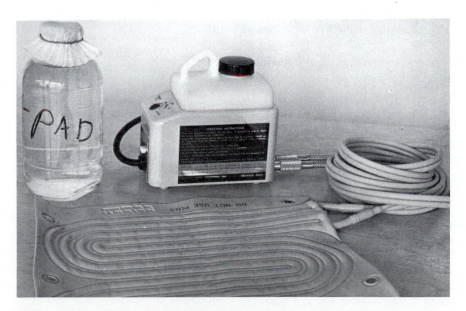

FIG 28-4 K-pad circulates distilled water through tubing in plastic pad at preset temperature. *(Courtesy Grossmont Hospital, La Mesa, Calif.)*

not be placed between skin surfaces or under the back.

A plastic pad that contains tubing through which warm water may be circulated at a preset temperature from a bedside heating unit is often used. A well-known appliance of this type is the K-pad (Fig. 28-4). Such an apparatus uses distilled water, which is periodically added to a reservoir at the top of the heating and circulating unit. Warm water is pushed out of the unit, flows through the continuous pattern of tubes embedded in the plastic pad, and returns to the heating unit. No pins should be used in stabilizing the position of the various-sized pads available. Pads may be tied or taped in place; however, if they are bent, the warm water may not circulate properly. Ideally, a pad should be neatly wrapped in a pillowcase or towel and the tubing covered with stockinette. Detailed operating instructions accompany the unit.

A commercially available chemical mixture contained within a waterproof envelope, activated by abruptly striking a premarked spot, represents another method of obtaining dry heat. These units are convenient, disposable, and efficient but somewhat expensive. In miniature form they may be used as infant heel warmers to enhance capillary dilatation before blood samples are obtained.

Moist heat. Moist heat therapy is more penetrating and faster-acting than dry heat therapy. Moist heat is usually applied locally in the form of hot soaks or compresses.

Hot soaks. If the condition of the young child permits such treatment, soaks of body parts when no open skin areas are involved may be carried out as part of a general bath, depending on the reason for the order. If this is not feasible, basins of water or other ordered solution may be provided at the bedside. If the area to be soaked involves an open lesion or wound that is not too extensive, a sterile container is provided for sterile water, tap water, or other solution. (Tap water from an approved water system is generally accepted as free from disease-producing microorganisms.) However, normal saline solution (properly called physiologic saline solution or sodium chloride, 0.9%) is often preferred because it contains approximately the same salt concentration as normal tissue fluid and therefore will not cause abnormal drying or bogginess in the body tissues. Because sterile physiologic saline solution is usually readily available in the hospital setting, it is often used for soaks involving small body areas. (Physiologic saline solution may be prepared in the home by adding 2 teaspoons of salt to 1 quart of water.) The temperature of hot soaks for children, unless otherwise ordered, is 105° F (40.5° C). The duration of the soak may vary according to orders, but the treatment is usually prescribed for 20 minutes. When the soak is terminated, any open skin area is dried and dressed as ordered.

Soaks involving large body areas are usually carried out in a bathtub. The tub is disinfected before and after use, but the procedure is not really sterile, just clean. Tepid (about 98° F [36.6° C]) body soaks are often ordered for severely burned patients. The soak, in these cases, is not administered as a heat treatment but for the cleansing and debriding action that occurs when the patient's inner dressings are removed in the water and the tub solution is agitated. Frequently such soaks, followed by the application of sterile dressings, are performed in a physical therapy department or special burn center using a whirlpool bath.

Hot compresses. Application of hot or warm compresses, however, is commonly part of a nurse's responsibilities. They may be applied to speed superficial abscess formation, promote wound drainage, or improve circulation. If the skin in the area to be compressed is broken, sterile gauze is used. The following are general suggestions for warm compress application (usually several alternatives are possible):

1. The procedure should be explained to patients according to their ability to understand and cooperate.
2. The area under the body part to be compressed should be protected by a clean, waterproof material overlaid by an absorbent towel or bath blanket.
3. The sterile gauze pads may be placed in a hot (110° F [43.3° C]) sterile solution as ordered (usually physiologic saline) and wrung with two sterile forceps until dripping stops. The pads may be placed on the designated area and replaced with new compresses about every 2 minutes.
4. In areas where the additional weight will not cause pain or injury, two or three warm compresses may be quickly covered by sterile, lightweight waterproof plastic, and the body part may be wrapped or covered by an insulating towel warmed by an overlying K-pad, hot-water bottle, or low-set electric pad.

Clean warm compresses are applied in much the same manner, except that sterile precautions need not be observed. Wriggly toddlers usually need to have the compresses gently tied in place and fairly constant nursing attendance to prevent the dismantling of the nurse's handiwork. Great care should be taken not to burn the child.

Children should not be left in a position in which they may come into direct contact with the hot water used for heating compresses.

Local application of cold

Effects. The local application of cold may also be therapeutic. Cold applied to the skin surface for brief periods (30 to 45 minutes) produces vasoconstriction of the treated area, which helps in the prevention (but not treatment) of swelling, the control of hemorrhage, and the retardation of any inflammatory process. Cold applied for a sufficient period will significantly cool muscles and other underlying organs, either directly or by reflex action. Cold also has an anesthetic quality that may sometimes become of primary importance. If applied to the skin for longer periods, cold may trigger a reverse reflex mechanism that results in vasodilatation.

Dangers. The local use of cold applications, like that of heat, is not without hazard. The skin surface must be frequently observed for mottling and tissue damage. Cold applied to areas in which circulation is inadequate may produce injury (frostbite) and lead to gangrene. The anesthetic quality of cold may make the patient unaware of injury inadvertently produced by other factors.

Methods. Like heat, cold is used therapeutically in dry or moist form. Moist cold is more penetrating than dry cold.

Dry cold. An example of the application of dry cold would be the typical ice bag or ice collar. Some of these, like the Freeze-A-Bag, are prefilled and sealed. Others must be filled. Small ice cubes and a small amount of cold water may be used to fill two thirds of the bag; all air is pressed out (it delays the transfer of cold), and the bag is capped. The bag should be wrapped in a cover to prevent condensation from wetting the patient or bedding. For effective local reaction an ice cap or ice bag should be removed approximately every 30 to 45 minutes to observe the skin and allow it to return to normal and to enable the cold to continue its process of vasoconstriction when reapplied.

Moist cold. Moist cold may be applied in the form of cold, damp compresses, cold soaks, or sponge baths.

Cold compresses. If the body part compressed can tolerate weight, clean, cold compresses are best made from washcloths or towels. If a delicate organ like an eye or an extremely tender body part is to be treated, gauze compresses may be used. The adjoining area is protected by a waterproof plastic or rubber sheet lined with an absorbent layer. A basin of water and ice, large enough to accommodate the compresses, should be at hand. The compresses should be well wrung out to prevent dripping, and once applied, they should be left exposed. Covering the compress would soon make it tepid, as a result of the heating capability of the body. The compresses must be changed frequently, depending on their size and density and the temperature of the body part to which they are applied.

It is difficult to apply sterile cold compresses because ice is not sterile. However, if a sterile technique is necessary, sterile cold solutions may be maintained in a refrigerator, and the sterile container may be packed in ice at the bedside during the treatment. Sterile compresses are handled in an aseptic manner with forceps or gloves. The use of forceps around the eyes and faces of young children in the usual bedside setting is not recommended. Their movements are too unpredictable. Wearing gloves is much less cumbersome and is safer.

Light gauze compresses usually must be changed about every minute to maintain their temperature. If any drainage or open skin area is present, the compress should not be reused but discarded.

Cold soaks. Cold soaks, often recommended to prevent the swelling of a twisted or sprained ankle, usually consist of a basin of cold water into which an extremity is placed for about 20-minute periods. Occasionally alternating cold and hot soaks are ordered to stimulate circulation.

The local use of heat or cold applications can be of strategic importance in patient care. The principles are old, but have proved worthy of study and application.

Key Concepts

1. Although the normal temperature range is variously defined, fever is usually indicated with oral temperatures of more than 100° F (37.8° C), rectal temperatures over 100.4° F (38° C), and axillary readings over 100° F (37.8° C).

2. Normal body temperature represents a balance between heat production and heat loss. Most body heat is inadvertently created in the process of normal body functions. Heat loss or conservation is controlled by vasoconstriction and vasodilatation, activity of the sweat glands, and involuntary skeletal muscle motion.

3. Elevated body temperature may be caused by three basic processes: (1) elevation of the body's temper-

ature set-point, (2) excessive heat production not involving an elevation in set-point, or (3) defective heat loss mechanism.

4. It may be desirable to cool the body to an extremely low temperature to slow down metabolism for patients undergoing cardiac and thoracic surgery. A less dramatic reduction in body temperature may increase metabolism and is an important factor to remember when caring for the neonate.

5. Body temperature may need to be maintained or raised to provide comfort, regulate metabolism, or combat exposure. This may be accomplished by various methods, including increasing room temperature, adding clothing or blankets, offering warm drinks, placing an infant in an incubator, or applying local heat.

6. There are six basic methods of reducing body temperature: increased fluid intake, reduced environmental temperature, administration of antipyretics, tepid tub bath, tepid sponge baths, and hypothermia blankets.

7. Local heat is frequently ordered to prevent chilling, to relieve pain, to hasten superficial abscess for-

mation or the drainage of an infected wound, and to relieve congestion in one body part by increasing blood supply to another.

8. Skin temperatures depend on the extent of the exposure to heat. Skin temperatures over 110° F (43.3° C) cause tissue damage; therefore the area receiving heat treatments should be observed frequently for signs of congestion and tissue damage.

9. Dry heat may be administered by an electric heating pad, a hot-water bottle, or a unit that circulates warm water through a plastic pad. Moist heat therapy is more penetrating and faster-acting than dry heat therapy. Moist heat is usually applied locally in the form of hot soaks or compresses.

10. Local application of cold helps to prevent swelling, to control hemorrhage, and to retard inflammatory processes. It produces an anesthetic effect. The skin must be freqently observed for mottling and tissue damage.

11. Dry cold may be administered with an ice bag or ice collar. Moist cold is more penetrating and may be applied in the form of cold, damp compresses, cold soaks, or sponge baths.

Discussion Questions

1. Why do infants and children experience wide swings in body temperature? What internal and external factors can contribute to elevated body temperature? To decreased body temperature?

2. Discuss the nursing measures that help to prevent rapid change in body temperature in infants and young children. What nursing measures are used to reduce elevated body temperature? What nursing measures are used to raise lowered body temperature?

3. What effects does localized application of heat have

on the body? What happens if large areas of the body are exposed to a heat source? Is time a factor in heat applications?

4. What effects does localized application of cold have on the body? What happens if large areas of the body are exposed to cold? Is time a factor in cold applications?

5. What special nursing precautions should be taken when utilizing either heat or cold to treat an infant or child?

UNIT
VIII

SUGGESTED SELECTED READINGS AND REFERENCES

General

Belson P: A plea for play, Nurs Times 83(26):16, 1987.

Betz CL and Poster E: Mosby's pediatric nursing reference, St Louis, 1989, The CV Mosby Co.

Birdsall C, Carpenter K, and Considine R: How is autotransfusion done? Am J Nurs 88(1):108, 1988.

DeBear K: Sham feeding: another kind of nourishment, Am J Nurs 86(10):1142, 1986.

Hahn K: Monitoring a blood transfusion, Nursing '89 19(10):20, 1989.

Joyner M: Hair care in the black patient, J Pediatr Health 2(6):281, 1988.

Lipson ER: New York Times parents' guide to the best books for children, New York, 1988, Time Books.

McGrath BJ: Fluids, electrolytes and replacement therapy in pediatric nursing, MCN 5(1):58: 1980.

Mitiguy JS: A surgical liaison program; making the wait more bearable, MCN 11(6):388, 1986.

Newman LN: A side-by-side look at two venous access devices, Am J Nurs 89(6):826, 1989.

Rae WA and others: The psychosocial impact of play on hospitalized children, J Pediatr Psychol 14(4):617, 1989.

Schaefer CE and Reid SE: Game play: therapeutic use of childhood games, Somerset, NJ, 1986, John Wiley & Sons, Inc.

Schmidt A and Williams D: The amazing Hickman and its easy home care, RN 45(2):57, 1982.

Smith J: Big differences in little people, Am J Nurs 88(4):459, 1988.

Smith L: Reactions to transfusion, Am J Nurs 84(9):1096, 1984.

Stevens MS: Which adolescents breeze through surgery? Am J Nurs 87(12):1564, 1987.

Thompson JM and others: Mosby's manual of clinical nursing, St Louis, 1989, The CV Mosby Co.

Trelease J: The new read-aloud handbook, New York, 1989, The Penguin Group.

Preparing Children for Procedures

Bates TA and Broome M: Preparation of children for hospitalization and surgery: a review of the literature, J Pediatr Nurs 1(4):230, 1986.

Carter JH and Hancock J: Caring for children; how to ease them through surgery, Nursing '88 18(10):46, 1988.

Doroshow ML and London DL: Surgery and children, a colorful way to introduce children to surgery, AORN J 47(3):696, 1988.

Eichelberger KM and others: Self-care nursing plan: helping children to help themselves, Pediatr Nurs 6(3):9, 1980.

Evans ML and Hansen BD: Administering injections to different-aged children, MCN 6(3):194, 1981.

Fassler D and Wallace N: Clinical essay: children's fear of needles, Clin Pediatr 21(1):59, 1982.

Gross S: Pediatric tours of hospitals—positive or negative? MCN 11(5):336, 1986.

Hansen BD and Evans ML: Preparing a child for procedures, MCN 6(6):392, 1981.

Lutz WJ: Helping hospitalized children and their parents cope with painful procedures, J Pediatr Nurs 1(1):24, 1986.

Mills GC: Preparing children and parents for cerebral computerized tomography, MCN 5(6):403, 1980.

Waidley E: Timely teaching: show and tell, preparing children for invasive procedures, Am J Nurs 85(7):811, 1985.

Diagnostic Tests

Engler MB and Engles MM: The hazards of magnetic resonance imaging, Am J Nurs 86(7):650, 1986.

Fischbach FT: Laboratory diagnostic tests, Philadelphia, 1988, JB Lippincott Co.

Kaplan J and others: Modern electrodiagnostic studies in infants and children, Pediatr Ann 13(2):150, 1984.

Kuhn JP: CT of the body in children, Pediatr Ann 15(5):367, 1986.

McFarland MB and Grant MM: Nursing implications of laboratory tests, ed., 2, Somerset, NJ, 1988, John Wiley & Sons, Inc.

Merten DL and Grossman H: Diagnostic imaging in pediatrics: the state of the art, Pediatr Ann 15(5):355, 1986.

Narchette L and Holloman F: A first-hand report on the new body scanners, RN 48(11):28, 1985.

Shetler MG and Bartos H: Culture specimens: how to collect, what to expect, RN 43(9):65, 1980.

Shetler MG and Bartos H: Stool specimens: key to detecting intestinal invaders, RN 43(10):50, 1980.

Shetler MG and Bartos H: Collecting synovial fluid and wound drainage cultures, RN 44(2):50, 1981.

Shetler MG and Bartos H: Eye and ear cultures, RN 44(3):58, 1981.

Suri S: Simplifying urine collection from infants and children without losing accuracy, MCN 13(6):438, 1988.

Tucker JB and others: Throat culturing techniques in the family practice model unit, J Fam Pract 12(5):925, 1981.

Orthopedic Procedures

Advantages of Hoffmann fixators, Am J Nurs 84(2):178, 1984.

Agee BL and Herman C: Cervical logrolling on a standard bed, Am J Nurs 84(3):314, 1984.

Brunner NA: Orthopedic nursing: a programmed approach, St Louis, 1983, The CV Mosby Co.

Evers JA and Werpechowski D: Dealing with fractures, RN 47(11):53, 1984.

Howard M and Corbo-Pelaia SA: The psychological aftereffects of halo traction and a review of acute care, Am J Nurs 82(12):1839, 1982.

Lane PL and Lee MM: Special care for special casts, Nursing '83 13(7):50, 1983.

Mulley DA: Harnessing babies' dysplastic hips, Am J Nurs 84(8):1006, 1984.

Nursing care of a patient in traction: programmed instructions, Am J Nurs 79(10):1771, 1979.

Rodts MF: An orthopedic assessment you can do in 15 minutes, Nursing '83 13(5):65, 1983.

Schaming D and others: When babies are born with orthopedic problems, RN 53(4):62, 1990.

Swagonan A: Caring for limb-deficient children and their families, MCN 11(1):46, 1986.

Swanson VM: The school-age traction patient: toward better behavior patterns, J Assoc Care Child Health 9(2):12, 1980.

Wise L: A comparison of orthopedic casts: breaking the mold, MCN 11(3):174, 1986.

Supporting Cardiopulmonary Functions

Carroll P: Safe suctioning, Nursing '89 19(9):48, 1989.

Carroll PF: What you can learn from pulmonary function tests, RN 49(7):24, 1986.

Crow S: Tips for successful respiratory suctioning, RN 49(4):31, 1986.

Colford L and Briglia F: Myths and facts . . . about pediatric resuscitation, Nursing '88 18(9):106, 1988.

Cuzzell JZ and Rodriquez LA: How to use a bag-valve-mask device for artificial ventilations, Am J Nurs 89(7):932, 1989.

Ehrhardt BS and Graham M: Pulse oximetry: an easy way to check oxygen saturation, Nursing '90 20(3):50, 1990.

Erickson RS: Mastering the ins and outs of chest drainage, Part 1, Nursing '89 19(5):36, 1989.

Erickson RS: Mastering the ins and outs of chest drainage, Part 2, Nursing '89 19(6):46, 1989.

Harrison LL: Teaching parents to provide home-care for ventilator-dependent children, MCN 14(4):281, 1989.

Hoffman LA, Mazzocco MC, and Roth JE: Fine tuning your chest PT, Am J Nurs 87(12):1566, 1987.

Jones S: Use ABGs to fine-tune resuscitation, RN 48(5):35, 1985.

Mapp CS: Trach care: are you aware of all the dangers? Nursing '88 18(7):34, 1988.

Miracle VA and Allnutt DR: How to perform basic airway management, Nursing '90 20(4):55, 1990.

Mofenson H and Greensher J: Management of the choking child, Pediatr Clin North Am 32(1):183, 1985.

Schessi EC: Learning the basics of cardiac monitors, Nursing '84 14(10):42, 1984.

Thompson SW: How to use the Heimlich maneuver on choking infants and children, Pediatr Nurs 9(1):13, 1983.

Willens JS and Copel LC: Performing CPR on children, Nursing '89 19(2):57, 1989.

Willens JS and Copel LC: Performing CPR on infants, Nursing '89 19(3):47, 1989.

Pain Prevention and Control

American Pain Society: Relieving pain: an analgesic guide, Am J Nurs 88(6):815, 1988.

Facing pain: How much does a child hurt? Am J Nurs 88(2):155, 1988.

Forlini J, Morin DM, and Treacy S: Painless peds procedures, Am J Nurs 87(3):321, 1987.

Kleiman R and others: PCA vs regular IM injections for severe post-op pain, Am J Nurs 87(11):1491, 1987.

Leduc Elly: The healing touch, MCN 14(1):41, 1989.

McCaffery M and Beebe A: Pain: clinical manual for nursing practice, St Louis, 1989, The CV Mosby Co.

McGrath PA and DeVeber LL: Helping children cope with painful procedures, Am J Nurs 86(11):1278, 1986.

O'Brien SW and Konsler GK: Alleviating children's postoperative pain, MCN 13(3):183, 1988.

Page GG: How well do we evaluate and control infant's pain? Am J Nurs 89(3):317, 1989.

Too little, too late, Nursing '88 18(4):33, 1988.

Zahourek RP, editor: Relaxation and imagery: tools for therapeutic communication and intervention, Philadelphia, 1988, WB Saunders Co.

Temperature Control and Therapies

American Academy of Pediatrics: Aspirin and Reye's syndrome, Pediatrics 69(6):810, 1982.

Foster RL, Hunsberger MM, and Anderson JJT: Family-centered nursing care of children, Philadelphia, 1989, WB Saunders Co, pp 824-826.

Griffin JP: Fever—when to leave it alone, Nursing '86 16(2):58, 1986.

Hasler MI and Cohen JA: The effect of oxygen administration on oral temperature assessment. Nurs Res 31(9):265, 1982.

Kilmon CA: Parents' knowledge and practices related to fever management, J Pediatr Health Care, 1(4):173, 1987.

Maheady DC: Reye's syndrome: review and update, J Pediatr Health Care 3(5):246, 1989.

McCance KL and Huether SE: Pathophysiology: the biological basis for disease in adults and children, St Louis, 1990, The CV Mosby Co, pp 400-406.

Reeves-Swift R: Rational management of a child's acute fever, MCN 15(2):82, 1990.

Relieving pain with heat or cold 18(7):64K. In Patient Teaching Nurse Reference Library, Springhouse, PA, 1984, Springhouse Corporation Book Division.

Schmitt BD: Fever in childhood, Pediatrics 74(5):929, 1984.

Common Pediatric Problems
and Their Nursing Care

29

Conditions Involving the Integumentary System

CHAPTER OBJECTIVES

After studying this chapter, the student should be able to perform the following:

1 Cite three ways in which the appearance and condition of the skin may reveal significant information regarding a person's physical and emotional status.
2 Define these terms often used to describe skin conditions: macule, papule, vesicle, pustule, petechia, contusion, excoriation, laceration, and ulcer.
3 State seven factors to be considered when describing a skin lesion.
4 Discuss the causes, preventions, signs and symptoms, treatments, and nursing implications of these common infant skin problems: miliaria rubra (prickly heat), seborrheic dermatitis (cradle cap), and diaper rash.
5 Describe the typical appearance of infantile eczema, frequent factors associated with its onset, and four objectives that must be considered as treatment is begun.
6 Explain the use of wet compresses in the treatment of weeping, crusted-type lesions of eczema and how the compresses should be applied.
7 Describe impetigo and indicate why systemic antibiotics are often prescribed as part of its treatment.
8 Compare tinea capitis, tinea corporis, and tinea pedis, as to location, description, treatment, and nursing care.
9 Discuss the identification, incidence, treatment, and nursing implications of infestations of pediculosis capitis (head lice) and the itch mite (scabies) in the young school-age population.
10 Respond to the questions of teenagers related to the causes, treatments, and typical duration of acne vulgaris.
11 Explain why the "rule of nines" used in the evaluation of the extent of a burn injury cannot be used without modification in evaluating an infant or young child.
12 Describe minor, moderate, and major burn injuries and indicate the first-aid care of burn victims.
13 List five main aims of burn therapy.
14 Define these terms associated with burn injury and therapy: eschar, debridement, granulation tissue, isografts (autografts), allografts (homografts), Curling's ulcer, and flexion contractures.
15 Discuss how members of a staff who are caring for a burned child may provide emotional support to the patient and his family.

The integumentary system consists of the skin as well as the hair, nails, sweat and oil glands, and superficial sensory nerve endings. These organs form the first line of defense against body injury. The integumentary system prevents both excessive loss of fluid from the body and the entry of certain poisons and microbes into the body. It is of special importance in the regulation of body temperature, principally through capillary dilatation and constriction and the formation of cooling perspiration. The skin can be an important avenue of fluid loss. However, it has only limited powers of absorption. It is of considerable aid in the evaluation of environmental conditions and therefore in the determination of individual safety. Embedded within the tissues of the integumentary system are nerve endings that relay to the brain sensations of pressure, touch, hot, cold, and pain.

The health of the skin is often a reflection of the health of the individual. Skin color, hydration, surface irregularities, and disturbances in sensation may reveal significant information about an individual's health habits and status. The skin may also give clues to a patient's emotional reactions. Involuntarily a person may blush with embarrassment or pale with fright.

LAYERS OF THE SKIN

The epidermis is paper thin and consists of several microscopic layers. The uppermost layer consists of dead cells ready to be shed from the body's surface. They are constantly being replaced by new cells, which are formed in the lower layers. The lower layers of the epidermis secure their nourishment from the dermis, or true skin, over which they lie.

The dermis, also called the *corium,* is a dense layer of connective tissue well supplied with blood vessels and nerves. It also contains sweat and oil glands and hair follicles, some of which may extend into the deeper subcutaneous tissue. Small muscle fibers may be attached to the hair follicles.

The subcutaneous layer is chiefly fatty tissue in a framework of elastic and fibrous tissue. It serves multiple functions, including those of lipid storage and insulation.

The observation of the skin and the description of its condition are often the nurse's responsibility. Her patients might not be hospitalized primarily because of skin problems. Skin difficulties may be of secondary importance in the diagnostic picture. However, the condition of the

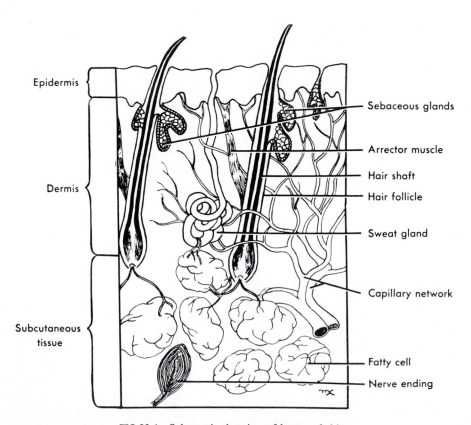

FIG 29-1 Schematic drawing of layers of skin.

skin is always of significance as the nurse views her patient's total needs.

KEY VOCABULARY

Physicians commonly use certain terms to describe the condition of the skin. Some of these words the nurse may wish to use in her own recording. Others she may not employ, but she should be able to interpret their meanings. These terms are simply defined as follows:

abrasion (adj., abraded) Loss of superficial tissue by friction (chafing).

contusion (adj., contused) A bruise; a black-and-blue mark.

crust (adj., crusted) Temporary covering of a lesion formed primarily by dried blood or serum (scab).

ecchymosis (adj., ecchymotic) Black-and-blue mark.

erosion (adj., eroded) Moist, circumscribed, often depressed lesion.

erythema (adj., erythematous) Reddened areas of the skin.

excoriation (adj., excoriated) Superficial laceration; a scratch.

jaundice or **icterus** (adj., jaundiced or icteric) Yellow tinge to the skin or sclerae.

laceration (adj., lacerated) Jagged cut or tear.

lesion Any change or irregularity in tissue caused by disease or injury.

macule (adj., macular) Flat spot or stain; the typical measles rash is macular.

papule (adj., papular) Small, solid elevation on the skin; the typical early stage of a pimple is papular.

petechia (adj., petechial) Small bluish purple dot caused by capillary hemorrhage.

pruritus (adj., pruritic) Itching.

pustule (adj., pustular) Pus-filled vesicle; a superficial cutaneous abscess.

ulcer (adj., ulcerated) Raw area often depressed or forming a cavity, caused by loss of normal covering tissue.

urticaria (*wheals* and *hives*) (adj., urticarial) Large, slightly raised, reddened or blanched areas, usually accompanied by intense itching.

vesicle (adj., vesicular) Small elevation of the skin obviously containing fluid, such as a blister.

A skin lesion should be described so that the following information is included:

1. Size (described in metric measurements, such as 1 cm in diameter)
2. Elevation (raised, flat, depressed)
3. Quality (smooth, rough, scaly, moist)
4. Color
5. Distribution (localized, scattered, and so on)
6. Associated sensory disturbances (numbness, itching, pain, burning, and so on)
7. Type of any drainage or exudate noted

COMMON SKIN PROBLEMS

Infant and toddler

Miliaria rubra (prickly heat or heat rash). Miliaria rubra is a common problem caused by blockage of the sweat pores. The exits of the sweat ducts are plugged, causing sweat to seep into the dermis or epidermis. This produces a red, pinhead-sized vesicular-papular rash that is associated with underlying erythema, especially in areas where perspiration is common or friction is frequent. It may be accompanied by considerable itching. Occasionally the rash may include pustular lesions. Prevention is easier than treatment. For instance, do not overdress children. Any procedure that reduces the need for perspiration helps improve the condition. Careful light dusting of the skin with a fine cornstarch or baby powder may be beneficial. Some dermatologists recommend the use of a skin lotion containing hydrocortisone. In the event of secondary infection an antibiotic drug may be prescribed.

Intertrigo. Intertrigo, often simply called *chafing,* is commonly found in the folds of the skin where friction is frequent and hygiene may be lacking. Examples of problem areas include the creases in the neck and the folds of the groin and gluteal muscles where the skin may become inflamed. As in miliaria rubra, prevention is simpler than a cure. Meticulous hygiene and keeping the area dry and lightly powdered are of great importance.

Seborrheic dermatitis (Fig. 29-2). Seborrheic dermatitis is a common dermatitis of infants up to 3 months of age. It is probably caused by a lipophilic, skin surface–dwelling yeast. The organism thrives in the oily environment induced by maternal transplacental hormone stimulation of the oil glands. The condition is usually benign and self-limiting, but it can be chronic and is often confused with atopic dermatitis. Seborrheic dermatitis is characterized by a scaly eruption (scales may be dry or greasy) on an inflammatory base; it chiefly affects the scalp, eyebrows, eyelids, and pubic regions. It is managed best with the topical agent, ketoconazole cream 2% (Nizoral), which kills the lipophilic yeast organism.

In infants seborrheic dermatitis is seen most commonly as "milk crust" or "cradle cap," yellowish, slightly adherent large scales found principally on the top of the head. It sometimes is related to a parent's reluctance to wash the soft spot on the baby's scalp for fear of causing injury. It also develops fairly often in the groin and may become secondarily infected with yeast (*Candida* or *Monilia*) or bacteria. Frequent shampooing and the use of mild medications containing sulfur, salicylic acid, or hydrocortisone are often prescribed for seborrheic derma-

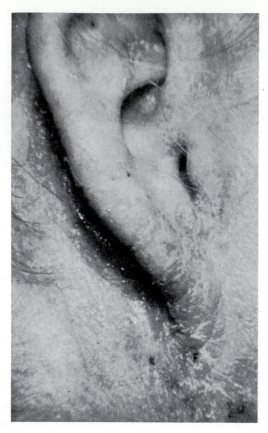

FIG 29-2 Seborrheic dermatitis. *(Courtesy W.W. Duemling, MD, San Diego, Calif.)*

titis. In adolescents it is often associated with acne. When the condition involves the scalp, the common name is dandruff.

Some children are affected by another form called intertriginous seborrhea, which is usually moist and involves areas behind the ears and the axillary and inguinal regions.

Diaper rash. Infants with diaper rash are believed to have an irritant dermatitis, but seborrheic dermatitis and eczema are other considerations. The rash may take multiple forms, from simple erythema to blisters and ulceration, depending on the causes. As a group, children with irritation of the diaper area usually have sensitive skin—a hereditary predisposition. Unfavorable conditions quickly trigger an unfavorable response. Situations that often set the scene for skin problems are poorly washed and rinsed diapers, infrequent diaper changes aggravated by prolonged use of plastic diaper covers, and incomplete or infrequent washing and drying of the diaper area. Careful attention to cleanliness is necessary. However, overzealous ministrations can cause problems, too.

To reduce the formation of irritating ammonia produced by the action of bacteria on urine, every effort is made to cut down the bacterial population on the diaper area. The use of gentle antiseptic final rinse, such as methylbenzethonium chloride sometimes may be recommended. The use of antiseptic rinses by diaper laundries is standard practice.

The cautious application of dry heat to diaper rash often improves the skin condition. A gooseneck lamp with a 25-watt bulb may be positioned over the prone infant. Precautions against burning should be observed. The lamp should be out of the child's reach and away from the bed linens. The bulb should be at least 12 inches (20.3 cm) from the child's buttocks. During heat treatments the diaper area should be free from medications. If the application of heat is difficult, simply exposing the area to the air is frequently helpful. Sunshine, if present, can be used for brief periods, but an infant should be carefully watched for overexposure.

Desitin, hydrocortisone, and certain antimicrobial agents, such as Polysporin and nystatin cream, may be ordered, depending on the needs of the particular patient. In general occlusive medications should be avoided (for example, nystatin cream is preferred to nystatin ointment).

Infantile eczema (atopic dermatitis) (Fig. 29-3). Infantile eczema most often appears after the second month of life. It often subsides considerably after the second year. It is characterized by skin lesions, which first appear as localized, scaling, red areas, usually on the head, neck, wrists, flexor surfaces of the elbows, and knees, although involvement may become progressively more extensive. Small vesicles, which break and weep serum (a yellow, sticky fluid), develop in these reddened areas fairly rapidly. The fluid dries, forming crusts on the skin. Lesions on various parts of the body may be in different stages of development—some moist, others dried and scaling. The skin may become thickened and fissured. Since itching is intense, the child invariably scratches the lesions; thus secondary infection is usually present. For this reason different types of topical medications may be applied to the affected parts of the body, depending on the aims of the treatment. Seborrheic dermatitis and fungal infections may be associated with atopic dermatitis. Permanent scarring does not occur unless the lesions become secondarily infected or deeply excoriated.

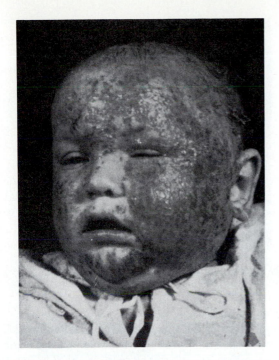

FIG 29-3 Infant with severe eczema. *(Courtesy R.B. Pappenfort, MD, San Diego, Calif.)*

Infantile eczema is considered to be essentially an allergic response. It is more properly a symptom of a disorder rather than a disorder itself. Infantile eczema has been called the most common manifestation of the allergic state in infancy. It is not always clear, however, just what agents, or *allergens*, cause the dermatitis. Exposure to allergens may occur in any of the following ways:

1. By ingestion (common foods causing difficulties in infancy are cow's milk, egg whites, wheat products, and citrus juices)
2. By inhalation (dust, pollen, and animal dander)
3. By skin contact with some medications and materials (rubber, plastic, and wool)

Many investigators believe that child-parent relationships and emotional stress play a significant role in the initiation and course of the disease. There is often a family history of allergy manifested by eczema, asthma, or hay fever. Eczema usually improves during the summer months and worsens during the winter.

Many factors must be considered in the treatment of eczema. If possible, the offending allergens should be identified and eliminated from the infant's environment. Secondary infection, if present, should be treated, and

itching, scratching, and exposure to known infections should be prevented. Treatment of the lesions to clear scaling, minimize discomfort, and improve appearance is continued. Psychologically, supportive care for the child and the family is of great importance.

To identify substances that may initiate the dermatitis, a careful history is taken by the physician. For the infant or toddler an elimination diet is often prescribed in which the foods that are allowed are listed in detail. If the baby is not breast-fed, goat's milk or soybean milk may be prescribed. The importance of rigidly following the diet must be impressed on the parents. As time goes on, more foods are added, one by one, to the diet. The child is carefully observed for changes in skin condition and general health after each addition.

The home environment of the infant must be carefully controlled also. Since many children with allergic symptoms of the respiratory tract show sensitivity to dust, their nurseries are stripped of all drapes, rugs, and fuzzy toys. The crib mattress is encased in a nonallergic cover, and wool blankets or clothing are eliminated. Although infants do not usually have pets, the presence of a dog or cat in the household may cause significant problems, and pets must sometimes find new homes. (Fish generally do not cause allergies.) The house should be frequently vacuumed with special attention to the child's sleeping quarters. Skin testing with special patch and scratch techniques in an effort to determine allergens is usually reserved for older children.

The child with eczema should be protected against contact with people who have staphylococcal, streptococcal, or viral infections, such as herpes simplex (cause of the common fever blister).

To help reduce scratching, which increases the possibility of secondary infection, various methods are used. Efforts are made to decrease the itching by using a minimum of clothing, all softly textured. Diapers are changed frequently. Fingernails and toenails are trimmed short. Formerly the baby's arms were restrained. Restraints are no longer recommended unless all other methods of control fail.

Different types of medications are used. Systemic antihistaminic drugs may ease itching. Sedation allows the infant to sleep. Erythromycin is useful in combating secondary infection. Bacitracin and neomycin are recommended for local application for the same reason. Various topical creams containing hydrocortisone are used to reduce inflammatory response if infection is not present.

If coal tar preparations are used, care should be taken

not to expose the areas to sunshine, which causes a chemical reaction that in itself is irritating to the skin. Jars containing coal tar preparations should be tightly closed to prevent deterioration. Coal tar ointment should be removed in special baths or with liquid petrolatum before a new application is made.

Medications are applied with clean hands or a finger cot or glove. They are generally used on a small area on a trial basis to test skin reaction. Many of these medications are expensive and should not be wasted.

Sometimes special baths or soaks are prescribed for the infant to remove crusts and reduce pruritus and weeping. Common ingredients added to the bath water are cornstarch, oatmeal preparations (such as Aveeno), or bicarbonate of soda solutions. The water should be tepid, about 95° F (35° C). If possible, a small baby bathtub should be used. Sometimes the skin of the infant is so dry that the physician restricts bathing. In routine bathing a soap substitute is regularly used.

Continual, tepid, wet medicated compresses are sometimes employed to dry weeping crusted lesions. Therapeutic compresses must be *kept wet* to accomplish the aim of the treatment. This type of compress or gauze bandage is not covered by waterproof material but is left exposed to cool the area by evaporation.

Older children may undergo so-called desensitization procedures. Through the injection of small but gradually increasing amounts of allergen, the body is sometimes eventually able to tolerate the substance without untoward reaction.

The course of infantile eczema is usually not steady improvement. The child improves, has a relapse, and improves again. The parents should be told to prepare themselves for a rather long siege of skin difficulty. However, the child over 2 years can usually expect a respite. Unfortunately, as eczema disappears other types of allergy manifestations, such as asthma or hay fever, may develop. The child with eczema is infrequently hospitalized because of the increased exposure to infection (despite precautions), the emotional upset that may occur in the child as a result of the change of environment, and the need for the "maternal figure." However, parental exhaustion and tension may be a factor in obtaining an admission to the pediatric unit of a hospital.

Preschool-age and young school-age child

Impetigo (Fig. 29-4). Impetigo is a skin infection caused by either coagulase-positive staphylococci or group A beta-hemolytic streptococci. It is highly contagious and serious in newborn infants and fairly con-

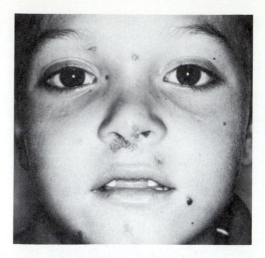

FIG 29-4   Impetigo. *(Courtesy David Allen, MD, San Diego, Calif.)*

tagious but less serious among children and adults. It is often associated with poor hygiene. Inflammation begins with the appearance of reddish spots on the skin, which develop into small blisters that become pus-filled and break, causing thick yellow-red crusts on older children but few crusts on infants. When the crusts are removed, small superficial erosions are seen. The face and hands are most frequently affected, but other areas may become involved. In the hospital, contact precautions are used.

Treatment includes careful cleansing and removal of the crusts, with compresses if necessary, and a small amount of the topical antibiotic, mupirocin ointment 2% (Bactroban) applied to the affected area three times daily until clear. Bactroban is highly effective but expensive. A course of penicillin or erythromycin administered systemically may be recommended because of the demonstrated association of certain strains of group A beta-hemolytic streptococci and nephritis. Also, a more rapid improvement of the lesions is seen when systemic therapy is used. The nurse should be especially cautious in the care of the lesions and disposal of infected material because the infection spreads easily. The child's fingernails should be clipped short. The dermatitis usually responds well to treatment.

Furuncles and carbuncles. Furuncles and carbuncles are deep infections of the hair follicles. They may occur singly or in groups. If the furuncles run together, forming one sore with several draining points, the resulting lesion is called a carbuncle. Carbuncles are uncommon in small children but seen with greater frequency among adolescent boys. A furuncle begins as a single papule associated

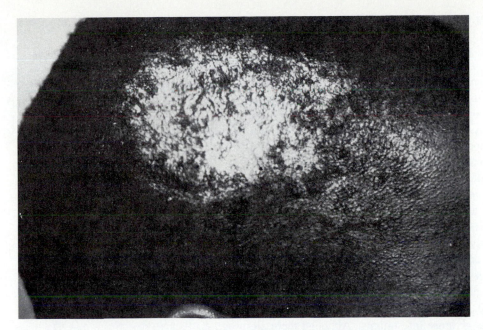

FIG 29-5 Tinea capitis (ringworm of scalp). *(Courtesy W.W. Duemling, MD, San Diego, Calif.)*

with a hair. The papule becomes a pustule, which enlarges and forms a head. Mupirocin ointment 2% (Bactroban) may stop progression of the lesion and preclude the need for systemic antibiotics or incision and drainage by the physician. If multiple furuncles are present, systemic antibiotic therapy will be prescribed.

Sty (hordeolum). A sty, an infection involving an eyelash follicle, usually clears spontaneously or may be incised.

Ringworm of the scalp, skin, and feet (Fig. 29-5). Ringworm of the scalp, or *tinea capitis,* used to be fairly common among school-aged children and is still seen from time to time, particularly in urban areas. It can be caused by several kinds of fungi. Some types of fungi are contracted from human beings, whereas others are contracted from animals. The fungus attacks hairs at their bases, causing them to break off close to the skin and leave circular balding areas. The scalp in the area of the hair loss may become red and scaly. Mild itching may be present. Diagnosis is usually made on the basis of the clinical history, observation with an ultraviolet light called *Wood's lamp,* or a microscopic examination of the affected hairs. Some fungi that commonly cause ringworm of the scalp fluoresce brightly when exposed to the rays of Wood's lamp.

In the past, treatment of ringworm was difficult, and the disease had a tendency to become chronic, usually healing spontaneously at puberty. Treatment included shaving the head. Boys and girls wore little stocking caps in an effort to cover the hair loss and prevent the spread of the disease. X-ray treatment was sometimes prescribed. The oral administration of the antibiotic griseofulvin has been succcessful. The medicine does not kill the fungus but prevents its spread into uninfected cells. As the infected cells are shed or removed, they are replaced by healthy cells. Clipping of the affected hair after a few weeks of treatment is also desirable. In addition, a local antifungal ointment may be ordered.

Ringworm of the skin, *tinea corporis,* may involve various areas, including the face, neck, arms, and hands. Although there are exceptions, the classic lesion of ringworm of the skin is rounded or circular with a gradually extending, small, raised vesicular border and with central healing. The lesion may vary considerably in size, but it is usually about the size of a quarter. Treatment consists of prevention of scratching and application of one of several topical remedies such as Tinactin (tolnaftate 1%), haloprogin (Halotex), Monistat-Derm and clotrimazole (Lotrimin). Local treatment is combined with systemic use of griseofulvin in some cases.

Ringworm of the feet, *tinea pedis,* or so-called athlete's foot, is essentially limited to postpubescent children. Younger children with scaling of the feet usually have some form of eczema. However, it is discussed here with the other types of ringworm. Ringworm of the feet is most often characterized by itching or burning of the feet, blisters, and painful cracks between the toes. At times it may extend to involve other areas and become serious if secondarily infected. It is caused by several kinds of fungi. Treatment consists of the use of griseofulvin or Nizoral. Better ventilation of the feet and the reduction of sweating in the area are helpful. Frequent changing of socks is a necessity. If the infection has been intense and tends to recur, the advisability of discarding shoes worn during the infection should be considered. Anti-fungal preparations such as Desenex or Whitfield's ointment, in addition to those already mentioned, are often used locally but are ineffective unless combined with griseofulvin. The feet should be carefully dried. A prophylactic antifungal dusting powder is often advised for susceptible persons. For the protection of other people, victims should not use public showers or swimming pools.

Pediculosis or louse infestations. Although there are three types of lice—head lice, body lice, and pubic lice—only one type is of significance to children, *pediculosis capitis,* or infestation of the hair of the head by lice. This condition is often seen in neglected children of lower socioeconomic levels. However, children who are well cared for may inadvertently become exposed and contract the infestation, much to their parents' shock.

The parasitic head louse causes itching as it travels on the scalp. Small, grayish, oval eggs called *nits* are laid and attached to the base of the hair shafts with a type of mucilage that is produced by the louse (Fig. 29-6). As the hair grows, the nits become more visable; they resemble tiny flakes of dandruff except that they do not brush out. New lice hatch within 1 week, and the cycle repeats. Pediculosis is often accompanied by excoriation and secondary infection caused by scratching.

Old-style treatment involved the local use of crude oil or kerosene. More acceptable and highly effective is the current use of shampoos of lindane (Kwell) or crotamiton (Eurex). Because of the potential systemic absorption of lindane and potential nervous system toxicity causing seizures if product directions are not observed, some clinicians are prescribing crotamiton for children under 50 pounds. At the end of the treatment, the hair should be combed with a fine-tooth comb to remove the devitalized nits. Warm vinegar solution also aids in the mechanical detachment of nits. The entire family of an affected person should be treated, if possible.

Scabies. Scabies is a superficial infestation by the itch mite *(Acarus scabiei,* or *Sarcoptes scabiei).* The female

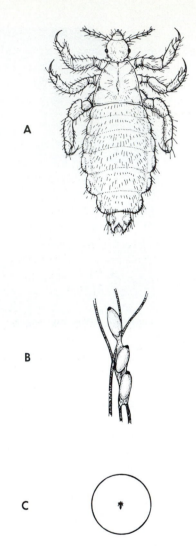

FIG 29-6 A, The female head louse (enlarged). **B,** Enlargement of nits on hair shafts. **C,** Life-sized louse.

mite burrows under the skin, making a tunnel about ½ inch (1.2 cm) long, which is visible as an elevated line from the skin's surface. The insect is so small that it is rarely visible to the naked eye. Scabies usually involves those body areas where the skin is moist and thin— between the fingers and toes, in the axillae, and on the groin and abdominal areas. The itch mite causes itching, as the name indicates. Various treatments are available. Lindane (Kwell) may be applied in cream form to cool, dry skin.

In the past there has been the question regarding the use of Kwell because of neurotoxicity. The new pyrethrin-containing pediculicides and scabicides have a much greater margin of safety and are at least as effective as some of the previously mentioned medicines. Instructions for application and removal should be carefully followed. The entire family of an affected person should receive therapy, if possible.

Adolescent

Acne vulgaris. Vulgar means "common," and acne vulgaris is a skin inflammation that is exceedingly common among teenage boys and girls. It may exist in a very mild form, or it may be extremely severe. There are probably several causes that, appearing together, produce the problem. Acne first appears, almost without exception, at the time of puberty. Hormone levels in the body are believed to play a role. Many times the parents of the affected child also experienced similar difficulty; therefore hereditary factors are not discounted.

The production of sebum, or fatty secretion of the oil glands, is stimulated by certain hormones during adolescence, and several types of skin microorganisms utilize sebum as a food source and change it into irritating fatty acids that cause acne. The pores clog, and blackheads (plugs of keratin, sebum, and microorganisms, also called *comedones,* the primary lesions of acne) form. The pores may also be clogged with dirt; however, blackheads are not commonly caused by dirt particles but by oxidation of the top of the plug, a process that may occur no matter how carefully the adolescent washes. Plugging of the oil ducts may lead to papules, pustules, and, at times, cyst formation and permanent scarring.

Since acne most often occurs on the face, shoulders, and back, it is of great cosmetic and psychologic concern. The teenager should be given professional help during this distressing period so that the interval is as short and free from complications as possible. Acne fosters a sense of inferiority and social insecurity at an already difficult period in life.

Treatment includes a review of general health habits. Little emphasis is placed on avoidance of carbohydrates and fatty foods, such as chocolate, nuts, and peanut butter, but a well-balanced diet is stressed. Lack of sleep, nervous tension, and menstrual problems may lead to a flare-up. Mild cases are treated with topical measures such as antibacterial detergent soaps or skin cleansers (Fostex or Acne-Aid) and lotions containing *keratolytic* compounds (salicylic acid, resorcin) or other agents (Benzoyl Peroxide, tretinoin [Retin-A]). Girls are advised to avoid oily makeup and moisturizers, but numerous tinted antibacterial creams or lotions are available

that help heal and mask the lesions—a very important pyschologic consideration. Frequent shampooing is often helpful. Patients should be instructed not to press or scratch the lesions, because this may break down tissue walls and spread infection. However, despite this advice, most patients find it extremely difficult not to tamper with the lesions they see in the mirror. The physician may remove comedones in the office with a special extractor or give careful instructions to the patient's family regarding the removal of comedones. The treatment of choice in advanced cases includes either tetracycline or erythromycin to kill the bacteria. Minocycline hydrochloride (Minocin) or isotretenoin (Accutane) may be necessary if these measures fail. (See teratogenic factors, p. 77.)

Usually acne is self-limiting and subsides in 3 or 4 years. However, severe cases may persist into middle age. The partial removal of scarred tissue may be accomplished, in selected cases, by superficial abrasion, a technique called *dermabrasion*. X-ray treatment is no longer recommended by dermatologists because of the possibility of causing skin changes later in life and the availability of other therapeutic alternatives.

Herpes simplex (type 1). Herpes simplex type 1, a viral infection, usually causes an irregular vesicular lesion on the margin of the lip (fever blister) or gums. The blister breaks, and a crust develops and eventually clears. These lesions have a tendency to recur in the same area, causing considerable annoyance, discomfort, and cosmetic concern. Occasionally herpes simplex takes on a more important aspect. It is serious when a newborn infant or very young child is involved because the lesions have a tendency to multiply, and when the eye is involved impairment of vision may result. Acyclovir, a recently developed antiviral agent, is vital to the management of severe herpes simplex (see p. 174).

Dermatitis venenata. Dermatitis venenata may be seen at any age; it is an inflammatory skin response to external contact with some irritating substance such as fibers, plants, synthetics, or adhesive tape. However, it is most often observed in those groups who hike in the midst of poison oak or poison ivy. Signs of skin irritation usually occur several hours after exposure and consist of redness, swelling, and small blisters at the point of contact. Itching is intense. If patients know that they have been exposed, the best immediate treatment before the appearance of symptoms is washing the area well. The best course of action is an initial proper identification of the offending plants and a prudent detour. After the blisters have developed, the urge to scratch must be resisted to prevent spreading. Calamine lotion and cortisone preparations applied locally may help relieve itching.

BURNS

Another problem, which primarily involves the skin but may finally affect many organs and processes of the body, is burns. Burns may be caused by exposure to hot liquids, strong chemicals, direct flame, radiation, sunlight, or electric current. Toddlers and young children are most often scalded by hot coffee, grease from frying pans, or hot water from unguarded bathroom faucets. Older children are frequently burned when their clothes catch fire while they are playing with matches, using kerosene, or standing too close to household heaters. In the United States approximately 500 children are hospitalized each day because of burns, and about 1,500 die each year from burns.

Classification

Burns are classified into four categories, depending on the depth of penetration of the body's surface.

A *first-degree* (partial-thickness) burn involves only the epidermis. It is very superficial; a tender, slightly swollen redness results. A common illustration of a first-degree burn is the typical summer sunburn. A *second-degree* (partial-thickness) burn involves the epidermis and dermis. This category is further divided into superficial and deep dermal burns. Some epidermal appendages must be intact for these burns to heal spontaneously. Deep dermal burns may change from partial-thickness to full-thickness wounds by infection, trauma, or obliteration of the blood supply to the affected part. A second-degree burn is characterized by blister formation or a reddened, discolored region with a moist, weeping surface. A *third-degree* (full-thickness) burn involves the entire dermis and portions of the subcutaneous tissue. The region affected has a brown, leathery appearance with little surface moisture. A *fourth-degree* (full-thickness) burn involves subcutaneous tissue, fascia, muscle, and perhaps bone. The tissue appears blackened and contracted. Partial-thickness burns can heal without grafting. Full-thickness burns must be grafted for healing to occur. Evaluation of the depth of a burn is not always easy immediately after the injury.

It is not only the degree of burn that is significant but also the amount of body surface affected. A person can usually survive a rather extensive superficial burn but may tolerate a deep burn only if a small area is involved. In evaluating the extent of a burn on an adult, the so-called rule of nines can be applied; it gives a certain percentage value to each part of the body—a percentage that is almost always nine or a multiple of nine. This method of calculation, unless modified, is not helpful when working with children because of the relatively

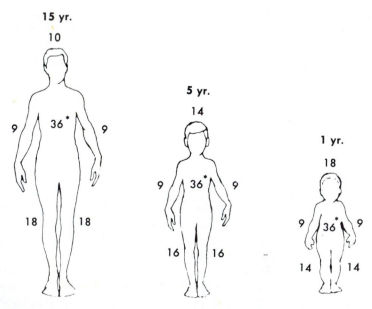

FIG 29-7 Modification of "rule of nines." (*Courtesy Burns Institute, Galveston Unit, Shriners Hospital for Crippled Children, Galveston, Texas.*)

large size of a baby's or a young child's head and the reduced length of the legs. (One example of modification based on size differences is illustrated in Fig. 29-7.)

The area, extent, and depth of a burn determine its severity, and treatment is planned according to severity. *Minor burns* are described as partial-thickness first- or second-degree burns covering less than 15% of the body surface and not involving strategic areas such as the face, hands, feet, or genitalia. Minor burns are treated on an outpatient basis. *Moderate burns* are described as partial-thickness second-degree burns covering over 15% but less than 30% of body surface or as full-thickness burns involving less than 10% of body surface. Moderate burns usually require hospitalization. *Major burns* are described as partial-thickness second-degree burns covering at least 30% of the body surface or as full-thickness third-degree burns involving more than 10% of the body surface. Most burns—either partial- or full-thickness—that involve a large part of the face, hands, feet, or genitalia are considered major burns. Children with major burns always require hospitalization, and children with critical burns are transferred to a major burn center if possible.

Therapeutic management and nursing responsibility

Initial considerations. Any person who is at the scene when someone is burned should first extinguish the fire if the victim's clothes are aflame. If an abundant source of water from a hose or bucket is readily available, it should be used; if not, handy blankets or throw rugs may be employed to smother the flames, since fire cannot continue in the absence of oxygen. If neither water nor blankets are available, the victim should be rolled on the ground or floor to smother the flames. When the fire has been extinguished, the burned area should be rinsed with cold water. The victim should be taken immediately to a physician's office, or, preferably, a hospital for evaluation and care. The victim should be transported wrapped in a clean sheet and blanket. No time should be expended on trying to remove the child's clothes unless they are smoldering. No medication of any type should be administered.

When a burned child is admitted to an emergency room or other hospital receiving area, the child's clothes should be removed gently, cutting along the seams of the garments if necessary. The child should be placed on and covered by sterile sheets in a room with good lighting. All those in attendance should wear face masks and should be provided with sterile gowns and gloves. The severity of the burns is estimated by the attending physician, and the need for hospitalization is determined.

Minor burns. The technique of immediately immersing the area briefly in cold water or holding an ice cube on the injured surface to reduce pain and edema has become popular. Care of minor burns usually consists of cleansing the area with mild soap and water, Iodophor soaps are currently used for their antibacterial effect. The area may be covered with a fine-mesh gauze, lightly lubricated with water-soluble antimicrobial cream (for example, nitrofurazone, neomycin, or bacitracin) and wrapped with a bulky, protective dressing. Depending on the condition of the dressing, the condition of the patient, and the physician's preference, this dressing may be left in place for 4 or 5 days. The child's tetanus immunization should be validated and, if not documented as up to date, should be given. Acetaminophen (Tylenol) may be prescribed for pain, and the patient should return to be seen by the physician in 48 hours.

Moderate or major burns. The first phase of therapy when moderate or major burns are present includes maintenance of an airway and prevention of shock. The airway is not a problem in all cases, but occasionally, because of the location of the external burn, the inhalation of fumes, or internal burning of the respiratory tract, it is of great importance. Blood gas analysis is mandatory, and a complete blood count, electrolyte determination, and blood typing provide a baseline that is vital for evaluating the child's state of health on admission. An endotracheal tube may be needed. Humidified oxygen should be administered and the airway suctioned as necessary.

A nasogastric tube (double-lumen sump) may be inserted to prevent tachypnea, associated with acute gastric dilatation and vomiting. Paralytic ileus, a complication associated with circulatory problems in small children, may also be prevented by nasogastric drainage.

Intravenous fluid therapy is the most important aspect of the early care of the burn patient. Loss of plasma into the burn area and evaporation of water from the burn results in a rapid decrease in plasma volume, a concentration of red blood cells, and ultimately an increase in hematocrit. Fluid replacement must be initiated immediately and continued at a high rate for about 24 hours, after which a plasma shift occurs. Fluid that has leaked into the burn area returns to the vascular area. In young children a peripheral cutdown is performed, or a central venous line is inserted.

An indwelling urinary catheter is usually also necessary. The amount and type of urine formation is observed and recorded hourly to determine the rate of intravenous therapy and to provide an index of the patient's general condition. An initial specimen should be sent to the laboratory for a baseline urinalysis and specific gravity and electrolyte studies. A dwindling urinary output may serve as a warning of developing hypovolemia and possible circulatory collapse. A urinary output of 1.0 to 2.0 ml/kg/hr for a child is desirable (approximately 10 to 30 ml/hr). Signs of overhydration revealed by excessive output require a reduction in fluids given intravenously. Electrolyte, specific gravity, and BUN/creatinine levels are followed regularly and frequently. It is extremely important to report irregularities in the urinary output, loss of a urine specimen, or an error in the measurement of a urine specimen because of the danger of miscalculating the rate and amount of intravenous fluids needed.

Overloading the circulatory system is a real possibility unless great care is exercised. The patient is weighed to provide a baseline for subsequent weight loss or gain. Vital signs are checked frequently, although meaningful blood pressure readings may be difficult to secure because of the age of the child and the location of the burn area. Some children need central venous pressure determinations.

Hospitalized children with serious burns are sometimes treated with low doses of parenteral penicillin to prevent infection by the staphylococci and streptococci present on the skin. Although prophylactic antibiotics are controversial, they are given as indicated by the patient's clinical course and specific cultures of the wound. Pain medication is administered intravenously to control shock. The child should be made comfortable but should not be oversedated. More pain accompanies a partial-thickness burn than a full-thickness burn, because in the partial-thickness burn, some nerve endings are still intact. The shock phase of the body's response to extensive burns usually lasts from 48 to 72 hours. Many hospitals routinely isolate their burn patients in an effort to prevent or reduce infection.

After 48 hours, the initial ileus that may be seen with major burns has passed, and either oral or nasogastric feedings should be initiated. Hypermetabolism is seen in all patients with extensive burns and continues until the wound is covered. Calorie and protein intake must be increased to facilitate wound epithelialization and graft acceptance. Increased nutritional requirements often necessitate tube feedings to supplement oral feedings. An antacid is given either orally or through the tube to prevent Curling's ulcer, which is a stress ulcer associated with serious burns. Frequent milk feedings, which chil-

dren usually take well, provide greatly needed calories and fluid. Children usually require about 80 calories per kg of body weight and 3 g of protein per kg of body weight daily. Adequate nutrition maintains basal weight and enhances wound healing, helping to prevent infection.

The vocational nurse should not be assigned the total bedside responsibility of a severely burned child during this critical period, although she may skillfully assist the registered nurse in important aspects of the care. The vocational nurse must understand the principles of the patient's treatment, and as the patient's condition becomes more stable, she aids more fully in the patient's care.

Wound care

After the patient is initially stabilized, the burn wound is treated. Hair adjacent to the burn wound should be shaved carefully and the burned area cleansed with water and small amounts of iodophor soap or saline solution. Cleansing is preferably performed in a hydrotherapy tub. At the time of admission the loose skin and blisters of partial-thickness burns are surgically removed by the physician in a procedure called *debridement*. Gradually a thick black crust (eschar), composed of the drying wound secretions and nonviable tissue, forms. An escharotomy may be necessary to relieve compression from circumferential burns. For the little girl in Fig. 29-8, an incision through the eschar was required to release pressure and to permit adequate respirations.

A modified exposure treatment is used for the immediate care of moderate and major burns. Partial-thickness burns are prepared for spontaneous healing by covering the area with fine-mesh gauze that is impregnated with antibacterial ointment or cream. The gauze is held in place by elastic netting or a Surgifix dressing. A sterile blanket may be applied to prevent chilling, and burned extremities should be elevated to minimize accumulation of edema.

The surface of the burn wound must be kept clean by vigorous daily cleansing in the form of povidone-iodine (Betadine) tub baths, whirlpool treatment, or local soaks. All dressing materials should be ready to reapply in a sterile manner after the soak. Soaking in the hydrotherapy tub facilitates removal of loose, sloughing tissue, exudate, and the topical medication.

Days later, as the eschar begins to separate, the physician cuts away portions of the dried crust, revealing new granulation tissue. When the granulation tissue is

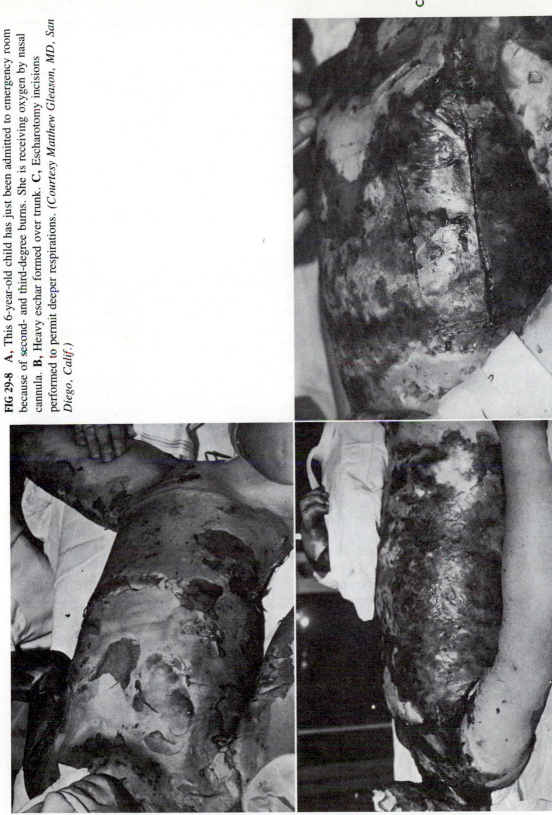

FIG 29-8 A, This 6-year-old child has just been admitted to emergency room because of second- and third-degree burns. She is receiving oxygen by nasal cannula. B, Heavy eschar formed over trunk. C, Escharotomy incisions performed to permit deeper respirations. (*Courtesy Matthew Gleason, MD, San Diego, Calif.*)

exposed (by removal of the eschar), antibiotic gauze is usually laid over the open granulation areas. Through soaks and redressings or intermittent surgical debridements, the burned areas are cleaned and the developing granulation tissue is prepared for elective grafting, which saves time and gives a better end result. Granulation tissue is a deep-pink, fragile tissue that bleeds easily. When the tissue is sufficiently prepared, the child undergoes grafting. Donor sites are selected on the patient's body. The donor site is usually covered with fine gauze and a pressure dressing. Later, when bleeding has been controlled, the outer pressure dressing may be removed. Donor sites heal in about 2 weeks. The newly grafted area is kept covered. The dressing should be observed for amount and type of drainage and odor. Exposed adjacent areas are observed for edema and circulatory problems. Grafts are usually firmly attached by the 12th day after the grafting procedure.

Full-thickness major burn wounds are currently being treated soon after admission by primary (tangential) excision. In the operating room under hypotensive anesthesia, which minimizes bleeding, devitalized burned tissue is cut down to the live tissue, and skin grafts are immediately applied. The primary objective of wound care is to reduce the size of the wound as rapidly as possible, thereby increasing the patient's chance for survival. When the wound is reduced to less than 20% of the body surface area, the chance for survival approaches 100%. Full-thickness major burns are, preferably, covered with the patient's own skin. These *autografts* from undamaged parts of the patient's own body provide permanent coverage (see box at right). Unfortunately, often too little skin remains, and homografts, heterografts, and synthetic grafts are used as temporary surface coverings. Donations from other persons (other than an identical twin) may "take" temporarily but are later rejected. These biologic dressings are used to cover the wound and prevent infection in preparation for skin autografts.

Immediate coverage of the burn wound with grafts or medication following debridement or primary excision is very important to the child's recovery. Such treatment should forestall pain, fluid loss, and infection and provide the best environment for wound healing.

After surgery the child is placed in protective isolation. Twenty-four-hour personalized nursing care is essential, with particular attention given to respiratory therapy, nutrition, the newly grafted area, and prevention of complications. The use of biologic dressings in the treatment of deep dermal and full-thickness burns has revo-

lutionized the treatment and rehabilitation of burn patients.

Topical medications. Because systemic antibiotics cannot reach the damaged area because of thrombosed or burned vessels, topical medication is an essential method of therapy. A thin layer of medication may be applied directly to the injured area with a sterile glove or tongue blade, or the medication may be embedded in sterile gauze strips that are positioned as needed. A spray form may also be available (Table 29-1).

Mortality caused by infection has declined as a result of the effectiveness of new and improved topical antimicrobial agents. The most desirable topical agent should be inexpensive, painless, nonallergenic, easy to apply, and effective against all microbial contaminants. It should also penetrate the wound without causing systemic effects or harm to viable tissue. Unfortunately, although several topical agents have led to excellent results, no single agent offers all these characteristics.

Mafenide hydrochloride (sulfamylon cream), povidone-iodine (Betadine) ointment, and silver sulfadiazine cream are useful for exposure treatment, combined with frequent hydrotherapy and reapplication of the agent.

Continuing concerns. No matter which burn therapy methods are selected, all treatment is intended to accomplish the following aims:

1. Preserve life
2. Promote healing
3. Prevent infection
4. Prevent deformity
5. Provide emotional and physical rehabilitation

Types of skin grafts

Permanent

Isografts (autografts)	Undamaged tissue from the patient's own skin (may also be from patient's identical twin)

Temporary

Allografts (homografts)	Tissue taken from a member or cadaver of the same species
Xenografts (heterografts)	Tissue taken from another species, for example, pigskin (porcine xenograft)
Synthetic grafts (Epigard)	Man-made grafts

Table 29-1   Comparison of three common topical antimicrobials

Agent	Cost	Advantages	Disadvantages
Mafenide cream 10% (Sulfamylon)	Least expensive	Penetrates eschar Easy application Effective against all gram-positive and gram-negative organisms	Tendency to cake; should be removed by tub bathing Burning pain on application May cause metabolic acidosis Requires a minimum of two applications daily Patient may develop sensitivity rash
Povidone-iodine (Betadine) ointment 10%; also available in foam preparation (Helafoam)	More expensive	Very wide spectrum Effective against gram-positive and gram-negative organisms, fungi, yeasts, protozoa, and viruses Sensitivity is infrequent	Ointment becomes liquid and runs off surface, staining linen Mild burning on application Foam dries out rapidly to a thick powder Inactivated by wound exudate
Silver sulfadiazine cream 1% (Silvadene)	Most expensive	Painless Effective against gram-positive and gram-negative organisms and *Candida albicans* Sensitivity is infrequent No discoloration	Poor penetration Supplemental systemic therapy usually needed

Maintaining good nutrition is essential for the survival and satisfactory healing of extensively burned children. An important aspect of the nurse's responsibility is the provision of a good nutritional intake. Initially the child with extensive burns is probably maintained on tube feedings, but fairly soon the patient may be fed orally with or without a nasogastric tube, depending on the child's progress. It is very important for the nurse to keep an accurate record of all nourishment and fluids taken. Many physicians request that a detailed daily intake record be kept for analysis by the dietitian for caloric and foodstuff (protein, fat, carbohydrate, vitamin, and mineral) content. Protein consumption is particularly important. Usually supplemental vitamins and iron are ordered. Vitamin C and zinc are substances believed to be particularly helpful in aiding tissue healing.

Frequent milk feedings and the prophylactic administration of antacids may prevent a Curling's ulcer, but the nurses should be alert for any signs of blood in the stool or nasogastric tube. The child's appetite should not be discouraged with servings that are too large. Feedings should be judiciously planned. The patient should not be expected to eat directly after an exhausting dressing change. A different schedule for the kitchen on some days or better planning of procedures on other days may be necessary, but patients should receive their meals when they can *best* eat. Likes and dislikes should be noted. The foods selected should be high in calories and protein. Sometimes permission to bring food from home brings forth happy cooperation by both parents and patients. Children must be weighed periodically to determine their nutritional status.

The immediate and long-term positioning of a seriously burned patient is critical in preventing extensive deformity. Although the position of flexion may be the position of greatest comfort to the patient, it also may become the cause of crippling contractures. The posture of extension may at first appear "heartless," but in the final analysis such placement of the head and extremities may save the patient weeks, if not months, of needless hospitalization and additional pain. The neck splint pictured in Fig. 29-9, *A* is made of a type of plastic, "Orthoplast" Isoprene, which, when molded and fitted to the individual patient, has been successful in preventing deformities that had previously been difficult to prevent (Fig. 29-9, *B*).

Active and passive exercises of the affected body parts, if neglected when ordered, may retard convalescence significantly. It is the responsibility of the nurse (and the physical therapy staff) to see that these important movements, which the patient often resists, are carried out. Appropriate exercises plus good positioning to prevent flexion contractures can contribute greatly to the early rehabilitation of the patient.

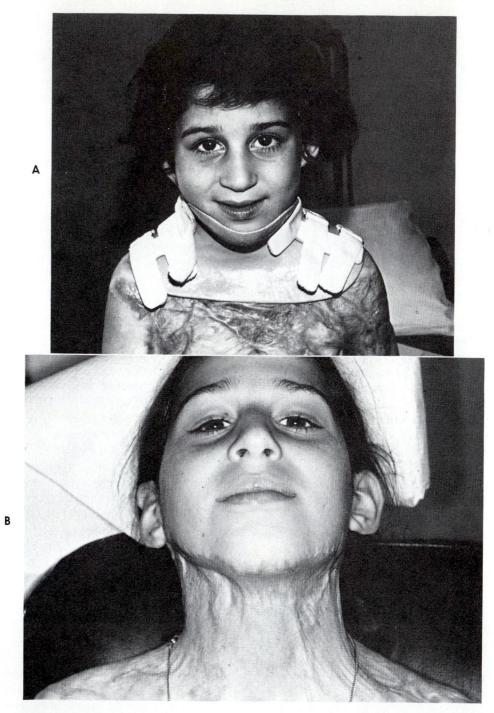

FIG 29-9   A, Same patient as in Fig. 29-8; splint to prevent neck contractures. **B,** Same child 5 years later; Treatment included skin grafting and splinting. *(Courtesy Matthew Gleason, MD, San Diego, Calif.)*

During the entire period of treatment and observation of the extensively burned patient, the morale of the parents and their child is of tremendous importance. Often the parents feel guilty concerning their child's accident. They may be appalled at the condition and appearance of the child. Some will be overly protective; others may hardly be able to make themselves approach the child. All will be extremely upset, whether they appear so or not. Children may feel extreme guilt if they consider themselves responsible for the injury. Children who have extensive burns characteristically regress in their behavior. Frequent and consistent parental visits are extremely important. Some children who have had a history of emotional disturbance before their accident develop extreme hostility toward their parents and others involved in their care.

Good communication among the physician, the nursing staff, the parents, and the burned patient is essential. Parents need to be informed of the child's progress and helped in their efforts to cope with their feelings while providing support to the child. A feeling of acceptance and freedom to talk without being criticized are important for both the child and his parents. Simple explanations of treatments take time at the beginning, but they save much time and anguish later on.

Play therapy, availability of toys and television, and an empathetic approach to painful procedures are all helpful. Often additional specialized assistance is required to meet the needs of the patient and family. The social worker, psychologist, or psychiatrist should be called upon to help maintain a healthy support system whenever necessary.

Rehabilitation. The rehabilitation of a burned child may be long and exhausting, but despite the pain and fatigue, the end result is worth the continued effort. Fortunately, with the greater availability of specialized burn care units or centers and the use of new surgical techniques, the time needed for rehabilitation promises to be much shorter. Splinting, traction, and frequent visits to the physical therapy department's pool or exercise room may be necessary. Plastic surgery is needed in some cases to relieve contractures or remove keloid formation (exaggerated scar tissue). Special tutoring may be required to prevent educational loss, and social contacts must be maintained, particularly for older children. A positive, constructive attitude toward therapy should be encouraged.

Patients who have been seriously burned are among the nurse's most challenging and difficult responsibilities. They are also among her most rewarding.

Key Concepts

1. Skin color, hydration, surface irregularities, and disturbances in sensation may reveal significant information about a person's health habits and status.

2. The description of a skin lesion should include the following information: size, elevation, quality, color, distribution, associated sensory disturbances, and type of any existent drainage or exudate.

3. Common skin problems in infants and toddlers include miliaria rubra, intertrigo, seborrheic dermatitis, diaper rash, and infantile eczema.

4. Infantile eczema is considered to be essentially an allergic response. Care should include identifying the allergens, eliminating them from the infant's environment, treating secondary infections, preventing scratching and exposure to known infections, treating the lesions, and providing psychologically supportive care to the parents.

5. Common skin problems in preschool- and young school-age children include impetigo, furuncles and carbuncles, sty, ringworm, pediculosis, and scabies.

6. Impetigo is a skin infection often associated with poor hygiene. Treatment includes careful cleansing, removal of crusts, and application of topical antibiotic ointment. Systemic antibiotics result in more rapid improvement of lesions.

7. Ringworm may be found in the scalp *(tinea capitas),* skin *(tinea corporis),* or feet *(tinea pedis).*

8. Treatment of head lice includes shampoos of lindane or crotamitron and manual removal of devitalized nits with a fine-tooth comb.

9. Common skin problems in adolescents include acne vulgaris, herpes simplex type 1, and dermatitis venenata.

10. Acne first appears at puberty, is usually self-limiting, and subsides in 3 to 4 years. Treatment includes ensuring a well-balanced diet and adequate rest, thorough cleansing, application of medicated lotions, and antibiotic therapy.

11. Burns are classified into four categories, depending on the depth of penetration of the body's surface: first-degree, second-degree, third-degree, and

fourth-degree. The area, extent, and depth of a burn determine its severity and treatment.

12. Initial burn therapy includes the following: maintenance of an airway, prevention of shock, replacement of fluids, insertion of a nasogastric tube, monitoring vital signs and laboratory values, controlling pain, and providing adequate nutrition.

13. Care of a burn wound includes cleansing, debridement, and application of dressings and topical medications. Treatment may also include skin grafts.

14. The goals of burn therapy are to preserve life, promote healing, prevent infection, prevent deformity, and provide emotional and physical rehabilitation.

15. Rehabilitation of a burned child may include splinting, traction, physical therapy, plastic surgery, and special tutoring.

Discussion Questions

1. Which skin problems would you expect to see in infants and toddlers? Develop a chart that lists the problem, its etiology, and the nursing care involved. Which skin problems are seen most often in preschool- and early school-age children? Expand the chart as described above.

2. Why are preschool- and young school-age children at increased risk for skin diseases of a contagious nature? What are the implications for the nurse working in a school setting?

3. Why is a condition like acne vulgaris a major problem and concern in adolescence? What can the nurse do to help an adolescent troubled by this or other skin conditions?

4. Identify the major causes of burns in the various age groups. How can the nurse help in the prevention of burns? How are the extent and severity of burns measured? What are the recommended methods for assisting a person whose clothes are on fire?

5. How does medical and nursing treatment differ in relation to minor and major burns? What nursing measures, both physiologic and psychosocial, are most significant in the treatment of burn victims?

30

Infection Precautions and Childhood Communicable Diseases

CHAPTER OBJECTIVES

After studying this chapter, the student should be able to perform the following:

1 Define the terms listed in the key vocabulary.

2 Describe the so-called chain of infection.

3 Explain how to break the chain of infection, listing six methods that could be used.

4 State how gowns, gloves, and masks can be used effectively as barriers during nursing care.

5 Contrast the three systems of isolation precautions recommended by the CDC: category-specific and disease specific, or "design your own."

6 Describe the CDC's "universal precautions" to reduce the risks of transmission of blood-borne infectious agents.

7 Describe and demonstrate how a nurse properly washes her hands.

8 Discuss how the nurse can reduce the anxiety level of the isolated child and his family.

9 Using the headings provided in Table 30-1, describe the following childhood contagious diseases: chickenpox (varicella); 2-week measles (rubeola); German measles (rubella); infectious parotitis (mumps); and whooping cough (pertussis).

10 Indicate three infectious agents mentioned in Table 30-1 for which, as of yet, there is no active immunization.

Infection precautions in the hospital are necessary for the safety of patients, visitors, students, and staff. The rationale for using certain barriers or techniques should be based on knowledge of how a contagious disease is transmitted, the chain of infection (Fig. 30-1). If the chain is broken, no new incidence of disease develops as a result of an infectious person's presence. Breaking the chain of infection is a critical responsibility for all health personnel.

It is also important that barrier techniques be as physically and psychosocially nontraumatizing as possible for all concerned. The pediatric patient particularly, depending on his stage of development, is already undergoing considerable stress. The burden of hospitalization and isolation techniques is particularly heavy for small children and their families.

With greater knowledge of the transmission modes of most infectious diseases and of methods for stopping

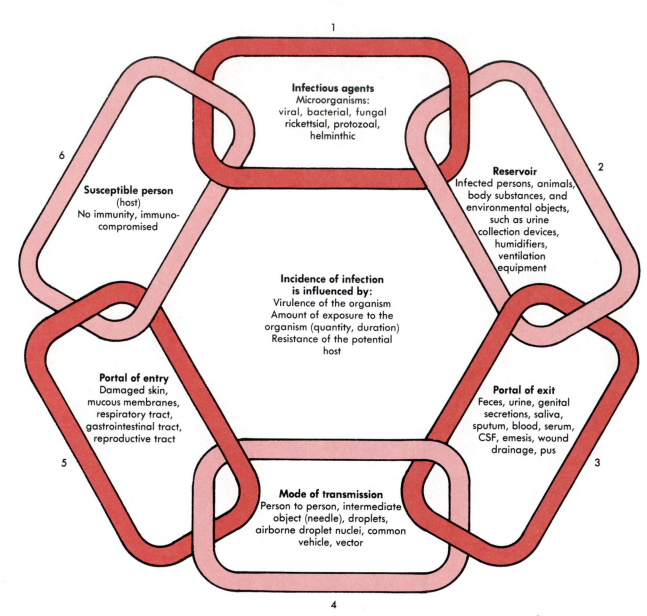

FIG 30-1 How to break links in chain of infection. *Link 1.* Microorganisms—wash hands; use disinfectants, antiseptics, sterilization, and antimicrobial medications. *Link 2.* Reservoir—identify, isolate, and control or eliminate reservoirs. *Link 3.* Portal of exit—control exit; consider all body substances potentially infectious; wash hands and wear gloves. *Link 4.* Mode of transmission—wash hands; wear gloves when handling body substances; control ventilation, sterilization, and disinfection procedures; use sterile technique. *Link 5.* Susceptible person—maintain intact skin and mucous membranes; keep hands away from nose and mouth; wash hands. *Link 6.* Portal of entry—strengthen natural body defenses (nutrition, rest, exercise, good hygiene); if possible, participate in immunization programs.

contagion, many old concepts involving communicable disease control are changing. As this knowledge influences the activities and attitudes of health care personnel, it benefits the nursing care of all patients. Currently, numerous hospital policies and procedures are undergoing such transition.

In many ways the newer recommended guidelines are less rigid, encouraging nurses to use independent judgment. Certainly guidelines are less ritualistic, as well as more logical and encompassing. Change simply for its own sake should not be endorsed; however, it would be unwise to fail to change when sound study and research indicate that certain patterns of care are unsafe, are wasteful of financial resources or personal energies, or cause needless patient distress.

In this regard the growing role of the infection control practitioner (ICP) in the hospital setting is especially welcome. This professional (usually a nurse with specialized training and certification) keeps records of infection rates; she proposes investigations to determine reasons for difficulty in patient care practices associated with infection risk; and she initiates examinations of appropriate interventions to reduce those risks. The ICP helps interpret and prepare protocols for many hospital practices, including infection precautions, and is a valuable consultant and educational resource for practicing nurses.

KEY VOCABULARY

During clinical assignments the student encounters certain terminology associated with infection risk or isolation precautions that may need to be reviewed. The following key vocabulary and brief discussions are designed to help in that review.

body substances A general term used to describe body products that are characteristically moist and that support the growth of organisms. Examples are feces, urine, emesis, wound drainage, pus, saliva, sputum, genital secretions, blood, serum, and cerebral spinal fluid.

carrier A person or animal capable of transmitting a disease without having any signs or symptoms of the disease.

colonization The presence and multiplication of organisms in body substances or on the body that do not cause tissue invasion or damage.

contagious (communicable or transmissible) disease Illness caused by living microorganisms or their toxins, which may be transmitted to susceptible persons by contact with persons carrying the organisms, their infected body substances, or other reservoirs. Transmission may occur by direct, indirect, or droplet contact or by airborne route.

I. Contact transmission
  A. Direct (person to person)
  B. Indirect (requires intermediate object, such as hands of nurse or needle, as in needlestick injuries)
  C. Droplet (Droplets usually do not travel more than 3 feet; droplets rapidly settle on horizontal surfaces.)
II. Airborne transmission (from residue of evaporated droplets [droplet nuclei] that can remain suspended in air for long periods or from dust particles in the air that contain infectious agents. Pulmonary tuberculosis is a major disease transmitted by droplet nuclei.)
III. Common vehicle transmission (such as contaminated potato salad at a picnic)
IV. Vector-borne transmission (such as mosquito-transmitted malaria)

contamination The presence of disease-producing agents on a person or in or on inanimate objects (for instance, clothing, water, food, or medical supplies).

epidemiology The study of the occurrence, distribution, and causes of disease and other conditions.

hyperimmune globulin Human immune globulin that contains a high titer of antibodies designed to prevent or lessen the impact of specific contagious disease (such as rubeola or hepatitus B).

immunity The ability to protect oneself against development of a contagious disease by the action of antibodies. Immunity may be active or passive.

I. Active immunity is relatively long-lasting but takes longer to achieve than does passive immunity. It is attained when a person's own body produces protective antibodies in response to exposure to an infective organism or its toxin. This occurs under the following conditions:
  A. By having had the disease
  B. By receiving specially prepared materials (toxins or vaccines) that stimulate the immune system to produce antibodies
  In these instances, the body *actively* protects itself.
II. Passive immunity is comparatively short-lived but may be achieved relatively quickly. It is attained under the following conditions:
  A. By receiving a prepared injection of antibodies (antitoxin), which are manufactured in the body of another person or, rarely, by an animal
  B. By an unborn baby receiving antibodies from his mother across the placenta
  C. By a nursing baby receiving antibodies from his mother's breast milk
  In these instances, the body *passively* receives the protection

incubation period Time that must elapse between the infection of a person at a time of exposure and the appearance of signs or symptoms of the disease. The incubation periods of most infectious diseases have two phases: (1) the period between exposure and communicability and (2) the period of communicability before the appearance of clinical signs and symptoms. This second phase is often called the prodrome of the infection, and during this phase the patient is usually most infectious to others. This phenomenon explains why childhood diseases such as chickenpox spread so efficiently— the infected person passes the infection to others during his prodromal period. By the time he becomes ill, others are already infected.

infection The presence and multiplication in the body of microorganisms that cause tissue invasion and damage. Mild or low-grade infections are not always recognized.

infectious diseases Those illnesses caused by microorganisms. (Any microorganism has the potential for producing disease, but many are prevented from causing illness by the person's own body defenses: the health condition of the body tissues may stop the entry or significant multiplication of an organism, or the activity of the immune system may form protective antibodies.)

isolation precautions Observance of barrier techniques that are designed to interrupt transmission of infectious agents from a reservoir (usually an infected patient) to a susceptible host (either the caregiver or another patient). Which barriers are employed depends on the portal of exit, modes of transmission, and portal of entry characteristic of the infection. Hand washing is always used, but gloves, gowns, masks, goggles, or special room assignments may also be used.

nosocomial infection (NI) An infection associated with hospitalization. Over half of these infections are not considered to be preventable because of the poor condition of the patient's body defenses. As a result, usually benign microorganisms normally resident in a patient's body may become pathogenic. Potentially preventable NIs are usually associated with invasive devices or procedures, many of which are performed by nurses (for example, IV placement and maintenance, urinary catheterization, wound care).

portal of entry The way in which microorganisms gain entrance into a person's body (for example, broken skin or mucous membranes in the nose, mouth, and urethra).

portal of exit The way in which microorganisms leave the body (for example, feces, emesis, urine, semen, water, blood).

reservoir of infection Place where microorganisms live and multiply (for example, in people, animals, plants, soils).

toxoid A preparation containing a toxin or poison produced by a pathogenic organism capable of providing active immunity against a disease but too weak to cause the disease itself.

vaccine A preparation containing killed or weakened (attenuated) living organisms that, when introduced into the body, causes the formation of antibodies against that type of organism.

ISOLATION PRECAUTIONS: BACKGROUND

In 1983, the Centers for Disease Control (CDC) published *Guideline for Isolation Precautions in Hospitals.** This booklet (along with additional recommendations for the prevention of transmission of blood-borne diseases issued in 1987/1988) is the current official governmental guide for shaping infectious disease control in hospitals in the United States.

To help meet the needs of many kinds of health care providers, the CDC offered the possibility of choosing one of three alternative isolation systems. The first is based on a modification of the previously used *category-specific isolation precautions*, which are primarily influenced by the mode and ease of transmission of an illness. The second is a system that describes *disease-specific isolation precautions*. Institutions were invited to study and select one of the two systems described or choose the third alternative by designing their own system for consistent use within their own setting.

The isolation system based on categorization of diseases is more likely to overisolate and to use supplies unnecessarily. However, it is thought to be easier to administer and to teach personnel and may be more practical when a possible infectious patient is not yet diagnosed. The disease-specific system requires more understanding of each illness and calls for increased judgmental skill but allows more individualized care and saves on supplies.

The possibilities presented by the third alternative have stimulated a thoughtful, fundamental critique of the problems associated with diagnosis-driven isolation practices as described in the first two systems and an emphasis on the danger of unidentified, undiagnosed infectious contacts. Indeed, it is the unknown contagious person who is potentially the most dangerous to his caregivers and other patients.†

---

*Garner JS and Simmons BP: CDC guideline for isolation precautions in hospitals, 1983, US Department of Health and Human Services, Centers for Disease Control, Center for Infectious Disease, Hospital Infections Program, Atlanta, Ga.
†Jackson MM and others: Why not treat all body substances as infectious? Am J Nurs 87(9):1137, 1987; Jackson MM: Implementing universal body substance precautions, State Art Rev Occup Med 4:39 (special issue), 1989.

Category-specific isolation precautions (system A)

Seven categories have been described in the 1983 CDC guideline for category-specific isolation precautions. (See Table 30-1 for a description of each.) Each category is represented by a different-colored instruction card that is placed outside the patient's door or at the bedside. The card for Enteric Precautions is reproduced, front and back, in black and white in Fig. 30-2. This category is often represented by diagnoses in pediatric settings.

A category included in former CDC recommendations and conspicuous by its absence in the 1983 guidelines is that of Protective or Reverse Isolation. The absence of this category does not mean that hospitals should never employ special protective techniques, particularly for the care of patients who, for a predictable, temporary period, are very vulnerable to infection (for example, those receiving total body irradiation or those with severe burns or dermatitis). However, it has been recognized that Protective Isolation, as it was previously outlined and practiced, may fail to reduce the risk of infections. Many persons at risk (immunocompromised patients) are infected by their own (endogenous) microorganisms or flora, or they are colonized or infected by microorganisms transmitted by the inadequately washed hands of personnel or nonsterile items used routinely within the former protective isolation protocol. Gowns, gloves, and masks are usually not the most effective protective devices for these patients' safety. Private rooms, conscientious hand washing, and careful instruction of all personnel and visitors seem to be more appropriate, except in special periods of high risk for specific patients.

Disease-specific isolation precautions (system B)

The disease-specific isolation precautions are based on the mode of transmission of the individual disease. Table B in the CDC guideline indicates suggested precautions, which material is considered infective, and how long isolation precautions are appropriate. A black-and-white instruction card should be completed (front and back) and displayed near the patient, indicating what precautions should be observed (Fig. 30-3).

Universal precautions. In 1987, Category VII in System A, entitled Blood/Body Fluid Precautions, was extended to include *all* patients (not merely those diagnosed or suspected of having blood-borne disease). This extension was primarily developed to reduce the risks of transmission of the HIV virus, which causes AIDS, and

the hepatitis B virus (HBV)*; however it would reduce the spread of all blood-borne disease. The term "Universal Precautions," as employed by the Centers for Disease Control, refers to the application of certain limited precautions to all caregiver/patient contacts within the health care setting.

"Universal Precautions" may require the use of barrier equipment such as gloves, plastic aprons, gowns, eyeglasses, goggles, face shields, masks, and leak resistant bags. Such precautions also mandate careful hand washing and thoughtful patient room assignment. They are always to be implemented when there is a risk of contact with blood, specific body tissues, or fluids or other body products containing visible blood (see Table 30-1).

Application of these precautions has significantly changed methods of performance. For example, maternity nurses wear eyeglasses (even if they don't need them) to protect themselves from splashing blood-contaminated fluid during intimate patient care at the time of labor and delivery. Some also wear plastic aprons or gowns. Gloves now cover the hands that clean and dry the newborn after birth. The principle behind "Universal Precautions" is the realization that all blood is potentially infectious and that the caregiver cannot know whose blood is or is not infected.

The universal precautions principle has been more broadly applied to all body fluids, excretions, and secretions in the "body substance isolation" (BSI) system, an alternative to the category-specific and disease-specific systems for isolation precautions. The BSI system is conceptually simple because the nurse plans the use of barriers based on the interaction with *every patient's body substances* rather than on the patient's diagnosis. The BSI perspective stresses the critical nature of hand washing and involves increased use of gloves in patient care. It minimizes the possibility of disease transmission from dry surfaces while emphasizing the precautions needed in caring for body substances that are moist or wet. BSI is now being evaluated clinically.†

---

*US Department of Health and Human Services, Public Health Service, Centers for Disease Control, Recommendations for prevention of HIV transmission in health-care settings, MMWR 36(2S):Aug 21, 1987; update of above recommendations, MMWR 37(24):June 24, 1988.

†Lynch P and others: Implementing and evaluating a system of generic infection precautions: body substance isolation, Am J Infect Control 18(1):1, 1990.

Text continued on p. 622.

Table 30-1   Summary of category—specific isolation precautions*

Precautions	Situation	Hand washing	Room arrangements	Masks†
I. Strict isolation	Highly contagious or virulent infection spread by air or contact	Always	Private—door closed	Yes—if entering room
II. Contact isolation	Highly transmissible—epidemiologically important infection or colonization not needing strict isolation	Always	May usually be shared by patients infected with same organism	Yes—if close to patient
III. Respiratory isolation	Infection transmitted over short distances through droplets (3 feet or less) and infrequently through indirect contact	Always	May usually be shared by patients infected with same organisms	Yes—if close to patient
IV. Acid-fast bacillus—tuberculosis (TB) isolation	Patients with pulmonary or laryngeal TB with active disease (positive sputum smear or chest x-ray strongly suggestive)	Always	Special ventilation, door closed—usually may be shared by patients infected with same organism	Yes—if patient, is coughing and does not reliably cover mouth

Based on Garner JS and Simmons BP: CDC guideline for isolation precautions in hospitals, 1983, US Department of Health and Human Services, Public Health Service, Centers for Disease Control, Center for Infectious Diseases, Hospital Infections Program, Atlanta, Ga.

US Department of Health and Human Services, Public Health Service, Centers for Disease Control, Recommendations for prevention of HIV transmission in health care settings, MMWR 36(2S): Aug 21, 1987; Update of above recommendations, MMWR 37(24): June 24, 1988.

*The category care of contaminated articles has been eliminated since special handling of all waste is recommended throughout the hospital.

†The need for masks or other face coverings must be carefully evaluated although not all categories require them.

‡All body substances need to be handled carefully—evaluate need of gloves regardless of whether isolation precautions are in place.

Plastic aprons or gowns	Gloves‡	Comments	Examples of specific diseases in category
Yes—if entering room	Yes—if entering room		Pharyngeal diphtheria Varicella (chickenpox) Zoster (localized in immunocompromised patient or disseminated)
Yes—if soiling likely	Yes—if touching infective material or likely to contaminate hands	Tends to promote over-isolation	Acute respiratory diseases in infants and young children (croup, bronchitis, URI) Gonococcal conjunctivitis of newborn Rubella—congenital and other types Major wound, skin infection (drainage not adequately covered)
No	No		Epiglottitis, *Haemophilus influenzae* Rubeola (measles) Meningitis—*Haemophilus influenzae;* meningococcal Mumps Pertussis (whooping cough)
Only to prevent gross contamination of clothing	No	Many children with pulmonary TB are not infectious	Specific for pulmonary or laryngeal TB patients

Continued.

Table 30-1 Summary of category—specific isolation precautions—cont'd

Precautions	Situation	Hand washing	Room arrangements	Masks†
V. Enteric precautions	Infection transmitted by direct or indirect contact with feces	Always	Private—if patient hygiene poor; may usually be shared by patients infected by same organism (Note: Define as on category card.)	No
VI. Drainage/secretion precautions	Infection transmitted by direct or indirect contact with purulent material or drainage from an infected body site	Always	No private room	No
VII. Universal blood/body fluid precautions (**Note: The application of category VII to all patients is now recommended. This extension of use is called "Universal Precautions"**)	Infection transmitted by direct or indirect contact with infected blood or body fluids as defined by CDC apply to blood and to other body fluids containing visible blood and semen, vaginal secretions, body tissues, and the following fluids: cerebrospinal, synovial, pleural, peritoneal, pericardial, and amniotic fluids	Always	Private—if patient hygiene poor; may usually be shared by patients infected by same organism	Depends on risk of situation

Plastic aprons or gowns	Gloves‡	Comments	Examples of specific diseases in category
Yes—if soiling likely	Yes—if touching infective material or likely to contaminate hands	Most infections in this category primarily cause GI symptoms. Exceptions are polio and coxsackieviruses.	Amebic dysentery Any diarrhea with suspected infectious origin Gastroenteritis with numerous infectious origins (*Giardia, Salmonella, Shigella*) Hepatitis—type A Typhoid
Yes—if soiling likely	Yes—if touching infective material or likely to contaminate hands	A new category—includes many infections formerly included in wound and skin precautions and discharge/secretion precautions. More serious infections of this type that are difficult to contain with dressings are placed in contact isolation.	Skin and wound infections, minor or limited
Yes—if soiling likely	Yes—if touching blood or body fluids or likely to contaminate hands	Care should be taken to avoid needle stick injuries—used needles should *not* be recapped; they should be placed in special, labeled, puncture-resistant containers that are kept nearby. Blood spills should be promptly treated with an appropriate disinfectant.	AIDS Hepatitis B, non-A, non-B hepatitis Syphilis, primary and secondary with skin and mucous membrane lesions

(Front of Card)

Enteric Precautions

Visitors—Report to Nurses' Station Before Entering Room

1. Masks are not indicated.
2. Gowns are indicated if soiling is likely.
3. Gloves are indicated for touching infective material.
4. **HANDS MUST BE WASHED AFTER TOUCHING THE PATIENT OR POTENTIALLY CONTAMINATED ARTICLES AND BEFORE TAKING CARE OF ANOTHER PATIENT.**
5. Articles contaminated with infective material should be discarded or bagged and labeled before being sent for decontamination and reprocessing.

(Back of Card)

Diseases Requiring Enteric Precautions*

Amebic dysentery
Cholera
Coxsackievirus disease
Diarrhea, acute illness with suspected infectious etiology
Echovirus disease
Encephalitis (unless known not to be caused by enteroviruses)
Enterocolitis caused by *Clostridium difficile* or *Staphylococcus aureus*
Enteroviral infection
Gastroenteritis caused by
    Campylobacter species
    Cryptosporidium species
    Dientamoeba fragilis
    Escherichia coli (enterotoxic enteropathogenic, or enteroinvasive)
    Giardia lamblia
    Salmonella species

Shigella species
Vibrio parahaemolyticus
Viruses-including Norwalk agent and rotavirus
Yersinia enterocolitica
Unknown etiology but presumed to be an infectious agent
Hand, foot, and mouth disease
Hepatitis, viral, type A
Herpangina
Meningitis, viral (unless known not to be caused by enteroviruses)
Necrotizing enterocolitis
Pleurodynia
Poliomyelitis
Typhoid fever (*Salmonella typhi*)
Viral pericarditis, myocarditis, or meningitis (unless known not to be caused by enteroviruses)

*A private room is indicated for Enteric Precautions if patient hygiene is poor. A patient with poor hygiene does not wash hands after touching infective material, contaminates the environment with infective material, or shares contaminated articles with other patients. In general, patients infected with the same organisms may share a room. See Guidelines for Isolation Precautions in Hospitals for details and for how long to apply precautions.

FIG 30-2   Sample instruction card for enteric precautions.

(Front of Card)

Visitors—Report to Nurses' Station Before Entering Room

1. **Private room indicated?**
   - _____ No
   - _____ Yes

2. **Masks indicated?**
   - _____ No
   - _____ Yes for those close to patient
   - _____ Yes for all persons entering room

3. **Gowns indicated?**
   - _____ No
   - _____ Yes if soiling is likely
   - _____ Yes for all persons entering room

4. **Gloves indicated?**
   - _____ No
   - _____ Yes for touching infective material
   - _____ Yes for all persons entering room

5. Special precautions indicated for handling blood?
   - _____ No
   - _____ Yes

6. **Hands must be washed after touching the patient or potentially contaminated articles and before taking care of another patient.**

7. Articles contaminated with _____ should be
   infective material(s)
   discarded or bagged and labeled before being sent for decontamination and reprocessing.

(Back of Card)

Instructions

1. On Table B, Disease-Specific Precautions, locate the disease for which isolation precautions are indicated.
2. Write disease in blank space here: _____
3. Determine if a private room is indicated. In general, patients infected with the same organism may share a room. For some diseases or conditions, a private room is indicated if patient hygiene is poor. A patient with poor hygiene does not wash hands after touching infective material (feces, purulent drainage, or secretions), contaminates the environment with infective material, or shares contaminated articles with other patients.
4. Place a check mark beside the indicated precautions on front of card.
5. Cross through precautions that are *not* indicated.
6. Write infective material in blank space in item 7 on front of card.

FIG 30-3 Sample instruction card for disease-specific isolation precautions.

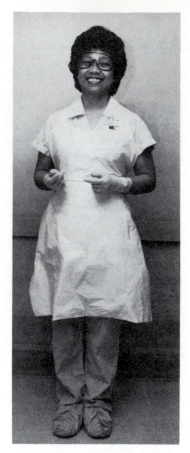

FIG 30-4 This maternity nurse works in a single-room maternity care setting. During the delivery phase, masks, plastic aprons, and goggles or glasses (as here) are available and recommended. Clean gloves are mandatory for immediate newborn care (see p. 139) and maternal perineal care. Immediate predelivery perineal care may entail the use of sterile gloves, depending on the method used.

BARRIER PROCEDURES AND CONCEPTS

Isolation procedures may differ in various settings; the hospital infection prevention manual and patient care nursing manual (PCN) should be consulted. Before specific barrier techniques are described, one should also consider the concepts discussed here.

Desirable characteristics of caregiver

The nurse working with any patient should be:

A. Free from communicable infections (of importance when caring for *any* patient)
B. Knowledgeable regarding possible special need to reevaluate assignment
   1. Pregnancy—fetus especially vulnerable in early trimester to teratogens: rubella, cytomegalovirus (CMV), and others
   2. Open wounds—may become infected
   3. Increased susceptibility
      a. Type of medications taken
      b. No record of chickenpox infection
      c. Appropriate immunization not current
C. Cognizant of the need to maintain good general health habits such as
   1. Proper nutrition
   2. Adequate rest
   3. Good personal hygiene, neatness
   4. Use of stress reduction techniques
D. Knowledgeable and dependable regarding infection precautions needed

Routine hand washing. The most important procedure for preventing the spread of infection is appropriate hand washing. Hand washing has been defined as a vigorous, systematic, brief rubbing together of *all* surfaces of lathered hands, followed by rinsing under a stream of water. When washing, the hands should be kept lower than the elbows so that contaminated water does not soil the arms. Faucets are closed with a paper towel after hand washing is completed. The ideal duration of hand washing is not specific, but for most activities (excluding special, longer presurgical, predelivery, or nursery hand scrubs), a vigorous wash of about 10 seconds is needed. If hands are visibly soiled, more time is required. Many transient microbes representing recent contaminants and about 80% of resident microbes are effectively removed with plain soaps or detergents and running water. Resident microorgnisms in the deep skin layers usually can be killed or inhibited by hand washing with products containing antimicrobial agents. Transient microorganisms, especially in hospital settings, may be pathogenic and cause nosocomial infections. Resident flora are more likely to cause infections when a patient is severely immunocompromised.

The fingernails of all health care personnel should be short and clean (body secretions and stool may collect under nails and be difficult to remove). The indications for hand washing depend on the type, intensity, duration, sequence, and area of activity. Except for emergencies, hands should always be washed in the following situations:

Before:

A. Initiating individual patient nursing care
B. Performing any sterile or invasive procedures or touching a wound
C. Pouring medications or touching food

After:

A. Complete individual patient nursing care
B. Touching wounds, mucous membranes, or body substances and using the bathroom
C. Touching inanimate objects that are likely to be contaminated, such as used urine measuring devices and catheters
D. Removing sterile or clean gloves

If health care personnel wonder if their hands need to be washed, they need to be washed.

Gloves. Disposable, single-use gloves, clean or sterile, depending on the patient's needs, are recommended to protect patients from microorganisms from personnel and to protect personnel from patient's microorganisms. Unless a careful "no touch" technique is employed, gloves are recommended when contact with body substances (excretions, secretions, blood, and body fluids) is possible.

Isolation gowns. The use of isolation gowns formerly was combined with considerably detailed protocol. This is chiefly because the definition of contamination often was "touching anything in the room of a patient with a contagious disease" and because of the now obsolete practice of reusing gowns for the same patient unless they became visibly soiled or damp. Currently, gowns are less frequently used and seldom reused. Gowns or aprons are used primarily to protect against splashing body fluids. They are stored in a clean area and put on with clean hands. After use, they are carefully removed and usually placed in a laundry bag or the trash. Then the nurse washes her hands.

Masks. Unfortunately, there is no proof that even high efficiency disposable masks protect the caregiver from airborne droplet nuclei. (Air travels the path of least resistance and may get behind a mask through gaps between the face and the mask at the sides.) However, masks, like gowns, may help prevent splashes from reaching skin, mouth, or nose. A mask also may be of some value in preventing disease because it keeps the wearer from touching his own nose or mouth. Masks should be replaced when moist and never reused.

Eye protection. Protective eyewear (glasses, face shields, and goggles) should reduce the risk of contamination of the mucous membranes of the eyes. However, sometimes they are a nuisance and may fog over, impairing vision.

Needle safety. Needles and sharps (knife blades, razors) should be deposited immediately after use in rigid puncture-resistant receptacles. Syringe needles should not be separated from disposable syringes nor should they be recapped, unless a proper receptacle is not readily available. In that case, a one-handed recapping technique may be used. Place the correctly sized cap on a flat surface and with one hand slide the needle into it. Keep your other hand behind your back. Do not place the cap over the needle with your free hand. Secure the cap covering the needle by pressure on its sides (see also p. 506).

Bagging of articles. Articles that are possibly contaminated should be enclosed in sturdy bags impervious to moisture. If there is a possibility that the outer surface of the bag is also contaminated the CDC recommends double-bagging. Most trash from a hospital room may be single-bagged for routine disposal. However, there are many different kinds of trash. Consult your hospital regulations regarding the disposal of different types of waste.

Food service. The use of paper plates for certain isolation patients is thought to be unnecessary. Emphasis should be placed on patient hand washing after use of the bedpan or toilet and before eating.

Discharge housekeeping. Methods of cleaning a patient's room should be standardized and the same methods used for all hospital rooms. The use of fogging devices is not recommended.

ADMISSION OF A PEDIATRIC PATIENT NEEDING ISOLATION PRECAUTIONS
Parental needs and fears

Almost without exception, admission to the hospital is a stressful period for parents and child. The anxiety and feeling of helplessness often experienced by parents are increased considerably when the admission necessitates the use of certain barrier techniques and entry into a special room labeled "Isolation." The sight of the medical and nursing staff wearing gowns or gloves and perhaps masks and the sound of alarming terms such as "contaminated" and "contagious" do not reassure parents. Everything seems strange and disquieting and not always accurate deductions often disturb their peace of mind. Many parents worry, "If Johnny has to be here, he must be terribly ill. I wonder what the other children here have. Couldn't Johnny catch something else from them?" Parents need much support and instruction at such a time. Physicians and nurses may find the assistance of the infection control practitioner expecially useful. Fortunately, isolation in a single room, complete with a nurse in gown and mask is not encountered often in pediatrics today. For example, if strict isolation is needed, it is typically limited to the first 24- to 48-hour period until antibiotics are able to render the patient noncontagious.

Text continued on p. 638.

Table 30-2 Communicable childhood diseases

Disease	Infectious agent and general description	Importance	Mode of transmission	Communicable period
Acquired immuno-deficiency syn-drome (AIDS) and human im-munodeficiency virus (HIV) in-fections	Human immunodefi-ciency virus (HIV-1)—a human retro-virus. Diagnosis of AIDS is based on clinical, immunologic, sero-logic, and virologic findings and exclu-sion of primary or secondary immuno-deficiency states.*	Relentlessly progres-sive, devastating disorder of extraor-dinary morbidity and mortality	Body secretions and contaminated nee-dles and blood prod-ucts Perinatal transmission from infected mother (Universal Precautions)† At-risk groups include male homosexuals, intravenous drug users, sexual part-ners of patients with AIDS or HIV infec-tion, and children born to infected mothers, (multi-in-fused hemophiliacs, other recipients of blood products, now have minimal risk)	Potentially infectious for indeterminant period before symptoms and dur-ing duration of dis-ease
Bacillary dysentery (shigellosis)	*Shigella sonnei* (most common), *S. flex-neri,* and *S. dysen-teriae* Acute inflammation of colon	Extremely widespread in areas with poor sanitary facilities and hygiene prac-tices Disease often severe in infancy but mild after 3 yr of age	Direct or indirect con-tact with feces of infected patients or carriers Contaminated food, water, and flies play important role (en-teric precautions)‡	As long as patients or carriers harbor organisms (until three consecutive stool or rectal swab cultures are negative) Healthy carriers un-common
Chickenpox; see varicella Chlamydia infec-tion, see pp. 174 and 307 Cytomegalovirus (CMV) infection, see pp. 306 and 307				

*Centers for Disease Control: Recommendations for prevention of HIV transmission in health care settings, MMWR 36(25):1, 1987; Centers for Disease Control: Update: Universal Precautions for the prevention of transmission of HIV, HBV and other blood born pathogens in Health care settings, MMWR 37(24):377, 1988.
†New Universal Precautions (see pp. 618-619).
‡Indicates Category-Specific Isolation Precautions recommended by CDC guideline for isolation precautions in hospitals, US Department of Health and Human Services, Public Health Service, Center for Infectious Diseases, Hospital Infections Program, Atlanta Ga 30333, 1983.
§Centers for Disease Control: Protection against viral hepatitis, MMWR 39(RR2):1,1990.
‖American Academy of Pediatrics: Report of the Committee on Infectious Diseases. In The red book, ed 21, Elk Grove Village, Ill, 1988.

Incubation period	Symptoms	Treatment and nursing care	Prevention
Highly variable ranges from months to years, thought to be present for years, in some cases, before onset of symptoms	Opportunistic infections or unusual forms of malignancy Early signs and symptoms: recurrent otitis media, sinusitis or pneumonia, failure to thrive, persistent thrush, fever of unknown origin, chronic unexplained diarrhea, hepatomegaly, generalized lymphadenopathy, and developmental delay	Antiretroviral therapy may soon be available to reverse cell-mediated immunodeficiency that results in infections with opportunistic agents Antimicrobial, antitumor therapy and nutritional support have prolonged lives	Exclusion of blood donors with a positive antibody test for HIV Transfusions and plasma infusions should be avoided whenever possible. The use of clotting factor concentrate should be restricted to hemophiliacs with essential clinical indications Deglycerolized RBCs for other blood product recipients Abstaining from high-risk sexual practices and from intravenous illicit drug abuse Use of autogenous transfusions
1 to 7 days (usually 2 to 4 days)	Mild to severe diarrhea; in severe cases blood, mucus, and dehydration Abdominal pain, fever, and prostration may be present	Treatment depends on severity of infection Trimethoprim, sulfamethoxazole (Septra) drug of choice Keep patient warm; oral fluids may be restricted; intravenous therapy may be necessary to prevent dehydration	Attack appears to confer limited immunity No preventive known other than improved individual and community hygiene

Continued.

Table 30-2   Communicable childhood diseases—cont'd

Disease	Infectious agent and general description	Importance	Mode of transmission	Communicable period
Diphtheria	*Corynebacterium diphtheriae* (Klebs-Löffler bacillus) Severe, acute infectious disease of upper respiratory tract and perhaps skin Toxins produced may affect nervous system and heart	Rarely seen because of routine childhood immunization, more comprehensive public health regulations, and enforcement of milk standards and carrier control 5% to 10% mortality Serious complications include neuritis, paralysis, and myocarditis	Direct or indirect contact with secretions from respiratory tract or skin lesions of patient Skin lesions (Contact Isolation)‡ Pharyngeal diphtheria (Strict Isolation)‡	Variable: 2 to 4 wk in untreated persons, or 1 to 2 days after antibiotic therapy initiated Isolation until two negative cultures 24 hr apart, from both nose and throat or skin lesions, obtained after end of antimicrobial therapy; contacts may be isolated
German measles (rubella, 3-day measles)	Rubella virus Acute infectious disease characterized chiefly by rose-colored macular rash and lymph node enlargement	Very common, frequently occurring in epidemic form Complications rare for victim but may cause deformities of fetus if contracted by pregnant woman during first trimester—nonimmune persons should avoid persons known to have this disease	Usually direct contact with secretions from mouth and nose May be acquired in utero (Contact Isolation for both forms of infection)‡	From 1 wk before rash appears until approximately 7 days after its onset For discussion of congenital rubella syndrome see pp. 306 and 393; affected infants may be infectious up to 1 yr of age unless nose, pharynx, and urine cultures are negative 3 months following birth
Gonorrhea (pp. 174 and 640)				
Hepatitis, viral; several types identified: Type A (infectious); Type B (serum); non-A, non-B	All types manifest similarities and differences; may vary with age and general condition of person infected	Hepatitis of all types represented third most commonly reported communicable disease in 1989		
(1) Type A (infectious) (HAV)	Hepatitis A virus (HAV): usually abrupt onset	HAV: Highest incidence in civilian populations in persons under 15 years, typically subclinical in children (very common in mentally retarded children)	Person-to-person; generally through fecal-oral route Transmission is facilitated by poor sanitation and close contact; ingestion of fecally contaminated food and water (e.g., shellfish, milk) (Enteric Precautions)‡	Uncertain; probably infectious 2 wk before onset of jaundice; minimal risk 1 wk after onset of jaundice

Incubation period	Symptoms	Treatment and nursing care	Prevention
2 to 5 days (occasionally longer)	Depend on type and part of upper respiratory area inflamed Formation of fibrinous false membrane, which may or may not be visible in throat or nose Nausea, possible muscle paralysis, and heart complications	Administration of antitoxin, analgesics, erythromycin, or penicillin Prednisone lessens incidence of myocarditis in severe disease Absolute bed rest; gentle throat irrigations; bland, soft diet; humidification Possible need for tracheostomy Watch for muscle weakness	Immunity after one attack, but person may be immune without history of disease Immunity determined by Shick test Routine primary schedule—Td (tetanus-diphtheria toxoids) booster injection recommended at 10-yr intervals
14 to 21 days (usually 18 days)	Rose-colored macular rash occurring first on face, then on all body parts; enlargement and tenderness of lymph nodes; mild fever	Supportive nursing care with good personal hygiene	Rubella vaccine Immune after one attack
	Jaundice for three types may be inapparent, fleeting, or persistent with or without itching	No specific therapy available; supportive care, rest, and high-calorie diet	
15 to 50 days; average 25 to 30 days	Fever, malaise, anorexia, nausea, enlarged liver, abdominal discomfort, dark urine, weight loss, jaundice Children usually have less severe clinical manifestations, and illness may not be accompanied by jaundice	Supportive care	HAV attack confers immunity for HAV IG‡ recommended for HAV contact; IG is protective if given before exposure or during incubation period; best if given within 72 hours after exposure IG immune globulin (formerly called "immune serum globulin," ISG, or "gamma globulin")§

Continued.

Table 30-2 Communicable childhood diseases—cont'd

Disease	Infectious agent and general description	Importance	Mode of transmission	Communicable period
(2) Type B (serum) (HBV)	Hepatitis B virus (HBV): characterized usually by insidious onset	HBV common in young adults; more often complicated by relapse and prolonged liver dysfunction; typically more severe in infants and debilitated patients	HBV reported more frequently; transmitted through inoculation of contaminated blood products, needles, and syringes; close and intimate contact, including sexual contact also transmitted from infected mother to infant during perinatal period (Universal Precautions)‡	Potentially infectious for indeterminate period before and after active symptoms; carrier state possible Neonates acquire illness from infected mother and have high risk of developing chronic active hepatitis
(3) Non-A, non-B viral hepatitis (NANB)	Causative agent or agents have not been identified Clinical features resemble HBV, insidious onset	Acute hepatitis, neither HAV or HBV, affects all age groups; common among low socioeconomic groups, such as commercial blood donors; most common type of hepatitis associated with blood transfusion (70% to 80%)	Most common cause of posttransfusion hepatitis Parenteral exposure to blood or illicit drugs (Universal Precautions)‡	Potentially infectious for indeterminate period before and after active symptoms; carrier state possible
Herpes simplex infections, see p. 174				
Measles (rubeola, or 2-week or red measles)	Measles virus Acute infection characterized by moderately high temperature, inflammation of mucous membranes of respiratory tract, and macular rash	Very common, highly infectious disease frequently occurring in epidemic form Possible serious complications include pneumonia, otitis media, conjunctivitis, and encephalitis	Direct contact with secretions from nose and throat, airborne (Respiratory Isolation)‡	From time of "cold symptoms" (about 4 days before rash) until about 4 days after rash appears

Incubation period	Symptoms	Treatment and nursing care	Prevention
45 to 160 days; average 120 days	Urticaria and arthralgia more characteristic of HBV Various combinations of anorexia, malaise, nausea, vomiting, abdominal pain, and jaundice Occasionally a rapid, severe (fulminating) type characterized by mental confusion, emotional instability, restlessness, coma, and internal bleeding; usually progresses to a fatal outcome within 10 days	Bed rest for symptomatic patients; well-balanced diet as desired; supplements of all vitamins, especially B complex Infants born to infected mothers should be given HBIG (within 12 hr of birth) and the first dose of hepatitis B vaccine as soon as possible (may be given at same time as HBIG, or within 7 days)	HBV attack confers immunity for HBV; Hepatitis B vaccine (Heptavax) confers immunity after 3 doses; second injection 1 month after first, third 6 months after first§; hepatitis B—immune globulin (HBIG) primarily for those exposed to HBV-contaminated blood (i.e., by needle stick); optimal effect if given within 48 hours after exposure; results of IG given to HBV contacts have been inconsistent, but it may be helpful, at least to attenuate the disease Effective screening of blood donors; absolute sterilization of equipment used for drawing blood, or use of disposable equipment
Mean range 2 to 12 wk	Same as HBV; symptoms may not be as severe	Same as HBV	Hepatitis B vaccine available for health care workers Avoid high risk per cutaneous exposure IG not known to be beneficial, but may offer some protection
8 to 12 days from exposure to onset of symptoms	Catarrhal symptoms like a common cold; conjunctivitis; photophobia Fever followed by maculopapular rash, which starts behind the ears and at the hairline and forehead, and moves progressively down the body, becoming more confluent over the face. Koplik's spots (eruption on mucous membrane of mouth) diagnostic, best seen before the rash	Antibiotics (for treatment of secondary bacterial infections) Acetaminophen (Tylenol) and tepid sponge baths for severe cases; various soothing lotions Boric acid eye irrigations; protection from bright lights—eyeshade Observation for onset of pneumonia or ear infection	Live measles vaccine; IG immune globulin will prevent or modify disease if given within 6 days of exposure. Usually immune after first attack

Continued.

Table 30-2   Communicable childhood diseases—cont'd

Disease	Infectious agent and general description	Importance	Mode of transmission	Communicable period
Meningitis (*Haemophilus influenzae* and *Escherichia coli* see pp. 663-666)				
Meningococcal meningitis (cerebrospinal fever)	*Neisseria meningitidis (N. intracellularis)* Meningococcus Serious, acute disease caused by bacteria that invade bloodstream and eventually meninges, causing fever and central nervous system inflammation	Occurs fairly often where concentrations of people are found (army bases, schools) because of healthy carriers Very severe or relatively mild Mortality depends on early diagnosis and treatment Complications include hydrocephalus, arthritis, blindness, deafness, impairment of intellect, and cerebral palsy	Direct contact with patient or carrier by droplet spread (Respiratory Isolation)‡	As long as meningococci are found in nose and mouth Usually not infectious after 24 hr of antibiotic therapy
Mononucleosis, infectious (glandular fever)	Epstein-Barr (EB) virus Mildly contagious disease characterized by increase in monocyte-type white cell in blood, splenomegaly, lymph node enlargement, fever, and fatigue Heterophil agglutinin studies positive fairly late in course of disease	Typically, disease of teenagers or young adults Trauma may rarely cause ruptured spleen; hepatitis in 8% to 10% of cases May involve prolonged convalescence	Probably droplets from nose and throat, saliva, or intimate contact (No Isolation)‡	Not known Probably only during acute stage
Mumps (infectious parotitis)	Virus Acute infectious disease causing inflammation of salivary glands and, at times, testes and ovaries	Possible serious consequences for male after puberty when an attack is more severe; sterility can be complication Meningitis or encephalitis occurs infrequently Mild pancreatitis may be encountered	Direct or indirect contact with patient by droplet spread (Respiratory Isolation)‡	From 1 to 7 days before parotid swelling until up to 9 days after onset

Incubation period	Symptoms	Treatment and nursing care	Prevention
1 to 10 days (usually 4 days)	Sudden onset of fever, chills, headache, and vomiting (convulsions fairly common in children) Cutaneous petechial hemorrhages, stiffness of neck, opisthotonos; joint pain, possibly delirium, convulsions	Spinal tap and culture needed to confirm diagnosis Temperature control; penicillin G cefuroxime or ampicillin, analgesics, and sedatives Watch for clinical signs of increasing intracranial pressure or meningeal irritation and eye and ear involvement Maintain dim, quiet atmosphere; turn gently; watch for constipation and urinary retention; attention to fluid balance	Meningococcal polysaccharide vaccines for group A and C meningococcal infections Extent of immunity after attack unknown Rifampin should be given to any person having intimate contact with secretions
Unknown (probably 4 to 7 wk)	Sore throat, malaise, depression, enlarged spleen, liver, and lymph nodes Possible jaundice with liver damage	Symptomatic, no specific therapy known Bed rest, high carbohydrate and protein intake Possible use of corticosteroids with severe throat involvement and airway obstruction	No immunization available
14 to 21 days (usually 18 days)	Tender swelling chiefly of parotid glands in front of and below ear Headache; moderate fever; pain on swallowing	Bed rest; bland, soft diet; analgesics; warm or cold applications to swollen glands Watch for tenderness of testes—scrotal support may be necessary	Mumps vaccine Usually immune after first attack

Continued.

Table 30-2   Communicable childhood diseases—cont'd

Disease	Infectious agent and general description	Importance	Mode of transmission	Communicable period
Rabies (hydrophobia)	Virus Only two nonfatal cases reported, acute infectious encephalitis, causing convulsions and muscle paralysis	Exceedingly dangerous Household pets may acquire rabies through bite of rabid wild animals All dogs should be immunized periodically; cats may also be carriers, but impractical to insist on immunization	Bite of rabid animals or entry of infected saliva through previous break in skin or mucous membrane (Contact Isolation)‡	Throughout clinical course of disease plus 3 to 5 days before appearance of symptoms (as demonstrated in dogs and cats)
Staphylococcal infections	Coagulase-positive staphylococci (*Staphylococcus aureus*); coagulase-negative (*s. epidermidis*); pus-producing coccus Descriptions variable	Found almost everywhere; causes many hospital infections; does not respond well to usual antibiotic therapy; extremely difficult to control; anyone may be carrier at intervals Complications include skin lesions, pneumonia, wound infections, arthritis, osteomyelitis, meningitis, and food poisoning	Depends on body area infected Via hands of hospital personnel Asymptomatic nasal carriers common Open suppurative lesions May be airborne Direct or indirect contact with infected secretions (Type of isolation depends on area infected—Contact, Drainage/Secretion, or Enteric Precautions)‡	As long as lesions drain or carrier state persists
Group A Streptococcal infections (GAS)	Strains of group A beta-hemolytic streptococci Diseases include septic sore throat, scarlet fever (scarlatina), erysipelas, impetigo, puerperal fever	Interrelated group of infections; septic sore throat probably most common Early complications include otitis media May cause serious complications not contagious in themselves—nephritis and rheumatic fever, with possible arthritis and carditis	In septic sore throat and scarlet fever, direct or indirect contact with nasopharyngeal secretions from infected patient; probably airborne In erysipelas, impetigo, and puerperal fever, direct or indirect contact with discharges from skin or reproductive tract (Type of isolation depends on area infected—Respiratory, Contact Isolation)‡	Variable

Incubation period	Symptoms	Treatment and nursing care	Prevention
Usually 2 to 6 wk	Mental depression, head-aches, restlessness, and fever Progresses to painful spasms of throat muscles, especially when attempting to drink Delirium, convulsions, and coma	No effective treatment known Supportive nursing care to help prevent convulsions; analgesics Death usually occurs in about 7 days	Vaccination of dogs; 10-day confinement of any dog who has bitten human Laboratory investigation of brain of dog that dies during this period; if rabies is diagnosed, person bitten must receive rabies vaccine; consult Red Book for specific treatments‖
Variable; 1 to 10 days to several wk	Depend on area infected Fever and characteristic signs of inflammation typical	Antibiotics according to drug sensitivity pattern of organisms; methicillin, ox-acillin, cephalosporins, vancomycin Topical antibiotics: bacitra-cin, neomycin, polymyxin, mupirocin	Good hygiene and aseptic technique best preventive
2 to 5 days pharyngitis 7 to 10 days impetigo	Depends on manifestations Septic sore throat, severe pharyngitis, and fever Scarlet fever, pharyngitis, fever, fine reddish rash, and strawberry tongue Erysipelas, tender, red skin lesions, and fever often recurrent Impetigo, refer to p. 598 Puerperal fever, refer to p. 5 and 216	Depends on manifestation Penicillin for at least 10 days to prevent rheumatic fever (erythromycin for persons allergic to penicillin)	No artificial immunization available Penicillin prophylaxis may be used with special groups Good asepsis important

Continued.

Table 30-2   Communicable childhood diseases—cont'd

Disease	Infectious agent and general description	Importance	Mode of transmission	Communicable period
Group B strepto-coccal infections (see p. 306) Syphilis (see pp. 172 and 640)				
Tetanus (lockjaw)	*Bacillus Clostridium tetani* Acute infectious disease attacking chiefly nervous system Wounds deprived of good oxygen supply especially vulnerable	Always considered in event of burns, automobile accidents, or puncture wounds Mortality of about 35%	Entrance of spores into wounds through contaminated soil Direct or indirect contamination of wounds (No isolation recommended except possibly gloves for wound care)†	None
Tuberculosis (TB) (see p. 175)	*Mycobacterium tuberculosis* (tubercle bacillus) Typically chronic infection that may affect many body organs Human type most often causes pulmonary infection Bovine type causes much of tuberculosis affecting areas outside lungs	Serious world health problem, particularly in economically deprived areas Infants and young children highly susceptible Pulmonary complications, hemoptysis, spontaneous pneumothorax, or spread to other organs with varied symptoms; possible orthopedic problems	Pulmonary TB Direct or indirect contact with infected patient's respiratory secretions in the form of droplet nuclei Other types of TB Transmission depends on lesion Bovine type may result from drinking milk from infected cows (now rare in US) (AFB Isolation for pulmonary or laryngeal TB; Drainage/Secretion Precautions for draining lesions)‡	Children with uncomplicated primary TB are usually noninfectious because of minimal pulmonary lesions. Communicable as long as organism is discharged in sputum or other body excretions Communicability may be reduced by anti-TB therapy Body often walls off a primary infection, controlling spread and preventing active disease

Incubation period	Symptoms	Treatment and nursing care	Prevention
3 to 21 days (usually 8 days)	Irritability, rigidity, painful muscle spasms, and inability to open mouth Exhaustion and respiratory difficulty	Specific—tetanus immune globulin (human; TIG preferred over tetanus antitoxin) Parenteral Pen G is effective in reducing the number of vegetative forms of the organism Sedation plus muscle relaxant Quiet, dim room Possible suction and tracheotomy Observation of fluid balance; watch for constipation and respiratory distress; protect from self-injury during convulsions	Routine primary immunization; booster at school age and Td every 10 yr (see p. 392)
From infection to primary lesion, 2 to 10 wk Time of appearance of active symptoms variable	Active pulmonary tuberculosis: anorexia, weight loss, night sweats, afternoon fever, cough and dyspnea, fatigue, and hemoptysis; in children dyspnea and cough often absent Diagnosis based on symptoms and microscopic studies of sputum, gastric washings, CSF, tissue; bronchoscopy; PPD skin test; chest x-ray exam	Specific—ioniazid (INH) plus ethambutol or rifampin Nursing care includes provision for mental and physical rest; nutritious diet; observation for toxic drug reactions and increasing respiratory distress; provision for and instructions in personal hygiene	Early detection and control of known cases through periodic x-ray examination, possible skin tests, and close medical supervision INH prophylaxis for neonate exposed to infected mother; separation from mother depends on mother's status Skin testing family members and case contact studies are paramount

Continued.

Table 30-2 Communicable childhood diseases—cont'd

Disease	Infectious agent and general description	Importance	Mode of transmission	Communicable period
Typhoid fever (enteric fever)	*Salmonella typhosa,* bacillus (one of many types have been identified) Relatively severe febrile systemic infection (sepsis) with symptoms involving lymphoid tissues, intestine, and spleen; may be accompanied by complete prostration and delirium Condition has prolonged course and convalescence	Always of potential public health importance when community hygiene breaks down Carrier states may persist Complications include intestinal hemorrhage and perforation, thrombosis, cardiac failure, and cholecystitis	Direct or indirect contact with urine and feces of infected patients and carriers Food and water supplies may be infected by contaminated flies or unsuspected carriers; community sewage facilities should be evaluated; excreta may have to be disinfected before being added to local system (Enteric Precautions)‡	As long as typhoid organism appears in feces or urine, 2% to 5% of those affected become permanent carriers
Varicella-zoster infections	Virus capable of causing varicella (chickenpox), or zoster (shingles)		Direct or indirect contact with respiratory secretions or moist skin lesions of varicella or zoster Special ventilation in room for outbreak control (Strict Isolation)‡	Approximately 1 to 2 days before rash appears until 6 days after its onset; dried crusts not contagious
Varicella (chickenpox)	Response to primary infection Mild, chiefly cutaneous infectious disease	Very common, highly contagious, usually mild disease Complications other than secondary infection from scratching rare; however, encephalitis possible	See precautions above	
Zoster (shingles)	Reactivation in debilitated persons or in persons receiving immunosuppressive therapy	Overwhelming severe infection seen in children receiving immunosuppressive therapy CAUTION: Contact!	Zoster less contagious, but susceptible children exposed to zoster lesions may develop chickenpox	

Incubation period	Symptoms	Treatment and nursing care	Prevention
1 to 3 wk (usually 2 wk)	In children symptoms may be atypical, may at first resemble upper respiratory tract infection; intestinal tract becomes inflamed and even ulcerated; spleen enlarges; fever mounts; pluse relatively slow; rash, or "rose spots," may be present	Ampicillin or chloramphenicol for typhoid fever Supportive nursing care; liquid to bland, soft diet as tolerated; bed rest Watch for abdominal distention and hemorrhage; small enemas may be ordered; observation of fluid balance	Immunity usually acquired after one attack Vaccine available
10 to 21 days (usually 14 days)	Zoster lesions confined to skin over sensory nerves preceded by local pain, itching, and burning	Keep fingernails short and clean to minimize secondary infections caused by scratching Calamine lotion, oral antihistaminics reduce pruritus	None; immune after one attack, OKA vaccine for high-risk patients Passive immunization of susceptible immunodeficient patients exposed to either varicella or zoster virus may be obtained with varicella-zoster immune globulin (VZIG) given within 96 hours of exposure; distributed by the American Red Cross Blood Services Regional Centers
	Slight fever; malaise; rapidly progressing papulovesiculopustular skin eruption in all stages of development, first appearing on trunk and scalp	Children with varicella should not be given salicylates because of potential development of Reye syndrome	None; immune after one attack, OKA vaccine for high-risk patients

Continued.

Table 30-2 Communicable childhood diseases—cont'd

Disease	Infectious agent and general description	Importance	Mode of transmission	Communicable period
Whooping cough (pertussis)	*Bordetella pertussis* (pertussis bacillus) Acute infection of respiratory tract characterized by paroxysmal cough ending in "whoop," often accompanied by vomiting	Severe disease in infants, may terminate fatally Complications include bronchopneumonia and convulsions, widespread hemorrhages, hernia, and possible activation of pulmonary tuberculosis	Direct or indirect contact with nasopharyngeal secretions of infected patients (droplet infection) (Respiratory Isolation)‡	From 7 days after exposure to 3 wk after onset of typical cough Greatest in catarrhal stage before onset of paroxysms

Unit preparation

Sometimes the admission of a new patient is anticipated, and an individual isolation unit can be set up before the child's arrival. Pediatric patients are not usually placed together in a room unless it is confirmed that their diagnoses are the same and the attending physicians involved grant permission. However, patients with diarrheal diseases or respiratory infections that appear to be caused by the same organism may sometimes share a room, having the same type of isolation while maintaining separate bed units. The room should be comfortably warm and well ventilated. In addition to a correctly sized bed or crib, a bedside stand, and the overbed table found in all standard patient units, a unit where a patient with an infectious disease is cared for should include the following:

1. Access to a sink, running water, and toilet
2. A box of gloves
3. A "hand-washing agent" in a dispenser that works for hand and arm care of personnel
4. Paper towels in a dispenser
5. Laundry hamper support and laundry bags
6. Plastic bags for collection of trash for discard
7. Other barriers, such as gowns or masks if care activities warrant their use. Some facilities put these items in a cart outside the door of the patient's room
8. All other articles needed for admission and daily care

It is important that all equipment be in readiness because much time is lost if the nurse must leave the patient to obtain equipment.

Admission modifications in isolation. Currently, in-room visitation by family members of isolated patients is much more liberal than in the past. Just who is allowed to enter depends on the type of infection and the visitor and patient being considered.

At admission, the child's clothes are usually placed in a clean bag and returned to the parents. Parents often ask, "What do we do with Johnny's clothes when we get them home?" and "What about all the things that Johnny used at home while he was sick?" Usually it is sufficient to suggest that the parents wash the child's clothes, using a hot water setting on an automatic washer and regular laundry detergent, and dry them in a dryer.

Parents should be encouraged and welcomed at the bedside. They should be shown where the supply of clean gowns is kept and taught to remove the gowns and place

Incubation period	Symptoms	Treatment and nursing care	Prevention
7 to 10 days (rarely more than 2 wk)	Early symptoms resemble typical common cold Cough worsens and may become violent and paroxysmal Vomiting may be caused by coughing or nervous system irritation; cough may linger after convalescence	Diagnosis confirmed with bacterial studies of mucus from the nasopharynx; immunofluorescent antibody technique will identify organism after it has been isolated Erythromycin antibiotic of choice; provision for rest and quiet; sedatives Light nutritious diet; judicious fluid intake to prevent dehydration; weight determinations Observed for onset of respiratory distress or other complications	Immunity usually produced after one attack Routine primary schedule plus boosters Erythromycin therapy shortens the period of communicability to 5 days or less

them in the laundry hamper and to wash their hands just before leaving.

Urine and stool specimens are collected in the usual way, and the outside of the container used to send them to the laboratory should be clean.

Psychosocial implications of isolation of pediatric patients

Much has been written about the impact of hospitalization on the child and his family. (See Chapter 19.) Less has been published regarding the additional stress experienced from various isolation precautions. One small study involving six children, aged 6 to 9 years, who had been isolated during their hospitalizations should offer nurses special food for thought.*

The first research question sought to discover whether the children understood the reasons for their hospitalizations. The 9-year-olds correctly expressed the reason for isolation, but the 6- and 7-year-olds did not. One of these children poignantly stated, "Because I was bad and got sick, I was supposed to stay in my room." Clearly, when possible, there needs to be exploration of the child's

*Broeder JL: School-age children's perceptions of isolation after hospital discharge, Matern Child Nurs J 14:153-174, 1985.

concept of the reason for his isolation and some of the procedures it involves. If children understand that punishment is not a part of the reason for isolation, more of their energy can be directed toward becoming well more quickly.

If the nurse must use a mask, letting the youngster see her face before she comes into the room may dispel some fears. A nurse's isolation regalia may be frightening. One of the children in the study explained that the nurse's gown was used "so she can operate on you." A number of children probably received the impression that the presence of people in gowns indicated impending unpleasant procedures because their nurses, trying to economize on time, always included a procedure when they came to see their patients. Perhaps nurses should consider the many different kinds of treatments that help children get better—playing games, talking, cuddling, and making friends or family members welcome to stay with the patient.

The familiar is usually soothing; little routines remembered may bring healing sleep. Significant contacts that are maintained bring a light to the patient's eyes. Nurses must remember the value of the caring touch, the encouraging voice, and the special toy as they seek to heal growing bodies and spirits.

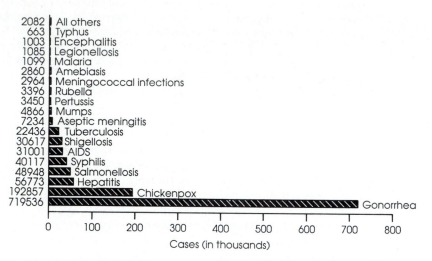

FIG 30-5 Cases of communicable diseases (in 1,000's) in the United States for 1988. Total number of reported cases of specified notifiable diseases, civilian cases only. *(From Centers for Disease Control: Summary of notifiable diseases, United States 1988, MMWR 37(54):10, 1989.)*

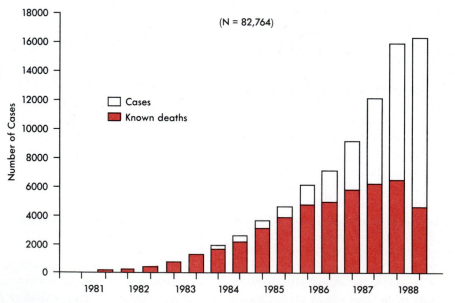

FIG 30-6 Acquired immunodeficiency syndrome (AIDS). Cases and known deaths, by 6-month periods of report to CDC, United States, 1981-1988. *(From Centers for Disease Control: Summary of notifiable diseases, United States 1988, MMWR 37(54):13, 1989.)*

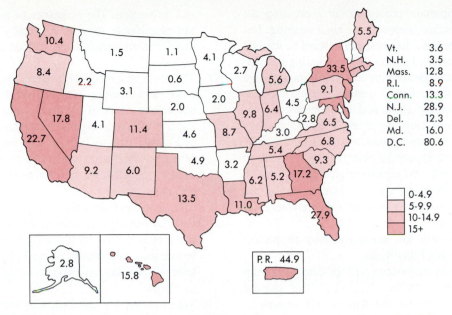

FIG 30-7 Reported AIDS patients per 100,000 population by state of residence United States 1989. *(From Centers for Disease Control: Summary of notifiable diseases, United States 1988, MMWR 39(5):81, 1990.)*

SIGNIFICANT COMMUNICABLE DISEASES OF CHILDHOOD AND THEIR NURSING CARE

Descriptions of some of the communicable diseases seen or mentioned most often in pediatrics are included in Table 30-2. Also summarized are nursing points to remember in each case. Fortunately, not all the diseases described are encountered by nurses today. However, all those described, and some not included, pose a potential threat to communities (Figs. 30-5 through 30-7). Diseases such as diphtheria, typhoid, and polio, for which proved preventives exist, could again ravage the population if public health standards decline and public education and support for immunization programs are not constantly maintained.

=== **Key Concepts** ===

1. The 1983 CDC guidelines offered the possibility of choosing one of three alternative isolation systems: category-specific, disease-specific, or a system designed for use within the particular institution.
2. The CDC guidelines describe seven categories for category-specific isolation: (1) strict isolation, (2) contact isolation, (3) respiratory isolation, (4) acid-fast bacillus–tuberculosis isolation, (5) enteric precautions, (6) drainage/secretions precautions, and (7) universal precautions.
3. Disease-specific isolation precautions are based on the mode of transmission of the individual disease.
4. In 1987 the CDC extended Category VII, blood/body fluid precautions, to include all patients. The term "Universal Precautions" refers to the applica-

tion of certain limited precautions to all caregiver/patient contacts within the health care setting.
5. The Body Substance Isolation (BSI) system is an alternative to the category-specific and disease-specific systems. With the BSI system the nurse plans the use of barriers based on the interaction with every patient's body substances, including body fluids, excretions, and secretions.
6. To minimize the spread of infection the care giver should be free of communicable infections, knowledgeable regarding possible special need to reevaluate assignment, knowledgeable about the need to maintain good general health habits, and knowledgeable and dependable regarding isolation precautions needed.

7. The most important procedure for preventing the spread of infection is appropriate hand washing. Except in emergencies, hands should always be washed in the following situations: before initiating individual patient care, performing any sterile or invasive procedure and touching a wound, pouring medications and touching food; and after completing individual patient care, touching wounds, mucous membranes, or body substances and using the bathroom, touching inanimate objects that are likely to be contaminated, and removing gloves.

8. Disposable, single-use gloves, clean or sterile, are recommended to protect patients and personnel from microorganisms.

9. Gowns or aprons are primarily used to protect against splashing body fluids.

10. Although masks may not protect the care giver from airborne droplet nuclei, they may help prevent splashes from reaching the skin, mouth, or nose.

11. Protective eyewear should reduce the incidence of contamination of the mucous membranes of the eyes.

12. Needles and sharps should be carefully and properly disposed of to prevent accidental puncture.

13. The parents of an isolated child need much support and instruction. The assistance of the infection control practitioner may be especially useful. Parents should be encouraged and welcomed at the child's bedside.

14. The room of an isolated pediatric patient should include the following: access to a sink, running water, and toilet; a box of gloves; a hand-washing agent; paper towels in a dispenser; laundry hamper support and plastic laundry bags; plastic bags for collection of trash for discard; barriers such as gowns and/or masks; and all other articles needed for admission and daily care.

15. The nurse can reduce the anxiety level of an isolated child by helping him understand that the isolation is not a punishment, by allowing him to see her face before she enters wearing a mask, by playing games, talking, cuddling, and welcoming friends and family members.

16. When caring for children with communicable diseases, the nurse should be knowledgeable about the infectious agent, mode of transmission, communicable period, incubation period, symptoms, treatment and nursing care, and prevention.

Discussion Questions

1. Identify the links in the chain of infection. Which nursing measures are able to "break" each link of the chain?

2. In addition to isolation technique, most health care institutions today use universal precautions. How are isolation technique and universal precautions used in a pediatric setting? What modifications are necessary due to the age and developmental stage of the child?

3. Why do reported cases of chickenpox exceed all other common communicable diseases of childhood? Why does chickenpox spread rapidly? Is there any risk to the parents of children with chickenpox?

4. It has recently been observed that some of the early measles vaccines did not give lifelong immunity. What problems and nursing concerns does this raise?

5. What implications does the growing number of AIDS cases and persons with HIV infection have for the pediatric nurse? What are the most common ways in which infants and children acquire HIV infection?

31

Conditions Involving the Neuromuscular and Skeletal Systems

All the systems of the body are intimately related. If a difficulty in one part of the body is severe enough or sufficiently prolonged, many body systems—in fact, the entire person—will react. The interdependence of the neuromuscular and skeletal systems is especially noteworthy.

Traumatic, infectious, or toxic injury to the nerve centers or nerve fibers that control the skeletal muscles often leads to wasting of those muscles and an inability to control or perhaps even initiate motion in related parts of the body. Poorly developed, abnormal, or damaged muscles may cause orthopedic deformities. Broken bones frequently cause muscle spasm and pain.

This chapter presents and reviews some of the more common neuromuscular and skeletal problems found in children, the methods of treatment, and the nursing care involved. Because of the amount of material, the presentation is divided into three parts. Part 1 discusses fractures, joint and extremity problems, and other conditions involving the bones and muscles; Part 2 considers

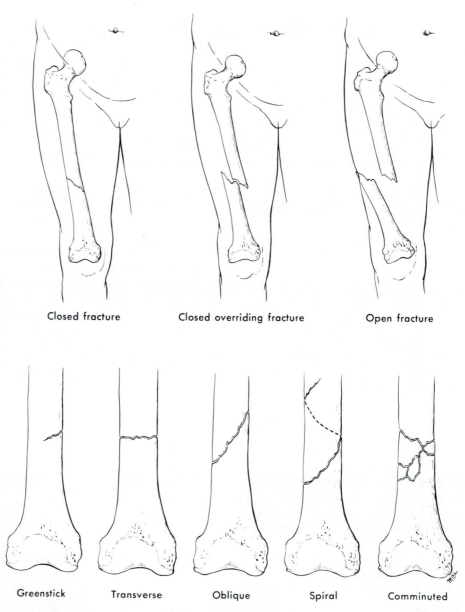

Closed fracture   Closed overriding fracture   Open fracture

Greenstick   Transverse   Oblique   Spiral   Comminuted

FIG 31-1 Types of fractures.

nervous system diseases that affect the bones and muscles; and Part 3 includes an assessment of vision, hearing, and related pediatric disorders.

A number of the problems affecting these interrelated systems are present at birth or are congenital in nature. The more common congenital defects were discussed in the chapter treating abnormalities of the newborn infant. For a brief description of hydrocephalus, cranial stenosis (craniosynostosis), microcephaly, spina bifida, clubfoot, congenital dislocated hip, syndactyly, and polydactylism, refer to Chapter 14.

Part 1: Fractures, and Joint and Extremity Problems

FRACTURES

A very common problem in childhood is a broken bone or fracture. Roller skates, skateboards, bicycles, and the rough-and-tumble life of youngsters contribute to the high incidence of fractures. Probably even more broken bones would occur in childhood if it were not for the relatively plastic condition of the child's skeletal system. Children's bones tend to bend rather than break. Frequently, if a bone does break, it is not completely severed; a portion of the bone remains intact. This type of fracture is called an incomplete or *greenstick fracture* (Fig. 31-1).

Classifications

Other common types of fractures described according to the course of the break sustained include *transverse*, *spiral*, and *oblique*. A *comminuted fracture* is especially difficult to repair because the bone is broken into more than two pieces. A *depressed fracture* is particularly important when the fractured bony area is the skull and abnormal pressure is exerted on sensitive brain tissue.

Fractures can result from excessive or sudden direct pressure, exaggerated muscular contractions, or an unsound bony structure. If an unsound bony structure is the case, the fracture is termed "pathologic." Some of the causes of pathologic fractures are osteomyelitis (infection of the bone marrow and surrounding bone cells), primary bone tumors (or metastases), and osteogenesis imperfecta congenita (congenital brittle bones), a disease of unknown origin in which bones may fracture even before birth, causing characteristic skeletal malformations occasionally accompanied by deafness. If a patient has an underlying bone disease, great care and gentleness must be practiced in turning and positioning the child (Fig. 31-2).

A careful note must be made of the general condition of a child who enters the hospital with a fracture of unknown origin, multiple fractures, or a repeated fracture. Sometimes these little patients are victims of abuse from their own parents, who are unable to meet the daily frustrations of parenthood in a mature manner or who have deep-seated psychologic problems. Such children usually exhibit bruises and suffer from malnutrition—battered child syndrome (Fig. 31-3 and pp. 407-408).

Every fracture, regardless of the course or extent of the break or its basic cause, may be placed in one or two main categories. If a bone is broken, but the skin overlying the fracture has not been pierced by the end of the

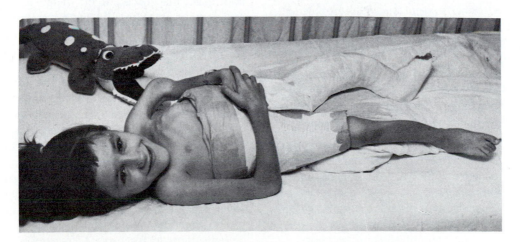

FIG 31-2 This alert young lady is a victim of osteogenesis imperfecta congenita. She was hospitalized for corrective surgery involving previous fractures. *(Courtesy Children's Hospital and Health Center, San Diego, Calif.)*

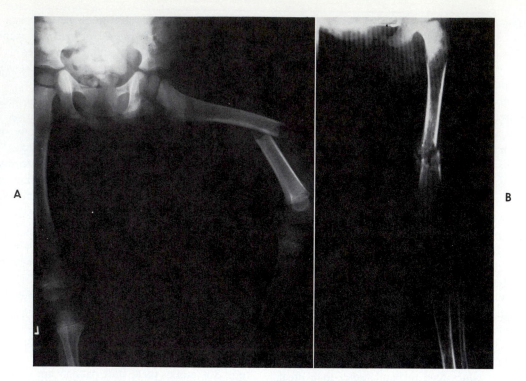

FIG 31-3 A, X-ray film of left femur of 19-lb, 2½-year-old child who entered hospital with multiple body bruises. Provisional diagnosis was "nonaccidental injury." **B,** X-ray film showing same leg after reduction of fractured femur. Shadowy outline around break is callus. *(Courtesy Naval Hospital, San Diego, Calif.)*

broken bone and no opening in the skin has occurred through which organisms could be introduced from the exterior to the bone, the result is called a *closed* (formerly *simple*) *fracture*. If, however, the skin has been broken, exposing the bone to infection, the resulting trauma is called an *open* (formerly *compound*) *fracture*. Open fractures are surgical emergencies because of the increased danger of infection and extensive soft tissue damage usually involved.

First-aid considerations

A nurse encountering an accident victim with unknown injuries should take the following action:

1. Evaluate the safety of the immediate environment (for example, turn off ignition of car, set out warning flares if on highway). Send someone for help if possible.
2. Establish an airway if respirations are not present.
3. Control hemorrhage if present.
4. Restore and maintain breathing if necessary.
5. Evaluate for spinal injury and fracture. Do not move victim until proper help is available.

6. Keep the patient warm and quiet to prevent and treat shock.

If a victim with spinal injury is moved improperly, the injury may be increased and permanent paralysis or even death may occur. If the victim is conscious but cannot move any extremity, the nurse must consider the possibility of a cervical fracture or a fracture of the thoracic spine. A patient with a possible broken neck should be moved by a team so that no twisting or injurious movement of the spine takes place. The individual should be securely positioned with sandbags and other restraints and carefully transported on a rigid support while supine with the chin up. Persons with suspected spinal injuries should be moved as little as possible. They should be frequently observed to detect the onset of respiratory difficulty and abdominal distention. The higher the injury on the spinal cord, the more body functions affected. Nonspinal fractures are less serious but still necessitate careful attention and first aid.

Indications of fracture. A fracture of an extremity may reveal itself early through the presence of the following:

1. Deformity in alignment and swelling
2. Pain or tenderness at the fracture site
3. Loss of function or abnormal mobility of the part
4. A "grating sensation" heard or felt at the suspected point of fracture (crepitus)
5. Black-and-blue areas caused by subcutaneous hemorrhage (ecchymosis)

However, the real proof of the presence of fracture is obtained by x-ray examination. Sometimes clinical symptoms are virtually lacking or inconclusive, but the x-ray film reveals a break. Every suspected skeletal injury should be treated as a fracture until proved otherwise.

Use of splints. First-aid treatment of a possible fracture includes limiting the movement of the injured part by stabilizing the part and the joint above and below the break to relieve muscle spasm and pain and to prevent further injury. A rolled newspaper, a cardboard box, or a magazine can be used for a splint. The splint should be applied in a position comfortable for the patient. The arm or leg should be splinted without an attempt to correct any deformity. No attempt should be made to straighten it because this may cause further damage. No attempt should be made to push back a broken bone protruding from the skin in the case of an open fracture. The area should simply be covered. If bleeding is present, direct manual pressure to obtain control should be used. A tourniquet should not be used because prolonged application can cause gangrene and loss of a limb. Rings and bracelets on a fractured upper extremity should be removed in the event of swelling. The application of icebags may decrease the possibility of swelling. Heat should not be applied. For bleeding from an arm or leg, the part should be elevated if possible.

When a fracture occurs involving the bones of an extremity, the muscles attached to the broken bone, which may have been under a certain amount of tension, usually contract as a result of loss of proper skeletal support. The muscles go into spasm in an effort to splint the injured part. If this spasm is exaggerated, the severed ends of the broken bone can be pulled farther out of alignment or can override, causing abnormal shortening of the limb.

Hospital care

Observation. When patients with possible fractures are first admitted to the hospital, their general condition is evaluated in detail. Vital signs (temperature, pulse, respiration, and blood pressure recordings) are obtained. Elevated blood pressure is important to report because

of the possibility of skull fracture. Low blood pressure is equally important because of the possibility of shock. The level of consciousness should be evaluated and the pupils of the eyes checked for abnormal pupil dilation or inequality of pupil size (other signs of possible skull fracture and brain injury). Depending on the patient's condition, intravenous solutions or blood may be given, but no food or fluid should be given by mouth because corrective surgery may be indicated. An x-ray examination of possible fracture sites should be made.

Reduction and casting. If overriding or angulation of a fractured bone has occurred, the displaced bone is pulled into alignment through some form of traction until the broken fragments are in proper position. The process of bringing the fragments into proper relationship is termed "reducing," or "setting," the fracture. If the fractured bone can be set without performing a surgical operation that actually exposes the involved bone, the procedure is called a *closed reduction*. If it is necessary to expose the site of the fracture to direct view to secure proper alignment and optimum healing or to use some method of internal immobilization, such as the installation of a nail, pin, or screws, the procedure is called an *open reduction*. Most children's fractures can be treated by closed reduction.

At times alignment may not be disturbed if the x-ray examination reveals a break, but the bony segments are still in proper relationship. If this is happily the case, no mechanical traction apparatus is needed. A plaster cast or protective splint is applied to maintain correct positioning to ensure proper healing. Occasionally only a relatively minor disturbance in alignment has occurred that can be reduced easily at the time the patient is first seen or may not even require reduction. In children a fracture often stimulates the formation of bone, and, curiously enough, at times the physician may desire a certain amount of overriding to prevent excessive growth of the fractured extremity.

If satisfactory alignment is difficult or impossible to achieve and maintain, some form of constant pull, or traction, must be exerted to reduce the fracture and bring the ends of the broken bone into proper alignment. The position of the bone and the progress of healing are intermittently checked by x-ray studies. When a sufficient amount of new bone (callus) is formed at the fracture site to help hold the bone segment in position, traction is discontinued and a protective cast is applied, allowing the patient more mobility. For a discussion of the basic nursing care involved in the hospitalization of a patient in traction or a cast, refer to Chapter 27.

Fractures involving the legs of infants and children are often treated by suspending both legs, wrapped in bandages, from a frame hanging directly above the bed. The infant's trunk almost entirely rests on the crib mattress, and only the pelvis is raised slightly from the surface of the bed. The legs are suspended at right angles to the mattress. Such an arrangement is called *Bryant's,* or *vertical traction* (see Fig. 27-3). It is useful in treating lower extremity fractures of infants and toddlers weighing under 30 pounds (13.63 kg). Even though only one leg is fractured, both are customarily placed in traction to stabilize the position and prevent undue twisting on the part of the child. When necessary, this traction device should be changed by the physician because this type of traction is potentially dangerous to the patient's circulation. The child should not be fussy in traction and toes should not be swollen; the physician should be notified if the child appears in distress. Older children usually are placed in types of traction similar to but smaller than those used for adults.

The healing of a broken bone, or *union* of a fracture, is accomplished through the deposit of new bone cells. In children, union is usually achieved in a relatively short time. Union is seldom delayed, and it is rare to see a case in which union never takes place.

Rehabilitation. After the bone has united, the weakened muscles attached to the bone may require gradual strengthening through a program of exercise as prescribed by the physician. This part of therapy is less necessary with young children because they start using the part immediately and usually do not need the encouragement required by many adults. The resources of the physical therapy department may be used on either an inpatient or an outpatient basis. The aims of treatment are return to function, freedom from pain, and normal appearance.

JOINT AND EXTREMITY PROBLEMS

The skeletal system can become distorted for reasons other than fracture. Some congenital deformities and intervening paralytic or inflammatory diseases of the skeletal system can cause muscular weakness or bone destruction, producing joint instability that prevents normal weight bearing. Some disorders reduce joint mobility so that the usefulness of a body part is greatly reduced. Other conditions affect the growth patterns of individual extremities. Various surgical procedures have been devised to increase the effectiveness of various body joints, either by increasing their ability to bear weight (increasing joint stability) or by permitting greater motion. If a

choice between motion and stability in the lower extremity must be made, the decision is made in favor of stability.

The following are a few of the more common procedures used to treat a wide variety of orthopedic problems.

1. *Arthrodesis* is the fusion of a joint to gain stability for weight bearing. It can be accomplished by removing the cartilage from the opposing ends of the bones that form a joint or by grafting bone into the area and then immobilizing it in a cast for a prolonged period to promote fusion. A *triple arthrodesis* is occasionally performed on a foot; as the name implies, it involves fusion of three joints. It prohibits some lateral movements of the foot itself but preserves ankle motion. Considerable bleeding can be expected after this type of surgery, and considerable pain may be involved. Weight bearing by the newly fused part is delayed until fusion is secure, in about 2 to 3 months.

2. *Arthroplasty* is the reconstruction of a joint to provide greater movement. The joints usually involved in the procedure are the hip and knee. Other procedures that involve total replacement of those joints have largely supplanted arthroplasty.

3. *Arthroscopy* is the visualization of a joint, most often the knee, by means of an arthroscope which can be inserted via a trochar through a tiny skin incision. Magnification allows diagnosis as well as some treatment procedures such as partial removal or repair of meniscal injuries.

4. *Osteotomy* is an opening into or a controlled fracture of a bone to correct a congenital or acquired skeletal deformity. In a *rotational osteotomy* the distal fragment of the bone is rotated to secure the desired correction.

5. *Tendon transplant* is a procedure in which a tendon from one part of the body is transplanted to another. It is performed for various reasons — to substitute the action of neighboring strong muscles for paralyzed or weak muscles, to replace badly damaged tendons, or to decrease a deformity caused by exaggerated muscle pull.

6. *Epiphyseal arrest* may be performed to slow the growth of one extremity that is unequal in length. A partial arrest can also aid in the correction of deformities such as knock-knees or bowlegs. It is accomplished by a bone block or by the placement

of stainless-steel staples into the epiphyseal area, where bone growth takes place. This procedure stops normal growth. The staples are removed when the desired results are obtained.

7. *Leg lengthening* is a difficult but possible alternative procedure for leg-length inequality. An osteotomy is performed followed by separation of the bone, bone grafting if necessary, and external fixation that allows gradual stretching over a period of several weeks.

8. *Open reduction and internal fixation* (ORIF) is the operative procedure used when a fracture requires open visualization to reduce it and stabilization by means of metal fixation. In children, fractures often heal as well and as quickly without this surgical procedure.

CONDITIONS INVOLVING THE BONES AND MUSCLES

Because many pediatric nursing courses are organized according to developmental sequence, the following conditions are presented according to the age group primarily affected. Such an approach is not without inconsistencies. Some conditions extend to children of all ages; moreover, many problems are present in infancy but are not diagnosed until later in childhood.

Infant

Torticollis (Fig. 31-4). Torticollis, or wryneck, is a congenital muscular abnormality often associated with birth trauma. Although the defect is minimal at birth, within 2 weeks a palpable fibrous tumor appears in the sternocleidomastoid muscle. The cause of these tumors is unknown. Within a few months the fibrous tumor gradually disappears, leaving behind a contracture (shortening) of the muscle. The head of the infant is tilted toward the side of the affected muscle, and the chin is rotated to the opposite side. When the condition is recognized early, treatment consists of passive stretching of the involved muscle. Parents are instructed in the exact maneuvers to be performed four or five times daily. The reward for faithful treatment is complete and permanent correction in at least 90% of the cases. When torticollis does not respond to conservative measures or when treatment is not consistent, surgery is indicated. The affected muscle is divided or partially excised. The head is immobilized in the correct position for a period of time. If surgery is delayed until the child is older, postoperative exercises are necessary to prevent a recurrence.

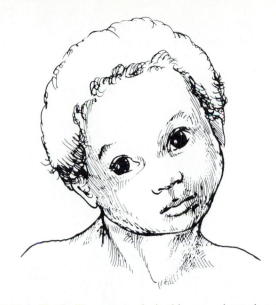

FIG 31-4 Torticollis or wryneck: in this case, shortening of right sternocleidomastoid muscle.

Childhood rickets. One disease resulting from nutritional disturbance is common childhood rickets. The name is misleading because nowadays a classic example of this disease is sometimes difficult to find in the United States. Rickets is always a potential health hazard in communities where there is little sunshine or little exposure of children to the outdoors and a diet deficient in vitamin D, calcium, or phosphorus. Vitamin D is crucial because it regulates the absorption and deposit of calcium and phosphorus. Most formulas are specially irradiated or fortified to provide adequate levels of vitamin D to infants and children. Other rich sources are the fish-liver oils. Sunshine, if it is not screened by window glass and clothing or rendered unavailable by air pollution, is the most inexpensive source of vitamin D. Of course, vitamin preparations can be purchased. Cases of rickets can be mild and pass undetected or very severe and remarkable. Classic manifestations are knock-knees or bowlegs, kyphosis (humpback) or scoliosis (an abnormal lateral spinal curvature), delayed closure of fontanels and protruding forehead (bossing), thickened wrists and ankles, enlargement of the cartilaginous area of attachment of the ribs to the sternum, forming the famous *rachitic rosary*, pigeon breast, and contracture of the pelvis. Treatment consists in greater intake of vitamin D, calcium, and phosphorus. It is possible but not likely for a person to have an excessive vitamin D intake. Discretion should be used in the selection and dosage of therapeutic vitamins.

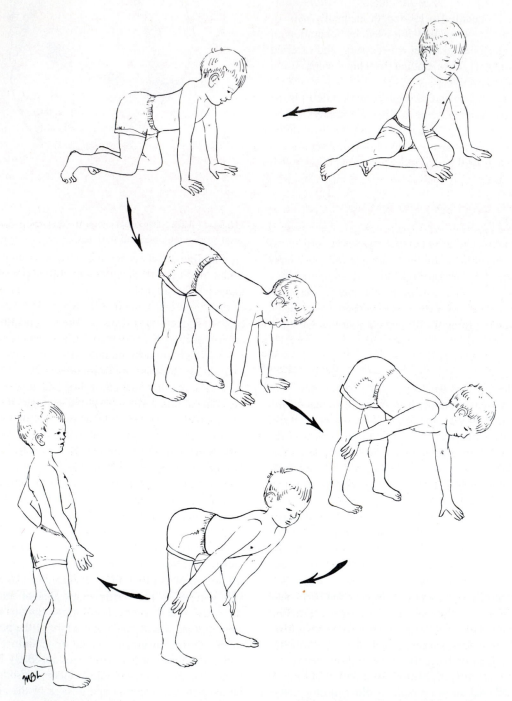

FIG 31-5   Gower's sign, "self-climbing procedure," characteristic of pseudohypertrophic muscular dystrophy.

Toddler

Duchenne's muscular dystrophy. A number of conditions are characterized by a progressive weakening of the musculoskeletal system and eventual wasting of muscle tissue. They differ in the main muscles affected, the course of the disability, and the typical age of onset. Duchenne's or (pseudohypertrophic) progressive muscular dystrophy is the most common form of the progressive types of muscle weakness. The onset of this disease usually occurs between the third and sixth years. It is a hereditary, sex-linked, recessive condition that affects males almost exclusively. Recently the gene that causes the disease was discovered. This genetic breakthrough allows for accurate carrier detection and even prenatal diagnosis and hopefully will lead to a successful treatment. In this type of dystrophy, a fatty infiltration of the muscle cells may produce a deceptively large muscle lacking strength, hence its title "pseudohypertrophic" muscular dystrophy. This condition is seen most often in the calf muscles. Intramuscular enzymes, creatine phosphokinase (CPK) and serum aldolase, leak into the blood serum as muscle tissue breaks down. Serum values of these enzymes are high in the early stages of the disease but decline as the disease progresses, and in the final stages they are only slightly above normal (apparently because so little muscle tissue is left). The affected young child has difficulty in walking and falls easily as the muscular weakness attacks, in sequence, the muscles of the legs, pelvis, and abdomen. A pronounced lordosis develops as the youngster struggles to remain upright. These children display a characteristic method of supporting themselves when attempting to rise to their feet from a seated posture on the floor. They rise to their knees, extend their legs and arms, grasp the lower part of their legs with their hands, and gradually push themselves upward in a self-climbing procedure. This maneuver is referred to as *Gower's sign* and is one of the most characteristic signs of muscular dystrophy (Fig. 31-5). The genetic background of the family, the history and examination of the child revealing the progressive nature of the disease, serum enzyme tests, electromyogram, and muscle biopsy confirm the diagnosis. Muscle biopsy is especially valuable in determining the exact type of muscular problem. It is currently possible to diagnose preclinical cases through determination of serum enzyme levels. Counseling of affected families and potential carriers is an important preventive measure.

A diagnosis of muscular dystrophy (no matter what type) is difficult for parents to accept. The term alone produces anxiety and fear in parents, so it must be emphasized that nonprogressive and indeed treatable muscle disorders may mimic Duchenne's. Only with confirmation by available techniques should parents be informed of this diagnosis.

Duchenne's muscular dystrophy is a tragic model of neuromuscular disease. Life expectancy is usually limited to the teenage period. Death often results from respiratory weakness and intervening infection. The course of the disease is downhill, and it is particularly disheartening for parents to see their child confined to a wheelchair and then bedridden to the extent that he needs help to turn over. Many times much can be gained if the parents of such children can meet together to share their common burdens and to learn from one another how certain problems can be met. The Muscular Dystrophy Association sponsors numerous clinics where those children can be cared for.

The nurse sees the child with muscular dystrophy in the hospital setting chiefly at the time of diagnosis. She may also see him when orthopedic appliances, such as braces and splints, are being evaluated or when the child is admitted for other health problems that make it difficult to nurse him at home.

Juvenile rheumatoid arthritis. The most common form of chronic arthritis encountered in pediatrics is juvenile rheumatoid arthritis (JRA). This disease is often grouped with the collagen vascular diseases and may affect a patient's entire health. Three major types of JRA are (1) a systemic form, characterized by fever, rash, internal organ involvement, and arthritis (though not always); (2) a polyarticular form (arthritis in numerous large and small joints); and (3) a pauciarticular form (arthritis in only a few joints). The arthritis manifests itself with joints that become swollen, stiff, painful with movement, and occasionally warm. The arthritis may involve just the knee or the ankle (as in the pauciarticular form), or nearly all joints, with the knees, ankles, wrists, and fingers more frequently affected. The fingers often assume a spindle shape, as a result of swelling of their middle joints (Fig. 31-6).

Signs and symptoms of JRA other than arthritis can occur, particularly in the systemic form, and may include enlargement of the liver, spleen, and lymph nodes, anemia, anorexia, pallor, and a salmon-colored, blotchy rash. Pericarditis and myocarditis are seen occasionally. Fever may be a significant manifestation of the disease. The patient's temperature may swing daily, reaching as high as 105° F (40.5° C) in the evening and return to normal by morning. The pattern on the temperature chart is usually characteristic and of great value in diagnosing systemic JRA.

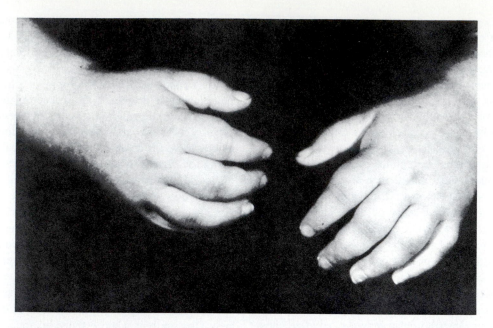

FIG 31-6   Juvenile rheumatoid arthritis. Spindle-shaped fingers in 2½-year-old boy. *(Courtesy Naval Hospital, San Diego, Calif.)*

Uveitis is a complication of juvenile rheumatoid arthritis in about 5% of patients. Inflammation in the anterior chamber of the eye can occur with no symptoms; therefore, patients with JRA need to be followed on a regular basis by an ophthalmologist. Uveitis can be so severe that blindness can result.

Anti-inflammatory medications, physical and occupational therapy, kind and understanding parental support, and promotion of general health all are important aspects of therapy. Nonsteroidal anti-inflammatory drugs (NSAIDs) are the drugs of choice to relieve pain, reduce swelling, and increase range of motion. When aspirin is used, it is prescribed four times daily at high doses. Blood salicylate levels are evaluated to ensure that proper doses are given. Children are carefully monitored and the parents cautioned about early signs of toxicity (p. 405). NSAIDs other than aspirin, such as ibuprofen, tolmetin, and naproxen, are beginning to be used more often because of their lower toxicity and less frequent dose requirements as compared with aspirin. These drugs can be just as effective as aspirin when used in significant doses and do not require blood level monitoring.

A second drug for treatment of patients with JRA is gold salts. This medication, often given in addition to an NSAID, can slowly relieve joint symptoms in difficult cases. It is given weekly usually by injection, although it is now available in oral form. Renal and hematologic complications can occur with gold therapy, so a complete blood cell count and urinalysis are performed before each dose of gold.

In rare instances, prednisone or other corticosteroids may also be used for the treatment of JRA, particularly in sytemic disease, refractory polyarticular disease, and uveitis. Steroids can greatly alleviate the symptoms of arthritis but do not affect the basic disease process. The usefulness of steroids is limited by their toxicity. Unwanted manifestations of such hormone therapy include decalcification of the skeleton, altered tissue response to infections and other injuries, personality changes, moon face, obesity, and excessive body hair (Fig. 31-7).

The JRA patient is likely to assume positions of comfort, which, if maintained for prolonged periods, can cause deformities that interfere with motions necessary for meeting the needs of daily living. Mobility should be encouraged as much as can be tolerated even during periods of active disease and inflammation. When pain and inflammation are suppressed by NSAIDs, children are then encouraged to ambulate and resume as close to normal activities as possible.

The most effective, continuous therapeutic exercise program is provided through the child's own play activities. Play activities should be directed to provide the maximum exercise for the joints most involved. The physical therapist can teach children and their parents

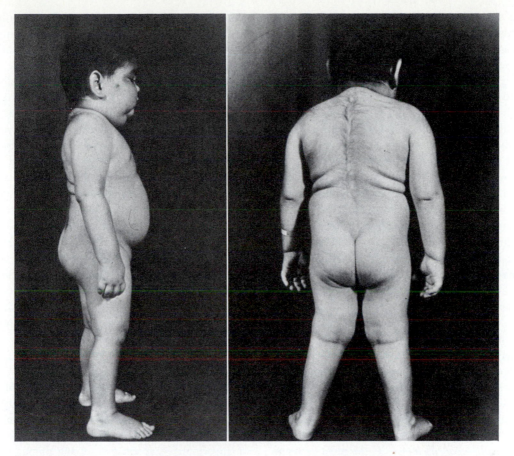

FIG 31-7 Hypercortisonism in 2½-year-old boy as result of intensive steroid therapy. Note moon facies, excessive growth of hair (hirsutism), prominent fat pads, buffalo hump, and marked weight gain. *(Courtesy Naval Hospital, San Diego, Calif.)*

exercises designed to give improved range of motion in each joint. Play activity and formal exercises help prevent the stiffness and deformity that result from inactivity.

JRA often gradually improves over a period of years, and usually subsides in the teen years. In rare cases, it may persist actively into adulthood. Even though JRA often "burns out" eventually, children can be left with difficult, lifelong joint deformities as a result of their years of active disease.

Orthopedic complications of hemophilia. The subject of damaged joints should not be completely closed without at least mentioning another interesting cause of joint difficulty. The child with hemophilia, the classic bleeder, may sustain considerable joint destruction because of "insignificant injuries" followed by hemorrhages into the joints of the knees and elbows. At times these patients

must be placed in traction and protective casts to treat this problem.

Preschool child

Legg-Calvé-Perthes disease (coxa plana). Legg-Calvé-Perthes disease is a self-limited disease of the hip produced by lack of circulation to the femoral head. The initial degeneration of the femoral head is followed by absorption and regeneration of bone. The entire process takes an average of 4 years.

This developmental disease of the hip is commonly seen in children between 4 and 8 years of age and has a much higher incidence in boys. Usually the initial complaint is a limp of several months' duration. Some children have a limp with pain (referred to the knee) that is aggravated by activity and relieved by rest. The primary cause of Legg-Calvé-Perthes disease is unknown.

Trauma and synovitis of the hip have preceded some cases. A great variety of treatments has been used, including 4 years of bed rest. Modern successful treatment of the disease centers around two basic principles: (1) maintaining a full range of motion and (2) keeping the femoral head deep in the socket during its period of healing. In this way the physician seeks to obtain a femoral head that fits well and to prevent the development of degenerative arthritis in the later years.

Treatment consists of traction until symptoms are resolved, followed by hip bracing in an abducted and slightly internally rotated position to maintain properly the femoral head in the acetabulum. Such bracing removes pressure from the avascular head of the femur. It helps to keep the child ambulatory with the least discomfort and limitation of activity during the years of necessary management. Surgery on the pelvis or femur may be indicated in the more severe cases of Legg-Calvé-Perthes disease. In general, the younger child at the time of diagnosis has a more favorable prognosis for development of a normal hip.

Osteomyelitis. Inflammatory bone conditions caused by disease-producing organisms were more common in the past. With the increased availability of different types of antibiotics, osteomyelitis (inflammation of the bone resulting from infectious agents) has decreased remarkably. Osteomyelitis can result from various types of infection, but *Staphylococcus aureus* is the most common invading organism. Less common causes are *H. influenzae*, group A beta-hemolytic streptococcus, and *Mycobacterium tuberculosis*.

Osteomyelitis is sometimes preceded by some type of local injury to the bone that either introduces the organism directly or weakens the bone so that it is more susceptible to any offending organisms brought to the area by the bloodstream from some distant source of infection.

Blood-borne infections are most common. Boys are more frequently affected than girls. Fever and pain near the end of a long bone are clinically associated with osteomyelitis. The characteristic pain is initially very severe and unremitting because pressure is building up in a closed space. Pseudoparalysis is a common presenting symptom in the young child who refuses to move the affected area because of pain. When pus begins to track out under the periosteum, the area is extremely tender, more so than a fracture. Treatment is started on the basis of the clinical examination alone. The child is placed on a regimen of bed rest, and the affected limb is immobilized. Analgesics are given to lessen the pain.

Although blood cultures are positive in only 50% of patients with osteomyelitis, they are taken immediately and during the first few days after examination in the hope of identifying the causative organism. Aspiration and culture of fluid at the suspected site of infection, and radionuclide bone scans may also aid in the specific diagnosis. Initially large doses of broad-spectrum antibiotics are given. X-ray evidence of osteomyelitis is not seen for 10 days following the onset of symptoms. Surgery is considered necessary if improvement is not seen within 36 to 48 hours after antibiotic therapy is instituted. The area of maximum tenderness is drilled to decompress the bone and to allow the pus to drain. The organism responsible for the infection is identified, and a cast may be applied to the affected limb. Intravenous antibiotic therapy is continued for another 3 to 6 weeks. During this time progress of the infection may be monitored by frequent sedimentation rates. When the results of this test are nearly normal, antibiotics can be stopped, and hopefully, the risk of chronic osteomyelitis and extensive bone damage has been minimized.

School-age child

Bone tumors. Some of the symptoms of infectious osteomyelitis are duplicated when the cause is not pathogenic organisms but the development of abnormal cells producing a tumor within the bone. Some of these masses of abnormal tissue are *benign* and of purely local importance. They may cause pain, at times accompanied by fever and deformity. The tumors may weaken the structure of the bone, but they do not spread (metastasize) to distant parts of the body. Other types of bone tumors grow rapidly and metastasize early through the bloodstream. These tumors are *malignant*. An osteosarcoma originates in connective tissue (of which bone is one example) and is the most common primary malignant tumor of bone. School-age boys are affected almost twice as often as girls. The most common sites are characterized by active epiphyseal growth (for example, the distal end of the femur and the proximal ends of the tibia and humerus). Initially the child complains of mild pain in the affected part, but in a matter of days to weeks, the pain is constant and severe. As the condition progresses, the tumor mass becomes obvious. Limitation of adjacent joint motion is common. Early diagnosis and immediate treatment are crucial.

X-ray studies are characteristic, but the diagnosis of bone tumor is made only after biopsy and pathologic studies of the tissue. Occasionally tumors of the bone in children may be secondary to tumors located elsewhere.

When a tissue of bony origin is malignant, aggressive anticancer chemotherapy and radical methods of treatment, including amputation, must be endorsed in an effort to save the patient. The prognosis has been vastly improved with recent advances in surgical treatment combined with multiple drug chemotherapy. Various limb salvage procedures have been developed to allow removal of bone tumors with maintenance of good form and function. The most recent development involves the use of an expandable internal prosthesis that can be lengthened as the child grows.

Spinal curvature. Scoliosis (S-shaped lateral curvature), kyphosis (humpback), and lordosis (exaggerated lumbar curvature) are abnormal types of spinal curvature.

Scoliosis. Of the three kinds of abnormal spinal curvatures, scoliosis (lateral curvature) is probably the most common spinal deformity encounted in childhood. Lateral curvature of the spine can be divided into two major

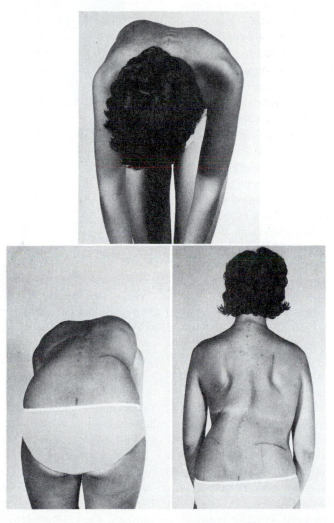

FIG 31-8 Idiopathic scoliosis in 14-year-old girl seen in first visit to orthopedist. Screening positions: standing and forward bend. Observe for (1) general posture and alignment of spine: (a) lateral angulation and (b) balance of head, neck, and shoulders over pelvis; and (2) asymmetry: (a) exaggerated flank crease—more prominent on opposite side, (b) high shoulder, (c) position of scapulae, (d) convexity on side of major curve (caused by protruding ribs), (e) prominent hip, and (f) one arm longer than other when hanging free in forward bend position. *(Courtesy Naval Hospital, San Diego, Calif.)*

groups: nonstructural (functional) and structural. The patient can voluntarily correct a nonstructural curve by altering position. In functional scoliosis, a condition outside the spine (such as poor posture, pain or muscle spasm, or short leg) can cause a temporary misalignment of the vertebrae. A structural scoliosis is an irreversible lateral curvature that leads to permanent anatomic changes unless early preventive measures are taken.

Three basic types of structural scoliosis are seen: congenital, paralytic, and idiopathic. Congenital scoliosis results when one side of the vertebral column grows faster than the other. Surgical correction at 1 or 2 years of age may be indicated to prevent greater asymmetric growth. Paralytic scoliosis may result from poliomyelitis, Duchenne type muscular dystrophy, myelomeningocele, or other neuromuscular disorders. To prevent respiratory complications, some type of stabilization of the spine must be considered either through external support or surgery. Idiopathic scoliosis is the most common type, accounting for 80% of the cases classified as structural. It is called idiopathic because the cause is unknown. However, there seems to be a definite familial tendency that suggests a dominant inheritance pattern. The condition is more common in girls and is most apparent during adolescence, although it usually begins much earlier. The level of the curve may be cervical, thoracic, lumbar, or a combination of these. The most important aspect of the deformity is its progression with skeletal growth. As the lateral curvature and rotation of the spine increases, permanent secondary changes develop in the vertebrae and ribs. Misalignment of the spinal joints worsens and eventually leads to painful degenerative spinal joint disease in adulthood. In addition to a "crooked back" with a high shoulder and prominent hip, the deformity of the spine may compromise cardiopulmonary function and shorten the patient's life expectancy. The progression of the curvature is slow and steady, seldom arousing the concern of the parent or child. Poor posture, an uneven hemline, and inability to get a proper fit in clothing are common complaints that cause the parents to bring the child in for evaluation. Because pain is not associated with the progressive curve, the deformity often reaches 30 degrees before it is detected. The deformity can be clinically evaluated in three positions (Fig. 31-8). Radiologic studies confirm the extent of the deformity. The primary (major) curve is greatest in angulation and is the least flexible. It is always more marked than would be expected from the physical appearance (Fig. 31-9).

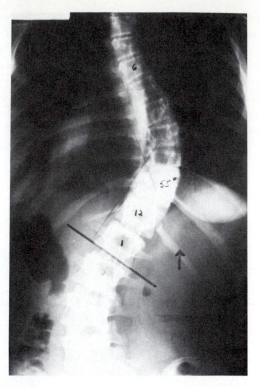

FIG 31-9 Radiograph of 14-year-old girl (same as in Fig. 31-8) shows 55 degree right thoracic curve of spine. *(Courtesy Naval Hospital, San Diego, Calif.)*

Screening. The only sure way of preventing the severe curvatures of idiopathic scoliosis, which usually involve major surgical procedures and their inherent risk, is by early recognition. The presence of a mild deformity allows the use of reliable, safe, effective nonsurgical treatment. Most children who demonstrate a curve at 11 or 12 years of age have almost always had it for a number of years. Therefore screening programs for lateral curvatures should begin before 10 years of age and include boys as well as preadolescent girls. Routine inspection of the spine by school nurses can be most rewarding.

Treatment. An orthopedist should determine the need for correction and examine the child with scoliosis at regular intervals to detect any progression of the curve. Curves up to 20 degrees can probably be left alone and watched. Curves between 20 and 40 degrees and progressing are stabilized with a brace. The *Milwaukee brace* (Fig. 31-10) is the standard device used in the nonoperative treatment of mild spinal curvatures. It is designed to provide dynamic correction that incorporates a vertical pushing force between the head and pelvis

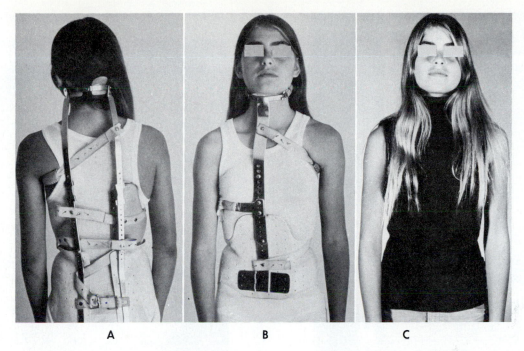

FIG 31-10 **A,** Thirteen-year-old girl wearing Milwaukee brace with right thoracic pad, left axillary sling, and left lumbar pad. Overall alignment is good. **B,** Same child, front view. Brace is contoured closely to body. **C,** Brace can be worn under clothing without being noticed.

through adjustable, rigid uprights, as well as a lateral corrective force directed toward the convex side of the major curve. The brace is well contoured and cosmetically acceptable. To prevent worsening of the scoliosis, it is necessary to wear the brace full time (for several years), except for brief periods needed for personal hygiene, until complete maturation of the spine has occurred. Prevention of progression of the curve is likely when treatment is begun at an early age. Normal activities (such as bike riding and skating) are encouraged while wearing the brace. In fact, an active exercise program is required to maintain good muscle tone. Most children learn to accept and live with the brace and have good results. Underarm braces are currently being considered as possible alternatives to the Milwaukee brace.

Surgical correction is usually considered for curves that are over 40 degrees. Surgery offers the best outcome for (1) curves that are cosmetically objectionable (over 60 degrees) in the preadolescent or postadolescent patient and (2) a growing child in whom conservative measures have failed. The operation consists of a spinal fusion supplemented by the insertion and spinal attachment of an internal apparatus. The Harrington rod serves to obtain correction and to provide an internal type of immobili-

zation (Fig. 31-11). After spinal fusion the patient may be placed in a body cast or brace postoperatively; then progressive ambulation in the cast or brace is encouraged (Fig. 31-12). Complete union and maturation at the fusion site takes about 1 year. However, newer surgical techniques and more refined instrumentation are allowing much earlier mobilization and a shorter time period for recuperation.

Halo traction. The halo traction is used in the treatment of a rigid spinal curvature associated with weakness or paralysis of the neck and trunk muscles. It also is employed in the care of cervical fractures and fusions. The halo consists of a metal ring attached to the skull by two posterior pins in the occipital bone and two anterior pins inserted into the temporal or frontal bones. It is attached to a weight while countertraction is exerted by weights connected to two Steinmann pins, which are inserted into the distal ends of both femurs. The weights are increased daily as tolerated by the child until maximum correction is obtained.

When maximum correction of the curve is evidenced by x-ray examination, a spinal fusion is usually done. Weighted halo traction may be continued to prevent loss of the correction, or a body cast or jacket is applied,

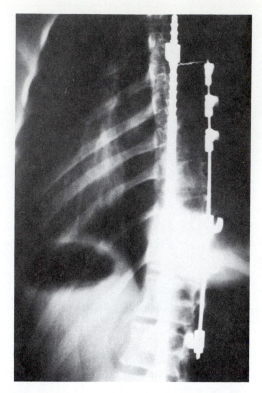

FIG 31-11 Radiograph of back of patient in Fig. 31-8, 6 months after spinal fusion and Harrington instrumentation. *(Courtesy Naval Hospital, San Diego, Calif.)*

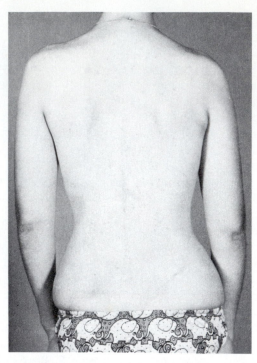

FIG 31-12 Postoperative standing position shows girl's spine reasonably well compensated (same girl as in Fig. 31-8). *(Courtesy Naval Hospital, San Diego, Calif.)*

incorporating the halo by means of an extended frame, to maintain the gains accomplished by the original traction and fusion.

Nursing care. The procedure should be explained step by step to children in words that they can understand. Their questions should be answered carefully. They may complain that the pins hurt. This usually indicates that the pins are loose, and it may be necessary for the physician to change one or more of the pins to a different site. The pins are cleaned daily with hydrogen peroxide, and the skin around each pin is painted with antiseptic.

Proper alignment of all equipment, especially the ropes, is necessary for effective traction. Young patients may prefer to remain in the supine position but should be turned at least every 2 hours, from back to side and side to back. Patients are encouraged to breathe deeply for a few minutes each time they are turned. Adequate ventilation of the lungs is extremely important because a respiratory deficit often accompanies advanced scoliosis. Treatment includes promotion of pulmonary function, which is accomplished by specific breathing exercises.

Active and passive range of motion helps maintain muscular strength. Careful attention is given to the skin, especially bony prominences and the heels. Neurologic and cardiac complications are not unusual. Appropriate notice should be given to these important considerations without frightening the child. Bowel and bladder difficulties are common. They may be lessened by adequate intake of fluids, foods rich in bulk, and occasionally laxatives. Remember that immobilization decreases appetite. Children should be given every opportunity to select their diets when a choice is possible. Their psychologic growth is just as important as their physical well-being.

Spinal fusion. Casts, which may be worn for an extended period after a spinal fusion, make turning the patient much simpler and safer. However, if a cast is not applied after a spinal fusion, care must be exercised so that the spinal column is not twisted during changes in position. The patient's bed should be kept flat unless specific permission has been granted to allow the patient to be on a slight incline while in *supine* position (on the back). A noncasted patient who is allowed to be turned should be gently log-rolled from back to side with the use of a turning sheet and at least two nurses (more if the size of the patient indicates that more hands are needed). Such a patient, casted or not, who is turned from the back to a side-lying position, should have a pillow between the thighs to prevent the adduction of the top leg and pull on the small of the back. Just how much motion is allowed a patient depends on the physician's wishes. Assessment for nerve damage from the surgery is important to consider, especially in the early post operative period.

Patients who have had a spinal fusion need the same basic preoperative and postoperative care required for all surgical patients. In addition, they need the special attention necessary for all casted patients (Chapter 27). Constipation is a particular problem; therefore the type of diet, fluid intake, and habit-times require special attention.

Therapy for severe scoliosis is usually long. It characteristically involves innumerable visits to the physician for evaluation, hospitalization at intervals for cast changes, brace adjustments or surgical interventions, and physical therapy. The parents and child (young woman or man) must be constantly encouraged to continue treatment faithfully until optimum, lasting results are achieved.

Part 2: Nervous System Diseases Affecting Bones and Muscles

INFANT

Seizure disorders

The term *convulsive seizure* denotes an excessive and disorderly discharge from nervous tissue, resulting in involuntary muscular activity or lapses in consciousness. It is really not a diagnosis but simply a description of a transient disturbance of the central nervous system (Fig. 31-13). As noted, seizures are caused by a number of conditions. Significant fever may be the precipitating cause, especially in children aged 6 to 36 months. Seizures also originate from congenital brain deformities or increased intracranial pressure caused by tumors, abscess formation, or edema of the brain. Cerebral irritation resulting from toxic or infectious agents may be implicated. A chronic or recurrent convulsive disorder may also be called *epilepsy*. Some writers reserve the term "epilepsy" for recurrent convulsions of the idiopathic variety (cases of unknown cause). Opinions differ regarding the role of heredity in idiopathic seizures. Some authorities believe that heredity may be a significant cause. Because

some states and communities have laws limiting the activities of those persons who have been diagnosed as epileptic and because the public does not always understand what the word means in a specific case, many physicians hesitate to use this particular term when describing the patient's problem. The nurse would also do well to use the word discreetly. It is estimated that approximately 1% of the population has some type of epileptic disorder. An additional 2% have had febrile seizures.

The two main types of seizures are partial and generalized (Table 31-1). Children with partial seizures experience focal symptoms such as motor, sensory, or experiential phenomena. Partial seizures are called simple partial if there is no loss of consciousness and partial complex if consciousness is impaired. Seizures are classified according to specific symptoms experienced or witnessed at the time of the event (p. 661). The generalized, tonic-clonic type represents one half of all seizure disorders, and the absence type, also known as petit mal represents about 10% of all seizure disorders. Twenty percent of epileptics have mixed seizure disorders, which manifest characteristics of more than one type. Generalized or tonic-clonic seizures affect the large muscle groups of the body. Usually the entire body becomes involved in dramatic, involuntary muscular contractions of considerable force. Absence seizures, on the other hand, are characterized by brief losses of consciousness revealed perhaps only by a prolonged blank stare or by minor tremors or the dropping of an object held in the hand. The frequency of either type of seizure can be variable. A child may experience a seizure rarely or many times during a 24-hour period. Diagnosis is aided by a study of the child's brain waves, or an electroencephalogram (EEG).

Children who have tonic-clonic seizures may experience a subjective warning of an impending episode. Such a warning is called an *aura*. It usually occurs a few minutes before the attack. It may come in the form of a vague feeling of uneasiness or as some type of sensory cue. For example, the patient may hear, see, or smell things in a particular manner. Such auras are useful to patients because they can seek out places of safety and privacy if they are forewarned of an attack. In small children the presence of an aura may only be detected through the awareness of a child's repetitive actions, such as climbing into mother's lap, preceding a seizure.

The tonic-clonic seizure usually begins with a period of rigidity and temporary respiratory arrest. The first sign of an attack may be involuntary movements of the eyeball

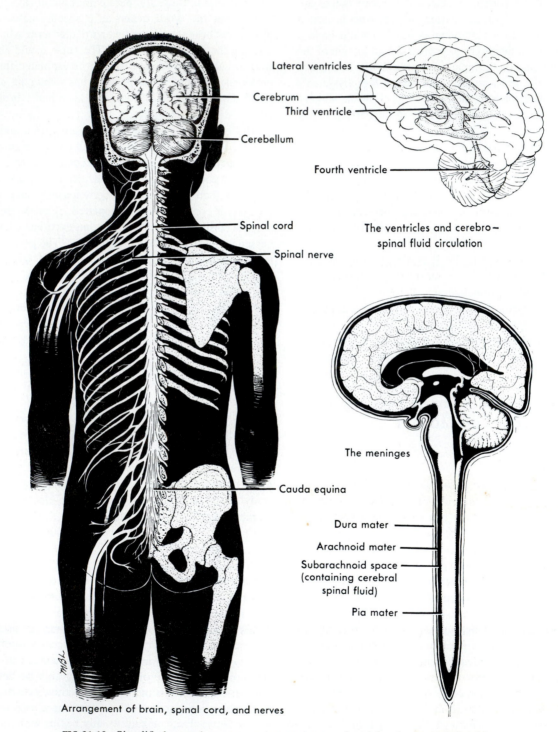

Lateral ventricles

Cerebrum

Third ventricle

Cerebellum

Fourth ventricle

The ventricles and cerebro—
spinal fluid circulation

Spinal cord

Spinal nerve

The meninges

Cauda equina

Dura mater

Arachnoid mater

Subarachnoid space
(containing cerebral
spinal fluid)

Pia mater

Arrangement of brain, spinal cord, and nerves

FIG 31-13   Simplified central nervous system anatomy and peripheral nerve relationships.

Table 31-1 Classification of seizures

Type of seizure	Clinical manifestation
Partial	Begins locally
1. Simple	Without loss of consciousness
a. With motor symptoms	Focal motor (Jacksonian seizure)
b. With somatosensory or special sensory	Abdominal disturbances or visual, auditory, and olfactory symptoms and/or dizziness
2. Complex	With impairment of consciousness (temporal lobe or psychomotor)
Generalized	Bilateral, symmetric onset
1. Absence	Brief loss of contact (petit mal)
2. Tonic-clonic	Major tonic-clonic motor activity (grand mal)
3. Infantile spasms	Myoclonic (brief symmetric flexion of head or trunk with mild clonus of arm and legs)

(eyes rolling upward or to the side) and a stiffening of body parts. The patient temporarily suspends respirations and may become cyanotic. Saliva is not swallowed, and the patient may drool. The patient may utter a high-pitched cry. This first period, called the *tonic phase,* is usually followed by intermittent contractions of the muscles. This secondary period is the so-called *clonic phase.* During this time the tongue and lips may be bitten, and saliva, as a result, may be blood-tinged.

The nursing care of a patient having a convulsion emphasizes the need to protect the patient from accidental injury and the importance of close observation and report. If possible, a patient should be placed on the side or lie with face turned to one side to prevent aspiration. He or she should be placed in an area where the possibility of personal injury due to uncontrolled muscular contractions is at a minimum: on the floor on a rug, if

possible, or in bed. The beds or cribs of patients who experience frequent seizures of tonic-clonic type should be equipped with side rails padded with folded blankets or pillows. In the hospital setting nurses previously have been taught to have a well-padded tongue blade at the bedside for insertion into the mouth between the back teeth before the onset of the clonic phase of the seizure to prevent mouth injury. However, in most instances a blade is not required; sometimes its use causes more problems such as loss of teeth or mouth lacerations than use of nothing at all. Nurses should not pry open a patient's mouth to insert a tongue blade. This can cause considerable injury and serves no practical purpose because the damage to the mouth in most cases has already occurred. Most hospitals have discontinued routine use of a tongue blade unless ordered by a physician, and the Epilepsy Society does not advise the general public to place anything into the person's mouth.

After first securing a safe position for the convulsing patient, the nurse should focus her powers of observation to later describe the circumstances and sequence of the attack. She should note the following:

1. When the seizure began and what type of activity immediately preceded its occurrence
2. What signs of difficulty were first noted, what part of the body was first affected, the position of the eyes, and how the convulsion progressed
3. How long the attack lasted and whether fever preceded or followed the attack
4. Whether the patient was incontinent
5. Whether prolonged cyanosis or profuse saliva appeared (may signal the need for the use of oxygen or possible suctioning)

In the majority of cases the seizure (ictus) subsides, and the child falls into a deep sleep called the *postictal state.* When awake again, the child may not remember the seizure but may feel tired and sore. Children should be reassured regarding the episode and be gently questioned to determine whether they had any warning, or aura, of the attack.

Almost all patients who suffer from idiopathic epilepsy and many with organically initiated seizures receive some type of anticonvulsant therapy. A number of medications are available, prescribed according to the individual needs of the patient. Some commonly used drugs to stop or control seizures are listed in Table 31-2. The time schedule established for taking anticonvulsants should be faithfully followed to prevent any interruption

NURSING CARE PLAN

The Child with a Seizure Disorder

Selected nursing diagnoses	Expected outcomes	Interventions

A. Potential for injury related to sudden loss of consciousness
Clinical manifestations:
Presence of seizure, disorientation.
	Child remains free from physical injury.	On admission, obtain seizure history and avoid situations known to elicit seizures.
		Keep siderails up.
		Pad head of bed and siderails.
		Keep area free of sharp and hard objects.
		Loosen any tight clothing.
		Do not restrain child's movements.
		Do not put anything in child's mouth.
		Place child on side or abdomen to prevent aspiration.
		Observe circumstances and sequence of seizure:
		  a. Time of onset and preceding activity
		  b. Location and type of movements
		  c. Duration of seizure
		  d. Incontinence
		  e. Salivation, cyanosis, respiratory distress

B. Ineffective airway clearance related to aspiration of saliva, foreign objects, or obstruction by tongue. Clinical manifestations: Increased salivation, coughing, cyanosis.	Child maintains patent airway.	Prevent known seizure activity, administer medication on time. Position child on side or abdomen to prevent aspiration. Observe for apnea and cyanosis. Suction as needed. Insert oral airway if indicated and administer oxygen as needed.
C. Anxiety related to loss of control during seizure and possible complications. Clinical manifestations: Verbalization of fears, embarrassment by loss of body control.	Child/parent verbalizes fear and concerns.	Stay with child after seizure. Discuss seizure events with child/parent. Listen to child/parent concerns and reassure as needed. Review medication protocol.

Table 31-2 Anticonvulsant guide

Medication and therapeutic blood level	Indication for use
Phenobarbital (15-40 μg/ml)	Tonic-clonic seizures Simple and complex partial seizures
Phenytoin (Dilantin) (10-20 μg/ml)	Tonic-clonic seizures Simple and complex partial seizures
Carbamazepine (Tegretol) (4-12 μg/ml)	Complex partial seizures Tonic-clonic seizures Simple partial seizures
Valproate (Depakene) (50-100 μg/ml)	Absence seizures Myoclonic seizures
Ethosuximide (Zarontin) (40-100 μg/ml)	Absence seizures
Clonazepam (Clonopin)	Absence seizures Myoclonic seizures (anticonvulsant not usually used)
Primidone (Mysoline) (4-12 μg/ml)	Complex partial seizures Tonic-clonic seizures
Clorazepate (Tranxene)	Partial and generalized seizures refractory to other medicines

in treatment and the possible appearance of a seizure. Other methods to prevent seizures stress a high-fat–low-carbohydrate (ketogenic) diet.

Complete or almost complete control can be obtained in approximately one half of cases. The condition of many patients can be well regulated with medical therapy, and these persons are able to live normal lives. A few types of epilepsy (for example absence seizures) may disappear after puberty; some change their form; others, unfortunately, persist throughout the patient's lives. The nurse should realize that fatigue, illness, excitement, hyperventilation, blinking lights, and especially failure to take anticonvulsants or a change in anticonvulsant therapy may bring on certain seizures.

The patient and family need continuous medical supervision and counsel. The patient should be encouraged to live life to the fullest within the limits of the disease as imposed by the community and the child's own sense of responsibility. The intelligence levels of people with epilepsy are similar to those found in the population as a whole.

The Epilepsy Societies have provided considerable public education regarding the disorder, attempting to remove false ideas and any legislation that unjustly limits the activities of affected persons.

Meningitis

Meningitis, simply stated, is inflammation of the meninges. Not all types of meningitis are infectious, but the infectious types are far more common. The *Haemophilus influenza* bacillus, meningococcus, and pneumococcus are common etiologic agents responsible for acute bacterial meningitis in children past 1 month of age. Meningitis usually affects children under 2 years of age, and *H. influenza* is by far the most common causative agent. Whatever the cause or age of onset, the treatment of meningitis is always considered a medical emergency. Early recognition and prompt treatment are essential for a favorable recovery. A long and severe infection may result in death or lingering neurologic damage (Fig. 31-14).

Typically the child is irritable and restless or drowsy. Previous upper respiratory tract infections and ear infections are frequently associated with *H. influenzae* meningitis. For this reason the nurse should impress on parents the importance of continuing medications (for otitis media or other inflammations) and all antibiotics prescribed for as long as ordered. Fever, vomiting, chills, headache, rigidity of the neck and back, and convulsions are common. In more severe cases the child may be in shock or may exhibit an involuntary arching of the back known as *opisthotonos* (Fig. 31-15). A high-pitched cry is characteristic. Meningococcal meningitis is usually accompanied by petechiae, a hemorrhagic skin rash caused by meningococcal invasion of the bloodstream. However, meningococcemia may occur without central nervous system involvement.

A lumbar puncture is performed at the slightest suspicion of meningitis. Both parents and children fear a lumbar puncture. Parents should be reassured of the importance, relative safety, and necessity of this procedure. Children, if conscious and old enough to understand, should be mentally prepared just before the procedure. They should be told what is going to happen and that they are likely to feel discomfort. Reminding them that it is important to lie still during the procedure can provide a sense of control and thereby reduce feelings of helplessness. During the procedure, the child should be told that it is okay to cry but that lying still is the best help. The assisting nurse must understand the importance of maintaining the position of the child. Several holds are possible, depending on the size of the child; however, positioning the child on the side (lateral decubitus) is usually preferred. The back of the patient is arched "like a kitten's" to provide greater room for the insertion of the needle between the vertebrae at the level of the iliac

NURSING CARE PLAN

The Infant/Child with Bacterial Meningitis

Selected nursing diagnoses	Expected outcomes	Interventions
A. Potential for spreading infection related to presence of infectious organisms. Clinical manifestations: Fever, irritability, crying, increased HR and RR.	Infection does not spread to others.	Maintain isolation for 24 hours after start of antibiotic therapy. Explain to parents reasons for isolation. Administer antibiotics as ordered by physician.
B. Altered cerebral tissue perfusion related to infectious process and increased cerebral edema. Clinical manifestations: Headaches; decreased LOC and pulse; bulging fontanel; increased head circumference and blood pressure; crying; irritability.	The child maintains adequate blood supply to brain. The child is free from seizure activity.	Elevate head of bed to facilitate venous return. Measure and record head circumference on infant. Assess neurologic status and vital signs every 2 hours and prn. Observe child for signs of ICP (increased head circumference, headache, bulging fontanel, increased blood pressure, decreased pulse, irritability, seizures, and high pitched cry.
C. Potential fluid volume deficit related to fever, vomiting, decreased level of consciousness and fluid restrictions. Clinical manifestations: Decreased urine output, increased urine specific gravity, poor skin turgor, no tearing, dry mucous membranes, sunken fontanel.	Child maintains adequate fluid and electrolyte balance.	Administer IV fluids as ordered by physician. Encourage oral fluids within ordered limits. Maintain strict I & O and check urine specific gravity every 8 hours. Assess child's hydration status every 4 hours (skin turgor, tearing, urine output. Weigh child daily.
D. Potential fluid volume excess related to inappropriate secretion of antidiuretic hormone. Clinical manifestations: Decreased urinary output, increased urine specific gravity, decreased serum Na, increased weight, nausea and irritability.	Child maintains adequate fluid and electrolyte balance.	Maintain fluid restriction as ordered by physician. Weigh child daily. Maintain strict I & O. Monitor serum electrolytes daily. Assess child for signs of fluid retention (decreased urine output, increased urine specific gravity, decreased serum Na, nausea, irritability).

crest. The skin is prepared with an antiseptic by the gloved physician. At the time of the lumbar puncture the pressure of the fluid within the meninges can be measured by attaching a measuring tube or manometer to the spinal needle.

Three specimens of spinal fluid are usually collected consecutively in specially numbered sterile specimen containers. All three containers are sent to the laboratory where they should be immediately examined for cellular and chemical content. From the contents of the first tube, Gram's stain and culture are done to identify any organisms that may be present. Gram's stain may identify the structure of an organism at once, before the culture report. Countercurrent immunoelectrophoresis may often identify an organism within a few hours. Culture results usually take 24 to 48 hours. The second tube is examined for chemical content, usually glucose and protein. The third tube is examined for blood cell content. The selection of the third tube for this procedure reduces the possibility that minor bleeding from insertion of the needle will alter the cell count. At the conclusion of the puncture procedure, care should be taken to remove iodine-containing preparations that were used to prepare the skin. This prevents the occurrence of serious contact rashes. A Band-Aid is placed over the site of the needle insertion.

The child is isolated for 24 hours after the start of antibiotic therapy. The purpose of isolation and why the nurse wears a gown should be explained to the parents. If they are not allowed to enter the room, the crib should be turned so they might at least see the child's face.

Intravenous fluids are started as soon as the lumbar puncture is completed. Fourth generation cephalosporins

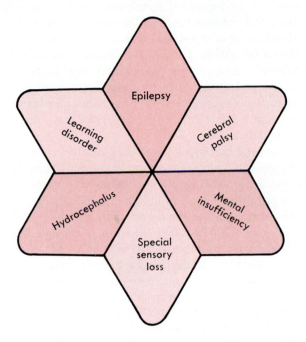

FIG 31-14 Residual complications of meningitis may include any one or all of these conditions.

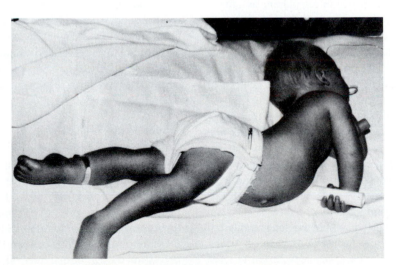

FIG 31-15 Victim of near-drowning showing marked opisthotonos. This posture may be assumed by anyone suffering from severe meningeal irritation. *(Courtesy Alan Schumacher, MD, San Diego, Calif.)*

are routinely started for broad-spectrum antibiotic coverage. When these are not available, ampicillin and chloramphenicol (Chloromycetin) are the treatment of choice for meningitis and should be started immediately. A reduction in the incidence of hearing loss has been demonstrated by the use of steroids introduced early in the management of some forms of bacterial meningitis. Good supportive care requires that dehydration be avoided but fluids may be limited to decrease the possibility of cerebral edema.

Effective restraints must be used to safeguard the infusion. The nurse should carefully position the restrained child on his side during intravenous therapy in case he convulses and aspirates vomitus. Constant nursing care and frequent observation of the child are necessary during the acute phase. Monitoring the vital signs is especially important when increased intracranial pressure is suspected. Slowed pulse, irregular respirations, and elevated blood pressure, which may be accompanied by an altered level of consciousness, are signs of increased intracranial pressure and should be called to the physician's attention at once. Cerebral pressure may be reduced by overventilating with a mask and bag, which decreases PCO_2, by infusion of drugs such as mannitol, or by surgical intervention. Such methods are often lifesaving.

The infant may be placed in an oxygen-enriched environment in an incubator. The older child may be placed in an oxygen tent. Other nursing responsibilities include control of temperature by sponging and maintenance of a quiet environment. Tylenol can be of great benefit to these very often irritable children, as long as care is taken not to interfere with monitoring the temperature response, which determines the length of antibiotic (ampicillin) therapy. Accurately recording the intravenous intake and the urinary output is important. (Urinary retention and fecal impactions are real possibilities.)

As the child progresses favorably, the nurse may safely encourage the parents to hold their infant or toddler during intravenous therapy, allowing for body contact and love, as well as position change. Granting as much freedom from restraint and provision for psychologic comforts (such as thumb-sucking) as is consistent with therapy and safety is very important.

The convalescent period should be long enough to permit the child to regain the previous physical status. Young children should be carefully reevaluated at intervals during the convalescence. Residual complications may include epilepsy, hydrocephalus, cerebral palsy (incoordination or weakness), mental insufficiency, special sensory loss, such as hearing and vision, and behavior or learning disorders (see Fig. 31-14).

Aseptic meningitis syndrome. The term "aseptic meningitis syndrome" includes a number of viral disorders that have an acute onset and usually a self-limited course with varying meningeal manifestations. Meningismus, meningeal irritation resulting in complications such as nuchal (neck) or spinal rigidity, is present. Lumbar puncture reveals abnormal numbers of blood cells and a sterile bacterial culture. To rule out other diseases, hospitalization for at least 48 hours for observation is necessary. Treatment is supportive and symptomatic. Like bacterial meningitis, follow-up should be provided, since residual complications can occur.

Neonatal meningitis. Newborns are frequent victims of meningitis. The organisms most often affecting these babies are group B streptococci followed by *Escherichia coli* and *Listeria*. Mixed infections in meningitis are almost always confined to the neonatal age group. About 1 in every 1,000 to 2,000 newborns is affected. These infections are often associated with low birth weight. Maternal infection, premature rupture of membranes, and complicated deliveries are often part of the obstetric history. Signs of meningeal irritation are minimal. The infant characteristically is lethargic and irritable and refuses to suck. Vomiting, respiratory distress, convulsions, and temperature instability, including hyperthermia and hypothermia, are common symptoms. Fourth generation cephalosporins, ampicillin, gentamicin, and other medications are given intravenously, usually by scalp vein. Abundant hair should always be shaved in advance. Intensive supporting nursing care is essential. Because of the difficulty in recognizing the disease early and the inability of the debilitated small infant to respond to treatment, survival may be as low as 60%, and children who do survive have a high incidence of residual complications.

Cerebral palsy (Fig. 31-16)

Cerebral palsy is a nonprogressive disorder of motion and posture resulting from brain injury or insult during a period of early brain growth. It is not in itself a disease but a condition that may result from numerous diseases that damage those parts of the brain responsible for voluntary muscular coordination. Such causes may include pressure on the brain or oxygen deprivation to the brain before or during birth (cerebral anoxia), direct injury, embolus or hemorrhage, arrested hydrocephalus, and infection or toxicity occurring any time after birth. Cerebral palsy is usually diagnosed in infancy, since it is com-

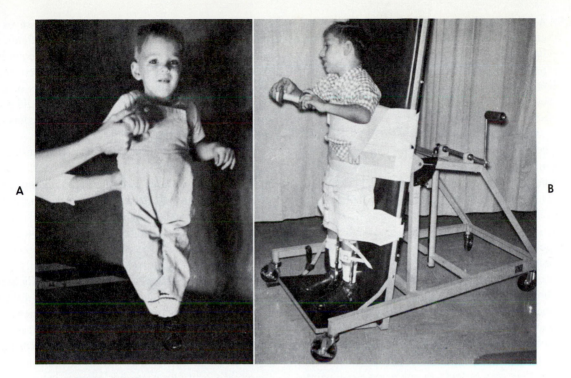

FIG 31-16 This little fellow cannot walk without support. **A,** With support, scissors gait is present (one foot crossing the other caused by adductor spasticity). **B,** Many hours on tilt table and consistent work and concern of therapists and parents have greatly strengthened this child's legs. *(Courtesy Crippled Children Services, Department of Public Health, San Diego, Calif.)*

monly caused by events associated with the prenatal or perinatal period. Treatment is directed toward limiting the disability and may continue throughout the affected person's life. The disorder may be limited and mild or severe and far-reaching, involving many body functions. There are approximately 1.3 cases of cerebral palsy per 1,000 persons in the general population.

The child with the disorder of movement called cerebral palsy may have injuries to the brain involving other functions. Some patients with cerebral palsy have associated seizures, mental insufficiency, behavior problems, special sensory difficulties, especially related to vision or hearing, and learning disturbances. The muscles of the mouth, tongue, and throat may be affected, influencing the ability to receive, chew, and swallow food, as well as to speak.

Therapists usually refer to the following main types of cerebral palsy:

1. The spastic type, the most common form, affecting 65% of the patients, is characterized by increased muscle stiffness or tone, exaggerated contraction of affected muscle groups when stimulated (stretch

reflex), jerky motions, and a tendency to have contractures. The lower extremities are most often involved. A scissors gait is common. The following body patterns of spastic cerebral palsy are:
   a. *Hemiplegia,* involving two limbs (an arm and a leg) on the same side
   b. *Double hemiplegia,* involving arms and legs on both sides, with one side more severely involved
   c. *Quadriplegia,* involving all four limbs, with the legs slightly more affected
   d. *Diplegia,* involving all four limbs, with the legs affected to a significantly greater degree
2. Extrapyramidal (nonspastic) types, comprising about 15% of cases, are characterized by a variety of emotional, postural, and sleep states. This type includes the following:
   a. *Athetoid,* characterized by involuntary, uncoordinated, purposeless movements involving joint motion rather than single muscle action (The upper extremities are more often involved.)

b. *Ataxic,* characterized by loss of a sense of balance and problems in evaluating spatial relationships and the relative positions of body parts
3. Mixed type of cerebral palsy combines features of types 1 and 2 and represents about 20% of affected patients.

It can be readily appreciated that the care of a cerebral-palsied child and his family cannot be the responsibility of just one practitioner. The problems are usually too extensive. A team approach is necessary, including pediatrician, orthopedist, physical therapist, occupational therapist, speech therapist, psychologist, medical-social worker, public health workers, office and hospital nurses, and schoolteachers.

These children and their families often have considerable emotional problems, which may be expressed in the way the parents treat the child and in their aspirations for the child's future. Parents may be overprotective and do too much for their child, making it difficult for him to master the skills of which they are capable. On the other hand, they may expect too much and cause painful frustrations. Parents may need help in establishing realistic goals and in providing an environment conducive to good mental and physical health. That the problem is not inherited should be clarified early to decrease parental feelings of guilt.

Association with other parents with similar problems and psychiatric assistance is often very rewarding. A hopeful aspect of cerebral palsy is that the initiating cause is not progressive in character, and so the neuromuscular involvement, with treatment, does not worsen. Cerebral palsy is not a degenerative disease like, for example, the muscular dystrophies, and considerable improvement can usually be gained. Through physical and occupational therapy, surgical techniques, and medication, youngsters with cerebral palsy are able to meet their daily personal needs and, in some cases, to prepare for self-supporting occupations. Special public school programs especially geared to meet the needs of such handicapped children may be available in the community. Children may attend some regular public school classes as well as special sessions designed to meet their individual needs during the school day.

When children with cerebral palsy are hospitalized, it is very important that the hospital staff know their capabilities as individuals. Information regarding successful feeding and dressing techniques, toileting practices, communication aids, and special problems saves hours of frustration and distress. The care of patients whose total neuromuscular involvement is slight requires little modification. The care of others requires considerable study and adjustment. Children with a history of seizures or upper extremity or head involvement should not have their temperatures taken orally until the safety of the procedure is evaluated.

Each child's diet must be evaluated to ensure that it is appropriate for his age, nutritional needs, and ability to handle and swallow. Although self-feeding may take considerable time and cause some disorder, these children should feed themselves as much as possible, using techniques they have been taught. Aids, such as swivel spoons, plate guards, training cups, and rocker knives, are invaluable (Fig. 31-17). Occasionally, special weights can be attached to the child's arms to help control involuntary motion. Children who because of their condition must be fed should be assisted with patience. Since severely affected children may require the occasional use of suction, an apparatus should be available. During feedings, the nurse should hold the child in such a way that the child's arm closest to her extends behind her. This often causes the child's head to rotate comfortably to the same side (tonic neck reflex). Gentle support of the chin or stroking the neck on either side of the esophagus may help lip closure and swallowing. Some children who have difficulty swallowing find carbonated drinks a problem. Waiting until the carbonation is minimal or serving other types of liquid is helpful.

Children with this condition should receive gentle, deliberate care. Excessive stimulation, sudden jarring movements, and the pressure of "having to hurry" induces greater tenseness and makes performance of relatively simple tasks extremely arduous. These children find it very difficult to relax, and they become fatigued easily. The simplest kind of controlled movement may require a tremendous amount of concentration and energy.

Whenever possible, the cerebral-palsied child should have contact with other boys and girls and should not be socially deprived. Contact with other youngsters is frequently limited. However, even those who have moderately severe muscular involvement often enjoy working with modeling clay, finger paints, large blocks, and hand puppets. Many enjoy music, television, and reading. An occupational therapist can work with the children to improve skills needed to meet everyday needs. These are presented to the young child in the form of games or special projects. Progress, though at times seemingly

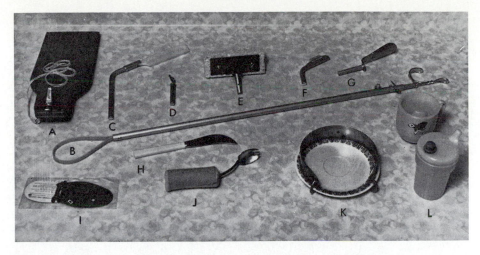

FIG 31-17 Various aids for everyday activities for handicapped. **A,** Nail clippers on wooden base, operated by string and foot action; **B,** gadget stick with hook attachment; **C,** comb attachment; **D,** clip attachment; **E,** mop or sponge attachment; **F,** magnet attachment; **G,** shoehorn attachment; **H,** rocker knife; **I,** elastic shoelaces; **J,** built-up handle on swivel fork (Spork); **K,** plate and plate guard; **L,** two types of weighted "trainer cups." *(Courtesy Children's Hospital and Health Center, San Diego, Calif.)*

small, should be recognized and praised. The child usually responds to this recognition and continues efforts to improve.

Although it may seem to some critics that a tremendous amount of time, effort, and financial expense is expended in community programs to help cerebral-palsied youngsters, such programs are rewarding from many points of view. In the long run it is less expensive to educate individuals to achieve their potentials than to provide the type of state-supported custodial care offered in the past. It often brings a measure of independence and a feeling of self-respect and personal worth to the individual patient. It brings hope and aid to concerned and burdened parents and inspiration to those who observe and help when they can.

TODDLER
Encephalitis

Encephalitis is an inflammation of the brain (encephalon). When the inflammation involves both the meninges and the brain tissue, the condition is referred to as *encephalomyelitis*.

Encephalitis is characterized by personality change, headache, drowsiness, fever, and often convulsions. Cranial nerves may become paralyzed, affecting speech, swallowing mechanism, and protective airway reflexes. Double vision may also be reported. Encephalitis may produce the same complications as does meningitis (see Fig. 31-14).

Encephalitis is caused by infectious agents, most often viral. Probably the most common epidemic viral encephalitis is due to enteroviruses and the most common sporadically occurring viral encephalitis is due to herpes simplex. Some types of encephalitis are caused by viruses spread by vectors, such as mosquitoes, ticks, or mites. Encephalitis following rubeola (2-week measles) was relatively common before immunization programs were available, occurring once in every 600 to 1,000 cases of "hard" measles.

Symptoms of encephalitis caused by toxins contacted by ingestion or inhalation are more properly referred to as *encephalopathy*. Lead poisoning in children, though not as common as formerly, is still reported every year. All furniture and toys used by young children (who consider tasting at least as important as feeling or smelling) should be protected by nontoxic, lead-free paint.

The nursing care of a child with encephalitis is much like that of a child with meningitis. Lumbar punctures may be performed to relieve intracranial pressure, and recently intracranial monitoring of pressure has been frequently used. The difference between encephalitis and meningitis may not always be clinically demonstrated by symptoms. Differentiation is then made on the basis of the results from laboratory examinations.

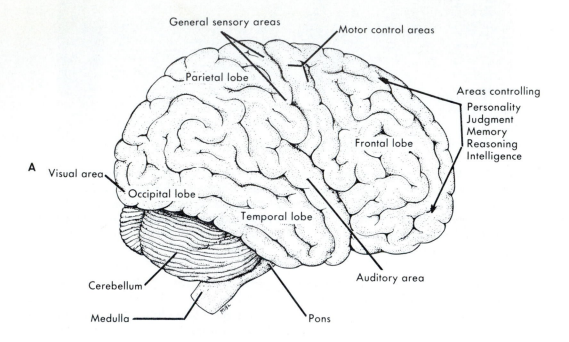

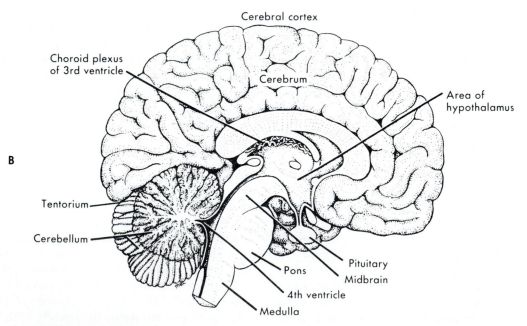

FIG 31-18 A, Surfaces of brain showing cerebrum, cerebellum, pons, and medulla with identification of specialized areas of cerebral function. **B,** Simplified sagittal section of brain showing internal relationships. Brain tumors in children often involve the cerebellum.

PRESCHOOL CHILD

Brain tumors (Fig. 31-18)

Although brain tumors are not found as frequently in children as in adults, nervous system tumors are the second most common malignancy in children. Pediatric brain tumors are situated rather deeply within the brain structure, making it difficult to ensure complete removal of the abnormal cells. About three fourths of brain tumors occurring in childhood involve the supportive connective tissue of the brain, called *glial cells*. The two most common gliomas are astrocytomas and medulloblastomas. Total resection of an infiltrating cerebral astrocytoma is seldom possible, but a cystic cerebellar astrocytoma is relatively slow-growing, usually encapsulated, and easier to remove.

Early symptoms of a developing brain tumor may appear gradually in the case of a slowly progressing lesion. However, some tumors (for example, medulloblastomas) grow rapidly and cause remarkable signs and symptoms rather soon. The signs and symptoms are caused by increased intracranial pressure. They include headache, dizziness, lethargy, indifference, and irritability. Emesis occurs typically in the morning. This is the result of fluid and pressure shifts as the child moves from a recumbent to a standing position. After vomiting the child can eat a normal breakfast because there is no nausea. Double or blurred vision and speech problems are reported fairly often. The pupils may be abnormally or unequally dilated or slow to react to changes in light intensity. Balance and gait may be affected because 60% of childhood brain tumors are subtentorial and often involve the cerebellum, a part of the brain that plays a significant role in the maintenance of equilibrium (Fig. 31-18, *B*). Rigidity, tremors, or convulsions occasionally occur. Local muscle weakness may be present. (Periodic testing of the handgrip is sometimes ordered.) In children younger than 2 years of age, when the cranial suture lines are not completely knit, there may be considerable enlargement of the head and fontanel because of the enlarging tumor or its obstruction of cerebrospinal fluid drainage. The blood pressure may be elevated, and the pulse may be slowed when compared with the normal values for the patient's age group. Respirations may be of the Cheyne-Stokes variety. Fever or wide swings in temperature occasionally occur. Diagnosis is confirmed through various procedures: skull radiographs (x-ray films), brain scans, electroencephalograms (EEGs), ventriculograms, and arteriograms, as well as clinical observation. Some of these procedures, though often necessary, are uncomfortable. Newer procedures, computed tomography (CT) and magnetic resonance imaging (MRI), cause the patient much less discomfort and risk (p. 516).

If a nurse is responsible for the care of a patient with a possible brain tumor, she must carefully access the child's capabilities before attempting to ambulate the child. She should ensure that she has sufficient assistance to prevent falls because some of these patients have poor balance. The patient should be observed for any of the signs and symptoms previously described. Observation of vital signs including blood pressure and eye reactions should always be part of the nursing care.

Surgery, radiation, and chemotherapy are the treatments currently available. Surgery, of course, is preferred. The complete removal of a well-confined tumor almost always produces a more optimistic prognosis. When only incomplete removal is possible, radiation and chemotherapy are often employed to retard tumor progression.

Nursing care in the days immediately following a craniotomy (surgical opening of the skull) is usually a complex affair. The vocational nurse may assist the registered nurse, but she should not have the responsibility of the child's complete bedside care because the child's condition is too unstable. The patient must be turned slowly and gently to prevent dizziness, nausea, vomiting, and a rise in blood pressure. Because crying elevates the blood pressure, all measures designed to prevent fear or distress are especially important. The head dressings may become damp from cerebrospinal fluid drainage and require reinforcing until they can be changed by the physician. The face, especially the eyes, may be bruised and swollen. Special eye irrigations may be necessary to prevent infection or ulceration resulting from disturbances in tear formation and drainage because of trauma. Frequent suctioning may be necessary. The child may appear unconscious but may be able to hear well; so conversations at the bedside should be prudent.

As patients with brain tumors improve, efforts to rehabilitate them should be made. Although the patients may eventually die, they may be able to live relatively satisfying lives for many months. Both patients and parents need much physical and emotional support to make the most of this indeterminate and occasionally prolonged period.

Neuroblastoma

A neuroblastoma is an undifferentiated malignant tumor arising during embryonic development from the adrenal medulla or from any of the nervous system's sympathetic ganglia located in the head, neck, chest, abdomen, or pelvis. It is the most common of all solid cancers of children. Both sexes are equally affected, and although the tumor may be recognized at various ages, a preponderance is diagnosed during the first 4 to 5 years of life.

Four common clinical manifestations of the neuroblastoma are (1) a mass usually involving the abdomen or lymph nodes; (2) neurologic signs, such as weakness in an extremity or paraplegia; (3) pain, usually in the bone or joints; and (4) orbital signs, such as local ecchymosis or proptosis (protruding eye). In addition, children with neuroblastoma often come to the hospital with varied constitutional symptoms, including weight loss, fever, anorexia, and anemia.

When a neuroblastoma is suspected, a number of diagnostic studies must be performed at once because the neuroblastoma is a highly malignant tumor with tendencies to produce widespread metastases. The sequence of studies includes a complete blood cell count; electrolyte, glucose, and other blood chemistry determinations; a urinary assay for catecholamines; intravenous pyelogram; radioactive bone scan; chest x-ray examination; computed tomography (CT); and bone marrow aspiration. In seven out of ten cases the tumor secretes excess quantities of catecholamines or metabolites or both into the blood. Urine measurements of their metabolic end products, vanillylmandelic acid (VMA) and homovanillic acid (HVA), make the 24-hour VMA and HVA urine determinations a valuable diagnostic test (p. 510). A good prognosis has generally been associated with diagnosis in children under 1 year of age with localized tumor. Staging of this tumor is important for planning treatment and estimating prognosis.

Stage I. Localized tumor, well encapsulated

Stage II. Tumor extended to regional lymph nodes

Stage III. Extensive tumor spread across the midline

Stage IV. Tumor with distant metastases and bone involvement

Stage IVS (S for *special*). Small primary tumor with metastases to the liver, skin, or bone marrow with no bone involvement

The cure rate decreases as the extent of disease increases. Unfortunately, more than 50% of cases have metastasized at the time of initial diagnosis. However, an aggressive therapeutic approach, combining surgical excision, irradiation, and chemotherapy is used in an attempt to save a significant portion of these children. Surgery alone is probably acceptable in Stages I, II, and IVS. Spontaneous resolution of residual tumor in stages

II and IVS is a common event with high cure rates (75% to 90%) in these children. Because neuroblastoma is radiosensitive, x-ray therapy to the tumor site and to any areas of local extension may be an indicated addition in other cases. Palliative x-ray therapy is used for metastatic lesions in bones, lungs, liver, and brain. Chemotherapy has improved survival and is useful in shrinking previously unresectable tumors. It is especially indicated in patients with bone involvement, when the urinary catecholamines remain elevated after all identifiable tumor has been removed, or when recurrence or late metastases are detected. Currently, multidrug chemotherapy is employed, using vincristine (Oncovin), cyclophosphamide (Cytoxan), doxorubicin (Adriamycin), cisplatin (Platinol), and VM-26, in addition to surgery and radiation therapy. No single chemotherapeutic agent or combination of drugs has been uniformly effective. When chemotherapy is given, control of anemia, specific antibiotic therapy for infections, and prevention of high blood levels of uric acid are necessary. Liberal fluids and allopurinol (Zyloprim) should be given to prevent uric acid kidney damage.

After surgery, children with neuroblastomas should be reevaluated often because, in spite of the use of chemotherapy and radiotherapy, results to date have been poor. Although an increasing number of long-term survivors are receiving chemotherapy, this tumor often has a rapid downhill course despite all therapy that is currently available. Preliminary investigations into bone marrow transplantation for neuroblastoma have begun.

SCHOOL-AGE CHILD
Head injuries

About 200,000 children are hospitalized annually with head injuries. Although most of these children have simple, closed head injuries, about 17% have skull fractures. One out of ten has active intracranial bleeding, and two out of ten have other body injuries associated with head injury. Identifying children with active intracranial bleeding and those with other injuries is a significant role of the nurse. The patients are typically boys between the ages of 4 and 9 years.

Concussion. The term "concussion" implies a loss of consciousness with a temporary neuronal dysfunction caused by jarring but with no pathologic evidence of damage to the underlying brain. The period of unconsciousness is usually brief and is measured in terms of minutes to hours. The period of memory loss that surrounds a concussion is termed *posttraumatic amnesia*

(PTA). It is important to be aware of the PTA phenomenon because it explains why the patient often cannot provide information about the injury. Usually the longer the PTA period, the greater the likelihood of brain injury rather than simple concussion. PTA is divided into retrograde amnesia, loss of memory for the period of time preceding the actual injury, and anterograde amnesia, the loss of memory for the period of time following the injury. Most patients display some persistent residual loss of memory surrounding the period of injury. A long retrograde amnesia is particularly significant in evaluating the extent of a head injury. Any head-injured child who loses consciousness or shows any neurologic deficit should be admitted to the hospital for observation.

Contusion and laceration. A contusion is an actual bruising of the brain. A laceration involves tearing of cerebral tissue. This bruising or tearing of cerebral tissue is frequently accompanied by hemorrhages or bleeding into the brain substance. Contusions and lacerations, in contrast to concussion, are characterized by specific (focal) findings. Changes in motor function, speech, and vision are important clues for determining the area of damage; for example: the left side of the brain controls the arms and legs on the right side of the body, speech is most often generated by the left side of the brain, and a visual center is located at the back of the brain. When disruption of brain tissue is associated with bleeding, intracranial pressure may begin to rise. Since the cranium containing the brain, cerebral blood vessels, and cerebrospinal fluid is rigid, any enlargement of one of these three components results in compression of the others. The brain substance is more vulnerable to compression than are blood and cerebrospinal fluid, and when no further compensation is possible, intracranial pressure begins to rise. Like other tissues, when the brain is subjected to injury, it becomes edematous. This swelling also causes intracranial pressure. Increasing intracranial pressure (ICP) is manifested by a deterioration in the state of consciousness, rising systemic blood pressure associated with slowing of the pulse rate, and irregularity of breathing. These are the classic neurologic signs indicating that the head-injured child is in trouble. A basic neurologic check (see box, p. 674) is used for observing a child who is beginning to manifest subtle signs of increasing intracranial pressure or who is admitted to the hospital for observation after a head injury. Consciousness is a bihemispheric and brainstem function. Nerve centers in the brainstem also control vital functions, such as respiration, heart rate, and blood pressure. The brainstem may be directly injured, or it may be compromised by potentially reversible lesions that cause compression, such as intracranial pressure and brain shifts or lesions that cause cerebral oxygen deprivation (ischemia).

The brainstem centers that help control vital functions are anatomically close to those that regulate pupil responses. Observations of changes in pupil size therefore aid in detecting damage to the brainstem.

Intracranial hematomas. Intracranial hematomas are space-occupying lesions that produce signs of intracranial pressure. They should be suspected in every case of head injury with coma or one-sided weakness. Short-term intracranial pressure may occur because of an expanding hematoma, or long-term pressure may occur because of cerebral edema caused by the injury. Unless the intracranial pressure is reduced, neurologic deterioration follows, which can prove to be fatal.

Epidural hematoma. About 75% of epidural hematomas are associated with a skull fracture (Fig. 31-19). This lesion, located between the skull and the outer covering of the brain (dura), results from a torn high-pressure arterial system. It characteristically demonstrates a relatively rapid downhill course unless identified and treated. Since the expanding hemorrhage cannot get through the bone, the hematoma presses down on the substance of the brain. Usually a brief period of unconsciousness is followed by a lucid interval of variable duration, after which the child is progressively confused, lethargic, difficult to arouse, and finally, comatose.

Pulse and respirations become slow, and blood pressure rises. A dilated pupil and hemiparesis of the opposite side of the body, accompanied by a deterioration in state of consciousness and vital signs, indicate a prompt need for surgical intervention. The high mortality from this kind of injury usually results from a failure in recognition and a delay in operation.

Subdural hematomas. Subdural hematomas are usually caused by rupture of low-pressure bridging veins in the space under the dura and may be associated with severe brain injury. Subdural hematomas are divided into three categories, depending on the time interval from onset of the injury to the course of symptoms. *Acute subdural hematomas* usually cause immediate unconsciousness with a rapid, downhill, progressive deterioration, resulting from massive bleeding and fatal brain compression. *Subacute subdural hematomas* develop slowly because bleeding is less profuse. Clinical manifestations usually appear between 2 and 14 days after injury. *Chronic subdural hematomas* manifest them-

Neurologic check

Assessment	Technique or observation used

Assessment

I. Level of consciousness
  A. Alert, oriented, responsive to
    1. Person
    2. Time
    3. Place

  B. Lethargic—drowsy
  C. Disoriented—confused
  D. Responsive to verbal stimuli
  E. Responsive only to painful stimuli
    1. Purposeful
    2. Nonpurposeful
      a. Flexor response
      b. Extensor response

  F. Coma

II. Pupil response
  A. Appearance
    1. Shape
    2. Size
    3. Equality

  B. Reaction to light
    1. Direct light reflex

    2. Consensual light reflex
  C. Extraocular movements

III. Motor function
  A. Facial symmetry
  B. Movement
    1. Upper extremities
    2. Lower extremities

  C. Strength
    1. Upper extremities
    2. Lower extremities
  D. Babinski reflex

IV. Vital signs
  A. Temperature
  B. Pulse
  C. Respiration
  D. Blood pressure

Technique or observation used

Ask the following questions:
  1. "What is your name?"
  2. "What is your favorite TV show? What day is today?"
  3. "Where are you? Where do you go to school?"
Patient responses are delayed.
Patient gives inappropriate responses.
Patient answers simple commands, e.g., "Open your eyes."
Pinch patient's upper arm.
Patient withdraws from stimulus—pushes it away.
Patient may only grimace.

Patient gives no response of any kind.

Observe both pupils simultaneously; pupils should be round (constricted in bright room and dilated in dark room) and equal in size.

Shine light directly into one eye; pupils should constrict briskly.
Shine light into one eye to note alternate pupil constriction.
Ask patient to follow your finger from side to side and up and down with eyes to detect limitation in movement.

Ask patient to show teeth—to make a "funny face."

Ask patient to raise arms and extend both arms forward.
Ask patient to move each leg individually upward and laterally.

Ask patient to squeeze examiner's hand or two fingers and to pull against resistance of examiner.
Stroke outside sole of each foot with tongue blade. Normally toes, especially big toe, turn down. Reflex is present when big toe rises (dorsiflexion) and other toes fan out. Reflex is normally present up to about 18 months of age.
Elevation is usually associated with infection elsewhere unless hypothalamus (temperature-regulating center) has been damaged.
Slowed pulse and irregular respirations associated with rising systolic pressure indicate increased intracranial pressure.

It is important to note the degree of alertness when the child is admitted to the emergency department or pediatric unit and to note the vital signs exactly. Changes in these important parameters as indicated above are classic signs that the patient is in need of prompt medical assistance. The physician should be notified at once.

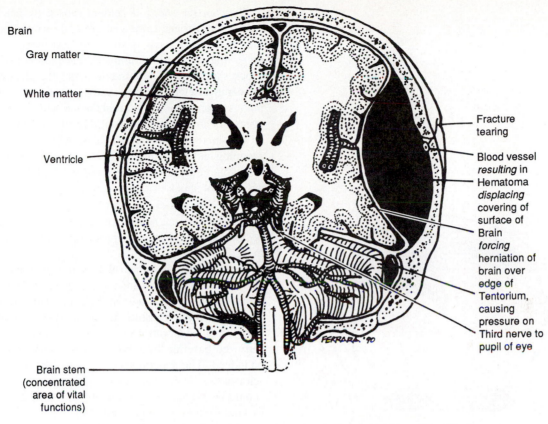

Brain

Gray matter

White matter

Ventricle

Fracture tearing

Blood vessel *resulting* in Hematoma *displacing* covering of surface of Brain *forcing* herniation of brain over edge of Tentorium, causing pressure on Third nerve to pupil of eye

Brain stem (concentrated area of vital functions)

FERRARA '90

FIG 31-19 Epidural hematoma located between skull and outer covering of brain.

selves weeks or months after the injury (Fig. 31-20). This condition occurs most frequently in infancy. A vascular membrane forms around the blood as the mass slowly enlarges because of leakage of plasma protein from the capillaries. Intracranial pressure mounts over a period of weeks to months and is manifested by vomiting (especially projectile type), a tense fontanel, and separation of the cranial sutures. Because chronic subdural hematomas are usually bilateral, the skull may become deformed and broad with a high forehead. The infant becomes irritable and is often underweight and anemic. Bilateral subdural taps confirm the diagnosis, and the fluid is removed. If the fluid is removed in time, repeated subdural taps can provide a complete cure; otherwise, a shunting procedure is necessary for the more persistent hematomas.

Skull fracture. Separate from but nevertheless associated with many injuries of the brain is skull fracture. A *linear skull fracture* (lengthwise) may often cause an underlying hematoma. This is particularly true if the fracture line crosses the normal distribution of blood vessels. In children 50% of skull fractures are in the parietal bone,

and these usually are evident on x-ray examination. A *depressed skull fracture* occurs when the bone is displaced or is pressing on the brain tissue. Debridement and surgical restoration of normal contour are required. Basal skull fractures are not always seen on x-ray examination. However, the nurse may suspect the presence of a basilar skull fracture by a variety of special findings not always initially present when the child is admitted. On the second day the nurse may notice black-and-blue marks around the eyes (raccoon sign) or ear (battle sign). A third finding is watery fluid that runs out of the ear (cerebrospinal fluid otorrhea) or a watery discharge from the nose (cerebrospinal fluid rhinorrhea). Cerebrospinal fluid leaking from the ear or nose causes increased concern because of the danger of infection and meningitis.

Continued assessment and nursing care. *Cerebral anoxia* is the most frequent cause of death in those with skull fracture. Therefore the establishment and maintenance of an adequate airway, accompanied by proper ventilation and circulation, are critical. Obstruction of the airway not only causes atelectasis and infection but also produces a serious abnormality in the gaseous ex-

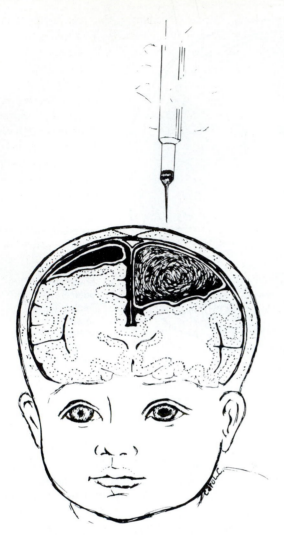

FIG 31-20 Bilateral, chronic subdural hematomas. Subdural taps are performed on infants by insertion of special subdural needle through lateral suture line.

change that can increase cerebral flow and cerebral edema, thus increasing intracranial pressure. When possible, blood gases should be periodically checked to validate the adequacy of ventilation. Tracheal suction may be essential to clear secretions, and a tracheostomy may be necessary to maintain a patent airway. Because vomiting frequently accompanies intracranial pressure, insertion of a nasogastric tube and removal of stomach contents may prevent aspiration pneumonitis. These patients should be kept in a lateral, slightly elevated position, unless contraindicated, because of the potential for aspiration. They should be turned and suctioned hourly.

Hypotensive shock is seldom caused by head injury unless hemorrhage from a severe scalp wound occurs or the brain injury itself is so severe that the vital centers are failing and death is imminent. The presence of clinical shock should alert the nurse to notify the physician and to search elsewhere in the body for hemorrhage. Scrupulous examination of the abdomen and extremities is necessary to detect the possibility of a ruptured spleen or fractured long bone. Blood should be obtained for grouping and cross-matching because replacement of lost fluid volume by intravenous route may be lifesaving. The presence of shock usually means injuries involving other organs: With the exception of a life-threatening lesion, such as hematoma, neurosurgical management should be postponed until other injuries are investigated and treated, if necessary.

Disturbances in cerebral function. A detailed neurologic examination is included with the initial medical examination of the head-injured child. This not only allows for a more accurate diagnosis of the extent of the injury, but observations made during the examination form the baseline from which subsequent progress can be judged. The general state of the patient, level of consciousness, heart rate, blood pressure, and breathing should be evaluated immediately with primary attention to vital circulatory and ventilatory functions on which life depends. Headache, vertigo, vomiting, increasing irritability, and restlessness often characterize the response of young children to head injury. These factors may or may not be evidences of intracranial pressure. Restlessness can be caused by cerebral hypoxia or by an overdistended bladder. An indwelling catheter should be inserted to relieve an overdistention of the bladder. Other causes of restlessness include extensive soft tissue injuries, fracture, and improperly applied cast or dressing. Seizures also frequently accompany head injuries in small children. Careful systematic serial observations and recordings of changing factors and physical signs are constantly compared with the baseline. In addition to the nurse's responsibility for the care of the child, the nurse must report at once any significant change in the patient's condition. Problems associated with raised intracranial pressure demand solution before irreparable brain damage is inflicted. A *neurologic check,* which includes evaluation of level of consciousness, pupillary signs, extremity movement, strength, and sensation, as well as vital signs, should be done every 15 to 30 minutes as necessary. Careful observation of the child, especially the level of consciousness, yields by far the most important information for further management. (See box on p. 677.)

Glasgow coma scale

Response	Score*
Eye opening	4 Spontaneous
	3 To speech
	2 To pain
	1 None
Best verbal	5 Oriented
	4 Confused
	3 Inappropriate
	2 Incomprehensible
	1 None
Best motor	6 Obeys commands
	5 Localizes pain
	4 Withdraws
	3 Flexion to pain
	2 Extension to pain
	1 None

*Eye + Motor + Verbal = 3 to 15. Any combination equal to 7 or less defines coma.

A child who is alert or is improving does not require any therapeutic measures. However, when serial examinations suggest that intracranial pressure is increasing significantly, various measures are employed to minimize this complication. Administration of dehydrating agents, such as mannitol, can be given over a 4- to 6-hour period every 12 hours to control cerebral edema. Dexamethasone (Decadron) and methylprednisolone sodium succinate (Solu-Medrol) are two glucocorticoids commonly used to prevent cellular decompensation and increasing cerebral edema. Anticonvulsant drugs may be necessary to control seizures. Normal daily maintenance fluids should be given at a uniform rate over a 24-hour period. An accurate record of fluid intake and output is essential and should be followed closely because lethargy, confusion, and convulsion can result from electrolyte imbalance and not an intracranial hematoma. Hematomas can be differentiated from cerebral edema by computed transaxial tomography (CT scan). This technique permits identification of hemorrhage and cerebral edema and clearly outlines ventricular cavities. The CT scan is the safest, fastest, and best initial study for the child who exhibits further neurologic deterioration or who is comatose. If scanning is not available, cerebral angiography is used to diagnose intracranial hematomas that may need to be evacuated by craniotomy.

Coma. Coma is defined as the inability to open the eyes, obey commands, or speak. Various degrees of impaired consciousness occur with head trauma. Recognition of the depth of responsiveness is essential in determining the initial severity of the patient's brain insult.

The Glasgow Coma Scale (GCS) is a reliable instrument designed to define the degree of responsiveness. Scoring of responsiveness depends on the ability to open one's eyes, obey commands, and speak in response to verbal or tactile stimuli. The worst score obtainable is 3; the best is 15. Patients who do not spontaneously open their eyes within 24 hours of head trauma have the poorest prognosis. (See box at left.)

In summation, the nurse must remember that intracranial monitoring remains the single most important aid in determining when the previously mentioned therapeutic measures should be initiated. Although children have a remarkable capacity to survive even the most severe type of head trauma, the management of each child remains a challenge.

Part 3: Vision, Hearing, and Related Disorders

VISION

Fortunately only a small percentage of children are totally blind—that is, visually unable to distinguish light from darkness. The majority of blind children have significant visual impairment but retain some measurable or functional vision. Common causes of visual impairment in infancy and childhood are (1) trauma, (2) strabismus (malalignment of the eyes), and (3) refractive error (image not clearly focused on the retina). In fairly recent years four factors have contributed to the reduction of visual disability:

1. Recognition of the cause of retrolental fibroplasia
2. Prevention and control of rubella
3. Early diagnosis and treatment of developmental eye problems
4. Technologic advances in eye examination and surgery

Pediatric eye examination

The gift of sight is indeed precious. Proper care of the eyes should be taught to growing children and to parents. Prevention of eye disease is the ideal, but early recognition of eye disorders with proper definitive treatment is the ultimate goal. Children should be observed

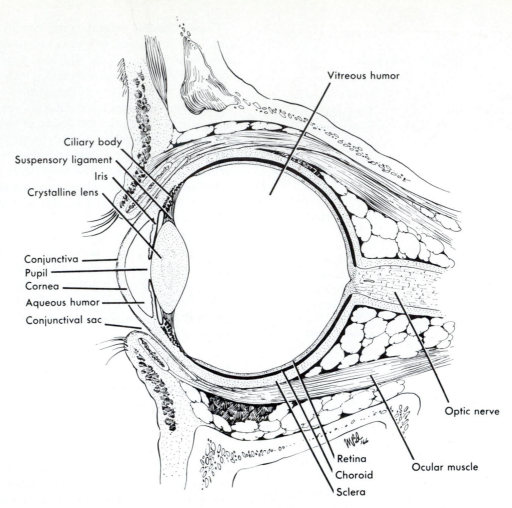

Ciliary body
Suspensory ligament
Iris
Crystalline lens

Conjunctiva
Pupil
Cornea
Aqueous humor
Conjunctival sac

Vitreous humor

Optic nerve

Retina
Choroid
Sclera

Ocular muscle

FIG 31-21   Basic anatomy of eye.

for signs and symptoms of the following possible visual difficulties:

1. Poor vision: inability to follow objects visually or visual inattentiveness to the environment in infants and preschoolers; difficulty with near or distant reading in school-age children
2. Strabismus: intermittent or persistent crossing of the eyes; squinting, blinking, or closing one eye in bright light or during visual tasks; head turning or tilting
3. Uncorrected refractive error: irritability with near or distant visual tasks or avoidance of these tasks; tearing, rubbing, or squinting of the eyes; recurrent eyelid inflammations

To identify and treat visual problems as early as pos-

sible, a professional eye examination should be performed for every child immediately after birth, at 6 months, and once in the preschool years between ages 3 and 5. Annual follow-up visual screening in the schools is recommended. The examination should include measurement of visual acuity, estimation of ocular alignment by corneal light reflexes or alternate cover testing, and examination of ocular structures for pathologic findings (Fig. 31-21).

Children with the following findings should be referred to an ophthalmologist:

1. Possible strabismus
2. Poor visual fixation preference (demonstrated by infants) *or* a visual acuity difference between eyes of two lines or more on the eye chart or vision in

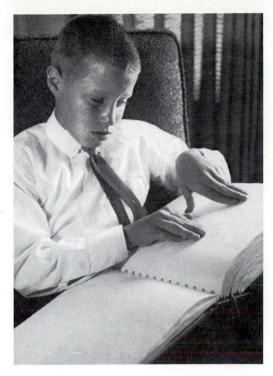

FIG 31-22 This industrious boy, reading from his Braille Bible, is blind as result of retrolental fibroplasia.

either eye of 20/40 or less (in preschool- or school-age youngsters)

3. Evidence of structural deformity of the eye
4. Family history of retinoblastoma, congenital cataracts, or genetic or metabolic eye diseases

Retrolental fibroplasia (retinopathy of prematurity)

Administration of oxygen, which saves the lives of numerous premature low birth weight infants, may also cause development of abnormal retinal vascularizations. Ultimately a contraction of this retinal scar tissue can result in a detachment of the retina and the appearance of a white fibrous sheath on the posterior surface of the lens. The incidence of retrolental fibroplasia (RLF) has decreased, but it is reemerging as the use of oxygen therapy rises in the salvage of high-risk infants (Fig. 31-22).

Specific language disability (developmental dyslexia)

Vision is important in gathering the large amount of data demanded by our learning processes; however, provision of proper eye care for children cannot be expected to eliminate all learning problems. Developmental dys-

lexia can occur in children in the presence or absence of visual deficit, even in children of normal intelligence. Therefore those best qualified to deal with learning disorders are educators and not vision specialists.

Amblyopia and strabismus

Strabismus (malalignment of the eyes) affects about 4% of the population. This imbalance of the extraocular muscles can lead to amblyopia (decreased vision in one eye resulting from disuse), poor binocular vision (decreased depth perception), and an unacceptable appearance ("cross-eyed," "wall-eyed"). Although strabismus is the most common cause of amblyopia, the next leading cause is a notable difference in refractive error (the eye most out of focus "turns off"). Specific treatment of amblyopia may include glasses or occlusive (patching) therapy. Patching the nonamblyopic eye stimulates the increased visual maturation of the amblyopic eye. Specific treatment of strabismus depends on the cause and may include glasses, occlusive therapy, orthoptics (visual exercises), or surgery (Fig. 31-23). Surgical treatment of a congenital strabismus in the first year of life significantly improves changes for binocular vision and an acceptable appearance.

Strabismus surgery involves either shortening or repositioning the extraocular muscles controlling the position of the eyeball. Postoperative care is usually dictated by physician preference and the patient's needs. Although restraints have been used frequently in the past, there is no substitute for an attentive parent or nurse. Parents have usually been instructed by the surgeon to expect that the child will have red eyes. The child may become needlessly frightened by occlusive eye dressings or the inability to open the eyes because of crusted secretions on opposing lid margins. Proper postoperative care can prevent both these situations.

Refractive errors

Poor visual acuity in one or both eyes may be the result of myopia (nearsightedness), hyperopia (farsightedness), or astigmatism (Table 31-3). Astigmatism is an irregularity in the curvature of the cornea or lens that blurs focal points; it may be associated with either myopia or hyperopia. When there is a significant difference in the ability of the eyes to focus—in their refractive powers—the condition is known as *anisometropia*. Refractive errors usually do not cause difficulties until the child reaches school age. Vision usually can be corrected to a normal level in both eyes with proper glasses. Only

Table 31-3 Refraction: three common defects in children

Normal refraction			Normal eye
Emmetropia (no refractive error) Light is focused on retina			Emmetropic eye

Abnormal refraction	Cause	Optical defect	Corrected with lens
Myopia (nearsightedness) Sees near objects more clearly than distant objects	Elongated eyeball Parallel rays are focused anterior to the retina	Myopic eye	Corrected with concave lens
Hyperopia (farsightedness) Sees objects more clearly at a distance	Shortened eyeball Parallel rays are focused posterior to the retina	Hyperopic eye	Corrected with convex lens

Table 31-3 Refraction: three common defects in children—cont'd

Abnormal refraction	Cause	Optical defect	Corrected with lens
Astigmatism (may be associated with myopia or hyperopia) Sees distorted image	Irregular corneal curvature Rays entering eye are not refracted uniformly in all meridians	Myopic astigmatism Corrected with myopic cylinder Axis 90°	

if amblyopia is present do uncorrected or poorly corrected refractive errors cause permanent loss of vision.

Children who wear glasses must be carefully taught to keep their glasses in a case when they are not being worn. Proper methods of handling and cleaning the lenses should also be demonstrated. When a young patient wearing glasses or contact lenses is admitted to the hospital, a note concerning them should be included in the child's admission record.

Cataracts

Congenital and early developmental cataracts constitute one of the most important causes of visual impairment in children. A cataract is an abnormal opacity of the crystalline lens, located just in back of the pupil. By obstructing the pathway of light to the retina, cataracts can cause partial or total blindness. Cataracts may be congenital, such as those caused by maternal rubella. Some cataracts are hereditary—the most commonly autosomal dominant. Nonhereditary cataracts may develop as a result of trauma, infection, retrolental fibroplasia, retinitis pigmentosa, or prolonged administration of corticosteroids. Surgical removal of the cataract lens is the only effective method of treatment available for all but

a few infants and children. The postoperative period is usually short. It usually requires a sterile eye pad and protective shield and occasionally involves some limitation of activity. Every effort should be made to reduce crying and prevent vomiting, because they increase intraocular pressure, strain on the sutures, and possible bleeding. Occasionally the child's eyes are bandaged. Before touching a child who cannot see, the nurse should speak so that he is not startled. A radio is a comfort when vision is limited by bandages and movement is restricted. Again, orientation to the hospital setting, preparation for the postoperative period, and parental support are extremely important.

Retinoblastoma

Retinoblastoma is a malignant tumor arising from retinal tissue. The tumor may be familial or sporadic and may be identified by thorough eye examination at birth. Frequently the diagnosis is made because of the presence of a white reflex from the pupil (leukokoria), strabismus, or ocular inflammation. Retinoblastoma is the most frequent ocular malignancy of childhood. Early recognition and immediate treatment are essential to prevent the rapid metastasis of this foreboding tumor.

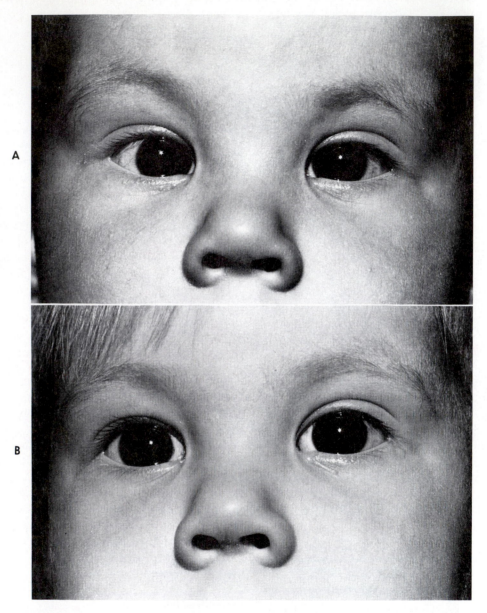

FIG 31-23 Infantile esotropia. **A,** Age 7 months—preoperative; **B,** age 12 months—postoperative (strabismus surgery at age 11 months). Note that although postoperative alignment is straight (that is, true strabismus has been eliminated), there are still typical facial characteristics for pseudostrabismus (flat nasal bridge, wide epicanthal skin folds, narrow interpupillary distance, and greater nasal than temporal scleral visibility). *(Courtesy David G. Martin, MD, San Diego, Calif.)*

Trauma

Serious injury may be associated with a decrease in vision. Nearly one third of monocular blindness follows trauma in childhood years. Arrows and other pointed objects are the chief instruments of blinding injuries in children under 15 years of age.

Of all possible injuries to the eye, traumatic *hyphema* (hemorrhage within the anterior chamber of the eye) is probably the most common ocular injury necessitating hospitalization. Bleeding usually arises from a tear or laceration in the anterior ciliary body rather than in the iris itself.

Prognosis for normal vision decreases as the amount of bleeding in the anterior chamber increases. This is the primary reason for the classic preventive regimen of bed rest, bilateral eye patches, and sedation. Patients should *not* be placed on the affected side. Long-term evaluation should include careful examination of the peripheral retina for tears and periodic evaluation for development of glaucoma. *Glaucoma,* a condition that results from high intraocular pressure, ultimately can lead to loss of optic nerve function and blindness.

Children with a visual loss are confronted with complex, interrelated problems throughout their childhood years. These problems are by no means exclusively personal. The burden is far-reaching, presenting major challenges to parents, teachers, and physicians and to nurses caring for such children in the hospital setting. Those who share this responsibility should be committed to assisting these children in achieving both physical and psychosocial well-being so that they can develop the skills necessary to live safely and happily in our society.

HEARING

The auditory system is the primary channel through which children learn speech and language, develop educationally, and dynamically adjust to the challenges of their environment. The importance of the integrity of the auditory system is both that simple and that complex. The degree of auditory dysfunction (hearing impairment), the developmental time at which hearing impairment occurs, and the duration of the impairment all determine to what extent the child develops normal speech, language, and educational and psychosocial skills. Because hearing impairment itself is generally physically invisible and manifests itself in problems of communication, learning, and psychologic and social behavior, it is sometimes misdiagnosed and subsequently managed as childhood autism, emotional disturbance, and mental retardation. As a result of such errors in diagnosis and treatment, hearing-impaired children can be denied the opportunity to realize their potential and take their places as contributing members of society. For children with congenital hearing loss, it is important to identify the loss and initiate intervention within the first 6 months of life in order to minimize the effect of the hearing loss on their communication and psychosocial development.

Types of loss

It is important to remember that the auditory system is divided primarily into two parts: the peripheral auditory system and the central auditory system (see Fig. 32-5, *A*).

The peripheral auditory system is composed of the outer, middle, and inner ears. The central auditory system is composed of afferent and efferent neurons connecting the sensory end organs of the inner ear to the brainstem and cortical structures.

The three main categories of hearing disorders are as follows: (1) *peripheral impairments,* resulting from lesions to the outer, middle, and inner ears and 8th cranial nerve; (2) *central impairments,* resulting from lesions to the brainstem and auditory cortex; and (3) *functional impairments* nonorganic, which are psychologic with no physiologic basis. There may, of course, be combinations of any or all of these in a given individual.

Disorders of both the peripheral and central auditory systems can be either congenital or acquired. Congenital and acquired losses can be *conductive* (caused by medically treatable pathologic conditions of the outer or middle ears); *sensory* (caused by permanent damage to the cochlea); *neural* (caused by damage to the 8th nerve); *mixed* (combination of conductive and sensori-neural); or *central* (caused by neural disease in the central auditory nervous system). Since the cochlea is composed of both sensory and neural structures, hearing loss secondary to cochlear damage is frequently referred to as *sensori-neural hearing loss.*

Incidence of hearing loss

Total deafness is relatively rare, but partial hearing impairment is not uncommon. The incidence of significant hearing impairment is 1:50 in neonates discharged from intensive care nurseries, and about 1:1,000 in well neonates. Most of these losses occur within the cochlea—that is, sensorineural hearing losses.

Common causes of hearing impairment and deafness

Hearing loss can occur during the prenatal, perinatal, or postnatal stages of a child's development. The most common prenatal factors associated with hearing loss are of genetic origin or occur as a result of maternal rubella in the first trimester.

The most common perinatal factors include prematurity, low birth weight (less than 1,500 g), hyperbilirubinemia (indirect bilirubin of 15 mg or greater), anoxia, and infection, for example, TORCHES disorders (see p. 306).

The most frequent postnatal factors are otitis media, meningitis, and other types of bacteriologic and viral infections (for example, scarlet fever, measles, mumps, and meningitis), and head injury.

An increasingly common cause of sensorineural hearing loss in the adolescent is exposure to excessively loud noise or music. In preschool, kindergarten, and elementary school children, otitis media is by far the most common cause of hearing loss (see p. 705). Although otitis media is a disease of the middle ear that can result in conductive loss of fluctuating severity, it appears from more recent research that the reoccurrence of otitis media in young children can have an irreversible effect on the development of the entire auditory system. Children with significant hearing loss associated with persistent or episodic otitis media before age 2 may have impairment in cognitive, language, and emotional development.

The following criteria are suggested as indications of significant hearing loss in young children (see also box on this page).

1. Hearing levels of 15 dB HL or greater for one or more of the speech frequencies (500, 1K, 2K, 4K Hertz)
2. Indications of otitis media during more than half the time for a period of 6 months in a child under 18 months
3. Fluctuating hearing levels from less than 15 dB HL to over 15 dB HL 6 months or more during the first year of life

Early detection of hearing loss. Early detection and treatment of hearing loss are the key to reducing its damaging effects. All newborns meeting one or more of the following *high-risk criteria* should be tested and followed up for the presence of hearing loss:

1. History of hereditary childhood hearing impairment
2. Rubella or other intrauterine infections (TORCHES)

Parameters of stimuli used to test hearing

Intensity levels—"loudness"

Hearing levels (HL)* for pure-tone hearing testing are measured *decibels* (dB). Zero dB HL is the threshold at which sounds are normally first detected. The levels used to measure human hearing thresholds range from 0 dB to 110 dB HL. Normal hearing levels for children for all frequencies tested are considered to be 0 to 15 dB.

Pure-tone frequencies—"pitch"

Pure-tone frequencies are measured in cycles per second, or *hertz* (Hz). Hertz refers to the number of vibrations per second that a sound source makes to produce each pure tone. The fewer the vibrations per second, the lower the frequency—"pitch"; the greater the number of vibrations, the higher the frequency. The human ear (fully intact) can usually hear frequencies from 20 Hz (very low) to 20,000 Hz (very high), but hearing tests usually monitor frequencies of 250, 500, 1,000, 2,000, 4,000, and 8,000 Hz (frequencies most important for hearing speech and most environmental sounds).

*From American National Standards Institute (ANSI): Specifications for audiometers, New York, 1970, American National Standards Institute.

3. Defects of ear, nose, throat, or larynx (malformed, low-set, or absent pinnae, cleft lip or palate, including submucous clefts, preauricular tags or pits)
4. Birth weight of less than 1,500 g
5. High serum bilirubin concentrations associated with jaundice that appear in the first 24 hours after birth

An infant meeting any of these criteria should be referred for an in-depth audiologic evaluation within the first 2 months of life. Even if hearing seems normal at that time, the child should receive subsequent regularly scheduled hearing evaluations. Regular evaluations are important because many genetically related hearing impairments and hearing losses resulting from ototoxic drug therapy do not appear until some time after birth.

Currently audiometric evaluation can begin in the neonatal nursery. Audiometric procedures that allow for the testing of very young children and children previously thought untestable include: (1) the auditory brainstem-evoked response (BAER) test, which objectively measures brainstem neural responses to auditory stimulation in relaxed or sleeping subjects (cortical-evoked responses to auditory stimulation can also be recorded; however, this must be done with an awake and cooperative subject); (2) the crib-o-gram, which is a completely automated crib assembly designed for auditory signal presentation and recording of infant response; and (3) the impedance test battery, which objectively measures tympanic membrane mobility, middle ear pressure, eustachian tube patency, and the presence of a functioning acoustic reflex (seventh to eighth cranial nerve reflex arc); this test is most reliable for children who are 7 months of age or older; (4) screening for the presence (normal) versus absence (abnormal) of evoked cochlear emissions.

Also included in the test battery are the more traditional behavioral tests of sensitivity to pure tones (see box), calibrated noises, and speech. Reflex responses to sound and classic conditioning methods are used to obtain this information from young children.

With previously undiagnosed or newly developing hearing impairment, certain behaviors may alert the observant nurse to the presence of peripheral or central hearing dysfunction in a child. Examples of these are as follows:

1. Better responses in quiet than in noisy environments
2. Hyperactivity
3. Disinterest in or lack of attention to sounds in the environment
4. Absence of a startle reflex in neonates and infants in the first 6 months of life
5. Difficulty following verbal instructions unless accompanied by visual demonstrations
6. Inadequate vocabulary
7. Defective sentence structure
8. Problems maintaining concentration
9. Social isolation
10. Inadequate reading or spelling
11. Poor reading comprehension
12. Discrepancy between achievement level and potential for learning
13. Significant discrepancy between verbal and performance IQ scores

Peripheral hearing loss is commonly measured using pure tones. Each pure tone has a single frequency of vibration that is perceived as a particular pitch and can be presented to the listener at a variety of levels of intensity or loudness. Presentation of pure tones at different intensity levels to a listener's ears is called the *pure-tone hearing test*. The purpose of this test is to find the intensity level for each frequency at which the listener can "just barely" detect that the tone is present. This hearing

level for each pure-tone frequency is called the listener's *threshold* for that tone.

For young children, mild hearing loss is considered to be hearing threshold levels of 15 dB or greater for *any one* or all the frequencies considered important for the ability to detect and understand speech (500 Hz, 1,000 Hz, 2,000 Hz, 4,000 Hz). Thresholds of 40 dB to 65 dB HL are moderate losses; 70 dB to 85 dB HL are severe losses; and 90 + dB HL are profound losses. An individual with thresholds of greater than or equal to 90 dB HL for a particular frequency is generally classified as being "deaf" for that frequency.

Conventional hearing aids should be considered at the first detection of sensorineural of hearing impairment for all children with mild to profound degrees of hearing loss. The earlier that hearing aids are applied, the better is the prognosis for development of speech and language skills. For a congenital sensorineural hearing loss, hearing aids ideally should be in place by 6 months of age. A joint referral to an otolaryngologist and an audiologist should be made. Cochlear implants are currently being developed to help children and adults who cannot use more traditional hearing aids or who have essentially no cochlear function with intact central auditory systems. These "hearing aids" are surgically implanted electric devices that run on batteries; they stimulate eighth nerve fibers directly rather than cochlear sensory cells, as do traditional hearing aids. (Contact an audiologist or otolaryngologist for further information and referral.)

Before speaking to hearing-impaired children, one should face them directly and obtain their visual attention. This allows them to supplement their limited sound perception with visual cues from your lips and face. Parents and nurses should take every opportunity to expose these young children to meaningful auditory stimulation in order to help improve their use of their residual hearing. With abundant and early exposure to meaningful speech and environmental sound, hearing-impaired children have a much better prognosis for maximum utilization of their auditory systems.

The fact that a child has a hearing defect or wears a hearing aid on admission to the hospital is an important nursing observation. If the child is scheduled for surgery, permission should be sought to allow the child to wear the aid until he is anesthetized in the operating room. The aid should be reapplied as soon as the child has awakened from surgery. Such permission reduces the fear of the young patient and facilitates the entire procedure.

It is important for the nurse to remember that she may well be the first health care professional to suspect the presence of a hearing loss in a child. Sensitivity to the potential of hearing loss and swift and appropriate referral and follow-up can be critical factors in the child's attainment of his full potential.

• • •

This chapter covers a great deal of information—perhaps too much. It treats no subject in depth. However, it is hoped that the student has been challenged to do further study of the needs of children with neuromuscular, skeletal, and sensory problems.

Key Concepts

1. Types of fractures are greenstick, transverse, spiral, oblique, comminuted, and depressed. Every fracture may be placed in one of two main categories: closed fracture, in which no opening in the skin has resulted; and open fracture, in which the skin has been broken, exposing the bone to infection.

2. The fracture of an extremity may be indicated by the presence of deformity in alignment and swelling, pain or tenderness at the fracture site, loss of function or abnormal mobility of the part, a "grating sensation" heard or felt at the suspected point of fracture, and black-and-blue areas caused by subcutaneous hemorrhage.

3. First-aid treatment of a possible fracture includes limiting the movement of the injured part by stabilizing the part and the joint above and below the break to relieve muscle spasm and pain and to prevent further injury.

4. The process of bringing the fragments of a broken bone into proper relationship is termed reducing or setting the fracture. Alignment may be restored surgically or through the application of traction. Casting or splinting is done to maintain correct positioning to ensure proper healing.

5. Various surgical procedures have been devised to increase the effectiveness of various body joints either by increasing their ability to bear weight or by permitting greater motion. Some of the more common procedures are arthrodesis, arthroscopy, osteotomy, tendon transplant, epiphyseal arrest, leg lengthening, and open reduction and internal fixation.

6. Torticollis, or wryneck, is a congenital muscular abnormality often associated with birth trauma.

7. Childhood rickets is a potential health hazard in communities in which there is little sunshine or little exposure of children to the outdoors and a diet deficient in vitamin D, calcium, or phosphorus.

8. Duchenne's muscular dystrophy is the most common form of progressive type muscle weakness. Onset usually occurs between 3 and 6 years of age; life expectancy is usually limited to the teenage period.

9. The most common form of chronic arthritis encountered in pediatrics is juvenile rheumatoid arthritis (JRA). There are three major types: (1) systemic, characterized by fever, rash, internal organ involvement, and often arthritis; (2) polyarticular, characterized by arthritis in numerous large and small joints; and (3) pauciarticular, in which arthritis affects only a few joints.

10. Therapy for JRA includes anti-inflammatory medications, physical and occupational therapy, kind and understanding parental support, and promotion of general health. Mobility should be encouraged as much as can be tolerated to avoid lifelong joint deformities.

11. Legg-Calvé-Perthes disease is a self-limiting disease of the hip produced by lack of circulation to the femoral head. Treatment consists of traction until symptoms are resolved, followed by hip bracing to properly maintain the femoral head in the acetabulum.

12. Osteomyelitis, or inflammation of the bone resulting from infectious agents, has decreased remarkably with the increased availability of antibiotics. Treatment includes bed rest, immobilization of the affected limb, analgesics, and broad-spectrum antibiotics.

13. An osteosarcoma originates in the connective tissue and is the most common primary malignant tumor of bone. Early diagnosis and immediate treatment are crucial. When a tissue of bony origin is malignant, aggressive anticancer chemotherapy and radical methods of treatment, including amputation, must be endorsed in order to save the patient.

14. Abnormal types of spinal curvature are scoliosis, kyphosis, and lordosis. Scoliosis, S-shaped lateral curvature, is the most common spinal deformity encountered in childhood. Idiopathic scoliosis is the most common type.

15. Screening is the only sure way of preventing the severe curvatures of idiopathic scoliosis. Screening programs should begin before 10 years of age and should include both boys and girls.

16. Treatment for scoliosis depends on the stage in which scoliosis is diagnosed and the severity of the curvature. Curves up to 20 degrees are usually left alone and watched. Curves between 20 and 40 degrees and progressing are stabilized with a brace. Surgical correction is usually considered for curves that are over 40 degrees.

17. When maximum correction of the spinal curve has been achieved, a spinal fusion is usually performed. Patients who have had a spinal fusion need the same basic pre- and postoperative care required for all surgical patients. In addition, they need the special attention necessary for all casted patients.

18. The two main types of seizures are partial and generalized. The nursing care of a patient having a convulsion emphasizes the need to protect the patient from accidental injury and the importance of close observation and thorough reporting.

19. Meningitis is always considered a medical emergency; early recognition and prompt treatment are essential for a favorable recovery. Diagnosis is confirmed by the results of a lumbar puncture. The nurse assisting with this procedure must understand the importance of maintaining the position of the child.

20. Nursing care of the child in the acute phase of meningitis includes correction of dehydration, restraints to safeguard intravenous infusion, frequent monitoring of vital signs, control of temperature, and recording of intake and output.

21. Cerebral palsy is a nonprogressive disorder of motion and posture resulting from brain injury or insult during a period of early brain growth. Treatment is directed toward limiting a disability and may continue throughout the affected person's life.

22. The three main types of cerebral palsy are spastic type, extrapyramidal (nonspastic) type, and mixed cerebral palsy, which combines the spastic and extrapyramidal types.

23. A team approach is necessary for the care of a cerebral-palsied child and his family. Through physical and occupational therapy, surgical techniques, and medication, youngsters with cerebral palsy are able to meet their daily personal needs and, in some cases, to prepare for self-supporting occupations.

24. Encephalitis is an inflammation of the brain caused by infectious agents. The nursing care of a child with encephalitis is much like that of a child with meningitis.

25. Signs and symptoms of brain tumors are headache, dizziness, lethargy, indifference, irritability, morning vomiting, double or blurred vision, speech, balance, and gait problems, and local muscle weakness. Care of the patient with a possible brain tumor includes observation for any of these signs and symptoms in addition to assessment of vital signs and precautions to prevent falls during ambulation.

26. Four common clinical manifestations of the neuroblastoma are (1) a mass usually involving the abdomen or lymph nodes, (2) neurologic signs, (3) pain, usually in the bone or joints, and (4) orbital signs. Because the neuroblastoma is a highly malignant tumor with tendencies to produce widespread metastases, aggressive therapy usually includes surgical excision, irradiation, and chemotherapy.

27. The term concussion implies a loss of consciousness with a temporary neuronal dysfunction caused by jarring with no pathologic evidence of damage to the underlying brain. The period of memory loss that surrounds a concussion is called post-traumatic amnesia (PTA).

28. Contusions and lacerations are characterized by specific findings, and are frequently accompanied by hemorrhages or bleeding into the brain substance. A basic neurologic check includes assessment of level of consciousness, pupil response, motor function, and vital signs.

29. Intracranial hematomas should be suspected in every case of head injury with coma or one-sided weakness. Unless the intracranial pressure is reduced, neurologic deterioration follows that can prove to be fatal.

30. Epidural hematomas result from a torn high-pressure arterial system and characteristically demonstrate a relatively rapid downhill course unless identified and treated.

31. Subdural hematomas may be associated with severe brain injury and are divided into three categories (acute, subacute, and chronic), depending on the time interval from injury to onset of symptoms.

32. Skull fractures are either linear or depressed. Symptoms that may alert the nurse to a skull fracture after the child's hospital admission include black-and-blue marks around the eyes or ears on the second day and watery fluid or discharge from the ear or nose.

33. Nursing care of patients with skull fractures includes

establishment and maintenance of an adequate airway and proper ventilation and circulation. Patients should be kept in a lateral, slightly elevated position and should be turned and suctioned hourly.

34. Initial examination of the head-injured child consists of a detailed neurologic examination to facilitate a more accurate diagnosis of the extent of injury and to form the baseline from which subsequent progress can be judged. The nurse is responsible for careful systematic serial observations and recording of changing factors and physical signs.

35. Recognition of the depth of responsiveness is essential in determining the initial severity of the comatose patient's brain insult. The Glasgow Coma Scale (GCS) is a reliable instrument designed to define the degree of responsiveness.

36. Common causes of visual impairment in infancy and childhood are trauma, strabismus, and refractive error.

37. A professional eye examination should be performed on every child immediately after birth, at 6 months, and once between ages 3 and 5. Annual follow-up screening in the schools is recommended.

38. Children with the following findings should be referred to an ophthalmologist: possible strabismus; poor visual fixation preference or a visual acuity difference between the two eyes of two lines or more on the eye chart; vision in either eye of 20/40 or less; evidence of structural deformity of the eye; and family history of retinoblastoma, congenital cataracts, or genetic or metabolic eye diseases.

39. The incidence of retrolental fibroplasia (RLF) has decreased, but is reemerging as the use of oxygen therapy rises in the salvage of high-risk infants.

40. Developmental dyslexia can occur in children in the presence or absence of visual deficit; therefore, educators are best qualified to deal with such learning disorders.

41. The imbalance of the extraocular muscles in strabismus can lead to amblyopia, poor binocular vision, and an unacceptable appearance. Specific treatment of strabismus depends on the cause and may include glasses, occlusive therapy, orthoptics, or surgery. Specific treatment of amblyopia may include glasses or occlusive therapy.

42. Refractive errors are myopia, hyperopia, and astigmatism, and usually do not cause difficulties until the child reaches school age. Vision usually can be corrected to a normal level with proper glasses.

43. Surgical removal of cataracts is the only effective method of treatment for all but a few infants and children. The postoperative period is usually short and requires a sterile eye pad, protective shield, and some limitation of activity. Every effort should be made to reduce crying and prevent vomiting.

44. Retinoblastoma is the most common ocular malignancy of childhood. Early recognition and treatment are essential to prevent rapid metastasis.

45. Traumatic hyphema (hemorrhage within the anterior chamber of the eye) is probably the most common ocular injury necessitating hospitalization. Treatment includes bed rest, bilateral eye patches, and sedation. Patients should not be placed on the affected side.

46. The degree of auditory dysfunction, the developmental time at which hearing impairment occurs, and the duration of the impairment all determine to what extent the child develops normal speech, language, and educational and psychosocial skills.

47. The three main categories of hearing disorders are (1) peripheral impairments, (2) central impairments, and (3) functional impairments.

48. Hearing loss can occur during the prenatal, perinatal, or postnatal stages of a child's development. The following criteria may indicate significant hearing loss in young children: hearing levels of 15 dB HL or greater, indications of otitis media during more than half the time for a period of 6 months in a child under 18 months, and fluctuating hearing levels from less than 15 dB HL to over 15 dB HL 6 months or more during the first year of life.

49. All newborns meeting one or more of the following criteria should be tested and followed up for the presence of hearing loss: history of hereditary childhood hearing impairment; rubella or other intrauterine infections; defects of ear, nose, throat, or larnyx, birth weight of less than 1,500 g; and high serum bilirubin concentrations associated with jaundice that appear in the first 24 hours.

50. Behaviors that may alert the nurse to the presence of peripheral or central hearing dysfunction in a child include the following: better response in quiet than noisy environments, hyperactivity, disinterest in or lack of attention to sounds in the environment, difficulty following verbal instructions unless accompanied by visual demonstrations, inadequate vocabulary, problems maintaining concentration, and social isolation.

Discussion Questions

1. Why are fractures a common problem in childhood and adolescence? How does this correlate to the developmental stages? Identify the types of fractures and their medical treatment, and review the nursing implications for care of the child with a cast or in traction.

2. Discuss how chronic musculoskeletal problems such as rheumatoid arthritis, scoliosis, Duchenne's muscular dystrophy, cerebral palsy, and osteomyelitis can make an impact on a child's growth and development. What is the role of the nurse in caring for children with these conditions?

3. What are the major causes of head injuries in infants and children? How are head injuries classified? How are cranial checks performed on a child? What signs indicate increased intracranial pressure?

4. Seizure disorders are frequently diagnosed during childhood. Identify the major seizure disorders. What should the nurse record regarding seizure activity? What safety precautions should be taken if a major seizure is witnessed? What is involved in the treatment of seizure disorders?

5. List two of the most common vision problems that occur in childhood. How can these be detected? What are the medical treatment and nursing concerns for each condition? What are the most common causes of hearing loss in infants and children? What can the nurse do to aid in the detection and prevention of hearing loss?

32

Conditions Involving the Respiratory and Circulatory Systems

CHAPTER OBJECTIVES

After studying this chapter, the student should be able to perform the following:

1 Define the terms listed in the key vocabulary.

2 Discuss pneumonia in the pediatric patient: its types, causes, general signs and symptoms, possible treatments, and nursing care.

3 Indicate the basic genetic hereditary pattern of cystic fibrosis, type of glands the disease affects, two body systems most involved, signs and symptoms, tests used, nutrition, typical treatments, and nursing care.

4 Compare croup (LTB) and epiglottis, considering typical patients, anatomy affected, symptoms, and types of treatment and care.

5 Describe the first-aid treatment of nosebleeds.

6 Define the terms "otitis media" and "myringotomy" and discuss two possible dangers of such infections.

7 List five nursing considerations to remember when caring for a 4-year-old child recently returned from the recovery room after "T and A" surgery.

8 State why the identification of a strep throat is important in the prevention of disease.

9 List five nonimmunologic factors that can trigger an attack of asthma in susceptible persons.

10 Outline the treatment of an 8-year-old child suffering from a severe asthmatic attack; include the definition of status asthmaticus and care in a hospital setting.

11 Describe four nursing concerns present when nursing a 2½-year-old who has just returned to his hospital room after a cardiac catheterization.

12 Indicate five signs of cardiac-related difficulty that infants with congenital heart disease frequently manifest.

13 Give a brief description of the following congenital heart defects: patent ductus arteriosus, atrial and ventricular septal defects, tetralogy of Fallot, complete transposition of the great vessels, and coarctation of the aorta.

14 List six observational aspects that the nursing care of a child with a moderately severe heart defect should include.

15 Discuss iron-deficiency anemia: definition, importance, ages of greatest incidence, prevention, and therapy.

16 Discuss sickle cell anemia, sickle cell trait, and the circulation problems that can occur in children having the disease.

17 Indicate four special safety considerations for children with a diagnosis of hemophilia.

18 Describe five signs or symptoms associated with leukemia and how their appearance relates to the primary bone marrow abnormalities characteristically present.

19 Discuss the supportive care of the leukemic patient

690

If one speaks of the respiratory system without mentioning the circulatory system, only part of an important story is told, because these two body systems are intimately related. One might say that the respiratory system begins and ends the story, but the circulatory system contributes the bulky middle chapters. To put it another way, the respiratory system is responsible for so-called *external respiration*, whereas the circulatory system includes in its duties responsibility for *internal respiration*.

For this reason pediatric disorders of the respiratory and circulatory systems are considered here in the same general section, although for convenience they are also presented in separate units. The respiratory system comprises Part 1 and the circulatory system Part 2 of this chapter.

KEY VOCABULARY

A brief review of basic terminology used in describing respiratory and circulatory action and problems may be helpful.

anemia Condition in which hemoglobin in the blood is reduced.

apnea Absence of breathing.

atelectasis Airless segment of lung; collapse of lung.

bronchiectasis Abnormal dilation of the bronchi in response to inflammation, which, if prolonged, leads to associated structural changes and a chronic, productive cough.

Cheyne-Stokes respiration Irregular, cyclic breathing characterized by a period of increasing respiratory action followed by an interval of apnea.

dyspnea Difficult breathing.

edema Abnormal, excessive amount of fluid within the body tissues.

emphysema Abnormal dilation and loss of elasticity of the microscopic air sacs, or alveoli, of the lung.

empyema Collection of pus in a body cavity, especially the pleural cavity.

eupnea Normal breathing.

leukocytosis Excessive increase in the number of white blood cells circulating in the blood.

orthopnea Condition in which breathing is possible by the patient only when in a standing or sitting position.

pneumothorax Abnormal collection of air or gas in the pleural cavity.

remission Lessening of severity or abatement of symptoms.

stenosis Abnormal narrowing of a passage or opening.

Part 1: The Respiratory System

In conjunction with the study of disorders of the respiratory system, the student should review Chapter 26, which briefly outlines the basic anatomy and physiology of the respiratory system and discusses methods of aiding respiration and oxygenation.

Respiratory difficulties (such as respiratory distress syndrome, tracheoesophageal fistula, and diaphragmatic hernia) that are particularly associated with the newborn period are discussed in Chapters 14 and 15. This presentation of respiratory pathology begins with a brief anatomic review, followed by a consideration of those common problems affecting children in various stages of development.

ANATOMIC REVIEW

Nose. The nose is an interesting structure; although for some people it may not be an aesthetic asset, it performs certain important functions. First of all, it prepares air for entry into the interior of the body. It filters, warms, and moistens the air. Humans also breathe through their open mouths, and except during the period of infancy, they do so fairly often. However, large amounts of air that enter the throat through the mouth are not properly warmed to body temperature or 100% humidified. The nose is also involved in the identification of different odors because the olfactory nerve endings are located within the nasal cavity. Many of the finer perceptions of the palate are influenced by the sensitivity of these nerves. Consider how uninteresting food seems when one has a cold and the proper ventilation of the nose is disturbed. A normal nose is also necessary for proper vocal response.

Pharynx and trachea. The pharynx is a passageway shared by both the respiratory and digestive systems. It extends from the back of the nasal cavity down past the posterior portion of the oral cavity to the level of the larynx and esophagus. Consequently the pharynx is divided descriptively into three parts: nasal, oral, and hypopharyngeal. The larynx and trachea extending from the hypopharynx complete the upper respiratory system.

Lower respiratory tract. The lower respiratory tract is usually considered to include the bronchi, bronchioles, alveoli, which form the tissues of the lungs, and pleurae, or coverings of the lungs. Infectious conditions involving these structures are, for the most part, more difficult to cure and more threatening to general health than those involving the passages of the upper respiratory system.

RESPIRATORY DISORDERS
Infant

Bronchiolitis. Bronchiolitis is a viral respiratory illness with clinical manifestations attributed to inflammatory narrowing of the small airways. The bronchioles are partially or completely obstructed as a result of mucosal swelling and exudate. The condition is more common in young infants and is seldom seen in children over 2 years of age.

Bronchiolitis begins as a simple cold. After a few days the infant develops a low-grade fever, shallow, rapid respirations, a cough, and an expiratory wheeze. Air can usually enter the bronchioles, but expiratory narrowing causes it to be trapped distal to the obstruction. Suprasternal and subcostal retractions are noted on inspiration. The infant is fatigued, irritable, anxious, and unable to eat or sleep. In severe cases some infants even become cyanotic.

Some physicians believe that a trial of bronchodilator therapy is warranted in severe cases, but in most cases of pure bronchiolitis, it is not effective. Intravenous aminophylline, subcutaneous epinephrine, or aerosol therapy with albuterol can be used once a trial of bronchodilator therapy is decided. If benefit is achieved, this therapy is continued.

Acute bronchiolitis in infants presents a frightening picture. Parents feel helpless, anxious, and fearful that the life of their child is in jeopardy. Fortunately mortality is very low, and the most severe period lasts only a few days. Recovery is almost always complete within 2 weeks. This information is most welcome by the worried parents. Their questions should be answered simply, and they are encouraged to stay at the crib side. The infant should be observed closely because apnea can occur. Color, respirations, and pulse need close observation.

Rest, oxygen, and hydration are most important. Nasal suctioning is usually necessary before feeding. Fluids should be urged frequently and in small amounts.

Pneumonia. Inflammation of the lung parenchyma is called pneumonia. Many microbiologic agents, as well as certain noninfectious agents and conditions, are known to cause pneumonia. The anatomic and pathologic changes may involve the lobar, lobular, interstitial, or bronchial areas. Pneumonia, most commonly seen in infants and young children, can be a potentially grave condition, and one of the major causes of mortality in the age group of 1 to 14 years. Early recognition and prompt treatment spare lengthy hospitalization and reduce the incidence of complications. Common causes of pneumonias in infants and children are

I. Primary pneumonias (no underlying predisposing condition diagnosed)
  A. Bacterial
    1. Pneumococcal
    2. Staphylococcal
    3. Streptococcal
    4. *Haemophilus influenzae*
  B. Nonbacterial
    1. Viral
    2. *Mycoplasma*
    3. *Chlamydia*
II. Secondary pneumonias (other predisposing conditions diagnosed)
  A. Hypostatic—caused by stasis of respiratory secretions resulting from lack of adequate inflation and drainage
  B. Asthmatic—caused by narrowed airways and increased mucus
  C. Associated with cystic fibrosis—caused by the presence of viscid respiratory secretions
  D. Aspiration pneumonias—involving accidental inhalation of
    1. Hydrocarbons—petroleum distillates, such as gasoline, kerosene, and furniture polish
    2. Foreign bodies—popcorn, peanuts, buttons, and other objects
    3. Gastric contents—associated with gastroesophageal reflux (GER) and other congenital anomalies of the esophagus or trachea and neuromuscular disorders

Signs and symptoms. The onset and clinical manifestations of pneumonia vary with the age of the child and the etiologic agent. The disease occurs most frequently in winter and spring. Bacterial pneumonias are often preceded by a viral upper respiratory tract infection, which alters the defense mechanisms of the lower respiratory tract. The classic signs and symptoms are fever, anorexia, listlessness, and cough. At first the cough is wet and loose, but soon it becomes dry and painful. The pain associated with lower lobe pneumonia is frequently referred to the abdomen. Therefore, one should think of pneumonia when a child presents with abdominal pain and fever because the abdominal pain can be due to a lower lobe pneumonia.

In the young child the temperature mounts rapidly, and seizures frequently occur. Respirations become rapid and shallow and are accompanied by flaring of the nostrils, grunting, and retractions. The pulse rate is extremely rapid (it may be doubled). Meningeal irritation, such as stiff neck, is sometimes present with upper lobe pneumonia, and a spinal tap is necessary to rule out coexisting meningitis. Cyanosis coupled with a rapid, weak pulse is always a grave sign. Since proper therapy depends on knowledge of the causative agents, the common pneumonias are discussed according to their cause.

Types

Bacterial primary pneumonias. Pneumococcal pneumonia is the most common type encountered in infants and young children. Typically, after symptoms of a mild cold, the infant suddenly refuses his milk or formula and becomes listless. His temperature rises rapidly, and respiratory distress is soon apparent. Fortunately, the pneumococcus is responsive to antibiotic therapy. A good response to penicillin usually takes place within 24 to 48 hours in uncomplicated cases. Response to therapy is delayed in cases that are complicated by fluid in the pleural space (pleural effusion), empyema, otitis media, or meningitis.

Staphylococcal pneumonia is the most serious of the pneumonias in infancy. It may follow an upper respiratory tract infection, or it may spread to the lungs by way of the bloodstream from a staphylococcal infection elsewhere in the body. Unless recognized and treated early, the disease characteristically progresses rapidly, causing severe respiratory distress, and may be associated with the formation of abscesses and air cysts (pneumatoceles). Antibiotic therapy with nafcillin or oxacillin is continued for a few weeks. Antistaphylococcal cephalosporins are also effective. Isolation technique is observed. Pneumothorax can occur resulting in sudden deterioration of respiratory status and is treated with chest tube insertion and continuous closed-suction drainage. Mortality is high in untreated infants.

Streptococcal pneumonia is more common in young children than in infants. It is usually preceded by a viral infection, such as rubeola, rubella, or varicella. The onset of chills and pleuritic pain may be sudden, or the pneumonia may start with a gradual rise in temperature, accompanied by cough. Streptococci cause an interstitial type of pneumonia, and occasionally abscesses and pneumatoceles can develop. Empyema usually requires closed-suction drainage. Penicillin G is the antibiotic of choice and is highly effective.

Pneumonia caused by *Haemophilus influenzae* type b is a serious disease. The onset of illness is usually acute, and the clinical course cannot be distinguished from other bacterial pneumonias. Infants and children under 5 years of age are most often affected and seem susceptible to bacteremia and empyema. There is a high incidence of associated infections such as URI, otitis media, epiglottitis, and meningitis. To prevent serious complications, chloramphenicol is given in large doses as soon as the disease is diagnosed and is continued until the drug sensitivity studies are completed. Lately, the cephalosporins are being used more frequently than chloramphenicol.

Nonbacterial primary pneumonias. Viral pneumonia can be caused by many viruses. A low-grade fever and coryza precede this interstitial pneumonia, which appears suddenly with the onset of tachypnea and a nonproductive, tight cough. Treatment is symptomatic, since antibiotics are of no value unless secondary bacterial complications occur. One exception is respiratory syncytial virus pneumonia, which is treated with ribavirin aerosol.

Mycoplasmal pneumonia is an atypical pneumonia caused by a pathogenic "filterable" microorganism known as *Mycoplasma pneumoniae* (Eaton agent). It is a tiny, free-living microorganism that has properties between those of bacteria and viruses. Infection usually results in a self-limited, interstitial pneumonia. Mycoplasmal pneumonia occurs most commonly in the adolescent. The onset is abrupt, and symptoms include fever, headache, malaise, chills, and a characteristic dry, hacking cough. Later the cough becomes productive, sometimes producing blood-streaked mucus. Erythromycin is the antibiotic of choice in treating this type of pneumonia in children.

Chlamydia pneumonia is caused by *Chlamydia,* which is transmitted to the infant in the birth canal. It can also cause conjunctivitis. The age of onset is 2 to 12 weeks and onset is gradual. The infected infants are afebrile. The most prominent symptom is staccato cough; it can be very severe and paroxysmal. Physical examination reveals rales and chest x-ray shows hyperexpansion with infiltrates. The antibiotic of choice is erythromycin or sulfisoxazole.

Secondary aspiration pneumonias. Infants and children have been known to aspirate not only their formula but all kinds of foods, poisons, and objects. The right upper lobe is frequently involved. Mucosal swelling and obstruction can occur. Symptoms vary depending on the child, the substance, and the amount aspirated. Treatment is supportive and aimed at preventing intercurrent infections. Of course, prevention of these incidents is the best therapy.

Aspiration of petroleum distillates, such as kerosene, gasoline, lighter fluid, and furniture polishes, causes a severe chemical pneumonitis, characterized by edema and inflammation. Some petroleum distillates are absorbed from the intestines and then excreted through the lungs. Treatment is symptomatic and may include steroids to reduce inflammatory changes or antibiotics to combat secondary infections.

A number of foreign bodies, including seeds, coins, nuts, popcorn, safety pins, and bones, have been removed from the respiratory passages of young children. (Young children who do not have their molar teeth yet must not eat peanuts or popcorn because of this common problem.) Foreign bodies inhaled into the lungs occlude the bronchi, causing atelectasis or hyperinflation. The young child manifests dyspnea, cyanosis, and asymmetric respirations. Incomplete obstruction causes wheezing, and, if it is untreated, fever and cough-producing purulent sputum soon develop. Delay in removal of the foreign object by bronchoscopy seriously alters the prognosis. Usually the foreign body becomes embedded, injuring the tissues and causing infection. Larger foreign bodies can get lodged in and obstruct the larynx and trachea, causing acute suffocation.

Diagnosis of the pneumonias. A high white blood cell count (WBC) of over 10,000 with increased polymorphonuclear cells and a shift to young forms (bands) is suggestive of bacterial infections. A low WBC (5,000 or less) is more typical of viral infections in general; therefore a differential white blood cell count is routinely requested on these patients. Blood cultures obtained before antibiotic therapy is initiated are helpful in the identification of specific organisms if septicemia is present. Nasopharyngeal cultures are not of great value because pneumococci, streptococci, *H. influenzae,* and staphylococci can be isolated from healthy children. Tracheal cultures obtained by suction techniques are more helpful in identification of organisms. X-ray films are perhaps the most valuable diagnostic tool in evaluating the extent or type of the pneumonia. Bronchoscopy (visualization of the tracheobronchial tree) may be performed when other procedures have failed to make an adequate diagnosis of the problem but is done only in special circumstances. Fluid or tissue may be removed by this method for a culture or for cytology studies. Lung biopsy is sometimes necessary when protracted pulmonary disease cannot be diagnosed by other means and when the clinical situation is very serious.

Treatment and supportive nursing care. Specific therapy is important in the treatment of pneumonia. Differentiating viral and bacterial infections initially is difficult.

Pneumococcal pneumonia is the most common pneumonia seen in infants and young children and can be treated adequately by any one of a variety of antimicrobial agents. Penicillin is the preferred drug. When the cause of the pneumonia is established, a specific drug can be given. Most nonbacterial pneumonias are viral in origin and are not influenced by antimicrobial therapy. Chlamydia pneumonia and mycoplasmal pneumonia are exceptions.

Supportive care is as important as antibiotic therapy in lessening the severity of the child's illness. Fluids are encouraged, and acetaminophen or aspirin is given for fever. Rest in bed is recommended during the febrile stage. Humidification and increased amounts of fluid are necessary for liquefaction of bronchial secretions. Saturated solution of potassium iodide (SSKI) or guaifenesin syrup (Robitussin) can help loosen secretions and initiate a productive cough. In general cough suppressants, such as codeine, are not recommended in pneumonia because a valuable mechanism used to help clear the bronchial tree would be lost. Respiratory therapies are important in the hospital setting. Bronchial drainage is carried out three or four times daily (before meals and at bedtime). Viscid secretions do not drain from the bronchi by gravity alone, but deep breathing, reinforced coughing, and respiratory therapy techniques, such as chest percussion and vibration, assist in their removal. Oxygen administration is used for children with hypoxia.

When the child's appetite improves, a nutritious diet of foods that are appealing should be ordered. Before feeding an infant, the nurse should remove nasal secretions. One or two drops of saline solution may be ordered, followed by gentle suctioning. A restless infant who cannot breathe does not eat.

Nursing care involves careful observation of respiratory patterns, pulse, color, and the general condition of the patient. Observance of the attending physician's

NURSING CARE PLAN

The Child with Pneumonia

Selected nursing diagnoses	Expected outcomes	Interventions
A. Ineffective airway clearance related to inflammation and obstruction of the respiratory tract. Clinical manifestations: Increased respiration rate, dyspnea, cough, elevated temperature, retractions, nasal flaring, grunting, and cyanosis.	Child regains/maintains normal respiratory function.	Assess child's respiratory status (lung sounds, color, respirations, rate, presence of nasal flaring and retractions, use of accessory muscles) every 4 hours and prn. Monitor IV antibiotics as ordered. Encourage clear oral fluids/IV hydration as needed. Monitor I & O. Assure respiratory treatments are given as ordered and assess child's response. Suction nares prior to feeding and prn. Elevate head of bed/place infant in infant seat to facilitate air exchange.
B. Fluid volume deficit related to decreased oral intake and fever. Clinical manifestations: Poor skin turgor, dry mucous membranes, no tears, decreased urinary output, increased urine specific gravity.	Child maintains adequate hydration.	Assess child's hydration status every shift (mucous membranes, skin turgor, tearing, urine output, urine specific gravity). Encourage clear oral fluids/IV hydration as needed. Maintain strict I & O. Administer antibiotics and antipyretics as ordered.
C. Anxiety related to respiratory distress and unfamiliar environment. Clinical manifestations: Verbalizes fear/anxiety, crying, restlessness.	Child and parents cope effectively and decrease level of anxiety.	Provide a quiet, restful environment. Remain with child when he is in distress. Explain procedures and treatment to child (age-appropriate) and parents. Encourage parents to participate in care of child. See Nursing Care Plan for The Hospitalized Child (p. 695).

positioning orders and frequent modification of body position within the prescribed limits are also important. Patients often breathe better with their heads and chests elevated; babies are often placed in infant seats. On the other hand, unresponsive or neurologically impaired patients should be positioned on their sides so that pharyngeal secretions can be drained out of their mouths and prevented from being aspirated into their airways with inspiration.

Isolation techniques are observed, mainly for contagious conditions such as staphylococcal pneumonia. Convalescence should not be rushed; adequate time for recuperation is important to allow the child to regain strength and weight.

When a child with pneumonia is treated at home or on an outpatient basis, the parents should be carefully instructed about the therapeutic and nursing measures. They should understand that medicines must be taken on time and in the correct amount. In general young children should be cared for by their parents in the familiar, comforting environment of their own homes. Nevertheless, hospitalization may be advisable during the first 2 or 3 days of illness to provide respiratory therapy and parenteral administration of drugs and fluid. Infants with pneumonia who are under 6 months of age are always hospitalized. Other children are hospitalized when they become too sick to take fluids, when they require intensive supportive measures (such as intravenous or oxygen therapy or surgical drainage) because of their diagnosis or condition, or when the family cannot or does not adequately care for them.

Although currently the diagnosis of pneumonia does not produce the same alarm in the hearts and minds of parents that it once did, it is still a potential threat to the life and future health of the child. Patients affected by this disease must be frequently evaluated and expertly nursed.

Cystic fibrosis (mucoviscidosis). Cystic fibrosis (CF) is a hereditary, multisystem disorder in which generalized dysfunction of the exocrine glands occurs, especially involving the mucous and sweat glands. It is usually characterized by the triad of chronic, severe pulmonary disease, pancreatic insufficiency, and abnormally high concentrations of electrolytes in the sweat.

Cystic fibrosis is transmitted as an autosomal recessive trait. There is no efficient, cost-effective way to identify persons in the general population who are carrying the gene. However, it is now possible to identify carriers of the CF gene (located on the long arm of chromosome 7) within affected families. Analysis of blood samples and chorionic villi for the presence of specific DNA markers linked to the CF gene allow for prenatal diagnosis. The immunoreactive trypsin (IRT) test of blood spots indicates whether the unborn child has the disease.

If one child has CF, the risk for each subsequent pregnancy is one in four. That is, each conception has the same 25% chance of producing an affected child (see p. 321 for genetic discussion). The incidence of cystic fibrosis in the United States is 1 per 1,600 to 2,000 live births. Boys and girls appear to be equally affected. Five percent of the white population and less than 1% of the black population are estimated to be genetic carriers of this hidden trait. Although the survival rate is steadily improving, cystic fibrosis remains a serious condition.

Couples who have a child with cystic fibrosis should be made aware of the genetic implications of the disease and appropriate counseling should be provided.

Symptoms. Clinical expression of the disease varies because of individual variation in age at onset and severity of involvement of the various organs and systems. However, the altered function of the exocrine glands leads to clinical manifestations, primarily in the respiratory and digestive systems (Fig. 32-1).

Almost all patients with cystic fibrosis have some degree of chronic pulmonary disease. The degree of pulmonary involvement and rate of progression usually determine the prognosis. Involvement occurs through a progressive sequence of events that are experienced by all patients sooner or later. Secretions of the mucus-producing glands become extremely thick and tenacious in the bronchi and bronchioles, causing coughing, wheezing, respiratory obstruction, emphysema, and frequently infection. As a result the defense in the lungs against microbes is severely compromised. In severe cases the chronic respiratory disease causes a barrel-like chest deformity, cyanosis, and clubbing of the fingers and toes. As hypoxemia and secondary pulmonary arterial hypertension develop, dilation of the right side of the heart and thickening of the right ventricular wall occur. When untreated, this process can result in heart failure and death. Cardiac disease secondary to pulmonary disease is termed *cor pulmonale* (Fig. 32-2).

Approximately 85% of patients with cystic fibrosis have digestive system problems. Since the pancreatic digestive enzymes in these patients are reduced or absent, foodstuffs (fats and proteins especially) may be poorly digested and assimilated. As a result the infant or child fails to thrive. Because much of the food eaten does not undergo the normal process of digestion and assimilation, the child will pass large amounts of feces and develop a protuberant abdomen. This bulky stool has a foul smell, and greasy appearance. It also floats in the toilet bowl because of undigested fat.

In a small percentage of cases (about 10%), the disease is recognized in the newborn nursery because of the detection of meconium ileus. In this condition the meconium, or stool formed in utero by the newborn infant, is thicker and stickier than normal meconium because of the absence or reduction of normal pancreatic digestive enzymes. The abnormal stool sticks to the walls of the ileum like paste and obstructs the lower digestive tract. The obstructed intestine becomes distended, and abdominal distention, or bloating, is noted, and no passage of stool occurs. Vomiting and dehydration may ensue. Any

CLINICAL MANIFESTATIONS OF CYSTIC FIBROSIS IN A CHILD

CF is a multi-system disorder of children

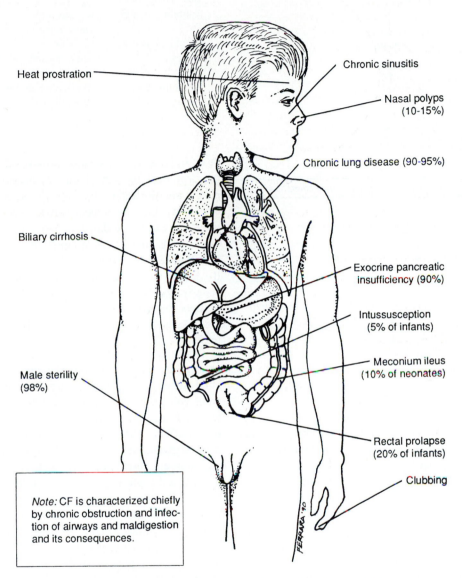

Heat prostration

Chronic sinusitis

Nasal polyps
(10-15%)

Chronic lung disease (90-95%)

Biliary cirrhosis

Exocrine pancreatic
insufficiency (90%)

Intussusception
(5% of infants)

Meconium ileus
(10% of neonates)

Male sterility
(98%)

Rectal prolapse
(20% of infants)

Clubbing

Note: CF is characterized chiefly
by chronic obstruction and infection of airways and maldigestion
and its consequences.

FERRARA '90

FIG 32-1   Clinical manifestations of cystic fibrosis in a child.

newborn infant who does not pass stool within 24 hours after birth should be carefully evaluated and examined for possible obstruction (see pp. 746-747 for management). Other clinical conditions in infancy that indicate the possibility of cystic fibrosis include obstructive jaundice, hypoproteinemia, prolonged bronchiolitis, and rectal prolapse.

Diagnosis. A high degree of clinical suspicion is usually the first step in the diagnosis of cystic fibrosis. Infants and children who suffer from recurrent respiratory tract infections or fail to thrive should be especially evaluated. The diagnosis is confirmed by laboratory evidence of abnormally elevated sweat chloride levels. A positive reaction implies an elevation of the concentration of chlo-

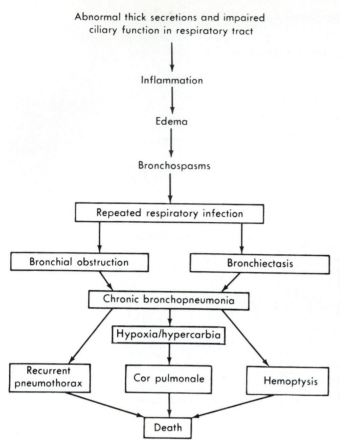

Abnormal thick secretions and impaired
ciliary function in respiratory tract

↓

Inflammation

↓

Edema

↓

Bronchospasms

↓

Repeated respiratory infection

Bronchial obstruction　　Bronchiectasis

Chronic bronchopneumonia

Hypoxia/hypercarbia

Recurrent pneumothorax　　Cor pulmonale　　Hemoptysis

Death

FIG 32-2 Pathologic sequence characteristic of cystic fibrosis.

Table 32-1 Pulmonary therapy

Treatment	Purpose
Intermittent aerosol therapy	To deliver medications and water to the lower respiratory tract
Antibiotic therapy	To treat infection and minimize progression of lung disease
Chest physical therapy	To facilitate the removal of secretions and prevent mucus accumulation
Breathing exercises	To establish and maintain a good breathing pattern

death in patients with cystic fibrosis is directly related to the degree of lung involvement, maximum therapeutic efforts are directed to the lungs (Table 32-1). Thick mucus obstructing the lungs leads to recurrent pulmonary infection and tissue damage. Early in the course of the disease, the mucus that accumulates in the bronchi and bronchioles is so viscid that the cilia are unable to expel it. As the mucus stagnates, it becomes contaminated, usually by *Staphylococcus aureus* and *Pseudomonas aeruginosa*. Resultant infection intensifies mucus production, and the accumulation leads to airway obstruction.

Control of pulmonary infection requires the use of appropriate antibiotics and adequate drainage of bronchial secretions by respiratory therapy. During sleep some children still use a fine-mist environment, but clinical investigations have failed to demonstrate any beneficial effect. The use of a continuing home pulmonary care program from the time of diagnosis to prevent progression and complications as much as possible has improved the life expectancy of children with cystic fibrosis. Children with advanced and steadily increasing pulmonary disease or severe pulmonary infections usually must be hospitalized for intensive parenteral antibiotic therapy. However, intravenous administration of antibiotics to inpatients and outpatients with acute and chronic infection can be accomplished by use of the heparin lock IV. In fact, many hospitalizations can be avoided by teaching selected children or parents this convenient method of parenteral antibiotic therapy. The heparin lock IV consists of a venous catheter attached to a small plastic tube that is sealed by a plastic cap in such a way as to protect sterility and patency. It facilitates frequent high intravenous doses of antibiotics without limiting activity. The patient can move about freely with only the lock in place, and the other equipment needed

ride above 60 mEq/L. This feature is so pronounced that mothers have noted that their affected children seem to have a "salty taste" when they are kissed.

The quantitative sweat test by pilocarpine iontophoresis is definitive for confirming the diagnosis of cystic fibrosis at all ages. Because of the seriousness of the disease and to ensure reliability, at least two positive tests are required before the final diagnosis is made.

When the diagnosis has been established, further tests may be performed to determine the extent of system involvement and to establish a baseline for future assessment of treatment and disease progress. Chest x-ray examinations and pulmonary function tests are performed to assess respiratory involvement. Abdominal x-ray examinations, stool analysis, and pancreatic function tests are performed to assess gastrointestinal involvement.

Treatment. Treatment of patients with CF is directed toward the organs involved and designed to meet the needs of the individual patient. Since the chief cause of

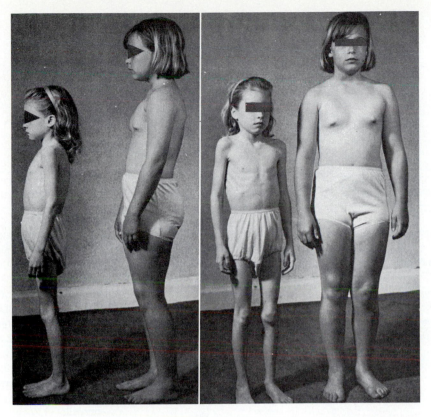

FIG 32-3 Both these girls are 10 years old. Youngster on left demonstrates effects of severe cystic fibrosis.

for the intravenous administration of medications remains at the bedside until the next dose is due. Postural drainage and percussion treatments vital in combating these infections can also be performed. For details of heparin lock IV maintenance, see p. 482.

Currently, an implantable intravascular access, the medi-port, has been used in CF patients. This allows for the administration of intravenous medications without venipuncture almost indefinitely. The medi-port has been valuable for children who require very frequent and prolonged intravenous antibiotic therapy as well as intravenous hyperalimentation. In severe cases, long-term intravenous antibiotics are used and in selected cases, heart-lung transplant has recently been done.

Nutrition. Maintaining nutritional goals becomes increasingly difficult as CF progresses. However, initially the aim is to encourage 100% of the recommended dietary allowance (for age) plus extra calories to make up for the calories lost because of malabsorption. Pancreatic insufficiency limits the patient's capacity for digesting

fats and proteins. The child usually has an eager appetite; however, because in an untreated case he is unable to digest much of the food he eats (and respiratory complications may interfere with nutrition), his arms and legs are characteristically spindly, his buttocks are emaciated, and his growth is retarded (Fig. 32-3). Fortunately the digestive problems usually improve with the addition of pharmaceutical preparations of pancreatic enzymes given with each meal. A major advance in this area is the enteric-coated enzyme, Pancrease, which allows for delivery of predictable levels of enzymes to the duodenum at the same time as food. Other products include Creon and Pancrease MT 16. The enzymes are taken by mouth with meals; the dosage varies, depending on the amount of food, the kind of food (particular fat content), and the degree of pancreatic insufficiency. The goal of pancreatic enzyme therapy is to increase intestinal absorption of foodstuffs and allow the patient as nearly normal a diet as possible while decreasing the number of bulky, foulsmelling, loose stools. Fat restriction is generally un-

NURSING CARE PLAN

The Child with Cystic Fibrosis

Selected nursing diagnoses	Expected outcomes	Interventions
A. Ineffective airway clearance related to thick secretions, inflammation and infection of lung tissue. Clinical manifestations: Rales/rhonchi, increased cough, change in sputum characteristics, cyanosis, tachypnea, fever, decreased activity tolerance, retractions, and nasal flaring.	Child regains/maintains baseline respiratory function. Child is relatively free from respiratory infection.	Assess child's respiratory status (color, lung sounds, respiratory rate, use of accessory muscles) every 4 hours and prn Administer IV antibiotics as ordered. Observe and document amount, color, and quality of sputum. Assure respiratory treatments (vigorous chest physiotherapy) are given as ordered and assess child's response. Administer oxygen prn. Encourage oral fluids/IV hydration as needed.
B. Altered nutrition: less than body requirements related to decreased respiratory function, inadequate enzyme secretion and food digestion. Clinical manifestations: Poor weight gain and anorexia.	Child maintains adequate caloric intake to promote growth.	Give child small, frequent meals. Administer vitamins and enzymes with meals and snacks. Assist child/parent in selecting food choices. Supplement with high-caloric snacks (Sustacal Shakes). Assess need for and administer nasogastric tube/gastrostomy feedings, if ordered.
C. Activity intolerance related to increased respiratory effort, decreased caloric intake, and presence of infection. Clinical manifestations: Tires easily, frequent naps, unable to perform ADLs.	Child regains/maintains baseline activity level.	Provide adequate rest periods throughout the day. Allow child to participate in planning daily schedule (children with CF tend to have more energy in the afternoon.) Ensure adequate caloric intake for age and activity level. Administer respiratory treatment and antibiotics as ordered to facilitate return to baseline activity level.

necessary, with the exception of the fat load of whole milk and excessive grease in food. Children should be encouraged to use skimmed or 2% milk rather than homogenized milk.

Recent studies demonstrate that better nutrition has a positive effect on the overall prognosis of the patient with CF. Nutritional supplements such as nasogastric tube, jejunostomy, and gastrostomy feedings, and even long-term intravenous hyperalimentation have been advocated.

Medium-chain triglycerides (MCTs) are more easily absorbed than other fats and provide an important source of calories. The MCT oil enables the preparation and digestion of fried foods, salad dressings, and mayonnaise. The diet should also be supplemented with twice the recommended daily dose of vitamins, prepared in such a way that they can be combined with water (water-miscible) because of malabsorption of the fat-soluble vitamins in cystic fibrosis. The water-miscible vitamins make supplementation of vitamins A, D, and K accessible to the patient. Supplementary vitamin K is recommended, especially for infants, to prevent blood clotting problems. In hot weather extra salt intake is necessary because of the large amounts lost in the perspiration. The prescribed amount can be incorporated in the preparation of food and need not be given separately. Heat prostration caused by salt depletion is a real danger to these children, especially on hot summer days and during periods of exertion. If excessive sweating is anticipated, sodium chloride intake should be increased.

Cystic fibrosis centers. Because cystic fibrosis is chronic and many organs and systems are involved, care is complex and requires a team effort to coordinate the services of many specialists. Comprehensive, coordinated services are the key to good management, and all children with cystic fibrosis should be referred to a cystic fibrosis center, where a team of experts in all aspects of the disease can design an individualized treatment plan. In addition to a specific treatment plan that includes instructions on medication, diet, and exercise, the patient and family are trained in techniques of postural drainage. Cystic fibrosis centers can also provide initial and continuing psychologic, psychosocial, genetic, and vocational counseling.

Nursing care. Nursing care entails a careful observation of the dietary intake and its effect on the child with CF and on elimination. Every effort should be made to offer a variety in meals within the limitations imposed and to make eating a pleasant experience.

Provision for frequent changes in position to prevent pneumonia and reduce skin problems is an important consideration in sick, malnourished patients with cystic fibrosis. Some of these children are very emaciated, and the skin over bony prominences is in special need of care. The rectal area must be meticulously cleaned. Rectal prolapse may be a complication occasionally. A soothing, local ointment may prevent irritation from the bulky stools. Any material soiled by feces should be removed immediately from the child's room. Appropriate air fresheners may be useful. Stools should always be described regarding their size, color, consistency, and odor.

The observation and report of respiratory distress is of paramount importance. Every effort should be made to protect the child from persons with any type of respiratory tract infection.

Because of the chronic nature of the disease, the severe strain it may place on the family finances, and the psychologic needs of the child, home care is recommended, except when the child's condition is such that appropriate care can be provided only through hospitalization. Parents may need much counseling and practical assistance to help meet their child's social and emotional requirements, as well as the child's physical needs. They also must be cautioned against becoming so preoccupied with the sick child that the needs of other family members are neglected.

Early diagnosis and improved methods of therapy have reduced the morbidity and greatly increased the longevity of children with cystic fibrosis. These children currently have a greater than 50% chance of living past the second decade.

Only rarely is a young man with cystic fibrosis fertile, since the same mechanisms that typically obstruct other glandular ducts of the body probably interfere with sperm transport.

Female patients have borne children, but their ability to conceive seems to be below normal because cervical mucus is abnormal.

The nurse caring for the child with cystic fibrosis must realize the strain under which the parents may be operating and their feelings of fatigue and frustration. Many families have lost other children because of this disease and have traveled almost the same road to final farewells before. Such a journey is no easier just because it has been traveled before.

Toddler

Croup (laryngotracheobronchitis). Acute obstructive subglottic laryngitis, or laryngotracheobronchitis (LTB), commonly known as croup, is a viral respiratory disease that involves the larynx, trachea, and bronchi. Mild to severe forms of LTB typically occur in children between 6 months and 3 years of age during cold weather. Croup is characterized by a sudden onset of inspiratory stridor, hoarseness, and a barklike cough following a 1- to 3-day history of a "cold." These manifestations are the result of inflammatory edema of the vocal cords and subglottic area, causing varying degrees of laryngeal obstruction. Sometimes, spasm accompanies the process. Most children are awakened without warning in the middle of the night by an acute attack. The child appears extremely anxious and frightened by this respiratory distress. Treatment is symptomatic. High humidity (running hot water in the bathroom) and gentle reassurance are important. If there is a spasm, it usually subsides in a few hours with high humidity therapy but may recur for 1 or 2 nights.

A more severe form of croup results when the inflammatory involvement of the trachea and bronchial tree produces a thick, viscous, purulent exudate. Edema and exudate lead to both inspiratory and expiratory difficulties. As the degree of severity of respiratory distress increases, suprasternal, intercostal, and substernal retractions occur. The child becomes hypoxic, restless, and desperately anxious. Impending suffocation is a real threat and a terrifying experience for both the child and the parents. This child needs immediate medical management and possible endotracheal intubation or tracheostomy.

During the admission procedure, every effort should be made to prevent aggravation of respiratory distress. The parents should remain at the cribside as the child is gently and calmly placed in an atmosphere of high humidity with oxygen. Maximum humidification is best accomplished with cool mist in the tent. The moist vapor helps allay irritation of the mucosa and promote liquefaction of the thick secretions. Clear fluids are encouraged if the respiratory distress is not severe and are also important in mobilizing respiratory exudate. Refusal to take fluids orally or severe respiratory distress necessitates intravenous therapy.

Increased pulse rate, restlessness, severe stridor, and use of the accessory muscles for breathing must be reported immediately. If the signs and symptoms of acute airway obstruction increase, emergency airway intervention must be considered before the child is exhausted. This is achieved in most hospitals by the insertion of an endotracheal tube or tracheostomy. In recent years endotracheal intubation has become the preferred method.

Arterial or arterialized capillary blood gases are helpful in assessing the clinical situation and determining the need for emergency airway intervention. Unfortunately, this procedure can upset the child to such a degree that the child may be more hypoxic during the blood drawing.

Nebulized racemic epinephrine (Vaponefrin) has been used with success in many cases of LTB. At first the child struggles against the aerosol, but after a short time the child relaxes and the labored breathing subsides as the therapy is continued over 10 to 15 minutes. The procedure may be repeated at 3 to 4 hour intervals. Racemic epinephrine is used for its topical vasoconstrictive effect, resulting in decreased mucosal edema. This treatment is extremely helpful in providing immediate, temporary improvement in patients with croup. However, the obstruction can recur in 1 to 2 hours as a result of a rebound phenomenon in severe cases. Therefore severe cases should be observed closely for recurrence even after a remarkable improvement.

Acute LTB should not be confused with epiglottitis (acute supraglottic laryngitis), a more serious acute airway problem that can lead to complete respiratory obstruction and death in several hours (Fig. 32-4).

Foreign bodies in the nose or throat. Children frequently push objects other than their fingers into the nasal cavity, probably as the result of natural curiosity. If the object does not spontaneously drop out or is not dislodged by sneezing and the episode is not reported by the child, it may be indicated by a bloody or purulent, foul nasal discharge originating from one nostril only. Such a discharge should make one suspect the presence of a foreign body. Removal of such an object should be attempted only by a physician who has the necessary instruments.

If a child is discovered choking, but still is conscious and able to cough, he should be encouraged to cough. If the child develops complete obstruction, four short, controlled blows on the back with the hand may dislodge the object. If the problem still persists, CPR should be initiated. If respiratory distress continues, the child should be seen immediately by a physician who may have to schedule a chest x-ray examination and perform a bronchoscopy. For discussion of aspiration pneumonia see p. 690 and for emergency CPR procedures see pp. 550-555.

Bronchitis. Bronchitis is most often caused by the same virus that has invaded other areas of the respiratory tract. Bronchitis is usually preceded by an upper respiratory tract infection and is a common problem in toddlers. It may remain mild or become progressively severe, leading to pneumonia. A disturbing, productive

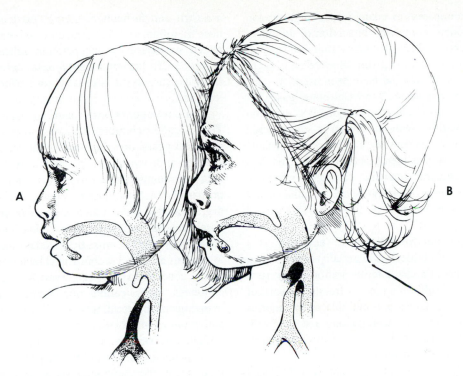

FIG 32-4 Anatomic difference between acute subglottic and acute supraglottic obstruction. **A,** Laryngotracheobronchitis (LTB), an acute inflammation particularly involving subglottic area of larynx, trachea, and bronchial tree, most commonly occurring in toddlers. **B,** Epiglottitis, an acute inflammatory swelling involving structures above opening of trachea (glottis), most often seen in preschoolers.

cough appears as the disease develops. Paroxysms may occur, particularly when the position of the child is altered, such as in the morning on rising or when first lying in bed after sitting for a period. Vomiting as a result of gagging when the secretions are thick is not uncommon. Cool moisture is sometimes helpful. A generous intake of fluids thins bronchial secretions, and aspirin or acetaminophen (Tylenol) may be necessary to lessen discomfort or fever. Unless the condition worsens, acute bronchitis is generally a self-limited infection that improves spontaneously in a few days.

Preschool child

Epiglottitis (Fig. 32-4). Acute obstructive supraglottic laryngitis, commonly known as epiglottitis, is usually caused by the *H. influenzae* type b bacteria. It is characterized by acute respiratory distress, high temperature, difficulty in swallowing, drooling, and a "cherry red" epiglottis on physical examination. The signs and symptoms of supraglottic obstruction result from inflammatory edema of the epiglottis. Children between 3 and 7 years of age are most frequently affected. The condition is usually seen in the winter months, and the onset is sudden. The child first complains of a severe sore throat and difficulty in swallowing (dysphagia). Soon the child is anxious, unable to eat or drink, prostrated, in a toxic condition, and drooling. Rapidly increasing dyspnea and drooling are the most important signs of impending disaster. Once the diagnosis is made, one should not be lulled into hopeful, watchful waiting. The child must have his airway secured, either by endotracheal tube or tracheostomy. Endotracheal intubation or tracheostomy should not be deferred in the hope that it will not be necessary. Epiglottitis can lead to complete respiratory obstruction and death in just a few hours.

It is important not to disturb the child unduly or to separate the child from his parents. The diagnosis is confirmed by visualization of the inflamed epiglottis or by a lateral neck x-ray film, and the child is moved from the emergency room to the operating room, where an elective endotracheal intubation or tracheostomy can be performed in a controlled setting. One should be aware that physical examination to visualize the epiglottis can precipitate a sudden, complete obstruction of the upper airway. Intravenous therapy with ampicillin and/or chloramphenicol and fluids is given. More recently cephalosporins such as cefuroxime have been used.

After the airway is secured, arterial blood gases are assessed to ensure adequate oxygenation. It is essential that warm mist with or without oxygen is administered through the artificial airways by a T-piece or tracheostomy collar. The child is then placed in a mist tent and returned to the pediatric intensive care unit, where an experienced staff can give constant care. No child should die from epiglottitis when it is diagnosed and treated promptly.

Epistaxis. Bleeding from the nose (epistaxis) is a common disorder of childhood, especially in boys from 4 to 10 years of age. On the anterior portion of the nasal septum, called Kiesselbach's area, a fragile network of capillaries subject to drying and multiple minor injuries is found. Traumas, such as nose picking and nose rubbing, forceful blowing, and insertion of foreign bodies, are the usual causes of bleeding.

Placing the child in a sitting position with the head tilted forward while compressing the nares with the thumb and forefinger is often sufficient to facilitate clot formation and stop the bleeding. This posture also prevents blood from dripping down the posterior pharynx, possibly leading to aspiration. Ice packs to the nasal area or to the back of the neck are of little or no value. If bleeding is persistent, an anterior nasal pack consisting of ½ inch of petrolatum-impregnated gauze or an application of agents such as aqueous epinephrine solution (1:1,000) or thrombin may be useful.

Any condition that contributes to vascular congestion of the nasal mucosa, such as nasal allergy or sinusitis, increases the frequency of epistaxis. Bleeding from the posterior region of the nasal cavity is uncommon. At times such nosebleeds may be a symptom of underlying blood dyscrasias, such as purpura, leukemia, or conditions associated with a rise in blood pressure. Frequent nosebleeds may or may not be significant. Parental fears can best be allayed by not only stopping the bleeding but also identifying and treating the underlying causes of the disorder.

Deviation of the septum. In some instances the cartilaginous and bony wall, or septum, that divides the nose into two lateral chambers does not occupy the midline. It may deviate toward one side or another as a result of natural development or, more commonly, as an aftermath of trauma. This may indirectly cause occlusion of

a nostril and difficult breathing, particularly when the nose is inflamed. This structural anomaly can be corrected surgically by an operation called a *submucous resection*. To prevent external nasal deformity resulting from the surgery, it is usually not performed until adolescence.

Acute nasopharyngitis (acute coryza, common cold). The so called common cold has plagued humanity for countless years. Preschool and young school-age children average approximately six colds a year. The common cold is probably caused by several viral organisms that primarily attack the nose and throat. Symptoms include dry, scratchy, sore, inflamed pharynx and an inflamed nasal mucosa, which produces a clear mucoid nasal discharge that later becomes thick and purulent. These local symptoms are often accompanied by headache, muscular pains, general malaise, and fever. As the viral infection continues, complications often arise from the intrusion of pathogenic bacteria, which may prolong the congestion and promote the extension of the inflammation to the middle ear, sinuses, larynx, trachea, and even to the bronchi and lungs. It is mainly the possibility of extension that makes the common cold a potentially dangerous condition.

A common cold is probably contagious for a number of hours before symptoms are observed by the patient. It is currently believed that the cold sufferer remains contagious for about 8 hours after the onset of visible signs. Contamination by spread of droplets is most common. It is very important to protect infants from exposure to colds because they are affected more seriously than older children. An infant may have a high temperature of 104° F (40° C), and febrile seizures are possible. Ears are almost always affected. Nasal congestion causes difficulties in breathing, nursing, and eating. It is impossible to prevent a child from ever having a cold, but everything possible should be done to protect a baby.

Because nasopharyngitis is caused entirely by viruses, no specific therapy is recommended. Supportive treatment consists of rest, relative isolation, increased fluid intake, and a bland, soft diet. Nasal obstruction in infants can be partially relieved by humidification or instillation of 1 or 2 drops of physiologic saline solution in each nostril, followed by gentle suction with an infant's nasal (or ear) syringe. Phenylephrine (Neo-Synephrine) hydrochloride nose drops (⅛% for infants and ¼% for older children) may also relieve nasal symptoms. Nasal vasoconstrictors should not be used for more than 3 or 4 days because of "rebound phenomena." (When the use of such vasoconstrictors has been prolonged and is suddenly stopped, congestion greatly increases, or "rebounds.")

Mild systemic symptoms and fever may be relieved by proper dosage of aspirin or nonsalicylate acetaminophen (Tylenol or Tempra). Aspirin can be extremely dangerous to a child whose intake of fluids has declined significantly. Remember, both the amount of aspirin given and the interval and duration of treatment must always be considered. Many children suffer from salicylate poisoning every year. A rule of thumb for a nurse to remember is that a child of average weight should be given only 1 grain (60 mg) of aspirin per year of age up to 5 grains and should not be given aspirin more than five times at 4-hour intervals without medical consultation. Dosages for babies under 1 year of age must be carefully determined. Children over 5 years of age but less than 12 years can usually be given 5 grains at a time if administration is not repeated more often than every 4 to 6 hours for a brief period.

To protect the nares or upper lip from excoriation caused by the fairly constant nasal discharge, cold cream or petrolatum is applied. Antibiotics are indicated in viral infections when secondary bacterial invaders become a problem.

Sinusitis. Acute sinusitis is often precipitated by an upper respiratory infection. Headache and a mucopurulent discharge from one or both nostrils, cough, and a diffusely red pharynx with mucopurulent discharge clinging to the posterior wall are indications that bacteria have invaded the sinuses. Improved ventilation and drainage are primary goals in the treatment. Hot compresses over the painful areas and increased humidification provide some comfort. Pain and fever are lessened by use of acetaminophen or aspirin. Instillation of nasal vasoconstrictors, preferably by spray, is helpful in shrinking the nasal mucosa and opening the airways. Each nostril should be sprayed once while the child is in a sitting position. About 3 to 5 minutes later the spraying should be repeated to reach the posterior part of the nose. Oral decongestants, such as pseudoephedrine hydrochloride (Sudafed), Triaminic, or Actifed, may be useful when local therapy is difficult.

Although most acute sinus infections are self-limited, appropriate antibiotic therapy (culture-sensitive) shortens the course of illness and usually prevents any further complications. However, children are occasionally seen with the complication of periorbital cellulitis. This condition follows a severe bout of ethmoid sinusitis and must be treated vigorously to prevent ocular and central nervous system (CNS) complications.

Otitis media. Otitis media, or inflammation of the middle ear, is a common, difficult problem related to malfunction of the eustachian tube that connects the middle ear to the nasopharynx (Fig. 32-5, *A*). Normally this tube protects the middle ear from nasopharyngeal secretions, provides drainage of secretions produced within the middle ear into the nasopharynx, and equalizes the air pressure in the middle ear with that of the atmosphere. Persistent obstruction of the eustachian tube caused by infection, allergy, and enlarged adenoids eventually leads to middle ear disease.

Acute otitis media is a common complication of upper respiratory tract infection in young children. Respiratory mucosa damaged by viral infection is readily colonized by pneumococci, *H. influenzae,* group A beta-hemolytic streptococci, and *Branhamella catarrhalis*. Bacteria usually gain access to the middle ear by way of the eustachian tube. Purulent fluid accumulates in the middle ear, causing severe pain, fever, and irritability. When the eustachian tube becomes inflamed, it may swell shut, and the purulent material produced by the infection builds up within the middle ear, causing earache, ringing of the ears, elevated temperature, occasional vomiting, and perhaps spontaneous rupture of the eardrum that may result in a "running ear."

Infants are especially susceptible to otitis media and may announce their discomfort by crying, fussy behavior, or pulling at the affected ear. Definitive diagnosis can be made only by visualization of the tympanic membrane and adjacent structures. Antibiotics are the mainstay of therapy. A successful outcome depends in large measure on early treatment. Parents should be encouraged to notify the pediatrician promptly when the child has an earache. Aspirin, acetaminophen, and Auralgan ear drops may be given for pain, although it usually subsides in 12 to 24 hours after antibiotic therapy has been initiated. Antihistamines and decongestants are often prescribed for the first 7 to 10 days in an attempt to clear nasal pharyngitis and inflammation of the eustachian tubes.

Specific antibiotic therapy is usually effective in the prevention of such complications as mastoiditis, meningitis, and the incidence of eardrum perforation. Amoxicillin, trimethoprim with sulfamethoxazole (Septra), and the cephalosporins are effective against both gram-positive and gram-negative bacteria, and any of these drugs can be used alone. Widely accepted is combined therapy, such as erythromycin or penicillin with sulfisoxazole. Therapy should be continued for at least 10 days. The nurse must forewarn parents that a follow-up visit to the physician is essential. The child's ear must

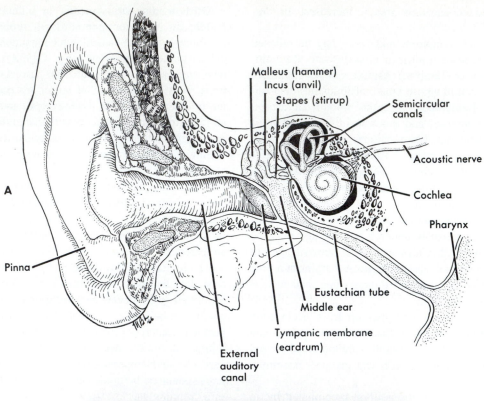

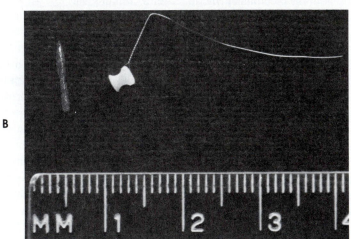

FIG 32-5   **A,** Basic anatomy of ear. **B,** Tympanostomy ventilating tube.

be inspected and evaluated after 10 days of treatment, since the appearance of the eardrum dictates the duration of therapy. No child is considered cured until the signs of middle ear disease have been resolved. Partially treated otitis media is a major cause of meningitis in young children.

In the past a myringotomy (surgical incision of the eardrum) was commonly performed to relieve pressure and evacuate fluid. Because most children respond well to antibiotic therapy, myringotomies currently are usually reserved for those few patients whose improvement at follow-up examination has not been satisfactory.

Serous otitis media. Recurrent attacks of acute otitis media characteristically precede serous, or "secretory," otitis media, a sterile middle ear effusion. The fluid varies greatly in its viscosity. When it is very thick, the condition is called "glue ear." Serous otitis is the most common complication of acute otitis media, and since no significant symptoms are present, the development of a conductive hearing loss is a real possibility. Unless definitive measures are instituted to open the eustachian tube, permanent hearing loss can result. Learning difficulties often signal such a hearing loss in school-age children. Children with conductive hearing loss caused by serous otitis media should be referred to an otologist. Surgical drainage (myringotomy) is often necessary. The aspirated fluid is cultured, and specific antibiotic therapy may be started. Placement of tiny middle-ear ventilating tubes through the eardrum seems to be the best treatment for serous otitis media (Fig. 32-5, *B*). The success of tympanostomy tubes is due to the artificial tubes providing equalization of air pressure on both sides of the tympanic membranes. Children with tympanostomy tubes must be protected when swimming or showering by wearing custom-made earplugs; otherwise, suppurative otitis media is a common sequel.

The most important aspect of long-term management is to relieve the basic cause. Allergies must be investigated and treated, and hypertrophied adenoids must be removed if they truly are obstructing the eustachian tube. A significant advance in the identification of middle ear disease has resulted from the use of the electroacoustic impedance bridge. A small probe in a rubber cuff is placed in the external canal and attached to the impedance meter. A tympanogram, which reflects the dynamics of the entire tympanic membrane—middle ear and eustachian tube system—is produced. For detecting otitis media and common conductive defects in children, tympanometry is far more reliable than otoscopic examination. Tympanometry is a simple procedure that can be easily carried out in a short time by nonprofessional personnel.

Hygiene of the ear. In some instances damage to the ear may follow ill-advised probing of the external auditory canal with implements such as toothpicks and matchsticks. It is wise to follow the old saying, "Never put anything in your ear except your elbow." The outer auditory canal should be cleaned by using a washcloth or a tightly rolled piece of cotton. If a collection of hardened wax, or cerumen, is suspected, the ear should be examined, and a physician or nurse trained in the technique of irrigating the ears should carry out the procedure.

Any body opening seems to offer a challenge to some children. Boys and girls occasionally push foreign bodies into the external ear canal. When foreign bodies are detected, they should be removed by a physician because the general public hasn't the knowledge, skill, nor instruments necessary to perform such a task. An irrigation should never be attempted before the child is taken to a physician. If the object is made of vegetable matter, it can swell with the liquid and become more difficult to extract.

School-age child

Adenoids and tonsils. Located in the pharynx are several structures of particular interest to the pediatric nurse. Situated in the nasopharynx are the nasopharyngeal tonsils, more often called the adenoids. Farther down on the lateral walls of the oral pharynx are the palatine, or faucial tonsils, which are the structures indicated when one whispers, "I've just had my tonsils out." These two kinds of tonsils are composed mainly of lymphoid tissue and play a role in the formation of immunoglobulins. In addition, they act as a respiratory tract defense mechanism by filtering microbes, thereby helping to prevent microbial invasion of the lower tract. These lymphoid tissues serve a useful purpose and should be preserved unless the problems caused by their continued presence outweigh their possible usefulness. Tonsils and adenoids are present at birth and achieve their maximum size by the time the child is 5 years of age. Significantly, at 2 years the tonsils are normally large, and the adenoids occupy one half of the nasopharyngeal cavity. The peak of adenoid size is reached by puberty, after which they cease to grow and begin to shrink. When adenoids are removed in very young children, they usually regrow. In the past tonsils and adenoids were thought to be the cause of many ills and were removed without much hesitation. However, much disillusionment has resulted from failure of surgery to achieve expected results. Moreover, this lightly regarded "minor" procedure has taken the lives of many children. In the United States alone reliable evidence shows that over 100 deaths a year result from cardiac arrest, hemorrhage, and infection that follow tonsillectomy.

Indications for removal. Because the adenoids are located close to the opening of the eustachian or auditory tube, enlarged adenoids may also be an underlying cause of frequent middle ear infections, or otitis media. The eustachian tube is more horizontal and is broader and shorter in infants and young children than it is in adults; thus ascending ear infections are fairly common in children.

Indications for an adenoidectomy are obstructive adenoids with recurrent acute purulent otitis media or chronic serous otitis media with conductive hearing loss. Children with the latter condition require surgical drainage to remove the fluid and placement of tympanostomy tubes in the eardrum to promote ventilation and prevent reaccumulation of fluid.

A tonsillectomy need not be done with an adenoidectomy, since these are two independent procedures with very different indications. The best results from a tonsillectomy are obtained when the symptoms have been clearly referable to the tonsils and not to problems such as frequent colds, sore throat, poor appetite, failure to gain weight, postnasal drip, or allergies. Definite indications for a tonsillectomy include a history of peritonsillar abscess (to prevent a second attack), chronic recurrent group A beta-hemolytic streptococcal tonsillitis (culture-proved), and hypertrophied tonsils that are causing chronic airway obstruction and pulmonary hypertension.

Contraindications and postponements. Tonsillectomy and adenoidectomy (T and A) surgery is contraindicated in children who have hematologic conditions, such as hemophilia, leukemia, aplastic anemia, or purpura. Routine laboratory screening of candidates for this surgery is particularly important to discover the potential postoperative "bleeder." Bleeding times (usually simplate method) and prothrombin levels may indicate the need for specific treatment or operative delay. Vitamin K is administered for prothrombin deficiencies. When severe systemic disorders, such as diabetes and cardiac or renal disease, are problems, surgery usually can be safely managed if a real need exists. However, T and A surgery is always postponed if a child is beginning to show signs of an upper respiratory tract infection.

Because of the numerous blood vessels in the operative area and the character of the procedure, the most common complication of either a tonsillectomy or an adenoidectomy is hemorrhage. For this reason the nurse should very carefully watch for symptoms of excessive bleeding and shock. If bleeding occurs, it usually occurs within the first 24 hours following surgery. The physician must be called to the bedside to evaluate the seriousness of the situation and to locate the source of bleeding. Minor bleeding usually stops when any associated clot, which inadequately obstructs a bleeding vessel yet impedes its constriction, is removed gently by suction. A sponge moistened with lidocaine (Xylocaine) and epinephrine is held firmly against the area for a few minutes. In the event of major hemorrhage from the tonsillar fos-

sae, or bed, reanesthetizing and resuturing may be necessary. Bleeding from the adenoid area is more common. Again, any clot must first be removed, and if the bleeding does not stop, the patient must be returned to surgery for another general anesthetic and cauterization with an electric bovie. If this treatment is not successful in curtailing bleeding, then a postnasal pack or Foley-type catheter with inflatable bag can be inserted and left in place until the next day (Fig. 32-6). Transfusions may be required if bleeding continues.

Postoperative care. Since the advent and use of recovery rooms, the burden of the immediate postoperative care of the surgical patient carried by the "floor" staff nurse has been lightened. However, it has not been eliminated. After having been gently suctioned and observed for immediate signs of cardiorespiratory distress, the T and A patient returns from the recovery room to the unit. The child is best positioned on his side with his anterior chest at a 45-degree angle to facilitate oronasal drainage, prevent aspiration, and provide easier observation. The nurse frequently checks pulse and respirations. She notes the child's level of consciousness and any pronounced restlessness. She observes the skin for color and moisture. She carefully evaluates the amount and kind of oronasal drainage, always asking herself, "Is it profuse? Is it a constant drip or ooze? Is the child swallowing frequently, perhaps swallowing blood? (If so, the patient soon vomits coffee-groundlike secretions.) Does the child need suctioning? Approximately how many tissues have been used? What is the color of the discharge?" Persistent, bright red drainage indicates active bleeding. Sometimes it is difficult for a student nurse to evaluate the amount of bleeding considered normal after T and A surgery. She should never feel apologetic for asking a more experienced nurse to help her judge the condition of her patient. Unless special indications develop, blood pressure is not routinely determined on a young child after T and A surgery.

As soon as the patient is conscious and responding, he should be given sips of water to ascertain his tolerance of oral fluids. The early introduction of clear, bland fluids helps prevent dehydration and elevated temperature. It also eventually helps to ease the sore throat. By the second day the child is ready for a soft, bland diet. About 50% of children who have had their tonsils or adenoids removed are discharged the same evening as the surgery.

Discharge planning should include written instructions for care. Parents and child should be told that his throat will be decreasingly sore for several days. Complaints of earache (referred pain from the throat) are common.

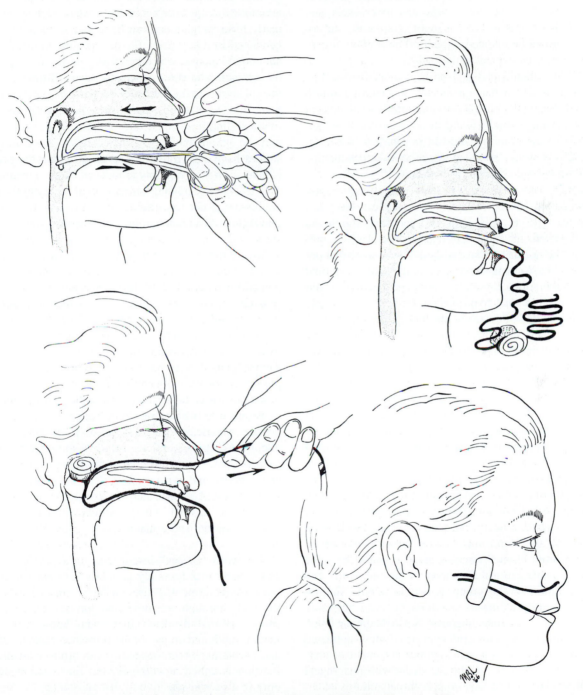

FIG 32-6 Insertion of postnasal pack to stop bleeding from adenoid area.

Acetaminophen with or without codeine may be prescribed for this discomfort. The child should be told not to blow his nose forcefully. A soft, bland diet should be continued for several days. The child should be encouraged to drink and eat and open his mouth widely. Fluids and food should be given at room temperature. Crisp or hard foods such as popcorn, chips, and dry crackers, and acid foods such as pickles, oranges, grapefruit, and tomatoes should be avoided. About 10 days after surgery children may eat whatever they wish.

Children should rest and be kept quiet for the first days at home. They may go outside on the third or fourth day and resume their usual activities after 1 week, except for swimming, which should be avoided for 2 weeks. School-age children are allowed to return to school at the end of 1 week, provided there are no infectious diseases among the children in their class.

Signs and symptoms that should be reported promptly by the parents to the physician include fresh bleeding, fever over 101° F, chest pain, and persistent cough. As already stated, the most common postoperative complication is hemorrhage. Parents should understand that occasional blood-streaked nasal or oral mucus is normal during the first two days; but if increased bleeding should occur, the child must be returned to the hospital promptly (if possible, without causing the child anxiety) for easier and more rapid care. No surgery is without risk. T and A surgery is not a minor operation, nor is it the answer for all ear, nose, and throat problems. It is an effective therapeutic procedure for selected patients.

Streptococcal pharyngitis (strep throat). Occasionally a severe pharyngitis develops from an infection by the group A beta-hemolytic streptococcus. Such a condition is commonly called a "strep throat." Streptococcal pharyngitis is uncommon before a child is 2 years of age and almost nonexistent in a child less than 1 year. Classically strep throat has sudden onset; the child has a high temperature, severe sore throat, tender cervical lymph nodes, exudate, a beefy, red pharynx, and petechiae on the soft palate. Unfortunately strep throat cannot be diagnosed from clinical findings alone because the same clinical manifestations accompany viral infections. The demonstration of the group A beta-hemolytic streptococcal organism by means of a throat culture is therefore essential for an accurate diagnosis. Since rheumatic fever, heart disease, and glomerulonephritis follow untreated streptococcal infections in a significant number of children, patients coming to the physician with pharyngeal inflammations should have routine throat cultures taken.

The patient's telephone number should be written on the laboratory slip, and those whose culture reveals a beta-hemolytic streptococcus should be notified and treated. While awaiting culture results, patients can be treated symptomatically with saline gargles, lozenges, and aspirin or acetaminophen. The 48-hour delay in starting antibiotic therapy does not increase the incidence of rheumatic fever or glomerulonephritis but is thought to be beneficial in that it gives the patient time to develop an antibody response, which helps prevent future infections by that particular strain of streptococcus. If time is taken to explain this to the patient or the parents, they are most grateful. The patient who is in a toxic state and has physical findings suggesting streptococcal pharyngitis may be given antibiotics immediately, but controlled studies have shown that the speed at which the patient recovers is not appreciably influenced by such treatment. The reason for treating streptococcal pharyngitis with antibiotics is not for a more rapid recovery but for the prevention of complications. Numerous studies have shown that this can be done if the child is treated within 7 days of onset of the illness. The American Heart Association recommends that streptococcal infections be treated for a period of 10 days with penicillin (or erythromycin if the child is allergic to penicillin). Streptococcal organisms are extremely sensitive to an oral course of penicillin, but since many patients stop their medication prematurely, one intramuscular injection of benzathine penicillin G has been recommended by some physicians as the treatment of choice. It is also advisable to take throat cultures of asymptomatic family contacts.

Respiratory disease resulting from allergy. About 24 million Americans (1 in 10) suffer from some sort of allergy. Allergic conditions include respiratory problems such as "hay fever" (rhinitis) and asthma as well as eczema, hives, and hypersensitivity to foods, venoms, and medications. Approximately 75% of these have hay fever, asthma, or both. Allergy is the leading chronic disease in children and a major cause of lost work days in adults.

The word "allergy" describes an unfavorable reaction of the body to a normally harmless substance from the outside environment. These substances may be taken into the body through the nose and lungs (pollens, mold spores, animal danders, mites, and house dust), the mouth (foods and drugs), or the skin (insect bites or stings and injections). A substance that can produce an allergic reaction is called an *allergen,* but the reaction occurs only in a person sensitive to that substance.

The tendency to become sensitive, or allergic, to some otherwise harmless substance is usually inherited. People vary greatly not only in their susceptibility to allergic diseases but also in the kind of allergic diseases they have. The organs or tissues in which the allergic reactions occur (lungs, asthma; nose, rhinitis; eyes, conjunctivitis; skin, eczema, urticaria, or hives; gastrointestinal tract, diarrhea) may change during a person's lifetime. These organs are frequently referred to as *target, organs*.

Although the tendency to become sensitive to a substance may be inherited, the allergic response develops only *after* exposure to that substance. This exposure can happen in utero, during childhood, or later in life. The development of a sensitivity to a particular substance depends on the *amount* and *frequency* of exposure to that substance. Sensitization may follow the first exposure or may not occur until after repeated exposures. Penicillin allergy is a well-known example of the latter phenomenon.

A general outline of the allergic process follows:

1. A person contacts a substance and produces sensitizing antibodies (immunoglobulin E) to that material.
2. These antibodies are then deposited on special cells (mast cells and basophils) in the body.
3. The allergen (substance to which a person is sensitive or allergic) contacts the antibody E attached to these cells in a subsequent exposure.
4. A reaction occurs whereby chemicals, or "allergic mediators," such as histamine, are released from these cells and cause the symptoms of allergy. These symptoms may include nasal congestion, sneezing and itching, wheezing, hives, or, in the most serious reactions, anaphylactic shock.

Diagnosis of allergy. The best way to find the sources of allergic symptoms is by a carefully taken history of what exposures preceded symptoms as well as the seasonal occurrence of symptoms. Specific potentially sensitizing allergens can then be documented through skin tests. When the test allergen meets antibodies sensitive to that substance in the skin, the chemical mediators are released, resulting in a positive reaction that resembles a mosquito bite (hive). Tests that indicate inhaled allergens are reliable and commonly agree with the patient's symptoms. Although they can be helpful, skin tests cannot always determine a food allergy. Therefore different trial diets are sometimes suggested to further evaluate foods as the source of the patient's symptoms.

Treatment of allergic rhinitis. The best way to treat an allergy is to prevent it by separating the patient from the allergen. For example, a fur-bearing pet should not be kept in a home with a person having a history of allergic problems. Dust and mite exposure in a patient's bedroom can be minimized by removing cloth draperies and fiber rugs and using special hypoallergenic pillows and nonporous mattress encasements. A second method of treatment consists of desensitizing patients to their allergens by injections of these substances in gradually increasing amounts. This regimen is used when allergens (such as pollens) cannot be adequately avoided. The process is called desensitization, hyposensitization, or immunotherapy.

Medications of various types are also employed for relief of symptoms. To be effective for this purpose, medication is often prescribed on a regular daily basis. Regular maintenance doses of medication should be taken as long as objective evidence exists of a symptomatic allergic state. Antihistamines such as tripelennamine hydrochloride (Pyribenzamine) and chlorpheniramine maleate (Chlor-Trimeton maleate and Teldrin) are often effective for the control of allergic rhinitis. They may be combined with a decongestant such as pseudoephedrine (Drixoral) or phenylpropanolamine (Duravent-A). A new class of antihistamines appears to be effective without causing drowsiness. A representative of this group is terfenadine (Seldane). Another allergic rhinitis and asthma medication is cromolyn sodium (Nasalcrom, Intal). It is administered in nasal spray prophylactically and as an adjunct to the treatment and control of chronic symptoms. A number of nasal cortisone sprays (Nasalide, Beconase, Vancenase) are very effective in improving and controlling nasal symptoms.

The xanthine drugs, theophylline and aminophylline, are valuable in counteracting the bronchospasm in asthma. Epinephrine is a rapid-acting, injectable bronchodilator and vasoconstrictor and is the most useful drug for the relief of anaphylactic shock, acute asthma, hives, and edema. More frequently used in chronic asthma are the beta-adrenergic sympathomimetic agents, such as metaproterenol, terbutaline, and albuterol. The symptom threshold can be increased with various bronchodilator combinations of theophylline and beta agents. However, such useful combinations may increase the side effects of these drugs. Thus, treatment with inhaled cromolyn or corticosteroids such as beclomethasone dipropionate (Vanceril, Beclovent) and triamcinolone (Azmacort) can offer prophylactic treatment for asthma symptoms.

Improvements in allergic symptomatology can occur without significant side effects. Often, exercise ability and irritant tolerance are also increased. However, there may be a continued need for medication. Follow-up care is important with emphasis on prevention of allergy attacks.

Corticosteroids are the most potent group of respiratory medications. In addition, they are effective anti-inflammatory agents in all allergic diseases. Their main drawback is that they can produce multisystem, major adverse side effects when taken orally or parenterally over a prolonged period. These negative effects can be reduced by administering the total dose required for symptom control in the form of prednisone on alternate mornings rather than in a daily regimen. Substantial reduction in these untoward generalized responses occurs with the topical application of the steroid medication— using aerosols for asthma and rhinitis, and drops, creams, and ointments for conjunctivitis and eczema.

Rhinitis is one of the most common allergic manifestations in children. It is characterized by sneezing, a profuse, watery nasal discharge, swelling and itching of the nasal mucosa, and often conjunctivitis. Allergic nasal obstruction is unpleasant for the child, parents, and teacher. Frequently it leads to constant mouth breathing, snoring, abnormal midface development with associated orthodontic problems, and a nasal voice. Associated problems are sinusitis and otitis media. Allergic rhinitis is commonly classified as seasonal (hay fever) or nonseasonal (perennial). Seasonal allergic rhinitis results most often from plant pollen sensitivity. House dust, animal danders, mold spores, and foods, in addition, are causes of nonseasonal allergic rhinitis in children. A careful history, physical examination, laboratory aids (such as nasal cytology to identify increased eosinophil counts), and skin testing all are important etiologic diagnostic measures. Treatment depends on the results of the diagnostic procedures. Most children with severe allergic rhinitis require specific treatment.

Asthma. Asthma is the most common major allergic manifestation in childhood. It affects from 1% to 5% of all children. Asthma accounts for 23% of school absenteeism, and in the United States causes numerous deaths annually. It is characterized by difficulty in breathing as the result of spasm of the small bronchi, obstructive edema of the bronchial mucosa, and the production of tenacious secretions all of which tend to obstruct air flow (Fig. 32-7). More difficulty is experienced in exhaling than inhaling. A pronounced expiratory wheeze is usually present. Rapid, shallow respirations are characteristic.

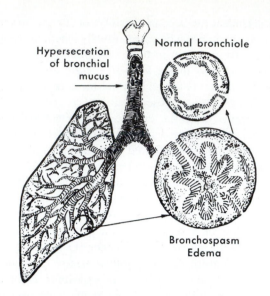

FIG 32-7 Cardinal anatomic changes in asthma occur at bronchiole level. Bronchospasm, edema, and hypersecretions of mucus cause severe dyspnea and wheezing.

Milder obstruction is frequently manifested by nocturnal or exertional coughing.

Asthma is the result of hyperreactivity of the bronchial airway. The lungs are clinically referred to as "twitchy." Although often the spasm, edema, and mucus that create this reversible obstruction are caused by an allergic reaction, many nonimmunologic precipitants can also initiate or compound the problem. These include infections, irritants, exercise, emotional stress, cold air, and weather changes. The clinical course of asthma therefore varies in different children as a result of its being such a multifactorial process.

Treatment of asthma. The treatment of asthma is usually divided into (1) specific measures, such as elimination of offending allergens and specific desensitization, and (2) nonspecific measures, which include medications, fluids, and supportive treatment.

Acute attacks of asthma can occur at any time and are related to multiple factors. There may be no single cause. Children exhibit symptoms when they reach a certain level or threshold of exposure to certain offenders. The cardinal feature is airway obstruction; patients' shoulders are hunched, their thoracic soft tissues retract as they inspire, and their accessory muscles of respiration bulge with the effort of breathing. Their respiratory rates are initially increased but may be normal or decreased if the obstruction is very severe, and their breathing is punctuated by spasms of coughing and audible wheezes.

NURSING CARE PLAN

Young Child with Croup

Selected nursing diagnoses	Expected outcomes	Interventions
A. Potential for suffocation related to inflammation and obstruction of upper respiratory tract. Clinical manifestations: 　Barking cough, stridor, retractions, prolonged inspiration, pallor, cyanosis, nasal flaring, restlessness or lethargy.	Child regains normal respiratory function.	Assess child for presence of barking cough, stridor, retractions, cyanosis, restlessness, lethargy, disorientation and notify physician of worsening condition. Keep child in cool mist tent and monitor mist and oxygen content every 2 hours. Assure respiratory treatments (racemic-epinephrine) are given as ordered and assess child's response. Keep child in upright position/helps ease motion of diaphragm in breathing. Maintain calm, quiet environment.
B. Anxiety related to respiratory distress, unfamiliar surroundings.		See Nursing Care Plan for The Hospitalized Child (p. 422).
C. Fluid volume deficit related to respiratory distress.		See Nursing Care Plan for The Child with a Fluid Volume Deficit (p. 478).

These children may be diaphoretic, restless, and fatigued. Difficulty in breathing always produces anxiety, and the patients' anxiety and that of their parents tends to compound the respiratory problems.

Treatment of acute attacks of asthma usually includes the administration of epinephrine (Adrenalin) by injection and then inhalation therapy with isoetharine, metaproterenol, or albuterol. Epinephrine suspension (Sus-Phrine) is often used to achieve more lasting effects. Adequate fluid intake is very important. Following the acute phase, postural drainage after inhalation therapy is highly effective in assisting removal of bronchial secretions or mucus plugs.

A potentially life-threatening situation, *status asthmaticus,* exists when the patient's respirations do not clear after three consecutive doses of epinephrine 1:1,000, given at 20-minute intervals or after a combination of epinephrine and inhalation therapy. This re-

quires aggressive medical treatment and close follow-up. Many patients with status asthmaticus require hospitalization.

Children with status asthmaticus may be dehydrated because they have been too ill to eat or drink and have lost fluids by hyperventilating, coughing, and perspiring. Vomiting also adds to the child's dehydrated state. Intravenous administration of fluids should be started to correct any fluid imbalance, maintain liquefied bronchial secretions, and serve as a vehicle for important medications. The nurse should carefully check the amount and time prescribed to prevent overhydration.

Thereafter, aminophylline, a compound of theophylline and a highly effective bronchodilator, is given intravenously over a 15- to 30-minute period and then at 4- to 6-hour intervals or as a maintenance drip after a loading bolus. Signs of theophylline intoxication include headache, restlessness, irritability, vomiting, and abdom-

NURSING CARE PLAN

The Child with Asthma

Selected nursing diagnoses	Expected outcomes	Interventions
A. Ineffective airway clearance related to edema, bronchospasms and excess mucus. Clinical manifestations: Coughing, wheezing, increased RR and HR, retractions, moist breath sounds, nasal flaring, lethargy, and pallor.	Child maintains patent airway. Child regains normal respiratory pattern.	Assess child for signs of respiratory distress: increased respirations and pulse, wheezing, nasal flaring, and retractions. Elevate head of bed, place infant in infant seat. Assure aerosol treatments given as ordered and assess child's response. Administer medications as ordered and assess response, presence of side effects. Ensure adequate hydration—see Nursing Care Plan for The Child with Fluid Volume Deficit (p. 478). Check for significant allergies (i.e., food or medication).
B. Impaired gas exchange related to inadequate respiratory function. Clinical manifestations: Agitation, audible wheezing, lethargy, grunting, stridor, tachycardia, tachypnea, cyanosis.	Child regains/maintains normal respiratory function.	Monitor respiratory rate, heart rate, blood pressure every 2 hours and prn. Anticipate change in IV medications. Assess child's response to therapy. Administer oxygen as needed. Obtain ABGs and blood work ordered. Be prepared for transfer to ICU.
C. Anxiety related to respiratory distress and hospitalization.		See Nursing Care Plan for The Hospitalized Child (p. 422).
D. Potential theophylline toxicity related to therapy. Clinical manifestations: Increased irritability, Increased HR, RR, and arrythmias, Nausea/vomiting/diarrhea Headache, restlessness, Insomnia, muscle twitching, Flushing, hypotension	Child maintains theophylline level between 10 and 20 μg/L.	Assess for clinical manifestations of toxicity. Monitor carefully aminophylline IV drip and blood serum levels. Monitor vitals signs every 4 hours and prn.

inal pain and should not be confused with increased severity of the asthma attack. Theophylline levels should be monitored and kept within the therapeutic range of 10 to 20 μg/ml.

Isoetharine (Bronkosol), metaproterenol (Metaprel, Alupent), or albuterol (Ventolin, Proventil) by inhalation are effective in further relieving bronchospasm and dyspnea in children. They are generally given every 4 hours.

Hydrocortisone sodium succinate (Solu-Cortef) or methylprednisolone (Solu-Medrol) is given intravenously to children who do not respond to bronchodilators, who have recently had corticosteroids, or who are receiving maintenance doses of steroids. It is important to note that the therapeutic effect of hydrocortisone sodium succinate is often not seen until 8 to 12 hours (frequently longer) after administration. If the patient improves, corticosteroids may be stopped abruptly after a short (less than 7 days) course. Although necessary for control of symptoms in severe cases, long-term use of steroids may have serious side effects, which include growth suppression, increased susceptibility to infection, and osteoporosis.

Antibiotics are indicated in the presence of bacterial infection. However, asthmatic flareups are more often associated with viral infections; in these instances antibiotics are not helpful. Oxygen is given to relieve hypoxemia. Since cyanosis is an unreliable sign of hypoxia, arterial blood gas levels may need to be determined and observed carefully. Oxygen may be administered if blood arterial oxygen is not within normal range.

Parents should be encouraged to stay at the child's bedside. They need to see what is happening to their child as well as to receive explanations about what is being done.

In patients with significant bronchitis or infection, chest physical therapy may be helpful. This consists of vibration, clapping, and coughing in various positions. Chest physical therapy and postural drainage are ordered as soon as the acute phase subsides. It is significant therapeutic aid for children whose excessive mucus is a problem. It is most effectively performed after bronchodilation is obtained from aminophylline and the aerosol treatment.

The nurse who is caring for the child with status asthmaticus must constantly but calmly evaluate the progress and changes that occur. Although most children demonstrate significant improvement after administration of aminophylline, inhalation therapy, and intravenous fluids, others do not respond for 12 to 24 hours. During this time, corticosteroids, antibiotics, and oxygen may be added to their therapeutic regimen. The foregoing measures are usually effective in time. Chest x-ray may be necessary when symptoms do not respond to therapy or when unusual signs are present, such as asymmetric breath sounds. Atelectasis, with or without pneumonia, mucus plugs in the bronchi, and spontaneous pneumothorax account for the major complications and must be treated separately.

However, sometimes response is not satisfactory: Labored breathing persists; the child becomes exhausted, incoherent, and no longer coughs or wheezes; and inspiratory retractions and cyanosis increase. These are the clinical signs of impending respiratory failure. Blood gas determinations exhibit a decreasing level of oxygen, rising carbon dioxide retention, and acidosis. This situation can be reversed if the danger is recognized and the child is moved to the intensive care unit where adequate equipment and personnel experienced with the grave complication are available. Delivery of 100% humidified oxygen, continuous nebulization treatments, infusion of isoproterenol and sodium bicarbonate, and mechanical ventilation may be necessary.

 ## Part 2: Circulatory Disorders

This section introduces some of the more common pediatric problems involving the heart and its vessels and circulating blood (Fig. 32-8). Although some of the frequently encountered congenital heart defects were briefly described in Chapter 14, no mention was made of the surgical possibilities of repair of such defects or the nursing care of the cardiac patient. The following paragraphs supply these omissions.

Varied abnormalities of the heart and large blood vessels can occur. Some cause little inconvenience. Others are incompatible with life or produce severe problems.

DIAGNOSTIC PROCEDURES

To evaluate heart function and detect cardiac abnormalities, an accurate history of the patient's complaints is sought, a complete physical examination is carried out, and various tests and specialized procedures are ordered.

Common noninvasive tests include permanent recording of the size and shape of the heart by x-ray examination, external pulse and heart sound recordings by phonocardiography, tests of the activity of the heart by electrocardiography, and sonar recordings (echocardiography), which allow examination of human fetal car-

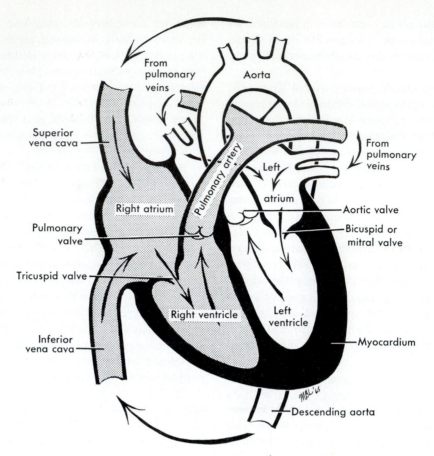

FIG 32-8   Structure and circulation of normal heart. Shaded area represents blood with low oxygen content.

diac development and when combined with *Doppler ultrasonography* techniques, provide diagnostic accuracy of most of the major congenital heart defects in infancy.

Laboratory tests of special significance include a complete blood cell count and hematocrit and hemoglobin determinations. Patients with a cyanotic type of heart disease either may have an excessive amount of circulating red blood cells (polycythemia) manufactured in an attempt to deliver more oxygen to the deprived body cells or may suffer from anemia. If polycythemia is present, the blood thickens and circulation slows down, occasionally causing the development of abnormal clots in the bloodstream—always a dangerous situation.

A special procedure called *angiography* is occasionally arranged. It involves the injection of a contrast medium into the circulation and observation of its flow by x-ray examination or fluoroscopy. When a contrast medium is injected directly into a heart chamber, it is termed *angiocardiography*. Such visualization of the aorta is termed *aortography*. Special procedures may also include the performance of right or left side of the heart catheterizations, which involve the introduction of a small catheter seen by fluoroscopy into a vein or artery and its gentle manipulation into various chambers of the heart and large associated vessels. This procedure is performed on an anesthetized or sedated patient and, although it is not without risk, yields considerable information. If possible, children are sedated, not anesthetized, so that they can cooperate during the procedure.

It is important for an anesthesiologist to be available in the catheterization laboratory for any possible needs for anesthesia support. Heart catheterizations reveal the pressure in various areas of the cardiocirculatory system and the amount of oxygen in the blood at different sites. The presence of abnormal openings can be demonstrated by direct passage of the small catheter through the defects or by evaluation of oxygenation patterns.

Therapeutic catheterization is a term used to describe

treatment approaches during the heart catheterization. These include balloon atrial septostomy to create a large interatrial communication and facilitate mixing of pulmonary and systemic venous blood in infants with a transposed aorta and pulmonary artery (transposition of the great vessels); balloon valvuloplasty to widen the obstructive and narrowed valve in patients with pulmonary stenosis; and balloon angioplasty to widen a narrowed blood vessel in patients with peripheral pulmonary stenosis or coarctation of the aorta.

Children returning to the nursing unit after cardiac catheterization should be treated as postoperative patients. Vital signs—pulse, respirations, and blood pressure—should be noted every 20 minutes until stable. Children should have blood pressure determinations on the arm that is not used for the catheter insertion. A mist tent or oxygen mask should be in readiness as ordered or indicated. Any dressing applied should be noted and observed. It is important to note skin color, temperature, and character of the pulse in the extremity catheterized, because this may detect blood vessel occlusion resulting from thrombus formation.

Infant

Congenital anomalies of the heart and great vessels. About 30,000 infants are born with recognizable heart disease every year in the United States. Formerly, about half of these infants died within 6 months. Currently, early diagnosis and treatment (through palliative or curative surgery) are effective in approximately 90% of cases.

Congenital heart disease refers to a structural abnormality present in the circulation at birth. These defects create at least three problems related to blood flow within the heart and circulatory system. A *volume overload* occurs when more blood than normal enters a ventricle. A *pressure overload* occurs when the outflow of blood is impeded or obstructed. Ventricular hypertrophy and finally congestive heart failure can result. *Desaturation,* low oxygen content of circulating arterial blood, occurs when unoxygenated blood returning from the body mixes with the oxygenated blood returning from the lungs. Acidosis can occur as the result of poor oxygenation of the various organs. Acidosis leads to decreased cardiac performance and still more acidosis. Some congenital anomalies of the heart illustrate all three types of blood flow problems. Early diagnosis and treatment are important (Fig. 32-9).

Signs and symptoms. Infants with serious congenital heart disease often manifest common signs and symptoms that reflect the underlying anomaly. *Cyanosis*—blueness of the lips, nail beds, and mucosal surfaces—may be caused by shunting of unoxygenated blood into the left side of the heart or may be associated with pulmonary edema. *Tachypnea* is defined as an excessive resting respiratory rate, 45 breaths per minute in the full-term infant or over 60 breaths per minute in the premature infant. Retractions and flaring of the nares occur with each breath. Rapid breathing is a response to heart failure or low oxygen content in the blood and is often precipitated by mild exercise. *Tachycardia,* an excessively rapid heart rate, can be difficult to evaluate in the infant, particularly if the child is moving and crying. A heart rate greater than 180 beats per minute when the infant is at rest is significant and should be reported at once, because infants quickly develop cardiac decompensation (inability to maintain the necessary blood flow). *Effort intolerance* is chiefly manifested by feeding problems. The infant usually starts feedings eagerly but soon becomes fussy and fatigued and stops feeding. The cycle is often repeated, but the infant seldom finishes a bottle. *Failure to thrive* is also common. Episodes of congestive heart failure and intercurrent pulmonary infection are common causes of retarded growth. *Murmurs,* or abnormal heart sounds, occur when flow of blood across a defect is turbulent or when valvular surfaces are irregular. They are the most commonly detected physical findings associated with congenital cardiac defects in infants.

Congestive heart failure (CHF) occurs when the heart can no longer pump blood sufficiently to meet the body's needs. When infants develop CHF in the early months of life, it is usually secondary to structural defects, which produce a pressure or volume overload. In an effort to preserve cardiac output and accommodate the larger volume of residual blood, cardiac dilation occurs. CHF is typically recognized by a combination of tachypnea and tachycardia associated with hepatomegaly caused by circulatory congestion. The development of CHF warrants prompt cardiac consultation and diagnostic studies. Frequently surgery offers the only chance of life.

Left-to-right shunts (acyanotic)

Patent ductus arteriosus (PDA). Patent means "open." The condition called patent ductus arteriosus refers to a holdover from the fetal circulation pattern. Review Fig. 4-4. You will remember that the ductus arteriosus is a short blood vessel that connects the pulmonary artery with the aorta, making it unnecessary for the blood circulating through the pulmonary artery to continue on to the nonfunctioning lungs of the fetus. Normally this arterial duct closes soon after birth and within a few weeks becomes a ligament.

If the ductus arteriosus does not close, the higher

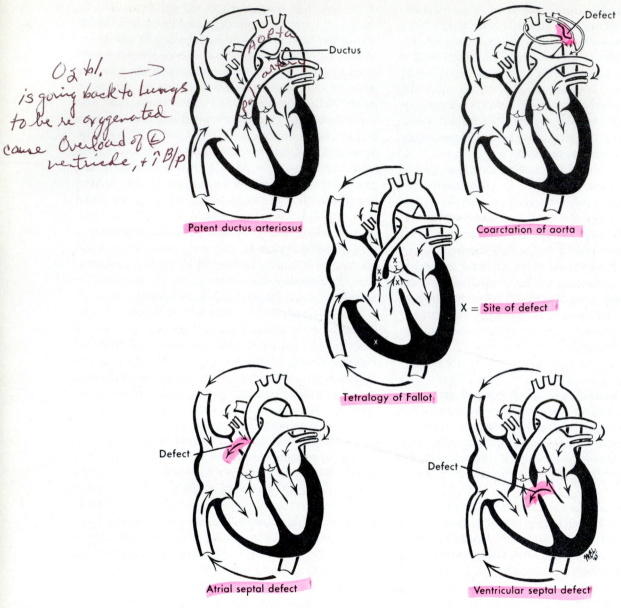

O₂ bl.
is going back to lungs
to be re oxygenated
cause Overload of L
ventricle, + ↑ B/p

FIG 32-9 Common congenital defects of heart and great vessels.

blood pressure in the aorta, which results after birth, forces well-oxygenated blood from the aorta back into the pulmonary circulation for a return trip to the lungs. This puts an abnormal workload on the left ventricle and can cause a significant elevation of the blood pressure in the pulmonary circulation. The growth of children suffering from this defect can be impaired if the duct remains large. They may experience dyspnea when they are ac-

tive, and without appropriate treatment their life expectancy is often reduced. The defect does not characteristically produce cyanosis unless pressures in the aorta and pulmonary artery are changed as the result of excessive pulmonary blood flow, which can increase pulmonary vascular resistance. Some premature babies with respiratory distress syndrome have delayed, spontaneous closure of the ductus or reopening of the ductus as a

NURSING CARE PLAN

The Infant/Child with Congestive Heart Failure Secondary to Congenital Heart Defects

Selected nursing diagnoses	Expected outcomes	Interventions
A. Decreased cardiac output related to structural defects and cardiac dysfunction. Clinical manifestations: Tachycardia, tachypnea, pallor, cyanosis, sudden weight gain associated with signs of dependent edema.	Child's heart rate will be within normal limits for age with strong and regular apical pulse. Child maintains normal serum K^+. Edema subsides, weight loss, increased voiding.	Assess heart rate 1 minute every 4 hours and before administration of digoxin. Administer digoxin as ordered (second nurse check dosage). Monitor serum K^+ daily. Adjust oral K^+ intake in diet as ordered. Assess child for presence of edema. Maintain strict I & O. Obtain daily weights. Administer diuretics as ordered. Maintain fluid and diet restrictions. Check other serum electrolytes as ordered.
B. Impaired gas exchange related to pulmonary congestion and anxiety. Clinical manifestations: Dyspnea, chest retractions, grunting, tachypnea, weak cry, restlessness.	Child maintains pink, warm skin. Child develops normal respiratory pattern.	Auscultate lungs every 4 hours and assess child for cyanosis, dyspnea, tachypnea. Position child in semi-Fowler's, position infant in cardiac chair to allow easier movement of diaphragm. Avoid restrictive clothing. Administer oxygen as ordered. Monitor oxygen saturation with pulse oximetry and blood gases as ordered.
C. Activity intolerance related to imbalance of oxygen supply and demand. Clinical manifestations: Tires with feedings and ADLs, fatigue, lethargy.	Child maintains balance between cardiac demands and oxygen consumption.	Provide quite, restful environment. Include periods of rest in daily care. Offer child small, frequent feedings; low salt formula (i.e., Lonalac or Similac PM), Use soft nipple with large hole. May need to gavage feed with supplementary oxygen source. Protect infant from sudden changes in temperature. Respond promptly to crying.
D. Anxiety related to perpetual dyspnea. Clinical manifestations: Restlessness, unhappiness, anxious face, perplexed frown, anorexia, breathlessness during feeding.	Evidence of peaceful, contented baby.	Feed early. Allow frequent rest periods. Limit sucking time to 45 minutes per bottle. Handle gently. Cuddle when possible. Consolidate nursing procedures. Provide uninterrupted sleep. Encourage parents to participate in care.

response to poor oxygenation in the lungs. Often this prevents weaning the baby from a mechanical ventilator unless the ductus is closed by medication or ligation.

Diagnosis is usually made on the basis of several findings. The detection of a continuous murmur or an abnormal sound accompanying heart action is only one. A thrill may be noted; the word "thrill" in this case refers to a vibration felt over the cardiac area. Blood pressure determinations may reveal a wide range between the systolic and diastolic readings—termed a *wide pulse pressure*. The appearance and stamina of the patient are noted. The patent duct may be visualized by echocardiography, aortography, or direct passage of a small catheter through the duct during fluoroscopy.

This condition may be treated surgically, usually with excellent results. The duct is tied off (ligated) or divided. Medicines that inhibit the synthesis of prostaglandins by the body's tissues are being used effectively in premature infants to close the ductus; they have no effect in older patients.

Atrial septal defect (ASD). An abnormal opening in the wall, or septum, that separates the right and left atria may be the result of the persistence of the foramen ovale, which during fetal life shunts some of the blood from the right to the left side of the heart. It may also be caused by the presence of a septal opening unassociated with normal fetal circulation. Cyanosis does not characteristically occur, since the blood pressure is higher in the left side of the heart and unoxygenated blood does not enter the systemic circulation. However, if some other abnormality is present (for example, pulmonary valve stenosis), right-to-left flow may occur, and cyanosis may result. Children with ASD usually have an overworked right side of the heart and congested pulmonary circulation because the extra flow through the defect reaches the lungs by way of the right ventricle. They may demonstrate cardiac enlargement, a systolic murmur, decreased resistance to respiratory tract infections, lowered exercise tolerance, and physical underdevelopment. A decision to attempt surgical correction is based on the condition of the individual child. If the shunt is small, patients do well without operative intervention. Surgery itself presents a minimum of risk. During surgery the defect is repaired either by direct closure with sutures only or by the incorporation of a plastic patch into the repair. The patch is eventually penetrated by growing heart fibers and becomes part of the septum.

Ventricular septal defect (VSD). The presence of an opening between the two ventricles is always an abnormality, whether it occurs in the fetus or the newborn infant. How seriously such an opening disturbs normal heart function depends on the position and size of the defect and the presence of other abnormalities in the heart or large vessels leaving the heart. If a large defect is found in the membranous portion of the septum, symptoms are usually severe. The blood generally travels through the opening from the left to the right ventricle. However, in some cases the shunt reverses as resistance in the pulmonary arterial bed increases, and the pressure in the right side of the heart mounts. Diagnosis is made on the basis of clinical symptoms, a characteristic heart murmur, and the results of x-ray examination, electrocardiograms, echocardiography, and, when indicated, cardiac catheterization. Specific treatment may be recommended for the individual child and consists of surgical repair by open heart surgery similar to that employed for ASD. Surgical risk is somewhat increased with VSD repair.

Right-to-left shunts (cyanotic)

Tetralogy of Fallot. The word element "tetra" means "four." Tetralogy of Fallot is a heart condition that is characterized by the presence of four classic features: an interventricular septal defect, a narrowing of the opening of the outflow tract of the right ventricle (pulmonary stenosis), an aorta situated above the septal defect (overriding aorta), and an enlarged, thickened right ventricular wall (right ventricular hypertrophy). Because the narrowed outflow of the right ventricle causes the pressure to rise in that chamber, hypertrophy of the right heart wall results, and the shunt of blood through the septal defect goes from right to left, usually causing considerable cyanosis. The infant suffering from tetralogy of Fallot has been called a "blue baby." The moderately to severely affected young child with this diagnosis typically has blue lips and nail beds and dusky-tinted skin, which becomes more cyanotic on exertion. Clubbing of the fingers and toes is often a feature (Fig. 32-10). A thrill and chest deformity may be noted. A child may have hypoxemic spells with respiratory distress, deep cyanosis, loss of consciousness, and a seizure. An affected child is small for his age.

When young children with cyanotic heart disease are fatigued, they often squat (Fig. 32-11). This position reduces the right-to-left flow of unoxygenated blood across the ventricular septal defect, traps desaturated blood in the lower extremities, and improves oxygenation.

Management of hypoxemic spells can be difficult and complex. Initially, when the infant is *excitable,* with respiratory distress, one can use a knee-chest position and administer oxygen. Morphine may be used for sedation. If the infant is flaccid or unconscious, morphine

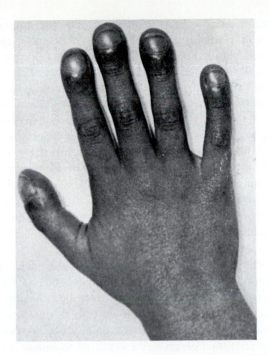

FIG 32-10 When ends of fingers become wide and thick, they are termed "clubbed." These fingers are also cyanotic. *(Courtesy Naval Hospital, San Diego, Calif.)*

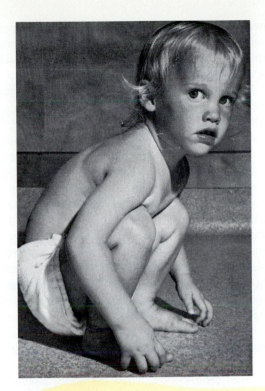

FIG 32-11 Squatting position improves oxygenation of some children with congenital heart defects.

is contraindicated. If metabolic acidosis occurs, sodium bicarbonate is sometimes given intravenously. If these measures fail, phenylephrine (Neo-Synephrine) or propranolol should be administered intravenously with proper monitoring of vital signs.

Diagnosis depends on clinical manifestations, x-ray examinations, electrocardiograms, echocardiograms, angiocardiograms, and cardiac catheterizations. Treatment can be medical or surgical, depending on the condition of the patient. In very blue newborns with tetralogy of Fallot, prostaglandin E_1 is given intravenously to dilate the ductus arteriosus, thereby increasing the flow of blood to the lungs, and improving the supply of oxygen to the body's tissues. This medication can be life-saving and must be followed by surgery. Before open heart surgery was available, surgical techniques were devised to improve the pulmonary circulation by creating an artificial ductus arteriosus, which recirculated poorly oxygenated blood to the lungs for oxygen enrichment. The Blalock-Taussig operation and the Waterston operation are such techniques. This type of palliative surgery is still useful when the child is considered too small for total correction but is experiencing life-threatening hypoxemic spells. Currently open heart surgery with total correction is

preferred, because the sources of difficulty can be viewed and repaired directly. Without surgical intervention the typical patient with tetralogy of Fallot faces a brief future.

Complete transposition of the great vessels. Transposition of the great vessels is a serious cyanotic congenital heart defect. In this condition the pulmonary artery originates from the left ventricle, whereas the aorta arises from the right ventricle. Life is possible as long as the foramen ovale or ductus arteriosus remains open or an interventricular septal defect exists. Prominent features are extreme cyanosis and congestive heart failure. Diagnosis is made on the basis of electrocardiogram, x-ray examination, echocardiogram, angiocardiogram, and cardiac catheterization. Usually a special balloon catheter (balloon septostomy) is used to create or enlarge an ASD without the risk of palliative surgery. Total correction is possible by switching the venous inflows to the heart. In the Mustard procedure, a "baffle," or partition made of pericardium, is placed in such a manner as to redirect the pulmonary venous return within the left atrium to the right ventricle and the systemic return to the left ventricle.

Immediate results have been excellent, with an overall mortality of less than 10% in patients without additional complicating cardiac anomalies. Some centers currently advocate as the operation of choice a switching of the great arteries and reimplanting of the coronary arteries in the aorta.

Obstructive lesions

Pulmonary stenosis. The pulmonary artery carries poorly oxygenated blood from the right ventricle through the pulmonary valve to the lungs, where it is reoxygenated. Narrowing of the valve itself or the areas immediately above or below it causes obstruction to the right ventricular outflow. The condition may be so mild that the infant has no symptoms, or it may be so severe that the infant is dyspneic, has effort intolerance, severe cyanosis, and congestive heart failure. A loud murmur is heard. The condition is diagnosed by electrocardiogram, x-ray film, and cardiac catheterization. Balloon valvuloplasty or open heart surgical repair is indicated if the right ventricular pressure is high. An incision in the pulmonary artery exposes the dome-shaped valvular stenosis, which is then incised (pulmonary valvotomy). If the primary obstruction is below the valve, the obstructing muscle can be resected. The results of this operation are usually excellent, and the risk is low, except in an infant.

Coarctation of the aorta. The aorta is the largest blood vessel in the body. As it leaves the heart, it normally arches to the left. The coronary arteries and three major vessels sprout from the aortic arch before it starts its descent into the lower thorax and abdomen. The innominate, left carotid, and left subclavian arteries are the three vessels that supply the head and upper extremities with oxygenated blood. The ductus arteriosus joins the aorta in the general area of the left subclavian artery before normal postnatal circulation develops. Sometimes the aorta is abnormally narrowed in the area of the arch, usually involving the segment just past the subclavian artery. Often smaller "collateral" vessels (usually branches of the subclavian and intercostal arteries) develop and bypass the narrowed portion to help supply circulation to the lower extremities. The narrowing of the aorta is often called "coarctation," since a narrowed figure results when two arcs are drawn side by side, like two Cs back to back. The resulting symptoms depend on the severity and location of the coarctation and whether any other cardiac or blood vessel abnormalities exist.

The presence of coarctation is suspected when forceful arterial pulses are present in the upper extremities but weak or absent pulses in the lower extremities and a systolic murmur is heard. Severe coarctation in the infant, especially if associated with another congenital heart anomaly, may precipitate profound congestive heart failure and require surgical intervention. The older patient may have few complaints, although occasionally headache, leg cramps, excessive fatigue, and frequent nosebleeds are reported. Diagnosis is confirmed by blood pressure measurements, x-ray examination, electrocardiogram, and aortogram.

Without appropriate treatment the life span is often shortened because of the onset of complications, such as hypertension, cerebral hemorrhage, subacute bacterial endocarditis, or heart failure.

Definitive treatment for coarctation is surgical. The narrowed portion may be cut out and the adjoining normal-sized segments sewn together. Occasionally the repair involves the insertion of a prosthesis or the use of the subclavian artery to widen the aorta. If stenosis occurs again after the operation, the preferred treatment is balloon angioplasty performed during cardiac catheterization.

Cardiac surgery. Assuming that facilities and skilled physicians are available, surgical treatment of large blood vessel or heart defects depends on the extent of incapacity suffered by the patient, the possibility of a satisfactory repair, and the risk involved. Surgery on the aorta, pulmonary artery, or other associated blood vessels is similar in some respects to heart surgery. However, when the malformations exist in the interior of the heart and cardiac circulation must be interrupted, the difficulty of the procedure and the risk to the patient increase significantly. A heart-lung machine was introduced in 1955. Before that time it was impossible to discontinue the beating of the heart long enough to make a lengthy repair without seriously depriving some vital structure (for example, the brain or kidneys) of carbon dioxide—oxygen exchange, thus causing tissue damage.

The heart-lung machine receives blood from the patient's venous circulation through tubes inserted into the inferior and superior venae cavae. It removes the carbon dioxide, instills oxygen, regulates blood temperature, and pumps the blood back into the systemic circulation in most cases by way of the aorta or femoral artery (called a *cardiopulmonary bypass*). Needless to say, this is a highly complex procedure, requiring a team of skilled physicians, nurses, and technicians.

A patient with a congenital heart defect may undergo

surgery as an infant, toddler, or child. To simplify organization, the following discussion includes more than the treatment and nursing care of the infant in its scope. Any child who is to have any type of surgery must be carefully prepared for the event. This is especially true in the case of scheduled chest or heart surgery because of the seriousness of the operation and the many procedures that must be carried out that require the trust and cooperation of the child to achieve optimum results.

Preparation of the child presupposes that the parents are prepared. This does not mean that the parents must feel totally calm and serene or that they and their child must know all the details of the procedure. The former would be unnatural; the latter would be both impossible and undesirable, probably causing more anxieties than it would ease. How much the child is told depends on age, expressed concerns, and intellect. How much the parents are told depends on their expressed concerns, intellects, and familiarity with the sciences involved. Whatever information is given, however simple, should be truthful.

Children who are scheduled for heart surgery are usually admitted to the hospital in advance of the procedure to enable them to learn about the hospital, to become acquainted with some of the nurses who will be caring for them, and to be introduced to some of the equipment and techniques that will be used after surgery. This preliminary period is also used as an opportunity to evaluate the child. It is a time when the child's general condition is observed and nutritional needs noted and, as far as possible, met. Weight is recorded each morning; scheduled blood pressure, respiration, and pulse checks are particularly important. The nurses should be alert for and should report any signs of fever, respiratory tract infection, or rash, which may indicate the presence of other diseases. Such signs can necessitate a postponement of surgery.

It is usually helpful to demonstrate some of the equipment that will be used with the child before its use under more stressful conditions is needed. Children can be shown an oxygen tent with humidifier and can get inside to see how the "small house" feels. They can "practice" their breathing exercises with the intermittent positive-pressure machine or learn how to cough with the nurse holding their chests. Explanations should be calm, factual, and geared to the child's level of understanding. Play therapy techniques are often helpful in explaining anticipated events to the child.

Treatment and nursing care of the cardiac patient
Postoperative nursing care. The postoperative nursing

care of open heart surgery patients is a nursing specialty in itself. A patient usually remains in the intensive care unit for several days. While the child is in the intensive care unit, his condition is usually monitored by machines that graphically record heart action, arterial and venous blood pressures, respirations, and temperature. In some cases heartbeat may be stimulated by the use of a mechanical pacemaker. The rate and quality of respirations are evaluated; the color and feel of the skin are noted. Chest suction is maintained to prevent a buildup of fluid or air in the thorax, which causes respiratory distress and atelectasis. Humidified oxygen is often administered by an oxygen tent or mask. The urinary catheter is checked frequently to determine kidney output. Intravenous fluids and blood transfusions are calculated and maintained according to order. Wound drainage and dressings must be checked. Turning and encouraging the patient to cough are extremely important. Intermittent positive pressure may be prescribed. Tracheal and nasopharyngeal suctioning may be ordered. Initially the patient's temperature may be subnormal, but later, temperature-reducing procedures may be necessary, including the use of the hypothermia blanket. A relatively high temperature after open heart surgery is fairly common. In some cases it can be a reaction to the massive blood transfusion received. However, the possibility of infection must not be discounted when a patient's temperature rises abnormally.

Continuing care. The patient needs constant, expert nursing observation and care. Many important nursing evaluations must be made during this critical postoperative interval. Caring for this type of patient in the immediate postoperative period is not within the scope of the vocational nurse. However, at times she may be called on to "lend a careful hand," with supervision, during a treatment or to help change the patient's position, depending on the child's needs and condition. The vocational nurse should know how important it is for the chest tubes to remain intact and the drainage bottles and suction machine to remain undisturbed. The bottles containing drainage from the chest should always be maintained lower than the lowest level of the child's chest to prevent backflow. To prevent such backflow, the bottles should be fastened to the floor or to a correctly positioned holder. In the event that a chest bottle breaks or the tube becomes disconnected, the part of the tube coming from the patient's chest must be immediately clamped off near the chest wall to prevent pneumothorax. Symptoms of pneumothorax include cyanosis, dyspnea, and chest pain.

As the patient's condition improves, chest suction is discontinued and the tubes removed. If temporary heart pacing wires were attached to the heart during the operation, they are withdrawn if the heart rhythm is normal. As the patient's condition becomes stable, the child may be assigned to the care of a licensed vocational nurse under the supervision of a registered nurse. The vocational nurse should know that the child is usually weighed while undressed each morning before breakfast to determine fluid retention. The child may be on a diet that limits sodium and carefully spaces a certain maximum oral fluid intake. The patient's pulse and respirations should be noted and recorded before and after any new activity. During periods of ambulation the child should be carefully evaluated for fatigue and given periods of rest as respirations, pulse, and color dictate. The pulse of these young children and infants is always taken over the heart with a stethoscope—that is, apically—for 1 minute. This technique requires training, since there are normally two sounds to each cardiac cycle. Older children may have radial pulse determinations for 1 minute. The quality, as well as the rate, should be noted. Occasionally apical-radial pulse determinations are ordered. These pulse rates are taken simultaneously and then compared; for example, they may be written 110A/100R. There may be more apical beats than radial beats (pulse deficits), but there is never an excess of radial beats. Blood pressure determinations are routinely made with the patient's pulse and respiration at scheduled intervals. Care must be taken in the selection of the size of cuff—it should cover two thirds of the distance from the shoulder to the elbow or should be 20% wider than the diameter of the patient's arm.

Ambulation and activity privileges are gradually increased. Many times conferences must be arranged with physician-nurse-parent participation to help parents adjust to the new capabilities of their children and to prevent the hazards of overprotection. Help regarding school responsibilities and even vocational planning may be sought.

Nonsurgical treatment and care. Sometimes patients' cardiac problems cannot be helped by surgery, or they must wait until they are in better condition or older before surgery is attempted. In these cases the children are treated by medicines, planned diets, and general health supervision. The nurse should be aware of the types of medications the child is receiving and the expected accomplishments, side effects, and toxic reactions of these medications. Sodium restriction is common. Often patients with cardiac defects are weighed daily, and ac-

curate intake and output records are maintained. Signs of developing heart failure, cardiac irregularities, or possible respiratory tract infection should be promptly reported. Limitations of activity can be necessary, although many pediatric patients with congenital cardiac defects automatically limit themselves to only the activities they can best tolerate. Quiet play is often more restful than enforced, resented "complete bed rest." The child who must be in an oxygen tent or who demonstrates susceptibility to fatigue should be disturbed as little as possible. When the child is disturbed, several procedures should be carried out at the same time to allow relatively long uninterrupted periods of sleep or rest. (For example, temperature, pulse, respirations, and blood pressure determinations, offering fluids, changing the child's gown or diapers, and shifting position can all be accomplished during one interruption.) Changes of position are important in preventing hypostatic pneumonia and skin breakdown. However, no *vigorous* back rubs should be performed on a patient with a cardiac defect. Proper positioning helps to ward off contractures and other deformities and assists proper body functions.

Possible complications of congenital cardiac defects
Cardiac decompensation—congestive heart failure (CHF). Certain complications that may develop in patients with congenital heart defects before, during, or after surgery should be mentioned. Probably the most common is the failure of the heart to continue the circulation of the blood in sufficient volume to meet body needs and prevent abnormal congestion of the blood in certain areas. Sometimes the heart can maintain an adequate blood flow by gradually increasing its size or altering its rate. If this occurs, the heart is said to be in *compensation*. If the heart cannot maintain the necessary blood flow, it is said to be in *decompensation,* or failure. Cardiac failure in infants, whatever the cause, is always a medical emergency.

Pulmonary congestion resulting from the inability of the left ventricle to pump effectively is characterized by pooling of blood in the lung capillaries, causing coughing, tachypnea, wheezing, and dyspnea. Blood-tinged froth may be expectorated. Acute pulmonary edema is a grave emergency. Immediate action is necessary. The following measures can be life-saving: placement of the infant in a sitting position and administration of oxygen by a ventilator and possibly parenteral morphine, digitalis, and diuretics.

Congestion of blood in the systemic venous system as the result of inefficient right ventricular contraction can cause nausea and vomiting, enlargement of the liver, and edema. In infants edema is often best demonstrated by a weight gain. Cyanosis, tachypnea, dyspnea, and tachycardia are major indications for diagnostic studies. However, studies are usually performed only after congestive heart failure is controlled, since the baby becomes fatigued by the work of breathing and may have an annoying cough and therefore difficulty with eating and sleeping. Prompt treatment with digoxin, oxygen, and diuretics decreases heart and respiratory rate and improves color, appetite, and disposition. Digoxin slows and strengthens the heartbeat and induces diuresis. A digitalizing dose (high dose) is given over a period of 16 hours, and a maintenance dose of 10% of the digitalizing dose is usually given every 12 hours. However, digoxin should be withheld and the physician notified if the apical pulse rate in the infant is less than 100 beats per minute. Signs and symptoms of toxicity include anorexia, vomiting, and excessive slowing or irregularity of the pulse rate. Diuretics especially help in relieving the pulmonary congestion that accompanies congestive heart failure if response to other forms of treatment is insufficient.

Nursing measures center around making infants more comfortable and conserving their energy. A sitting position in a cool, humidified oxygen tent is beneficial. Early feeding with soft nipples and allowing for frequent rest periods reduces fatigue. Uninterrupted sleep should be encouraged by bathing infants when they are awake and only when absolutely necessary. The recording of accurate, current vital signs, intake and output determinations, and weight is critical. As soon as the child's condition is stable, he is prepared for surgery or discharge until a surgery appointment can be made. The parents should be increasingly involved in care while their child is hospitalized so that they are not unprepared when the child comes home. The help of a public health nurse or hospital home visitor can be valuable in this setting.

Subacute bacterial endocarditis. Any damage to cardiac tissue or a congenital heart or blood vessel anomaly can set the stage for inflammation of the lining of the heart (endocarditis) and arteries (endarteritis). The inflammation usually results from a blood-borne infection, originating at some other body site. It may have its onset after surgical procedures, such as dental extraction, tonsillectomy, or adenoidectomy, or it may be spread from an abscess or infection elsewhere in the body. Signs and symptoms include temperature elevation, weight loss, fatigue, anemia, leukocytosis, the presence of petechiae, an enlarged spleen, and perhaps even partial paralysis or other central nervous system symptoms caused by the presence of emboli in the brain that originated in the inflamed heart tissue. Prophylactic antibiotics must be prescribed before and during certain procedures that can introduce bacteria into the bloodstream.

Cerebral thrombosis. Cerebral thrombosis can develop when an excess of circulating red blood cells is called into action to increase the oxygen-carrying capacity of the blood. Dehydration can result in a thicker, slower-moving fluid in the blood vessels. Clots, or thrombi, can form, and a cerebral vascular accident can take place. Maintenance of adequate fluid intake, the use of oxygen to relieve episodes of cyanosis, and possibly the cautious use of anticoagulants in patients likely to develop such a complication are suggested means of reducing the risk.

Disorders of the blood and blood-forming organs. The cardiovascular system (heart and blood vessels) is designed so that nutrients, hormones, and oxygen reach the individual body tissue cells and so that waste products from those cells are properly transported for elimination by the kidneys, lungs, or skin. To do this efficiently, the circulating fluid within the cardiovascular system—blood—contains many substances. Of particular interest are the three types of structures called the "formed elements." The red blood cells, or *erythrocytes,* help transport oxygen and carbon dioxide in the blood to and from the lungs. The white blood cells, or *leukocytes,* and antibodies of various types help protect the bloodstream and surrounding body tissues from the intrusion of disease-producing microorganisms and foreign proteins. The platelets, or *thrombocytes,* assist in the formation of clots to repair any leak in a damaged blood vessel. Any lack or defect in the normal makeup of the blood is likely to cause symptoms of disease. It is impossible and of little practical nursing value to describe within the pages of this text all the various problems that can occur when the blood is abnormal. However, four kinds of disorders that are seen with some frequency in pediatric service are briefly discussed. They are the *anemias, hemophilias, leukemias,* and *purpuras.*

Anemias. When the term "anemia" is used, it indicates a condition in which the total hemoglobin content of the blood is abnormally reduced, either because of lack of sufficient hemoglobin in the red blood cells or lack of red blood cells. Hemoglobin is the substance in red blood cells necessary for the normal transport of oxygen to the body cells. The most common cause of anemia in children is iron deficiency. Another anemia that has received much attention is sickle cell disease.

Iron-deficiency anemia. The most common type of

anemia in the world, found especially in the pediatric population, is iron-deficiency anemia. Pallor, irritability, anorexia, and listlessness direct attention to this disorder. The anemia is usually discovered secondarily to the problem that brought the child and his parent to the physician. Hemoglobin concentrations of less than 11 g/100 ml and a hematocrit level of less than 33% in a healthy infant strongly suggest iron deficiency. Insufficient iron for synthesis of hemoglobin is the cause of this problem. Children under 3 years of age and adolescent girls have the highest incidence of this disorder. The major cause of iron-deficiency anemia is insufficient dietary intake of iron to meet the demands of body growth (especially of low birth weight and premature infants and adolescents). Infants with iron deficiency commonly have a diet of large amounts of cow's milk, which is low in iron. Causes of anemia other than dietary deficiency include (1) acute or chronic blood loss and (2) impaired absorption (severe prolonged diarrhea). Treatment consists of oral administration of iron preparations, preferably ferrous iron, a revision of diet to include iron-rich foods (muscle meats, liver, eggs, wheat, green leafy vegetables), and if the condition is particularly severe or unresponsive as a result of parental failure to provide the items above, intramuscular injections of iron-dextran complex may be ordered. Packed red cells are rarely given. Since the highest incidence of iron-deficiency anemia is in infancy (6 to 18 months), the best and cheapest preventive measure against this form of anemia is the widespread use of iron-fortified formulas during the entire first year of life in bottle-fed infants. Recent studies have shown that breast-fed infants are able to maintain good iron levels because more iron is absorbed from breast milk than from cow's milk. Premature, breast-fed infants require iron supplementation because of their greater growth requirements. The increased utilization of breast-feeding and iron-fortified formulas have led to significant reductions in iron-deficiency anemia in preschool children. According to some experts this improves growth, learning, and resistance to disease.

Sickle cell disease. Sickle cell disease is a collective term that embraces several hereditary disorders whose clinical and laboratory features are related to the presence of sickle hemoglobin (Hb S) in red cells. Although a few cases have been reported in the white race, sickle cell disease is found primarily in blacks. About 75,000 black Americans have the disease. Chronic illness of increasing severity and reduction of life span result from hemolytic anemia with its intermittent crises.

The sickling abnormality is attributed to a mutant gene responsible for the synthesis of a type of hemoglobin different from the normal. The abnormal change in the shape of the red blood cell from a biconcave disk to a crescent, or sicklelike, shape becomes apparent following exposure to low oxygen tensions or low pH. The basic defect in sickle hemoglobin is in the alteration of only one amino acid of the 574 that make up normal hemoglobin. This single change is responsible for all the clinical manifestations of sickle cell disease.

Sickle cell anemia. Every person possesses a pair of genes that governs the synthesis of hemoglobin. One gene is inherited from each parent. Sickle cell anemia (SCA) is expressed in those persons who receive the mutant sickle cell gene from both parents (homozygous inheritance, SS) (Fig. 32-12).

SICKLE CELL TRAIT (SCT). The sickle cell trait is probably the most common defect in hemoglobin found in the United States. It is present in those persons who have received a Hb S gene from one parent and a normal Hb A gene from the other parent (heterozygous inheritance, AS) (Fig. 32-13). The most important consideration in SCT is the genetic risk of SCA for the offspring. Although persons with SCT have as much as 40% Hb S under normal conditions, no clinical signs of disease or hemoglobin abnormalities are typically present. Rarely someone with sickle cell trait manifests symptoms of stress when exercising excessively or traveling at high altitudes in nonpressurized airplanes. SCT confers some degree of protection against the lethal effects of malaria, which may account for the major distribution of Hb S in central Africa and the very fact that SCA exists. The presence of a gene for another abnormal type of hemoglobin, or the gene for thalassemia, should be suspected in a child with sickle cell disease when the blood of only one of the parents shows the sickle cell trait. These other sickle cell types (Hb SC and Hb SB thalassemia) cause the same problems as Hb SS disease.

Young infants are usually spared the severe symptoms of SCA because of the temporary presence of fetal hemoglobin (Hb F). Hb F is gradually replaced with the Hb S. As the proportion of Hb S increases, the symptoms of anemia may appear—usually when the baby is between 6 and 12 months of age.

HEMOLYTIC ANEMIA. This anemia is caused by intravascular sickling that occurs diffusely throughout the body. Sickling red cells often form spontaneously during venous circulation when the red blood cells give up oxygen to the tissues. They also form when there are changes in pH or electrolyte balance associated with infection, acidosis, or dehydration. The body acts quickly to re-

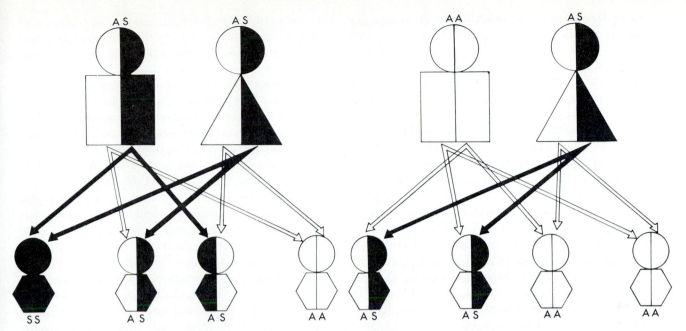

FIG 32-12 Sickle cell anemia (homozygous inheritance). When both parents carry sickle cell gene *(AS)*, possibilities for inheritance in offspring are that one child in four will inherit sickle cell anemia *(SS)*; two children in four will inherit sickle cell trait *(AS)*; one child in four will be normal *(AA)*.

FIG 32-13 Sickle cell trait (heterozygous inheritance). When only one parent is carrier of sickle cell gene *(AS)*, possibilities for inheritance in offspring are that two children in four will be normal *(AA)*; two children in four will carry sickle cell trait *(AS)*.

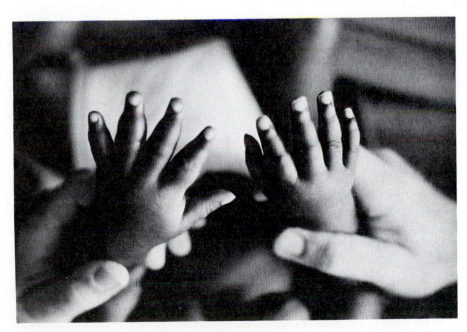

FIG 32-14 Dactylitis—swelling of the hand—sickle cell interference in circulation. *(Courtesy of CDR Alton L Lightsey, MC, USN, Naval Hospital, San Diego, Calif.)*

move these abnormal sickled cells from the bloodstream, and this causes the severe degree of anemia that occurs.

VASOOCCLUSIVE CRISIS. The exact events leading to the onset of painful crises are not clearly known. Many of these crises are preceded by infections. The basis of the painful crisis appears to be occlusion of blood vessels by sickled red cells. This interferes with normal tissue blood supply, resulting in subsequent cellular death and damage of the organs involved. Before an individual reaches 2 years of age, dactylitis, or the "hand-foot," syndrome commonly occurs (Fig. 32-14). The symmetric, painful swelling of the hands and feet results from interference with circulation to the metacarpals and metatarsals. If the child's pain is not too severe, increased fluids, application of warmth, and acetaminophen relieves the pain. In other children the pain is unbearable and is relieved only by stronger analgesics. Occlusive episodes after the first or second year of life most frequently occur during the preschool period. Episodes of acute abdominal pain can be severe, accompanied by fever, muscle spasm, nausea, vomiting, and leukocytosis.

SEQUESTRATION CRISIS. A crisis associated with shock is called "acute splenic sequestration crisis" (ASSC). The mother notes a rather sudden increase in pallor accompanied by abdominal distention and thirst. By the time these children arrive at the hospital, they have become notably dyspneic and weak. Left-sided abdominal (splenic) pain is present, and the pulse and respirations are elevated. Prompt diagnosis and treatment are essential to ensure survival. Transfusion of packed erythrocytes and plasma expanders should be started immediately on admission. The nurse who recognizes the situation should hasten the admission procedure, but be sure to check the child's weight and height accurately. It is imperative to take blood specimens and urine samples immediately and to have ready special equipment for transfusions. Because reduced oxygenation increases sickling, an atmosphere of well-humidified oxygen is used. The nurse also must keep in mind that parents often fear censure or reproach by those in authority and, in their effort to gain approval, may hide their feelings or hold back information regarding the child. The nurse must give these parents every opportunity to examine their feelings about themselves and the child. She should listen carefully as she works with and encourages the parents, because if she is to really help the child, she must first help the parents. Because of the rapidity with which a sequestration crisis can occur (and even recur) and its threat of fatality, a splenectomy may be performed.

APLASTIC CRISIS. Since children with SCA have a continuing hemolytic anemia, they must produce increased numbers of new red blood cells each day. Conditions that suppress the bone marrow production of red blood cells can lead to a life-threatening anemia termed "aplastic crisis." This commonly occurs following infections or as a result of a deficiency of materials needed to produce red blood cells (for example, iron or folic acid). Treatment for aplastic crisis involves transfusions of packed red cells until the cause of the decreased production can be determined and corrected.

INFECTIONS. Children with SCA develop irreversible damage to the spleen after numerous occlusive crises involving this organ. Since a normal spleen is needed to fight certain bacterial infections, children with SCA do not handle these infections well. Pneumococcal infection, which often complicates upper respiratory infections, has been a leading cause of death in children with SCA. Prompt diagnosis and aggressive antibiotic therapy is essential for these children. Parents should be instructed in the early signs and symptoms of infection, and children should have immediate access to medical care. All children with SCA should receive immunization with the pneumococcal vaccine and Hemophilus B (HbCV) vaccine, which are protective against the common strains of pneumococcus and hemophilus that can cause life-threatening infections in these children. The National Sickle Cell Care Study has demonstrated reduced mortality in children with sickle cell anemia who were given daily prophylactic penicillin. Currently, all children with sickle cell anemia should receive penicillin daily to prevent infectious death.

The therapy for SCA and its frequent crises remains one of the major clinical problems in pediatric hematology. There is no cure for SCA or even a completely satisfactory treatment for its crises.

DETECTION OF SICKLE HEMOGLOBIN AND COUNSELING. Screening programs for SCA or SCT should not be set up unless a genetic counseling service can be provided to those found to carry the trait. Otherwise, the benefits of the screening are largely lost, and anguish can be created over an essentially benign condition. Screening programs must incorporate meaningful education about the nature of SCA and its mode of inheritance, as well as individual counseling. In mass screening, Sickledex (sickle-turbidity tube test) or the sickle cell slide test is adequate, but positive reactions must be followed by hemoglobin electrophoresis to confirm results. Newborn infants can be screened in the hospital for both the condition and the trait. Such hospital programs facilitate optimum infant care and early diagnosis of crises and provide counseling for the parents.

Nursing care. The nursing care of children with anemia, whatever its basic cause, must take into account the excessive fatigue experienced by most of these boys and girls. Their energy must be conserved. They especially need help and encouragement to build good habits in nutrition. Frequent small feedings are more successful than large infrequent meals. The enlarged liver and spleen and tender muscles of some of these patients all demand gentle care. Attention to signs of bleeding (external or internal) is important. Signs of jaundice, increased pallor, increased lethargy, or irritability should be reported. Patients receiving blood transfusions should be carefully observed and protected against possible infiltration of the blood (a potentially serious event). Signs of toxic reactions, complaints of chest or back pain, itching hives, or elevated temperature with or without chills should be noted and reported early. The rate of administration should be closely watched to ensure that the circulatory system is not overloaded.

Hemophilias

Hemophilia A–factor VIII deficiency. Classic hemophilia, antihemophilic globulin (AHG), or factor VIII deficiency, is an uncommon but not rare disorder involving a defect in the clotting mechanism of the blood. Hemophilia results from a defect in a gene on the X chromosome concerned with blood clotting. It is a sex-linked, recessive condition confined almost exclusively to males and can pass from one generation to another from a carrier mother to her son. A male receives only one X, from his mother, which impairs his blood clotting process. Since the female receives two X chromosomes, one normal gene ensures normal blood clotting. A girl inherits the condition only if her father is a hemophiliac and her mother is a carrier. Because of its hereditary feature, it has figured prominently in the history of royal families and has been called the disease of kings.

The defect in clot formation is caused by the lack of antihemophilic globulin, or factor VIII, in the blood plasma. A wide range of factor VIII values (50% to 200%) exists, but in most healthy persons the average is 100%. A severe hemophiliac has less than 1% of factor VIII. Hemophiliac patients are susceptible to spontaneous, unprovoked hemorrhage. Moderate hemophiliacs have from 2% to 5% of factor VIII and may bleed excessively with minor trauma. Mild hemophiliacs have 10% to 20% of factor VIII and may, with care, live free from bleeding episodes. Surgical procedures, dental extractions, and even the normal rough-and-tumble existence of young children are especially hazardous for a hemophiliac patient.

Current treatment consists of administration of factor VIII concentrate in an amount necessary to control hemorrhage. However, protection afforded from one infusion rapidly disappears, because the concentration of factor VIII falls to one half of its original level in 8 to 10 hours. Because of this, it may be necessary to repeat administration of factor VIII within 10 hours if bleeding continues. The precise level of factor VIII needed to control bleeding is not known, but the amount of factor VIII given should be related to the seriousness of the bleeding. In central nervous system bleeding the goal is to maintain 100% factor VIII activity until the site of bleeding is completely healed. In joint bleeding, 50% factor VIII activity is usually sufficient for optimum results. The combination of immobilization and a level of 10% to 20% is usually adequate to control soft tissue bleeding. Efforts to control bleeding by using local measures (pressure, cold, or applications of thrombin) should be attempted if possible. Some cities have hemophilia centers that are prepared to render intravenous therapy to these patients on an outpatient basis. Many patients and families are taught to administer the concentrate at home. This allows faster therapy for bleeding episodes and the maintenance of a more normal lifestyle.

FACTOR VIII INHIBITORS. A small number (about 5%) of patients with classic hemophilia develop inhibitors (antibodies that block factor VIII). The presence of a circulating inhibitor is usually detected by the lack of response to a dose of factor VIII that normally would control the bleeding. Inhibitors may develop in young children after a few exposures to factor VIII, but no evidence shows that the inhibitors are related to the number of transfusions a patient receives. Without exposure to plasma products, the amount of inhibitor may gradually decrease, and factor VIII can then be given again with temporary benefit. Effective control of bleeding in patients is very difficult when the inhibitor is circulating.

Hemophilia B–factor IX deficiency (Christmas disease). Factor IX plasma thromboplastic component (PTC) deficiency accounts for about 15% of patients with hemophilia. The causes and symptoms are similar to those of hemophilia A. A factor IX concentrate has become available for treatment and is used in the same manner as factor VIII.

Hemophilia C–factor XI deficiency. Factor XI plasma thromboplastin antecedent (PTA) deficiency differs from hemophilias A and B. It is usually a mild disorder and may appear in either boys or girls as the result of an autosomal recessive trait in which bleeding occurs only in the homozygote. Bleeding episodes in factor XI deficiency are best treated with infusions of fresh plasma. The nursing care of all patients with bleeding problems is similar except that the type of intravenous therapy ordered differs, depending on the kind of replacement needed.

The parents of a patient with hemophilia are under considerable strain. They must constantly observe the environment of their adventuresome toddler or growing child. With the help of their attending physician, they must progressively educate the child to make choices in activity with consideration for the degree of hazard it entails. They do not want their child to be a psychologic cripple, unable to live an interesting, creative life, nor do they want him to be a reckless rebel.

Supervision and nursing care. The nursing care of children with hemophilia must emphasize prevention. The sides of infants' cribs should be padded. Toddlers should be denied toys and objects with sharp edges or objects that are easily broken. Rubber toys are very satisfactory for play. Children learning to walk can be fitted with knee-pads. Bleeding into the joints may produce considerable pain and deformity. Every effort should be made to prevent stiffening of the joint and loss of function. The nurse must provide her charge with interesting but safe diversion and watch for any signs of increasing bruises or internal or external blood loss. She must observe the child for untoward reaction during transfusion and check whether the intravenous infusion is flowing as ordered. Her care must be gentle and thoughtful.

Home care program. Currently patients are taught to self-administer replacement factors at home. It has been demonstrated and proved that prompt treatment at home can reduce the amount of factor needed and can save the patient time-consuming trips and hospital costs. In addition, early treatment of bleeding episodes has been shown to prevent the crippling complications caused by recurrent spontaneous bleeding into the joints.

In an effort to accomplish the goal, selected patients or their parents are instructed to administer cryoprecipitate and plasma concentrates as necessary at home. Whenever therapy becomes necessary to control minor bleeding episodes, the physician is contacted for advice about the proper dosage. Antihistamines and steroids are kept on hand to be taken by the patient if a transfusion reaction occurs.

Nurses often follow the progress of the patient at home, instructing the family about the importance of accurate records and emphasizing the need for periodic outpatient physical evaluations. The home care program spares patients the expense of frequent hospital visits and the burden of travel and waiting; most of all, it promotes a more normal life, utilizing the maximum intellectual and social potential of the hemophilic child.

Toddler and preschool child

Leukemias. Although cancer is the leading cause of death from disease in children, and leukemia is the most common childhood malignancy, the outlook can no longer be considered hopeless. Leukemia is a primary malignant disease of the bone marrow characterized by an abnormal increase of immature white blood cells or undifferentiated blast cells. This uncontrolled proliferation of leukemic cells prevents production and development of normal blood cells (hematopoiesis), which leads to infections, anemia, and bleeding. These abnormal white blood cells invade the various tissues of the body, causing pressure symptoms. (For example, infiltration of the bone marrow produces severe pain in bones and joints; mediastinal nodes can cause tracheal compression that in turn causes respiratory difficulty and cough.) The predominating symptoms depend on the area of the body invaded by the leukemic cells. Diagnosis is suspected on the basis of discovery of immature white blood cell forms in the circulating blood. An unequivocal diagnosis is confirmed by microscopic examination of the bone marrow, usually obtained from the posterior iliac crest. At times the number of circulating white blood cells is extremely elevated. Some cases demonstrate total white blood cell counts above 100,000 per mm^3. In some children the number of white blood cells in the peripheral circulation is relatively low, and proportionately few immature forms are seen; the disease is said to be *aleukemic*. However, at the same time the bone marrow can be packed with abnormal cells.

Incidence. Leukemia is the most common form of cancer in children. A slightly increased incidence occurs in boys, and the peak age of onset in children is 3 to 4 years of age. Certain children have been clearly identified as being at increased risk for developing leukemia (Table 32-2). Although there seems to have been a decline over the past 15 years in the occurrence of acute leukemia, it accounts for almost 32% of the malignant diseases in children under 15 years of age.

Types. The different types of leukemia are classified according to the kind of white cells principally involved and the relative speed of the disease process. The most common leukemic cell observed in pediatric practice is the undifferentiated form called a "blast," or stem cell,

Table 32-2 Incidence of leukemia*

Goups affected	Number affected
Nonwhite American children under 15 years of age	1 in 5,500
White American children under 15 years of age	1 in 3,000
Siblings of leukemic children	1 in 720
Children with Down syndrome	1 in 95
Children exposed to atomic irradiation	1 in 60
Monozygotic twin sibling (with one diagnosed in infancy)	1 in 5 (both will get it)

*Peak: white children, 3 to 4 years; nonwhite children, younger.

an immature form of white blood cell, usually of the lymphocytic cell line. Acute lymphoblastic leukemia (ALL) accounts for the majority of cases. Acute granulocytic or myelogenous leukemia (AML) accounts for about 20% of cases. This form, however, does not respond as favorably as ALL to the antileukemic agents currently available.

Signs and symptoms. The signs and symptoms of leukemia may be rather slow and insidious in onset or rapid in their development. These children may complain of fatigue and weakness, and lose weight. They may be pale and bruise easily. Fever, with a persistent respiratory tract infection, is a common complaint. The child's liver and spleen, infiltrated with abnormal cells, may be enlarged. Before the era of modern treatment—"Total Therapy" with central nervous system (CNS) prophylaxis—central nervous system involvement developed in approximately 50% of children during the course of their illness. A smaller number of children (8%) initially have central nervous system leukemia at the time of diagnosis. Central nervous system leukemia causes increased intracranial pressure, which is typically manifested by headache, nausea and vomiting, slowed pulse, and elevated blood pressure. The child is highly irritable and tired. Spinal fluid examination confirms the physician's diagnosis.

The course of the disease usually involves several hospitalizations and many trips to the outpatient clinic to receive therapy or to be treated for complications of therapy.

Complete remissions of the disease for extended periods have been induced with specific drug combinations (treatment protocol). The major objectives of chemotherapy are the induction of a complete remission and the maintenance of patients in a state of remission for the longest possible time, with the expectation that a significant percentage of children with ALL (50% to 80%) can be cured of their disease. A complete remission is defined as "restoration to normal health and clinical well-being." Physical and laboratory examinations are negative, blood and bone marrow are considered normal, and all evidence of disease is absent. Best results to date have been achieved with intensive courses of drug combinations and with optimum supportive care, including transfusions of platelets and antibiotic therapy.

Since 1947, when the first brief, temporary remission was induced with aminopterin, antileukemic drug therapy has greatly improved.

Treatment. Although intensive research continues in an attempt to unravel the origin and development of the disease, there is no doubt that the disease is treatable. In fact, the word "cured" is being used to describe long-term survivors no longer receiving chemotherapy.

Modern treatment currently consists of intermittent administration of high doses of several drugs in combination (Table 32-3). The duration of remissions has been increased by the addition of prophylactic therapy to the central nervous system by radiation or spinal canal (intrathecal) injections of methotrexate. Use of this therapy has reduced the incidence of central nervous system leukemia from 50% to less than 5%. In an attempt to prevent the immunosuppressive effects of continuous chemotherapy, the maintenance schedules currently used involve intermittent doses of multiple agents in combination, followed by rest periods without therapy or moderate daily dose schedules periodically reinforced with "induction" agents. Children with acute leukemia should be referred to specialized centers where the optimum opportunity for effective therapy is available (Fig. 32-15).

Complete remissions for long periods have been induced in almost all patients with acute lymphoblastic leukemia. Children in remission must have regular medical supervision, including frequent hematologic studies. Relapse is marked by falling hemoglobin levels, thrombocytopenia, severe decreases in the white blood cells called "neutrophils," and the reappearance of immature or "blast" cells in the blood and bone marrow.

Prognostic factors. The major prognostic determinants in children with acute lymphoblastic leukemia (ALL) are age and white blood cell count at the time of diagnosis. Children between the ages of 2 and 10 years with white blood cell counts of less than 25,000 per mm^3 have the best prognosis. Young infants, older children,

Table 32-3 Drugs currently used in the treatment of leukemia

Agent	Routes of administration	Signs of toxicity
Induction		
Prednisone	Oral	Moon-shaped face, osteoporosis, acne, fluid retention, ulcers, increased susceptibility to infection, personality changes
Vincristine (Oncovin)	IV	Peripheral neuropathy, hair loss
Daunomycin	IV	Bone marrow depression,* alopecia, nausea, vomiting, oral ulceration, congestive heart failure
L-Asparaginase	IV, IM	Chills, fever, nausea, vomiting, hypersensitivity reactions
Adriamycin	IV	Bone marrow depression,* alopecia, nausea, vomiting, oral ulceration, congestive heart failure
Thioguanine	Oral	Bone marrow depression*
Cytarabine (Cytosar)	IV SQ	Bone marrow depression, nausea, vomiting
Methotrexate	{ IV Intrathecal	Anorexia, abdominal pain, oral and gastrointestinal tract ulceration, bone marrow depression, hair loss (rare)
Maintenance		
6-Mercaptopurine	Oral	Bone marrow depression,* nausea, vomiting, oral and gastrointestinal tract ulceration
Methotrexate	{ Oral IV Intrathecal	Anorexia, abdominal pain, oral and gastrointestinal tract ulceration, bone marrow depression,* hair loss (rare)
Cyclophosphamide (Cytoxan)	Oral IV	Bone marrow depression,* skin rashes, hair loss, hemorrhagic cystitis, oral ulceration, diarrhea
Cytosine arabinoside (Cytosar or ARA-C)	{ IV SQ Intrathecal	Bone marrow depression,* nausea, vomiting

*Bone marrow depression is characterized by leukopenia, thrombocytopenia, and anemia.

and children with white blood cell counts greater than 50,000 per mm³ have a worse prognosis. The length of the first remission is also considered to be a prognostic indicator of length of survival. The longer the remission continues, the more optimistic is the prognosis. In general, chemotherapy for acute lymphoblastic leukemia is discontinued after 3 years of continuous complete remission.

Subgroups of Acute Lymphoblastic Leukemia (ALL) with a poor prognosis have recently been identified. In infant ALL, which occurs in children 1 year of age or younger, patients more often have a high initial white blood count, an increased incidence of extramedullary disease (CNS and renal), and a much lower 2-year, event-free survival rate (20%).

Children over 10 years of age, especially those with a high leukocyte count at diagnosis, have a poor prognosis. Many of these children have a mediastinal mass, organomegaly, and T-cell markers on their lymphoblasts.

Similarly, children with Burkitt's (B-cell) leukemia have had a rapidly fatal course. Fortunately, newer intensive chemotherapy protocols appear to be improving the outlook in these children.

Various cytogenetic abnormalities of the leukemic cell have been associated with a poor prognosis. Patients whose lymphoblasts exhibit hypoploidy (less than 46 chromosomes) or those that possess a reciprocal translocation of chromosome 4 and 11, 8 and 14, or 9 and 22 have had a poor outcome. These children should be treated aggressively in the hope of preventing relapse.

Intensive research ultimately designed to control completely the growth of leukemic cells continues. In the meantime a real effort is being made to develop a long-range therapeutic plan for each patient so that treatment can be largely conducted in cooperation with the physician in the patient's hometown.

Supportive care. Platelet transfusions have reduced the number of deaths caused by hemorrhage and in-

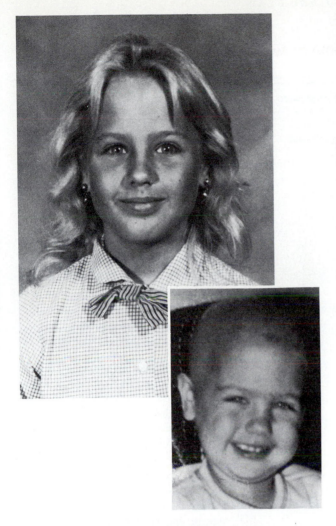

FIG 32-15 Stephanie, age 11, was originally diagnosed with acute lymphocytic leukemia at age 2 years *(insert)*. Her chemotherapy was discontinued after 3 years.

creased the opportunity to use effective drugs that depress platelet production. Corticosteroids increase capillary resistance and are useful adjuncts in the control of bleeding. Bleeding from accessible areas is occasionally controlled by the local application of thromboplastin and Gel-foam.

Infection poses the greatest threat to the life of the leukemic child. Although fever can result from the primary disease, it is important to search for infection in all patients with an elevated temperature. Cultures should be taken from blood, urine, rectum, throat, and nasopharynx. Drugs used in the control of bacterial infection, until cultures are available, include oxacillin or a ceph-

alosporin for staphylococci, streptococci, and pneumococci; ampicillin is used against *Haemophilus influenzae.* Amikacin or piperacillin or both are used against gram-negative organisms, such as *Pseudomonas, Escherichia coli,* and *Proteus.* Children who are in relapse are particularly at risk for fungal, viral, and protozoal infections. Oral moniliasis is seen frequently and is treated with oral nystatin (Mycostatin). A susceptible leukemic child who is exposed to chickenpox should receive zoster immune globulin (see p. 637 for availability and use of serum immune globulin). Interstitial pneumonia caused by the protozoal organism *Pneumocystis carinii* is a major cause of illness and death. Trimethoprim-sulfamethoxazole (Septra) is the drug of choice for this condition. Recent studies show that prophylactic Septra administration prevents the development of *Pneumocystitis carinii* pneumonia. Other methods that are currently available in some institutions to assist in the prevention and treatment of infection include granulocyte (white blood cell) transfusions and germ-free environments (laminar-flow rooms). These methods remain investigational, expensive, and not readily available to all patients.

Antileukemic drugs can cause a rapid breakdown in the malignant cells, which in turn raises the uric acid load that must be handled by the kidneys. This increased load, especially combined with a state of dehydration caused by poor fluid intake and vomiting, causes renal injury. Allopurinol helps accelerate the excretion of uric acid and reduces the risk of kidney stone formation. Parenteral fluid therapy also lessens this risk.

Almost all patients on cancer chemotherapy experience moderate to severe nausea and vomiting. Recently the introduction of new antiemetic agents and a better understanding of dosages and scheduling has led to better control of chemotherapy-induced nausea and vomiting. Reglan, Benadryl, and Lorazepam, used in combination, provide better antiemetic control of these unpleasant side effects than any other single drug.

Another side effect of some of the antileukemic drugs is that of alopecia, or hair loss, a nondangerous but distressing development. The child and the parent can be consoled by the fact that the hair will grow back.

Children with leukemia who are admitted to the hospital because of recurring symptoms are usually very uncomfortable and irritable. Pressure from the large number of white blood cells infiltrating the various body organs makes those organs tender. These children usually do not like to be moved, although changes in position are necessary to prevent respiratory tract infection and skin breakdown. Their lowered platelet counts lead to

The Child with Leukemia

Selected nursing diagnoses	Expected outcomes	Interventions
A. Potential for infection related to immunosuppression. Clinical manifestations: Fever, increased respiratory and heart rate.	Child is free from infection.	Place child in room with noninfectious child. Screen visitors for illness. Provide good skin care and oral hygiene. Maintain aseptic technique with procedures. Monitor vital signs every 4 hours for signs of infection. Avoid rectal temps, suppositories, enemas and IM injections.
B. Potential for injury (hemorrhage) related to decreased platelet count chemotherapeutic agents. Clinical manifestations: Tachycardia, decreased blood pressure, pallor, diaphoresis.	No bleeding present.	Handle child gently; institute age-appropriate safety measures. Assess skin daily for petechiae and bruising. Provide meticulous but gentle oral hygiene and skin care. Test stool, urine, and emesis for presence of blood. Monitor platelet level daily and IV administration of platelets.
C. Altered nutrition: less than body requirements related to anorexia, nausea, vomiting, altered taste sensations. Clinical manifestations: Weight loss, decreased appetite, weakness/fatigue, delayed wound healing, nausea/vomiting.	Child has sufficient caloric intake to meet body needs.	Offer small, frequent high-caloric meals. Allow child to assist with food selection. Provide oral care before meals. Administer antiemetics before meals. Avoid hot, spicy, and rough foods and others which the child finds unpleasant. Monitor parenteral feedings as ordered.
D. Body image disturbance related to side effects of steroids and chemotherapeutic agents. Clinical manifestations: Verbalizes negative feelings toward self, decreased interest in self-care, withdrawal from peers.	Child will acknowledge and express acceptance of body changes.	Discuss with child what changes will occur. Be accepting of child's body changes. Provide opportunities for child to discuss concerns. Encourage early and consistent peer visits. Stress that hair will regrow 3-6 months after therapy and hair loss will decrease with future therapy. Stress that "moon face" appearance is temporary. Discuss options for wigs, scarves, and hats. Reassure that appearance is temporary.

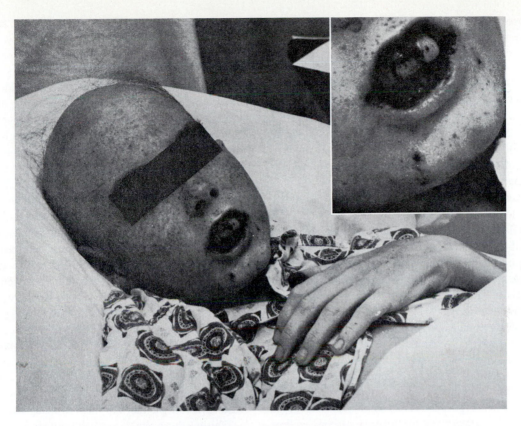

FIG 32-16 This young boy with leukemia demonstrates typical mouth lesions. Loss of hair resulted from therapy. *(Courtesy Naval Hospital, San Diego, Calif.)*

easy bruising and spontaneous hemorrhages in many parts of their bodies. Their anemia contributes to their fatigue and pallor. Because of the frequent ulceration of their mucous membranes, oral hygiene must be gentle (Fig. 32-16). Only soft toothbrushes, gauze, or applicators should be used. Mouthwashes of equal amounts of hydrogen peroxide and saline and the application of viscous lidocaine (Xylocaine) before meals are helpful local measures that often provide comfort. To maintain the child's nutritional needs during this difficult period and to lessen painful injections, a Hickman catheter is inserted. This catheter facilitates venous access and serves as a vehicle for intravenous medications and hyperalimentation (see p. 481).

Fever is often present, and measures to reduce temperature elevation (Chap. 28) frequently must be employed. Rectal temperatures are contraindicated because of the fear of inducing perirectal abscesses in children with low neutrophil counts. The presence of a member of the family at the bedside at frequent intervals is a great help to the patient, and often the child responds by taking fluids offered by the parent when all other overtures are refused. The ability to minister to the needs of their child in these trying days is almost always a source of strength to the parents, who feel a need to do something for their child. Little routines and special ways of doing things that comfort the child are important to the parent and the patient. As much as possible, they should be followed. The nursing staff should not withdraw from the parents, thinking that there is little they can do. Nurses must continue to provide support throughout the illness.

Prognosis. In childhood approximately 97% of the leukemias are acute rather than chronic. Before current methods of treatment were available, the survival time for children with acute leukemia from the time of diagnosis until death was sometimes as brief as 3 to 4 weeks and rarely spanned 6 months. Currently 60% of children with acute lymphoblastic leukemia who get optimum treatment are in uninterrupted remission for at least 5 years. About 90% of these children will remain in remission indefinitely with only a rare relapse in the sixth or seventh year (Table 32-4).

Because most leukemic children experience long periods of remission and some indeed never suffer relapse, maintenance of the family's basic life-style is extremely important. Life should go on in as normal a fashion as possible. Discipline, consistent with developmental age, must be expected and maintained for the affected child just as it is for any sibling. Overly indulgent, permissive treatment usually leads to what becomes impossible demands, fails to make the child feel happier or more secure, and often creates resentment, jealousy, and increasing tension within the family.

The child should not be overprotected, and activity limits should be clearly spelled out by the physician. The child should participate in everything physically and mentally feasible that is desirable. Parents should emphasize what the child *can do*. Unless clarified, this one area may cause great dissension between parents. School is "where it's at" for this child. As soon as possible, the child should return to class. Through conferences with the school nurse and teachers involved, guidelines can be established. It is the parents' responsibility to make clear to the school staff from the beginning that special treatment is neither desired nor appreciated.

Idiopathic thrombocytopenic purpura. Idiopathic thrombocytopenic purpura (ITP) is a syndrome of unknown cause characterized by bruises, purpura, and petechiae resulting from a great reduction in the number of platelets (less than 100,000/mm³). A normal circulating platelet count is 250,000/mm³. Each normal thrombocyte has a life span of 8 to 10 days. In ITP the platelet may survive for only hours. Seepage of blood into the mucous membranes, subcutaneous tissues, and skin occurs. Epistaxis is common. A bone marrow sample reveals normal or increased thrombocyte formation, which rules out leukemia, the fear of many parents. ITP occurs in all age groups, with a maximum incidence in the preschool group. About half the number of cases are preceded by a febrile upper respiratory tract infection. In most younger patients the disease runs a benign, self-limited course, and most children experience a spontaneous remission within a period of 6 weeks to 4 months.

Children 10 years of age or over may have a more serious chronic type of ITP. In this age group girls are affected more frequently than boys, and the condition is likely to be associated with bleeding and the presence of an antiplatelet factor in the plasma. Steroids have been employed to help prevent bleeding and to suppress the synthesis of antiplatelet antibodies, but their use is not curative. Platelet transfusions have been given to control active bleeding, although platelet survival is short. Recently large doses of intravenous immune globulin have been shown to increase platelet survival and increase platelet counts to safe levels. When all treatments have failed and spontaneous recovery has not occurred within a year, splenectomy has been followed by a sustained restoration of platelet numbers in many cases.

During the acute phase, activity should be restricted and the child protected from the risk of increased injury. Children with very low platelet counts should be kept in bed if possible. Salicylates and other drugs that foster bleeding should be avoided because they may alter platelet function and trigger spontaneous hemorrhage. Other

Table 32-4 Life expectancy of the child with leukemia

Year	Treatment	Survival in months
Acute lymphoblastic		
1937-1953	Supportive	3-5
1954-1962	Prednisone, 6-mercaptopurine, methotrexate	12
1963-1965	Prednisone, 6-mercaptopurine, vincristine, methotrexate, cyclophosphamide	24
1966-1968	Same drugs used in combination	33+
1969-1990	Total therapy	60+ (5 years +)
	Prednisone, vincristine, 6-mercaptopurine, methrotrexate, cyclophosphamide, L-asparaginase, cytarabine (Cytosar)	
	Central nervous system prophylaxis	
Acute myelogenous		
1990	Daunomycin, thioguanine, vincristine, cytosine, arabinoside, prednisone, cyclophosphamide	12-36+*

*Improved chemotherapy protocols and bone marrow transplantation offer hope for cure in 30% to 50% of children with acute myelogenous leukemia.

nursing measures include careful observation of the progress of skin lesions and alertness for any signs of internal bleeding. A major complication, and the most serious risk to the child in the early course of the condition, is intracranial hemorrhage.

School-age child

Rheumatic fever (Fig. 32-17). Rheumatic fever is a disorder usually of childhood that can involve various organs of the body. However, because its most important complication is extensive cardiac damage, it is discussed here. Although rheumatic fever has dramatically decreased in incidence in the United States, it is still a recognized cause of acquired heart disease.

The mechanism of the disease is not completely known, but it is fairly certain that it is the result of abnormal immune response to a recent infection by group A beta-hemolytic streptococcus. This same organism causes the so-called strep throat, erysipelas, and scarlet fever. However, rheumatic fever itself is not communicable. It is not understood why some people develop rheumatic fever after group A beta-hemolytic streptococcus infections, whereas others do not. Rheumatic fever is most commonly found in the school-age child.

Signs and symptoms. The symptoms of rheumatic fever vary. However, a patient must exhibit certain minimal signs and symptoms for the diagnosis to be established (see Jones criteria in box below). The onset of the condition usually occurs about 2 weeks after the streptococcal infection. At times the infection is unapparent. The child may complain of leg aches and joint tenderness, which migrates from joint to joint—one time involving a knee, next an ankle, later a wrist (polyarthralgia). These pains occur during the day as well as the night. When the child begins to have migratory, hot, swollen, tender enlarged joints (polyarthritis), the diagnosis is quickly suggested. The child may fatigue easily and have a fever. The extent of the fever varies considerably, depending on the severity of the disease. He may also report abdominal pain, believed to be caused by lymph node enlargement. Epistaxis (nosebleed) may occur.

Carditis, or inflammation of the heart, occurs in about 40% to 50% of cases during the initial attack of rheumatic fever. Constant observation for rapid or irregular pulse, heart murmurs, increased heart size, and signs and symptoms of cardiac failure must be carried out. Carditis is the most important feature of rheumatic fever with the prognosis of the patient largely resting on the severity of this complication. One reason is that over an extended period of time, small inflammatory nodules or growths can form in the heart. Often they interfere with the action of the mitral or aortic valves, making it difficult for the valves to close properly or open sufficiently.

A sign that occasionally accompanies rheumatic fever is the development of painless *subcutaneous nodules* near the occiput, knuckles, knees, elbows, and spine. These

Jones criteria (revised) for guidance in the diagnosis of rheumatic fever*

Major manifestations

Carditis
Polyarthritis
Chorea
Erythema marginatum
Subcutaneous nodules

Minor manifestations

Clinical
   Previous rheumatic fever or rheumatic heart disease
   Arthralgia   Fever
Laboratory
   Acute phase reactions:
      erythrocyte sedimentation yrate
      C-reactive protein, leukocytosis
Prolonged P-R interval

Supporting evidence of streptococcal infection

Increased titer of streptococcal antibodies
   ASO (antistreptolysin O)
   Other antibodies
Positive throat culture for Group A streptococcus
Recent scarlet fever

*The presence of two major criteria, or of one major and two minor criteria, indicates a high probability of the presence of rheumatic fever. Evidence of a preceding streptococcal infection greatly strengthens the possibility of acute rheumatic fever. Its absence should make the diagnosis doubtful (except in Syndenham's chorea or long-standing carditis). From Jones criteria (revised) for guidance in the diagnosis of rheumatic fever, © 1967, American Heart Association. Reprinted with permission.

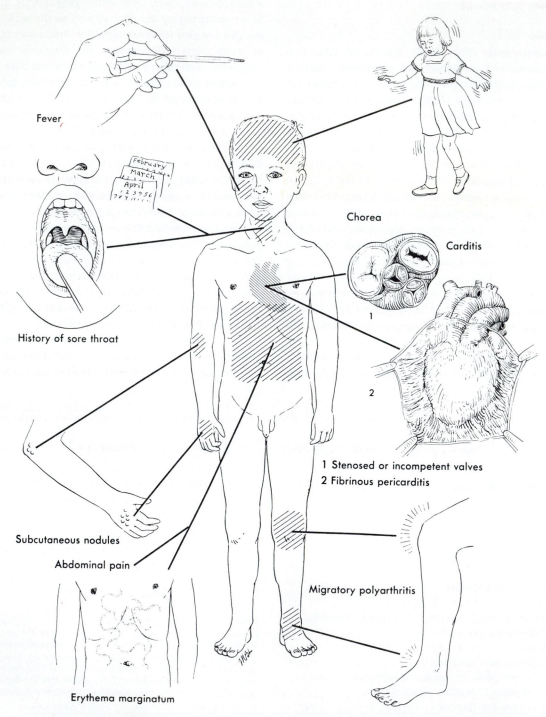

Fever

History of sore throat

Subcutaneous nodules

Abdominal pain

Erythema marginatum

Chorea

Carditis

1 Stenosed or incompetent valves
2 Fibrinous pericarditis

Migratory polyarthritis

FIG 32-17 Possible signs and symptoms of rheumatic fever.

nodules appear late in the course of the attack and are usually associated with severe carditis.

Another feature that is seen at times, especially in preadolescent girls, is Sydenham's *chorea* (known in earlier times as St. Vitus' dance). Chorea may be described as involuntary muscular twitching or movement. It sometimes manifests itself as grimacing. The child may seem exceptionally clumsy and may fail to accomplish muscle tasks involving concentration or fine control. The disorder is characterized by jerky, uncoordinated movements. It may be preceded by a period of emotional instability and behavior problems. It may be so mild as to escape the notice of the casual observer or so severe that it makes normal, daily activities dangerous or impossible. Speech may become slurred and handwriting difficult to decipher.

Still another diagnostic sign of acute rheumatic fever is the appearance of a highly distinctive rash known as *erythema marginatum*. This red-line eruption forms irregular patterns on the trunk and extremities but not on the face. However, it is rarely seen.

Diagnosis is made on the evaluation of the signs and symptoms present plus the reports of several laboratory tests. None of the laboratory tests is specific for rheumatic fever, but when made in conjunction with a clinical evaluation of the patient, they are valuable aids. An increased *blood sedimentation rate* and presence of *C-reactive protein* in the blood indicate the presence of an inflammatory process in the body that may be rheumatic fever. It is also possible to detect, with tests such as the *antistreptolysin O titer,* the presence of antibodies in the blood, formed in response to the invasion of streptococci. Sometimes a nose or throat culture returns a positive result for strep. Members of the patient's family should be checked for the presence of a streptococcal infection or the carrier state. Rheumatic fever, because of factors not yet completely determined, has a tendency to run in families.

Treatment. Treatment of rheumatic fever includes the administration of penicillin to eliminate any lingering residual streptococci and prevent a reinfection. Penicillin does not cure the symptoms of rheumatic fever, it only helps prevent further attacks. If the patient is allergic to penicillin, erythromycin can be used to eradicate the streptococcus. Sulfonamides or penicillin are equally useful in preventing reinfections. Aspirin is helpful in controlling the pain of arthritis and lowering the temperature. Prednisone is sometimes used in acute cases of carditis, with the hope of decreasing the possibility of permanent heart valve damage. Prednisone is often life-saving in overwhelming inflammation involving all the structures of the heart.

Nursing care. The nursing care of the child with rheumatic fever depends on the severity of the disease and the symptoms present. When laboratory tests and clinical features indicate that the disease is active and perhaps progressive, every effort should be made to reduce the workload of the heart by providing emotional and physical rest. However, "doing nothing" is not very restful for most children, especially if they do not really feel sick. The nurse and the patient's family need a great deal of ingenuity to provide rest that is acceptable and therefore therapeutic for the child. Good observation is essential. The pulse rate is taken for a full minute to determine quality and rhythm. Often the determination of the pulse while the patient is sleeping is requested. The nurse should review the signs and symptoms of rheumatic fever and check her charge for indications of them. Possible signs of cardiac failure are extremely important to report (p. 724). Careful positioning and skin care are necessary.

The child with symptoms of chorea needs special supportive care; careful explanation of the condition to the patient is a necessity. Chorea may appear as the sole symptom of rheumatic disease. In the event of moderate to severe disability, rest, prolonged warm baths under supervision, and tranquilizers can help. Patient nursing care is a must. The condition usually subsides spontaneously in 2 to 3 months.

When the signs of inflammatory activity subside, the electrocardiogram results are favorable, and the pulse rate is within normal limits, the child may be allowed more freedom. However, the child must continue to be carefully evaluated to discover individual tolerance for increased exercise. Because recurrences of the disease are fairly common and the possibility of permanent heart damage increases with each attack, it is imperative that the parents understand the importance of continued medical supervision. To prevent recurrences, the patient should avoid exposure to infections and receive either daily oral—or preferably, monthly intramuscular—long-acting penicillin therapy.

• • •

The lungs, heart, blood vessels, and blood are separate anatomic entities. However, if one of these is disturbed, the others invariably respond to meet the physiologic needs. The nurse who recognizes this interdependence is better able to serve the patient with the deformed heart, inflamed respiratory tract, or abnormal blood.

===== Key Concepts =====

1. Respiratory disorders in infants include bronchiolitis, pneumonia, and cystic fibrosis.

2. Pneumonia, whether primary or secondary, is a severe disease. In pediatrics it is most commonly seen in infants and young children; and it is a major cause of death in the 10- to 14-year age group.

3. Cystic fibrosis is a hereditary, multisystem disorder in which generalized dysfunction of the exocrine glands occurs. It is usually characterized by chronic, severe pulmonary disease, pancreatic insufficiency, and abnormally high concentrations of NaCl in the sweat. Treatment is directed toward the organs involved and designed to meet the needs of the individual patient. Good nutrition has a positive effect on the overall prognosis.

4. Respiratory disorders in the toddler include croup, foreign bodies in the nose or throat, and bronchitis.

5. Laryngotracheobronchitis (croup) is a viral respiratory disease characterized by a sudden onset of inspiratory stridor, hoarseness, and a barklike cough following a 1- to 3-day history of a "cold."

6. Respiratory disorders in the preschool child include epiglottitis, epistaxis, deviation of the septum, acute nasopharyngitis, sinusitis, and otitis media.

7. Symptoms of acute nasopharyngitis (common cold) are a dry, scratchy, sore, inflamed pharynx, an inflamed nasal mucosa resulting in nasal discharge, headache, muscular pains, general malaise, and fever. Supportive treatment consists in rest, increased fluid intake, a bland, soft diet, and relief of nasal obstruction.

8. Acute otitis media is a common complication of upper respiratory infection in young children. Symptoms include severe ear pain, fever, and irritability. Early administration of antibiotics is usually effective in preventing complications.

9. Respiratory disorders in the school-age child include problems with the adenoids and tonsils, streptococcal pharyngitis (strep throat), and respiratory disease resulting from allergy.

10. Postoperative nursing care of the T and A patient includes the following: position child on his side, check pulse and respirations, assess level of consciousness, observe skin for color and moisture, and carefully evaluate the type and amount of oronasal drainage.

11. Only through analysis of a throat culture can strep throat be diagnosed, because its symptoms are often the same as those seen with viral infections. Diagnosis is important because rheumatic fever, heart disease, and glomerulonephritis follow untreated streptococcal infections in a significant number of children.

12. Allergies may be treated by separating the patient from the allergen, immunizing the patient by the process of desensitization, or administering medications to relieve symptoms.

13. Asthma is the result of hyperreactivity of the bronchial airway. Although the spasm, edema, and mucus that create this reversible obstruction are often caused by an allergic reaction, nonimmunologic precipitants can also initiate or compound the problem. The treatment of asthma includes specific measures to eliminate allergens or desensitize the patient and nonspecific measures to relieve symptoms.

14. Treatment of acute attacks of asthma usually is injection of epinephrine followed by inhalation therapy with albuterol. Status asthmaticus exists when this therapy does not improve respiration. This potentially life-threatening condition requires aggressive treatment, and the patient will need to be hospitalized.

15. Diagnostic procedures to evaluate heart function and detect cardiac abnormalities are noninvasive tests, such as electrocardiography and echocardiography, laboratory tests such as a complete blood cell count and hematocrit and hemoglobin determinations, and special procedures such as angiography, angiocardiography, and cardiac catheterization. Children returning to the nursing unit after cardiac catheterization should be treated as postoperative patients.

16. Signs and symptoms commonly seen in infants with serious congenital heart disease are cyanosis, tachypnea, tachycardia, effort intolerance, failure to thrive, and heart murmurs.

17. Common congenital defects of the heart and great vessels include patent ductus arteriosus, coarctation of the aorta, tetralogy of Fallot, atrial septal defect, and ventricular septal defect.

18. A patient with a congenital heart defect may undergo surgery as an infant, toddler, or child. Preparation of these patients is particularly important because of the seriousness of the surgery and the many procedures that must be performed.

19. Complications that may develop in patients with congenital heart defects before, during, or after surgery

include congestive heart failure (CHF), subacute bacterial endocarditis, and cerebral thrombosis.

20. Anemia is a condition in which the total hemoglobin content of the blood is abnormally reduced. The most common cause of anemia in children is iron deficiency. Symptoms include pallor, irritability, anorexia, and listlessness. The primary cause is insufficient dietary intake of iron. Treatment consists in oral administration of iron preparations and increased dietary intake of iron-rich foods.

21. The sickling abnormality is attributed to a gene responsible for the synthesis of an abnormal type of hemoglobin. Children with this abnormality may experience hemolytic anemia, vasoocclusive crisis, sequestration crisis, aplastic crisis, and infections.

22. The nursing care of all patients with hemophilia is similar except that the type of intravenous therapy differs, depending on the kind of replacement needed. Prevention of bleeding is the primary goal.

23. Signs and symptoms of leukemia may be slow and insidious in onset or develop rapidly. They include fatigue and weakness, weight loss, pallor, easy bruising, and fever with a persistent respiratory tract infection. Current treatment consists in intermittent administration of high doses of several medications in combination.

24. Supportive care of the child with leukemia includes detection and treatment of infection, control of nausea and vomiting, careful positioning, gentle oral hygiene, fever reduction, and emotional support of both the child and family.

25. Currently 60% of children with acute lymphoblastic leukemia (ALL) who receive optimum treatment experience uninterrupted remission for at least 5 years. About 90% of these children will remain in remission indefinitely.

26. Signs and symptoms of rheumatic fever vary and usually occur about 2 weeks after a streptococcal infection. Treatment includes the administration of penicillin, aspirin, and sometimes prednisone. Nursing care depends on the severity of the disease and the symptoms present. Emotional and physical rest are essential while the disease is active or progressive.

Discussion Questions

1. What are the most common respiratory infections seen in infants and children? What symptoms are commonly seen with respiratory tract infections? What nursing interventions aid in the treatment of respiratory infections?

2. Why is the name mucoviscidosis very descriptive of the disease process seen with cystic fibrosis? Which body systems are involved in the disease process? What forms of therapy would you expect to use to assist children afflicted with CF? What is the prognosis for children afflicted with this disease? What can the nurse do to provide physical and emotional support to the child and the family?

3. Explain what is meant by an "allergy." How are specific allergies identified? What types of treatment are available to persons with allergies? What is the nurse's role in care of persons with allergies? How are allergies significant in the administration of food and medication?

4. What is asthma? What is the relationship of asthma to allergies? Why is asthma very frightening to the child experiencing an attack? How does caring for an asthmatic child affect the parents? What is the typical treatment for an acute asthmatic attack? Why is status asthmaticus a life-threatening condition? What are the nursing implications when providing care to an asthmatic child?

5. The fetal circulatory system differs from the postnatal circulatory system. Identify each of the circulatory changes that normally occur. Which abnormal condition occurs if each of these changes fails to happen? What symptoms are observed in each of these conditions? What nursing interventions are particularly important in caring for a child with cardiac conditions?

6. List three types of anemia observed in children. What is the most common cause of anemia in children? How does sickle cell anemia differ from other forms of anemia? Why is sickle cell disease a serious problem for the affected child?

7. Discuss the genetic nature of sickle cell anemia and hemophilia. What precautions must be taken when providing nursing care to children with these conditions? What special safety needs do these patients have?

8. What are the signs and symptoms of leukemia? How is it diagnosed? What treatments are currently used? What is the prognosis for children with leukemia? Discuss a nursing plan for a 4-year-old boy whose family has just learned of his diagnosis of acute lymphoblastic leukemia.

33

Conditions Involving Digestion and Associated Metabolism

CHAPTER OBJECTIVES

After studying this chapter, the student should be able to perform the following:

1 Indicate the agent that causes thrush, two ways that the problem may be acquired by an infant, and the usual treatment.

2 Describe the anatomic problem called pyloric stenosis; identify two possible signs of the condition and three important postoperative nursing considerations.

3 Discuss infant colic, including four possible causes and methods of treating this symptom.

4 Explain why *oral* intake is characteristically reduced and why hospitalization can be needed when an infant or young child is experiencing significant diarrhea.

5 Cite four nursing considerations included in the care of a child hospitalized for diarrhea.

6 Trace the life cycle of the pinworm; indicate how an infestation is diagnosed and what treatments and health education might be recommended.

7 Discuss the origin of umbilical hernia and possible indications for surgery when the condition persists beyond infancy.

8 Define the following pediatric digestive problems: Meckel's diverticulum, meconium ileus, intussusception, congenital megacolon.

9 Describe how to construct a Stile's dressing and why it is used.

10 Identify the basic endocrine problem faced by insulin-dependent diabetic patients (IDDM-1) and describe the signs and symptoms that are characteristically shown by such patients before treatment.

11 List four possible precipitating factors of diabetic ketoacidosis and four possible causes of insulin-induced hypoglycemia.

12 State the emergency procedure to follow when a patient shows signs of a hypoglycemic reaction and describe the administration of glucagon.

13 Describe how to prepare two different types of insulin in the same syringe for administration as ordered and tell why it is necessary always to proceed in the same way.

14 Outline the daily nutritional requirements for a 7-year-old boy with insulin-dependent diabetes who weighs 50 pounds. Discuss needed calories, daily percentage of required carbohydrate, fat, and protein, and possible caloric distribution during the day.

15 Explain the Somogyi phenomenon and its treatment.

A smoothly functioning digestive system can be a source of great pleasure. The digestive system can also initiate considerable distress, depending on its general condition and the amount of dietary discretion the person employs. This chapter briefly presents the malformations, infestations, infections, and foreign bodies commonly found in the digestive tracts of children (Fig. 33-1). Also, although it is not considered primarily a digestive problem, a review of diabetes mellitus is included because it influences the metabolism of digested glucose and because dietary regulation is required. For the convenience of nursing teachers and students, most of the material is presented according to the age group primarily affected.

ANATOMY AND PHYSIOLOGY

The digestive system is formed by the mouth, esophagus, gastrointestinal tract, and related organs, such as the liver, gallbladder, and pancreas. The adult alimentary canal is an unsterile tract of many shapes and turns that, if stretched out for its entire length, reaches about 30 feet. Although in children the size of the alimentary canal is greatly abbreviated, its importance is not. Hunger is a primary drive, and appetite, its educated twin, is soon acquired. Children may not know all about their digestive tracts, but they know that hunger represents a real need. Parents often rather despairingly speak of the "bottomless pit." The digestive tract and its accessory organs reduce foodstuffs (carbohydrates, proteins, and fats) to their smallest working chemical units. These chemical units are then absorbed through the mucous membrane of the intestinal walls and eventually reach the bloodstream to be distributed to the individual cells, providing the body with building materials, heat, and energy. To accomplish this, the digestive system works on food both *mechanically* (through the action of the teeth, tongue, cheeks, and muscular contractions of the tract, called *peristalsis*) and *chemically* (through the activity of various enzymes, emulsifiers, acids, and bacteria, which are normally active in different portions of the tract). The student is invited to review Chapter 18 if more details of the digestive process are desired. Substances not absorbed into the rest of the body by way of the bloodstream or lymphatic system are removed normally by periodic defecation, or bowel movement.

Disorders of the digestive system reveal themselves in several predictable ways. Anorexia, nausea, vomiting, constipation, abdominal distention and pain, diarrhea, and weight loss are common manifestations. The observation of a child's stool is of great importance in pediatrics. The amount, color, consistency, general appearance, and odor of a child's bowel movements can be of real diagnostic significance and aid in evaluating the condition of the digestive tract.

KEY VOCABULARY

An understanding of the following terms is necessary for a discussion of the digestive system and its disorders.

digestion Process by which food is broken down mechanically and chemically in the gastrointestinal tract and converted into absorbable forms.
endocrine gland Structure producing a hormone that is discharged into the bloodstream.
exocrine gland Structure that produces a secretion deposited in a particular area of the body via a duct.
glycosuria Presence of glucose in the urine.
hyperglycemia Excess of glucose in the blood.
hypoglycemia Deficiency of glucose in the blood.
ileus Obstruction or paralysis of the small intestine.
metabolism All energy and material transformations that occur within living cells.

DIGESTIVE AND METABOLIC PROBLEMS
Infant

For a discussion of cleft lip, cleft palate, and esophageal atresia with tracheoesophageal fistula see Chapter 14.

Oral moniliasis. Thrush, or oral moniliasis, mentioned earlier (p. 242) as a possible complication during the newborn period, results from contamination of the infant's oral cavity with vaginal secretion containing *Candida (Monilia) albicans* at the time of birth or, less often, from improper hygiene and feeding techniques after birth. White, curdlike plaques appear on the tongue and cheeks and adhere to the surface of the mucous membrane (Fig. 12-3). The mouth may be tender, and the desire to eat may be decreased. Thrush can be treated by nystatin (Mycostatin) oral suspension (1 ml) four times a day for 10 days. All objects that have entered the infected infant's mouth should be adequately sterilized. The condition usually responds well to therapy. Thrush is also a fairly common condition among children receiving long-term, broad-spectrum antibiotic therapy. The antibiotics destroy the normal flora of the alimentary canal and allow the ubiquitous fungus to multiply without competition. Most cases of moniliasis associated with antibiotic therapy resolve when the drug is discontinued.

Esophageal stenosis. The narrowing of a child's esophagus, esophageal stenosis, can be congenital in origin or due to incomplete development of the lumen

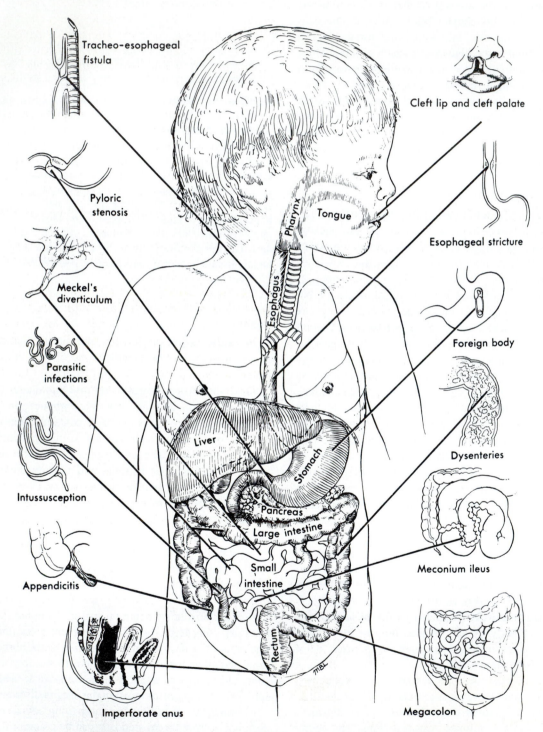

FIG 33-1   Summary of common pediatric problems involving digestive system.

(esophageal atresia). However, the condition can be acquired from prolonged peptic acid irritation, such as occurs with chronic reflux or vomiting. It can also be secondary to chemical burns from strong alkali or acid ingestion where inflammation and scar formation produces stenosis.

Patients often require periodic esophageal dilations and may need a gastrostomy, or artificial opening into the stomach, because of difficulty in maintaining nutrition. Surgical excision of the narrowed area and joining together of the remaining parts (anastomosis), replacement of the area by a bowel transplant, or esophageal reconstruction using tissue from the greater curvature of the stomach may be undertaken.

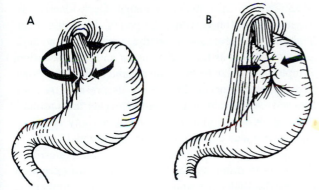

FIG 33-2 **A,** Preoperative GER. **B,** Nissen fundoplication—fundus of the stomach is wrapped around the distal end of the esophagus.

Gastroesophageal reflux. Infants and young children with gastroesophageal reflux (GER) can develop chronic bronchitis, recurrent pneumonia, bronchiectasis, atelectasis, or asthmalike symptoms as a result of the aspiration of gastric content, which is very toxic to the airways and alveoli (Fig. 33-2). The other common complications of reflux include failure to thrive due to excessive regurgitation and esophagitis with possible stricture. In most cases effective treatment is attained through a medically conservative regimen, with thickening of the formula with rice cereal, maintenance of the child in an upright position at a 30° to 40° angle, and, in some instances, administration of medications such as metoclopramide (Reglan) or bethanechol chloride (Urecholine). However, in severe or refractory cases a surgical intervention such as a Nissen fundoplication (in which a valvelike mechanism is created by wrapping the fundus of the stomach around the distal esophagus, reducing reflux) is necessary. Aspiration of gastric content can also occur in tracheoesophageal fistula and in children with spastic neurologic problems.

Congenital pyloric stenosis. Abnormal narrowing of the pyloric sphincter, which forms the exit of the stomach, can cause progressive vomiting and malnutrition in the infant (Fig. 33-3). This narrowing is caused by spasm of the sphincter, local edema, and an overgrowth of the circular muscle fibers of the pylorus. The symptoms do not usually begin until the child is approximately 2 to 3 weeks old and rarely have their onset after 2 months

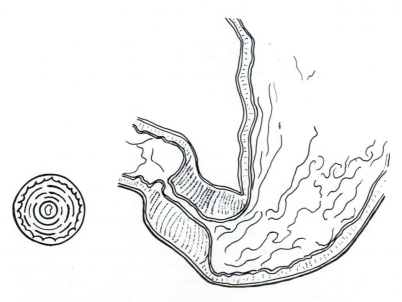

FIG 33-3 Congenital hypertrophic pyloric stenosis. Abnormal narrowing of pyloric sphincter—sagittal and cross-sectional view.

of age. This disorder seems to have a slight hereditary tendency and occurs more often in male than in female infants.

At first the vomiting is only occasional. However, if the stenosis is unrelieved, vomiting becomes more frequent, forceful, and projectile. If this situation persists, the child loses weight and begins to show signs of dehydration, electrolyte imbalance, and malnutrition. The emesis contains no bile because the opening to the duodenum is too small to allow such staining. Despite the frequent vomiting, the infant continues to have a good appetite and takes fluids when they are offered. The physician makes a diagnosis on the basis of the history, the clinical examination, x-ray studies that use a contrast medium, or ultrasound studies of the pylorus that demonstrate abnormal hypertrophy of the pylorus. A hard, olive-shaped tumor (hypertrophied pylorus) may be palpated, and visible, left-to-right peristalsis may be noted as the stomach tries to force the swallowed milk or formula into the duodenum. When this effort proves ineffective, the peristaltic waves reverse themselves, and emesis results.

In the United States, treatment of pyloric stenosis is usually surgical. A nasogastric tube is inserted before surgery to ensure that the stomach is empty and to prevent aspiration during the surgery. The procedure is called the Fredet-Ramstedt operation. The surgeon cuts down through the enlarged muscle of the pylorus to the mucous membrane, relieving the constriction. This operation, when performed on infants well prepared for the procedure, is highly successful in relieving the cause of the persistent vomiting. Postoperative care consists of observation of the surgical site or dressing and careful introduction of glucose water in small amounts at fairly frequent intervals as ordered. The infant should be held at a steep incline while being fed, burped well before, during, and after a feeding, and placed in an infant seat or propped on his right side after feedings. When the baby is in the infant seat, gravity aids the drainage of the offered fluid. Placing the infant on his right side also aids drainage and helps bubbles come to the top of the stomach, where they can be expelled with less formula loss. A side or upright position also helps prevent aspiration. After drinking, the infant should be disturbed as little as possible. It is important not to overfeed the child; this can lead to vomiting and strain on suture lines. If three or four glucose-water feedings are well tolerated, the infant is given progressive amounts of diluted formula, beginning with 30 ml. When 75 ml feedings are reached, the child is started on his usual formula or begins

monitored breast-feeding. If the feedings are retained, the infant is discharged to the care of his parents. This can be as early as the second postoperative day.

Meckel's diverticulum. A structural remnant from embryonic life is a pouch in the ileum called *Meckel's diverticulum*. During intrauterine life a duct joined the umbilicus with the intestine and led to the yolk sac, allowing temporary nourishment of the developing fetus. In the course of normal development this duct closes. However, remnants persist in a small percentage of people, and sometimes these remnants cause difficulty. An open tract, capable of discharging the contents of the small bowel onto the abdominal wall, can endure. More often a blind pouch with no connection or only a cord attachment to the umbilicus remains. Occasionally gastric mucosa is found within the pouch. Meckel's diverticulum can ulcerate and hemorrhage massively and painlessly or can act as the lead point for an intussusception. Symptoms similar to those of appendicitis or intestinal obstruction can occur. Frequently its presence is undiagnosed until exploratory surgery reveals the problem. Nursing care is similar to that involving any condition that necessitates exploration of the abdominal cavity.

Meconium ileus. Obstruction of the small intestine in the newborn infant caused by the presence of exceptionally thick, sticky meconium is called meconium ileus. The meconium is so viscous that it cannot pass normally through the bowel. Obstruction often occurs near the ileocecal junction. This condition virtually always indicates the exocrine disorder called cystic fibrosis of the pancreas, although it is not present in all cases of cystic fibrosis. Meconium ileus results because the pancreas fails to produce the enzymes that normally help liquefy the meconium. (See pp. 696-701 for discussion of cystic fibrosis.)

Symptoms are those of small bowel obstruction and include bile-stained emesis, abdominal distention, and absence of the normal meconium stool. This is a difficult pediatric problem because of the type of malfunction, the young age of the patient, and other aspects of the total disease process. In mild cases the treatment can be medical, with reliance on special enemas that help dissolve or mechanically clear the impaction and on oral administration of pancreatic enzymes. A therapeutic enema of diatrizoate meglumine (Gastrografin) is frequently a successful nonoperative method of relieving the impaction. Intravenous fluid therapy is imperative during this procedure, because diatrizoate meglumine draws fluid and serum from the intravascular compartment into the lumen of the bowel in an effort to release

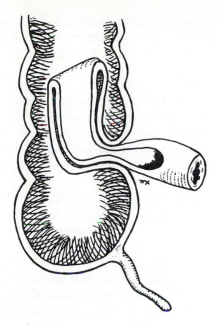

FIG 33-4 Ileocecal intussusception—telescoping of adjacent parts of bowel.

the firm bind of sticky meconium. Many cases, however, require surgery to clear the obstruction. Resection of the intestine and a temporary ileostomy may be necessary. The child is usually very ill, and the prognosis is guarded.

Intussusception. A telescoping of adjacent parts of the bowel is called intussusception (Fig. 33-4). Meckel's diverticulum or polyps can lead to intussusception. When intussusception occurs, it most frequently involves the area of the ileocecal valve. Such an abnormal relationship of parts of the intestine can disturb circulation to the involved portions and result in gangrene, perforation, and obstruction of the bowel. This condition most often affects infants and toddlers. The onset is usually sudden. At first the child may draw up the legs and cry out intermittently. Later the discomfort is intensified by progressive vomiting of bile-stained and even fecal emesis. Stools, at first loose, become scanty and characteristically assume a color and consistency of currant jelly because they are formed at this time largely of mucus and blood. If the condition is unrelieved, the child rapidly becomes prostrate. A high temperature develops, and the child's life is endangered. A favorable prognosis depends on early detection and treatment of the condition.

Diagnosis is made by considering the history, physical examination, and plain survey films of the abdomen. Treatment of choice in all cases, except those in which peritonitis or frank intestinal obstruction is suspected, is the barium enema. The pressure of the inflowing enema

can reduce an intussusception. In some cases reduction comes only after raising the height of the barium or by giving repeated enemas after each evacuation. A small number of intussusceptions recur after primary barium enema treatment. When surgery is indicated, the intussusception is identified and usually "milked" gently backward until the telescoping is completely relieved. Resection of the damaged segment of intestine is necessary in other cases.

Congenital megacolon (Hirschsprung's disease or aganglionic megacolon). Classic congenital megacolon, or Hirschsprung's disease, is characterized by lack of normal peristaltic activity in the distal segment of the colon, usually the sigmoid, because of improper *innervation* (lack of the necessary nerve ganglia in the musculature of the affected bowel or lack of coordination between the parasympathetic and sympathetic divisions of the nervous system). It is seen more often in males than in females. Signs and symptoms of congenital megacolon appear early in infancy. Failure to pass a meconium stool within 24 hours in a term newborn should arouse suspicion. Constipation (sometimes interrupted by small amounts of stool), progressive abdominal distention (which may be sufficiently severe to cause respiratory embarrassment), anorexia, and occasional vomiting all may suggest the diagnosis. Pronounced abdominal distention can grossly distort the appearance of the child. Diagnosis is made after a review of the patient's history, palpation and auscultation of the abdomen, rectal examination, x-ray examination, and a rectal biopsy for microscopic examination of the tissue (mandatory for the definitive diagnosis). The biopsy is painless and is obtained surgically by securing three to four small fragments of tissue, with a suction capsule 3 to 4 cm inside the rectum. (Complications are almost unheard of with the present method of biopsy.)

Megacolon is treated surgically through resection of the aganglionic length of colon. In a small percentage of patients the entire colon can be involved, and rarely a portion of the small bowel needs inclusion in the resected intestine. The type of procedure performed depends on the age and individual needs of the child. The most satisfactory treatment appears to be an abdominoperineal removal of the abnormal section of bowel with an anastomosis of the remaining normal colon to the anal canal (Swenson's pull-through). A variation of this is the Soave procedure. Afterward, the child is fed parenterally. Gastric suction and an indwelling urinary catheter may be continued for an indefinite period. The anal sphincter may be dilated daily. The presence of bowel sounds and normal stool are eagerly awaited. At times this procedure is inadvisable, and a colostomy is performed.

More common than classic aganglionic megacolon is pseudo-Hirschsprung's disease, which has a psychogenic basis. Its onset is not in the newborn period; x-ray studies and biopsy studies are negative. Investigation of family living patterns and stresses by qualified personnel is necessary.

Colic. Although colic is often spoken of as a disease entity, it is not a disease but a symptom. In the dictionary it is defined as "acute abdominal pain." However, when parents and nurses speak of "the colic," they are usually referring to the intermittent abdominal distress in the newborn infant that is fairly common in the early months of life. Fortunately the problem does not always last 3 months, in spite of the frequent use of the phrase "3-month colic." Children and their parents seem to be troubled most in the early evening and night. Infants suddenly draw up their legs on their abdomens, clench their fists, become red in the face, and start to cry. This goes on intermittently as though they were troubled with periodic intestinal cramping. During these episodes they may pass gas by mouth or rectum.

Various explanations for the abdominal discomfort have been advanced. Probably there are multiple causes. Infants troubled with colic tend to have a low birth weight (5 to 7 pounds [2270 to 3180 g]). It may be caused basically by an immaturity of the gastrointestinal system. Most explanations of the pain experienced involve the presence of excessive gas in the digestive tract. Excessive air can result from the following:

1. Poor bottle-feeding techniques, including failure to tip the bottle sufficiently to ensure a full nipple at all times, too-rapid feeding, the use of nipples with very small holes, which necessitates considerable suction (and air swallowing) to obtain the formula, and failure to burp the infant often enough
2. Excessive use of carbohydrate in the formula, which may cause increased fermentation and gas formation
3. A tense, nervous infant fostered by a tense, nervous mother

Attempts to remedy colic consider these possible causes. Various types of bottles and nipples are marketed as anticolic devices, some of which merit a try if the infant does not respond to other techniques. Different units using presterilized plastic-bag bottles are available. The physician may recommend a change in formula. Antispasmodics, tranquilizers, or phenobarbital are not generally effective and rarely prescribed. The explanation for etiology and improvement is not understood. It should be remembered that true colic is self-limited and eventually clears in all infants; therefore reassurance is an essential part of treatment.

In rare instances an infant requires hospitalization because of colic. When the nurse cares for colicky infants, the importance of proper feeding techniques is readily apparent. A child who is not well burped usually eats poorly and is more susceptible to regurgitation, vomiting, and colic.

Diarrheas. Any diarrheal disease causing profuse fluid loss is a particular threat to the very young person, the very old person, or the debilitated person, regardless of the initial cause of the diarrhea. Subsequent dehydration and electrolyte imbalance is a significant danger. Fortunately, with the improvement in community sanitation and hygiene, the increased availability of refrigeration, and the adoption of the disinfection techniques used in infant formula preparation, infectious types of diarrheas are currently not as common in the United States as they were in the past.

The infant who becomes dehydrated because of diarrhea or diarrhea and vomiting is admitted to the hospital. The infant should be weighed and a stool culture obtained immediately.

Diarrheal disease of early childhood is a syndrome, the course of which varies with age, severity, nutritional status, and cause. Some of the common causes of diarrhea include infection, anatomic abnormalities, malabsorption syndromes, and disease outside the gastrointestinal tract. Most acute diarrheas appear to have a viral cause and frequently accompany acute upper respiratory tract infections. Bacterial causes of infectious diarrheas most often include staphylococci, pathogenic *Escherichia coli*, *Shigella*, *Salmonella*, *Yersinia*, and *Campylobacter*. An increasingly common cause of diarrhea in toddlers and preschoolers is the parasite, *Giardia lamblia*.

General nursing care. Whatever the cause, acute diarrheal disorders need immediate treatment. The disturbance in intestinal motility and consequent malabsorption causes dehydration and fluid and electrolyte imbalances. Usually severe diarrhea subsides when fluid and electrolyte therapy is administered intravenously and oral intake is briefly reduced. Oral intake may be briefly restricted initially to rest the gastrointestinal tract and make it less irritable. Enteric precautions (see Table 30-1) and antibiotic therapy may be indicated for treating diarrheas caused by pathogenic *E. coli* and staphylococci and for severe infections caused by *Salmonella* and *Shigella*-type organisms. (See pp. 624 and 636.) Daily calculations of the child's fluid intake and output and weight must be accurately recorded. It may be necessary to weigh the infant's diaper to assess output accurately. Because of the frequency of stools, a special medicated ointment may be prescribed for application after each cleansing of the perirectal area. Of course, the color, consistency, general appearance, and amount of the stool should be regularly noted and recorded. Taking temperatures rectally is contraindicated to prevent stimulation and to reduce trauma to the rectum.

Abdominal hernias. A hernia is an abnormal protrusion of a portion of the contents of a body cavity through a defect in its surrounding wall, commonly causing abnormal swelling or pressure. The general public calls the condition a "rupture." Common in infancy and childhood are inguinal and umbilical hernias. They are usually congenital.

Inguinal hernia. Hernia repair in the inguinal region is a common surgical procedure. Such hernias are found most often in males. They can be unilateral or bilateral and are usually on the right side when unilateral. When the testes originally descend into the scrotum from the abdominal cavity, they are surrounded by a small sac or tube of peritoneum that is continuous with the abdominal lining. Usually this sac soon closes off, making any further communication with the abdominal cavity impossible. However, occasionally the closure is incomplete or does not take place, and the intestine can slip down the open inguinal canal, causing a swelling in the area.

This prolapse of the intestine is not important in itself. However, a possibility exists that the misplaced loop of intestine can become trapped (incarcerated) in the inguinal canal or scrotum, and the circulation to the trapped segment can become impaired (strangulated), causing intestinal obstruction and gangrene of the bowel. Early clinical signs are vomiting and colicky abdominal pain.

Inguinal hernia also develops in girls. The anatomy is different but parallel. The inguinal canals, which are occupied by the round ligaments, can allow loops of intestine to enter the area of the groin. Only 10% of inguinal hernias involve females.

To prevent incarceration, all inguinal hernias should be corrected soon after diagnosis. In infants and small children up to 2 years of age, the hernia is repaired in a simple procedure (herniotomy). In older children a slightly more complex procedure is used. A surgical incision is made in a natural skin crease where the scar will not be seen. The hernia sac is carefully tied off. For boys an abnormal collection of fluid may be found in the scrotal area surrounding the testes (hydrocele). This fluid is aspirated, and the abnormal peritoneal sac is excised. The child usually tolerates the entire procedure very well, and in most cases minimal postoperative analgesia is required. A protective spray dressing is applied over the new incision. This allows direct observation of the area.

Diapers are usually not applied in a routine fashion until 24 hours after surgery. One approach to the diaper problem is the use of Stile's dressing (Fig. 33-5). A small bed cradle is placed over the legs of the infant. The diaper is brought upward between the legs and fas-

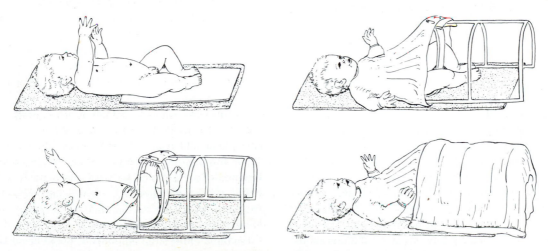

FIG 33-5 Steps in constructing Stile's dressing. Be sure that gown is pulled tightly when attached to cradle. At times cradle must be tied to crib.

tened to the frame of the cradle. A long infant gown, securely tied in back, is drawn tightly up over the frame and also fastened with pins. The cradle is then draped with a small blanket.

Hospitalization for inguinal hernia repair is not always necessary. A simple hernia repair can be done as an outpatient procedure. Parents are instructed to bring the child to the hospital in a fasting state about 1 hour before the scheduled procedure. The parents remain until the child is taken to the operating room and are present when the child awakes. In 2 to 3 hours and when able to take fluids, the child may be discharged from the hospital. Parents should be reminded to return in 4 days to have the sutures removed from the infant's incision. Older children's sutures are removed on the sixth postoperative day.

Umbilical hernias. Umbilical hernias in infancy are thought to be caused by severe localized abdominal stress brought about by crying, coughing, and vomiting. Umbilical hernias often close spontaneously when the child learns to stand and walk and the abdominal muscles are strengthened through use. However, umbilical defects greater than 1.5 cm in diameter in children seldom close spontaneously. (Umbilical hernias are particularly common in black children.) If an umbilical hernia is not closed during childhood the defect often becomes more serious in pregnant women, and the multiparous woman is subject to the dangerous threat of incarceration. To prevent this serious problem in adulthood, a more aggressive approach is urged. Prophylactic umbilical hernia repair is recommended for all girls over 2 years and all boys over 4 years of age.

Imperforate anus. The problem of imperforate anus has already been mentioned in Chapter 14. Fig. 14-15 depicts the common types of the malformation encountered. Usually surgery for correction must be performed very early to prevent complications and ensure a better possibility of success. If a male newborn infant has a rectourethral fistula, surgery must be prompt to prevent the development of serious ascending urinary tract infection. For infant girls with an associated posterior vaginal anus, corrective surgery can be delayed until the child is 4 to 6 months of age.

Whether an abdominal or perineal surgical approach is necessary depends on the type of defect and the distance of the terminal end of the colon from the perineum. A temporary colostomy may be necessary. After creation or repair of the anorectal area, frequent dilation of the canal may be ordered.

Galactosemia. One metabolic defect that has dietary significance and has received considerable attention in the literature recently is *galactosemia*. If this congenital error in the metabolism of the sugar galactose is untreated, it may cause physical and mental retardation, cataracts, enlargement of the liver and spleen, and cirrhosis. The body is unable to change galactose to glucose, a chemical reaction that normally takes place primarily in the liver. An enzyme needed to accomplish the task is deficient or missing. Galactose builds up in the bloodstream and spills over into the urine, where it is identified by appropriate tests.

Early signs of galactosemia in the infant are vomiting, listlessness, and failure to thrive. These signs are not apparent until at least 1 or 2 weeks after birth. Since galactose is present in milk sugar, it is important that the defect be diagnosed early and that a milk substitute such as Nutramigen or a meat-base formula be used. Like those of children with phenylketonuria (PKU), the diets of galactosemia patients must be closely supervised to prevent the ingestion of the offending food. Also, like the young patient with PKU, the child with galactosemia may be able to expand dietary horizons gradually after a period of several years on a rigid, restricted regimen.

Toddler and preschool child

Foreign body ingestion. Children do not limit their experimental tasting and swallowing to articles that are meant to tempt an appetite or even to digestible items. All kinds of objects have gone down the "little red lane." Fortunately most complete the entire journey without incident if they make it through the esophagus into the stomach. Most objects pass in 4 to 7 days but are allowed 2 to 3 weeks if no symptoms such as pain or blood in the stools are present. Objects hanging up in the esophagus should be treated as a medical emergency and promptly removed.

One can carefully examine the stool for small round objects that have been ingested. However, sharp or long pointed objects can pose the threat of perforation. If the object is detectable by x-ray examination, it is viewed and periodically watched. If trauma to the tissue seems likely, an operation to retrieve it may be necessary. The abdomen of a child who has swallowed a foreign object should not be palpated. One physician even suggests placing a small sign on the child, cautioning would-be investigators to avoid such maneuvers.

Giving a child large amounts of bread or potato after ingestion of a foreign object is of doubtful value. A

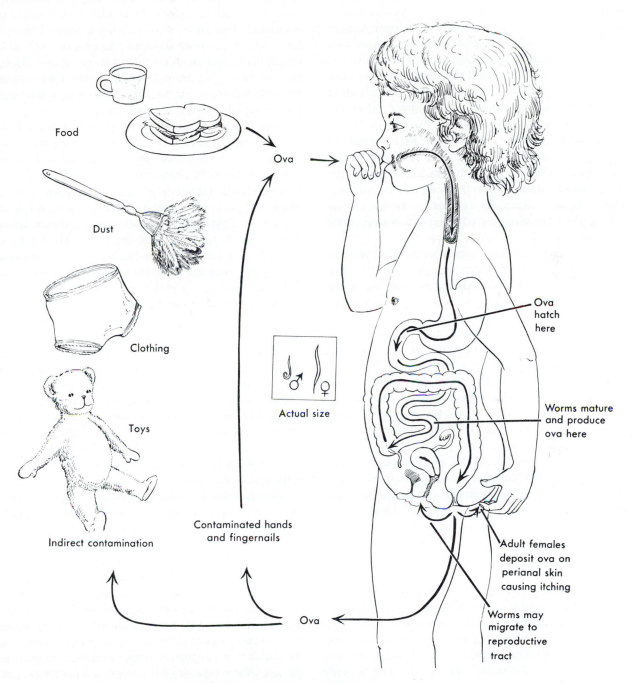

Food

Dust

Clothing

Toys

Indirect contamination

Contaminated hands and fingernails

Ova

Ova

Actual size

Ova

Ova hatch here

Worms mature and produce ova here

Adult females deposit ova on perianal skin causing itching

Worms may migrate to reproductive tract

FIG 33-6 Life cycle of pinworm *(Enterobius vermicularis).*

laxative should never be given in such circumstances.

Parasitic infestations. All bacteria are parasites; however when one speaks of *parasitic infestations,* one is usually referring to organisms that are multicellular in their adult form and large enough to be seen with the naked eye. Many kinds of parasites in this category trouble human beings. Many of them are found in abundance in tropical areas of the world and represent tremendous public health problems. This text mentions only those found fairly frequently in the United States: pinworms, roundworms, and *Giardia.*

Oxyuriasis (pinworm, threadworm, or seat-worm infestation). Although the official name of the pinworm is *Enterobius vermicularis,* the name of the disease this small, white, threadlike worm causes is known as oxyuriasis, or enterobiasis, an extremely common infestation. It does not always produce symptoms and often goes undiagnosed.

The pinworm eggs are ingested or possibly inhaled. Most often children introduce the eggs into their own mouths by their contaminated fingers. Fingers become contaminated by touching objects used by affected children who have not carried out proper toilet hygiene. When the infestation becomes established, children can easily reinfect themselves. The eggs are swallowed and hatch in the intestine. They mature in and near the cecum. When the adult female worms are ready to lay their eggs, they migrate down the intestinal tract to the anus. During the night the female worms leave the anus and lay their eggs in the folds of the anal sphincter and the perineum. Occasionally the worms migrate to the vagina and cause a vaginitis in a little girl. All this activity usually causes considerable local irritation and itching. The child usually scratches the area, contaminating the fingers with the eggs laid in the region. In the course of time, fingers travel to the mouth again, and the cycle repeats (Fig. 33-6). The interval between the ingestion of an egg and the appearance of the female pinworm at the anus is approximately 6 to 8 weeks.

Usually mild pinworm infestations cause few symptoms other than anal itching and secondary complications caused by scratching. However, sometimes pinworms cause sleep disturbances, restlessness, irritability, and occasionally secondary vaginal or periurethral irritation from scratching. Abdominal pain and grinding of teeth is not a part of the typical clinical picture, despite lay opinion to the contrary. With large infestations inflammation of the appendix rarely occurs.

Diagnosis is made if small worms are seen around the anus 1 to 2 hours after the child is asleep, if they are expelled on the surface of a stool, or if eggs are detected microscopically. Since the female lays her eggs in the skin folds outside the body of the child, ova are rarely found in the stool. Usually a so-called Scotch tape test is ordered. The nurse or parent takes a piece of Scotch tape, which has been fastened "sticky side out" to a tongue blade, and presses it against the rectal area. Some microscopic eggs adhere to the tape. The tape is then carefully secured to a glass slide "sticky side down" and sent to the laboratory for examination.

In the past when a child was affected, the entire family was treated. Currently, only the family members who have symptoms are treated, and a more pleasant form of therapy is available. Mebendazole (Vermox), a single-dose, chewable tablet for all ages, is effective in most cases, or pyrvinium pamoate (Povan) can be given in one or two doses. The nurse and parents should know that pyrvinium pamoate colors the stools red, and if the child has an emesis while the medication is still present in the gastrointestinal tract, the emesis may also be reddish.

Other measures must be followed to help ensure a cure. Personal toilet hygiene should be stressed. The necessity for hand washing after using the toilet is not understood by children unless it is taught. Frequent cleansing of the rectogenital area is required. The toilet seat must be cleaned often. Because of the intense itching that can occur at night, an affected child should have very short fingernails. Many children are infested without the nurse's knowledge; therefore, it is always good technique to refrain from shaking used bed linen. Instead, it should always be rolled. Waving the child's linens only helps scatter the eggs.

Ascariasis (roundworm infestation). Ascaris lumbricoides, the worm that causes ascariasis, looks like a pink or white earthworm. It is usually 6 to 15 inches long. The eggs are found in the soil or on objects contaminated by soil containing involved feces. The disease is perpetuated by poor sanitary facilities and poor hygiene practices.

The microscopic egg is swallowed and hatches in the duodenum. The small intermediate stages of the worm (larvae) pass through the wall of the intestine to penetrate the venules or lymphatics. They commonly migrate to the liver, the right side of the heart, and the lungs. The small larvae then penetrate the alveoli and ascend the bronchioles, bronchi, and trachea. On reaching the glottis they are swallowed. These same larvae develop into adult male and female forms in the small intestine. The adult male is approximately 6 to 10 inches long. The female

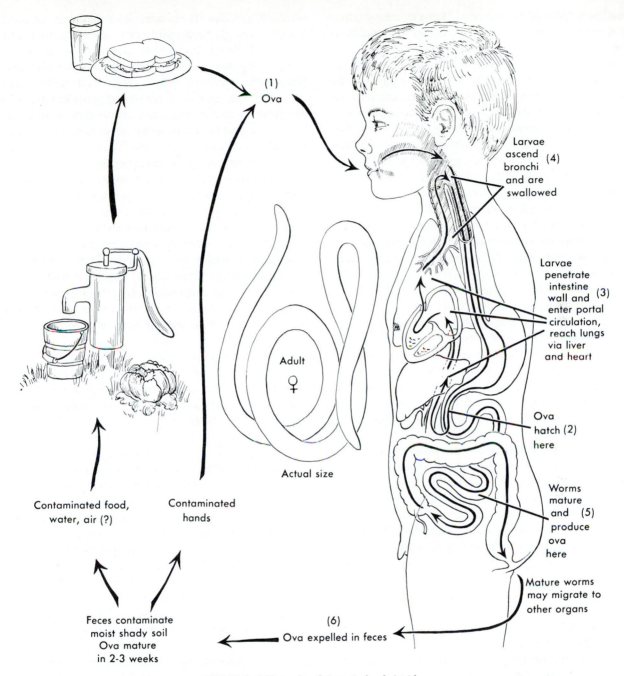

FIG 33-7 Life cycle of *Ascaris lumbricoides*.

is about 8 to 15 inches long and about the diameter of a pencil. The adult worms subsist on the semidigested food in the intestinal canal. Fertilized eggs expelled in feces must undergo a 2- to 3-week period of maturation in the soil before becoming capable of producing disease (Fig. 33-7).

This parasite, because of its migratory habits (even the adult worm can travel up and down the digestive tract, occasionally making an alarming appearance at either end), can cause a variety of symptoms if the infestation is of some intensity. The larval migrations can cause nausea and vomiting or initiate symptoms of pneumonitis or intestinal obstruction. They can even produce perforation. Allergic reactions, skin rash, nervousness, and irritability are not uncommon.

Positive diagnosis is made on the basis of finding the ova in the stool or seeing the worms emerge from the gastrointestinal tract. Treatment by piperazine citrate (Antepar) is effective for *Ascaris* infestation, provided that reinfection caused by poor hygiene practices does not occur. Mebendazole (Vermox) can also be used when ascariasis is associated with other worm species. All infected persons must be treated for successful control of the disease. Public education programs teaching general hygiene are a must. Turning infested topsoil under is also believed helpful. The prognosis is good unless secondary complications such as pneumonia, intestinal obstruction, or perforation develop. The outlook then becomes more guarded.

Giardiasis. After pinworms, *Giardia lamblia* is the most common parasite in the United States and the most common cause of chronic diarrhea in children in day care programs past the age of 2 years. It is predominantly spread by hand-to-mouth transmission, that is, poor hygiene; however, it can be spread by contaminated water or animals. The cysts are swallowed and develop in the duodenum as adult trophozoites with adherence to the intestinal mucosa. In addition to the most common presentation diarrhea, weight loss, and failure to thrive are common. Suspected cases are diagnosed by collecting three stool specimens on separate days as the eggs (cysts) are shed intermittently. If the stools are negative and the diagnosis still highly suspected, fluid from the duodenum can be obtained by way of a swallowed string test (Entero-test) or a tube aspirate of duodenal fluid. The duodenal fluid samples are 95% accurate but obviously more invasive than stool testing, which is 40% to 60% accurate in good laboratories. Treatment for children is usually metronidazole (Flagyl) for 7 to 10 days or Furoxone.

Appendicitis. Inflammation caused by local obstruction or infection of the vermiform appendix, located at the base of the cecum, is a common indication for abdominal surgery. However, appendicitis is not always easy to diagnose in young children. Other problems mimic the condition, and the young child is not often very descriptive regarding general discomfort. Pain may first be felt in the umbilical area. Later it may be localized in the lower right-hand abdominal quadrant. Restlessness, mild constipation or diarrhea, and anorexia followed by nausea and vomiting are often reported. A low grade fever is characteristic. The white blood cell count

is usually elevated. If the inflamed appendix is removed before it has ruptured, recovery is usually prompt and uneventful. However, delay or the use of laxatives can result in the rupture of the appendix. Peritonitis complicates the condition. Recovery is then slower, and the risk to the patient is multiplied considerably. The campaign to educate the public not to give laxatives or enemas to persons complaining of abdominal pain has not yet been won.

The patient with a ruptured appendix, related abscess, or peritonitis is very ill. This person usually cannot be sent to surgery immediately but must wait until the administration of antibiotics, intravenous fluids, and possible cooling measures are completed so that the patient is in the best condition possible for the appendectomy. A nasogastric tube is often passed to relieve flatus and prevent vomiting. At the time of surgery, a drain is usually placed in the abdominal wound, and drainage may be significant. A high Fowler's position is maintained to prevent the spread of infective material in the abdomen. Intravenous feedings are continued for several days postoperatively, and only ice chips or sips of water are allowed by mouth. Intake and output determinations are important. Currently, more and more of these patients are recuperating satisfactorily, and the phrase "ruptured appendix" is no longer as dreaded as it was formerly.

School-age child

Diabetes mellitus. Diabetes mellitus is the most common metabolic disorder of children. It is not a true digestive problem, since carbohydrates are reduced to glucose by the digestive system and the glucose is absorbed into the bloodstream. The difficulty arises because the islets of Langerhans in the pancreas fail to produce the hormone insulin. In the absence of sufficient insulin, utilization of glucose is impaired, and hyperglycemia with its acute and long-term manifestations results.

About 1 in 600 school-age children has a form of diabetes that requires insulin replacement throughout life. Males and females appear to be equally affected. No correlation with socioeconomic status has been found. Because varied etiologic and pathologic factors cause the different types of hyperglycemia, the term "insulin-dependent diabetes mellitus" (IDDM-1) is used most commonly to describe the disease exhibited by children and adolescents. In these patients diabetes usually begins before age 15. The young people eventually demonstrate an absolute deficiency of insulin.

Although diabetes mellitus can manifest itself any time during a person's lifetime, the earlier the disease appears, the earlier that complications of the disease are encountered. During the first year following diagnosis of IDDM-1, the islets of Langerhans hypertrophy, causing an erratic production of insulin. As the condition progresses, the islets atrophy, finally becoming entirely incapable of insulin production. This is the main difference between IDDM-1, formerly called "juvenile diabetes," and maturity-onset diabetes (IDDM-2), in which disturbed carbohydrate metabolism can be the result of many factors that together cause a relative decrease in the endogenous supply of needed insulin.

Etiologic factors. The exact cause of diabetes mellitus is not known, but inheritance plays an important role. Evidence also indicates that certain environmental factors such as toxins and viral infections may precipitate the condition in susceptible persons through autoimmune destruction of the islet cells. Therefore it can be hypothesized that a genetic predisposition to developing IDDM-1 exists and that some unknown factor or insult can occur that precipitates the condition.

Pathophysiologic factors. Insulin is important in the metabolism of carbohydrates, fats, and proteins. It is also required for efficient entry of glucose into skeletal muscle and fat cells. In insulin-dependent diabetes, glucose is unavailable for cellular metabolism. It cannot be converted to glycogen for storage in the liver and muscles nor can it be burned properly. Hyperglycemia and other compensatory symptoms occur as glucose utilization by tissue is impaired. When glucose concentration reaches approximately the level of 180 mg/100 ml, glucose spills over into the urine (glycosuria), causing diuresis to occur (polyuria). Large amounts of water and electrolytes are lost, with subsequent dehydration. This is associated with excessive thirst (polydipsia).

When the amount of glucose available is insufficient to provide fuel to meet the body's needs, protein and fats are broken down and used to help furnish these necessities. However, metabolism of fat is not complete without the concurrent metabolism of carbohydrate. This incomplete fat metabolism produces ketone bodies (acetone, diacetic acid, and oxybutyric acid) that accumulate abnormally in the blood (ketonemia). Diacetic acid and oxybutyric acid must be neutralized in the body by bases, or alkalies. As the ketones are excreted, sodium, potassium, and neutralizing bases are also lost in the urine. The body's supply of base is depleted, the sensitive electrolyte balance is upset, and metabolic acidosis gradually develops (diabetic ketoacidosis).

Signs and symptoms. The classic clinical symptoms of diabetes are polyuria, dehydration despite polydipsia, and weight loss despite polyphagia. Most children initially have a brief history of lethargy, weakness, and weight loss. Daily loss of water and glucose occur. Improper metabolism of fats and protein also occurs. Unexplained weight loss and polyuria or the resumption of nocturnal enuresis are indications for testing. Glycosuria, hyperglycemia, and ketonuria are diagnostic of insulin deficiency. No further tests are necessary to confirm the diagnosis.

Acute care. A serious complication of this disease is diabetic ketoacidosis (DKA). Severe dehydration, confusion, coma, and even death can occur unless the condition is reversed promptly by insulin and appropriate fluid replacement. DKA is truly a medical emergency requiring the close attention of a physician and a nurse at the bedside.

The goal of initial therapy is to improve circulation and then to correct the acidosis. Dehydration is often of the magnitude of 10%. An intravenous line is placed, and fluids are started immediately. Adequate insulin is administered, usually as a bolus in normal saline, followed by an infusion to provide a constant steady insulin concentration in plasma. When acidosis is corrected (serum bicarbonate of 14 mEq/L or greater), insulin infusion is discontinued, and insulin is given subcutaneously. Blood glucose levels are monitored as often as needed by means of the Dextrostix or chem-strips with or without the assistance of a glucose meter. Hypoglycemia must be prevented. When the blood sugar falls below 300 mg/dl, the intravenous fluids should contain enough glucose to keep up with the insulin. Since the urinary output is good, an acetest can be performed on a regular basis to give an indication that DKA is resolving. Intake and output are carefully plotted; vital signs—particularly the pulse—should be monitored often; and any significant change should be reported promptly.

Precipitating factors of diabetic ketoacidosis include trauma, infection, pregnancy, vomiting, or emotional stress. This life-threatening condition is relatively uncommon because of increased recognition of the classic symptoms of diabetes. However, a small number of children demonstrate repeated episodes of DKA, which can represent treatment failure or inadvertent or deliberate error by the patient in the administration of insulin.

Management during the period following control of DKA consists of establishing appropriate nutritional intake while discontinuing intravenous fluids and converting to subcutaneous insulin administration.

Insulin. One of the essentials in the management of the child with diabetes is to provide a dosage of insulin

Table 33-1   Insulins commonly used in the management of children with insulin-dependent diabetes mellitus (IDDM-1)

Type of insulin	Appearance	Onset (hours)	Peak (hours)	Duration (hours)
Rapid action—short duration				
Regular	Clear	½-1	2-4	6-8
Semilente	Cloudy	½-1	2-4	8-10
Intermediate action—longer duration				
Globin	Clear	1-2	6-8	12-14
NPH	Cloudy	1-2	6-8 +	12-14
Lente	Cloudy	1-2 +	6-12	14-16

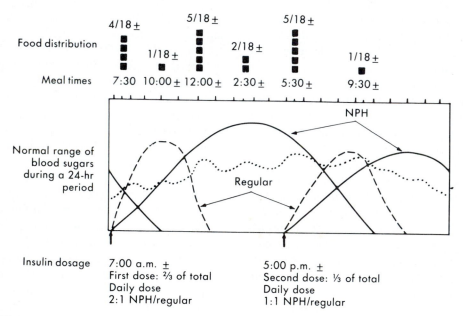

FIG 33-8   Twenty-four-hour insulin schedule using 2-dose regimen of regular and NPH insulins. *(From Guthrie RA and Guthrie DW: Nursing management of diabetes mellitus, ed 2, St Louis, 1982, The CV Mosby Co.)*

that can effectively cover a 24-hour period. Approximately five types of insulin are available that are commonly used in the management of the child with IDDM. Table 33-1 describes their activity. U-100 insulin is the standard concentration used. Special low-dose syringes are available to make doses more accurate. To maintain normal blood glucose levels, twice-a-day injections of a combination of rapid- and intermediate-acting insulins are often needed. For the prepubertal child, the total insulin dose generally does not exceed 1 unit per kg body

weight per day and is generally divided as follows: Two thirds of the dose is given before breakfast with longer-acting insulin and short-acting insulin in a 2 to 1 ratio; the predinner dose is comprised of the remaining third of the total daily dose, with the longer- and short-acting insulins in equal doses (see Fig. 33-8 for sample schedule). When both rapid-acting and intermediate-acting insulin are prescribed together, the two insulins should be drawn up in the same syringe and always in the same sequence, with the rapid-acting insulin drawn up first followed by the intermediate-acting preparation. This procedure ensures that any residual insulin in the "dead space" remains constant, and that there is greater stability of the patient after a therapeutic dose has been established.

The "honeymoon" period. During the initial presentation of IDDM-1, insulin requirements are 0.5 to 1.0 U insulin/kg/day, but after stabilization, insulin requirements decline as a result of partial recovery of the islet cells. This period (which lasts for up to 1 year) is characterized by easy control and general well-being, and is known as the "honeymoon" period. During the honeymoon period, normal blood sugar levels can usually be obtained with administration of a small daily dose of insulin.

When children are regulated in the hospital, they are often placed on regular insulin coverage in addition to the two-dose schedule. Regular insulin has a rapid but relatively brief action. The amount of insulin that patients receive depends on the level of blood sugar and the presence or absence of urinary ketones. The sites of injection should be changed each day to prevent hypertrophy of subcutaneous fat. Children should be taught to keep a record of the daily placement of their insulin. Children 7 and 8 years of age often express curiosity about the process of preparing the dosage, and some (who are more dependable and composed) are even capable of injecting themselves. Children must have considerable practice in preparing dosages with adequate supervision. They also should be taught about the actions of the different insulins to understand the relationship between regular, good dietary habits and insulin injections. Children and their parents need to know when the onset and the peak of the prescribed insulin occur, as well as its duration.

At the onset of diabetes or following recovery from ketoacidosis, the total daily dose of insulin should range between 0.5 to 1 International Units (IU) of insulin per kilogram of body weight per day. The insulin dose can be adjusted at home so that the diet and exercise can be varied. This is done by adjusting the short-acting insulin, keeping in mind anticipated exercise and food.

Exercise. An integral component of growth and development is exercise, and children with diabetes should be encouraged to participate in any activity they like, including competitive sports. However, exercise decreases insulin requirements by increasing the sensitivity of skeletal muscle to insulin. Appropriate adjustments in food intake and insulin dosage must be considered. If exercise is increased or decreased, food intake must be adjusted accordingly.

Nutritional intake. The nutritional intake of a child with diabetes should be comparable to that of the healthy nondiabetic child of the same age, sex, weight, and level of activity. Since the amount and type of insulin prescribed depends on caloric intake, regularity of caloric intake for the fixed dose of insulin becomes vital (see Fig. 33-8).

Total calories should be adjusted to meet the individual child's needs in growth, activity, and appetite, including foods of their own culture, social group, and ethnic background. Because weighing each food imposes rigidity and a burden on the child and family, the American Diabetic Association has prepared a simplified method of calculating food intake based on the concept of food

Daily nutritional requirements
This suggested guide should be modified if additional exercise is planned or if the child becomes ill

Prepubescent

65 kcal/kg
(30 kcal/lb)

Pubescent and postpubescent

35 kcal/kg
(16 kcal/lb)

Composition of calories

Should supply sufficient calories to meet the needs of exercise, growth, and appetite

Carbohydrate	50%-55%	(Avoid sucrose)
Fat	30%	(Use polyunsaturated fats)
Protein	15%-20%	

Meal plan

Caloric intake should be divided into 3 meals and 2 or 3 snacks based on the individual's life style and on the dynamics of insulin

Breakfast	4/18
Midmorning	1/18
Lunch	5/18
Midafternoon	2/18
Dinner	5/18
Bedtime	1/18

Nutritional intake should be evaluated annually to compensate for growth. Referral or consultation with the nutritionist should be made whenever necessary.

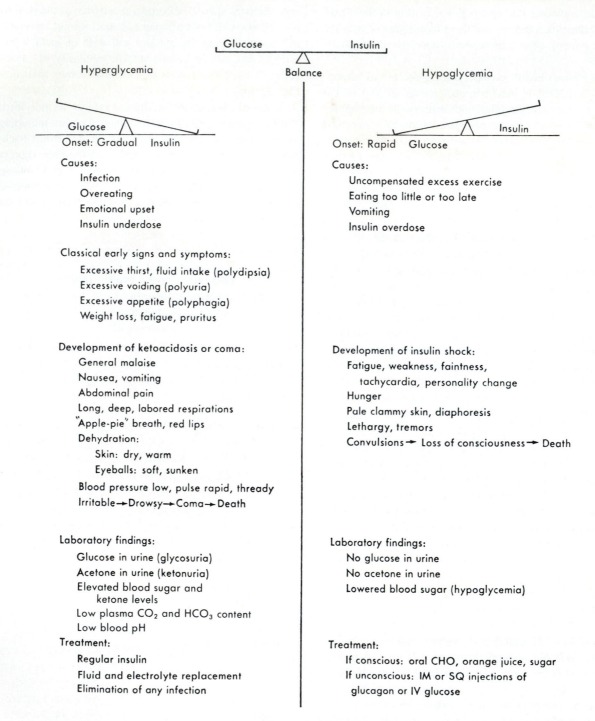

FIG 33-9   Glucose-insulin balance chart.

exchanges. Six basic exchanges are listed, and within each exchange a wide variety of foods can be substituted or exchanged. Common foods should be used that can be modified to meet the tastes and economic needs of the child and family. Emphasis should be placed on regularity of food intake and on the constancy of carbohydrate intake, avoiding simple sugars (see box on p. 757).

Insulin-food relationships. In the hospital the patient's nutritional intake is carefully measured to establish a baseline; then, using the blood glucose patterns and the child's appetite, it is modified as needed. No food or liquids should be given, with the exception of water, without a physician's authorization. The patient should be encouraged to eat all the food served on the tray on time. (Before serving a tray, the nursing staff should determine whether the child has received any ordered insulin. The type of insulin the patient receives dictates when the meal should be served.) The glucose content of any uneaten portion is calculated, and a replacement (usually a drink) that must be finished is sent to the patient. Any inability to eat or emesis should be promptly reported. The way in which the young patient is adhering to the nutritional intake should be carefully reported and recorded. Conferences in which the physician and nutritionist work along with the older child may be arranged and are often profitable. Sometimes when youngsters feel they have made some of the rules, these rules are easier to keep.

Hypoglycemia (insulin-induced hypoglycemia). Insulin itself can cause problems. Too much insulin can be more disastrous than too little. A balance between the insulin needed and the insulin available must be maintained to prevent either hyperglycemia or the other extreme, known as hypoglycemia (Fig. 33-9).

Unlike hyperglycemia, hypoglycemia can develop rapidly, within minutes or hours. The first signs of insulin-induced hypoglycemia are diaphoresis and personality change. This change can take various forms, depending on the patient; each person usually reacts in a way that is particularly characteristic for that individual. If the condition is not relieved, the patient can develop deep shock, become unconscious, and possibly experience convulsions. Intractable hypoglycemia can cause severe brain damage.

Nurses and patients should be familiar with the early signs of hypoglycemia so that it can be easily counteracted (Fig. 33-9). Children usually learn to recognize their symptoms well. All persons with diabetes should carry some rapidly available source of glucose in the event they feel the beginning of an insulin reaction. A

sugar lump followed by a small protein or fat snack is recommended. In the hospital a small glass of orange juice or crackers are usually given. If no improvement is obtained in 15 minutes, additional food should be given. If the child has difficulty taking the necessary oral glucose, an intramuscular or subcutaneous injection of glucagon is ordered. Glucagon activates liver enzymes that break down liver glycogen to produce glucose. It must be remembered that glucagon does not work in the glycogen-depleted child. However, when the hypoglycemia is caused by excess insulin, the liver glycogen stores should be generous, since such storage is enhanced by insulin. The family needs to know that glucagon should be given one time only for each episode, and that the child should be fed immediately. Glucagon is available in 1 mg vials. The typical dose is 0.5 mg (or one-half vial) for children under 1 year of age and 1 mg for older children. The intramuscular route is preferred because of more rapid absorption. It usually takes 10 to 20 minutes for glucagon to work. Sometimes intravenous administration by the physician of a 20% to 50% solution of glucose is required. If the patient has been given a slow-acting, long-duration insulin, response to therapy for hypoglycemia can be slow and treatment more complex. The physician should always be notified of the occurrence of insulin reactions. When a patient complains of symptoms of possible reaction or the nurse is suspicious that such a process is occurring, blood glucose should be evaluated immediately using one of the quick assays. At times it is difficult to determine clinically whether the complaints and appearance of the patient are caused by the lack of glucose or too much glucose in the blood. If no laboratory test is feasible, glucagon or intravenous glucose is often ordered. If the difficulty is caused by insulin reaction, the patient responds. If it is not, no real harm has been done. Hypoglycemia should be treated promptly. Prolonged, severe hypoglycemia can cause brain damage and subsequent mental deterioration, impaired motor coordination, and even death.

As can be seen from Fig. 33-9, a number of causes exist for insulin excess and resulting reactions. Probably the most common cause is uncompensated excessive exercise. Exercise causes sugar to be metabolized more effectively because of increased efficiency of insulin. Unless insulin dosage is reduced or glucose is increased, hypoglycemia is likely in the presence of unplanned exercise. Thus, it is important for the child with diabetes to have periods of regular exercise suitably spaced after meals and to recognize the possibility of short-acting insulin adjustment to compensate for special activities.

Another cause of hypoglycemia is failure to eat, to eat enough, or to space the food intake appropriately. Midmorning, midafternoon, and bedtime snacks are essential for small children but can be impractical for teenaged children, who feel odd eating a snack at school. In a hospital setting the nurse should be sure snacks are given to and are consumed by the patient. If the child is nauseated or has an emesis, this should be immediately reported because this condition can also lead to hypoglycemia. Meals must be served on time; a long delay after the injection of regular insulin also sets the stage for an episode of hypoglycemia.

Difficulties in determining appropriate doses of insulin are also a source of glucose-insulin imbalance. The patient may not respond to the dosage as expected. Errors in insulin administration resulting in an overdose are also a real possibility. Great care must be taken in reading the orders and in preparing the injection. One strength (U-100) of insulin is available in both rapid-acting and intermediate-acting insulin. When mixing the two types of insulin in the same syringe, the nurse must be sure of her technique.

1. Just enough replacement air must be injected into the bottle of cloudy (e.g., NPH) insulin without dipping the injecting needle into the insulin. The needle is then removed from the bottle.
2. The rapid-acting insulin should be withdrawn into the syringe, using the proper scale.
3. The intermediate insulin is then withdrawn into the syringe, using the proper scale.
4. An air bubble is put into the syringe and the syringe rocked back and forth to mix the two insulin types.

This technique must be followed to prevent the conversion of rapid-acting insulin into an intermediate-acting type by inadvertent injection of intermediate insulin into a vial of regular insulin.

Hyperglycemia. Hyperglycemia, the opposite body condition from hypoglycemia, occurs when the insulin available in the blood is insufficient to metabolize the glucose present.

The most frequent cause for development of hyperglycemia is the onset of infection or illness. Infection greatly intensifies the body's need for insulin, and unless insulin dosage is adjusted, hyperglycemia can result. Prompt and proper attention to even minor infections in the child with diabetes can prevent progression to a serious metabolic disturbance.

Failing to follow the prescribed meal pattern or "snitching sweets" can be a possible problem. It takes a great deal of self-understanding and self-discipline to refrain from eating some of the tempting but forbidden foods available, especially if one feels hungry. Development of self-direction and self-control is paramount for the young child and particularly for the adolescent. Nutritional discipline should be encouraged by allowing the child to participate in its planning, and possibly making provision for special occasions. The availability of so many 1-calorie soft drinks has made the social lives of teenagers with diabetes mellitus a bit less strained. However, they should be cautioned that the label "dietetic foods" does not necessarily mean "foods for the diabetic." These foods are expensive, and children can have regular dessert items in conservative amounts now and then. Children should be made to believe that the only persons they ultimately cheat are themselves when they knowingly choose foods unwisely or try to falsify blood or urine tests.

Emotional upset also increases the possibility of hyperglycemia. The insulin requirement rises in periods of stress. The emotionally stable child is much easier to regulate with insulin than a child with many emotional problems. Emotional problems are the most common cause of hyperglycemia in adolescents. Possible errors in the administration of insulin that can result in an underdose, as well as an overdose, must be prevented.

The need for insulin progressively increases as the child reaches sexual maturation and adolescence. Failure to increase insulin dosage leads to the development of hyperglycemia and ketosis. Under these circumstances, the daily dose of insulin may exceed 1.0 IU/kg/day. However, caution must be exercised in preventing rebound hyperglycemia (Somogyi effect).

Somogyi phenomenon. Children receiving high doses of insulin, 1 to 2 IU/kg/day, are likely to experience behavior changes, early morning sweating, restless sleep, or headaches. Other children can be asymptomatic but rapidly develop glycosuria and ketosis. This is the rebound phenomenon first described by Somogyi (repeated periods of unapparent hypoglycemia followed by rebound hyperglycemia). Treatment for the Somogyi phenomenon is frequent blood glucose checks and immediate reduction of insulin dosage.*

Blood glucose self-monitoring. Long before children are ready to give themselves insulin injections, they are able to test their own blood using reagent strips and a meter to determine the glucose level. Blood testing is accomplished by using specially designed lancets for ob-

*Somogyi M: Exacerbation of diabetes by excess insulin action, Am J Med 26:169, 1959.

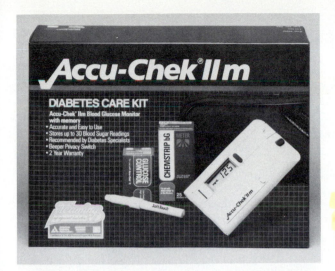

FIG 33-10 AccuChek II-m is a battery-powered meter that uses test strips to measure blood sugar. It gives blood sugar results immediately, thus allowing home blood glucose monitoring and an accurate way to plan diet, exercise, and medication changes. *(Courtesy Boehringer Mannheim Corporation, Indianapolis, Ind.)*

taining fingerstick samples or by an automatic finger-pricking device. The drops of blood are placed on a reagent strip, and the resultant color change correlates with the blood sugar. This can be accomplished visually or by using a reflectance meter, such as the Accu-Chek II m (kit shown in Fig. 33-10). When using a blood glucose monitor, the instrument must be carefully programmed with the correct programming strip. The manufacturer's directions must be followed, especially the "timing" during the procedure. Blood glucose testing is one of the best ways to help control diabetes.

Testing should be done 30 minutes before eating and at least twice daily, before breakfast and the morning insulin and before dinner and the evening insulin. These results, when looked at in terms of 2- to 4-day trends, give enough information to justify or change the current insulin dosage. In addition blood glucose levels should be done once per week before lunch to ensure that the morning short-acting insulin is appropriate and at bedtime to evaluate the evening short-acting insulin. It is also important to measure the blood glucose at 2 or 3AM at least once a week because blood glucose concentration is lowest and insulin reactions may occur. Blood glucose measurements should not be less than 70 mg/dl to avoid hypoglycemia.

When the blood sugar exceeds 200 mg/dl on two successive occasions, the patient should check urine for ketones. If ketones are negative, the acute hyperglycemia should *not* be managed with more insulin. Only when the ketones are positive with a simultaneous elevation in blood sugar should extra insulin be given. The parents should contact the child's physician or health care provider to get advice and to provide advance notice that DKA may be in the offing.

Long-term goals and prognosis. Long-term care begins immediately after the initial hospitalization and control of ketoacidosis. The goals of long-term care are (1) promotion of normal growth and development both physically and emotionally; (2) maintenance of a high level of metabolic control; (3) instruction of the child (and parent) in the skills of self-care; and (4) development of a happy, useful, and productive citizen.

Advances in the therapeutic use of insulin have provided a reasonably acceptable approach to the treatment in children. Vascular disease follows within the second decade after diagnosis. The vascular lesions are of two main types: (1) premature atherosclerosis leading to a high morbidity and mortality from cardiovascular, cerebrovascular, and renal disease and (2) microangiopathy or peripheral vascular insufficiency (caused by thickening of capillary basement membranes), leading to retinopathy and blindness, progressive renal failure, and various neuropathies. Poorly controlled IDDM in children is associated with earlier vascular complications.

Recent advances in the care of children with IDDM-1 indicate that consistent improvement in life expectancy can be accomplished when plasma-glucose levels are maintained as close to normal as possible. To date this is approximated in most children by the split-dose insulin regimen and a multiple feeding plan. However, vascular complications continue to occur in all children sooner or later.

Scientific efforts continue in the search for the exact cause and prevention of diabetes. In the meantime technologic advances in the monitoring of IDDM-1 continue to be sought in an effort to prevent or reduce the long-term complications. Among the most recent developments is the introduction of a portable insulin pump that is designed to mimic the release of insulin by the pancreas. This development shows promise but as yet is not suitable for children or adolescents. It is also costly and does not provide an easy method of monitoring.

Review of nursing responsibility. The nursing care of the diabetic patient is discussed throughout this section; however, the following questions should be of assistance in aiding the nurse to organize and evaluate her care of the patient:

NURSING CARE PLAN

The Child with Insulin-Dependent Diabetes Mellitus I (IDDM-I)

Selected nursing diagnoses	Expected outcomes	Interventions
A. Potential for injury related to insulin deficiency (hyperglycemia). Clinical manifestations: Blood glucose elevated (180 mg/ml), glucosuria, polydipsia, polyphagia, polyuria, weight loss, dehydration, and dry skin.	Child maintains blood glucose level between 70 and 120.	Monitor blood glucose levels before meals and at bedtime. Administer/Supervise child's administration of insulin as ordered by physician before breakfast and dinner. Monitor child's food intake and encourage child to eat planned meals. Offer snack between meals and at bedtime, and encourage child to eat snack. Record foods not eaten and give replacement as needed. Encourage regularity of daily activity and excercise.
B. Potential for injury related to insulin excess (hypoglycemia). Clinical manifestations: Blood glucose level below 70, fatigue, personality change, weakness, hunger, shakiness, drowsiness, pallor, and diaphoresis.	Child maintains blood glucose level between 70 and 120.	Check blood glucose level and report to physician. Administer orange juice or other sugar substitute or glucagon as ordered by physician. Evaluate feeding schedule and feed if appropriate. Evaluate insulin dosage. Evaluate activity.
C. Knowledge deficit related to home management of child. Clinical manifestations: Need for information. Request for information.	Child/parent describes and demonstrates understanding of condition: dietary management; insulin injections; exercise needs and blood glucose monitoring.	Review/Teach child and parents: a. Dietary exchange plan b. How to mix insulin c. How to administer injections d. Action and adverse side effects of insulin e. Exercise need to maintain physical fitness f. Use of blood glucose monitor and interpretation g. Signs of hyperglycemia and hypogylcemia Provide practice sessions to ensure understanding of lesson.

1. **Insulin requirement.** Do you know the type of insulin your patient is receiving and when the patient receives injections? Do you know how the injections are being rotated?
2. **Nutrition.** Do you know the amount of calories the physician has prescribed? If a strict diet is ordered (usually the case), have you made sure that your patient eats everything or receives a replacement? Do you evaluate his meals for variety and interest? Do you watch for and limit the possibility of the patient obtaining food not calculated in the diet? Does the patient have a scheduled interval nourishment?
3. **Blood glucose testing.** Do you know the method to be used? Are you collecting the specimens properly? Where are the results recorded?
4. **General hygiene.** Is the patient getting as much exercise as possible so that his insulin requirement (because of differences in amounts of exercise taken) will not change greatly on the patient's discharge? Is his skin in good condition? Are there any signs of infection anywhere in the body?
5. **Glucose-insulin imbalance.** Do you know the signs and symptoms of developing hypoglycemia and hyperglycemia?
6. **Patient-parent education and participation.** Are you assisting the patient and parents in learning more about the disease and its treatment and control, depending on their level of understanding? Are you helping the patient to develop attitudes of self-control and feelings of achievement and well-being? Does the child keep records of insulin intake, blood glucose tests, and general health? How much is the patient able to participate in his care?
7. What special interests and aspirations does this patient have?
8. What has this patient taught you?

For diabetic patients to become contributing citizens in the community and to enjoy life to its maximum, they must understand their disease, accept the limitations it imposes, and learn to function in a relatively independent setting. The alert, intelligent, warm-hearted nurse can do much to help them meet these goals.

It is very helpful for patients with diabetes mellitus to be able to room together. They usually are mutually supportive and learn from one another. (Most of the time such learning is positive and beneficial.) Children with this disorder should be encouraged to participate in school, church, and community activities and not look on their metabolic problem as an excuse for difficult behavior or special privileges. The fact that they have diabetes mellitus should not be hidden. Teachers, schoolmates, and employers should be aware of the presence of the condition. In many states special summer camping experiences are set up for children with this disorder. These 2-week sessions have been of great help to many youngsters.

• • •

A source of much pleasure and occasional pain, the digestive system continually struggles to meet the challenges of unskilled cooks, individual abuse, and emotional stress. Nurses should be able to help prevent or ease some of the difficulties faced by this sensitive body servant. In so doing, they fulfill part of their obligation to the person whose total well-being is their concern.

Key Concepts

1. Thrush results from contamination of the infant's oral cavity with vaginal secretions containing *Candida albicans* at the time of birth or, less often, from improper hygiene and feeding techniques after birth. Thrush can be treated with nystatin oral suspension.
2. Congenital pyloric stenosis is the abnormal narrowing of the pyloric sphincter, caused by spasm of the sphincter, local edema, and an overgrowth of the circular muscle fibers of the pylorus. Symptoms include progressive vomiting and malnutrition. Treatment is usually surgical.
3. Most explanations of the pain experienced with colic involve the presence of excessive gas in the digestive tract. Excessive air can result from poor bottle-feeding techniques, excessive use of carbohydrate in formula, or a tense, nervous infant. In attempts to remedy colic, consider these possible causes.
4. Dehydration and electrolyte imbalance are significant dangers when diarrheal disease causes profuse fluid loss in a young child. Severe diarrhea usually subsides when fluid and electrolyte therapy is administered intravenously and oral intake is briefly reduced.
5. Inguinal and umbilical hernias are common in infancy and childhood. Ninety percent of inguinal hernias are found in males. Repair is a common surgical procedure. Umbilical hernias often close spontaneously when the child learns to stand and walk. If

this does not occur, repair is recommended for girls over 2 years and boys over 4 years of age.

6. Oxyuriasis, the disease caused by pinworms, causes few symptoms other than anal itching and secondary complications caused by scratching. Mebendazole is an effective treatment in most cases. Thorough cleansing and good personal toilet hygiene must be stressed.

7. Round worm infestation causes ascariasis, which is perpetuated by poor sanitary facilities and poor hygiene practices. Treatment by piperazine citrate is effective. Public education programs teaching general hygiene are a must.

8. Diabetes mellitus is the most common metabolic disorder of children. Insufficient insulin is produced, utilization of glucose is impaired, and hyperglycemia with its acute and long-term manifestations results.

9. Insulin-dependent diabetes mellitus (IDDM-1) describes the disease exhibited by children and adolescents. The classic clinical symptoms are polyuria, dehydration despite polydipsia, and weight loss despite polyphagia.

10. Diabetic ketoacidosis (DKA) is a serious complication of IDDM-1. Precipitating factors include trauma, infection, pregnancy, vomiting, and emotional stress.

11. Approximately five types of insulin may be used in the management of a child with IDDM-1. Activity of these insulin types varies in onset, peak, and duration.

12. The amount of exercise and nutritional intake of a child with diabetes should be comparable to that of a healthy, nondiabetic child of the same age and sex. Exercise level, food intake, and insulin requirements are interdependent.

13. The first signs of insulin-induced hypoglycemia are diaphoresis and personality change. A source of glucose such as orange juice, a sugar cube, or crackers should be given. If the child has difficulty taking oral glucose, an intramuscular or subcutaneous injection of glucagon is ordered.

14. Causes of hypoglycemia include uncompensated excessive exercise, failure to eat enough or to space food intake appropriately, and difficulties in determining appropriate doses of insulin.

15. Hyperglycemia occurs when the insulin available in the blood is insufficient to metabolize the glucose present. The most common cause is the onset of infection or illness. Other precipitating factors may include failure to follow the prescribed meal pattern, emotional upsets, and errors in insulin administration.

16. The Somogyi phenomenon involves repeated periods of unapparent hypoglycemia followed by rebound hyperglycemia. Treatment includes frequent blood glucose checks and immediate reduction of insulin dosage.

17. Blood glucose testing is one of the best ways to help control diabetes. Children are able to test their own blood to determine the glucose level using reagent strips and a meter.

Discussion Questions

1. What nursing observations could indicate problems with the gastrointestinal tract? Why are vomiting and diarrhea particularly significant in an infant or young child? What nursing interventions are used in these situations?

2. What is a hernia? Describe the different types of hernias seen in children. Do all hernias require surgical repair?

3. Discuss the significance of metabolic disorders such as galactosemia and phenylketonuria. When and how are these diagnosed? Discuss the dietary considerations related to these diseases. How can you help the child and the family to deal with the dietary restrictions?

4. Identify the most common parasitic and bacterial diseases of the intestine. How are these diseases most often acquired? How are they spread? How can they be recognized? What diagnostic tests are used? What is the typical treatment? How can the nurse reduce the spread of these parasites?

5. Describe the etiology and pathophysiology of diabetes mellitus. What are the signs and symptoms? Diagnostic tests? What is the current treatment? What are nursing responsibilities when caring for a diabetic child in a hospital setting?

6. Control of diabetes involves careful balance of diet, insulin, and exercise. Why is this particularly difficult in the child? Consider the developmental tasks of adolescence. Why might the adolescent diabetic rebel and deviate from his treatment plan? What can the nurse do to help?

34

Conditions Involving the Genitourinary System

CHAPTER OBJECTIVES

After studying this chapter, the student should be able to perform the following:

1 Define the terms listed in the key vocabulary.
2 List three congenital abnormalities of the genitourinary tract and name three possible signs of unseen structural genitourinary problems in the newborn.
3 Discuss the need for surgical correction of significant hypospadias and the postoperative observation and care required.
4 Discuss the need for correction of cryptorchidism and the methods that may be employed to treat it.
5 Indicate three factors or conditions that may be associated with an increased incidence of urinary tract infections.
6 Identify four possible signs of urinary tract infection in the child under 3 years of age and three signs and symptoms characteristic of school-age children.

7 Emphasize the importance of treating pediatric urinary reflux and indicate three significant postoperative nursing considerations when ureteral reimplantation is performed.
8 Describe the common relationship between kidney disease and the possible development of definite hypertension in children.
9 Outline the nursing needs of the hospitalized child with generalized edema associated with childhood nephrotic syndrome.
10 Discuss enuresis, describing its incidence in the pediatric population, the physical, maturational, and psychologic considerations that may be involved, and the therapies that can be used.

URINARY SYSTEM

The urinary system consists of two kidneys, two ureters, the bladder, and the urethra (Fig. 34-1). The primary function of these organs is to excrete metabolic waste products. The kidneys perform additional functions, such as the production of renin, which controls blood pressure, and erythropoietin, which stimulates red blood cell synthesis.

To regulate the composition of blood, the kidneys perform the complex task of producing urine. The ureters, bladder, and urethra are involved in the transportation, storage, and elimination of the urine.

Kidneys

The kidneys are paired organs located on each side of the vertebral column, just above the waistline. They

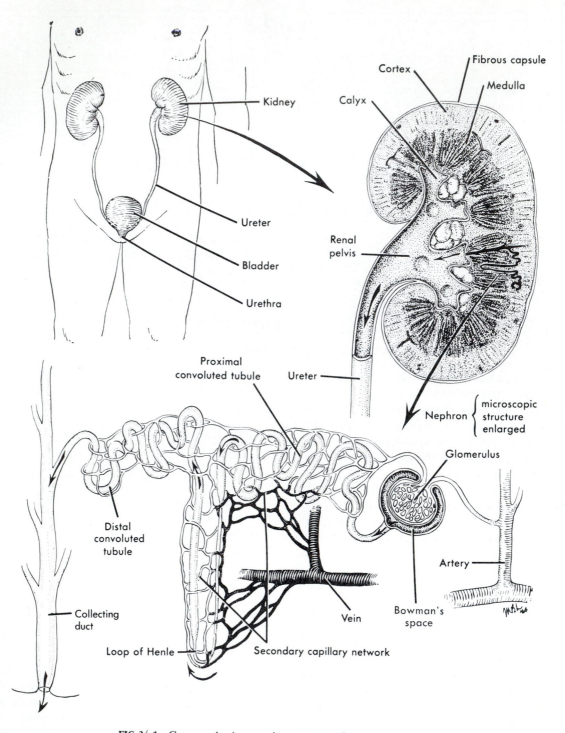

FIG 34-1 Gross and microscopic structures of urinary system.

lie outside the peritoneal cavity against the muscle of the posterior abdominal wall.

In the adult the kidneys are about 4½ inches (11.5 cm) long and 2½ inches (6.4 cm) wide; they are somewhat bean-shaped. On the medial border of each kidney is a concave notch called the "hilus." The renal artery, renal vein, nerves, and ureter join the kidney at the hilus.

When describing the internal structure of the organ, one may speak of two areas: the functioning portion, the *parenchyma,* and the collecting portion, the *pelvis.* A longitudinal section of the kidney reveals that the parenchyma in turn is composed of two parts: an outer portion called the *cortex* and an inner portion called the *medulla.* The pelvis is formed by the expansion of the upper end of the ureter. The pelvis subdivides to form the major and minor *calyces* (singular, calyx).

The parenchyma of each kidney consists of approximately 1 million functional units called *nephrons.* Each nephron has two parts: the glomerulus and the tubule. The glomerulus is a collection of specialized capillaries. The tubule has three main parts: the proximal convoluted tubule, the loop of Henle, and the distal convoluted tubule. Each nephron unit is linked by a connecting segment to the collecting duct, which drains urine into the renal pelvis. The glomeruli and the convoluted tubules are in the cortex. The medulla contains the loop of Henle. The collecting duct begins in the cortex and traverses the medulla.

The kidneys perform the complex task of removing toxic metabolic wastes, such as urea and uric acid, and excessive amounts of substances, such as water and electrolytes, from the blood. In this way the kidneys regulate the composition and volume of blood.

Three processes are involved in the production of urine: filtration, reabsorption, and secretion.

1. *Filtration* occurs in the glomerulus. As blood flows through the lumen of the glomerular capillary, some of the water, salts, and other small molecules are filtered through capillary walls and enter Bowman's space. Blood cells, platelets, and most plasma proteins are not filtered but remain in the capillary lumen because of their large size. The liquid that has passed into Bowman's space is called the *filtrate.* The filtrate flows down the lumen of the tubule, where it is modified by reabsorption and secretion. The modified filtrate eventually becomes urine.

2. *Reabsorption* occurs through the walls of the convoluted tubules, the loop of Henle, and the collecting duct. By means of a very complex process, the tubular cells reabsorb water, glucose, electrolytes, and other molecules from the filtrate. This reclamation process is vital to the maintenance of the fluid and electrolyte balance of the body.

3. *Secretion* takes place in the tubules. In the proximal convoluting tubules, penicillin, iodopyracet, phenolsulfonphthalein, and hippuric acid are among the substances secreted. In the distal convoluting tubule, hydrogen ions and ammonia are secreted in the varying amounts necessary to control and maintain the acid-base balance of the body. Sodium is exchanged for either potassium or hydrogen ion by a pump that is stimulated by the hormone aldosterone.

The modified filtrate first passes from the distal convoluting tubule into the straight collecting duct, where water is reabsorbed. From there it enters the renal pelvis as urine. In the normal adult the amount of filtrate is very great—generally 190 L per day. Large amounts of water and salt must be reabsorbed to keep the body fluids in balance. The tubules reclaim about 188.5 L, the remaining 1.5 L is excreted as urine. The average daily urinary output of urine varies greatly with the size of the child and the fluid intake.

Ureters

In the adult the ureters are small tubes about ⅕ inch (0.5 cm) in diameter and 12 inches (30 cm) in length. (The size varies with age.) The expanded upper end of the ureter collects the urine from the kidney, and peristaltic waves convey the urine down the ureters and into the bladder. The ureters lie behind the peritoneum and descend from the kidney to the posterior bladder wall. They enter the bladder in an oblique manner, preventing reflux, or backflow, of urine.

Bladder

The bladder is a dome-shaped, hollow, muscular sac that stores urine. It is located directly behind the symphysis pubis. Intertwining muscle bundles form the bladder wall. These muscular layers are collectively called the *detrusor muscle.* The internal sphincter is composed of smooth muscle bundles at the bladder outlet. The bladder outlet and the two ureteral openings outline a triangular area called the *trigone.*

The detrusor muscle is usually relaxed, allowing the bladder to expand as needed to accommodate urine storage. After a certain volume of urine is collected, the urge to void is felt. The desire to void is recorded by the sensory parasympathetic endings in the detrusor muscle. If the child decides to void, the detrusor muscle contracts, the internal sphincter opens, and urine enters the urethra. In the child who has developed neurologic bladder control (2-3 years of age), voiding may be postponed, but when the bladder becomes very full, a point is reached at which even the most desperate efforts can no longer retain the urine.

Urethra

The urethra is a small tube that serves as a passageway for the elimination of urine from the bladder. The external outlet of the urethra is called the *urethral meatus*.

The urethra is a comparatively short tube in the woman; it is about 1½ inches (3.8 cm) long. In the midportion of the female urethra is a circular striated muscle that forms the external sphincter.

The male urethra is about 8 inches (20 cm) long and also serves as part of the reproductive tract. It is divided into three sections: prostatic, membranous, and penile. The prostatic urethra is about 1 inch (2.54 cm) long and extends from the internal sphincter of the bladder through the prostate gland to the pelvic floor. The membranous urethra is about ½ inch (1.3 cm) long and lies between the prostatic and penile sections of the urethra; it is surrounded by the external sphincter. The penile urethra is about 6 inches (15 cm) long and extends through the penis, terminating at the urethral meatus.

Urine

Urine is a transparent, amber-colored liquid with a characteristic odor. It is usually acid in reaction. The specific gravity of urine ranges from 1.003 to 1.030. Approximately 95% of urine is water. The remaining 5% consists of wastes from protein metabolism and inorganic components, such as sodium and potassium chloride.

The examination of urine is the keystone in diagnosing disorders of the urinary system. A properly collected specimen can yield a wealth of information about renal function and the nature of kidney disorders. Urinalysis also reveals much information about infections and toxic and metabolic disorders. Proteinuria, hematuria, pyuria, bacteriuria, and casts are important clues to the presence of renal disease.

KEY VOCABULARY

anuria Lack of urine formation.
albuminuria Presence of albumin in the urine.
bacteriuria Presence of bacteria in the urine.

enuresis Involuntary discharge of urine in daytime or nighttime, after the age by which bladder control should have been established.
frequency Number of repetitions of a periodic process in a unit of time; when speaking of urinary function, the term implies an abnormal increase in the number of voidings.
hematuria Presence of blood in the urine.
nocturia Excessive urination during the night.
oliguria Diminished amount of urine production with subsequent scanty urination.
polyuria Abnormally increased urinary output.
proteinuria Finding of protein, usually albumin, in the urine.
pyuria Abnormal white blood cells in the urine.
reflux The regurgitation of urine from the bladder into the ureter.
uremia Toxic condition associated with renal insufficiency and the retention in the blood of nitrogenous substances normally excreted by the kidney.
urgency Patient cannot wait to void, must urgently run to bathroom.
vesicoureteral reflux Regurgitation of urine from the bladder into the ureter.

ANOMALIES OF THE GENITOURINARY TRACT
Infant

The embryologic development of the urinary system is closely related to the development of the genital organs in both sexes. Because of this factor, genital and urinary tract deformities are discussed together. Genitourinary deformities comprise 30% to 40% of all congenital anomalies. A deformity of the genitalia may be accompanied by a deformity of the upper urinary tract. Deformities are multiple in approximately 20% of cases, and often they accompany anomalies in other systems (for example, imperforate anus). Improved prenatal ultrasound has identified many anomalies before birth, often allowing treatment to be instituted shortly after birth.

Malformations of the genitourinary tract may lead to death. When the anomaly can be recognized early, surgical correction or treatment may be life-saving. This is true because many anomalies are obstructive and lead to hydronephrosis, which, if bilateral, may ultimately result in renal failure.

External deformities are obvious and readily detected. However, there is little physical evidence of internal disease unless it is far advanced. The nurse should be aware of this and know the few signals demanding close observation. It is important to note the number and amount of voidings in the newborn infant. Failure to void within the first 24 hours after birth is a danger sign and should be reported to the physician immediately. Abdominal enlargement or swelling in the area of a kidney also warrants immediate attention. A poor urinary stream may be a sign of a pathologic disorder in the genitourinary tract. About 7% of neonates with nonspecific signs of illness (such as sepsis and failure to gain weight), have a urinary tract infection.

The signs and symptoms of urinary problems in older children are more easily detected. Crying on urination, urgent and frequent urination, straining to void, and dribbling all point to genitourinary system difficulties. Unexplained fever, lassitude, weight loss, and failure to thrive are nondescript symptoms but may relate to advanced disease. Serious kidney infections may run a silent course. It is always wise to investigate any of the preceding signals, since renal failure can be the result of a hidden anomaly.

Renal agenesis. Bilateral renal agenesis is incompatible with life. Autopsy studies have revealed that it is more common in males than in females. Lack of fetal urine causes a severe reduction in amniotic fluid (oligohydramnios). Since amniotic fluid is required for normal lung development, these patients have pulmonary hypoplasia. Oligohydramnios also causes the uterus to exert pressure on the fetus for prolonged periods of time, thus interfering with normal growth and development. The combination of renal agenesis, pulmonary hypoplasia, and facial and limb abnormalities is frequently called *Potter's syndrome*.

Unilateral renal agenesis is a survivable condition, but the single kidney is more likely to be diseased and associated with other malformations, especially of the ureter.

Double kidney. Duplication of the kidney and ureter is the most frequently encountered anomaly of the urinary tract and is more common in girls than boys. The ureters from each double kidney may enter the bladder at different points (complete duplication) or may unite to enter the bladder as one ureter (partial duplication). Sometimes the ureter from the upper kidney enters the genitourinary tract ectopically and causes incontinence. Duplication of the kidney and ureter is clinically significant only when other anomalies causing incontinence, obstruction, reflux, or infection exist.

Horseshoe kidney. A horseshoe kidney results when the lower ends of both kidneys fuse, forming a single mass shaped like a horseshoe. These kidneys lie closer to the spine and usually lower than does separate kidneys. A horseshoe kidney may be asymptomatic, but complications, especially obstruction, infection, and reflux, are common.

Polycystic kidney. True polycystic disease is always hereditary and always bilateral. Polycystic kidneys are larger than normal and sometimes are huge, filling the entire abdomen. They contain innumerable cysts, compressing the parenchyma. Such kidneys are constantly susceptible to infection, obstruction, and stone formation. Treatment can only be palliative. The prognosis varies with the type of polycystic kidneys. Some patients survive only a few months, but others live into the third or fourth decade. Inheritance can be autosomal recessive or autosomal dominant. The autosomal recessive form is associated with hepatic fibrosis.

Ureterocele. A ureterocele is a ballooning of the lower end of the ureter because of an abnormally narrow ureteral orifice. Ureteroceles are usually unilateral. Double ureters are commonly associated with the anomaly. When an extra ureter is present, the one that enters the bladder normally is often distorted by the enormous ureterocele. As a result, it becomes obstructed, and kidney infection may ensue. Treatment consists of excising the redundant portion and reconstructing the opening so that obstruction is eliminated. The portion of kidney adjacent to the ureterocele is usually so destroyed as to require removal. If an obstruction does not exist, treatment is symptomatic.

Exstrophy of the bladder. Exstrophy of the bladder, fortunately, is a rare condition. It ranks with the most severe human anomalies. Because of a defect in midline closure associated with incomplete development of the pubic arch, the interior of the bladder lies completely exposed through an opening in the lower abdominal wall. A number of severe genital anomalies (for example, epispadias) usually accompany the defect.

Children who have exstrophy of the bladder become foul-smelling because they are constantly soaked in urine. Often the surrounding skin becomes excoriated, causing great pain. Early in life the exposed bladder mucosa becomes inflamed, bleeds readily, and is acutely sensitive. Infection is frequent but can usually be controlled by antibiotic therapy.

Treatment is surgical. An anatomic reconstruction of the bladder is the operation of choice. The most desirable time for this operation is at birth. After this operation the child is totally incontinent for a period of years, during which time the bladder grows sufficiently to make antireflux operations possible. When the bladder (vesicle) sphincters are made more complete and function somewhat normally, efforts can be directed to make the child continent. Dilation of the ureter, reflux, and chronic infection often occur when the child is rendered continent too early.

If the exstrophic bladder is deemed unsuitable for reconstruction or has failed prior attempts at closure, other methods of draining, especially ileal bladder or conduit procedures, are employed. It is currently popular to "augment" small exstrophic bladders with intestinal segments to render them suitable for reconstruction.

Exstrophy of the bladder is a survivable condition; however, the prognosis depends in great measure on the extent of renal damage resulting from defective drainage and infection.

Hypospadias. Hypospadias is a common deformity in which the urethra terminates at some point on the ventral (under) surface of the penis (Fig. 34-2). The position of the urethra on the penis or perineum determines the type of treatment. Because the prostatic urethra is never involved in hypospadias, the sphincters function normally, and the child has good urinary control. Often a meatal stricture is associated with varying degrees of hypospadias. When such a stricture is recognized, it is easily corrected by dilation or meatotomy.

In the more severe types, a cordlike anomaly causes the penis to arc downward (chordee). These more extensive deformities all require surgical repair to establish normal control of voiding and make normal reproduction possible later in life. Boys with hypospadias should not be circumcised without prior urologic consultation, because the foreskin is needed in the repair.

Treatment. Operative repair is usually accomplished in one stage at about 1 year of age. In this way the child avoids ridicule from peers and lasting psychologic problems from genital surgery.

Various plastic techniques are employed to correct hypospadias, and the procedures are constantly being improved. The difficulties encountered in achieving a successful correction of hypospadias are considerable. The parents should be aware that more than one operation may be required. They should also know that after a successful urethroplasty the penis may be scarred, although appearing normal to the casual observer.

Postoperative care. When surgery is completed, the penis is wrapped in petroleum gauze and then covered with a dry gauze bandage. Some surgeons use a clear Tegaderm wrapping. This helps to prevent postoperative swelling, pain, and bleeding. Unless this precaution is taken, failure of the repair can occur. A catheter drains the bladder while the incision is healing. The nurse must observe the patient carefully to detect swelling, bleeding, or obstruction of the catheter. In many pediatric centers hypospadias surgery is now performed on an outpatient day-surgery basis. However, the child is often hospitalized for repair of more serious forms of hypospadias.

After the operation the child is kept on his back. A bed cradle helps to prevent pressure on the operative area. Many times Stile's dressing is used (see Fig. 33-5).

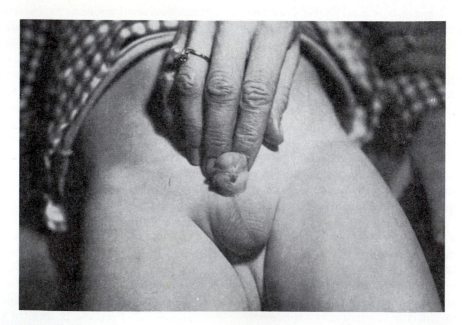

FIG 34-2 Hypospadias (meatus located on undersurface of penis). *(Courtesy Matthew Gleason MD, San Diego, Calif.)*

On the second postoperative day the child may be allowed freedom of movement in his crib, provided the nurse can take time to sit, talk, and play with him. She should attempt to keep his hands occupied lest he busy them with his dressing. Parents should be encouraged to stay with their children because they are best able to keep them constructively occupied.

Epispadias. When the urethra opens on the dorsal (upper) surface of the penis, the condition is called epispadias. Various degrees of epispadias can occur. However, the deformity is uncommon, except when associated with exstrophy of the bladder. Treatment is the same as that for hypospadias or exstrophy.

Intersexual anomalies. A semiemergency exists when simple inspection of the newborn infant's genitalia does not reveal the sex of the child. Chromosome and endocrine studies are usually helpful in these cases. Exploratory abdominal surgery for gonadal biopsy can also be undertaken to identify the sex of the sexually indeterminate child and decide upon the most appropriate sex for rearing.

Pseudohermaphroditism. When a person possesses external genitalia resembling those of one sex and the gonads of the opposing sex, the condition resulting is termed "pseudohermaphroditism." Sometimes a severe hypospadias with undescended testicles or a hypertrophied clitoris and malformed labia cause problems in sex identification. Female pseudohermaphrodites possess ovaries, but their external genitalia mimic those of the male. Such masculinization of the female infant results from an overdeveloped adrenal cortex (congenital adrenal hyperplasia) and subsequent increased production of male sex hormones (androgens) by the adrenal glands. Male pseudohermaphrodites are chromosomal males, but because of some testicular dysfunction or the existence of other problems, sexual ambiguity is present.

Whatever the condition, it should be corrected—but only after the true sex has been determined. Treatment usually consists of corrective plastic procedures on the external genitalia or the administration of appropriate missing hormones.

Mixed gonadal tissue and ambiguous genitalia. An extremely rare condition exists when a child possesses gonads of both sexes. Prompt attention to this problem reduces the possibilities of serious emotional sequelae. Gender assignment should be performed as soon as possible so that the child has an opportunity for a normal, happy, and successful life. Treatment is not often an emergency, but sex assignment is crucial.

Hydrocele. As the testis descends through the ingui-

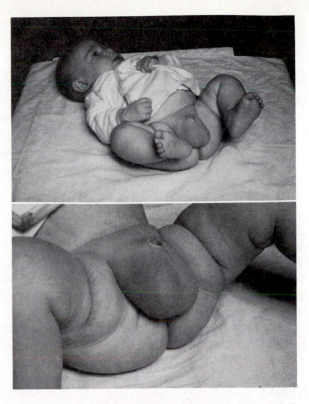

FIG 34-3 Five-month-old infant with bilateral congenital hydroceles.

nal canal to the scrotum, it is preceded by a fingerlike projection of the peritoneal cavity called the *processus vaginalis*. This processus obliterates shortly after birth in the majority of boys. If the processus persists, peritoneal fluid may travel to the scrotum causing a fluid collection or hydrocele around the testis (Fig. 34-3). Intestine may also pass into the processus as an indirect inguinal hernia. When an infantile hydrocele persists beyond 1 year of age, surgical correction is recommended to prevent hernia formation and correct the cosmetic abnormality. If a clinically detectable hernia develops, it is repaired as soon as it is diagnosed because of a tendency for bowel to become trapped and strangulated within the processus in infants.

Cryptorchidism. Failure of the testes (singular, *testis*) to descend into the scrotum occurs in about 1% to 5% of full-term newborns and more frequently in premature infants. This cryptorchid condition is usually unilateral and frequently associated with an inguinal hernia.

Testicular maldescent is rarely associated with symptoms. It is associated with an increased incidence of testicular injury, torsion, and cancer. Other concerns are impaired fertility and a possible increased incidence of malignancy in the undescended testis. Though a predisposition to malignancy may exist with a nonscrotal testis, early surgical correction may prevent this.

If spontaneous descent is to occur for a crypt-orchid testis, it is usually complete by 1 year of age. Human chorionic gonadotropin (hCG) can be a therapeutic aid in the management of bilateral cryptorchidism. Its use can aid descent, help differentiate between a retractile or a truly cryptorchid testis, or establish the presence or absence of bilateral intraabdominal testes.

If the testes do not descend spontaneously or in response to HCG, surgical correction, or orchiopexy, is indicated. Although an optimum age for this step is not agreed on universally, most pediatric urologists feel it should be performed between the ages of 1 and 2 years. Further delay accomplishes little and can result in impaired fertility in the individual or increased danger of eventual testicular malignancy.

Early scrotal placement of the testes or placement of testicular prostheses for congenital absence is important for the child's healthy emotional and social development.

Toddler

Infections of the urinary tract. The diagnosis of urinary tract infection requires demonstration of significant bacteriuria, usually over 100,000 bacteria per ml of urine on a culture of a properly collected urine specimen. Infection may be confined to the bladder (cystitis) or may spread to the upper urinary tract (pyelonephritis). In patients with pyelonephritis, the kidney can undergo irreversible damage as the result of bacterial invasion. Pyelonephritis can cause hypertension and chronic renal failure. Urinary tract infections are always considered serious and can be difficult to eradicate. Such infections are thought to rank second in frequency only to infections of the respiratory tract.

Etiologic factors. There are many causes of urinary tract infections. Urinary stasis, which occurs when urine flow is obstructed, is associated with infection. Obstruction can occur at several sites: The ureteropelvic junction is one of the most common sites. Posterior urethral valves can cause obstruction in males. Kidney stones, vesicoureteral reflux, and urinary bladder dysfunction predispose to infection.

In most patients bacteria enter the urine via the urethra. Because the female urethra is much shorter than the male's, females tend to have more urinary tract infections than males.

Incidence. Urinary tract infections are relatively com-

mon in children. About 5% of all females have such infections during the school-age years.

Anatomic abnormalities of the urinary tract. Most children with proven infection should be screened for anatomic abnormalities of the urinary tract with sonographic or radiographic procedures. Both an intravenous pyelogram or renal ultrasound and a voiding cystourethrogram are necessary to assess the anatomy of the urinary tract. These studies detect a wide variety of urinary tract abnormalities, including reflux, obstruction, renal anomalies, and stones. Radiographic studies should be performed when the infected patient is male, regardless of the patient's age. All infected females under 3 years of age and older girls with repeated or febrile infections must also be screened.

Clinical symptoms. Symptoms vary considerably in urinary tract infections. In children under 3 years of age the onset is likely to be abrupt and severe, accompanied by a high temperature, which can reach 104° F (40° C). Pallor, anorexia, vomiting, diarrhea, and convulsions may occur. These *acute* symptoms usually disappear in a few days with appropriate treatment.

Older children complain of sharp or dull pain in the flank. Gross hematuria or pyuria may be present. Bladder symptoms such as frequent, urgent, and burning urination are common complaints. Chills and fever may also be present. Occasionally urinary tract infection may be asymptomatic.

Some patients whose upper tract infections continue for a long period develop chronic pyelonephritis. Chronic pyelonephritis progresses slowly over many years. As the result of continuous low-grade infection, the patient characteristically has a history of recurrent bouts of nonspecific symptoms such as nausea, vomiting, diarrhea, fever, irritability, headache, and transitory urinary abnormalities. Poor general health, anemia, failure to grow, or failure to thrive are typical findings. The child may appear very pale or pasty-looking. This condition suggests the late stages of renal damage and the development of uremia. Hypertension frequently appears as the end result of advanced renal scarring.

Treatment. Urinalysis and a culture of a properly collected specimen are the key to successful treatment. Therapy depends primarily on identification of the causative organism in a carefully collected urine culture. Detection and correction of anatomic abnormalities in the urinary tract are also essential to prevent progressive renal destruction (see p. 781).

A clean, midstream voided specimen is collected and sent to the laboratory for culture and sensitivity studies.

If it is impossible to obtain an adequate specimen by such means, a catheterized specimen is ordered. Prompt therapy is indicated. Sulfonamides or broad-spectrum antibiotics are administered until the laboratory studies are complete. Specific medications are ordered and continued for at least 10 days to 2 weeks.

The patient should be placed in bed in a cool, quiet environment until the fever has subsided. A tepid sponge bath may also be ordered. Fluids are encouraged to ensure adequate hydration and a good urine output. An accurate account of the fluid intake and urinary output is essential. Although it is not necessary to insert a catheter for accurate output, a simple check mark is not sufficient for the information needed. Weighing the diaper or an estimation of the amount of diaper saturation is far more valuable. After removing the diaper, the nurse should carefully wash and dry the child's genitalia before applying the clean diaper. This prevents further contamination and also protects the skin from becoming irritated and excoriated.

An adequate diet is important, and every attempt should be made to offer food that the child is able and willing to eat. A good milk intake supplies the needed protein, carbohydrate, fat, and most important, water. The parents should be encouraged to visit during mealtime. Parents are best able to understand the sick child's desires, and usually the child is more likely to eat for Mom or Dad. A daily check of weight, blood pressure, and vital signs offers valuable clues in the early detection of complications.

Reflux. In 20% to 30% of children with proven urinary tract infections, urine refluxes from the bladder into the ureters (vesicoureteral reflux) during voiding. This abnormality is detected by a radiographic procedure called a voiding cystourethrogram. The persistence of reflux encourages infection. Vesicoureteral reflux is caused by anatomic defects in the urinary tract or by infection. The junction between the bladder and the ureter is only mildly abnormal when reflux is caused by infection. The abnormality improves if the patient's urine is kept sterile by administration of antibiotics for prolonged periods. Surgery is usually unnecessary when reflux is caused by infection alone, provided the infection can be controlled.

Anatomic defects in the connection between the ureter and the bladder or obstruction to urine flow in the urethra can also cause reflux. Patients with anatomic defects often require surgery. The functional anatomy of the vesicoureteral junction can be improved by surgically reimplanting the distal ureter into the bladder wall.

Nursing care. The general postoperative care of this patient is much the same as for any surgical patient. The nurse should recognize the importance of changing surgical dressings that have become saturated with urine. Urine is an excellent medium for the growth of bacteria. However, the nurse should be aware that some surgical drains can be purposely attached to the dressings, and special care is therefore required. Some physicians wish to change the dressings themselves for this reason. Drainage tubes must be carefully checked for patency. These postoperative patients can return to the nursing area with as many as three urinary catheters, depending on the extent of the surgery (one suprapubic cystotomy tube empties the bladder of any urine not drained via the ureteral tubes, and two ureteral catheters act as splints for the newly implanted ureters). Drainage from each of the tubes should be closely observed and recorded separately. These catheters are never clamped. When the patient is able to sit up in a wheelchair, the catheters should be arranged so that they do not kink. The collection bottles must hang below the level of the kidneys, draining freely. Water intake is always encouraged and recorded, particularly in young children, who quickly dehydrate. Dehydration promotes the growth of bacteria.

Pain is commonly associated with this type of surgery. Narcotics should be given as ordered on time. Antispasmodic drugs such as oxybutynin chloride (Ditropan), propantheline bromide (Pro-Banthine), or methantheline bromide (Banthine bromide) are also ordered. These drugs usually relieve the immediate postoperative colicky pain.

Reflux associated with renal involvement is also caused by lower tract congenital obstructions. Unless the obstruction is corrected by reconstructive surgery when indicated, pyelonephritis can progress, leading to severe renal impairment.

Prognosis. When the disease is recognized early and treated properly (long-term antibiotic therapy for infection or surgical removal of obstructions), the prognosis is excellent. Chronic infections present a much more serious and difficult problem because severe renal damage is the ultimate result.

Wilms' tumor. Wilms' tumor is one of the most common abdominal neoplasms of childhood. It is a congenital, mixed renal tumor that develops from abnormal embryonic tissue; occasionally (5% - 10%) occurs bilaterally. Composed of varying proportions of abnormal glomerulotubular structures, connective tissue, muscle, and blood vessels, the tumor initially grows within the renal capsule. As it grows larger it distorts the kidney in a bizarre manner and can occupy as much as one half of the abdominal cavity. Unfortunately, the tumor often invades the renal veins and metastasizes through the bloodstream to vital organs, especially to the lungs. Extension of the tumor through the renal capsule into surrounding tissues can occur and is associated with a poorer prognosis. Cure rates for even Stage II or III tumors are excellent.

Etiologic factors. Like other forms of cancer, the exact cause of Wilms' tumor is unknown. Recent evidence suggests that chromosomal abnormalities may play an important role.

Incidence. Wilms' tumor accounts for approximately 7% of all cancer in children. Boys and girls are equally affected. About two thirds of all children with Wilms' tumor are diagnosed before they are 3 years of age. The tumor can be present at birth and is rare after 7 years of age.

Clinical features. The initial manifestation of Wilms' tumor is a mass in the region of the kidney that is usually discovered by the parents in the course of daily care or accidentally during a routine examination. As the tumor grows, the child's abdomen becomes very large, and pressure symptoms arise. Constipation, vomiting, abdominal distention, and even dyspnea can occur. Weight loss, pallor, and anemia are common in the late stages. Pain, hematuria, and hypertension are uncommon, but, if present, they support the diagnosis of a renal tumor.

Treatment and nursing care. When Wilms' tumor is suspected, both parent and nurse must be careful not to feel or touch the child's abdomen because handling can cause rupture of the tumor through the renal capsule and metastasis via the bloodstream. Diagnosis is usually confirmed by intravenous pyelography and renal ultrasound. Occasionally, computed tomography or an MRI is necessary to evaluate the extent of the tumor. The choice of therapy is guided by the age of the child, extent of the tumor, and metastatic considerations at the time of diagnosis. Treatment usually consists of prompt radical nephrectomy. Radiation therapy has a limited role in treatment since the advent of more effective chemotherapy.

The kidney, tumor, and perirenal fat are removed through a transabdominal approach. Blood transfusions may be given to replace blood lost during the surgical procedure and to correct preexisting anemia. Intravenous administration of fluids is continued for 24 hours. If bleeding occurs, it is easily detected when the child's pulse rate, respirations, blood pressure, and color are checked often. The dressings should be changed only if necessary, since little or no drainage occurs from the incision.

Actinomycin D has a significant antitumor effect and is particularly useful in the prevention of pulmonary metastases. Vincristine is also a highly effective drug in the treatment of Wilms' tumor. When both drugs are used in combination, the survival rate is significantly greater. Actinomycin D potentiates radiation. When indicated, courses of combination drug therapy are given at the time of resection, 6 weeks later, and then every 3 months. Length of treatment depends on the stage of the disease as well as "favorable" or "unfavorable" histology. Side effects from the administration of chemotherapy and radiation therapy include nausea, vomiting, anorexia, malaise, diarrhea, and loss of hair. During the interval between medication and radiation therapy, the child's hair usually grows back. Bone marrow depression, ulceration of the mucous membranes, and peripheral neuropathies are manifestations of acute toxicity associated with the administration of actinomycin D and vincristine. Drug therapy can be temporarily discontinued to allow the child to recover from the toxicity of the treatment.

Complications. The most serious complication in Wilms' tumor is metastasis. Characteristically, Wilms' tumor metastasizes through the bloodstream to the liver, lungs, brain, and other vital organs. The tumor can also spread by direct extension or by the lymphatics.

Prognosis. Wilms' tumor is always fatal if not treated and until recently has had a high mortality rate despite treatment. However, with major therapeutic advances in the last decade in surgery, radiation therapy, and combination chemotherapy, 90% of children with Wilms' tumor are currently expected to be cured of their disease. Although the prognosis is better when the tumor is discovered early, the use of combined therapy offers children with metastatic disease a good chance for cure. Follow-up care includes frequent x-ray examinations of the lungs and other areas of potential tumor involvement and close monitoring of the remaining normal kidney. As the child progresses favorably, less frequent examinations are required, but annual examinations are recommended to follow normal development and to detect any late effects of treatment.

Hypertension and renal disease. Measurement of blood pressure in children can be difficult and time-consuming. The patient should be as quiet as possible. The blood pressure cuff should cover at least two thirds of the upper arm. Repeated measurements may be required to establish an accurate average reading of the patient. Normal blood pressure is related to age and

NURSING CARE PLAN

The Young Child with Wilms' Tumor

Selected nursing diagnoses	Expected outcomes	Interventions
A. Anxiety related to diagnosis of Wilms' tumor and treatment protocol. Clinical manifestations: Crying, multiple questions, verbalized anxiety, and restlessness.	Child and parents cope effectively and decrease level of anxiety.	Assess present knowledge base and reinforce previously given information. Explain procedure and treatments to child and parents in age-appropriate manner. Listen to child's and parents' fears and concerns and reassure as needed.
B. Alteration in comfort related to presence of tumor, surgical removal of kidney, and chemotherapy. Clinical manifestations: Crying, grimacing, guarding, not moving in bed, increased respiratory and heart rate.	Relief from discomfort.	Assess child's level of pain. Observe child for nonverbal responses to pain. Administer analgesics as ordered. Utilize nonpharmacological methods of relief. Provide diversionary activities as needed. See Nursing Care Plan for The Child in Pain (p. 525).
C. Potential constipation related to presence of abdominal tumor. Clinical manifestations: Abdominal discomfort; no stool; firm abdomen; dry hard stool.	Child has soft, formed stools.	Obtain child's baseline stool pattern. Observe stools and note color, amount and consistency. Encourage oral fluids and roughage. Administer stool softeners as ordered.

weight. Technically, high blood pressure, or hypertension, is defined as a blood pressure over 2 standard deviations above the mean for the age in question. For a child of 5 years of age, the upper limit of normal is 112/78.

The two basic categories of hypertension are borderline hypertension and definite hypertension. Patients with blood pressure over 140/90 are said to have definite hypertension. Patients with blood pressure elevated for age but less than 140/90 have borderline hypertension. Thus a 5-year-old with a blood pressure of 125/82 has borderline hypertension.

Investigators are currently collecting data on patients with borderline hypertension. From early studies it appears that these patients rarely have a known underlying cause for their hypertension. Borderline hypertension is thus "essential," or idiopathic, and a diagnostic workup is deemed unnecessary. Dietary salt restriction may be recommended for control of borderline hypertension. Use of antihypertensive drugs in these patients is controversial. Long-term followup is recommended.

Children with definite hypertension usually have an underlying disease causing the hypertension. The most common cause of hypertension in children is renal disease. Renal tumors, renal vascular disease, hydronephrosis, and glomerulonephritis can cause hypertension. Occasionally, excessive secretion of catecholamines or aldosterone by a tumor can cause hypertension in a child.

Careful diagnostic workups are mandatory in children with definite hypertension.

Patients with definite hypertension tend to develop target organ disease. Congestive heart failure can occur. Blood vessels can also be damaged. Children with severe hypertension—blood pressure over 160/110—can suddenly develop hypertensive encephalopathy. Common signs and symptoms are headache, visual disturbance, tinnitus, seizures, and coma. In typical cases the neurologic problem is reversible; occasionally, a stroke may occur. Sometimes hemorrhages, exudates, and arterial spasm can be viewed in the retinal vessels with an ophthalmoscope. These changes are called hypertensive retinopathy. Severe symptomatic hypertension is a medical emergency requiring prompt treatment.

Treatment of hypertension depends on its cause. Tumors should be surgically excised. Renal artery stenosis can be corrected by angioplasty or surgery. In other cases, medications are effective. Propranolol (Inderal), hydralazine (Apresoline), and diazoxide (Hyperstat) are commonly used. Diuretics also help lower blood pressure. Newer agents such as captopril (Capoten) and minoxidil (Loniten) are helpful in severe hypertension. The patient must be carefully monitored for adverse side effects. Aggressive medical management is important in an effort to lower the risk of stroke and other types of vascular injury.

Preschool child

Nephrotic syndrome of childhood (minimal change nephrotic syndrome). Nephrotic syndrome is a chronic renal disease characterized by anasarca (severe generalized edema), heavy proteinuria, low serum albumin levels, and high serum cholesterol values.

Etiologic factors. In 80% of children with nephrotic syndrome, the renal biopsy shows only a minimum of abnormalities. This disease is also called lipoid nephrosis, idiopathic nephrotic syndrome of childhood, or minimal change nephrotic syndrome. In these patients the cause of nephrotic syndrome is unknown. In the remaining 20%, renal biopsies may show abnormalities such as glomerulonephritis.

Incidence. Minimal change nephrotic syndrome is more common in boys than in girls and occurs most frequently between 2 and 6 years of age. The incidence of nephrotic syndrome in childhood is 7 per 100,000.

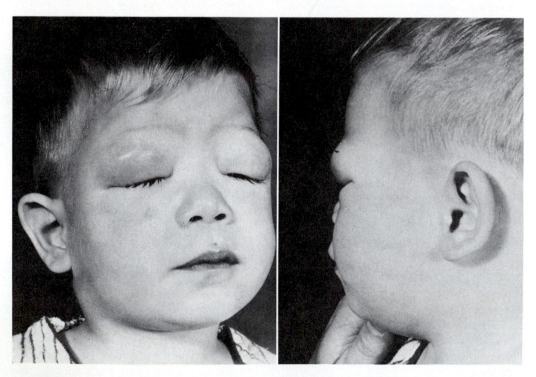

FIG 34-4 Two-year-old child with nephrotic syndrome. Progressive periorbital edema. *(Courtesy Naval Hospital, San Diego, Calif.)*

Clinical symptoms. Onset of nephrotic syndrome is insidious. Periorbital puffiness may be the first sign. In severe cases, it progresses steadily until the eyes are closed (Fig. 34-4). As the edema increases, the arms, legs, and abdomen may reach massive proportions. At the peak of the edema, the child can weigh almost twice as much as normally (Fig. 34-5). Anorexia and varying degrees of diarrhea are commonly found. Discomfort from massive edema causes the child to be irritable and easily fatigued. Anasarca can lead to inadequate ventilation. Gross hematuria and hypertension are unusual in minimal change nephrotic syndrome and suggest the possibility of glomerulonephritis.

Complications. The nephrotic child is vulnerable to infections, probably because of the loss of gamma globulin in the urine (proteinuria). Bacteremia associated with

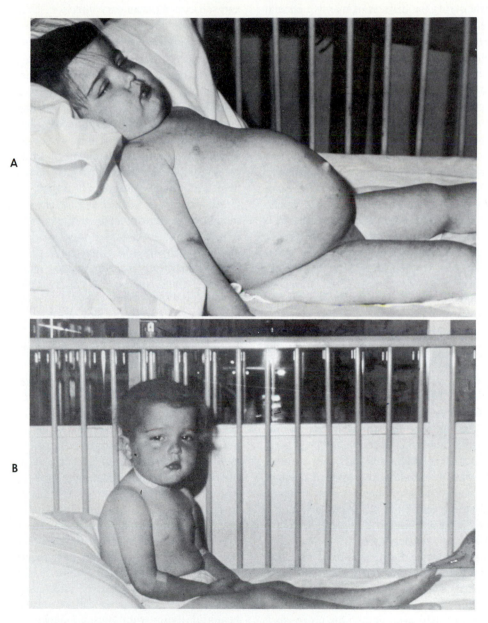

FIG 34-5 Two-and-one-half-year-old child with nephrotic syndrome. **A,** Before therapy. **B,** After therapy. *(Courtesy Naval Hospital, San Diego, Calif.)*

peritonitis is common. Encapsulated organisms such as pneumococci and *Haemophilus influenzae* are frequently identified. Infections are the leading cause of death in patients with minimal change nephrotic syndrome. Hypercoagulability and vascular thrombosis may also occur.

Treatment and nursing care.. The goal of treatment for nephrotic syndrome is a child as nearly normal as possible, judged by both clinical well-being and laboratory findings. The aims of nursing care include comforting the patient during the distress of massive edema, maintaining good nutrition, and preventing intercurrent infections. Edema can be controlled in many patients with a low sodium, fluid-restricted diet. If the edema is severe, intravenous albumin and diuretics may be administered to increase urine production.

Most patients with minimal change nephrotic syndrome respond to steroid therapy. Prednisone, 2 mg/kg/day, reverses the proteinuria, usually by 10 to 14 days. When proteinuria ceases, urine output improves, serum albumin normalizes, and edema disappears. During remission the steroid therapy is gradually withdrawn. Some patients stay in remission on no medication; other patients require maintenance therapy. Maintenance prednisone is usually given every other day to minimize side effects. Alkylating agents such as cyclophosphamide or chlorambucil can produce a prolonged remission in some patients but are not used routinely because of the risks of serious complications.

Relapses of nephrotic syndrome are often associated with intercurrent infections, especially those involving the respiratory and urinary tracts. Immediate intensive antibiotic therapy is mandatory if infection arises.

In selecting a hospital room for the nephrotic child, the nurse must remember the child's increased susceptibility to infection. Placing the child in a double room with another child of the same age who also has nephrotic syndrome is most desirable.

Weighing the child on admission and each morning thereafter is one way of evaluating the amount of edema present. A daily abdominal girth measurement, taken in a flat position at the level of the umbilicus just after a breath is exhaled, is also helpful. If massive edema is present, the child's self-concept is likely to be greatly distorted. It is important for the parents to be reassured and to be given whatever information is necessary about the condition and its outcome so that they in turn can reassure their child. They should particularly realize the seriousness of the disorder, even though the prognosis is better than ever before. Fever or signs of respiratory distress should be reported to the physician.

Massive edema is uncomfortable. The skin is stretched thin and easily broken. Keeping the child's body dry and clean helps prevent skin infections. Application of powder between skin surfaces and in skin folds is soothing and protective. If the child is not toilet-trained, the nurse must take great care to prevent excoriation of the buttocks and genitalia. Medicines are given orally or intravenously but never intramuscularly or subcutaneously. Great care must be taken to protect the edematous skin from injury and subsequent secondary infection. Usually the child is most comfortable in a semi-Fowler's position to reduce respiratory embarrassment. This position can also reduce periorbital edema.

Maintenance of good nutrition is essential because beneath the edema exists a thin, poorly nourished body. The child should be given a well-balanced, high-protein diet. Salty foods such as potato chips and pickles should be avoided. Restriction of fluid intake may be necessary to control edema. Allowing the child some choice encourages appetite and helps prevent severe nutritional depletion, which often readily occurs.

An accurate account of fluid intake is important when the output is scanty. Although the nurse may not be able to measure the exact output, she must record approximate amounts each time the child voids.

Limited activity is recommended until diuresis begins. During the active phase of the disease, the child is usually sluggish and therefore satisfied to rest most of the time. When massive edema is present, the child is content to rest all the time.

After discharge from the hospital, the child is periodically examined until the prednisone is gradually discontinued. Although infection is a common complication in these children while they are receiving prednisone, it is not necessary to interfere with their normal home and school activities. If an outbreak of an infectious disease such as chickenpox (varicella) should occur at school, it is wise to have the child remain at home. Any sign of intercurrent infection must be reported to the physician and treated immediately.

Prognosis. By controlling infection, antibiotic therapy has greatly reduced the death rate of these patients to <1%. About 90% of the children respond to steroid therapy. Many of the children have recurrent episodes of nephrotic syndrome. Each episode usually resolves with steroid treatment. Eventually, after many years of intermittent treatment, these children usually fully enjoy healthful living with normal kidneys and absence of medication. Progression to end-stage renal disease is unusual in minimal change nephrotic syndrome.

NURSING CARE PLAN

The Child with Nephrotic Syndrome

Selected nursing diagnoses	Expected outcomes	Interventions
A. Fluid volume excess (extravascular) related to depletion of serum protein. Clinical manifestations: Increased weight gain, pitting edema, firm and distended abdomen, edematous scrotum/labia, periorbital edema, respiratory distress.	Child regains and maintains fluid and electrolyte balance.	Asses child for presence of edema. Measure abdominal girth daily (same level and position). Maintain strict I & O (provide intake volume equal to output or as ordered by physician.) Weigh child daily (same time and scale). Check each void for specific gravity and for protein. Restrict salt and/or nutritional intake as ordered. Monitor BP and IV albumin and Lasix/diuretics as ordered and child's response to diuretic therapy. Monitor serum electrolytes daily.
B. Potential for infection related to bedrest, fluid excess; decreased immune response (from steroid therapy). Clinical manifestations: Fever, increase respiratory and heart rate, anorexia, abdominal pain, vomiting, diarrhea.	Child does not develop infection. Child shows no evidence of skin breakdown.	Place child in room with noninfectious children. Reposition child every 2 hours; cushion bony prominences and support edematous body parts (scrotum). Provide good oral hygiene and skin care. Utilize egg crate mattress. Bathe and dry skin carefully. Promote well-balanced "renal" diet. Observe child for signs of peritonitis (increased abdomen distention, pain, rigidity, vomiting and/or diarrhea). Monitor IV antibiotics (REMEMBER: LIMITED INTAKE!).
C. Altered nutrition: less than body requirements related to anorexia, loss of protein in urine. Clinical manifestations: Poor appetite, proteinuria	Child has sufficient caloric intake to meet growth needs.	Encourage high-calorie, high-protein, low-sodium diet. Allow child to assist with food selection. Offer small, frequent meals and snacks. Make mealtime pleasant and relaxed.

School-age child

Acute glomerulonephritis (nephritis or Bright's disease). Acute glomerulonephritis is an inflammatory disease of the glomeruli affecting both kidneys. The clinical manifestations include gross hematuria, often with cola-colored urine, edema, proteinuria, casts, hypertension, and elevated amounts of nitrogen products in the bloodstream (azotemia).

Etiologic factors. Streptococcal infection is the most common cause of acute glomerulonephritis. The infection precedes the onset of glomerulonephritis by 1 to 3 weeks. Other infectious agents such as pneumococcus, hepatitis virus, or Epstein-Barr virus can also cause acute glomerulonephritis.

Patients with acute glomerulonephritis should be carefully studied to determine the infectious etiology. Since group A streptococcus is the most common cause, streptozyme titer test, antistreptolysin titer test, and direct culture of the pharynx or skin lesions are essential.

Incidence. Glomerulonephritis is common in children, especially between 5 and 10 years of age. It seems to be more common in boys than in girls and is most frequently observed in the late winter months or early spring. This seasonal pattern is related to the peak incidence of streptococcal infections of the upper respiratory tract.

Symptoms. Gross hematuria, proteinuria, edema, periorbital puffiness, hypertension, weakness, pallor, anorexia, headache, nausea, or vomiting may be present. Rarely patients present with congestive heart failure or neurologic problems from hypertension (hypertensive encephalopathy).

Treatment and nursing care. Necessary bed rest is usually welcomed by the child during the acute phase of the disease. Activities can be resumed as soon as gross hematuria has cleared and signs of edema, hypertension, and other urinary abnormalities have subsided.

These children should be separated from other children who have infections (especially of the upper respiratory tract), but complete isolation is not indicated. They should be observed closely for any recurrences of upper respiratory tract infection. Exacerbations rarely occur with new strains of streptococcal organisms. Reinfection by the same nephritogenic strain is generally not possible by virtue of type-specific immunity after infection. Antibiotic therapy is indicated when evidence of infection is present. Long-term prophylactic use of penicillin in the prevention of recurrence of glomerulonephritis is not recommended. Treatment with furosemide diuretics controls edema in most patients. Antihypertensives such as

hydralazine are frequently used. Dialysis is occasionally necessary for severe electrolyte imbalance resulting from renal failure.

Severe renal failure. Severe renal failure is uncommon in children but serious complications of acute glomerulonephritis may occur in some children. When an imbalance of fluids and electrolytes persists, peritoneal dialysis or hemodialysis may be needed to control the uremia.

Prognosis. Acute glomerulonephritis is usually a self-limited condition, and most children recover completely. A few children present a more complex entity with persistent urinary abnormalities and hypertension, which ultimately results in chronic glomerulonephritis.

Chronic glomerulonephritis. Chronic glomerulonephritis is a major cause of chronic kidney failure in children. There are many causes of chronic glomerulonephritis. Systemic infections, hereditary diseases, drugs, and toxins are known causes. Renal biopsy can be helpful in defining the type and the prognosis of nephritis.

Gross hematuria, edema, severe hypertension, and anemia may be initial symptoms. The majority of untreated patients develop chronic renal failure and end-stage renal disease. The onset of end-stage renal disease varies in length from a few months to 10 to 20 years.

Treatment and nursing care. In general, chronic glomerulonephritis is difficult to treat; the nephrotic syndrome associated with chronic glomerulonephritis does not resolve with oral prednisone therapy. However, recent studies have shown that some forms of glomerulonephritis can be improved with new treatments. Removal of blood plasma, performed by an automated plasma exchange, can improve the conditions of certain patients. High-dose steroid therapy—methylprednisolone (Solu-Medrol) 30 mg/kg—given intravenously can also improve renal function. Sometimes treatments to reverse the destructive inflammation in the kidney are unsuccessful. These patients develop end-stage renal disease and require kidney transplants or dialysis.

Patients with chronic glomerulonephritis may be hospitalized for a course of treatment or for complications. They should be watched closely for hypertension. Daily weights are critical for estimating fluid balance. Frequently these children are anxious and benefit greatly from kind and understanding nursing care. Exposure to infectious illnesses should be avoided.

Acute renal failure. Acute, or temporary, renal failure can be caused by shock (acute tubular necrosis), toxins (such as aminoglycoside antibiotics or heavy metals), glomerulonephritis, or hemolytic uremic syndrome.

Hemolytic uremic syndrome is the most common form of acute renal failure to affect previously well children. Patients have a prodromal illness of vomiting and diarrhea, which is often bloody. The illness progresses quickly to severe hemolytic anemia, renal failure, thrombocytopenia and neurologic problems.

Recent studies have shown that hemolytic uremic syndrome is caused by the common bacteria *Escherichia coli*. Some strains of this bacteria are capable of producing a powerful toxin, called *verotoxin,* which is thought to cause the disease. Young children are susceptible to the illness if they lack immunity to the toxin. The outlook for children with acute renal failure is good. In most cases renal failure will resolve if good supportive care is provided.

Treatment and nursing care. Treatment for acute renal failure consists in specific correction of electrolyte imbalances. Hyperkalemia, which can cause dangerous and even fatal arrhythmias, can be treated with Kayexalate. Infusion of sodium bicarbonate, glucose, and insulin can be used to control hyperkalemia in an emergency situation. Acidosis is treated with sodium bicarbonate. Hyperphosphatemia can be treated with oral phosphate-binding agents such as calcium carbonate and aluminum hydroxide. Hypocalcemia is corrected by oral and sometimes intravenous calcium administration. Supplemental vitamin D is frequently required.

Fluid overload can cause congestive heart failure. Dialysis can be used to correct fluid overload and electrolyte imbalance. Both peritoneal dialysis and hemodialysis can be safely performed in children.

Hypertension can be a serious problem in children with renal failure. Accurate measurement of the blood pressure should be performed frequently with an appropriate size cuff that covers at least two thirds of the upper arm. Oral and intravenous antihypertensive medications may be required.

Infection and neurologic problems are common complications in renal patients. Fever should be promptly reported to the physician. Any changes in mental status should also be recorded and reported. Patients are at risk to have seizures from a variety of causes including hypocalcemia, hyponatremia, hypernatremia, hyperglycemia, hypoglycemia, and uremia. Hypertensive encephalopathy may also occur in these patients.

A restricted diet is frequently prescribed to help control hyperphosphatemia and hyperkalemia. Protein intake is adjusted on an individual basis depending upon the particular needs of the patient. Sodium restriction is frequently prescribed.

End-stage renal disease. The term end-stage renal disease refers to patients with severe failure of kidney function. This occurs when kidney function, as measured by creatinine clearance, is less than 10% of normal. It may be caused by congenital defects, toxins, glomerulonephritis, obstruction of the urinary tract, and pyelonephritis. Renal dialysis is necessary before the patient deteriorates from end-stage renal disease.

Patients with severe uremia are lethargic and anorexic. Confusion, seizures, and coma may also be observed. Pallor caused by anemia is often notable. Growth retardation is common.

Treatment and nursing care. There are three treatments for patients with end-stage renal disease: renal transplantation, peritoneal dialysis, and hemodialysis. Renal transplantation is the best treatment for children. Although the child's immune system may try to reject the transplant, steroids and cyclosporine (Sandimmune) usually reverse rejection. Home peritoneal dialysis is successful when intelligent, conscientious parents are involved. Children with severe renal failure can survive for many years. Almost all these patients attend school and participate in normal activities, with the possible exception of strenuous physical exercise. Nursing care for these patients is rewarding and challenging. Dialysis patients require special diets that are restricted in potassium, sodium, phosphorus, and protein.

Enuresis. Enuresis is defined as involuntary voiding of urine, occurring especially at night (nocturnal enuresis), after the child is 4 years of age. However, a wide age range is associated with the neuromuscular maturation of urinary sphincter control. Children with nocturnal enuresis usually have a normal urinary stream and good daytime bladder control. Enuresis can be primary or acquired. When bladder control has never been achieved, enuresis is said to be primary. If enuresis occurs after control has been achieved for at least 1 year, it is said to be acquired.

About 15% of pediatric patients are evaluated because of this disturbance. Enuresis is very common in childhood, and the condition is more prevalent in boys than in girls.

The exact cause of enuresis in most children is unknown. Psychologic or developmental disorders are found in some patients, but enuresis is also caused by an anatomic defect or a systemic disease. The most significant step toward solving the problem is an attempt to find the correct cause. Before a psychologic explanation is sought, anatomic abnormalities and organic disease must be ruled out.

Generally daytime wetting (diurnal enuresis) and other urologic symptoms are associated with organic disease. Diabetes mellitus, urinary tract infection, urinary tract anomalies, neurologic defects, and obstructions such as meatal stenosis are often responsible for the condition. Psychologic problems also account for some cases of enuresis. Improper toilet training, an unhappy environment, a poor parent-child relationship, immaturity associated with other infantile habits, and developmental disturbances such as jealousy and insecurity are examples of psychologic causes of enuresis. Whatever the cause, the correction of enuresis is highly important to both these children and their parents. It enables children to develop normally and to be like their friends, and it offers the parents peace of mind and a healthy child.

Every enuretic patient should have a careful medical history and physical examination performed to determine if renal enlargements, a distended bladder, a constriction of the external urinary meatus, or a neurologic change is present. An extremely careful urinalysis and urine culture are essential. Intravenous urography, cystography, and cystoscopy are sometimes necessary to diagnose organic causes but are unnecessary if the child has simple nocturnal enuresis without daytime symptoms and if the history and physical examinations are otherwise within normal limits.

Imipramine hydrochloride (Tofranil) controls the condition completely in some patients. This drug, however, has some potential toxic manifestations. Therefore a physician must carefully evaluate the problem before ordering imipramine hydrochloride, and if it is indicated, the child must be carefully watched for side effects such as facial tics, nightmares, and belligerent behavior. Large overdoses can prove fatal. Recently introduced for the treatment of nocturnal enuresis is DDAVP (Desmopressin) an antidiuretic hormone analogue administered as a nightly nasal spray. DDAVP reduces the volume of urine.

A condition often confused with enuresis is the presence in a girl of an ectopic ureter, which empties into the vagina or urethra beyond the sphincter. These children may void normally (from their normal ureters and bladder) but are always wet from constant drainage from the ectopic ureter. Surgery can correct this problem.

Enuresis may also diminish through the use of fairly simple techniques. Giving less fluids in the evening is helpful to a few children. Waking children and taking them to the toilet during the night saves embarrassment to school-age children.

Some children, principally those who have deep sleep patterns, benefit from the use of mechanical devices that wake them with lights or alarms when the bed becomes wet. Consistent use of these detectors and the associated programs recommended encourage lighter sleep, more awareness of bladder filling, and fewer accidents.

Parents should not threaten or punish their children because they wet the bed. This only increases the child's sense of inferiority and failure and can even deter the will to improve. Instead, every effort should be made to assure children that they can overcome the condition if they really want to. Encouragement comes in the form of rewards (for example, being allowed to go camping or sleep overnight at grandmother's house). Such rewards, together with the child's desire to stay dry, can achieve positive results. Enuretic children without any organic disease or severe psychologic problem usually gradually overcome the condition by age 10 to 12 years.

Torsion of the testicle. Contraction of the cremaster muscle not only elevates the testis but rotates it. Depending on the degree of twisting, torsion of the spermatic cord usually causes severe scrotal pain as the result of an interruption of the blood supply and ensuing necrosis of the testis. Torsion can occur at any age and is not uncommon in the adolescent. It can occur while sleeping, playing games, or jumping into cold water. Torsion of the testicle occurs in patients who have failure of fixation of the testicle to the bottom of the scrotum. The failure of fixation is usually bilateral.

Torsion is an acute emergency. Hope of saving the testicle depends on prompt diagnosis and immediate reduction by manipulative procedures or surgery. Isotope scans to determine blood flow to the testis are most useful diagnostic tools. Sonograms are very helpful in differential diagnosis to rule out acute epididymitis and tumor. If surgery is performed bilateral orchiopexy should be accomplished to prevent a future torsion of the opposite side.

Key Concepts

1. The urinary system consists of two kidneys, two ureters, the bladder, and the urethra. To regulate the composition of blood, the kidneys perform the complex task of producing urine. The ureters, bladder, and urethra are involved in the transportation, storage, and elimination of the urine.

2. Signs of genitourinary problems in infants include failure to void within 24 hours after birth, abdominal enlargement or swelling in the area of the kidney, and a scant urinary stream. In older children, signs include crying on urination, urgent and frequent urination, straining to void, and dribbling.

3. Hypospadias is a common deformity in which the urethra terminates at some point on the undersurface of the penis. Surgical repair is usually accomplished at about 1 year of age.

4. Cryptorchidism, testicular maldescent, is associated with an increased incidence of testicular injury and torsion. It may also be associated with infertility and possibly predispose the child to malignancies. If the testes do not descend spontaneously or in response to hCG, surgical correction is indicated.

5. Possible signs of a urinary tract infection in children under 3 years are high temperature, pallor, anorexia, vomiting, diarrhea, and convulsions. Older children experience sharp or dull flank pain, gross hematuria, or pyuria. Frequent, urgent, and burning urination are common complaints.

6. Urinalysis and a culture of a properly collected specimen are the key to successful treatment of a urinary tract infection. Therapy depends primarily on identification of the causative organism.

7. Vesicoureteral reflux is caused by anatomic defects in the urinary tract or by infection. Patients with anatomic defects often require surgery. Long-term antibiotic therapy may be effective when the condition is caused by infection.

8. Wilms' tumor is one of the most common abdominal neoplasms of childhood. The initial manifestation is a mass in the region of the kidney. Constipation, vomiting, abdominal distention, and even dyspnea can occur. Treatment usually consists of prompt radical nephrectomy, followed by chemotherapy.

9. The most common cause of definite hypertension in children is renal disease. Renal tumors, renal vascular disease, hydronephrosis, and glomerulonephritis can cause hypertension. Treatment depends on the cause.

10. Nephrotic syndrome is a chronic renal disease characterized by anasarca, heavy proteinuria, low serum albumin levels, and high serum cholesterol values. The aims of nursing care include comforting the patient during the distress of massive edema, maintaining good nutrition, and preventing intercurrent infections.

11. Acute glomerulonephritis is an inflammatory disease of the glomeruli affecting both kidneys. Clinical manifestations include gross hematuria, often with cola-colored urine, edema, proteinuria, casts, hypertension, and azotemia. Antibiotic therapy is indicated when evidence of infection is present. Nursing care includes providing bed rest, limiting activities, and protecting the child from infection.

12. Enuresis is defined as involuntary voiding of urine, and is very common in childhood. The condition may be caused by psychologic or developmental disorders, an anatomic defect, or a systemic disease. Treatment depends on the cause.

Discussion Questions

1. How do the structures and functions of the genitourinary tract of the infant and child differ from those of the adult? Identify some of the commonly occurring abnormalities of the genitourinary tract. What can be done in these conditions?

2. Why are urinary tract infections particularly common in infants and young children? Are they more common in boys or girls? Why is this the case? What can the nurse do to reduce the incidence of urinary tract infections?

3. Which renal diseases result in hypertension? How can you assess the blood pressure of an infant or young child? Discuss the two types of hypertension in children.

4. Streptococcal infections such as strep throat are common in childhood. What serious conditions can occur as a result of an untreated group A beta-hemolytic streptococcal infection? (You will also want to refer to Chap. 32.)

5. Nephritis and nephrotic syndromes affect the functioning of the kidneys. How do their clinical manifestations differ? What special nursing measures are instituted? What special precautions should you take in providing care to children with severe kidney involvement?

UNIT
IX

SUGGESTED SELECTED READINGS AND REFERENCES

Conditions involving the neuromuscular and skeletal system

Barker E and Higgins R: Managing a suspected spinal cord injury, Nursing '89 19(4):52, 1989.

Burgess KE: Increased ICP, Nurs Life 5(2):33, 1985.

Cohen FL: Neural tube defects: epidemiology, detection, and prevention, J Obstet Gynecol Neonatal Nurs 16(2):105, 1987.

DiChiara E: A sound method for testing children's hearing, Am J Nurs 84(9):1104, 1985.

Fode NC: Subarachnoid hemorrhage from ruptured intracranial aneurysm, Am J Nurs 88(5):674, 1988.

Geraniotis E, Koff SA, and Enrile B: The prophylactic use of clean intermittent catheterization in the treatment of infants and young children with myelomeningocele and neurogenic bladder dysfunction, J Urol 139(1):85, 1988.

Henneman EA: Brain resuscitation, Heart Lung 15(1):3, 1986.

Joseph B and others: Clean, intermittent catheterization of infants with neurogenic bladder, Pediatrics 84(1):78, 1989.

Joy C: Pediatric cerebral resuscitation, Crit Care Nurs Clin North Am 1(1):181, 1989.

Keen TP: Nursing care of the pediatric multitrauma patient, Nurs Clin North Am 25(1):131, 1990.

Kotecki J and others: The miracle of little Carlos (pediatric head injury), Nursing '90 20(5):52, 1990.

McCash AM: Controlling ICP after a craniotomy, RN 48(6):23, 1985.

Reilly AN and others: Head trauma in children: the stages to cognitive recovery, MCN 12(6):405, 1987.

Reimer M: Head-injured patients: how to detect early signs of trouble, Nursing '89 19(3):34, 1989.

Richardson K and others: Biofeedback therapy for managing bowel incontinence caused by meningomyelocele, MCN 10(6):388, 1985.

Scherer P: Assessment: the logic of coma, Am J Nurs 86(5):541, 1986.

Steffee DR, Suty KA, and Delcalzo P: More than a touch: communicating with a deaf and blind patient, MCN 15(4):36, 1985.

Sullivan J: Brain resuscitation: nursing interventions, Crit Care Nurs Clin North Am 1(1):155, 1989.

Tackenberg JN: Treatment for ICP barbituate coma, Nursing '89 19(3):32R, 1989.

Watkins S, Moore TH, and Phillips J: Clearing impacted ears, Am J Nurs 84(9):1107, 1985.

Wong D: Changing what children hear in the ICU can lower intracranial pressure, Am J Nurs 88(3):279, 1988.

Eye, ear, and throat

Barker-Stotts K: Action stat! Hyphema, Nursing '88 18(12):12, 1988.

Bluestone CD: Modern management of otitis media, Pediatr Clin North Am 36(6):1371, 1989.

Brodsky L: Modern assessment of tonsils and adenoids, Pediatr Clin North Am 36(6):1551, 1989.

Catalano JD: Strabismus, Pediatr Ann 19(5):289, 1990.

Friedman EM: Caustic infections and foreign bodies in the aerodigestive tract of children, Pediatr Clin North Am 36(6):1403, 1989.

Stager DR, Birch EE, and Weakley DR: Amblyopia and the pediatrician, Pediatr Ann 19(5):301, 1990.

Orthopedics

Alderman C: Outside fixation, Nurs Stand 3(12):24, 1988.

Bailey-Allen AM: Care plans, Orthop Nurs 7(3):51, 1988.

Button S: Rotation plasty for childhood osteosarcoma, Nurs Times 83(22):49, 1987.

Greipp ME: Anthropometric considerations in the orthopaedic assessment, Orthop Nurs 7(4):36, 1988.

Helmer FT and Halbert N: The development of a patient classification system for pediatric orthopaedic units—a case study, Orthop Nurs 6(6):32, 1987.

Johnson JB and Killman-Young J: Adolescence, anxiety, and adaptation: preparing for posterior spine fusion with instrumentation, J Pediatr Nurs 3(5):348, 1988.

Osborne LJ and DiGiacomo I: Traction: a review with nursing diagnoses and interventions, Orthop Nurs 6(4):13, 1987.

Swagman A: Caring for limb-deficient children and their families, MCN 11(1):46, 1986.

Conditions involving the integumentary system

Burns

Amon L: Updating the management of the burned child. Part II, Nurs Res 4(9):30, 1989.

Atchison N, Guercio P, and Monaco C: Pain in the pediatric burn patient: nursing assessment and perception, Issues Comp Pediatr Nurs 9(6):399, 1986.

Cunningham JJ, Harris LJ, and Briggs SE: Nutritional support of the severely burned infant, Nutr Clin Prac 3(2):69, 1988.

Dyer C and Roberts D: Thermal trauma, Nurs Clin North Am 25(1):85, 1990.

Forshaw A: Dispensary of hope, Nurs Times 83(46)28, 1987.

Forshaw A: Spotlight on children. Burns and aftercare, Nurs Times 83(1):51, 1987.

Garvin G: Wound healing in pediatrics, Pediatr Clin North Am 25(1):181, 1990.

Martin LM: Nursing implications of today's burn care techniques, RN 52(5):26, 1989.

Mikhail JN: Acute burn care: an update, J Emerg Nurs 14(1):9, 1988.

O'Neil CE, Hutsler D, and Hildreth MA: Basic nutritional guidelines for pediatric burn patients, J Burn Care Rehabil 10(3):278, 1989.

Wallace L: Abandoned to a "social death"? Nurs Times 84(10):34, 1988.

Common skin problems

Castiglia PT: Acne, J Pediatr Health Care 3(5):259, 1989.

Clore ER: Dispelling the common myths about pediculosis, J Pediatr Health Care 3(1):28, 1989.

Coody D: There is no such thing as a good tan, J Pediatr Health Care 1(3):125, 1987.

New technology: zapping port-wine stains, Nurs Life 6(1):17: 1986.

Nicol NH: Atopic dermatitis: the (wet) wrap-up, Am J Nurs 87(12):1560, 1987.

Putnam CD and Reynolds MS: Mupirocin: a new topical therapy for impetigo, Pediatr Health Care 3(4):224, 1989.

Quan Mand Strick RA: Management of acne vulgaris, Am Fam Physician 38(2):207, 1988.

Schmitt D: Lina had lost her looks and her will to live, Nurs '89 19(7):43, 1989.

Strohecker BA and others: Soft tissue expansion: plastic surgery takes a giant leap forward with this new skin-generating technique, Am J Nurse 88(5):668, 1988.

Isolation precautions and communicable diseases

Ando Y and others: Bottle feeding can prevent transmission of HTLV-1 from mothers to their babies, J Infect 19(1):25, 1989.

Bentler M and Stanish M: Nutrition support of the pediatric patient with AIDS, J Am Diet Assoc 87(4):488, 1987.

Castle M and Ajemian E: Hospital infection control, Somerset, NJ, 1987, John Wiley & Sons Inc.

Centers for Disease Control: Acquired immunodeficiency syndrome—United States, update 1989, MMWR 39(5):81, 1990.

Centers for Disease Control: Mumps—United States 1985-1988, MMWR 38(7):101, 1989.

Centers for Disease Control: Pertussis surveillance—United States, 1986-1988, MMWR 39(4):57, 1990.

Centers for Disease Control: Protection against viral hepatitis (ACIP), MMWR 39(RR-2):1, 1990.

Centers for Disease Control: Update: Tuberculosis elimination United States, MMWR 39(10):153, 1990.

Engel NS: Multiple drug therapy for pediatric tuberculosis, MCN 14(3):169, 1989.

Garrett JE: The AIDS patient: helping him cope and his parents cope, Nursing '88 18(9):50, 1988.

Grabbe LL and Brown LB: Identifying neurologic complications of AIDS, Nursing '89 19(5):66, 1989.

Grimes DE and Woolbert LF: Measles outbreaks: Who are at risk and why? J Pediatr Health Care 3(4):187, 1989.

Hamilton D: For A.I.D.S. patients, little things can mean a lot, Nursing '88 18(5):61, 1988.

Harrison L and others: Establishing and evaluating a children's sick room program, MCN 12(3):204, 1987.

Henderson, D: HIV infection: risks to health care workers and infection control, Nurs Clin North Am 23(4):767, 1988.

Ivey FD and Gerner HM: Adults do get chickenpox, Am J Nurs 87(12):1658, 1987.

Jackson MM: Infection prevention and control for HIV and other infectious agents in obstetric, gynecologic and neonatal settings, NAACOG Clin Issues 1(1):115, 1990.

Jager H: AIDS and AIDS-risk patient care, Somerset, NJ, 1988 John Wiley & Sons, Inc.

Kobert LJ: Are universal precautions changing the "nurture of obstetric nursing?" Am J Nurs 89(12):1609, 1989.

Kuhn JP: CT of the body in children, Pediatr Ann 15(5):367, 1986.

Lancaster E: Tuberculosis on the rise, Am J Nurs 88(4):485, 1988.

Laufman JK: Dilemmas in practice: AIDS, ethics and truth, Am J Nurs 89(7):924, 1989.

Lewis A: Nursing care of the person with AIDS, Rockville, Md, 1988 Aspen Publishers.

Madsen L: Tuberculosis today, RN 53(3):44, 1990.

McArthur J: AIDS dementia, your assessment can make all the difference, RN 53(3):36, 1990.

McConnell EA: What's safe to reuse? What's not?, Nursing '89 19(2):104, 1989.

Mettina SM: When patients with genital herpes turn to you for answers, Nursing '89 19(8):61, 1989.

Mitchel C and Smith L: If it's AIDS, please don't tell, Am J Nurs 87(7):911, 1987.

Molavi A: Pentamidine for the prevention and treatment of P. carinii pneumonia, Am Fam Physician 40(1):195, 1989.

Nattina SL: Syphilis, a new look at an old killer, Am J Nurs 90(4):68, 1990.

Pace NL: Combating the hidden epidemic: chlamydia, Nursing '89 19(4):32Z, 1989.

Peter G and others, editors: Report of the Committee on Infectious Diseases, ed 21, Elk Grove, Ill, 1988 American Academy of Pediatrics.

Sealander JY and Kerr CP: Herpes simplex of the nipple: infant to mother transmission, Am Fam Physician 39(3):111, 1989.

Shubin S: Caring for AIDS patients: the stress will be on you, Nursing '89 19(10):43, 1989.

Spies C: Should hospital patients be screened for AIDS? Nursing '88 18(2):49, 1988.

Tying and untying a surgical mask, Nursing '89, 19(7):65, 1989.

Ward-Wimmer D: Nursing care of children with HIV infection, Nurs Clin North Am 24(4):719, 1988.

Woodland DG, Larson J, and Hudson L: Screening for chlamydia trachomatis at a university health service, J Obst Gynecol Neonatal Nurs 18(2):145, 1989.

Conditions involving the respiratory and circulatory systems

Blue CL: Exercise induced asthma: the "silent asthma," J Pediatr Health Care 2(4):167, 1988.

Bone RD and others: The use of continuous infusion of factor concentrates in the treatment of hemophilia, Am J Hematol 32(1):8, 1989.

Bussel JB: Thrombocytopenia in newborns, infants and children, Pediatr Ann 19(3):181, 1990.

Catchpole A: Cystic fibrosis: intravenous treatment at home, Nurs Times 85(12):40, 1989.

Cohen MR: Action stat! Drug induced anaphylaxis, Nursing '85 15(2):43, 1985.

Everett D: For a child with pneumonia, there's no place like home, RN 53(3):85, 1990.

Goldson E: Bronchopulmonary dysplasia, Pediatr Ann 19(1):13, 1990.

Gregory-Addesa G: Helping your patient when nausea goes with the treatment, RN 49(4):43, 1986.

Hayman LL and others: Reducing risk for heart disease in children, MCN 13(6):442, 1988.

Hill MN and Cunningham SL: The latest words for high BP, Am J Nurs 89(4):504, 1989.

Huston CJ: Action stat! Epiglottitis, Nursing '88(4):59, 1988.

Kemp JP and Meltzer EO: Gaining control of the allergic child's environment, Pediatric Ann 18(12):801, 1989.

Lungmuss F: Meningitis and epiglottitis: a new immunization against haemophilus influenzae type b infections, Health Visitor 62(6):179, 1989.

MacMullen NJ and Brucker MC: Pregnancy made possible for women with cystic fibrosis, MCN 14(3):196, 1989.

McWilliams B, Kelly HW, and Murphy S: Management of acute severe asthma, Pediatr Ann 18(12):774, 1989.

Nederhand KC and others: Respiratory syncytial virus: a nursing perspective, Pediatr Nurs 15(4):342, 1989.

Nemes J, Schmidt E, and Kelly L: Epiglottitis: ED nursing management, J Emerg Nurs 14(2):70, 1988.

Sheahan SL: Chlamydia trachomatis infections: a health problem of infants, J Pediatr Health Care, 3(3):144, 1989.

Taylor B: Coughs and colds in children, Health Visitor 61(10):313, 1988.

Congenital heart disease

Friedman WF: Congenital heart disease in infancy and childhood, In Braunwald E, editor: Heart disease, Philadelphia, 1988, WB Saunders Co.

Hoffman JI: Congenital heart disease, Pediatr Clin North Am 37(1):25, 1990.

Pinsky WW and Arciniegas E: Tetrology of Fallot, Pediatr Clin North Am 37(1):179, 1990.

Radtke W and Lock J: Balloon dilation, Pediatr Clinics North Am 37(1):193, 1990.

Rotondi P, guest editor: Neonatal and pediatric cardiovascular nursing, Critical Care Nursing Clin North Am 1(2):195, 1989.

Cancer

Mitchell AD: Management of infections in the neutropenic child with cancer, Pediatr Ann 17(11):677, 1988.

Schlesselmann SM: Helping your cancer patient cope with alopecia, Nursing '88 18(12):43, 1988.

Suderman JR: Pain relief during routine procedures for children with leukemia, MCN 15(3):163, 1990.

Wickham RS: Advances in venous access devices and management strategies, Nurs Clin North Am 25(2):345, 1990.

Yeager AM: Bone marrow transplantation in children, Pediatr Ann 17(11):694, 1988.

Conditions involving digestion and associated metabolism

Aquilina SS: Gastroesophageal reflux problem or nuisance? J Pediatr Health Care 1(5):233, 1987.

Arnold WC: Parenteral nutrition, and fluid and electrolyte therapy, Pediatr Clin North Am 37(2):449, 1990.

Dedinsky GK and others: Complications and reoperation after Nissen fundoplication in childhood, Am J Surg 153(2):177, 1987.

Dick GE: Chest wall deformities in children, Pediatr Ann 18(3):161, 1989.

Englest DM and Guillory JA: For want of lactase . . . , Am J Nurs 86(8):902, 1986.

Harberg HJ: The acute abdomen in childhood, Pediatr Ann 18(3):169, 1989.

Hill LL: Body composition, normal electrolyte concentrations, and the maintenance of normal volume, tonicity, and acid-base metabolism, Pediatr Clin North Am 37(2):241, 1990.

Kallen RJ: The management of diarrheal dehydration in infants using parenteral fluids, Pediatr Clin North Am 37(2):265, 1990.

Katzman EM: What's the most common helminth infection in the U.S.? MCN 14(3):193, 1989.

Moore CC: Congenital gastric outlet obstruction, J Pediatr Surg 24(12):1241, 1989.

Stringel G and others: Gastrostomy and Nissen fundoplication in neurologically impaired children, J Pediatr Surg 24(10):1044, 1989.

Stroh SE, Stern HP, and McCarthy SG: Fecal incontinence in children: a clinical update, MCN 14(4):252, 1989.

Tunell WP: Gastroesophageal reflux in childhood, Pediatr Ann 18(3):192, 1989.

Diabetes

Anderson KM: Feeding practices for infants and young children with diabetes mellitus, J Pediatr Perinatal Nutr 2(1):1, 1988.

Crowe L and Billingsley JI: The rowdy reactors: maintaining a support group for teenagers with diabetes, Diabetes Educator 16(1):39, 1990.

Evans BS: The family as a unit in the management of diabetes, Home Healthcare Nurse 6(5):10, 1988.

Frey MA and Denyes MJ: Health and illness self-care in adolescents with IDDM: a test of Orem's theory, Adv in Nurs Science 12(1):67, 1989.

Kupper NS, Foster MB, and MacMillan DR: Treating children with type I diabetes mellitus: choosing an appropriate nutritional treatment strategy, Diabetes Educator 14(3):238, 1988.

Leach D and Erickson GL: Children's perspectives on diabetes, J School Health 58(4):159, 1988.

Lipman TH and others: A developmental approach to diabetes in children: birth through preschool (Part I), MCN 14(4):255, 1989.

Lipman TH and others: A developmental approach to diabetes in children: school age–adolescence (Part II), MCN 14(5):330, 1989.

Sabo CE and Michael SR: Managing D.K.A. and preventing a recurrence, Nursing 19(2):50, 1989.

Conditions involving the genitourinary system

Barry J: Continence. Night-time despair, Nurs Times 84(14):82, 1988.

Campbell JR: Inguinal and scrotal problems in infants and children, Pediatr Ann 18(3):189, 1989.

Dobson P: Continence. Easing childhood shame, Nurs Times 85(33):79, 1989.

Gartland C: Organ transplants. Looking after Jodi, Nurs Times 83(7):24, 1987.

Gibson LY: Bedwetting: a family's recurrent nightmare, MCN 14(4):270, 1989.

Hermann D: The pediatric acute scrotum, Pediatr Ann 18(3):198, 1989.

Hudson K and Hiott K: Coping with pediatric renal transplant rejection, ANNA J 13(5):261, 1986.

Jenkins B and Casbaugh C: Action stat! Testicular torsion, Nursing '89, 19(7):33, 1989.

Regensberg D: Objective: Social continence. Children—incontinent or enuretic? Nurs Res 3(2):31, 1988.

Glossary

KEY TO PRONUNCIATION

ā	āte	ȧ	sofȧ	ē	ēat	ī	"eye"	ō	ōh	ü	boot
ă	ăs	ä	ärm	ĕ	bĕt	ĭ	ĭt	ŏ	nŏt	ū	"you"
ȧ	ȧh			er	(ur)her			ȯ	saw	ŭ	bŭt

abduction (ăb-dŭk′shŭn) Movement away from the midline.

abortion (ȧ-bŏr′shŭn) Termination of a pregnancy before the fetus is sufficiently developed to live; may be spontaneous or induced.

abortus (ȧ-bŏr-tŭs) An aborted fetus (expelled from the uterus before sufficiently developed to live).

abrasion (ă-brā′zhŭn) Loss of superficial tissue, skin, or mucous membrane because of friction.

abruptio (ăb-rŭp′shē-ō) A tearing away from.

abruptio placentae (plȧ-sĕn′tē) Premature separation of a normally implanted placenta.

abscess (ăb′sĕs) Focus of suppuration within a tissue; pocket of pus.

abstinence (ab′stĭ-nents) Going without voluntarily; refraining from sexual intercourse.

acetabulum (ăs-ĕ-tăb′ū-lŭm) Rounded cavity on the external surface of the innominate bone that receives the head of the femur.

acidosis (as-ĭ-dō′sis) Abnormal increase in acidity of the blood and tissues.

acinus (ăs′ĭ-nŭs) (pl. acini) Smallest division of a gland, often referring to the mammary glands.

adenoids (ăd′ĕ-noyds) Grouping of lymphoid tissue located on the posterior wall of the nasopharynx (the pharyngeal tonsils).

adnexa (ăd-nĕx′ȧ) Accessory parts of a structure; uterine adnexa—oviducts and ovaries.

afebrile (ā-fĕb′ril) Without fever.

afibrinogenemia (ā-fī″brĭn-ō-jĕ-nē′mĭ-ȧ) Lack of the protein fibrinogen in the blood, causing problems in coagulation.

aggregate (ăg′grē-gāt) Total substances making up a mass.

airway Normal passageway for respired air or a device used to prevent or correct respiratory obstruction.

albinism (ăl′bĭn-ĭsm) Abnormal but nonpathogenic absence of pigment in skin, hair, and eyes.

albumin (ăl-bū′mĭn) One kind of protein.

albuminuria (ăl-bū′-mĭ-nū′rĭ-ȧ) Presence of albumin in the urine.

alignment (ă-līn′ment) Arranging in a line.

alimentation (ăl-ĭ-mĕn-tā′shŭn) General process of nourishing the body.

alkalosis (ăl″kȧ-lō′sĭs) Abnormal increase of alkalinity of the blood and tissues.

allergen (ăl′er-jĕn) Any substance that produces an allergic response.

alveolus (ăl-vē′ō-lŭs) (pl. alve′oli) Little hollow or cavity; the air sac or cell of the lung tissue.

ambient (ăm′bē-ȧnt) Surrounding.

ambivalence (ăm-bĭv′ȧ-lĕnts) Simultaneous feelings of attraction and repulsion, love and hate for a person, object, or action.

amblyopia (ăm-blĭ-ō′pē-ȧ) Reduction or dimness of vision in one eye without apparent associated organic abnormality.

amenorrhea (ā-mĕn-ō-rē′ȧ) Absence of menstruation.

amnesic (ăm-nē′sĭk) Capable of producing amnesia, or loss of memory.

amniocentesis (ăm′nē-ō-sĕn-tē′sĭs) Puncture of the intra-uterine amniotic sac usually through the abdominal wall to obtain sample of amniotic fluid.

amniotic (ăm-nē-ŏt′ĭk) Pertaining to the amnion, the innermost of the fetal membranes that secretes the fluid inside the bag of waters.

analgesic (ăn′ăl-jē′sĭk) Capable of producing analgesia, or relief from pain.

analogue (ăn′ă-lŏg) One of two organs in different sexes or species that are similar in function but different in structure.

anaphylactic (ăn″ă-fĭ-lăk′tĭk) **shock** Syndrome that occasionally occurs after the reintroduction of a substance (antigen) into a person or animal previously sensitized to it; characterized by circulatory collapse and shock.

anasarca (ăn-ă-sär′ka) Severe generalized edema.

anastomosis (ă-năs′tō-mō′sĭs) Natural or surgical joining of blood or lymph vessels, or a surgically created communication between different hollow organs or parts of the same organs.

ancillary (ăn′sĭ-ler-ē) Subordinate or auxiliary.

android (ăn′droyd) Manlike; adjective used to describe a male-type pelvis.

anemia (an-ē′mē-ă) Condition in which there is a reduction below normal of hemoglobin in the blood.

anencephalic (ăn-ĕn-sĕf′ă-lĭk) Lacking a cerebrum, cerebellum, and part of the cranium.

anesthetic (ăn′ĕs-thĕt′ĭk) Capable of producing anesthesia, that is, complete or partial loss of feeling.

angiocardiography (ăn″jē-ō-cär-dē-ŏg′ră-fē) Injection of contrast material into the pulmonary circulation and observation of its flow by radiography or fluoroscopy.

anion (ăn′ī-ăn) Particle of matter (ion) carrying a negative electrical charge.

ankylosis (ăn-kĭ-lō′sĭs) Abnormal immobility and consolidation of a joint.

anomalies (ă-nŏm′ă-lēz) Deviations from the normal.

anorexia (ăn-ă-rĕk′sē-ă) Loss of appetite.

anovulatory (ăn-ov′ū-lă-tō″rē) Not accompanied by production and discharge of an ovum.

anoxia (ăn-ŏk′sē-ă) Lack of oxygen.

antagonistic (ăn-tăg-ă-nĭs′tĭk) Acting with antagonism, that is, in opposition to an agent or principle; counteracting; hostile.

antenatal (ăn-tē-nā′tăl) Before birth; prenatal.

antepartal (ăn-tē-pär′tăl) Before delivery.

anteroposterior (ăn″tĕr-ō-pŏs-tīr′ē-ur) From front to back.

antiarrhythmic (ăn″tē-ă-rĭth′mĭk) Preventing (or effective against) arrhythmia, or irregular cardiac contractions.

antibody (ăn′tĭ-bŏd-ē) Protective protein substance formed by the body in the presence of pathogenic organisms or foreign materials.

antipyretic (ăn″tĭ-pī-rĕt′ĭk) A substance or procedure which reduces fever usually by lowering the thermoregulating set point in the hypothalamus.

antisepsis (ăn″tĭ-sĕp′sĭs) Literally "against infection or decay"; the use of procedures usually involving chemicals (antiseptics) that hinder the growth of microorganisms without necessarily destroying them.

antitoxin (ăn-tĭ-tŏk′sĭn) Protective protein formed by the body in response to the presence of a toxin; a preparation containing antibodies designed to produce passive immunization.

anuria (ă-nyur′ē-ă) Failure of kidney function; lack of urine formation.

apnea (ăp′nē-ă) Absence of respiration, temporary or permanent.

areola (ă-rē′ō-lă) (pl. areolae) Ring of pigment on the breast surrounding the nipple.

arteriogram (är-tĭr′ē-ō-grăm) X-ray procedure that reveals arterial pathways injected with special contrast materials.

artery (är′ter-ē) Blood vessel that carries blood away from the heart.

arthralgia (ar-thrăl′jĭ-ă) Pain in a joint.

arthritis (är-thrī′tis) Inflammation of a joint, usually accompanied by pain and frequently by changes in structure.

arthrodesis (är″thrŏd-ē′sĭs) Surgical fusion of a joint performed to gain stability for weight bearing.

arthroplasty (är′thrō-plăs-tē) Surgical formation or reconstruction of a joint.

asepsis (ă-sĕp′sĭs) Literally "without infection or decay"; refers to the absence of living disease-producing microorganisms or to procedures that produce such an absence.

asphyxia (ăs-fĭk′sē-ă) Lack of oxygen and excessive carbon dioxide buildup in the body resulting from an abnormal gaseous environment, disease, aspiration etc.; leads to death if uncorrected.

aspirate (also see aspiration.) Noun: that which is obtained by aspiration.

aspiration (ăs-pĭ-rā′shun) Process of drawing in or out as by suction.

assimilation (a-sĭm-ĕ-lā′shun) Processes whereby the products of digestion change to resemble the chemical substances of the body tissues, first passing through the lacteals and blood vessels.

astrocytoma (ăs-trō-sī-tō′ma) Tumor of the brain tissue.

ataxic (ă-tăk′sĭk) Pertaining to ataxia, or the incoordination of the voluntary muscles; one possible result of brain damage.

atelectasis (ăt-ĕ-lĕk′tă-sĭs) Lack of proper lung expansion; collapsed or airless segment of lung.

athetoid (ăth′ĕ-toyd) Pertaining to athetosis, or the presence of involuntary, purposeless weaving motions of the body or its extremities; one possible result of brain damage to the basal ganglia of the brain.

atopic (ā-tŏp′ĭk) Pertaining to allergic responses, particularly those having a hereditary tendency such as asthma.

atresia (à-trē′zhuh) Lack of a normal opening or canal.

atrium (ā′trē-ŭm) (pl. atria) Cavity or sinus; one of two upper chambers of the heart.

atrophy (ăt′rà-fē) Lack of nourishment; wasting or reduction of size of cells, tissues, organs, or regions of the body.

attenuate (à-tĕn′yōō-āt) To weaken the virulence of; to reduce in force; to make thin.

attitude (ăt′ĭ-tüd) In speaking of fetal position, refers to the degree of flexion of the baby's head and extremities in the uterus.

aura (är′à) Subjective warning of an impending epileptic seizure.

auscultation (aws-kŭl-tā′shŭn) Process of listening for sounds produced in some body cavity.

autoclave (aw-tŏ-clāv) Appliance used to sterilize objects by steam under pressure.

autoimmune (ah′tōh-ĭ-mū′n) Production in an organism of antibodies that react against its own tissues, with appearance of certain clinical and laboratory manifestations.

autonomy (aw-tŏn′à-mē) State of self-government or self-direction.

autosomal (aw′tō-sōhm-ŭl) Having the character of a non–sex-determining chromosome.

autosome (äw′tō-sōhm) Any chromosome except sex-determining X and Y.

bacillus (bà-sĭl′ŭs) (pl. bacilli) Rod-shaped bacterium.

barrier techniques Various forms of ways of preventing the spread of infection from one person to another.

basophil (bā′so-fĭl) One type of white blood cell.

bilirubin (bĭl-ĭ-rū′bĭn) Orange or yellow pigment in bile; a product of red blood cell destruction; elevated levels in the blood may cause jaundice.

biopsy (bī′ŏp-sē) Procurement of a specimen of tissue for microscopic examination.

blastocyst (blăs′tō-sĭst) Spherical mass consisting of a central cavity surrounded by a single layer of cells produced by the cleavage of the ovum.

bolus (bō-lŭs) A lump of food ready to be swallowed; a relatively large dose of medication or contrast material given at one time, usually intravenously.

booster injection Substance or dose used to renew or increase the effect of a drug or immunizing agent.

bossing Rounded protuberance, particularly on the skull, in the area of the forehead; one possible manifestation of rickets.

bradycardia (brād″ē-kär′dē-à) Slowness of the heartbeat; in adults, usually a rate of fewer than 60 beats per minute.

Braxton Hicks (brăx′ton hĭks) **contractions** Uterine contractions that occur throughout pregnancy and help enlarge the uterus to accommodate the growing fetus; during the last weeks of pregnancy they may become very noticeable; false labor contractions.

breech (brēch) **birth** Delivery of the child, feet or buttocks first.

bronchiectasis (brŏn-kē-ĕk′tà-sĭs) Abnormal dilatation of the bronchi in response to inflammation, which may lead to structural changes and chronic cough.

buffer Apparatus or substance serving to neutralize the shock of opposing forces.

bulbar (bul′bär) Pertaining to the "bulb," or medulla, of the brain and the cranial nerves.

calcaneus (kăl-kā′nē-ŭs) Heel bone, or os calcis; type of clubfoot in which only the heel touches the ground; patient may walk on inner side of heel.

callus (kăl′ŭs) New bone formation at the site of a healing fracture; also a thickening of the epidermis at sites of pressure or friction.

calyx (ka′lĭks) (pl. calyces) Small subdivision of the pelvis of the kidney.

Candida albicans (kăn′dĭ-dà ăl′bĭ-kănz) Formerly called *Monilia albicans;* a yeastlike fungus that may infect various portions of the body, causing a variety of symptoms (e.g., leukorrhea, dermatitis, stomatitis).

cannula (kăn′ū-là) (pl. cannulae) Small tube; large needle sheath used for insertion into a body cavity or tube.

canthus (kăn-thŭs) (pl. canthi) Corner at each side of the eye where the eyelids meet.

caput succedaneum (kă′pŭt sŭk-sē-dā′nē-ŭm) Abnormal collection of fluid under the scalp.

carbohydrate (kär″bō-hī′drāt) A compound of carbon combined with H_2 and O_2 that supplies heat and energy to the body.

cardiovascular (kär-dē-ō-văs′kūl-är) Pertaining to the heart and blood vessels.

caries (kăr′ēz) Dental decay.

carrier Person or animal capable of transmitting a contagious or hereditary disease but showing no outward sign of the disease.

cast Solid mold usually made of plaster to help protect, position, or immobilize a part; microscopic sediment that has been partially shaped by the kidney tubules; any other body discharge or excretion retaining the shape of a body part that held it.

catalyst (kăt′à-lĭst) Substance that speeds the rate of a chemical reaction without itself being permanently altered by the reaction.

catamenia (kăt-à-mē′nē-à) Menses, or menstruation.

cataract (kăt′à-răkt) Abnormal opacity of the crystalline lens of the eye.

catecholamines (kăt-ĕ-kōl′à-mēnz) Group of similar compounds that includes dopamine, norepinephrine, and epinephrine.

catheter (kăth′ĕ-ter) Hollow tube for insertion into a cavity or a canal for the purpose of discharging fluid contents or introducing other substances.

cation (kăt′ĭ-ăn) Particle of matter (ion) carrying a positive electrical charge.

cecum (sē′kŭm) Blind pouch that forms the first portion of the large intestine or colon; the attachment for the appendix.

celiac (sē′lē-ăk) **disease** Chronic intestinal indigestion.

cellulitis (sĕl-ū-lī′tŭs) Inflammation of the body tissues, most commonly the skin.

cephalhematoma (sĕf-ăl-hē-mà-tō′mà) Swelling on the head caused by a collection of bloody fluid under the periosteum of the skull as the result of trauma.

cephalic (sē-făl′ĭk) Pertaining to the head.

cephalocaudal (sĕf-à-lō-cawd′ăl) Moving from the head toward the base of the spine.

cephalopelvic (sĕf′-à-lō-pĕl′vĭk) The relationship of the fetal head to the maternal pelvis.

cerumen (sē-rü′mĕn) Ear wax.

cervical (sĕr′vĭ-kàl) Pertaining to the neck or cervix.

cesarean (sēz-ăr′ē-ăn) **birth** Abdominal delivery made possible by incising the uterine and abdominal walls.

Chadwick's (chăd′wĭks) **sign** Violet tinge of the cervical and vaginal mucous membranes; a presumptive sign of pregnancy.

chancre (shăng′ker) Craterlike lesion seen in first-stage syphilis.

chemotherapy (kē′mō-thĕr″ă-pē) Use of chemical agents in the treatment of disease.

Cheyne-Stokes (chān′stōks) **respiration** Irregular, cyclic-type breathing characterized by a period of increasing respiratory action followed by an interval of apnea.

chloasma gravidarum (klō-ăz′mà grăv-ĭ-dā′rŭm) Deepening pigmentation of skin during pregnancy, especially of the face; "mask of pregnancy."

chordee (kŏr-dē′) Abnormal downward curvature of the penis.

chorea (kō-rē′a) Involuntary muscular twitching or movement.

choriocarcinoma (kō-rĭ-ō-kär-sĭ-nō′mà) Rare malignancy associated with hydatidiform mole of pregnancy.

chorion (kō′rĭ-ŏn) Outermost membrane of the growing fertilized egg; one of two membranes that later form the "bag of waters."

chorionic gonadotropin (kō′rē-ŏn-ĭk gŏ-năd′ō-trō′pĭn) Gonad-regulating hormone produced by the chorionic villi (human chorionic gonadotropin [hCG]).

chorionic villi (vĭl′ī) Fingerlike tissue projections of chorion on the outer wall of the fertilized egg.

chromosomes (krō′mà-sōmz) Microscopic structures seen fairly easily in the nucleus of a cell during its reproduction, which contain the genes or determiners of heredity.

chronicity (krŏn-ĭs′ĭt-ē) State of being chronic.

cisternal (sĭs-tĕr′năl) **puncture** Puncture with a hollow needle between the cervical vertebrae, through the dura mater, into the cisterna at the base of the brain.

clavicle (klăv′ĭ-kàl) Collarbone.

clitoris (klĭ′tà-rĭs) Small, sensitive erectile structure located at the anterior junction of the labia minora.

coagulation (ko-ăg-ye-lā′shun) Process of clotting.

coccus (kŏk′ŭs) (pl. cocci) Spherical bacterium.

coitus (kō′ĭ-tŭs) Sexual intercourse.

colic (kŏl′ĭk) Intermittent pain caused by spasm of any hollow or tubular soft organ; abdominal cramping fairly common in first 3 months of infancy.

collagen (kŏl′à-jĕn) Protein substance existing in many of the body's connective tissues.

collateral (kà-lăt′er-àl) Situated at the sides; supplementary, reinforcing.

colonization (kŏl′ĭ-nī-zā′shun) Presence and multiplication of organisms without tissue invasion or damage.

colostrum (kŏl-ŏs′trŭm) Breast secretion produced by the mother the first few days after childbirth.

colporrhaphy (kŏl-pōr′ă-fē) Surgical repair of the walls of the vagina.

comatose (kō′mà-tōs) In a coma, or abnormally deep sleep, caused by illness or injury.

comedo (kŏm′ē-dō) (pl. comedones) Discolored, dried, oily secretion plugging the pores of the skin; blackhead.

comminuted (kŏm′ĭ-nŭt-ĕd) Broken into many pieces; comminuted fracture, a crushed bone.

compatible Able to work together; not in opposition; able to be mixed without destructive changes.

compression (kom-presh′un) Squeezing together; state of being pressed together.

conception (kon-sĕp′shŭn) Union of the male sex cell, spermatozoon, and the female sex cell, ovum; fertilization; beginning of a new being.

conduit (kŏn′dü-ĭt) Tube or other device conveying water or other fluid from one region to another.

condyloma (kŏn-dĭ-lō′ma) Wartlike growth usually found near the anus or vulva; the broad, flat form (c. latum) is characteristic of syphilis in its secondary stage.

congenital (kon-jĕn′ĭ-tàl) Existing at birth.

conjugate (kŏn′jū-gāt) Anteroposterior diameter of the pelvis.

conjunctiva (kŏn-jŭnk-tī′và) Mucous membrane that lines the inner surface of the eyelid and covers the anterior portion of the eye.

contaminated Soiled, stained, touched, or exposed in such a manner that the article in question becomes unsafe to use as intended or without barrier techniques.

continence (kŏnt′ĭ-nĕnts) Control of bladder or bowel function, or self-restraint, especially in regard to sexual intercourse.

contraception (kŏn-trà-sĕp′shun) Prevention of the fertilization of an egg or ovum.

contracture (kon-trăk′chur) Permanent contraction of a muscle resulting from spasm or paralysis causing limitation of motion; high resistance to the passive stretch of a muscle.

contusion (kŏn-tū′zhŭn) Injury that does not result in breaking the skin; black and blue area; bruise.

convulsion (kon-vŭl′shŭn) Violent, involuntary contraction or series of contractions of muscles; seizure.

corium (kō′rĭ-ŭm) Dermis layer of the skin; "true skin."

cor pulmonale (kōr pŭl-mŏn-āl′ē) Cardiac enlargement or failure secondary to respiratory disease.

cortex (kōr′tĕks) Outer or more superficial part of an organ.

coryza (kōrī′zà) "Common" head cold.

crepitus (krĕp′ĭ-tŭs) Grating sensation sometimes heard or felt at the site of a fracture; crackling sound heard in certain diseases.

cretinism (krē′tĭn-ĭzm) Infantile hypothyroidism characterized by mental retardation and other disturbances in mental and physical development.

crust (crustation) External protective layer; scab.

cryptorchidism (krĭpt-or′kĭd-ĭzm) Failure of the testicles to descend into the scrotum.

cul-de-sac of Douglas Blind pouch formed by the peritoneal lining of the abdominal cavity located between the uterus and rectum.

curettage (kä-ret′ăj) (uterine) Scraping with a curette to remove uterine contents (as in inevitable, incomplete, or early abortion), to obtain specimens for use in diagnosis, or to remove growths (e.g., polyps).

CVA Cerebrovascular accident.

cyanosis (sī-ăn-ō′sĭs) Bluish or grayish coloration of the skin caused by poor oxygenation of the blood.

cystitis (sĭs-tī′tĭs) Inflammation of the urinary bladder.

cystocele (sĭs′tō-sēl) Prolapse of the urinary bladder caused by the weakened tissue wall between the bladder and vagina.

cystourethrogram (sĭs″tō-ū-rĕth′rō-gram) X-ray film of the bladder and urethra.

cytology (sī″tŏl′ō-jē) Study of cells.

cytoplasm (sī′tō-plăz-ŭm) Portion of a cell inside the cell membrane but outside the nucleus.

debilitate (dē-bĭl′ĭ-tāt) To produce weakness; enfeeble.

debridement (dā-brēd-mŏn′) Surgical removal of dead, damaged, or contaminated tissue.

debris (dà-brē) Rubbish; ruins.

decalcification (dē-kăl-sĭ-fĭ-kā′shŭn) Removal or withdrawal of lime salts from bone.

decidua (dĭ-sĭd′ū-à) Pertaining to endometrium of pregnancy, which is cast off at parturition.

deciduous (dē-sĭd′ū-ŭs) **teeth** Primary or baby teeth.

decubitus (dē-kū′bĭ-tŭs) Bedsore.

dehydration (dē-hī-drā′shŭn) Condition in which the body tissues lack normal fluid content.

dentition (dĕn-tĭsh′ŭn) Process or time of teething.

dermatitis (dĕr-mà-tī′tĭs) **venenata** Skin disturbance caused by external irritants.

deterioration (di-tĭr″ē-à-rā′shun) Gradually worsening.

detrusor (dē-trü′sor) **muscle** Smooth muscle of the bladder wall.

diaphoresis (dī-ă-fō-rē′sĭs) Profuse sweating.

diaphragmatic (dī-à-frăg-măt′ĭk) **hernia** Protrusion of abdominal contents through an abnormal opening in the diaphragm.

diaphysis (dī-ăf′ĭ-sĭs) Shaft or middle part of a long bone.

diastolic (dī-ăs-tŏl′ĭk) Pertaining to diastole—the blood pressure at the time of greatest cardiac relaxation.

digestion (dī′jĕs′chĕn) Process by which food is broken down mechanically and chemically in the gastrointestinal tract and converted into absorbable forms.

digital (dĭj′ĭ-tàl) Pertaining to the digits; that is, the fingers or toes.

digitalization (dij′ĭ-tăl-ĭ-zā′shŭn) Administration of digitalis to slow and strengthen the heartbeat (particularly the initial administration of the drug).

dilatation (dĭl-à-tā′shŭn) Expansion of an organ or orifice; dilation.

diploid (dĭp′loyd) Having double the number of chromosomes found in the ova or sperm, the normal chromosome number for body cells.

disorientation (dĭs-ō-rē-ĕn-tā′shŭn) Inability to evaluate properly direction, location, time, surroundings, or personal role.

distal (dĭs′tàl) Farthest from the trunk of the body or from a specific point of reference.

distention (dĭs-tĕn′shŭn) (also distension) Inflation, stretching, ballooning.

diuresis (dī″ū-rē′sĭs) Increased urine output.

diuretic (dī-ū-rĕt′ĭk) Agent that increases the secretion of urine.

diverticulum (dī-ver-tĭk′ū-lŭm) (p. diverticula) Sac or pouch in the walls of a canal or organ, especially the colon.

ductus arteriosus (duk′tŭs är-tēr-ē-ō′sŭs) Short blood vessel located between the pulmonary artery and aorta in the fetus.

ductus deferens (dŭk′tŭs dĕf′ĕr-ĕnz) Excretory duct of the testicle; vas deferens.

dyscrasia (dĭs-krā′zhē-à) Undefined disease, malfunction, or abnormal condition, often used when speaking of abnormalities of the blood.

dysentery (dĭs′ĕn-tĕr-ē) Inflammation of the intestines, especially of the colon, usually characterized by mild to severe diarrhea.

dysmenorrhea (dĭs-mĕn-ō-rē′á) Painful or difficult menstruation

dyspnea (dĭsp-nē′á) Difficult breathing.

dystocia (dĭs-tō′shá) Difficult labor, particularly difficulty in the mechanics of childbirth.

ecchymosis (ĕk-ĭ-mō′sĭs) Black-and-blue mark caused by hemorrhage into the skin, usually a relatively large area.

eclampsia (ĕ-klămp′sē-á) Toxemia of pregnancy also known as preeclampsia or pregnancy-induced hypertension (PIH) may involve the serious complications of convulsion or coma. If it does, the condition is then called eclampsia.

ecology (i-kŏl aji) Interrelationships of organisms and their environment as manifested by natural cycles and rhythms.

ectopic (ĕk-tŏp-ĭk) **pregnancy** Pregnancy that develops in an abnormal place (e.g., in the uterine tube, abdomen, or ovary).

edema (ē-dē′ma) Abnormal, excessive amount of fluid within the body tissues.

edematous (ĕ-dĕm′ăt-ŭs) Characterized by the presence of edema, that is, an abnormal amount of fluid in the tissues.

effacement (ĕf-ās′mĕnt) (of the cervix) Shortening and thinning of the cervix or neck of the uterus.

efficacious (ef″á-kā′shus) Capable of producing an intended effect.

effleurage (ĕf-lü-rahzh′) Stroking movement used in massage.

effusion (ē-fū′shun) Escape of fluid into an area.

ejaculation (ē-jăk-ū-lā′shŭn) Ejection of the seminal fluid from the male urethra.

electroencephalogram (ē-lĕk-trō-ĕn-sĕf′á-lō-grăm) Tracing made by an apparatus designed to detect and record brain waves.

electrolyte (ē-lĕk′trō-līt) Substance that, in solution, conducts electric current.

embolus (ĕm′bō-lŭs) (pl. emboli) Foreign substance traveling in the circulatory system, e.g., a blood clot or air.

embryo (ĕm′brē-ō) Unborn young of any creature in an early stage of development when specific identification is difficult with the naked eye.

emesis (ĕm′ĕ-sĭs) Referring to vomiting or the substance vomited.

emission (ē-mĭsh′ŭn) Discharge (e.g., discharge of semen), especially involuntary.

emphysema (ĕm-fĭ-sē′má) Abnormal dilatation and loss of elasticity of the alveoli or air sacs of the lungs.

empyema (ĕm-pī-ē′má) Collection of pus in a body cavity, especially the pleural cavity.

encephalitis (ĕn-sĕf-a-lī′tĭs) Inflammation of the encephalon, that is, the brain.

encephalopathy (ĕn-sĕf″á-lŏp′á-thē) Any dysfunction of the brain.

endarteritis (ĕnd-är-tĕr-ī′tĭs) Inflammation of the lining of the arteries.

endocarditis (ĕn-dō-kär-dī′tĭs) Inflammation of the lining of the heart.

endocrine (ĕn′dō-krĭn) Pertaining to ductless glands that discharge their secretions (hormones) directly into the bloodstream.

endogenous (ĕn-dŏj′ĕ-nŭs) Originating or growing from within.

endometritis (ĕn-dō-mē-trī′tĭs) Inflammation of the endometrium, or lining of the uterus.

endotracheal (ĕn′dō-trā′kē-ál) Within the trachea.

engagement (ĕn-gāj′mĕnt) In obstetrics, refers to the entrance of the presenting part of the fetus into the true pelvis; the passage of the largest diameter of the presenting part into the true pelvis.

engorgement (ĕn-gŏrj′mĕnt) In obstetrics, refers to the swelling of the breasts because of local congestion of the veins and lymphatics associated with lactation.

enteric (en-tĕr′ĭk) Pertaining to the small intestine.

enterobiasis (ĕn″tĕr-ō-bī′a-sĭs) Disease caused by pinworm infestation.

enterostomy (ĕn-tĕr-ŏs′to-mi) The surgical creation of an opening into the small intestine through the abdominal wall.

enuresis (ĕn-ū-rē′sĭs) Bed-wetting at an age when urinary control should be present.

epicanthus (ĕ-pĭ-kăn′thŭs) Fold of skin extending from the nose to the median end of the eyebrow, characteristic of the Mongolian race.

epidemiologic (ep′ĭ-dē″mē-o-loj′ĭk) Pertaining to the study of epidemics, their origin, and prevention or, more broadly, the origins of any condition.

epididymis (ĕp-ĭ-dĭd′ĭ-mĭs) (pl. epididymides) Small oblong organ, situated on the testis, containing a coiled extension of the tubules of the testis, which eventually joins the vas deferens.

epiphysis (ĕ-pĭf′ĭ-sĭs) (pl. epiphyses) End of a long bone.

episiotomy (ĭ-pĭz-ē-ŏt′á-mē) Surgical incision extending from the soft tissue of the vaginal opening into the true perineum, performed to protect the perineum from laceration or help hasten the delivery of an infant.

epispadias (ĕp-ĭ-spā′dē-ás) Abnormal condition in which the urethral opening is located on the upper (dorsal) surface of the penis.

epistaxis (ĕp-ĭ-stăk′sĭs) Nosebleed.

epithelial (ĕp″ĭ-thē′lē-al) Pertaining to the outermost layer of the skin and/or the lining tissue of hollow organs and inner passages of the body.

equilibrium (ē-kwĭ-lĭb′rē-um) Equal balance, between powers; mental balance; equality of effect.

equinus (ē-kwī′nŭs) Condition characterized by a tiptoe walk affecting one or both feet, often associated with clubfoot.

Erbs' palsy (erbz pawl'zē) Injury to the brachial plexus causing partial paralysis of the arm.

erectile (ē-rĕk'tĭl) Capable of becoming erect.

erysipelas (ēr-ĭ-sĭp'ĕ-lŭs) Acute febrile disease, with localized inflammation and swelling of the skin and subcutaneous tissue accompanied by a systemic disturbance of a variable degree, caused by a streptococcus.

erythema (ār-ĭ-thē'mȧ) Redness of the skin; characteristic red blotches on the skin of the newborn infant.

erythema marginatum (märj-ĭ-nȧ'tŭm) Rash occasionally seen in cases of rheumatic fever.

erythroblast (ĕ-rĭth'rō-blăst) Immature, inadequate form of red blood cell normally found only in the bone marrow.

erythroblastosis fetalis (ĕ-rith″rō-blăst-ō-sĭs fē-tă'lĭs) Hemolytic disease of the newborn characterized by anemia, jaundice, enlarged liver and spleen, and the presence of erythroblasts circulating in the blood stream.

erythrocyte (ĕ-rĭth'rō-sīt) Red blood corpuscle or cell.

eschar (ĕs'kär) Thick crusts that may form over burned areas on the body, composed of hardened drainage.

esophageal (ĕ-sŏf″a-jē-ăl) Pertaining to the esophagus, or food tube, leading from the throat to the stomach.

estrogen (ĕs'trō-jĕn) Class name for a female sex hormone; more particularly, the hormonal secretion of the ovary that builds up the lining of the uterus and promotes feminine characteristics.

etiology (ē″tē-ŏl'ō-jē) Cause of a disease or any other phenomena.

euglycemia (ŭ-glī-sēm-ia) Normal or acceptable blood glucose levels.

eupnea (ūp-nē'ȧ) Normal breathing.

excoriation (ĕks-kō-rĭ-ā'shŭn) A raw exposed area on the body without skin cover as a result of injury.

excrete (ek-skrēt) To separate and eliminate from an organic body.

exocrine (ĕks'ō-krĭn) Term applied to glands whose secretion reaches an epithelial surface either directly or through a duct.

exogenous (ĕks-ŏj'-ĕ-nŭs) Originating or growing from without; resulting from external causes.

exstrophy (ĕks'trō-fē) Eversion or the turning inside out of a part with or without the abnormal exposure of the part.

exudate (ĕks'ū-dāt) Accumulation of a fluid in a cavity; drainage flowing from one body area to another; drainage from wounds.

fallopian (fă-lō'pī-on) **tubes** Uterine tubes, or oviducts, leading from the uterine cavity toward each ovary.

familial (fȧ-mĭl'ēȧl) Pertaining to or characteristic of a family.

fascia (făsh'ē-ȧ) Fibrous connective tissue found under the skin or covering, supporting, and separating muscles and other organs.

febrile (fēb'rĕl or fēb'rĭl) State of being feverish.

fertility (fertile) (fĕr-tĭl'ĭ-tē) Quality of being productive; capable of bearing children.

fertilization (fĕr-tĭ-lĭ-za'shŭn) Union of male and female sex cells; conception.

fetus (fē'tŭs) Later stages of the developing young within the uterus or egg when the species is distinguishable by the naked eye.

FHR Fetal heart rate.

fibrinogen (fī-brĭn'ō-jĕn) Protein in the blood plasma necessary for coagulation.

fistula (fĭs'tū-lȧ) (pl. fistulae) Abnormal tubelike passageway from a normal body cavity or canal to another body cavity or to the outside of the body.

flaccid (flă'sĭd) Soft, flabby, relaxed; lacking normal tension or tone.

flexion (flĕk'shŭn) Act of being bent.

follicle (fŏl'ĭ-kȧl) Small secretory sac or cavity; protective tissue envelope of the female sex cell, or ovum.

fontanel (fŏn'tȧ-nĕl) Soft spot found between the cranial bones of the skull of an infant, formed where sutures meet or cross.

foramen (fō-rā'mĕn) Small opening.

foramen ovale (ō-vā'lē) Normal opening between the atria in the heart of the fetus.

foreskin (fōr'skĭn) Prepuce, or fold of skin covering the glans penis.

fornix (fō'nĭx) (pl. fornices) Arch or fold.

fourchette (für-shĕt') Tense band of mucous membrane connecting the posterior ends of the labia minora.

frenulum (frĕn'ū-lŭm) (pl. frenula) Any small fold of mucous membrane or tissue that acts like a bridle; fold of mucous membrane extending from the underside of the tongue to the floor of the mouth at the midline; lower fold of the labia minora that surrounds the clitoris.

frequency (frē'kwĕn-sē) Number of repetitions of a periodic process in a unit of time; when speaking of urinary function, the term implies an abnormal increase in the number of voidings.

FSH Follicle-stimulating hormone.

fulminating (fŭl'mĭ-nā-tĭng) Occurring with great rapidity.

fundus (fŭn'dŭs) (pl. fundi) Part of an organ opposite its opening; top of the uterus.

furuncle (fū'rŭng-kȧl) Infected hair follicle; a boil.

fusion (fū'shŭn) Process of uniting.

galactosemia (gȧ-lăk″tō-sē'mē-a) Metabolic condition involving the metabolism of galactose, which may produce mental retardation and other symptoms.

gamete (găm'ēt) Male or female reproductive cell capable of entering into union with each other in the process of fertilization.

gamma globulin (găm'mȧ glŏb'ū-lĭn) Blood protein fraction containing most of the protective immune antibodies (immune globulin [IG]).

gastroenteritis (găs″trō-ĕn-ter-ī-tĭs) Inflammation of the mucosa of the stomach and intestines.

gastrostomy (găs-trŏ′sta-mē) Intentional establishment of an opening into the stomach through the abdominal wall, usually for artificial feeding.

gavage (gȧ-vazh′) Feeding through a stomach tube passed either nasally or orally.

gene (jēn) Hereditary determiner located on the chromosomes.

genetics (jĕ-nĕt′ĭks) Study of inheritance or genes.

genitalia (jĕn-ĭ-tal′ē-ȧ) Organs of generation, or reproduction.

gestation (jĕs-tā′shŭn) Period of intrauterine fetal development; pregnancy.

gingivitis (jĭn″jĭ-vī′tĭs) Inflammation of the gums.

glans penis (glănz pē′nĭs) Sensitive portion (tip) of the penis.

glioma (glī-ō′mȧ) Tumor involving the supportive tissue of the brain or glial cells.

glomerulus (glō-măr′ū-lŭs) (pl. glomeruli) Cluster or coil of connecting capillaries located at the top of the expanded end (Bowman's capsule) of the urinary tubules in the kidney.

glottis (glŏt′ĭs) Opening of the larynx including the associated vocal cords.

gluten (glü′tĕn) Protein found in wheat, rye, and oats.

gluteus (glü-tē′us) Any of the three muscles that form the buttocks.

glycosuria (glī-kō-sü′rē-ȧ) Presence of glucose in the urine.

gonadotropic (gō-năd-ō-trō′pĭk) Relating to stimulation of the gonads, that is, the ovaries or testes.

gravida (grăv′ĭ-dȧ) Pertaining to the number of pregnancies a woman has had; a pregnant woman.

gumma (gŭm′mȧ) Soft gummy tumor that may develop during third stage of syphilis.

gynecoid (gī′nĕ-coyd or jīn′ĕ-coyd) Womanlike; typical female pelvis.

gynecomastia (gī-nĕ-kō-măs′tĭ-ȧ or jĭn-ĕ-kō-măs′tĭ′ȧ) Swelling of the newborn or adult male breast tissue.

habilitate (hȧ-bĭl′ĭ-tāt) To teach skills needed for everyday living or prepare for a specific job or task.

hallucination (hȧ-lŭ-sĭ-nā′shŭn) False perception having no relation to reality and not accounted for by any external stimuli; may be visual, auditory, olfactory, etc.

Hegar's (hā′gärz) **sign** Softening of the uterine isthmus, the area between the cervix and body of the uterus; a probable sign of pregnancy.

helix (hē′-lĭks) A spiral or coil-like formation

hemangioma (hē-măn-jē-ō′mȧ) Blood vessel tumor.

hematocrit (hē-măt′ȧ-krĭt) **reading** The percentage of whole blood volume occupied by red blood cells after they have been separated through use of a centrifuge.

hematoma (hē-mȧ-tō′mȧ) Tumor composed of blood cells, resulting from tissue injury.

hematuria (hē-mȧ-tü′rĭ-ȧ) Presence of blood in the urine.

hemoglobin (hē-mō-glō′bĭn) Oxygen-carrying protein pigment found in the red blood cells.

hemolytic (hē-mō-lĭt′ĭk) Pertaining to or causing the breakdown of red blood cells.

hemoptysis (hē-mŏp′tĭ-sĭs) Presence of blood-stained sputum.

hemorrhoid (hĕm′ō-royd) Rectal varicosity; "pile."

heparinized (hĕp′er-rĭn-īzed) Containing heparin employed as an anticoagulant.

hermaphroditism (her-măf′rō-dĭt-ĭsm) Possession by one individual of the gonads and external genitalia of both sexes.

hernia (hĕr′nĭ-ȧ) Rupture; an abnormal protrusion of a portion of the contents of a body cavity because of a defect in its surrounding walls, frequently causing swelling, pressure symptoms, or other complications.

herpes (hĕr′pēz) **simplex** Viral infection characteristically causing an eruption of small, clustered blisters on the skin or mucous membranes.

heterozygous (hĕt″er-ō-zī′gŭs) Having the two members of one or more pairs of genes dissimilar.

homozygous (hō″mō-zī′gŭs) Having both of a given pair of genes alike.

hordeolum (hŏr-dē′ō-lŭm) Sty or infection involving the eyelash follicle.

hormone (hŏr′mōn) Internal secretions of thyroid gland, pancreas, etc.; chemical substance originating in an organ, gland, or part that is conveyed through the blood to another part of the body, helping to regulate body processes.

Hutchinson's (hŭch′ĭn-sŭnz) **teeth** Notched teeth characteristic of congenital syphilis.

hydatidiform (hī″da-tĭdĭ-fōrm) **mole** Condition in which the fertilized ovum becomes altered and an abnormal tissue develops instead of a baby and normal placenta.

hydrocele (hī′drō-sēl) Abnormal collection of fluid in the lining tissue (tunica vaginalis) of the testis.

hydrocephalus (hī-drō-sĕf′ȧ-lŭs) Collection of abnormal amounts of cerebrospinal fluid within the cranium, causing enlargement of the immature skull.

hydrophobia (hī-drō-fō′bē-ȧ) Rabies; fear of water.

hydrotherapy (hī-drō-thĕr′ȧ-pē) Scientific application of water to treat diseases (hot baths, etc.).

hymen (hī′mĕn) Membrane partially covering the vaginal opening; "the maidenhead."

hyperalimentation (hī″per-ăl′ĭ-mĕn-tā′shŭn) Term typically used to describe total parenteral nutrition (TPN) by vein.

hypercalcemia (hī-per-kăl-sē′mē-ă) Excessive amount of calcium in the blood.

hypercapnia (hī″per-kăp′nē-ȧ) (increased P_{CO_2}) Excessive amount of carbon dioxide in the blood.

hyperemesis gravidarum (hī-pĕr-ĕm′ĕ-sĭs grăv-ĭ-dā′rŭm) Persistent, exaggerated nausea and vomiting during pregnancy.

hyperextension (hī″pŭr-ĕck-stĕn′shŭn) Maximum extension or overextension of a limb or part.

hyperglycemia (hī-pĕr-glī-sē′mē-à) Excessive amount of glucose in the bloodstream.

hyperkalemia (hī-per-kà-lē′mē-ă) Excessive amount of potassium in the blood.

hypernatremia (hī-per-nà-trē′mē-ă) Excessive amount of sodium in the blood.

hypertension (hī-per-tĕn′shŭn) Abnormal elevation of the blood pressure, especially the diastolic pressure.

hyperthermia (hī-per-ther′-mē-à) Abnormally elevated body temperature caused by a breakdown of normal thermoregulating processes (such as in heat stroke) or rarely artificially induced in an effort to combat disease.

hypertonic (hī″per-tŏn′ĭk) Excessive or above normal in tone or tension; a solution containing excessive amounts of salts.

hypertrophy (hī-per′trō-fē) Increase in size or bulk; excessive development.

hyperventilation (hī-per-vĕn-tĭl-ā′shŭn) Overbreathing accompanied by a carbon dioxide deficit commonly causing dizziness as well as tingling and numbness in the hands.

hypnotic (hĭp-nŏt′ĭk) Medication that causes sleep.

hypocalcemia (hī-pō-kăl-sē′mē-ă) Abnormally low blood calcium level.

hypogastric (hī-pō-găs′trĭk) Pertaining to lower middle area of the abdomen.

hypoglycemia (hī-pō-glī-sē′mē-à) Deficiency of glucose in the blood.

hypokalemia (hī-pō-kà-lē′mē-à) Deficiency of potassium in the blood.

hyponatremia (hī-pō-nā-trē′mē-à) Deficiency of sodium in the blood.

hypospadias (hī-pō-spā′dē-às) Condition characterized by the abnormal opening of the urethra on the under-surface of the penis.

hypostatic (hī-pō-stăt′ĭk) Pertaining to the settling of a deposit or congestion in an area, caused by lack of proper activity.

hypotension (hī-pō-tĕn′shun) Abnormal decrease of systolic and diastolic blood pressure.

hypothalamus (hī-pō-thăl′à-mŭs) Area of heat control and other body regulation located near the base of the brain.

hypothermia (hī″pō-thur′mē-à) Pertaining to subnormal temperature of the body.

hypovolemia (hī″pō-vō-lē′mē-à) Diminished blood volume.

hypoxia (hī-pŏks′ē-à) Lack of adequate amount of oxygen.

hysterotomy (hĭs-tĕr-ŏt′ō-mē) Opening of the uterus; cesarean birth.

icterus (ĭk′tĕr-ŭs) Jaundice; a yellow tint to the skin.

idiopathic (ĭd-ē-ō-păth′ĭk) Adjective meaning that the cause of a condition is unknown.

ileostomy (ĭl″ē-ōs′tà-mē) Surgical formation of a fistula or artificial anus through the abdominal wall into the ileum, or an ileal pouch created as a part of the Bricker procedure.

ileum (ĭl′ē-ŭm) Lower portion of small intestine.

ileus (il′ē-ŭs) Obstruction or paralysis in the intestines.

iliopectineal (ĭl″ē-ō-pĕk-tĭnē-al) **line** Imaginary line dividing the upper or false pelvis from the lower or true pelvis; the linea terminalis forming the brim or inlet of the pelvis.

immunity (ĭ-mū′nĭ-tē) Ability to protect oneself against the development of infectious disease.

immunofluorescent (ĭm″mŭ-nō-floō-ō-rĕs′ĕnt) **antibody technique** Detection of antibodies using special proteins labeled with fluorescein to illuminate with fluorescent light source.

immunosuppressive (ĭm″yoò-nō-sŭh-prĕs′ĭv) Capable of interfering with a normal immune response.

impaction (ĭm-păk′shŭn) State of being lodged and retained abnormally in a part or strait; a large accumulation of relatively hard stool in the rectum or colon, difficult to move.

imperforate (ĭm-pĕr′fōr-āt) Without an opening.

impetigo (ĭm-pĕ-tī′gō) Contagious skin infection caused by coagulase-positive staphylococci or group A beta-hemolytic streptococci.

implantation (ĭm-plăn-tā′shŭn) Nesting of the fertilized ovum in the wall of the uterus; artificial placement of a substance in the body.

incarcerated (ĭn-kär′sĕr-à-tĕd) Trapped; confined.

incest (ĭn′sĕst) Sexual intercourse between close relatives.

incontinence (ĭn-kŏn′tĭ-nĕnts) Inability to retain urine or feces because of loss of sphincter control.

incubation (ĭn-kū-bā′shun) **period** Period of time that must elapse from the infection of an individual at the time of exposure until the appearance of signs and symptoms of the disease.

inertia (ĭn-ĕr′shà) Sluggishness; absence of activity; resistance to movement or change.

infanticide (ĭn-făn′tĭs-ī d) Killing of an infant.

infectious (ĭn-fĕk′shŭs) **disease** Disorders caused by organisms that invade tissue and cause symptoms of illness.

infecund (ĭn′fĕk-ŭnd) Unfruitful; infertile; unable to conceive.

infertile (ĭn-fer′til) Unable to conceive; may refer to a man or woman.

infusion (ĭn-fū′zhun) Introduction of a solution into a vein.

inguinal (ĭn-gwĭ-nal) Pertaining to the region of the groin.

inhibitor (ĭn-hĭb-ĭt-er) Agent that curtails or stops certain activity.

insemination (ĭn′sĕm-ĭ-nā-shŭn) (artificial) Injection of semen into the uterine canal by a process unrelated to intercourse.

integumentary (ĭn-tĕg-ū-mĕn′tà-rē) Referring to the integument, that is, the skin, including the hair, nails, oil and sweat glands, and superficial sensory nerve endings.

interstitial (ĭn-tĕr-stĭsh′al) **fluid** Body fluid found outside the bloodstream in the spaces between the tissue cells.

intertrigo (ĭn″ter-trē′gō) Reddened skin eruption produced by friction of adjacent parts; chafing.

intractable (ĭn-trăk′tĕbl) Not easily controlled, difficult to treat.

intrauterine device (IUD) Object placed into the uterus to avoid pregnancy by perhaps preventing or disrupting implantation or fertilization.

intravesical (in″truh-vĕs′ĭ-kul) Inside the urinary bladder.

intubation (ĭn″tü-bā′shŭn) Introduction of a tube into a hollow organ or passageway to keep it open.

intussusception (ĭn-tŭs-sŭs-sĕp′shŭn) Telescoping of adjacent parts of the bowel, usually in the ileocecal region.

in utero (ū′tĕr-ō) Inside the uterus.

inversion (ĭn-vĕr′shŭn or ĭn-vĕr′zhŭn) A turning upside down, inside out, or end to end.

involution (ĭn-vō-lū′shŭn) A turning or rolling inward; the reverse of evolution, a term especially used to describe the return of the uterus to approximately its prepregnant size and position after childbirth.

iodophor (ī-ō′dà-fōr) Antiseptic containing iodine combined with detergent or an agent or carrier that enhances its solubility.

ion (ī′ăn) One or more atoms carrying an electrical charge.

irrigation (irr″ĭ-gā′shŭn) Act of cleansing by a stream of water or other solution.

ischemia (ĭs-kē′-mē-à) Localized tissue anemia.

ischial (ĭs′kē-al) **spines** Two relatively sharp bony projections protruding into the pelvic outlet from the ischial bones that form the lower lateral border of the pelvis; used in determining the progress of the fetus down the birth canal.

jaundice (jawn′dĭs) Yellow tinge to the skin or sclerae; icterus.

karyotype (kăr′ē-ō-tīp) Total characteristics of the chromosomes of a cell nucleus including number, form, size, and grouping, usually photographed, cut out, and arranged on a card for study.

kernicterus (ker-nĭk′ter-ŭs) Yellow staining of the basal ganglia of the brain in the jaundiced newborn infant; a complication of severe hyperbilirubinemia.

ketogenic (kē-tō-jĕn′ĭk) **diet** High-fat, low-carbohydrate diet.

ketone (kē′tōn) **bodies** Group of compounds produced during the oxidation of fatty acids; one example is acetone.

kwashiorkor (kwash-ĭ-ōr′kōr) Disease resulting from protein deprivation in infancy and childhood, common in certain parts of Africa.

kyphosis (kī-fō′sĭs) Humpback.

labia majora (lā′bē-à mà-jō-ra) (sing. labium) Two fleshy, hair-covered folds located on both sides of the perineal midline, extending from the mons veneris almost to the anus in women.

labia minora (mĭ-nō′ra) Two small folds of tissue covering the vestibule located just under the labia majora in women.

laceration (lăs-er-ā′shŭn) Jagged cut or tear.

lacrimal (lăk′rĭm-al) **glands** Tear glands.

lactation (lăk-tā′shŭn) Process of milk production or the period of breast-feeding in mammals.

lactogenic (lăk-tō-jĕn′ĭk) Inducing the secretion of milk (e.g., the lactogenic hormone prolactin, or LTH).

lanugo (là-nü′gō) Soft, fine hair on the body of the fetus or newborn.

laparotomy (lăp-a-rŏt′ō-mē) Abdominal operation; surgical opening of the abdomen.

laryngospasm (lär-ĭng′gō-spă-zŭm) Spasm of the muscles of the larynx.

larynx (lär′ĭnks) Voice box.

lesion (lē′zhŭn) Any change or irregularity in tissue resulting from disease or injury.

lethargic (lĕth-är′jĭk) Drowsy; sluggish.

leukemia (lū-kē′mē-a) Disease characterized by overproduction of abnormal, immature, white blood cells; "cancer of the blood."

leukocyte (lü′kō-sīt) White blood cell.

leukocytosis (lü-kō-sī-tō′sĭs) Excessive increase in the number of white blood cells circulating in the blood.

leukopenia (lü-kō-pē′nē-à) Abnormal decrease of circulating white blood cells.

leukorrhea (lü-kō-rē′à) White or yellowish cervical or vaginal discharge.

levator ani (lĕ-vā′tōr ă′nē) Major muscle that helps form the pelvic diaphragm or floor.

ligament (lĭg′à-mĕnt) Strong, fibrous tissue that serves to connect bone to bone or to support an organ.

ligation (lī-gā′shŭn) Closing off by tying, especially arteries, veins, tubes, or ducts.

lightening (līt′ĕn-ĭng) Descent of the fetus into the true pelvis, which lessens pressure on the maternal thorax and abdomen.

linea nigra (lĭn′ē-à nī′gra) Dark line that develops during pregnancy extending from the pubis to the umbilicus.

lipoids (lĭp′oydz) Fatty-type substances.

lipoprotein (lĭp″ō-prō′tēn) Simple protein combined with a lipid or fatlike substance.

lithotomy (lĭth-ŏt′a-mē) Cutting operation for removal of a calculus, usually a urinary tract stone.

lochia (lō′kē-à) Vaginal drainage after childbirth.

lordosis (lōr-dō′sĭs) Exaggerated lumbar curvature; swayback.

lues (lū′ēz) Syphilis.

lumbar puncture Needle insertion into the subarachnoid space of the spinal cord between the lumbar vertebrae for diagnosis or therapy.

luteal (lü′tē-àl) **hormone** Progesterone.

lymphocyte (lĭm′fō-sīt) One kind of white blood cell.

macule (măk′ūl) Flat spot or stain.

magnetic resonance imaging (MRI) A noninvasive method of viewing the internal structures of certain body parts combining a strong magnetic field and radiofrequency waves plus computer technology to produce diagnostic images; the preferred technique to discover and evaluate CNS abnormalities.

malaise (ma-lāz′) General discomfort, uneasiness.

mandible (măn′dĭ-bŭl) Jawbone.

mastitis (măs-tī′tĭs) Inflammation of the breast.

maternicity (mă-tern-ĭs′ĭtē) Emotional attachment of mother to infant with bonds of affection.

maturation (măt-ū-rā′shŭn) Process of developing, ripening, or becoming more adult.

meatotomy (mē-ă-tŏt′ō-mē) Incision of the urinary meatus or opening to enlarge the passage.

meatus (mē-ā′tŭs) Passage or opening.

meconium (mĕ-kō′nē-ŭm) First feces of the fetus or newborn.

medium-chain triglyceride (MCT) (trī-glĭs′ŭr-ĭd) A glycerine ester combined with an acid and distinguished from other triglycerides by having 8 to 10 carbon atoms; easily digested, high-caloric in nature.

medulla (mĕ-dŭl′ă) Inner portion of an organ (e.g., the medulla of the kidney or adrenal gland).

megacolon (mĕg-ă-kō′lŏn) Abnormally large colon.

megaloblast (mĕg′ă-lō-blăst) Large, early form of red blood cell with a characteristic nuclear pattern, found in the blood where there is vitamin B_{12} or folic acid deficiency.

menarche (mĕ-när′kē) First menses, or menstruation, experienced by a girl.

meningitis (mĕn-ĭn-jī′tĭs) Inflammation of the meninges covering the spinal cord or brain.

meningococcemia (mĕ-nĭn-gō-kŏk-sē′mĭ-ă) Presence of meningococci in the blood.

meningococcic (mĕ-nĭn-gō-kŏksik) **meningitis** Cerebrospinal fever.

meningomyelocele See myelomeningocele.

menopause (mĕn′ō-pawz) Period that marks the permanent cessation of menstrual activity.

menorrhagia (mĕn-ō-rā′jē-ă) Excessive bleeding at time of the menstrual period.

menses (mĕn′sēz) Menstruation.

menstruation (mĕn-strū-ā′shŭn) Monthly elimination of a bloody vaginal discharge, the portion of the lining of the uterus that had been prepared for the fertilized egg in the event of pregnancy.

mentum (mĕn′tŭm) Chin.

metabolic (mĕt-ă-bŏl′ĭk) Pertaining to the physical and chemical changes that take place within a living organism.

metabolism (mĕ-tăb′ă-lĭz-ĕm) All energy and material transformations that occur within living cells.

metacarpal (mĕt″ă-kä′păl) Pertaining to one of the five bones of the palm of the hand.

metastasis (mĕ-tăs′tă-sĭs) Spread of disease (e.g., cancer) from its primary location to secondary locations; the colonizing element.

metrorrhagia (mĕ-trō-rā′jē-ă) Presence of bloody vaginal discharge between menstrual periods.

microcephaly (mī-krō-sĕf′ă-lē) Failure of the brain to develop to a normal size.

microgram (μg) One millionth of a gram (μ = mu; used for the prefix micro, which stands for multiplication of a gram by 10^{-6}).

microorganism (mī-krō-or′găn-ĭzm) Minute living body not perceptible to the naked eye (e.g., bacterium, protozoon).

milia (mĭl′ē-a) (sing. milium) Pinpoint white or yellow dots commonly found on the nose, forehead, and cheeks of newborn babies resulting from nonfunctioning or clogged sebaceous glands.

miliaria rubra (mĭl-ē-ā′rī-ă rü′bră) Heat rash; prickly heat.

miscarriage Spontaneous abortion.

mitosis (mī-tō′sĭs) Cellular division in which the chromosomes split longitudinally to reproduce an identical tissue cell.

mohel (moy′ĭl) Ordained Jewish circumciser.

molding Shaping of the baby's head as it travels through the birth canal.

Monilia (mō-nĭl′ē-ă) See moniliasis.

moniliasis (mō-nĭ-lī′ă-sĭs) Yeast infection of the skin or mucous membranes caused by *Candida albicans*, formerly called *Monilia albicans*; commonly found in the vagina; infection of the mouth is termed thrush.

monitrice (mōn′ă-trĭs) A monitor or adviser of a patient, especially during labor and birth.

monocyte (mŏn′ō-sīt) Type of white blood cell.

mortality (mŏr-tăl′ĭ-tē) State of being mortal, subject to death or destined to die; the death rate.

morula (mŏr′ü-lă) Mass of dividing cells resembling a mulberry, resulting from the fertilization of an ovum; an early stage of life.

mosaicism (mō-zā′ĭ-cĭzm) Presence of body cells with different genetic contents in the same individual.

motile (mō′tĭl) Capability of spontaneous movement.

mucosa (mū-kō′să) Mucous membrane.

mucous (mū′kŭs) (adj.) Secreting or containing mucus; slimy.

mucoviscidosis (mū-cō-vĭs-ĭd-ō′sĭs) Another name for cystic fibrosis, a genetic disease affecting the exocrine glands involving primarily the respiratory and digestive systems.

mucus (mū′kŭs) (n.) Slippery secretion produced by the mucous membranes.

multifactorial Caused by many factors; involving many genes or combinations of genes.

multiform (mŭl′tĭ-form) Having many forms or shapes.

multigravida (mŭl-tĭ-grăv′ĭ-dă) Woman who has had two or more pregnancies.

multipara (mŭl-tĭp′ȧ-ra) Technically, a woman who has completed two or more viable pregnancies.

musculature (mŭs′kū-lȧ-tūr) Arrangement and condition of the muscles in the body or its parts.

mutation (myoo-tā′shŭn) Process of change or alteration particularly involving hereditary potential (genes, chromosomes).

myelin (mi′lĭn) The white fatty sheath that covers some nerves.

myelinization (mī′lĭn-ī-zā′shŭn) Process of supplying or accumulating myelin during development, or repair, of nerves.

myelitis (mī-ĕl-ī′tĭs) Inflammation of the spinal cord or bone marrow (osteomyelitis).

myelomeningocele (mī″ĕl-ō-mĕ-nĭng′ō-sēl) Herniation of elements of the spinal cord and the meninges through an abnormal opening in the spine.

myocarditis (mī″ō-kär-dī′tĭs) Inflammation of the muscular tissue of the heart.

myomectomy (mī-ō-mĕk′tō-mē) Removal of a portion of muscle or muscular tissue.

myometrium (mī″ō-mē′trē-ŭm) Muscular layer of the uterus.

myopia (mī-ō′pē-ȧ) Nearsightedness.

myringotomy (mĭr-ĭn-gŏt′ō-mē) Incision into the eardrum.

nebulization (nĕb′ū-lȧ-zā′shŭn) Producing spray or mist-like particles from a liquid.

necrosis (nĕk-rō′sĭs) Death of tissue.

neonatal (nē-ō-nā′tȧl) Concerning the newborn infant or the first 4 weeks of life after birth.

neoplasm (nē′ō-plă-zŭm) Tumor.

nephron (nĕf′rŏn) Working unit of the kidney; the renal corpuscle and its tubule.

nephrosis (nĕf-rō′sĭs) Renal disease of unknown cause seen in children, characterized by massive edema and albuminuria.

neuropathy (nū-rŏp′ă-thē) Any disease of the nerves.

neutrophil (nū′trō-fĭl) One kind of white blood cell.

nevus (nē′vŭs) (pl. nevi) Mole, pigmented area, or vascular tumor on the skin.

nitrous oxide (nī′trŭs ŏk′sīd) Laughing gas (N₂O).

nocturia (nŏk-tū′rĭ-a) Excessive urination during the night.

nodule (nŏd′ūl) Small aggregate of cells.

nosocomial (nō′so-ko-mĭ-ȧl) Of or pertaining to a hospital; an infection associated with hospitalization.

nuchal (nū′kȧl) Pertaining to the neck.

nucleotide (nū′-klē-ō-tīd) The basic structural unit of nucleic acid.

nucleus (nū′klē-ŭs) Central point about which matter is gathered; controlling portion of a cell regulating metabolism and reproduction of the cell.

nulligravida (nŭl-ĭ-grăv′ĭ-dȧ) Woman who has never been pregnant.

nullipara (nŭl-ĭp′ȧ-rȧ) A woman who has never completed a pregnancy of viable age.

nurture (ner′cher) To feed, rear, foster, care for; nourishment, care, and training of growing children or things.

nystagmus (nĭs-tăg′mŭs) Constant, involuntary movement of the eyeballs.

oblique (ō-blēk′) Slanting; inclined.

obturator (ŏb′tū-rā″tōr) Small, curved rod with an olive-shaped tip that fits inside a tracheostomy tube to aid in its insertion.

occiput (ŏk′sĭ-pŭt) Occipital bone or back part of the skull.

occlude (ŏ-klūd′) To close or plug.

occluded (ŏ-klūd′ĕd) Closed up; obstructed.

occult (ŏ-kŭlt′) Obscure, hidden.

oligo (ŏl-ĭ-gō) Combining form meaning few, diminished, or scanty amount of.

oligohydramnios (ŏl′-ĭ-gō-hī-drăm-nē-ōs) Deficiency of amniotic fluid during pregnancy.

oliguria (ŏl-ĭ-gū′rē-ȧ) Diminished amount of urine production with subsequent scanty urination.

omphalocele (ŏm′făl-ō-sēl) Absence of the normal abdominal wall in the region of the umbilicus creating defects of varying sizes.

opaque (ō-pāk′) Lacking transparency.

ophthalmia neonatorum (ŏf-thăl′mē-ȧ nē-ō-nă-tōr′ŭm) Infection of the eyes of the newborn infant, particularly that caused by gonorrheal organisms.

opisthotonos (ŏ-pĭs-thŏt′ō-nŏs) Involuntary arching of the back because of irritation of the brain or spinal cord.

orchiopexy (or″kē-ō-pĕk′sē) Surgical fixation of a testis or testicle in the scrotum to correct undescent.

orthopnea (ŏr-thŏp-nē′ȧ) Condition in which breathing is difficult except when the patient is in a standing or sitting position.

orthostatic (ŏr-thō-stăk′ĭk) Concerning an erect position or related to a standing position.

osmosis (ŏs-mō′sĭs) Passage of a liquid (solvent), usually water, through a semipermeable partition separating solutions of different concentrations to equalize the concentration of any substance dissolved in the solutions.

ossification (ŏs-ĭ-fĭ-kā′shŭn) Process of bone formation.

osteomalacia (ŏs″tē-ō-mȧ-lā′shē-ȧ) Adult rickets or softening of the bone.

osteomyelitis (ŏs″tē-ō-mī-ĕ-lī′tĭs) Inflammation of the bone marrow and surrounding cells.

osteoporosis (ŏs″tē-ō-po-rō′sĭs) Deossification with decrease in bone tissue resulting in structural weakness.

otitis media (ō-tī′tĭs mē′dē-ȧ) Middle ear infection.

ovary (ō′vȧ-rē) Paired, almond-shaped gland that produces female hormones and female sex cells, or ova.

oviduct (ō′vĭ-dŭkt) Fallopian, or uterine, tube.

ovulation (ō-vŭ-lā′shŭn) Rupture of an ovarian follicle and the expulsion of the ovum.

oximeter (ŏks-ĭ′-mĕtr) Instrument used to measure O₂ concentrations (percentages).

oxytocic (ŏk-sē-tō′sĭk) Medication that stimulates the uterus to contract.

palliative (păl′ē-ă-tĭv) Alleviates without curing.

palpation (păl-pā′shŭn) Examination by touch or feel.

papule (păp′ūl) Small, solid elevation on the skin; the typical early stage of a pimple.

papulovesiculopustular (păp-ū-lō-vĕ-sĭk″ū-lō-pŭs′tū-lar) Adjective used to describe a rash; characterized by papules, vesicles, and pustules.

paracentesis (păr-ă-sĕn-tē′sĭs) Artificial withdrawal of fluid by puncture of a body cavity, especially the abdominal cavity.

paralytic (păr-à-lĭt′ĭk) Describes person suffering from loss of the ability to move a part or parts of his body.

parametrium (păr″à-mē′trē-ŭm) Outermost covering of the uterus formed in part by a portion of the peritoneum.

paraplegia (păr′à-plē″jà) Paralysis of legs and lower part of the body; both motion and sensation are affected.

parenchyma (pà-reng′kĭ-mà) Functioning portion of an organ as distinguished from supportive cells forming its framework.

parenteral (pà-rĕn′ter-àl) Pertaining to methods of drug or food administration other than through the use of the gastrointestinal tract (e.g., intravenous or subcutaneous routes).

paresis (pà-rē′sĭs) Partial or incomplete paralysis; term also used to describe neurologic deterioration associated with late stage syphilis (incoordination, paralysis, seizures).

paroxysmal (păr″ok-sĭz′màl) Of the nature of a sudden attack.

parturient (păr-tū′rē-ĕnt) Laboring or newly delivered mother.

parturition (păr-tū-rĭsh′ŭn) Childbirth; delivery.

patency (pā′tĕn-sē) State of being freely open.

pathogen (păth′ō-jĕn) Microorganism or substance capable of producing a disease.

pathologic (păth′à-lŏj′ĭ-kàl) Caused by or involving disease; concerning disease.

pediculosis (pĕ-dik-ū-lō′sĭs) Infestation of an individual by head, body, or pubic lice.

pelvimeter (pĕl-vĭm′ĕ-ter) Device used to measure the pelvis.

pendulous (pĕn′dū-lŭs) Hanging; lacking proper support.

percussion (per-kush′ŭn) Tapping the body lightly but sharply for diagnosis or therapy.

perinatal (pĕr-ĭ-nāt′àl) Associated with the period before or after birth.

perineum (per-ĭ-nē′ŭm) Area of the external genitalia in both male and female; specifically, the area between the vagina and the anus or the scrotum and the anus.

periorbital (pĕr′ē-or′bĭt′àl) Surrounding the socket of the eye.

periosteum (pĕr-ĭ-ŏs′tē-ŭm) Fibrous membrane that forms the covering of bones except at their articular surfaces.

peripheral (per-ĭf′er-āl) Located at the surface or away from the center of the body.

peristalsis (pĕr-ĭs-tăl′sĭs) Progressive, wavelike movement that occurs involuntarily in hollow tubes of the body, especially the alimentary canal.

peritoneum (pĕr″ĭt-o-nē′ŭm) Serous membrane lining the interior of the abdominal cavity and surrounding the contained internal organs.

peritonitis (pĕr-ĭ-tō-nī′tĭs) Inflammation of the peritoneum.

permeable (pur′mē-à-bàl) Capable of being penetrated.

per se (per sā) Essentially; by itself; of itself.

pertussis (per-tŭs′ĭs) Whooping cough.

petechiae (pà-tē′kē-ī) Small, bluish purple dots on the skin resulting from capillary hemorrhages.

petrification (pĕt″rĭ-fĭ-kā′shŭn) Process of turning into stone.

phagocytosis (făg″ō-sī-tō′sĭs) Ingestion and digestion of bacteria and microscopic particles by phagocytes, certain white blood cells.

pharynx (făr′ĭnks) Musculomembranous passageway at the back of the nose and mouth partially shared by both the respiratory and digestive systems.

phlebitis (flĕ-bī′tĭs) Inflammation of a vein.

phlebotomy (flĕ-bŏt′ō-mē) Withdrawal of blood from a vein.

photophobia (fō-tō-fō′bē-à) Unusual intolerance to light.

pica (pī′kà) Abnormal craving for substances not meant for consumption.

pigmentation (pĭg-mĕn-tā′shŭn) Coloration resulting from the deposit of certain substances in the skin.

pipette (pī-pĕt′) Narrow calibrated glass tube with both ends open, used to measure and trasfer liquids from one container to another by application of oral suction.

pituitary gland (pĭ-tū′ĭ-tàr-ē) Endocrine gland located at the base of the brain involved in many body functions; the "master gland."

placenta (plà-sĕn′tà) Flattened, circular mass of spongy vascular tissue attached to the inside of the uterine wall that serves as the metabolic link between the fetus and the mother; from its surface protrudes the umbilical cord that carries food and oxygen to the fetus and waste away from the fetus; also serves as a point of attachment for the bag of waters that encloses the fetus.

placenta previa (prē′vēà) Low implantation of the placenta near or over the cervix within the uterine cavity causing hemorrhage late in pregnancy.

placentae abruptio See abruptio placentae.

plantar (plăn′tär) Concerning the sole of the foot.

platelet (plā′lĕt) (blood platelet) Thrombocyte, a necessary element for blood clot formation.

platypelloid (plăt″ē-pĕl′oyd) Abnormal type of female pelvis, flattened from front to back.

pneumatocele (nŭ-mă′tō-sēl) Herniation of lung tissue; a sac or tumor containing gas.

pneumomediastinum (nŭ″mō-mē-dē-ăs-tī′nŭm) Air or gas in the mediastinal tissues located between the lungs.

pneumonia (nŭ-mō′nē-à) Inflammation of the lung tissue.

pneumothorax (nŭ-mō-thō′răks) Collection of air or gas in the pleural cavity (the potential space between the two coverings of the lungs).

polyarthritis (pŏl″ē-är-thrī′tĭs) Inflammation that involves more than one joint, often migratory in character.

polycystic (pŏl-ē-sĭs′tĭk) Composed of many cysts, that is, little sacs usually containing fluid.

polycythemia (pŏl″ē-sī-thē′mē-à) Abnormal condition characterized by an excess of red blood cells.

polydactylism (pŏl-ē-dăk′tĭl-ĭzm) Presence of extra fingers or toes.

polydipsia (pŏl-ē-dĭp′sē-à) Excessive thirst and fluid intake.

polyhydramnios (pŏl″ē-hī-drăm′nē-ōs) Excessive volume of amniotic fluid.

polymorphonuclear (pŏl″ē-mor-fō-nū′klē-er) Leukocyte having a lobated or segmented nucleus.

polyphagia (pŏl-ē-fā′jē-à) Excessive appetite.

polyuria (pŏl-ē-ū′rē-à) Excessive urinary output.

portal of entry Avenue by which an infectious agent gains entrance into the body.

precipitate (prē-sĭp′ĭ-tāt) **delivery** Birth that occurs with such rapidity that proper preparation and medical supervision are lacking.

preeclampsia (prē-ĕk-lamp′sē-a) Toxemia of pregnancy uncomplicated by convulsion or coma; pregnancy-induced hypertension (see eclampsia).

prehension (prē-hĕn′shŭn) Use of the hands to pick up small objects; grasping.

prepuce (prē′pŭs) Foreskin of the penis or hood of the clitoris.

presenting part Part of the baby that comes through or attempts to come through the pelvic canal first; often synonymous with "obstetric presentation."

primigravida (prĭ-mĭ-grăv′ĭ-dà) Woman who is having or has had one pregnancy.

primipara (prī-mĭp′à-rà) A woman who has carried one pregnancy to a viable age.

progesterone (prō-jĕs′tĕr-ōn) Female sex hormone manufactured by the corpus luteum of the ovary and, during pregnancy, by the placenta; aids in preparing the lining of the uterus for pregnancy and maintaining a pregnancy once established.

progestin (prō-jĕs′tĭn) Any progestational hormone; a synonym for progesterone.

prognosis (prog-nō′sĭs) Prediction regarding the course of a disease and the likelihood of recovery.

prolapse (prō-lăps′) Falling out of place (e.g., a rectocele).

prophylactic (prō-fĭ-lăk′tĭk) That which prevents disease.

prophylaxis (prō-fĭ-lăk′sĭs) Preventive treatment.

proptosis (prŏp-tō′sĭs) Forward displacement.

prostaglandin (prŏs′tă-glănd-ĭn) Group of fatty acid derivatives present in many tissues, including the prostate, involved in regulating many body processes.

prostate (prŏs′tāt) Exocrine gland found at the base of the male bladder that secretes an alkaline fluid stimulating sperm motility.

prosthesis (prŏs-thē′sĭs) Artificial body part.

proteinuria (prō-tē-ĭn-ū′rē-à) Finding of protein, usually albumin, in the urine.

prothrombin (prō-thrŏm′bĭn) Chemical substance found in the blood, necessary to coagulation.

protozoa (prō-tō-zō′à) (sing. protozoon) Simple microscopic animals, usually single celled.

protrusion (prō-trü′zhŭn) State or condition of being forward or projecting.

protuberant (prō-tōō′băr-ànt) Bulging.

pruritus (prü-rī′tŭs) Itching.

pseudohermaphroditism (sū″dō-hĕr-măf′rō-dīt-ĭzm) Condition in which an individual possesses external genitalia resembling those of one sex and the internal sex organs, or gonads, of the opposite sex.

psychosis (sī-kō′sĭs) Mental disturbance involving personality disintegration and loss of contact with reality.

psychosocial (sī″kō-sō′shàl) Involving both psychologic and social factors.

ptyalism (tī′à-lĭzm) Excessive salivation.

puberty (pū′ber-tē) Period in life when one becomes capable of reproduction.

puerperium (pū-er-pĭr′ē-ŭm) Six-week period following childbirth; the postpartal period.

purpura (pur′pū-rà) Purple discoloration that occurs as a result of spontaneous bleeding into the skin or mucous membranes.

pustule (pŭs′tŭl) Pus-filled papule; a superficial cutaneous abscess.

pyelogram (pī′ĕl-ō-grăm) Radiograph of the ureters and renal pelves.

pyelonephritis (pī″ĕl-ō-nĕf-rī′tĭs) Infection of the renal pelvis and the working units of the kidney, the nephrons.

pyogenic (pī-ō-jĕn′ĭk) Producing pus.

pyrosis (pī-rō′sĭs) Heartburn.

quickening (kwĭk′ĕn-ĭng) Maternal identification of fetal motion; felt by multiparas at about the sixteenth week of pregnancy and by primiparas 2 weeks later.

radiograph (rā′dĭ-ō-grăf) X-ray film.

rationale (răsh-ŭn-ăl′) Logical reason for a course of action or procedure.

rectocele (rĕk′tō-sēl) Prolapse or displacement of the rectum because of weakening of the rectovaginal wall.

reduction (rē-dŭk′shŭn) In orthopedics, refers to realignment of a broken bone or the correct placement of a dislocation.

reflux (rē′flŭks) Return or backward flow (e.g., regurgitation of urine from the bladder into the ureter).

regurgitation (rē-gŭr-jĭ-tā′shŭn) Return of solids or fluids to the mouth from the stomach; any abnormal backflow of fluid within the body.

remission (rē-mĭsh′un) Lessening of severity or abatement of symptoms.

reservoir (rĕz′er-vwár) Chamber or receptacle for holding fluid; store; reserve.

resorption (rē-sōrp′shŭn) Disappearance of all or part of a process, tissue, or exudate by biochemical reactions.

retinoblastoma (rĕt-ĭn-ō-blăs-tō′má) Malignant tumor of the eye.

retinopathy (rĕt″ĭn-ŏp′a-thē) Any disorder of the retina.

retraction (rē-trăk′shŭn) State of being drawn back.

retroflexion (rĕt-rŏ-flĕk′shŭn) Bending or flexing backward; an abnormal position of the uterus bent backward toward the rectum, forming an angle between the cervix and the body of the organ.

retrograde (rĕt′rō-grād) Moving backward; degenerating from better to worse.

retrolental fibroplasia (rĕ″tro-lĕn′tál fi″brō-plā′zē-á) Oxygen-induced separation of the retina of the eye behind the lens; characteristic of premature infants.

retroversion (rĕt-rō-ver′shŭn) Turning or state of being turned back; backward displacement of the body of the uterus so that the cervix points toward the symphysis pubis instead of toward the sacrum.

Reye syndrome A potentially life-threatening disease possibly associated with recent viral illness such as chicken pox or influenza and salicylate use, though its cause is unclear. It is characterized by nausea, vomiting, rash, liver function changes with typical fatty degeneration, and progressive brain dysfunction, coma, and seizures.

RH blood factor Blood protein found in approximately 85% of the American population; those persons who possess it are termed Rh positive.

rheumatism (rü′má-tĭzm) Any of numerous conditions characterized by inflammation or pain in muscles, joints, or fibrous tissue.

rhinitis (rī-nī′tĭs) Inflammation of the nasal mucosa.

rickets (rĭk′ĕts) Disturbance in skeletal development because of poor nutritional intake or absorption of vitamin D and/or calcium or phosphorus; characterized by abnormal softening of the bones.

rubella (rü-bĕl′á) German, or 3-day, measles.

rubeola (rü-bē′ō-lá) Red, or 2-week, measles.

sacrum (sā′krŭm) Fused bone that, with the coccyx, forms the lower portion of the spine and posterior surface of the pelvis.

salmonellosis (săl″mō-nĕl-ō′sĭs) Infection (including typhoid) caused by ingesting foods containing species of the genus *Salmonella*.

salpingitis (sal″-pĭn-jī′-tĭs) Inflammation of the oviduct or uterine tube.

sarcoma (sär-kō′má) Malignant tumor originating in connective tissue.

scabies (skā′bēz) Infestation of the skin by the itch mite *Sarcoptes scabiei;* "7-year itch."

sclera (sklĕ′rá) (pl. sclerae) White outercoating of the eyeball extending from the optic nerve to include the cornea.

scoliosis (skō-lĭ-ō′sĭs) Abnormal lateral spinal curvature.

scrotum (skrō′tŭm) Pouch forming part of the male external genitalia and containing the testicles and part of the spermatic cord.

scultetus (skŭl-tē′tŭs) **binder** Many-tailed abdominal binder.

seborrhea (sĕb-ōr-ē′á) Functional disorder of the sebaceous (oil) glands of the skin and/or scalp causing crusting and scaling; on the scalp it may be called dandruff, milk crust, or cradle cap, depending on the location and density of the scaling.

sedative (sĕd′á-tĭv) Medication that quiets and reduces tension.

semen (sē′mĕn) Fluid discharge from the male reproductive organs that contains the sperm to fertilize the female ovum.

sensitization (sĕn-sĭ-tĭ-zā′shŭn) Process of making a person reactive to a substance such as a drug, plant, fiber, or serum.

sepsis (sĕp′sĭs) Presence or state of contamination, putrefaction, or infection (adj., septic).

septicemia (sĕp-tĭ-sē′mē-á) Disease condition resulting from the absorption of pathogenic microorganisms and/or the poisons resulting from infectious processes into the blood.

sequela(e) (sē-kwē′lă) Condition following and resulting from a disease.

sequestrum (sē-kwĕs′trŭm) (pl. sequestra) Fragment of a diseased, decaying bone that has become separated from surrounding tissue.

serology (ser-ŏl′ō-jĭ) Study of blood serum.

serosanguineous (sē″rō-săn-gwĭn′ē-ŭs) Containing both serum and blood.

show In obstetrics, the blood-tinged mucoid vaginal discharge that becomes more pronounced and red as cervical dilatation increases during labor.

shunt (shŭnt) To turn away from; to divert; a normal or artificially constructed passage that diverts a flow from one main route to another.

sibling (sĭb′lĭng) One of two or more children of the same parents.

smegma (smĕg′má) Cheesy secretion of the sebaceous

glands found in the area of the labia minora and the clitoris of the female or the prepuce in the male.

spastic (spăs-tĭk) Type of muscular action characterized by stiff, uncoordinated movement.

spasticity (spăs-tĭs'ĭ-tē) Stiff, awkward, uncoordinated movements caused by hypertension of the muscles, usually caused by brain damage.

sperm Male sex cell, spermatozoon, carrying the male hereditary potential.

spermatozoon (sper″ma-tō-zō'on) (pl. spermatozoa) Male sex cell.

spermicide (sper'mĭ-sīd) Agent that kills spermatozoa.

sphincter (sfĭngk'ter) Circular muscle constricting or closing an opening.

spore (spōr) Protective form assumed by some bacilli (usage in bacteriology).

stasis (stā'sĭs) Cessation of flow in blood or other body fluids.

station (stā'shŭn) Depth of the presenting part in the pelvic canal as measured by the relationship of the presenting part to the ischial spines of the pelvis.

status asthmaticus (stăt'ŭs ăz-măt'ĭ-kŭs) Severe asthmatic condition that does not respond to usual treatment with epinephrine.

steatorrhea (stē-ăt-ōr-rē'à) Presence of excessive fat in the stool.

stenosis (stĕn-ō'sĭs) Abnormal narrowing of a passage or opening.

sterile (stĕr'ĭl) Free of living microorganisms, including spore forms.

stoma (stō'mà) Mouth or opening of a pore; a body opening, natural or artificial; term usually applied to a colostomy, ileostomy, or ileobladder opening.

strabismus (stră-bĭz'mŭs) Crossed or crooked eyes; squint.

streptococcus (strĕp-tō-kŏk'ŭs) (pl. streptococci) Spherical microorganism that forms a pattern resembling beads on a string.

striae (strī'ē) Stretch marks often seen on the skin of pregnant women.

stridor (strī'dōr) Harsh-sounding respirations.

subcostal (sŭb-kŏs'tàl) Lying beneath a rib or ribs or just below the last rib adjacent to the abdomen.

subinvolution (sub-ĭn-vō-lū'shŭn) Incomplete return of a part to its normal position or dimensions; term usually applied to an abnormal, incomplete return of the uterus to its prepregnant state after childbirth.

subluxation (sŭb″lŭk-sā'shŭn) Incomplete dislocation of a bone.

supine (sü-pīn') Positioned on the back or palm up.

suprapubic (sü″prà-pū'bĭk) Above the pubis.

suprasternal (sü″prà-stur'nàl) Above the sternum, adjacent to the neck.

surfactant (ser-făk-tănt) A secretion of lipoproteins produced in the lungs which reduces the surface tension of pulmonary fluids allowing more efficient respiration. Its

absence is a key factor in the incidence of infant respiratory distress syndrome.

syndactylism (sĭn-dăk'tĭl-ĭzm) Fusion or webbing of two or more fingers or toes.

syndrome (sĭn'drōm) Complete picture of a disease; all the symptoms of a disease considered as a whole.

synthetic (sĭn-thĕt'ĭk) Artifically prepared.

systolic (sĭs-tŏl'ĭk) **pressure** Pertaining to systole; blood pressure at the time of greatest cardiac contraction.

tachycardia (tăk″ē-kär'dē-à) Excessive rapidity of the heart's action.

tachypnea (tăk″ĭp-nē'à) Rapid rate of breathing.

talipes (tăl'ĭ-pēz) Any of a number of deformities of the ankle or foot, usually congenital; clubfoot.

telangiectasia (tel-ăn″jē-ĕk-tā'zē-à) Small reddened areas often found on the eyelids, midforehead, and nape of the neck of newborn infants, caused by superficial dilation of capillaries.

tendon (tĕn'dŭn) Fibrous tissue that connects muscle to bone or other structures.

teratogenic (tĕr″à-tō-gĕn'ĭk) Capable of causing a major or minor deviation from normal structure or function in the developing embryo or fetus.

testis (tĕs'tĭs) (pl. testes) Paired, oval, male sex gland that produces a male sex hormone and spermatozoa.

testosterone (tĕs-tŏs'tĕr-ōn) Male hormone produced by the testes.

tetanus (tĕt'ă-nŭs) Lockjaw; an acute potentially fatal infectious CNS disease caused by *Clostridium tetani* often found in the soil; immunization is critical.

tetany (tĕt'a-nē) Nervous disorder characterized by intermittent tonic spasms of the muscles that may be caused by inadequate calcium levels in the bloodstream.

therapeutic (thĕr'à-pū'tĭk) Having medicinal or healing properties; a healing agent.

thermal (ther'măl) Pertaining to heat.

thoracentesis (thō-răs-ĕn-tē'sĭs) Removal of fluids through the chest wall by the insertion of a special needle.

thrombocyte (thrŏm'bō-sīt) Blood platelet necessary for coagulation.

thrombocytopenia (thrŏm″bō-si″tō-pēn'ĭ-à) An abnormal decrease in the number of platelets in the blood.

thrombophlebitis (thrŏm″bō-flē-bī'tŭs) Inflammation of a vein in conjunction with the development of a blood clot.

thrombosis (thrŏm-bō'sĭs) Formation of a blood clot.

thrombus (thrŏm'bŭs) Blood clot formed in a blood vessel or cavity of the heart.

thrush (thrŭsh) Fungous infection caused by *Candida albicans* in the mouth or throat, especially in infants; characterized by white patches that adhere to the mucous membranes.

tincture (tĭngk'tūr) Substance that, in solution, is diluted with alcohol.

tinea capitis (tĭn'ē-à kăp'ĭ-tĭs) Ringworm of the scalp.

tinea corporis (kŏr′por-ĭs) Any fungous skin disease, especially ringworm of the body.

tinea pedis (pēd′ĭs) Fungous skin disease or ringworm of the foot; commonly called athlete's foot.

tocolytic (tō-kō-lĭ′-tĭk) Medication or regimen designed to stop labor.

torsion (tŏr′shŭn) Act or condition of being twisted.

torticollis (tŏr-tĭ-kŏl′ĭs) Wryneck or tilting of the head caused by the abnormal shortening of either sternocleidomastoid muscle.

toxemia (tŏk-sē′mē-à) Presence of poisonous products in the blood and body; disease of unknown etiology suffered by some pregnant women, characterized by high blood pressure, albumin in the urine, and edema (see eclampsia and preeclampsia [pregnancy-induced hypertension]).

toxoid (tŏks′oyd) Preparation that contains a toxin or poison produced by pathogenic organisms capable of producing active immunity against a disease but too weak to produce the disease itself.

tracheostomy (trā-kē-ŏst′ŏ-mē) Surgical opening of the trachea through the neck to help ensure an airway; a planned intervention usually of some duration or permanence.

traction (trăk′shŭn) Process of pulling.

transcutaneous (trăn″kū-tā′nē-ŭs) Performed through the skin.

transilluminated (trăns-ĭl-lŭ mĭ-nā′tĕd) Inspection of cavity or organ by passing light through its walls.

translocation (trănz″lō-kā′shŭn) Displacement of part or all of one chromosome onto another.

transverse (trăns-vĕrs′) Lying at right angles to the long axis of the body; crosswise.

transverse presentation Presentation in which the fetus lies crosswise in the pelvis and cannot be delivered vaginally unless turned.

trauma (träw′mà) Injury or wound; a painful emotional experience.

treponemal (trĕp″ō-nē′màl) Pertaining to a genus of spiral organisms, parasitic to man, with undulating or rigid bodies.

trichomonas vaginitis (trĭ-kŏm′ō′nàs vă-jĭ-nī′tĭs) Inflammation of the vagina caused by the parasitic protozoan *Trichomonas vaginalis* that results in itching and a profuse, bubbly, yellow discharge.

trigone (trī′gōn) Triangular space; triangular area in the urinary bladder formed by the urethral outlet and the two ureteral openings.

trimester (trī-mĕs′tĕr) Three-month period of time.

trisomy (trī′sō-mē) Occurrence of three of a given chromosome in a cell rather than the normal diploid number of two.

trophozoite (trŏf-ō-zō′ĭt) Animal spore during its developmental stage; motile form of the ameba.

turbidity (tûr-bĭd′à-tē) Cloudy or dense state; like a fog.

turgor (tur′gur) Normal tension in living cells; distention or swelling.

ubiquitous (ū-bĭk′wĕt-ŭs) Existing or seeming to exist everywhere.

µg See microgram.

ulcer (ŭl′ser) Raw area often depressed or forming a cavity by loss of normal covering tissue.

ultrasonography (ŭl″trà-sō-nŏg′rà-fē) Pulse echo diagnosis or technique using high-frequency, inaudible sound waves.

umbilicus (ŭm-bĭl′ĭkŭs or ŭm-bĭ-lī′kŭs) Site of the umbilical cord attachment; the navel.

uremia (ū-rē′mē-à) Toxic condition associated with renal insufficiency and the retention in the blood of nitrogenous substances normally excreted by the kidney.

ureter (ū-rē′tur/ūr′ĕ-ter) Long tubes conveying the urine from the kidneys to the urinary bladder.

ureterocele (ū-rē′ter-ō-sēl) Ballooning of the lower end of the ureter.

urethra (ū-rē′thra) Canal through which the urine is discharged.

urethroplasty (ū-rē′thrō-plăs-tē) Operation to correct hypospadias; surgical repair of the urethra.

urogram (ū′rō-gram) X-ray photograph of any part of the urinary tract.

urticaria (ur-tĭ-kā′rē-à) Wheals; hives; large, slightly raised, reddened or blanched areas often accompanied by intense itching.

uterine inertia (ū′ter-ĭn ĭn-er′shà) Abnormal relaxation of the uterus either during labor, causing lack of obstetric progress, or after childbirth, causing uterine hemorrhage.

uterus (ū′ter-ŭs) Hollow, muscular organ that serves as a protector and nourisher of the developing fetus and aids in his expulsion from the body; the womb.

vaccine (văk′sēn) Preparation containing killed or weakened living microorganisms that, when introduced into the body, cause the formation of antibodies against that type of organism, thereby protecting the individual from the disease.

vagina (và-jī′nà) Canal opening between the urethra and anus in the female that extends back to the cervix of the uterus.

varicella (văr-ĭ-sĕl′à) Chicken pox; acute contagious disease, commonly of childhood, characterized by a body rash seen simultaneously in all stages of development.

varicosity (văr-ĭ-kŏs′ĭ-tē) Abnormal swollen vein, the walls of which are thinned and weakened.

vas deferens (văs dĕf′er-ĕnz) Excretory duct of the testis.

vasodilator (văs-ō-dī-lī′tŏr) Drug that dilates the blood vessels.

vein (vān) Blood vessel that carries blood to the heart.

venereal (ven-ĭr′-ēàl) Pertaining to or caused by genital contact or sexual intercourse.

ventricle (vĕn′trĭk-ŭl) Small cavity or chamber; one of two lower chambers of the heart; one of several cavities in the brain where cerebrospinal fluid is formed or drains.

vernix caseosa (vĕr′nĭks cāz-ē-ō′sà) Yellowish, creamy protective substance on the fetus caused by the secretion of the sebaceous glands of the skin.

version (ver′shŭn) In obstetrics, the changing of the fetal presentation by internal or external manual maneuvers.

vertigo (ver′tĭ-gō) Dizziness.

vesicle (vĕs′ĭ-kĕl) Elevation of the skin, obviously containing fluid; a blister; or referring to the urinary bladder.

vesicular (vĕs-īk′ū-lar) Blisterlike.

vestibule (vĕs′tĭ-būl) Triangular space between the labia minora in which the openings of the urethra, vagina, and Bartholin's glands are located.

viable (vī′à-bŭl) Capable of life; capable of living outside the uterus; subject to legal definition.

virulent (vīr′ū-lĕnt) Highly poisonous; infectious.

virus (vī′rŭs) Submicroscopic infective agent.

viscid (vĭs′ĭd) Sticky.

viscosity (vĭs-kŏs′ĭ-tē) State of being thick, gummy, or sticky.

vulnerable Susceptible to being wounded; in an unfavorable condition.

vulva (vŭl′và) External female genitalia.

wheal (wēl) Large, slightly raised, reddened or blanched area, often accompanied by intense itching.

zygote (zī′gōt) Fertilized egg.

Appendix : Growth Charts

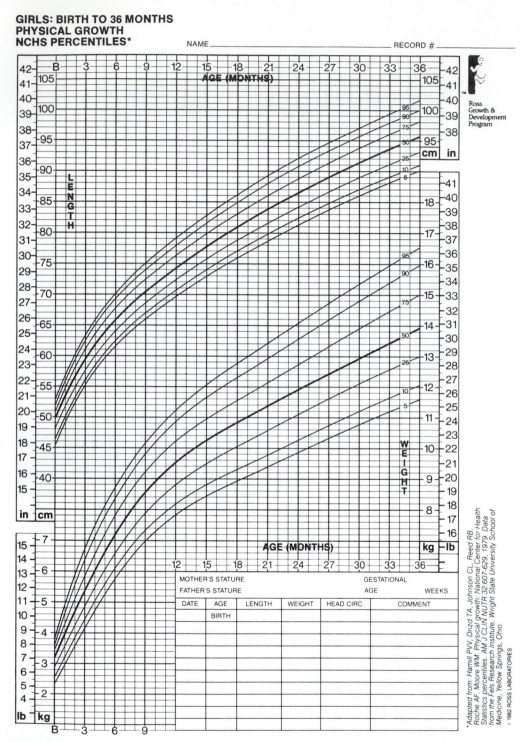

GIRLS: BIRTH TO 36 MONTHS
PHYSICAL GROWTH
NCHS PERCENTILES*

These charts were constructed with data from the National Center for Health Statistics, US Public Health Service. The data on these charts are considered representative of the general United States population. *(Reproduced with permission from Ross Laboratories.)*

GIRLS: BIRTH TO 36 MONTHS
PHYSICAL GROWTH
NCHS PERCENTILES*

NAME _____

RECORD # _____

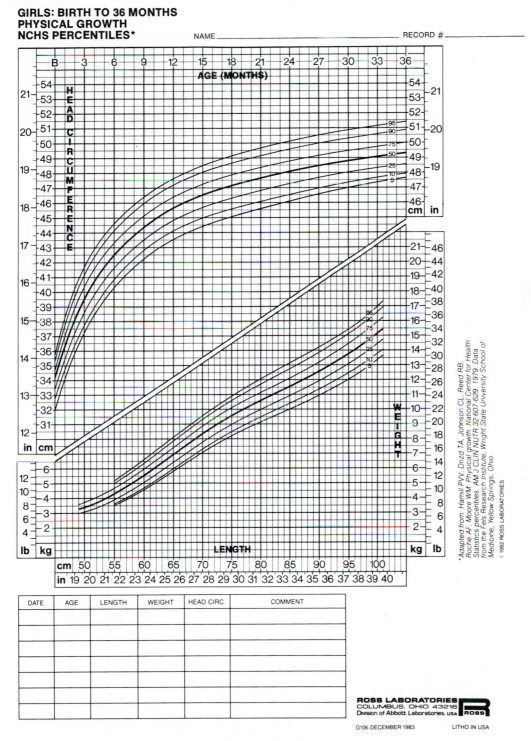

*Adapted from: Hamill PVV, Drizd TA, Johnson CL, Reed RB,
Roche AF, Moore WM. Physical growth: National Center for Health
Statistics percentiles. AM J CLIN NUTR 32:607-629, 1979. Data
from the Fels Research Institute, Wright State University School of
Medicine, Yellow Springs, Ohio.

© 1982 ROSS LABORATORIES

DATE	AGE	LENGTH	WEIGHT	HEAD CIRC.	COMMENT

ROSS LABORATORIES
COLUMBUS, OHIO 43216
Division of Abbott Laboratories, USA

G106 DECEMBER 1983   LITHO IN USA

For legend see p. 808.

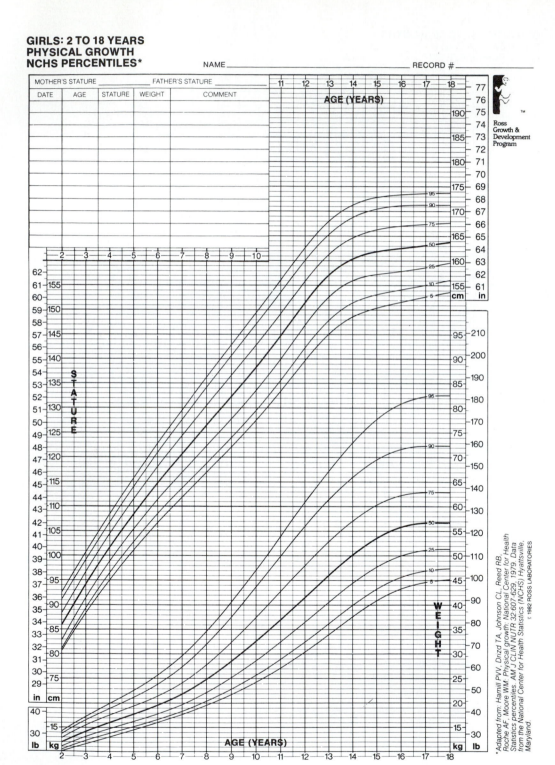

GIRLS: 2 TO 18 YEARS
PHYSICAL GROWTH
NCHS PERCENTILES*

NAME _____   RECORD # _____

For legend see p. 808.

GIRLS: PREPUBESCENT PHYSICAL GROWTH NCHS PERCENTILES*

NAME_____ RECORD #_____

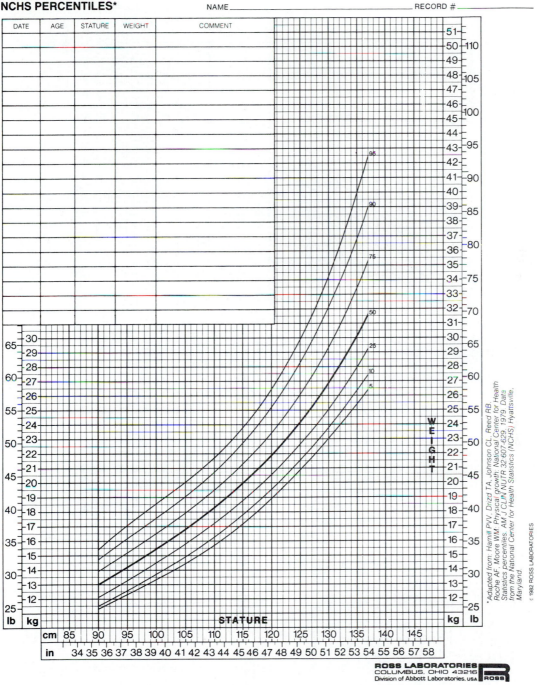

STATURE

*Adapted from: Hamill PVV, Drizd TA, Johnson CL, Reed RB, Roche AF, Moore WM. Physical growth: National Center for Health Statistics percentiles. AM J CLIN NUTR 32:607-629, 1979. Data from the National Center for Health Statistics (NCHS), Hyattsville, Maryland.

© 1982 ROSS LABORATORIES

ROSS LABORATORIES
COLUMBUS, OHIO 43216
Division of Abbott Laboratories, USA

G108/JUNE 1983   LITHO IN USA

For legend see p. 808.

BOYS: BIRTH TO 36 MONTHS
PHYSICAL GROWTH
NCHS PERCENTILES*

NAME_____   RECORD #_____

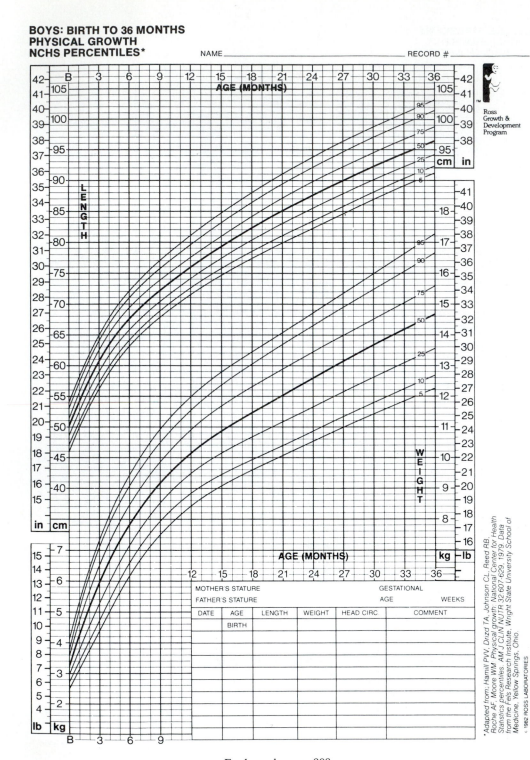

For legend see p. 808.

*Adapted from: Hamill PVV, Drizd TA, Johnson CL, Reed RB,
Roche AF, Moore WM. Physical growth: National Center for Health
Statistics percentiles. AM J CLIN NUTR 32:607-629, 1979. Data
from the Fels Research Institute, Wright State University School of
Medicine, Yellow Springs, Ohio.

© 1982 ROSS LABORATORIES

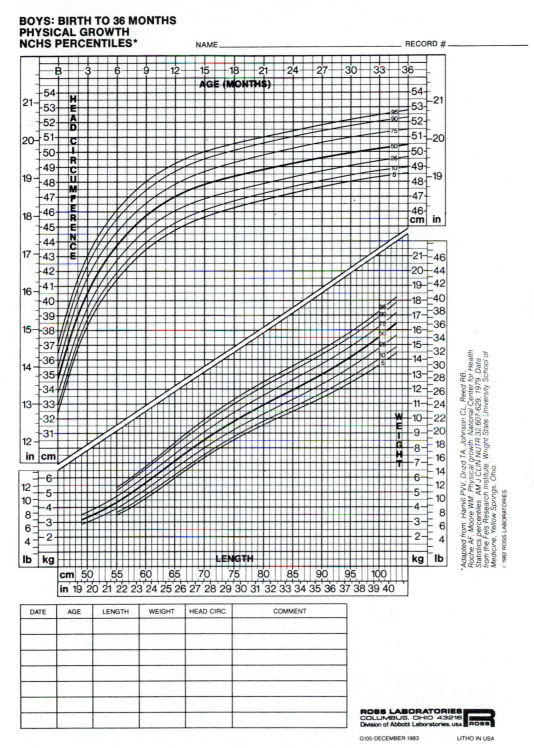

BOYS: BIRTH TO 36 MONTHS
PHYSICAL GROWTH
NCHS PERCENTILES*

NAME_____ RECORD #_____

*Adapted from: Hamill PVV, Drizd TA, Johnson CL, Reed RB, Roche AF, Moore WM: Physical growth: National Center for Health Statistics percentiles. AM J CLIN NUTR 32:607-629, 1979. Data from the Fels Research Institute, Wright State University School of Medicine, Yellow Springs, Ohio.

© 1982 ROSS LABORATORIES

DATE	AGE	LENGTH	WEIGHT	HEAD CIRC.	COMMENT

ROSS LABORATORIES
COLUMBUS, OHIO 43216
Division of Abbott Laboratories, USA

G105/DECEMBER 1983   LITHO IN USA

For legend see p. 808.

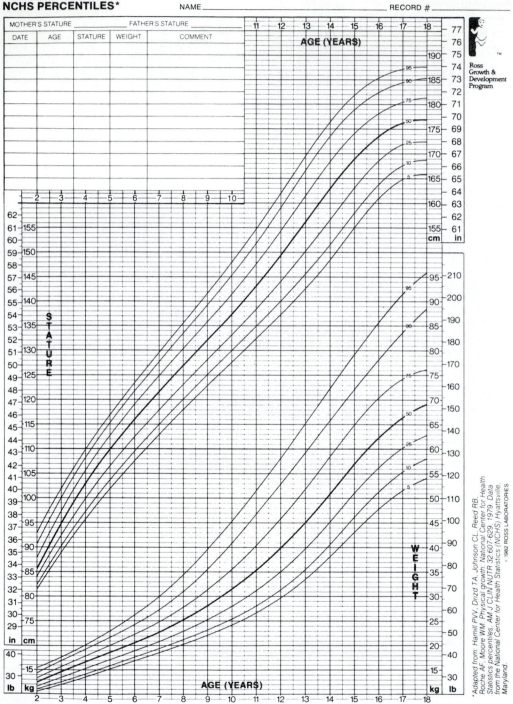

BOYS: 2 TO 18 YEARS
PHYSICAL GROWTH
NCHS PERCENTILES*

For legend see p. 808.

**BOYS: PREPUBESCENT
PHYSICAL GROWTH
NCHS PERCENTILES***

NAME _____ RECORD # _____

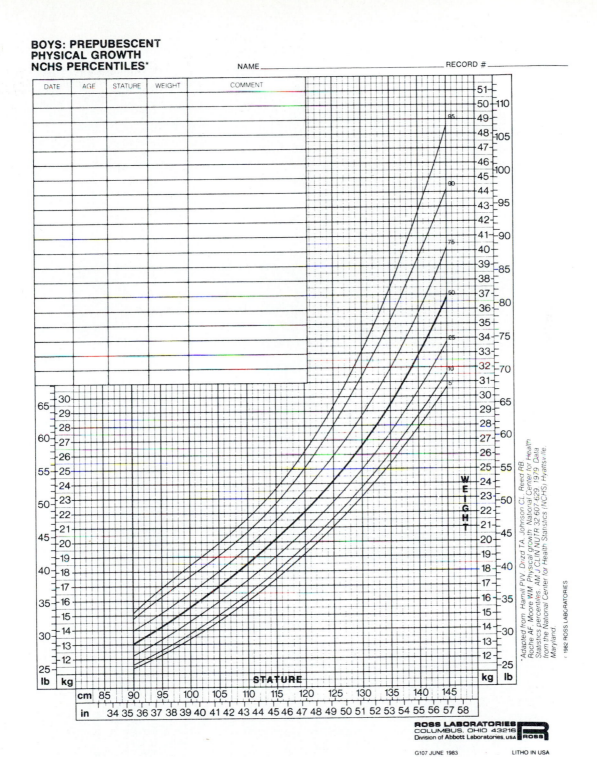

*Adapted from Hamill PVV, Drizd TA, Johnson CL, Reed RB, Roche AF, Moore WM. Physical growth: National Center for Health Statistics percentiles. AM J CLIN NUTR 32 607-629, 1979. Data from the National Center for Health Statistics (NCHS) Hyattsville, Maryland.

© 1982 ROSS LABORATORIES

ROSS LABORATORIES
COLUMBUS, OHIO 43216
Division of Abbott Laboratories, USA

G107 JUNE 1983   LITHO IN USA

For legend see p. 808.

Index